Human Nutrition and Dietetics

SIR STANLEY DAVIDSON

B.A. Cantab., M.D., F.R.C.P. Edin., F.R.C.P. Lond.,
M.D. (Hon. Oslo), LL.D. Edin. and Aberd.

Extra-Physician to Her Majesty The Queen in Scotland:
Regius Professor of Medicine, University of Aberdeen,
1930-1938;
Professor of Medicine and Clinical Medicine, University of
Edinburgh, 1938-1959;
Physician-in-Charge, Royal Infirmary, Edinburgh, 1938-1959.

REG PASSMORE

D.M. Oxon., F.R.C.P. Edin.
Reader in Physiology, University of Edinburgh;
Formerly Lieutenant-Colonel, Indian Medical Service.

JOHN F. BROCK

D.M. Oxon., F.R.C.P. Lond., D.Sc. (Hon. Natal), F.A.C.P.
(Hon.), F.C.P. (Hon. S.A.).

Emeritus Professor of Medicine, University of Cape Town;
Honorary Consulting Physician, Groote Schuur Hospital.

A. STEWART TRUSWELL

M.D. Cape Town, F.R.C.P. Lond., F.F.C.M.

Boden Professor of Human Nutrition,
Sydney University, Australia.
Head of Nutrition Section School of Public Health and
Tropical Medicine, Sydney.
Honorary Consultant in Nutrition, Royal Prince Alfred
Hospital, Sydney.

Human Nutrition and Dietetics

SIR STANLEY DAVIDSON
R. PASSMORE
J. F. BROCK
A. S. TRUSWELL

SEVENTH EDITION

CHURCHILL LIVINGSTONE
EDINBURGH LONDON AND NEW YORK 1979

CHURCHILL LIVINGSTONE
Medical Division of Longman Group Limited

Distributed in the United States of America by Churchill
Livingstone Inc., 19 West 44th Street, New York, N.Y. 10036,
and by associated companies, branches and representatives
throughout the world.

© Longman Group Limited 1979

First edition 1959
    Reprinted 1961
Second edition 1963
    Reprinted 1965
Third edition 1966
    Reprinted 1967
Fourth edition 1969
    Reprinted 1971
ELBS edition first published 1969
ELBS edition reprinted 1970
ELBS edition reprinted 1971
Fifth edition 1972
    Reprinted 1973
ELBS edition of fifth edition 1973
Sixth edition 1975
ELBS edition of sixth edition 1975
    Sixth edition reprinted 1976
Seventh edition 1979

ISBN 0 443 01765 4 (cased)
ISBN 0 443 01764 6 (limp)

British Library Cataloguing in Publication Data
Main entry under title:

Human nutrition and dietetics. – 7th ed.
    1. Nutrition
    I. Davidson, *Sir* Stanley
    641.1   TX353   79-40560
Printed in Great Britain by Pitman Press, Bath

Preface to the Seventh Edition

Knowledge of nutrition is of increasing importance in the world today. The number of undernourished and malnourished children and adults in the poorer countries is not diminishing as their populations grow. In the richer countries obesity, diabetes, heart diseases and cancers assume more and more clinical importance, and nutrition has major roles both in their treatment and prevention.

The excellent reception of this book since it was first published in 1959 has convinced us that the policy on which it was based remains sound. This is set out in the preface to the first edition, which is reprinted. For this edition every section has been carefully revised. The seventh edition has been completely revised. It has three new chapters (fuels of the tissues, food processing and consumer protection). The sections on dietary fibre, alcohol, zinc, vitamin D, ascorbic acid, dietary standards, wheat, meat science, infective agents in foods, food toxicity, anorexia nervosa, diseases of the gastrointestinal tract, diseases of the kidneys, community nutrition, food nutrition and cancer, and adult man have been rewritten.

This book is unique in several respects. It covers the whole field of nutrition at a moderately advanced level: nutritional biochemistry; energy metabolism and regulation; foods; deficiency diseases; nutrition in the cause and management of other diseases; public health nutrition; therapeutic dietetics. It is readable and has been regularly revised and kept up to date. Although based in Britain, it is internationally orientated. The authors live in three different countries, and have worked in many more; there is much material and many references from the USA and from numerous developing countries. Indeed there are few countries in the world that are not mentioned somewhere in the book.

The teaching of nutrition is made difficult by the reluctance of many to use the SI units of international science. The calorie and the pound are so much a part of our language that they are only dying slowly as nutrition units. More and more concentrations of nutrients are being expressed in molar units. We are convinced that ultimately these changes make for clarity, although inevitably there continues to be confusion during the changeover period. In most cases we express results in both the old and new units.

The move of A.S.T. from Queen Elizabeth College, London, to the new Boden Chair of Human Nutrition in Sydney University has made the mechanics of revision more complicated but full cooperation between the authors has been maintained. Sir Stanley Davidson continues to give support and encouragement though poor vision, which happily has not deteriorated, prevents him from taking an active part in revision. The work which J.F.B. could do was limited by a coronary bypass operation which has been successful. The authors have been assisted by Dr Joyce Baird and by Dr Martin Eastwood in the revision of the chapters on diabetes and gastrointestinal diseases. Large parts of the chapter on renal diseases have been rewritten by Dr Mike Bone. The new chapter on fuels of the tissues was written by Dr Philip James, who also contributed much of the material to the chapter on the control of body weight. We are grateful for all this help but, as some of their material has been altered to bring it into line with the rest of the book, we ourselves take full responsibility for the final versions. The diet sheets and glossary prepared for the sixth edition in collaboration with Miss Mary Ellen Collins of the Peter Bent Brigham Hospital and Dr Ruth Kay respectively are substantially unchanged. Their help has, we hope, resolved most of the difficulties that arise from the slightly different uses of the English language on the two sides of the Atlantic. Many others have helped us with advice on sections of the book, and we wish to thank especially Miss Susan Ash, Dr Darnton-Hill, Miss Alison Paul, Miss Cathie Hull, Dr J.A. Loraine, Dr D.B.L. McClelland, Dr D.J. Naismith, Miss Jean Robertson, Miss Marie Sardie, Dr D.A.T. Southgate and Professor A.G. Ward.

Our publishers, Churchill Livingstone, continue to give us kindly assistance and invaluable advice throughout the preparation of this book.

STANLEY DAVIDSON
R. PASSMORE
J.F. BROCK
A.S. TRUSWELL

Edinburgh, 1979

Preface to the First Edition

In 1940 one of us (S.D.), with Dr Ian Anderson, published *A Textbook of Dietetics*. This was based on lectures given to medical students at Aberdeen University and was designed to aid British general practitioners in treating and preventing disease by dietetic measures. Since then, great developments have taken place in the science of human nutrition. The application of this science has spread far beyond the field of clinical practice and is now recognised to be vitally important in many public health problems, as Lord Boyd Orr forecast in his foreword to the first edition of *A Textbook of Dietetics*.

Since many people now realise the importance of good food in adequate amounts for the preservation of health, and the value of suitable diets for the treatment of disease, it seemed to us that a new book on human nutrition and dietetics was needed. Our intention has been to set out the whole wide subject of human nutrition in proper perspective and to bring its many aspects together into one volume.

If asked 'Who is this book for?' we would reply: 'For anyone interested in applying modern scientific knowledge to the practical problems of human nutrition, both in health and disease'. This includes people in many different walks of life.

General practitioners, physicians and surgeons are responsible for seeing that their patients are provided with diets that are most suited for promoting health and aiding recovery from illness. Medical students may find that this book will help them to co-ordinate their knowledge of the physiological, biochemical, clinical and public health aspects of human nutrition. The doctor, in whatever branch of medicine he practises, ought to have a general understanding of the viewpoint of physiologists and food technologists, and *vice versa*. Dietitians and nurses must see that the doctor's dietary prescription is translated into a menu providing meals that are eaten and enjoyed by the patient. For this they need to maintain close and cordial co-operation with the hospital catering officer. Public health doctors and food administrators have the duty to ensure that supplies of food are available, adequate both in quantity and quality, for the needs of the people. Food technologists — chemists, millers, refrigerating engineers and others — must make certain that the methods they use for processing food do not spoil its nutritive value. Farmers and other food producers may well wish to know how the goods which they produce and sell contribute to essential human needs. For people in all of these categories some understanding of the modern science of human nutrition is invaluable.

In recent years nutritional science has advanced in many directions and has sometimes become so highly technical that it is often difficult for an expert in one particular field to view his work clearly in relation to other closely allied developments. There is thus a danger that misunderstandings and misdirected efforts may hinder measures for providing food adequate to sustain the health of mankind.

As doctors we have written this book in the language and style familiar to medicine; nevertheless we hope it will be intelligible to non-medical people professionally concerned with the subject. For this reason we have tried, as far as possible, to avoid obscure technical medical terms. Our aim has been to make most of the text understandable to any interested reader with a background of general scientific education.

The book is divided into six parts.

Part I gives an account of the physiology of nutrition. It is somewhat longer and more complete than the accounts found in most standard textbooks of physiology.

Part II gives a general description of the foods most commonly eaten by man. Their chemical and nutritive properties are described, as are the effects of food processing — milling, preserving and cooking. A short account is given of the various forms of food poisoning.

Part III describes in detail those diseases that are known to be primarily due to faulty nutrition.

Part IV deals with the role of defective diets in contributing to the onset of general diseases which are not primarily nutritional in origin. An account is given of the dietetic treatment of the principal diseases in which diet is of undoubted therapeutic value.

Part V is concerned with nutrition in relation to public health. The various measures available (especially in times of crisis) for ensuring an adequate supply of food are discussed. This part includes an account of the work of the Food and Agriculture Organization of the United Nations (FAO) and of other international bodies concerned with human nutrition. A chapter on the population problem is included.

Part VI deals briefly with the modifications necessary in normal diets to meet the special circumstances of pregnancy, lactation, childhood, athletic training and climatic extremes. Rations for expeditions and emergencies (such as shipwreck) are also discussed.

Numerous tables showing the nutritive values of different foods will be found in Parts I and II, while twenty diets recommended for the treatment of various diseases, and a table of suitable dietary exchanges, have been inserted at appropriate points in the text of Parts III and IV.

In presenting this book our hope is that we have been able to show that the business of feeding people now rests on a sound scientific basis, and that the study of human nutrition deserves recognition as a proper academic discipline.

STANLEY DAVIDSON
A. P. MEIKLEJOHN
R. PASSMORE

January, 1959

Contents

PART I

Physiology

1. Historical and Geographical Perspectives

Nutrition as a science can be said to have been founded by Lavoisier towards the end of the eighteenth century, but dietetics is a much older subject. Hippocrates frequently gave his patients advice about what foods they should eat and, since the days of ancient Greece, doctors in all countries have used dietetics as an important part of their treatment. Nutrition is an art and also a science, based on increasingly secure foundations. Only in the twentieth century did governments begin to assume responsibility for seeing that the poorer and underprivileged sections of society receive enough of the right types of food; to carry out this responsibility knowledge of the science of nutrition becomes of great practical importance.

From a nutritional point of view mankind can be divided into four types: (1) primitive hunter-gatherers, (2) peasant agriculturists and pastoralists, (3) urban slum dwellers, and (4) the affluent. There are not many primitive hunter-gatherers in the world today, but the major part of the human race are still peasant agriculturists, although increasing numbers are either joining the urban slum dwellers or becoming affluent. In no country is there only one type of community. Britain and the United States of America are affluent, but contain many urban slum dwellers and in each there are still a few peasant agriculturists. India has all four types of communities. She is still predominantly a country of peasants, but the rapidly growing towns have increasing numbers of poor urban slum dwellers and a sizeable affluent society; in the jungles a few primitive hunter-gatherers live their lives outside any civilisation.

In this book the problems of therapeutic dietetics and community nutrition are not sharply separated. Each depends on the same fundamental biochemical and physiological science. Before starting an account of this science, a brief description is given of the main nutritional problems in the four types of society.

HUNTER-GATHERERS

Homo sapiens and his predecessors *Homo erectus* and *Australopithecus* were primarily vegetarians but they have done some hunting for up to a million years. Hunting slowly developed as man moved away from the other primates; he became omnivorous (whereas other primates are largely vegetarian) skilled in toolmaking and developed social groups, such as large families and hunting bands. All these changes probably arose more or less simultaneously.

It was only 10000 years ago that the next stage, the technical development of agriculture, began. Thus for at least 99 per cent of the time that man has been evolving from his primate precursors, he has been a hunter-gatherer so that our bodies have presumably evolved well adapted for doing what hunter-gatherers do and eating what they eat.

It is a common misconception that our forebears lived in the cold and ate nothing but meat. The archaeological evidence indicates that man originated in the sunny parts of the world. Loomis (1967) has suggested that man's original skin colour was brown, giving protection from the sun, and that white men evolved after settlement in northern Europe where dark-skinned people would suffer more readily from rickets (p. 276). However, there must have been many differences in diets from place to place and from time to time. For example, Eskimos and Lapps obtain ample vitamin D from marine sources; in some coastal sites the relative amounts of shells in the middens compared with the numbers of bones indicate that shellfish provided the major part of the animal protein intake. Until recently the vegetable part of early man's diet was ignored. Remains of vegetable food in archaeological sites are far less spectacular and much more difficult to identify than the animal bones.

But what were the women doing while their menfolk went out hunting? In rock paintings in southern Africa man the hunter is shown stalking antelopes and shooting at animals with bow and arrow. But the women, with their secondary sex characteristics overemphasised, often have short sticks in their hands, which may be weighted with a stone towards the lower end. These are not weapons. They are sticks used for digging out roots and tubers to eat, the Stone Age forerunners of spade and plough. Thus archaeology gives some understanding of our early ancestors' way of life.

We can also study the hunter-gatherers who are living in the world today. There are only a few groups left and in another generation there may be even fewer. It is not that the people themselves are dying out but their technology is too limited and subtle to stand up to competition from industrial technology. At a symposium on contemporary hunter-gatherers Lee (1967) showed that most of them, except in the Arctic, obtain more food from gathering vegetables than from hunting animals. Lee and De Vore of Harvard made a study of Kung Bushmen in north-west Botswana. These Bushmen are isolated from the outside world of technology by a waterless belt around them, 80 miles wide. This area appears as a blank on the map, except for Mount Aha which when you get there is not a mountain at all. The strategy of the Harvard study was that two or three social anthropologists lived in their own camp near a Bushman camp for a year or more at a time. They learnt the click language, made friends with and observed the Bushmen while disturbing their way of life as little as possible.

One of us (A.S.T.) made three visits to assess their medical and nutritional states at different seasons (Truswell and Hansen, 1976). Our main conclusions were as follows. First, the Bushmen do not become obese, except for the few who live with Bantu primitive pastoralists in the neighbourhood. At the end of the dry season the Bushmen tend to become somewhat undernourished and energy deficient, and this may contribute to their short adult stature.

Secondly, they showed no malnutrition unless something had gone wrong, e.g. an illness or an injury. There were no clinical or biochemical signs of deficiency of any vitamin.

Thirdly, high blood pressure was not found, and both systolic and diastolic pressures fall with increasing age in male Bushmen. This is in striking contrast to the picture in affluent communities, in which mean systolic and diastolic pressures rise with age in both men and women. The explanation could be that the Bushmen do not eat salt (Truswell et al., 1972). There is no archaeological evidence that palaeolithic or mesolithic man undertook salt extraction or had any interest in salt deposits. This seems to have started in neolithic times, presumably when there were food surpluses, which had to be preserved and stored.

Fourthly, the Bushmen's plasma cholesterol concentration averaged 3.0 mmol/l (120 mg/100 ml), a figure among the lowest in the world. Much higher figures are found in most populations who eat meat, as the high proportion of saturated fatty acids in the fat of domestic animals tends to raise cholesterol concentration. But the meat of wild buck has no fat round it and the small amount of fat in the muscle of wild bovids contains mostly polyunsaturated fatty acids (Crawford, 1968). The Bushmen do not eat only meat; they obtain more than half their energy from vegetable foods. The largest single item in their diet is the mongongo nut, Ricinodendron rautanenii, which is a good source of protein and whose oil is rich in linoleic acid. The essential characteristic of the hunter-gatherer's diet is that it is mixed. The men go out hunting but the supply of meat is intermittent and more of it comes from hares and other small animals, than from the larger antelopes. The women, meanwhile, collect vegetable food. This often involves walking long distances carrying heavy loads of nuts, etc. on their backs, and sometimes a baby as well. The

old women stay behind in camp and do the chores like breaking up nuts and fetching water in ostrich egg shells from the well a mile away.

Fifthly, the Bushmen do not have carious teeth though their teeth get worn down by the hard food as they get older. They occasionally enjoy wild honey but have no other concentrated sugar.

Sixthly, their numbers are few and appear to be stationary; One reason for the wide spacing of births could be the delayed resumption of ovulation as breast feeding is continued for about three years. If they do not die from infections or accidents, they live to a good old age. The proportion over 65 years, approximately 7 per cent, is the same as that in Scotland in 1901.

These observations on the Bushmen and other studies on contemporary hunter-gatherers give some insights into nutritional and other aspects of early man, but care is needed in extrapolating because present-day hunter-gatherers may be regressive societies.

Some people would like to go back to the hunter-gatherer's way of life, but this is impossible; there are too many of us and hunter-gatherers need a lot of space.

PEASANT AGRICULTURISTS AND PASTORALISTS

How to grow crops and to domesticate animals was discovered independently in several widely separated centres from about 8000 or 9000 BC, first around Mesopotamia. It was then possible for people to stay in one place, to build homes and cities, and to store treasure. Distribution became uneven, societies became structured and jobs specialised. The population increased greatly. Wars and human epidemics became part of the pattern of life. Great civilisations like the Egyptian, the Mayan and the classical Greek were based on primitive agriculture.

In large areas of rural Africa, South America, Asia and Oceania the people are still at this stage of technical development and obtain their food from subsistence farming. Nutrition in this setting has five striking differences from that of hunter-gatherers.

First, with harvests once a year, food has to be stored. Hunter-gatherers do not store food; they share it.

Secondly, some of the wealthy overeat and become obese. Hunter-gatherers feast now and again after a successful hunt but not regularly.

Thirdly, alcohol is available, made from the ready supply of carbohydrate in cereals. Hunter-gatherers do not have this solace. Perhaps in smaller social groups they have less need for it.

Fourthly, the most dangerous nutritional effects have come from concentrating on a single crop that yields the most energy (calories per acre or joules per hectare). If this crop fails from drought or blight there is famine. The Irish potato famine of 1845–46 was the most terrible example in Europe (p. 500). The Irish peasants at that time had become completely dependent on potatoes. When the crop became infected by epidemic potato blight the effect was devastating. If a crop becomes contaminated with a toxin many people are likely to be poisoned. Ergotism and lathyrism are examples.

Fifthly, there is the liability to develop specific deficiency diseases, when a large proportion of the dietary energy comes from a single staple food, e.g. a cereal or starchy root. Children are more likely than adults to suffer from such a disease, because of their extra need of nutrients for growth and because the common infections of childhood increase rates of utilisation. The two most important of such specific deficiency diseases are kwashiorkor, principally due to lack of protein, and keratomalacia, where lack of vitamin A may lead to permanent blindness. Diets based on large quantities of a cereal from which most of the vitamin B_1 has been removed by milling may lead to beriberi, a disease once common amongst rice-eaters in the East. Pellagra is still an important disease amongst maize-eaters in Africa and elsewhere. It is due to a lack of nicotinic acid and its precursor, the amino acid tryptophan.

Most of the healthy and virile populations of the world have been peasant agriculturists. The Highlands of Scotland and Nepal have for generations produced famous battalions of fighting men, feared and respected by their adversaries throughout the world. Peasant agriculturists are healthy and feed well, as long as they have enough good land and favourable weather; but in Asia and Latin America and to a lesser extent in Africa increases in population, due to decline in mortality from infectious disease, have caused fragmentation of the holdings. It is difficult for a man to provide a good mixed diet for his family on less than 10 acres (4 hectares) of land.

Pastoralists

Pastoralists are at the same technical level as subsistence agriculturists but have a different way of life and are less numerous. In arid grasslands they follow their grazing animals with the seasons, travelling light and living in tents. The life of Lapps is based on reindeer, of Iranian nomads on sheep and goats, and of Tibetan nomads on yaks; in Africa the Tuareg depend on their camels, and the Fulani and Masai on their cattle. Pastoral tribes once had a military advantage with their horses over their sedentary neighbours. (Sedentary is used here in the anthropological sense to mean settled on an area of land, not inactive.) However, now the two groups usually coexist peacefully in a symbiotic relationship, trading animal for agricultural products. Pastoralists have fallen behind since sedentary groups, in tidy constituencies, have more voting power, more schooling and get on better with administrators.

Pastoral tribesmen do not show the usual relation between income and the quality of the diet (p. 460). Although they are poor in money yet they may eat a diet rich in animal protein. Some consume large quantities of sour milk even as adults; their intestinal lactase persists, as in northern Europeans. They may not eat this rich animal diet all the year round. Nutritionists know far less about the day-to-day way of life of these people than they do about sedentary groups, which are more comfortable to study. Pastoralists deserve sympathetic understanding by officials: there should be a place for them in the ecosystem.

URBAN SLUM DWELLERS

The industrial revolution produced multitudes of a new urban proletariat who were uprooted from their rural origins and packed round the factories in bad housing. Such conditions, so vividly described by Dickens and other novelists, are being repeated today in many countries. But the problems are bigger because the twentieth-century slum and shanty town dwellers have fewer resources and are more numerous. In the industrial countries the growing cities of 100 years ago, for all their grime and misery, had a solid basis of economic life. But, as Barbara Ward (1969) has described, the new migrant multitudes are pouring 'into an urban wilderness where opportunities grow less as the millions pile on top of one another and the farms do not feed them or the industries employ them'.

An increasing number of the world's population is crowding in and around the cities of Asia, Africa and Latin America. They tend to have the worst of both worlds. Traditions are lost but not replaced by education. Families are broken up, mothers go out to work and leave their babies inadequately cared for. The food which they buy is likely to be poor value for money and contaminated by pathogens. The problems are often compounded by alcoholism and violence.

In many towns in Africa, Asia and Latin America the infant mortality (defined on p. 473) is over 100, whereas in prosperous countries with good health services it is below 15. In 1900 infant mortality rates were over 100 in many towns in Europe and North America. A combination of poor hygiene and bad nutrition was and is responsible. In a slum, conditions are ideal for the spread of infections, notably gastroenteritis and respiratory infections. These illnesses diminish food intake and increase the need for nutrients, and so readily precipitate marasmus, a severe and often fatal state of undernutrition in children. Infants prematurely weaned are particularly susceptible. While the infant mortality in a poor community may be 10 times that in a prosperous one, in the 1 to 4 year age-group the mortality may be 50 times higher. Again infectious diseases may precipitate severe undernutrition in toddlers on a poor diet with little or no milk. Measles and whooping cough are ubiquitous. Nowadays in Britain these illnesses are usually mild and a death is exceptional. Yet 70 years ago large numbers of young children in Britain died of measles and whooping cough, as they still do in many countries.

In slum conditions adolescents and adults are much less susceptible to deficiency diseases than are children, but such diseases may follow severe infections. In adults a more important cause is drug dependence. Alcohol was the drug most commonly responsible in the past and still is in many places, but nowadays other psychotropic drugs may contribute. Persons dependent on drugs may become malnourished for four reasons: (1) they may spend so much money on the drug that they cannot afford a proper diet, (2) a drug may depress their appetites, (3) a drug habit may upset incentives to healthy living, and (4) a drug may interfere with metabolism in the tissues and organs, notably in the liver. Poor nutrition is but one aspect of urban poverty, albeit a very important one. It sets up a vicious circle, making its victim physically and mentally unfit for work and so driving him and his family deeper into poverty. All contemporary experience shows that programmes for better housing, for clean water, for the control of infectious diseases, for more and better food, and for education in health and nutrition, or the provision of better wages and more jobs, do not alone solve the problems of poverty. A coordinated attack simultaneously along these fronts is needed. Nutritionists cannot work effectively on their own. They require to be in a team with other health and social workers.

AFFLUENT SOCIETIES

Affluent societies, as in Britain today, present nutritionists with a new set of challenges. The whole picture is different. In place of undernutrition we are now more worried by overnutrition. The most malnourished segment of the community is no longer the babies, who tend to be obese, but some of the elderly, especially those who are lonely, depressed and failing physically or mentally. Some new varieties of malnutrition are appearing in patients whose lives have been saved by the miracles of modern medicine or surgery.

We are free of fear of crop failure and can eat our favourite dishes all the year round. Modern food industry uses foods imported from many parts of the world and preserves them mainly by refrigeration and canning. We are now worried about our foods being too refined— without sufficient fibre—or adulterated by fertilisers, insecticides and food additives. Instead of food taking much time and effort to prepare and being eaten formally with all the family, we have instant and convenience foods. The housewife may not be sure what is in them. The family tends to eat in a hurry in different places, and the mother may not know what her children are eating.

A feature of affluent societies is that they consume enormous quantities of pharmaceuticals. Many of these increase the needs for specific nutrients and interfere with nutrition in other ways. Patients receiving such drugs are at increased risk of nutritional disorders. Examples can be found by looking up the items under 'drugs' in the Index.

In Britain in the 1970s about 42 per cent of our energy came from fat and 20 per cent from sugar. There is a strong suspicion that diet has at least something to do with several of the chronic and degenerative diseases of later life. The relationship between diet and dental disease is fairly clear (p. 391) though what is to be done is not. Coronary heart disease, diabetes, gallstones, diverticulosis and some cancers may each be partly determined by diet.

Instead of lack of basic education and no nutritional advice, we find ourselves in a Tower of Babel of nutritional breakthroughs and threats. From newspapers, women's magazines, television, radio advertisements and supermarket shelves we are bombarded with information from competing interests in the food industry, from journalists and from some medical men. One can hardly blame the man or woman in the street if they conclude that all the advice and advertisements cancel each other out. 'It can't matter much what you eat, so I'll eat what I enjoy.'

For professional nutritionists there are two kinds of job to be done. First, we have to continue scientific research, and the biggest challenge is to try and work out the place of nutrition among the multiple and interacting causes of the chronic disease where we have epidemiological clues. Because little progress is being made in the prevention of chronic disease, life expectancy in men has now stopped lengthening in Western countries (Burch, 1972). The science of nutrition has achieved much in relating gross nutritional deficiency to certain acute diseases. But we have a long way to go in relating subtle nutritional imbalances to the increased risk of a chronic disease many years later. This is not a field in which quick results can be guaranteed and the situation is made difficult because of inadequate financial investment in this type of research.

The second big task is to discover how to give the people in an affluent society a better understanding of what they should aim to eat. And since an increasing proportion of our food is prepared by manufacturers, there is a responsibility to advise them on long-term planning of their products. The trouble is that to give any general advice at all one has to make a judgment on insufficient evidence, then simplify it and put it in a form that appeals to people. Professional nutritionists should have their arguments in professional societies and journals, not on the air or in newspapers. We should try a bit harder to reach a consensus for the benefit of the people as a whole.

School children, young adults and the elderly each require different nutritional advice. Food habits are acquired early in life and it is very difficult to change them. Nutrition education is considered on page 477.

This account of historical and geographical perspectives attempts to lay a basis for the application of nutritional science to the needs of a varied and evolving world population. The scientific principles are broadly the same whatever cultural group is being considered. The applica-tion through nutrition education is vastly different. If this universal science is to bring the best results for the world as a whole we must learn to apply it to all groups, using language and educational techniques which are adapted to regional cultures.

2. Composition of the Body

What are little boys made of?
What are little boys made of?
Slugs and snails and puppy-dogs' tails;
That's what little boys are made of.

What are little girls made of?
What are little girls made of?
Sugar and spice and all things nice;
That's what little girls are made of.

Many carcasses of small animals have been analysed chemically, but the results do not necessarily apply to man. A complete chemical analysis of the human cadaver is a formidable task which has been carried out on a number of occasions, but not sufficiently often to give the range of variations in people of different age and sex (Widdowson *et al.*, 1951). Nevertheless, enough is known to state that the data in Table 2.1 are representative of a normal man.

Table 2.1 A normal chemical composition for a man weighing 65 kg

	kg	Per cent
Protein	11	17.0
Fat	9	13.8
Carbohydrate	1	1.5
Water	40	61.6
Minerals	4	6.1

Most of the material listed in Table 2.1 is part of the essential structure of the body, but a portion represents reserves or stores. Of the 9 kg of fat not more than about 1 kg is essential; the remainder represents a store which can be drawn upon in times of need. In obese people this store may be very much larger and form up to 70 per cent of the body weight. Most of the protein is an essential component of the cells, but probably about 2 kg can be lost without serious results. By contrast, the body can be depleted at most by 200 g of carbohydrate. During starvation the store of carbohydrate is continually replenished by synthesis from the larger reserves of protein and fat. The body can lose up to 10 per cent of its total water and at least a third of the mineral content of the skeleton without serious risk to life. The size of the stores and the factors that determine deposits and withdrawals are important nutritional considerations, amplified in succeeding chapters.

COMPARTMENTS OF THE BODY

At a meeting of the New York Academy of Sciences in 1963 the Professor of Surgery at Harvard, Dr Francis D. Moore, went to the blackboard and wrote the following equation:

$$MAN = CM + EST + FAT$$

This is interpreted as follows. A man can be divided into three compartments. CM is the cell mass which is the active tissue, carrying out all the work of the body. EST is the extracellular supporting tissue which supports the cell mass. This again can be subdivided into two parts: the extracellular fluid, and minerals and protein fibres in the skeleton and other supporting tissue. The extracellular fluid comprises the blood plasma and lymph and the fluid which bathes the cells. The living skeleton is, however, very different from the dead specimens familiar in anatomy museums. It is a cellular organ in which the supporting mineral deposits are laid down. FAT is the energy reserve held in adipose tissue beneath the skin and around the internal organs.

In a healthy body the cell mass may contribute about 55 per cent of the total weight, the extracellular supporting tissue about 30 per cent and the fat reserve about 15 per cent. These proportions may be greatly altered by disease. Thus in starvation arising from lack of food or in the emaciation that results from any wasting disease, the cell mass is reduced and the fat reserve may be almost completely utilised. The extracellular supporting tissue is little altered in absolute size and so becomes relatively bigger and may comprise 50 per cent or more of the body weight. In obesity the fat reserve is greatly increased.

ELECTROLYTES

An important difference exists between the chemical constitution of the fluid within the cells and that of the extracellular fluid which surrounds them. Cell fluid is primarily a solution of potassium ions and extracellular fluid a solution of sodium chloride. The anions within the cell are provided mainly by phosphates, proteins and organic acids in varying proportions. Table 2.2 shows approximate concentrations of these and other ions in the two fluids. The difference between the concentration of the ions inside and outside the cells is only maintained by the expenditure of energy which is provided by the metabolic processes within the cells. Much of the energy expenditure of the resting body is used to maintain this electrolyte equilibrium. Cellular activity either in muscle, nerve or secretory cell is associated with local disturbances of ionic equilibrium at the cell wall and chemical energy is needed to restore resting conditions.

Table 2.2 A normal distribution of ions in intracellular and extracellular fluids

	Intracellular (mEq/1)	Extracellular (mEq/1)
Cations:		
Na+	10	145
K+	150	5
Ca²+	2	2
Mg²+	15	2
	177	154
Anions:		
Cl⁻	10	100
HCO₃⁻	10	27
SO₄²⁻	15	1
Organic acids		5
PO₄³⁻	142	2
Proteins		19
	177	154

CHEMICAL DISSECTION OF THE BODY

It is possible by chemical methods to determine the size of the chief compartments of the human body. The methods are of necessity indirect. Many of them are too complex and time-consuming to be of practical value in routine clinical medicine. They are, however, mostly within the competence of even a small research laboratory. The results obtained, using the methods now to be described, have had a profound effect on our understanding of the changes that take place in the body as a result of nutritional diseases. They make possible quantitative measurements of these changes. A fuller account of the chemical anatomy of the human body is given by Passmore and Draper (1970).

The dilution principle

It is possible to determine the volume (V) of a fluid in an irregular container by adding to it a measured quantity (Q) of a substance which diffuses freely and evenly throughout the fluid. After an interval to allow even distribution of the test substance, its concentration (C) in the fluid is determined. Then the volume can be calculated from the formula

$$V = \frac{Q}{C}$$

This principle has wide applications in human biology.

Total body water

In living man or any intact animal it is possible to estimate the total body water in the following way. A known weight of a substance which is freely diffusible in all the body fluids is given to the subject, either by mouth or by intravenous injection. After sufficient time has been allowed for the substance to diffuse throughout all the tissues, a sample of blood is withdrawn and the concentration of the substance in the plasma determined. The total body water can then be calculated as described above. Corrections have to be made for any excretion or metabolism of the substance during the period of diffusion. Many freely diffusible substances, e.g. urea, antipyrine and ethanol, have been used for this purpose. Today the isotopes deuterium and tritium are usually employed. Consistent results with each have been obtained by experienced workers. As there is the dual assumption not only that the test substance is freely diffusible into all cells of the body, but also that proper corrections have been made for any losses, the prudent sometimes express their results in terms of the size of the 'tritium space' or the 'antipyrine space'. A normal value for the total body water is 40 litres and varies from 50 to 65 per cent of the body weight, or even more widely according to the degree of fatness of the subject.

Extracellular water

A number of substances — sucrose, inulin (a carbohydrate derived from a plant root), sodium thiocyanate, sodium thiosulphate and the bromide ion, which can be labelled isotopically — when injected into the body appear to occupy a 'space' which is much smaller than the total body water and which is probably the same as the extracellular fluid. The 'thiocyanate space' can be measured conveniently in any laboratory without special equipment, and provides a useful measure of the extracellular fluid. (Thiocyanate enters the red blood corpuscles and a correction has to be made in calculating the extracellular fluid from the thiocyanate space.) The extracellular fluid normally comprises 18 to 24 per cent of the body weight. In patients with oedema from starvation or other cause, it may be increased to 50 per cent of the body weight. In dehydration it is markedly reduced.

Cell water and cell mass

If the total body water and extracellular water are measured as described above, the difference between the two can be taken as the cell water. Thus the reference man whose chemical composition is given in Table 2.1 has a total body water of 40 l. If the extracellular water is 15 l then

Cell water = 40–15 = 25 litres

Cells vary in their water content. Muscle cells are about 75 per cent water. Red blood corpuscles, brain cells and cells in tendons and connective tissue contain much less water. It is a reasonable approximation to say that 70 per cent of the whole cell mass is water. Hence in our reference man

$$\text{Cell mass} = \text{cell water} \times \frac{100}{70} = 35.7\,\text{kg}$$

This figure represents about 55 per cent of the total body weight of 65 kg. Thus in a healthy lean man the active metabolising tissue comprises little more than half the body weight. In an obese individual the proportion will be much less.

An estimate of the cell mass can also be made by measuring the amount of the natural isotope of potassium, ^{40}K, in the body, using a whole body counter.

Effects of age

The water content of the newborn baby is high and usually about 80 per cent of body weight. Fomon and Owen (1964) record values of 70 to 73 per cent at 4 to 6 weeks of age and below 65 per cent after 3 months of age. Most of this excess water is present in the extracellular fluid, but the water content of the cells may also be higher than in the adult.

The water content of old people is usually a little less on average than in young adults (McCance and Widdowson, 1951; Norris et al., 1963; Young et al., 1963). A drying up of the cells and shrinkage of the extracellular fluid with age is a fundamental feature of human biology. At first the process is rapid, but it soon slows down and thereafter cannot be readily detected. However, it is unusual to find a healthy man or woman in the nineties, who has not obviously shrunk, as Charles Dickens (1867) observed: 'Anyone may pass, any day, in the thronged thoroughfares of the metropolis, some meagre, wrinkled yellow old man.... This old man is always a little old man. If he were ever a big old man, he has shrunk into a little old man; if he were always a little old man, he has dwindled into a less old man.' To be able to dry up gracefully may be the secret of a happy old age.

Body fat

Determination by underwater weighing

Archimedes was set the problem of finding out how much silver was present in a crown of reputedly pure gold. He solved it by determining the density (mass/volume) of the crown and of pure gold and of pure silver. Then if x is the fraction of silver in the crown

$$\frac{1}{d(\text{crown})} = \frac{1-x}{d(\text{gold})} + \frac{x}{d(\text{silver})}$$

The proportion of fat in the human body can be determined using the same principle, for it is well known that fat floats. The density of human fat has been measured many times and does not differ significantly from 0.900. The density of the fat-free body, the lean body mass, cannot be accurately determined, but there is much evidence that in health it is close to 1.10. If x be the percentage of fat in the human body

$$\frac{100}{d(\text{body})} = \frac{100-x}{1.10} + \frac{x}{0.90}$$

$$x = \frac{495}{d(\text{body})} - 450$$

The density of the human body can be determined by weighing first in air and then in water. If M is the mass of the body and V the volume, then

$$d = \frac{M}{V}$$

The volume is obtained by displacement. The difference between the weight of the body in air and the weight when submerged in water is the weight of the water displaced. The volume corresponding to this mass of water can be obtained by dividing by the density of water at the time of underwater weighing. The underwater weight has to be corrected for the upthrust of the residual air in the lungs. This in a young person is about 1.2 litres, but increases as the lungs lose their elasticity with age. It can be measured using a nitrogen washout technique. It is impossible to measure the gas in the alimentary tract. The amount is usually small (about 100 ml) and can be neglected.

Attempts to assess the fat content of man from measurements of body density arose as a result of a practical problem. Some men on a draft for recruitment into the US Navy were marked unfit for service by a medical board because their weights exceeded the maximum permissible for their heights. As these men were professional footballers in civil life, it seemed unlikely that they were unfit for naval service because of obesity. A US naval surgeon, Behnke, and his associates (1942) examined the men. They were weighed in air and under water. Their density was thus calculated and found in some cases to be as high as 1.090 to 1.097, indicating a fat content of 4 per cent or less. From this it was concluded that the excess weight was mainly due to extra muscle and not fat.

The real difficulty in calculating the total fat from the density measurement and body weight in air arises from the impossibility of getting a direct measure of the density of the lean body mass (the body minus its fat content) owing to the varying density of the skeleton. As the bath is around 37^0C the procedure is not unpleasant for the subject (as we can vouch from personal experience) and is applicable to active people of either sex.

Table 2.3 gives some values for the fat content of both men and women. The range of values is wide, but young women appear to be twice as fat, on average, as young men. Physical training reduces body fat. In most forms of athletics a competitor would have little chance of reaching Olympic standards until he had trained so that his body fat was less than half that found in normal subjects (Pařízková, 1977). Whether the increase in the fat store with age is physiological is discussed on page 244.

Table 2.3 Some values for the amount of fat present in the human body obtained by underwater weighing

City	Age	Fat as a percentage of body weight		Reference
		Mean	Range	
Men—				
Prague (trained runners)	22.5	6.3	—	Pařízková (1977)
Edinburgh	18–22	11	5–27	MacMillan *et al.* (1965)
Tokyo	22	12	6–22	Arimoto (1957)
Minnesota	25	14	—	Keys (1955)
Minnesota	55	26	—	Keys (1955)
Women—				
Prague (Olympic gymnasts)	—	8	—	Pařízková (1977)
Edinburgh	18–22	26	18–35	MacMillan *et al.* (1965)
New York State	16–30	29	20–38	Young *et al.* (1963)
Tokyo	21	23	13–33	Arimoto (1957)
Minnesota	24	25	—	Keys (1955)
New York State	50–60	42	29–55	Young *et al.* (1963)
Minnesota	56	38	—	Keys (1955)

Determination using the dilution principle
A gas that is much more soluble in fat than in water and quickly dissolves in all the body fat could provide a means of measuring total body fat. Hytten *et al.* (1966) have used an isotope of krypton (^{85}Kr) and Halliday (1971) cyclopropane. However, the method is beset with technical difficulties when applied to man and, as yet, has not yielded reliable results.

Subcutaneous fat
A large proportion of the body fat is carried directly beneath the skin. Special calipers have been designed for measuring skinfold thickness. Measurements taken at several sites on the body can be combined to give an index of body fatness and correlate well with determination of total body fat from density measurements. Skin calipers, if carefully used, provide a simple and practical means of assessing the obesity. They are further discussed on page 244.

The skeleton
No reliable method for assessing the size or composition of the skeleton in the living body has been developed. Indeed there have not been sufficient direct analyses of human skeletons to allow accurate statements of the range of variation. It is known that in the USA Negroes have on average a slightly heavier skeleton than whites. Garn (1963) provides an excellent summary of what knowledge is available and points out how accurate studies of body composition in life are handicapped by lack of methods for study in this compartment. A brief statement on the chemical composition of the skeleton is given on page 91.

GROWTH

Many examples are given in this book of how growth and development may be impaired as a result of a failure of nutrition. A child does not grow like a crystal, and a newborn body is not a miniature adult. The internal organs notably the brain and liver, form a much larger proportion of total weight than in the mature body, and there is relatively much less muscle, bone and adipose tissue. Growth of some organs takes place in different stages of childhood. The brain grows rapidly in the first two years of life, when it reaches about 75 per cent of adult size; the uterus remains small for the first ten years and then grows to adult size in two or three years; the lymphatic organs, thymus, tonsils and lymph nodes are small at birth, grow rapidly in the first few years to a maximum size by the age of 10 and thereafter regress. These differential growth rates are controlled over the years by a metabolic clock, set to a timetable which is genetically determined but which may be slowed down for a period by a poor diet and severe or repeated infections. Early in fetal life the control system becomes centred in the brain and it operates principally through the hypothalamus, which itself regulates the trophic secretions of the anterior pituitary gland and hence other endocrine glands. These glands have a major role in the control of growth, and in early life disease affecting any one of them disrupts the pattern of growth in various different ways. Cretinism (p. 270) arising from a failure of the thyroid gland to secrete its hormones is a good example.

Growth can occur only if the organs and tissues receive the nutrients needed for the synthesis of their protein and other molecules. It is therefore dependent on an adequate diet. An insufficiency of energy and protein are the commonest causes in man of failure to grow or of disproportional growth except in affluent societies. The effects of this lack on body composition are described on page 259. In theory, a dietary deficiency of any one of the 35 or more nutrients known to be essential for mammals could be responsible for impairment of growth in man. Well-known examples are lack of iron, vitamin D and vitamin A, leading to failure of normal development of red blood corpuscles, bone and epithelial surfaces respectively.

Growth is also impaired when disease of the alimentary tract prevents adequate absorption of nutrients. Examples are repeated attacks of gastroenteritis and coeliac disease. Many disorders of metabolism prevent normal utilisation of nutrients and so retard growth or development. Diabetes and phenylketonuria are well-known examples. Chronic infectious diseases severely retard growth. They may do this by reducing appetite, by preventing normal absorption or utilisation of nutrients and by the increased need for nutrients brought about by fever.

Disturbances in growth occur most commonly in the period immediately after weaning. In the uterus the fetus normally receives an adequate supply of nutrients even if the mother's diet is far from satisfactory. Only when a mother's diet is grossly insufficient or if the placenta is abnormal is fetal growth impaired (p. 517). Similarly lactation supplies the needs of early infancy when the growth rate is most rapid. As a child gets older, growth rate slows and the need for nutrients is relatively less; stores of nutrients may have been built up and infectious diseases are in general less frequent and less severe owing to the buildup of immunity. However, insufficient food for a significant period at any time during childhood and adolescence may prevent an individual from reaching his full potential in height and weight, as judged by accepted standards (p. 470). Chronic undernutrition delays the onset of puberty and the menarche (Tanner, 1962).

Animal experiments, mainly on rats and pigs, by McCance and Widdowson (1974) show that severe distortions of the pattern of growth follow dietary restriction at various stages of development. Even if a newborn pig is prevented from growing for a year by this means, rapid growth follows when a normal diet is given, although the animal does not quite reach normal size and proportions. In man a short interruption of growth and development arising as a result of nutritional failure can be made good by **catch-up growth** (Fig. 2.1), provided a good diet is given. In general, children below the age of 5 years can make up for a period of retarded growth very well, but thereafter their capacity to do so declines. In urban slums and some peasant communities the usual diet of children may be barely adequate and in such communities a a severe nutritional illness may permanently impair growth and development. This is discussed in Chapter 29.

For further reading a short and practical textbook by Marshall (1977) on human growth and its disorders is recommended.

Cell growth

An organ or tissue may enlarge in two ways. The number of cells may increase by multiplication, **cell hyperplasia**, or the individual cells may get bigger, **cell hypertrophy**. In some tissues, hyperplasia ceases early in life. Thus in the brain the number of neurones reaches approximately the adult value during the second year of life. Thereafter if any are destroyed, they cannot be replaced by hyperplasia. During the period of rapid hyperplasia in early life the brain is especially susceptible to damage by any factor disturbing normal nutrition (p. 266). In adults both cardiac and skeletal muscle cells cannot divide. When an athlete goes into training and gains weight by 'putting on muscle' and this is due to cell hypertrophy. If the ventricles of the heart have to carry out extra work, either in health due to heavy physical activity or in disease, e.g. hypertension or aortic valve damage, they enlarge due to cell hypertrophy. By contrast the epithelial lining of the gut is replaced by cell hyperplasia every two or three days throughout life. Liver cells retain the power to regenerate and after severe damage with the death or **necrosis** of

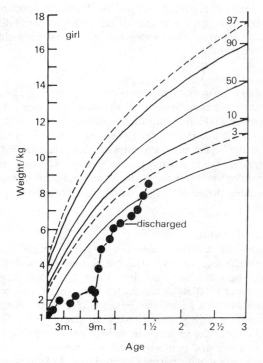

Fig. 2.1 Catch-up growth in a Baganda girl who was admitted to hospital when 9 months old weighing only 2.4 kg (McCance and Widdowson, 1974).

many cells, hyperplasia may restore liver function to normal levels (p. 415). Adipocytes also are capable of hyperplasia. As in health, adipocytes in fat depots are normally well loaded with fat, they have a limited capacity for hypertrophy and obesity is associated often with hyperplasia. If part of any organ is destroyed by trauma or disease, it is replaced by fibrous tissue formed by fibroblasts, connective tissue cells which proliferate in the damaged area.

The distinction between cell hyperplasia and hypertrophy is very important in considering the effect of nutritional factors on individual organs.

3. Energy

Just before the French Revolution Lavoisier and the physicist Laplace carried out experiments in which they placed a guinea-pig in a very small closed chamber surrounded by ice. They measured the amount of ice melted over a 10-hour period and at the same time the amount of carbon dioxide given out by the animal. They demonstrated that there was a relationship between the heat produced by the animal and the respiratory exchange. Lavoisier also measured the oxygen consumption of men, and showed that it increased after food and exercise.

Lavoisier has properly been considered the founder of the modern science of nutrition. For over a hundred years after his death on the guillotine, ingenious and learned men exercised their talents in designing calorimeters in which laboratory animals and men could live for many hours or even a few days whilst their metabolism was studied. In 1849 Reynault and Reiset in Paris carried out numerous experiments on small animals and planned to construct a large human respiration chamber in a hospital. They were unable to get the necessary funds and they had to drop their project. Pettenkofer and Voit were more fortunate. They acquired the patronage of King Maximilian II of Bavaria. By 1866 they had constructed at Munich a chamber in which a man could live for several days and have all his respiratory exchanges measured. After measurements on a fasting man lasting 24 hours, the protein 'burned' was calculated from the urinary nitrogen and the fat from the respiratory carbon dioxide (after deducting the carbon in the protein burned and assuming no change in the carbohydrate store of the body). A difference of only 6.2 per cent was found between the measured oxygen absorption and that calculated as necessary for the combustion of the body materials metabolised. This accuracy indicates both their experimental skill and the soundness of the assumptions on which their calculations were based.

Rubner in Berlin, Zuntz in Switzerland and Johansson in Sweden were others who from 1880 onwards extended the work of the Munich school and so laid many of the foundations of modern nutritional science. But it was the American, Atwater, a student of Voit in Munich, who carried out the experiments which have established the essential quantitative physiological knowledge on which all assessments of the energy needs of men are based. Atwater returned to the USA from Germany in 1892 and enlisted the help of Rosa, an engineer. Together they constructed a human calorimeter which could measure the heat produced by a man with an accuracy of 0.1 per cent. At the same time the chamber incorporated the respiration apparatus used by Pettenkofer and Voit. Table 3.1 illustrates how accurately Atwater was able to measure the energy exchange of man.

When in 1906 Hopkins at Cambridge carried out his experiments which demonstrated beyond doubt the existence of 'accessory food factors' (later known as vitamins), Atwater had completed his work. A chapter had been written in the textbooks of physiology which has needed no subsequent revision. After Hopkins' discovery, interest shifted sharply from the energy needs to the vitamin needs of both man and animals. The quality rather than the quantity of an individual's food became the foremost interest.

The first part of this chapter gives an account of the classical physiology of energy exchanges. It differs little from accounts written in the early part of the century and it

Table 3.1 An experiment of Atwater and Benedict (1899) (values in megajoules)

		Total 4 days	Average 1 day
(a)	Heat of combustion of food eaten	41.22	10.31
(b)	Heat of combustion of faeces	1.26	0.32
(c)	Heat of combustion of urine	2.25	0.56
(m)	Heat of combustion of alcohol eliminated	0.35	0.09
(d)	Estimated heat of combustion of protein gained (+) or lost (−)	−1.16	−0.29
(e)	Estimated heat of combustion of fat gained (+) or lost (−)	−2.26	−0.56
(f)	Estimated energy of material oxidised in the body $a-(b+c+m+d+e)$	40.78	10.19
(g)	Heat determined	40.06	10.02
(h)	Heat determined greater (+) or less (−) than estimated $(f-g)$	−0.68	−0.17
(i)	Heat determined greater (+) or less (−) than estimated $(h+f)$ (per cent)	–	−1.6

is extremely unlikely that any essential changes will be made in the future. Excellent accounts of the subject by writers personally associated with the classical experiments have been given by Graham Lusk (1906) and Magnus Levy (1907). All serious students of the science of nutrition should read carefully one or other of these books which describe in detail so much of the work that is fundamental to the science.

The second part attempts to appraise the energy needs of contemporary man. It is a guide for those responsible for food planning or for drawing up ration scales. In contrast to the former part it rests on a limited experimental and scientific basis. However, practical policies have often to be decided by judgments based on inadequate data.

PHYSIOLOGY

Forms of energy

The biologist is interested in energy in five forms: (1) solar, (2) chemical, (3) mechanical, (4) thermal, (5) electrical.*

In plants and animals the various forms of energy are quantitatively interchangeable. It has been frequently demonstrated that living creatures, like inanimate matter, can neither create nor destroy energy but can only transform it and so obey the first law of thermodynamics, which states the principle of the conservation of energy.

Animals differ from green plants in that they cannot utilise solar energy directly. Green plants are able to synthesise complicated organic substances such as carbohydrates, proteins and fats from simple inorganic materials, such as CO_2, H_2O, NH_3 and SO_4. In this process, photosynthesis, solar energy is used and converted into chemical energy which is stored by the plant. Plants, which are independent of other forms of life, are thus distinguishable from all animals, which are wholly dependent on plants. This is true now. It may not be so in the future, if chemists succeed in making synthetic foods on an adequate scale.

Animals get their energy from their food in a chemical form, which is derived directly or indirectly from plants. This energy is bound in molecules of carbohydrate, fat, protein and alcohol.

Energy taken in as food is used (1) to perform mechanical work, (2) to maintain the tissues of the body, and (3) for growth.

In the conversion of chemical energy into mechanical energy, man acts as an engine with a measurable thermodynamic efficiency. Most of the energy is dissipated as heat. At best a man can convert 25 per cent of the energy in his food into mechanical work. In this respect he is much more efficient than most steam engines and about on a par with a good internal combustion engine.

* The existence of powerful electric organs in some fish is a clear-cut demonstration that animals can generate electrical energy: most electrical organs in fish are modified muscle end plates. The processes of excitation in both muscle and nerve are dependent on electrical changes on the cell membranes.

Of the energy required for maintenance less than 10 per cent is used for internal mechanical work, e.g. the beating of the heart and the movements of respiratory muscles. Over 90 per cent is used either for the osmotic pumps which maintain the differences in electrolyte concentrations between intra- and extracellular fluids or for the synthesis of protein and other macromolecules. These syntheses take place continuously with the turnover of cell constituents, and at an increased rate in the growing child.

The energy in the food is ultimately converted into heat and its dissipation maintains the temperature of the body. Unless the environmental temperature is very cold, even a small amount of muscular activity produces enough heat to maintain the temperature, especially if the heat is conserved by adequate clothing. The extra heat developed when hard mechanical work is done represents waste that must be eliminated if the temperature of the body is to be kept normal. This is effected by means of sweating.

The unit of energy is the joule (J) and is the energy expended when 1 kilogram (kg) is moved 1 metre (m) by a force of 1 newton (N). Physiologists and nutritionists are concerned with large amounts of energy and the convenient units are the kilojoule ($kJ = 10^3 J$) and the megajoule ($MJ = 10^6 J$).

Rates of work or energy expenditure are conveniently expressed in watts ($W = J/s$). Twelve people sitting talking in a room produce heat at the rate of about 60 kJ/min and this is equivalent to a one kilowatt electric fire, as many hostesses know.

Formerly energy was always expressed quantitatively in units of heat, the unit used being the kilocalorie (kcal).

The calorie is a derived, not a basic unit. The International Table calorie was defined by the 1956 Steam Conference as 4.1868 J exactly. The 15° calorie is the amount of heat required to raise the temperature of water 1°C from 14.5° to 15.5°; it is approximately 4.1855 J. The thermochemical calorie is based on the heat of combustion of benzoic acid and is 4.184 J. All three conversion factors are in use in current authoritative reports on nutrition and there is some confusion. Either of the first two are appropriate for nutritional work but we follow the Royal Society (1972) and use the thermochemical calorie, i.e. 4.184 J (and 1 kcal = 4.184 kJ). In practice 4.2 is usually close enough as a conversion factor. The error from rounding off is less than the variation in energy content of foods. The calorie has become such a familiar unit that it will be some time before many people become accustomed to the use of the joule. Accordingly in many places in this book energy values are given in both joules and calories.

Energy content of food

If a foodstuff is placed in a small chamber or bomb (Fig. 3.1) and exposed to a high pressure of oxygen it can be ignited by a small electric current. All the organic material is burnt and the heat liberated can be measured. The heats of combustion of the three 'proximate principles'—carbohydrates, proteins and fats—and of alcohol are shown in Table 3.2. There are slight differences in the heats of combustion of the nutrients in different foods. In the animal body, the tissues are able to oxidise carbohydrate and fat completely to carbon dioxide and water, but the oxidation of protein is never complete. Nitrogenous substances derived from protein such as urea, uric acid and creatinine are excreted in the urine. Many observations of the heat of combustion of urine have shown that it contains unoxidised material equivalent to 33.1 kJ (7.9 kcal)/g of nitrogen or 5.23 kJ (1.25 kcal)/g of protein oxidised by the

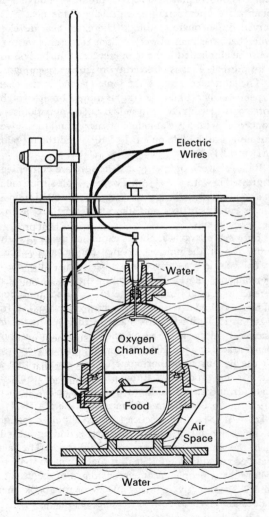

Fig. 3.1. The bomb calorimeter. The bomb is placed inside a vessel of water, the temperature of which can be accurately measured. The foodstuff is placed in a small crucible. The bomb is filled with oxygen at high pressure and the foodstuff ignited by means of electric leads. The material in the bomb burns and the heat produced leads to a rise of temperature in the surrounding water.

body. It is therefore necessary to subtract 5.23 kJ/g from the heat of combustion of protein. Further corrections are necessary to allow for the incomplete absorption of nutrients in the alimentary canal. Atwater, over 50 years ago, made a large number of experiments in which he analysed the faeces of three young American men for periods lasting for three to eight days, whilst on mixed diets typical of the time. He concluded that 92 per cent of protein, 95 per cent of fat and 99 per cent of carbohydrate were normally absorbed. From this the 'Atwater factors' for the available energy of the three different proximate principles (as given in Table 3.2) have been derived. It is important to remember that these factors make allowance for the energy in the food lost in faeces and urine. They are physiological approximations based on experiments on a limited number of subjects on one kind of diet. Experiments carried out in Glasgow on young and old persons of both sexes on diets containing varying amounts of vegetables and cereals confirmed that for most practical purposes the Atwater factors can be used to calculate metabolisable energy (Southgate and Durnin, 1970).

In practice, the energy values of diets are calculated from tables of food analyses, of which many are available (Chap. 16). These tables give figures for the carbohydrate, protein and fat content of each food as determined by chemical analysis; the energy value of the food is calculated by multiplying these figures by the Atwater factors or some variant of them. Differences may arise from the methods of calculating the results. The protein content of each food is always determined from its nitrogen content. Most proteins contain about 16 per cent of nitrogen. To calculate the protein content of foods, the nitrogen content has frequently been multiplied by 6.25, but this figure is only an approximation and certainly too high for cereals and too low for milk. For these 5.7 and 6.4 per cent respectively are better values, and have been used by some authors in the construction of their tables. The heat of combustion of the different carbohydrates varies significantly. In older tables of food analyses the carbohydrate content is calculated by difference, i.e. the carbohydrate content of the food is taken to be the difference between the total weight and the sum of the water, protein, fat and mineral content. It is then mostly starch, which has a higher value than the sugar. In some modern tables the amount of glucose, fructose, sucrose, dextrins and starch have been determined and the carbohydrate content expressed in terms of monosaccharide. It does not then include the cellulose and other unavailable carbohydrates (p. 27) and the best conversion factor is 15.7 kJ (3.75 kcal)/g.

In general all these differences and inconsistencies are small in comparison with the variations between different samples of the same food. In particular almost all animal foods have a very varying fat content and this may greatly affect their energy value. On the other hand the chemical

Table 3.2 The heat of combustion and the available energy in the three proximate principles in a mixed diet

	Heat of combustion kJ/g	kcal/g	Loss in urine kJ/g	kcal/g	Availability	Atwater factors kJ/g	kcal/
Protein							
Meat	22.4	5.35	5.23	1.25	92	17	4
Egg	23.4	5.58					
Fat							
Butter	38.2	9.12	—		95	37	9
Animal fat	39.2	9.37					
Carbohydrate							
Starch	17.2	4.12	—		99	16	4
Glucose	15.5	3.69					
Ethyl alcohol	29.7	7.10	trace		100	29	7

composition of a given variety of a cereal is relatively constant.

Despite all these uncertainties the energy values for foods given in tables of food composition are of practical use. They are unlikely to lead to any serious error in making up diets for an individual patient or for prescribing ration scales for institutions, service personnel, etc. They are well tried and practical guides. The intelligent user would, however, be well advised to find out exactly how the energy values in his particular table have been obtained and to keep an eye open for possible anomalies. An excellent account of the history of the various factors in use today with full references to the classical papers has been given by Widdowson (1955) and McCance and Widdowson (1967).

The uncertainties inherent in all tables of energy values of food make them of little use to the research worker who wishes to feed diets of accurately known energy content for metabolic balance studies on patients or laboratory animals. For such there is no escape from painstaking analyses of samples of the foods eaten and the urine and faeces excreted.

Alcohol can serve as a source of energy for man. The heat of combustion of ethyl alcohol is 29.7 kJ (7 kcal)/g and under favourable circumstances, as Atwater showed, all this energy can be utilised by man. How much of the alcohol ingested is actually used under different dietary circumstances is a difficult problem, which is considered in Chapter 7.

Sheep and other ruminants are able to derive energy from cellulose and other types of dietary fibre (except lignin), which are broken down by bacteria in the alimentary tract to short-chain fatty acids: these are subsequently absorbed into the circulation and metabolised. There is no evidence that man derives significant amounts of energy from cellulose but it is possible that, when fibre intake is very large, small amounts of energy from this source may be absorbed from the large intestine.

MEASUREMENT OF ENERGY EXPENDITURE

Direct calorimetry is easy in theory, though difficult and costly in practice. If an animal or man is put into a small chamber in which all the heat evolved can be measured, then the total energy expenditure is the sum of that heat plus any mechanical work performed (as on a stationary bicycle). Figure 3.2 is a diagrammatic representation of the Atwater and Rosa chamber. With this they established two quantitative relationships in human metabolism.

1. Total energy expenditure (the sum of the heat produced plus the mechanical work done) was equal to the net energy from the food consumed (the total chemical energy in the food minus the energy lost in the faeces and urine). They left no doubt that man obeys the fundamental law of the Conservation of Energy.
2. Total energy expenditure is quantitatively related to the oxygen consumption.

Indirect calorimetry is the measurement of oxygen consumption and technically a simpler procedure than the measurement of heat. It is based on the fact that when an organic substance is completely combusted either in a calorimeter or in the human body, oxygen is consumed in amounts directly related to the energy liberated as heat. The oxidation of glucose goes quantitatively as follows:

$$C_6H_{12}O_6 + 6O_2 = 6\,CO_2 + 6\,H_2O + \text{heat}$$

180g	6 × 22.4 litres	6 × 22.4 litres	6 × 18g	2.78 MJ

This equation states that 180 g of glucose yields 2.78 MJ of energy or that the heat of combustion of 1 g of glucose is 2.78/180 = 15.5 kJ (3.69 kcal). As 6 × 22.4 litres of oxygen are used, 1 litre of oxygen is equivalent to 2.78/(6 × 22.4) = 20.8 kJ (4.95 kcal). The ratio of the carbon dioxide produced to the oxygen used is known as the respiratory quotient (RQ). The RQ for the oxidation of glucose is 1.0.

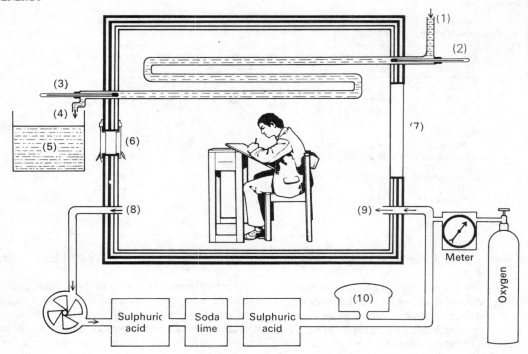

Fig. 3.2 The Atwater and Rosa respiration calorimeter. The walls of this chamber are insulated. Heat produced in it is absorbed by water passing in at (1) and out at (4), its temperature on entering and leaving being recorded on the thermometers (2) and (3). The volume of water that has flowed through the colling system is measured in the vessel (5). The subject may be observed through the window (7), while food may be introduced and excreta removed through the porthole (6). Air leaves the chamber at (8) and passes through a blower and over sulphuric acid and soda-lime to absorb water and carbon dioxide. Oxygen measured by a gas meter is added to the system before the air passes into the chamber at (9). (10) is a tension equaliser. (From Bell, G. H., Davidson, J. N. and Scarborough, H. (1968). *Textbook of Physiology and Biochemistry*, 7th edn. Edinburgh: Livingstone.)

Similar equations can be written for the combustion of a fatty acid or a protein. Table 3.3 gives values for the heat of combustion, RQ and energy equivalent of O_2 for fat, protein and starch (the chief carbohydrate in the diet). This table was first set out by the Swiss physiologist Zuntz over 80 years ago. As the energy equivalent of oxygen is much the same, whichever of the three foodstuffs is oxidised, a figure of 20 kJ (4.8 kcal)/litre of oxygen is a good approximation when, as is usual, a mixture of the three is being used.

It is also known that 1 g of urinary nitrogen arises from the metabolism of 6.25 g of protein. If, in addition to the oxygen used (O_{2m}), the carbon dioxide produced (CO_{2m}) and the urinary nitrogen (U_N) are also measured, it is then possible to calculate the amounts of carbohydrate, fat and protein metabolised. This is known as the **metabolic mixture.** The energy used can also be calculated more precisely. Four equations give the means of doing this.

Carbohydrate (g) $= 4.12\,CO_{2m} - 2.91\,O_{2m} - 2.54\,U_N$
Fat (g) $= 1.69\,O_{2m} - 1.69\,CO_{2m} - 1.94\,U_N$
Protein (g) $= 6.25\,U_N$
Energy (kJ) $= 15.8\,O_{2m} + 4.86\,CO_{2m} - 12.0\,U_N$

These equations are derived from the values presented in Table 3.3 and the value given above for the protein equivalent of urinary nitrogen. Any reader can check them by solving three simple, if cumbersome equations. They were first set out by Consolazio *et al.* (1963). Energy expenditure and the metabolic mixture can be calculated rapidly from the equations either by hand, using a pro-forma, or by a computer. Their use gives the same answer as the classical method described in most textbooks, based on a calculation of the non-protein RQ. The non-protein RQ is an abstraction which has no physiological meaning, as protein metabolism is never zero.

If neither the urinary nitrogen nor the carbon dioxide output have been measured, a useful approximation of the rate of energy expenditure (E) can be derived from measurements of the minute volume of expired air (V) and its oxygen content (O_{2E}) using Weir's (1949) formula

$$E \text{ (watts)} = 3.43\ V\ (20.93 - O_{2E})$$

Measurement of oxygen consumption

The oxygen consumption of man has been measured in respiration chambers, where there is the advantage of

Table 3.3 Energy yields from oxidation of foodstuffs (Zuntz, 1897)

1 g of —	O_2 required ml	CO_2 produced ml	RQ	Energy developed		Energy equivalent of 1 l of O_2	
				kJ	kcal	kJ	kcal
Starch	828.8	828.8	1.000	17.51	4.183	21.13	5.047
Animal fat	2019.2	1427.3	0.707	39.60	9.461	19.62	4.868
Protein	966.1	781.7	0.809	18.59	4.442	19.26	4.600

being able to record it over long periods. However, respiration chambers are expensive and difficult to manipulate (though far less so than calorimeter chambers) and, when within one, the subject's activities are necessarily limited. For these reasons most measurements of oxygen uptake are made when the subject is breathing into some form of apparatus, which can measure the total volume of gas expired (the minute volume) and provide a sample of expired air for analysis. This involves the use of valves which separate the inspired air from the expired air. These valves may be housed in a small metal or plastic box with a rubber mouthpiece which the subject grips between his teeth. Alternatively they may be housed in a rubber mask covering the face. The rubber mouthpiece is most frequently employed. Some people experience an initial difficulty in breathing through valves and require a period of practice or training before reliable results are obtained. Indeed all subjects need a few minutes practice before they breathe naturally through a strange apparatus. For most people such a short period is all that is necessary and, in our experience, the importance of prolonged training has often been exaggerated.

Many different types of apparatus have been designed. The Benedict Roth spirometer (Fig. 3.3) is a closed circuit system in which the subject breathes in oxygen from a metal cylinder about 6 litres in capacity, and the expired air passes back through a soda-lime canister (to absorb the carbon dioxide) into the same cylinder. The cylinder floats on water inside a second cylinder. As the oxygen is consumed the inner cylinder falls and the rate of fall is recorded by an ink-writer on a rotating drum. The Benedict Roth apparatus is used in hospitals for measuring the resting or basal metabolism, for which purpose it is eminently suitable. It is very simple to use and the direct reading of oxygen consumption avoids the necessity of gas analyses. As the carbon dioxide is not measured the RQ cannot be calculated and the heat equivalent of oxygen is assumed to be 20 kJ (4.8 kcal)/l. The apparatus is not portable so it can only be used when the subject is at rest either lying or sitting. The physiologist is usually interested in the carbon dioxide production as well as the oxygen consumption. To measure both, the subject after breathing in ordinary room air breathes out into a Douglas bag, which is made of rubber or plastic of 100 litres capacity. The expired air is collected for a period of 3 to 10 minutes. The air in the bag is then passed through a gas

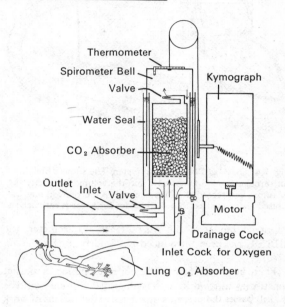

Fig. 3.3 Benedict Roth spirometer. The subject wears a nose-clip and breathes through a mouthpiece which is connected to the apparatus by two valves. He breathes in oxygen through the inspiratory valve and breathes out through the expiratory valve into the carbon dioxide absorber. The amount of oxygen used is recorded on the revolving drum by the pen attached to the counter weight.

meter, measured and a portion set aside for subsequent analysis of the carbon dioxide and oxygen content. The Douglas bag method is the simplest and most reliable means of measuring the respiratory exchanges. It is the method of choice in the laboratory. However, it is cumbersome and clumsy to use for experiments in the field or in industry. For measurements of energy expenditure during industrial work and everyday life, the procedure has been greatly facilitated by the development in Germany of the Max Planck respirometer (Müller and Franz, 1952). This apparatus (Fig. 3.4) is a light-weight portable respirometer, which can measure directly the volume of the expired air and simultaneously divert a small fraction into a plastic bladder for subsequent analysis. The instrument weighs only about 2.5 kg and can be worn on the back like a haversack. Its introduction made possible the systematic measurement of the energy used in a variety of normal occupations as diverse as housework and coalmining. An

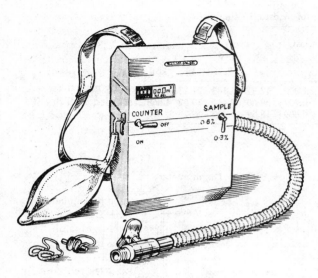

Fig. 3.4 The Max Planck respirometer. The subject breathes out through an expiratory valve and the volume is directly measured and recorded on the counter. A portion of the expired air is diverted into the bladder for subsequent analysis.

improved model of the Max Planck respirometer, the MISER, has been introduced by Goldsmith (Eley *et al.*, 1978).

There have been many differences of opinion as to what constitutes hard work. A physiological definition would be useful; Table 3.4 presents quantitative definitions of work intensities. It is based on a study by Christensen (1953) in the Swedish iron industry, but is generally applicable. The figures given are for men of about 65 kg.

Table 3.4 Energy expenditure in relation to intensity of muscular work (modified from Christensen 1953)

Grade of work		W	kcal/min
Very light	less than	170	<2.5
Light		170–350	2.5–4.9
Moderate		350–500	5.0–7.4
Heavy		500–650	7.5–9.9
Very heavy		650–800	10.0–12.5
Exceedingly heavy	over	800	over 12.5

Rates of energy expenditure

Many thousands of measurements of the energy expenditure of men and women undertaking a great variety of activities have been made by indirect calorimetry. These have been collected into a series of tables, which provide estimates of the energy output of man during his various activities in day-to-day life (Passmore and Durnin, 1955) and updated later (Durnin and Passmore, 1967). The tables are in some ways complementary to the well-known food tables which provide estimates of dietary energy

Table 3.5 Examples of the energy expenditure of physical activities

Light work at 170–350 W (2.5–4.9 kcal/min)

Assembly work
Light industry
Electrical industry
Carpentry
Military drill
Most domestic work with modern appliances
Gymnastic exercises
Building industry
Bricklaying
Plastering
Painting
Agricultural work (mechanised)
Driving a truck
Golf
Bowling

Moderate work at 350–500 W (5.0–7.4 kcal/min)

General labouring (pick and shovel)
Agricultural work (non-mechanised)
Route march with rifle and pack
Ballroom dancing
Gardening
Tennis
Cycling (up to 10 mph)

Heavy work at 500–650 W (7.5–9.9 kcal/min)

Coal mining (hewing and loading)
Football
Country dancing

Very heavy work at 650 W (> 10 kcal/min)

Lumber work
Furnace men (steel industry)
Swimming (crawl)
Cross-country running
Hill climbing

intake. Table 3.5 is a selection of figures giving the energy expenditure of various physical activites. There are naturally variations in individual efficiency in carrying out the same task, and these affect the energy expenditure. The major part of human work consists in moving the body about and in most activities energy expenditure is closely related to body weight. Obviously the grading of activities can only be approximate. Many measurements indicate that most jobs on a farm involve moderate physical activity, but some are heavy and others, perhaps an increasing number, are light. Similarly when most of us play tennis we are moderately active, but it requires heavy work to win a Wimbledon championship.

Resting and walking together make up a large proportion of the total daily energy expenditure. Each is now considered in more detail.

Energy expenditure at rest

When a subject is at complete rest and no physical work is being carried out, energy is required for the activity of the internal organs and to maintain the body temperature, as already discussed. This energy is called the basal or resting metabolism. The **basal metabolic rate** (BMR) is determined experimentally when the subject is lying down at complete physical and mental rest, wearing light clothing in a room comfortably warm and at least 12 hours after the last meal. Table 3.6 gives standard values for the BMR of people of both sexes and of all ages. It is based on a compilation of many hundreds of observations on people in many countries. It will be observed that the results are expressed in W/m². Surface area has long been used to standardise measurements of the BMR in individuals of varying size. Rubner showed many years ago that animals so diverse as the horse, man, the dog and the mouse had very different BMRs if expressed in W/kg of body weight, but the figures for each species are remarkably similar if expressed in W/m² of surface area. The surface area of a few men and women has been accurately determined by pasting small pieces of paper all over the body and measuring the area of the paper. From these measurements it was shown that surface area can be predicted from measurements of height and weight. A nomogram has been constructed for this purpose (Fig. 3.5).

While surface area provides a convenient standard for comparing the BMR of different species, it is not the best standard for assessing the BMR of individual members of the same species. In particular, in people whose body shape and composition depart markedly from the normal, the use of the surface area may mislead. This is certainly so in obese people. The BMR is more closely related to the 'lean body mass' than to the surface area. When the figures are expressed in relation to the lean body mass the differences between men and women recorded in Table 3.6 disappear. They are not the result of any fundamental differences in the metabolism of the two sexes, but reflect the fact that women are fatter than men (p. 9). Table 3.7 gives normal values for the resting metabolism of adults of different weights related to their body fat. This can be determined from skinfold measurements (p. 244) or assessed clinically. From this table standard values can be obtained more easily than from Table 3.6 and in our experience agreement with measured values obtained both from hospital patients and from students in their practical classes is equally good.

As Table 3.6 shows, the BMR is high in actively growing young children and falls rapidly in the first 12 years of life. Thereafter a steady slow decline sets in.

Natives of the tropics usually have a BMR about 10 per cent below the standards in Table 3.6. Most (but not all) immigrants to the tropics from Europe and North America show a similar fall. The higher BMR in cold climates is most likely an adaptation to the environment. There is no convincing evidence that there are any racial differences in the BMR.

When changing from the lying to the sitting or standing position the metabolism may rise by about 20 and 30 per cent respectively. When sitting quietly in a chair throughout the day, metabolism can be taken to be about 20 per cent above the basal rate plus an additional 10 per cent if a meal has been taken in the previous three hours.

When asleep throughout the night, the overall metabolic rate approximates very closely to the BMR. When sleep begins, the effect of the last meal may raise the metabolism slightly, but in the small hours of the morning it is usually a little lower than basal rates. This is probably due to a slight fall in body temperature. These two effects cancel each other and errors introduced in calculating total metabolism throughout the night from the BMR are negligible.

Thermogenic effect of food

This term is used to describe the effect of food in raising the metabolic rate above the value found when fasting. Previously known as the specific dynamic acid of food, this effect was much studied by Rubner and others between 1885 and 1910 and their work is summarised by Lusk (1928) in his textbook. They established that food might increase metabolism by as much as 30 per cent and 'that meat ingestion raises the metabolism most, fat next and sugar least of all the foodstuffs'.

Later investigators (Garrow and Hawes, 1972; Swindells, 1972; Bradfield and Jourdan, 1973) agree that it is

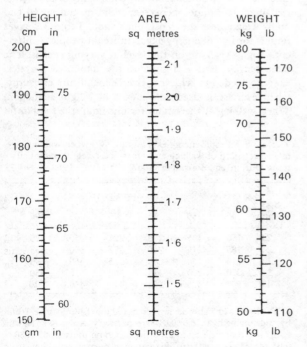

Fig. 3.5 Nomogram for calculating surface area. A line joining the height on the right-hand scale cuts the centre scale at the predicted surface area.

Table 3.6 Standards for basal metabolic rates (W/m²) (Fleisch, 1951)

Age (years)	1	3	5	7	9	11	13	15	17	19	20
Male	61.7	59.7	57.2	55.0	52.5	50.0	49.2	48.6	47.5	45.6	45.0
Female	61.7	59.4	56.4	52.8	49.7	48.9	46.9	44.2	42.2	41.4	41.1

Age (years)	25	30	35	40	45	50	55	60	65	70	75	80
Male	43.6	42.8	42.6	42.2	41.9	41.7	41.1	40.6	40.0	39.2	38.6	38.3
Female	40.8	40.8	40.8	40.6	40.0	39.4	38.6	38.1	37.5	36.9	36.4	35.8

Table 3.7 Normal values for the resting rate of energy expenditure of adults (watts)

Men	Women	Fat per cent	Weight (kg)							
			45	50	55	60	65	70	75	80
Thin		5–	—	68	73	78	83	88	92	97
Average		10–	—	65	70	75	80	85	88	93
Plump	Thin	15–	57	62	67	72	77	82	85	90
Fat	Average	20–	55	58	63	68	73	78	82	86
	Plump	25–	—	55	60	65	70	75	78	83
	Fat	30–	—	—	57	62	67	72	75	80

difficult to get consistent quantitative results and they give less emphasis to the specific nature of the effect of different nutrients. The size of the effect is not closely related to the size of the meal. On normal diets the overall effects amount to no more than 5 to 10 per cent of the basal metabolism over 24 hours. It is therefore not a phenomenon of much practical importance and, in particular, there is no case for attempting to adjust obesity diets, so as to maximise the effect.

The causes of the thermogenic effect remain uncertain. The fact that it can be demonstrated within 10 minutes of ingestion of a meal (Passmore and Ritchie, 1957) suggests that part of it can be accounted for by the work necessary for the secretion of gastric juice which may contain hydrogen ions at 10^6 times the concentration present in the plasma. However, this cannot account for its continuation, which may be for as long as five to six hours after a heavy meal. Clearly the absorption of food must in some way stimulate metabolism in the cells in general. The observations of Brooke and Ashworth (1972) are of interest; they showed that in malnourished Jamaican children a test meal had a maximum effect of 6 per cent; The effect with the same meal was 23 per cent when the children were growing rapidly during nutritional rehabilitation, but the value fell to 6 per cent when recovery was complete. This suggests that the effect is related in some way to protein synthesis but Garrow and Hawes (1972) found as much heat production after gelatin (of poor biological value) and sucrose as after milk protein. Perhaps in adults the ingestion of food may accelerate protein turnover.

Energy expenditure when walking

This has been extensively studied in many countries. There can be no doubt about the complexity of the factors that may determine energy expenditure, but speed and body weight are the most important. Table 3.8 gives figures for rate of energy expenditure for people of different weights walking on the level at varying speeds. The table can be used as a guide to the amount of physical exercise needed to achieve a given expenditure of energy, when exercise is used as a means of weight reduction. When walking at these rates for one hour, the food or fat

Table 3.8 Rates of energy expenditure (W) when walking related to speed of walking and gross body weight (modified from Durnin and Passmore, 1967)

Speed (mph)	Weight (kg)					
	45	55	65	75	85	95
2.0	150	185	200	225	250	275
2.5	185	215	240	275	300	335
3.0	215	250	285	315	360	390
3.5	250	290	325	360	410	450
4.0	285	325	365	415	460	510

The figures in Table 3.8 are converted into kJ/min or kcal/min by multiplying by 0.06 or 0.0144 respectively. A man of 65 kg who spends 30 min walking to his office at 4 mph utilises $365 \times 30 \times 0.06 = 6.57$ kJ or 158 kcal. This amount of energy could come from about 18 g of either dietary or adipose tissue fat. It is some four times more energy than he would have spent in 25 min in bed and 5 min driving to the office in his car.

stores have to provide from 550–1830 kJ (130–435 kcal). For a 65 kg person one hour's brisk walking the figures are unlikely to be in error by more than ± 15 per cent for any individual. They are not applicable to anyone who is lame and so walks at a mechanical disadvantage.

ENERGY REQUIREMENTS OF MAN

When in health and with food freely available, each individual meets his own energy needs with remarkable precision (p.76). In clinical practice the assessment of a patient's energy requirements usually requires a simple experiment which presents no difficulty. For instance, to find out whether 10.5 MJ (2500 kcal)/day will provide sufficient energy for an accountant with diabetes to carry out his business in the office and pursue his usual recreations, all that is necessary is to give him a diet providing 10.5 MJ and observe if he gains or loses weight. There are wide variations in the energy requirements of individuals, even of those following the same occupation and apparently leading similar kinds of lives. If exact knowledge of an individual's requirements is needed, resort to this simple experiment is necessary.

It is much more difficult to determine the energy requirements of large groups of people. Such information is needed by governments to provide a base for national food policies. It is also needed by those responsible for planning diets for the armed forces, schools and other institutions. The problem of assessing how much food is needed, neither too little nor too much, is an old one which presented itself even before Noah began to victual the Ark. It is ever-recurring.

METHODS OF ASSESSMENT

Dietary surveys
Voit in 1881 recorded the food consumed by labourers and artisans in Germany and concluded that the average man needs 12.8 MJ (3055 kcal)/day. Similarly Atwater in 1902 calculated the energy in the diets of farmers in Connecticut and Vermont; he found that they consumed 14.3 and 15.2 MJ (3410 and 3635 kcal)/day respectively. Since then dietary surveys have been carried out on a large scale in many countries and provide the basis of many estimates of human energy requirements. The technique of dietary surveys is discussed in page 474. Their use is subject to two inevitable drawbacks. (1) When food is available in abundance and there is nothing to restrict consumption, more food than is required may be eaten. On the other hand, when supplies are insufficient or purchasing power is low, consumption is likely to be less than optimal requirements. (2) A dietary survey can give no information of how the energy in the diet is expended, how much is needed for occupational activities and how much for off-work and recreational activities. With the changing patt-

erns of life brought about by mechanisation in industry and increased means of mechanical transport, these are often important questions.

On the practical side, the carrying out of family dietary surveys (measuring all the food consumed over a period in one household) is relatively simple. Individual dietary surveys, in which all the food consumed by a single person is measured and which provide much more detailed information, are technically more difficult; a high degree of co-operation on the part of the subject is necessary.

Surveys of energy expenditure
These attempt to overcome the drawbacks inherent in the methods of dietary surveys. Such surveys demand the collection of two distinct types of data, (a) the recording, often minute by minute, of the diverse physical activities in which the subject spends his time, and (b) the assessment of the energy cost of each activity either by direct measurement of oxygen consumption or from previously published tables. The sum of all the products (time spent in each activity multiplied by the energy cost of that activity) equals the total energy expenditure.

The first of such surveys was carried out in workers in all the major industries in Germany during World War II (Lehmann et al., 1950) and used as a basis for food rationing. The results of several surveys on men and women with different occupations carried out in the United Kingdom between 1950 and 1965 are given in Table 3.9. Such surveys are at least as accurate as individual dietary surveys, but somewhat more difficult to carry out.

RECOMMENDED INTAKES

Tables giving recommended intakes of energy have been drawn up by international and national committees in many countries. The use of these tables is discussed in Chapter 15, in which two of them are reproduced in full.

It is important to remember that the recommendations of all tables apply only to large groups of people. Individual requirements may depart markedly from the figures given. The recommendations are intended to provide a measure of the food sufficient to supply the energy required for a fully productive working life and for active recreations.

The energy requirements of individuals are dependent on four variables: (1) physical activity, (2) body size and composition, (3) age, and (4) climate and environment.

There are also extra needs for growth in childhood and adolescence and for pregnancy and lactation.

Effect of activity
In one of the first surveys of energy expenditure, the authors presented a summary of their results with the daily energy divided into three parts, one expended during

Table 3.9 Daily rates of energy expenditure by individuals with various occupations in the United Kingdom between 1950 and 1965 (Durnin and Passmore, 1967)

Occupation	Energy expenditure (MJ/day)		
	Mean	Minimum	Maximum
Men			
Elderly retired	9.7	7.3	11.8
Office workers	10.5	7.6	13.7
Colliery clerks	11.7	9.6	13.8
Laboratory technicians	11.9	9.3	15.9
Elderly industrial workers	11.9	9.1	15.6
Building workers	12.6	10.2	15.7
University students	12.3	9.4	18.5
Steel workers	13.7	10.9	16.6
Farmers	14.4	12.1	16.8
Army cadets	14.6	12.5	16.8
Coal miners	15.4	12.4	19.1
Forestry workers	15.4	12.0	19.2
Women			
Elderly housewives	8.3	6.5	10.1
Middle-aged housewives	8.7	7.4	9.6
Laboratory technicians	8.9	5.6	10.6
Assistants in department store	9.4	7.6	12.0
University students	9.6	5.8	10.5
Factory workers	9.7	8.2	12.4
Bakery workers	10.5	8.2	14.2

sleep, one during activities at work and one during non-occupational activities and recreations (Table 3.10). This approach proved useful and was the basis of the FAO (1957) and FAO/WHO (1973) recommendations for the requirements of adults. It is certainly convenient for

Table 3.10 Average daily expenditure of energy by 10 clerks (average age 28.3 years, weight 64.6 kg) and by 19 miners (average age 33.6 years, weight 65.7 kg) as measured over a whole week by Garry *et al.* (1955)

	Clerks		Miners	
	MJ	kcal	MJ	kcal
Asleep and day-time dozing	2.1	500	2.1	490
Activities at work	3.7	890	7.3	1750
Non-occupational activities and recreations	5.9	1410	5.9	1420
Total	11.7	2800	15.3	3660

considering the energy needs of men and women employed in industry, but less applicable to peasant agriculturists and to women whose main activities are domestic and in the home. Table 3.11 shows how the approach can be used to estimate the needs of adult men in the United Kingdom today.

Energy expenditure in bed approximates closely to the basal metabolic rate for 8 hours amounts to about 2 MJ.

The occupational energy is taken as 4.0, 5.5 and 7.5 MJ for men following sedentary, moderately active and very active occupations respectively. The difficulty lies in placing a particular group of workers into one of those categories. Many workers in the traditional heavy industries nowadays only do heavy muscular work for short periods and most of their time is spent in work which would be classified as light or moderate (Table 3.5).

Non-occupational energy varies very widely from 3.0 to 7.0 MJ. There is no evidence that those employed in sedentary work are more likely to choose recreations demanding physical activity than those in heavy industry (see Table 3.10). A figure of 4.5 MJ has been taken in calculating the recommended intake for each of the three groups. The figure is lower than the figure of 5.5 MJ previously used (DHSS, 1969). The reduction has been made not on the findings of surveys, but on a general impression that more time is being spent in watching television and spectator sports and less in active recreations and games.

For adult women figures of 1.75, 3.5 and 3.75 MJ may be taken as the energy expenditure resting in bed, in occupational activities and in recreations respectively, giving a total daily food requirement of 9.0 MJ.

All these figures are only applicable to large groups. Dietary energy requirements are determined in large part by the extent of the physical activity of individuals. This is continually changing in part by free choice and in part determined by changes in the nature of industrial and domestic work and the opportunities available for different types of recreation.

Table 3.11 is a useful guide for planning food supplies and prescribing diets for large groups in the United

Table 3.11 Energy expenditure and range of requirements of food for individuals and recommended intakes for groups of men in different occupational groups in the United Kingdom

	Sedentary	Moderately active	Very active
	MJ/8 hr	MJ/8 hr	MJ/8 hr
Energy expenditure			
In bed	2.0	2.0	2.0
At work	4.0	5.5	7.5
Non-occupational	3.0–7.0	3.0–7.0	3.0–7.0
	MJ/24 hr	MJ/24 hr	MJ/24 hr
Energy requirement from food	9.0–13.0	10.5–14.5	13.0–17.0
Recommended intake for a group	10.5	12.0	14.0

Kingdom. As the figures assume a way of life, the table does not set out general physiological standards. For other countries and for this country in the future modifications may be needed.

Effect of body size and composition

A big 80 kg man obviously needs more food than a small 40 kg woman. However, it is difficult to relate quantitatively food requirements and body size. Small animals eat much more food per unit of body weight than large ones. This is because the ratio of surface area to weight increases as size diminishes and consequently more energy is needed to meet heat losses from the relatively large surface. In mammalian species of varying size, food requirements are closely correlated with weight to the power of 0.73.

Durnin (1970) has discussed the relationship between energy expenditure and body weight for men and women and points out that over the normal range of variation of body weight metabolic rates are correlated directly with body weight as closely as with body weight to the power 0.73. The recommended intakes in Table 3.11 are designed for men and women weighing 65 and 55 kg respectively. For moderately active men requiring 12.5 MJ (3000 kcal)/day, this represents 190 kJ (46 kcal)/kg body weight, and for women requiring 9.0 MJ (2200 kcal)/day,

the figures are 165 kJ (40 kcal)/kg body weight. For men over the range of 50 to 70 kg it is sensible to relate energy requirements to body weight using the above figures.

Outside these ranges the use of these factors is not justified because of changes in body composition. Heavy people are likely to have a higher proportion of body fat, and light people a lower proportion. Indeed dietary surveys in Britain show that heavy people eat no more than those of normal weight (Thomson et al., 1961). Possibly big people are less physically active than small people.

Effect of age

Age may affect requirements in two main ways. First, as people become older they tend to engage in employment which demands a smaller expenditure of energy, and also to reduce physical exercise not connected with their work. For example, miners tend to leave the heavy jobs at the coal face after the age of 45 and by 60 few remain at this type of work. When older people take lighter employment they need less food. Secondly, in the basal metabolic state and in the 'resting' condition, the expenditure of energy per unit of body weight decreases slowly after the early twenties (Table 3.6). This decline with age is largely due to a reduction in the proportion of metabolically active tissue in the body.

Recommended intakes at various ages are given in Tables 15.1 and 15.2 (pp. 153 and 154).

Effect of climate

It is a common opinion that cold weather stimulates appetite and hot weather depresses it. There are, however, few observations of either food intakes or energy expenditures under comparable conditions to support this. Any effect of climate is mainly due to changes in physical activity, but also the basal metabolism is some 10 per cent lower in the tropics than in temperate climates as many studies have shown (Patwardhan, 1952; Mason et al., 1965). Both very cold and very hot weather tend to restrict outdoor physical activity and so food requirements. McCance et al. (1971) studied a group of British students and a group of Sudanese students first in Cambridge

Table 3.12 Mean daily energy intake and expenditure and weight change during 8 days by British and Sudanese male students in Cambridge in the winter (temperatures 1 to 12°C) and in Khartoum in the summer (temperatures 20 to 35°C)

	Energy intake		Energy expenditure		Weight change kg
	MJ/day	kcal/day	MJ/day	kcal/day	
10 British subjects					
in Cambridge	13.7	3280	13.7	3300	+0.57
in Khartoum	10.1	2420	11.2	2680	−0.73
8 Sudanese subjects					
in Cambridge	13.5	3240	11.5	2760	+0.99
in Khartoum	12.4	2970	10.3	2460	+0.88

during the winter and later in Khartoum during the summer. In both places the students had a similar programme of laboratory and education work which took up about four to six hours per day and ample opportunity for games and outdoor activities. Table 3.12 gives some of the results and shows that both food intake and energy expenditure were substantially less in Khartoum than in Cambridge. It is difficult to make recommendations for energy requirements in the tropics, but it seems sensible to reduce the recommended intakes given above by 5 to 10 per cent in places where the mean annual temperature exceeds 25°C.

Growth in childhood

The energy intake of children of different ages must obviously allow for satisfactory growth and physical development, and for the high degree of activity characteristic of healthy children. Recommendations are based on observed intakes of normally growing children and are related to body weight. Table 3.13 gives figures for infants at three-monthly intervals and Table 3.14 for children up to 5 years at yearly intervals. For information about older children and adolescents see Tables 15.1 and 15.2 (pp. 153 to 155). The energy requirement per kilogram of body weight is more than double that of the adult during the first year of life but falls slowly as the rate of growth per unit of body weight falls with age.

tions in activity. Studies of the food consumption of small groups show a range of intakes with a coefficient of variation of ±30 per cent of the mean. The energy expenditure of healthy active children can be extremely high. At the other end of the scale, that of inactive children can be so low that they will become obese even when their energy intake is below the recommended amount. In dealing with feeding problems involving small groups of children, account must be taken of activity as well as of size and age.

Clearly, it is not always desirable to adjust the energy allowances of growing children to their actual weight. Thus if children are below the standard weight for their age (p. 471) owing to malnutrition, they may need more than the recommended intake per kilogram of body weight to enable them to grow faster. There is however a limit to the extent to which a child can catch up after a period of undernutrition. If a child has been seriously undernourished for a long period, it is inevitable that he will develop into a small adult and giving large amounts of food only has the effect of making him obese.

Pregnancy

During pregnancy extra energy is needed for the growth of the fetus, the placenta and associated maternal tissues. The overall increase in resting metabolism during a pregnancy amounts to about 110 MJ (Emerson *et al.*, 1962). Additional energy is also required for movements and activities

Table 3.13 Recommended daily intakes for infants

Age range	Body weight kg	kJ/kg	MJ/day	kcal/kg	kcal/day
Birth up to 3 months	4.6	500	2.3	120	550
3 up to 6 months	6.6	480	3.2	115	760
6 up to 9 months	8.3	460	3.8	110	910
9 up to 12 months	9.5	440	4.2	105	1000

Table 3.14 Recommended daily intakes for children up to 5 years of age

Age range	Body weight kg	kJ/kg	MJ/day	kcal/kg	kcal/day
0 up to 1 year	7.3	450	3.3	110	800
1 up to 2 years	11.4	430	4.9	103	1170
2 up to 3 years	13.5	420	5.7	100	1350
3 up to 4 years	15.6	410	6.4	98	1530
4 up to 5 years	17.4	400	7.0	96	1680

The energy required for growth is difficult to assess. From various studies on rats and man in positive nitrogen balance, Payne and Waterlow (1971) estimate that the energy cost of 1 g of tissue gained is of the order of 20 kJ. They conclude that about 23 per cent of the dietary energy is used for growth by an infant in his first 3 months, the figure falling to 6 per cent at the end of the first year and to 2 per cent in the fifth year.

In children of all ages there are wide individual varia-

when the mother becomes heavier and for laying down a reserve store of fat. All of these factors add up to a requirement of an extra 330 MJ (80 000 kcal) spread out over the nine months of pregnancy. This additional energy need can be covered either by increased food intake or by reduced physical activities. The extent to which these two factors operate during pregnancy is determined by social and economic conditions. Thus a poor woman with several small children to care for needs extra food, whereas a well-to-do primipara with few domestic responsibilities may cut down physical activities and so not require additional food. With many women, both a reduction in activity and a modest increase in food intake are likely to take place.

Lactation

The quantity of breast milk produced by individual women varies widely and depends on many factors, including the social environment and the physical and mental health of the mother. For the purpose of estimating requirements for lactation for a period of six months, an average daily milk production of 850 ml (equivalent to about 2.4 MJ or 600 kcal) may be assumed. Satisfactory data for assessing the efficiency of human milk production do not exist, but it may be of the order of 80 per cent. To provide milk with a value of 2.4 MJ, a mother would therefore need additional 3.0 MJ/day from food if her body stores are not to be depleted. In fact very few women who are lactating eat an additional 3.0 MJ/day. It is normal for a woman to lay down about 4 kg of fat during pregnancy (p. 518) and this provides a reserve of some 150 MJ (36 000 kcal) for use in lactation. An additional dietary intake of 2.1 MJ (500 kcal)/day during lactation is recommended in the USA. This is above intakes of lactating Australian women six to eight weeks after the birth of their children, as recorded by English and Hitchcock (1968).

4. Carbohydrates

Carbohydrates provide most of the energy in almost all human diets. In the diets of poor people, especially in the tropics, up to 90 per cent of the energy may come from this source. On the other hand, in the diets of the rich in many countries the figure may be as low as 40 per cent. Neither of these extremes is generally desirable.

Green plants can synthesise carbohydrate from water and carbon dioxide under the influence of sunlight. Part of this carbohydrate goes to make the supporting structures of the plant—the fibre or wood which are largely composed of cellulose; a part provides energy for growth, and a part may be stored as sugars or starch. These stores provide for the energy needs of the plant during times when photosynthesis is dormant, and for its seeds, which contain a store of carbohydrate for the nutrition of the embryo until energy is again available from photosynthesis. Man and his ancestors have been remarkably successful in seeking out and latterly cultivating various seeds, fruits and roots which contain concentrated supplies of carbohydrate. Undoubtedly this has been a cardinal factor in his evolutionary development. Ruminants such as sheep have no particular powers of selecting or conserving vegetable foods rich in carbohydrates and so, to satisfy their energy needs, must spend the greater part of their life chewing grass—a food that is 80 per cent water. Man, on the other hand, by his successful cultivation, particularly of cereal grains, can lay up a store of food from which he can quickly obtain sufficient energy and have time left for other things.

Carbohydrates are a class of chemical compounds composed of carbon, hydrogen and oxygen. They contain two atoms of hydrogen for each atom of oxygen, the same ratio as in water. Carbohydrates in food are divided into two categories. The first comprises **available carbohydrates**, which can be digested in the upper gastrointestinal tract of man, absorbed and utilised. These are the sugars and certain polysaccharides such as starch. The second category or **unavailable carbohydrates,** consists of fibrous polymers like cellulose that do not provide significant nourishment to man. They are broken down by bacteria in varying degrees; this occurs in ruminants above the sites of nutrient absorption but in other animals and man only in the large intestine, distal to the absorptive sites.

Certain related compounds and close derivatives are conveniently considered with the polysaccharides although they are not carbohydrates in strict chemical terms. The polyols like sorbitol differ from sugars only in having an alcohol group in place of a keto group on one of the carbon atoms; they follow similar metabolic paths in the body. Lignins are considered with the unavailable carbohydrates because they are found together in plants and have biological effects similar to other forms of dietary fibre. It is convenient to discuss oligosaccharides along with other sugars but some of these are poorly digested.

Analysis of the different carbohydrates in foods by direct chemical methods has lagged behind that of proteins, amino acids, fats and fatty acids. Southgate (1976) has compiled a critical manual of the methods that can now be used. The different types of carbohydrate in common foods are shown in Table 4.1.

SUGARS

Sugars are subdivided into monosaccharides, disaccharides and oligosaccharides. A large monograph on their role in nutrition produced by the US Nutrition Foundation (Sipple and McNutt, 1974) is available.

Monosaccharides

These are the simplest sugars containing from 3 to 6 atoms of carbon in each molecule. They are called trioses, tetroses, pentoses, hexoses or heptoses, according to whether they contain 3, 4, 5, 6 or 7 carbon atoms.

Hexoses

Glucose (dextrose, grape sugar). This is the only hexose sugar known to exist in the free state in the fasting human body; it is present in the blood in a concentration of about 5 mmol/litre (90 mg/100 ml).

Because of the asymmetrical carbon atoms in the molecule, solutions of glucose rotate polarised light. The rotation is to the right, hence the alternative name—dextrose—which is often used in industry. This property can be used to distinguish glucose from fructose (see below). Glucose is a reducing agent; its power of reducing copper compounds from the cupric to the cuprous state is the basis of Benedict's and Fehling's tests for detecting glucose in the urine.

Few natural foods, except some fruits such as grapes, contain more than traces of free glucose. However, starch consists of glucose in combined form and glucose is also a principal constituent of sucrose and some other sugars (see overleaf).

Table 4.1 Dietary carbohydrates (based on Southgate, 1973)

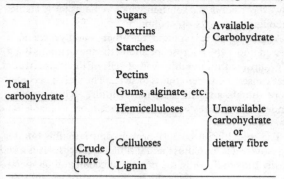

Total carbohydrate	Sugars, Dextrins, Starches	Available Carbohydrate
	Pectins, Gums, alginate, etc., Hemicelluloses	Unavailable carbohydrate or dietary fibre
Crude fibre	Celluloses, Lignin	

Glucose manufactured from starch is sold commercially in a variety of relatively expensive proprietary preparations as a dietary adjunct; there is no evidence, however, that they possess any advantage over sucrose as sources of energy for healthy people.

Fructose (laevulose, fruit sugar). This has the same empirical formula — $C_6H_{12}O_6$ — as glucose, but its structure is different. It is found in free form in some fruits, such as figs, and also in honey and it is a constituent of sucrose and some complex carbohydrates. It rotates polarised light to the left; hence its alternative name—laevulose. Fructose is slightly sweeter than glucose.

Galactose. This is a constituent of lactose (milk sugar) and of many plant polysaccharides.

Mannose. Mannose is a hexose of more interest to sugar chemists than nutritionists; small amounts are found in certain foods such as manna, from which it takes its name. Manna is the dried sap of certain species of ash and other trees, including the tamarisk which grows in the Sinai Desert. It is a component of several polysaccharide gums.

Hexose derivatives

Sorbitol (D-glucitol). Sorbitol is a polyol or sugar alcohol which is made commercially from glucose by hydrogenation. By this means the aldehyde (CHO) group in the glucose molecule is changed to an alcohol (CH_2OH) group. Though sorbitol is found in some fruits (such as rowan berries), it is chiefly the factory product that finds a use in dietetics. At least 90 per cent of ingested sorbitol is absorbed and metabolised, after conversion to fructose. However, its rate of absorption from the gut is slower than that of glucose so that it has less effect on the blood sugar. Sorbitol is used in the manufacture of 'diabetic' jams, marmalade, tinned fruits, fruit drinks and chocolate. Owing to its slow absorption and osmotic effect, large amounts of sorbitol cause diarrhoea and this limits its intake.

Mannitol and **dulcitol**. These are obtained by hydrogenation of mannose and galactose respectively, in the same manner as sorbitol from glucose. Mannitol is also extracted commercially from sea-tangle (*Laminaria*), the long, ribbon-like seaweed that grows just below the low-tide line round the coasts of Britain. These sugars have a variety of industrial uses and are sometimes employed in the manufacture of foods as improvers.

Inositol. This is a cyclic alcohol with six hydroxyl radicals allied to the hexoses. It occurs in many foods and especially in the bran of cereal grains. Inositol in combination with six phosphate molecules forms the compound phytic acid which hinders intestinal absorption of calcium and iron. Inositol has sometimes been classified as a vitamin because mice require traces of it in their diet; but there is no evidence that it is an essential nutrient for man.

Pentoses

Dietetically, the 5-carbon sugars are of little or no importance as a source of energy for the body. Yet they are present in small amounts in all cells, whether animal, plant or bacterial, since D-ribose and D-2-deoxyribose are components of nucleic acids. Pentoses are synthesised by all types of animals as well as man and are not essential in the diet.

The pentose sugars most commonly present in human foods are L-arabinose and D-xylose which are widely distributed in plant polysaccharides. These pentoses are normally found in human urine in small amounts, related to the dietary intake. Small amounts of ribose and another pentose, fucose, are also found in normal urine, but these are endogenous in origin.

Xylitol is the sugar alcohol corresponding to xylulose, manufactured from wood xylose. It is metabolised through the transketolase system. It is as sweet as sucrose and, although more expensive, is less prone to cause dental caries (Scheinin *et al.*, 1974).

Disaccharides and oligosaccharides

Sucrose (cane sugar, beet sugar). This is the familiar sugar in common domestic use. It is composed of one molecule of glucose combined with one molecule of fructose. These can be split apart by hydrolysis in the process of digestion and also by the action of acids in the laboratory or factory. Sucrose itself rotates polarised light to the right, but since fructose is more laevo-rotatory than glucose is dextro-rotatory, hydrolysis of a sucrose solution changes the rotation to the left. Hence the hydrolysis of sucrose (which takes place very readily) has been described in the past as 'inversion'. 'Invert sugar' is the commercial name for the product, which is a mixture of glucose and fructose. Sucrose is processed from sugar cane and sugar beet.

Lactose. Lactose is the principal sugar present in milk and is unique to mammals. Like sucrose it is derived from two monosaccharides linked together, one of which is glucose and the other galactose.

Maltose. This is a disaccharide derived from two

molecules of glucose with a 1-4 linkage. As its name suggests, it is formed from the breakdown of starch in the malting of barley.

Trehalose. This sugar is composed of two glucose molecules connected by a bridge between the two anomeric carbon atoms (1-1 linkage). It is present in many fungi and bacteria and is known as mushroom sugar. It is also present in many insects. Normally only very small amounts are ingested in the diet, and it is not known whether large quantities could be digested.

Raffinose. Raffinose is a trisaccharide of glucose, fructose and galactose; it is found in molasses.

Stachyose. This is a tetrasaccharide present in beans. The flatulence after consumption of large amounts of beans is probably due to stachyose and raffinose, which are not digested by the enzymes in the small intestine but pass to the colon where they are fermented by the resident microflora.

Sweetness

The tongue and oral mucous membranes contain taste buds, receptor cells responding to gustatory stimuli. The same cell can respond quantitatively to a stimulus which is sweet, bitter, salt or acid. Sugar was first introduced into European diets because its sweet taste was appreciated and this is the main reason why such large amounts are consumed today. Sugars and allied carbohydrates have varying degrees of sweetness as indicated in Table 4.2. Artificial sweetening agents are discussed on page 208.

AVAILABLE POLYSACCHARIDES

Starch

Starch is the form in which utilisable carbohydrate is stored in granules within the seeds and roots of many varieties of plants. The starch grain usually contains two polysaccharides derived from glucose. The first, comprising about 15 to 20 per cent of the total starch, is a long unbranched chain of several hundred glucose units and is known as amylose. Amylose is responsible for the intense blue colour resulting on the addition of a trace of iodine to suspensions or solutions of starch. The major component of starch is amylopectin; it is a highly branched glucose polymer and, if free from amylose, gives a brownish violet colour on the addition of iodine. Some varieties of grains, such as the 'waxy' variants of maize and rice, contain virtually no amylose. Starch grains, as obtained freshly

Table 4.2 The relative sweetness of sugars and allied carbohydrates

Sucrose	100
Fructose	170
Glucose	50
Glucose syrup	20–50
Sorbitol	50
Lactose	20

from plants, are completely insoluble in water. Heat, however, promotes a solution which remains fairly stable, although it may gel on cooling.

A section of raw potato or other starchy vegetable viewed under the microscope shows the starch grains lying in groups, within the thin-walled cells of the plant. Moist heat causes the starch grains to swell. The starch becomes more soluble and the cells may rupture. Thus cooking renders the starches in vegetable foods more available for digestion.

The starch molecule is broken down in the human digestive tract to maltose and ultimately glucose. It is also slowly broken down in the process of cooking, if temperatures considerably above the boiling point of water (100° C) are used. Thus when starchy foods are grilled or fried, or when barley is malted, some maltose and even glucose may be split off from the starch molecule.

Dextrins

These are degradation products of starch with varying numbers of glucose units per molecule. A proprietary preparation, Caloreen, is a mixture of dextrins averaging five glucose units per molecule. Liquid glucose is a mixture of dextrins, maltose, glucose and water. Both are used as a means of giving carbohydrate in an easily assimilated form to patients who are seriously ill. They are less sweet than glucose and Caloreen has one-fifth the osmotic pressure.

Glycogen

This is the animal equivalent of starch and is found in human tissues. The glycogen molecule is composed of 3000 to 60 000 glucose units built up in branching chains, each branch consisting of 12 to 18 glucose units. Unlike starch grains, glycogen dissolves in water; it is readily broken down by the appropriate enzymes to yield glucose. Animal livers and shellfish are the richest natural sources. An oyster (removed from its shell) usually contains about 6 per cent (wet weight) of glycogen.

UNAVAILABLE CARBOHYDRATE OR DIETARY FIBRE

These are interchangeable terms. The former has long been in use but, since lignin is not a carbohydrate, dietary fibre is now preferred—however, pectins are not fibrous. Roughage is a third alternative in common use.

Cellulose

This is the fibre on which green plants depend mainly for support and the most abundant organic compound in the world. Like starch, it is a polymer of glucose units in straight chains but their 1-4β linkages cannot be split by intestinal amylase, which is stereospecific for 1-4 α linkages. Celluloses from different sources differ in molecular weight and in their physical properties. Ruminants can digest cellulose because bacteria in the rumen contain the enzyme cellulase. In man a little bacterial fermentation of cellulose occurs but only in the large bowel.

Hemicelluloses

These are a heterogeneous group of polysaccharides which are closely associated with cellulose in plant tissues but can be separated from them by extraction with aqueous alkali. The largest chemical group are the pentosans, xylans and arabinoxylans; a second group consists of hexose polymers such as the galactans, and a third group are the acidic hemicelluloses which contain galacturonic or glucuronic acid. The hemicelluloses are not digested in the small intestine but are broken down by microorganisms in the colon more readily than cellulose.

Lignin

This is formed in plant tissues when they become woody. It is not a polysaccharide but an aromatic polymer based on coniferyl and sinapyl alcohols. It is totally indigestible even by ruminants.

Pectin

These are amorphous, but not fibrous, and found in the soft tissues of fruits and vegetables; they are soluble in hot water. Their principal constituent is galacturonic acid, together with varying amounts of other sugars. Varying proportions of their galacturonic acid units are present as methyl esters. In the presence of sugars and in a warm, slightly acid, dilute solution, they turn into a jelly. This useful property is responsible for the setting of jams.

Gums and alginates

Several gums, obtained from plants are used as thickeners in the food industry. Examples are guar gum, a very viscous galactomannan from the seeds of the Indian legume *Cyamnopsis tetragonolobus,* and locust bean gum, also predominantly a galactomannan, from the carob tree *Certonia siliqua,* a legume that grows in the Near East and Mediterranean.

Seaweed polysaccharides include *agar* (a polymer of galactose) used by bacteriologists and as a food by the Japanese and also alginic acid (a polymer of mannuronic and guluronic acids). Alginates are used as thickening agents and stabilisers in foods, especially in salad dressings, dairy products, e.g. whipped cream, and as a foam stabiliser in beer (Wood, 1975).

Chemical measurement of these different classes of substances in foods is difficult. Southgate (1969) has developed a sequence of selective extractions and hydrolyses which takes just over five days to complete. Van Soest's methods are quicker but do not give as much information. Neutral detergent fibre, the residue after boiling with neutral solutions of sodium lauryl sulphate and EDTA, contains hemicellulose, cellulose and lignin.

Acid detergent fibre, the residue after refluxing in sulphuric acid and cetrimide, is the cellulose and lignin (van Soest and Robertson, 1977). Van Soest's and Southgate's methods correspond fairly well (Southgate, 1977). Enzymatic methods are being developed (Hellendoorn *et al.,* 1975). In older food tables the only figures given are for 'crude fibre', which is the portion of the carbohydrate that resists extraction first with sulphuric acid and subsequently with sodium hydroxide. This method originated in the town of Weende in Germany in 1860; it includes all the cellulose and lignin but only small amounts of hemicelluloses.

CARBOHYDRATES IN DIETS

In agricultural societies the major portion of the dietary carbohydrate was and still is starch from cereal grains. In industrial societies, sugar provides a significant portion which appears to increase with prosperity. Thus in 1889 in the USA the yearly supply of cereal products was 358 lb/head and of sugar and syrups 53 lb/head. In 1961 the figure for cereals had fallen to 146 and that for sugar had risen to 115 (Antar *et al.,* 1964). A similar change occurred in the UK (Hollingsworth and Greaves, 1967). This is the greatest change in the national diets in the last 150 years. Consumption of cereal products continues to fall slowly in the UK, but that of sucrose has now ceased to rise.

In affluent communities some 60 per cent of dietary energy comes from separated fats and oils, sugar and refined carbohydrates, foods low or completely lacking in fibre. Crude fibre intakes are only 1 to 1.5 g/day from cereals (nearly all refined) and between 2 and 10 g/day from fruit and vegetables, in all 3 to 11 g crude fibre/day. In poorer countries the consumption of fruit and vegetables is of the same order, supplying 2 to 10 g crude fibre/day, but cereals are estimated to provide 10 to 15 g crude fibre/day (total 12 to 25 g crude fibre/day).

Total dietary fibre is difficult to determine, as explained above, and measurements of consumption in groups of people are only just starting. By Southgate's method average figures have been obtained of 17 g for urban Copenhagen and 31 g/day for rural Finland (International Agency for Research on Cancer, 1977) and in England 19 g/day on ordinary diets and 31 g/day in vegetarians (Gear *et al.,* 1978). In the Third World intakes are probably larger but measurements have not yet been reported.

Carbohydrates are probably not an essential part of a diet. The Arctic explorer Stefansson and a colleague lived for a whole year on a diet composed only of meat (McClellan and Du Bois, 1930) and so almost devoid of carbohydrate. They kept in good health. Members of some meat-eating tribes get little or no carbohydrate in their diet and it does not seem as if carbohydrate is a dietary essential — at least for adult man. Nevertheless from necessity most men are at least partial vegetarians and carbohydrates are a major component of their diets.

DIGESTION AND ABSORPTION

The first stage in the digestion of foods takes place in the mouth. Chewing breaks up the structure of vegetable foods and exposes their sugars and starch to the subsequent action of the digestive juices. Many vegetable foods, if not properly chewed, fail to be digested and may cause intestinal flatulence and colic. Unripe apples and chunks of raw turnip are familiar examples. Some substances, e.g. the pith of oranges, if not divided up by chewing, may occasionally coalesce in the stomach to form a ball or **bezoar** which can cause intestinal obstruction.

The digestion of starch begins almost at once, since the saliva contains ptyalin, a starch-splitting enzyme. This works best in a neutral medium and is inactive in the presence of acids. Its contribution to the digestion of starch is therefore limited by the time that the acid gastric juice takes to permeate the food entering the stomach. The acidity of the gastric contents may cause a little hydrolysis of sucrose.

The digestion of carbohydrates in the lumen of the small intestine is due chiefly to amylase secreted in the pancreatic juice. The optimum pH for this enzyme is slightly on the alkaline side of neutrality, so that its action is aided by the alkaline digestive secretions of the pancreas and small intestine. The starch and glycogen of the food are thus broken down to their component disaccharides. These together with sucrose, lactose and other dietary disaccharides are absorbed into the mucosa of the small intestine. In the brush border of the columnar cells of the intestinal epithelium they come into contact with the disaccharidases, lactase, sucrase and maltase, and are split into monosaccharides which are absorbed into the portal blood. If the function of the intestinal mucosa is impaired either for genetic reasons or as result of disease, patients become intolerant of dietary sugars which are lost in a watery diarrhoea. Lactase deficiency is discussed on page 407.

Cellulose and other polysaccharides are resistant to human enzymic digestion and so pass on to the large intestine where they contribute to the bulk of the faeces and may be fermented by the resident bacterial flora.

The hexose sugars are absorbed through the walls of the small intestine at a rate faster than could be accounted for by simple physical diffusion, and also against a concentration gradient. The sugars compete for a transport mechanism and so absorption takes place at different rates. Galactose and glucose are absorbed most rapidly, followed by fructose, mannose, xylose and arabinose in diminishing order.

An account of the general problems of intestinal absorption is given by Newey and Smyth (1967) and of carbohydrate absorption by Mansford (1967) and McMichael (1971).

DISPOSAL AND UTILISATION

The routes along which dietary carbohydrates may pass before utilisation in the tissues as a source of energy are shown in Fig. 4.1. After digestion and absorption as glucose into the blood stream carbohydrate may be utilised directly (A), temporarily stored in the form of glycogen (B), or converted into fat (C).

After a meal, the amount of glucose disposed of by each of these routes depends on the proportion of carbohydrate, fat and protein in the meal and also on the state of the energy stores in the body. The relative importance of the different fuels of the body is discussed in Chapter 8. Here only brief accounts are given of three important ways of disposal of glucose after absorption from the gut.

DIRECT UTILISATION

Glucose can be utilised by all the tissues of the body. Formerly it was held that most of the dietary carbohydrate was used directly and glucose was called 'the prime fuel' of the body. Now it seems certain that much, perhaps most, of the glucose absorbed from the intestines is converted into fat (see below). However, there is one organ, the brain, which is dependent mainly on glucose.

Glucose and the nervous system

Mental effort involves no measurable extra expenditure of energy, yet the nervous system as a whole uses large amounts of energy to maintain its mechanism in working order. Nearly one-fifth of the total basal metabolism takes place in the brain. Nervous tissue appears to derive its energy from carbohydrate, since, under normal circumstances, its RQ has always been found to be about 1.0 (Lambertsen *et al.*, 1953). It seems to be able to do this without glycogen as an intermediary. Although small amounts of glycogen are constantly present in nervous tissue, it is not apparently used as fuel and remains fixed in

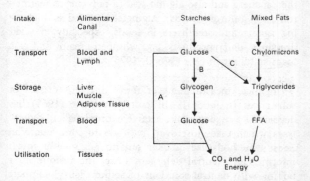

Fig. 4.1 The supply of energy to the tissues.

amount, even when the blood glucose is so low as to cause neurological symptoms. Nervous tissue seems to have no important store or reserve of energy and is therefore immediately dependent on the level of glucose in the blood for its continued activity. During starvation the blood sugar falls slightly but is still maintained with precision. If the glucose in the blood is suddenly reduced as by the injection of excessive amounts of insulin, changes in nervous activity quickly follow. Mental confusion is a frequent symptom of overdosage in diabetic patients which may even result in hypoglycaemic coma. However, in starvation the brain can utilise other fuels.

CONVERSION INTO GLYCOGEN

The synthesis of glycogen (animal starch) from glucose was demonstrated by the great French physiologist Claude Bernard (1850). This was the first demonstration of a chemical synthesis taking place in animals. Previously the orthodox view was that only plants could synthesise carbohydrates, fats and proteins. Animals were held to be able only to transmute and break down the chemical material present in their food.

Table 4.3 sets out figures giving the glycogen and sugar content of the body. The liver is the organ richest in glycogen; the concentration in skeletal muscle is much lower, but owing to the greater bulk of the muscles they contain the major part of the store.

The size of this carbohydrate store is undoubtedly small under normal circumstances. For instance nearly all is used up if a subject walks for two to three hours without food. Towards the end of the walk the RQ falls to 0.75 or lower, indicating that almost all the energy for the walk is being derived from fat. On occasions the store may be much bigger. Thus if the muscle glycogen is first depleted by prolonged exercise and then the subject is given a high carbohydrate diet, glycogen concentration in muscle may rise to 60 g/kg. The possible importance of this to athletes is discussed on page 537. There is a rare group of 'glycogen storage diseases', genetic in origin, in which there is a deficiency of one of the enzymes responsible for glycogen mobilisation. Concentrations as high as 120 g/kg skeletal muscle have been reported in this group of diseases.

It is possible that after overfeeding, large amounts of excess carbohydrate may be stored as glycogen. Human subjects given a dietary excess of carbohydrates did not show a rise of RQ to above 1.0, which is clear evidence of a net conversion to fat, before the excess intake was over 500 g (Passmore and Swindells, 1963). This excess may have been stored temporarily as glycogen. Some of this may have been in adipose tissue. Adipose tissue of rats normally contains little or no carbohydrate, but during refeeding after starvation it may contain as much as 10 g/kg (Mirski, 1942).

Glycogen, as it is stored in the muscles, is immediately available as a source of energy. This can be released in part

very rapidly without the need for oxygen. Lactic acid is the product of the anaerobic breakdown of glycogen. Given a sufficient supply of oxygen, the lactate thus formed is immediately oxidised, releasing further energy. If, however, the supply of oxygen to the muscle is temporarily insufficient, some of the accumulated lactate leaks out of the cells into the blood and so finds its way to the liver. The liver is able to convert this lactate back to glycogen. The sequence: liver glycogen → blood glucose → muscle glycogen → blood lactate → liver glycogen is known as the Cori cycle.

Table 4.3 Glycogen and sugar content of normal man. Body weight, 70 kg; liver weight, 1800 g; muscle mass, 35 kg; volume of blood and extracellular fluids, 21 litres (Soskin and Levine, 1952)

	g/kg	Total g
Muscle glycogen	7	245
Liver glycogen	60	108
Blood and extracellular fluid sugar	0.8	17
Total body carbohydrate		370

The accumulation of lactate through temporary shortage of oxygen in the muscles begins with moderate muscular effort such as walking at about 4 mph. After severe exercise it may reach 10 mmol/l in the blood. Excess of lactic acid in the muscles of a runner may explain why they are sometimes taut and tender after a race.

CONVERSION INTO FAT

Whenever the diet provides more glucose than the tissues require, the excess is ultimately turned into fat and deposited in the adipose tissues of the body. This was first clearly demonstrated by the classical experiment carried out over a hundred years ago by Sir John Bennet Lawes and Sir Joseph Gilbert (1853) at Rothamsted. They showed that young pigs put on four times more fat than their diet supplied, and concluded that fat is formed from starch within the body. Even when the dietary carbohydrate is not in excess of needs a large proportion of it may be converted into fat, which is then used by the tissues. Stetten and Boxer (1944), using deuterium as an indicator, showed that in rats on a high carbohydrate diet at least 10 times as much glucose was converted into fatty acids as into glycogen. Further isotopic studies have shown that the rate of turnover of glucose in the body is much slower than the rate of turnover of the free fatty acids (FFA). Dole (1965) has calculated that FFA can provide energy for the tissues at a rate two and a half times as fast as can glucose. Of the three routes indicated in Figure 4.1 by which glucose can supply energy to the tissues, it now seems probable that under normal circumstances the major part goes by route C

FRUCTOSE

Fructose, mainly derived from dietary sucrose by hydrolysis in the small intestine, is absorbed more slowly but utilised more quickly than glucose. In the liver it is converted by fructokinase into fructose 1-phosphate, which is broken down into the trioses dihydroxyacetone phosphate and glyceraldehyde; these can then serve as a source of energy for the tissues. As these processes are not dependent on insulin, fructose can be utilised by diabetics in limited quantities. As fructose is utilised more rapidly than glucose, it has been used in place of the latter in intravenous infusions, especially in the treatment of diabetes. However, intravenous fructose is liable to lead to the accumulation of lactic acid (lactic acidosis) and its value is now disputed.

In liver disease the rate at which fructose is removed from the blood may be reduced and a fructose tolerance test is sometimes used as a measure of liver function. Very occasionally there is a genetically determined lack of one of the enzymes responsible for fructose metabolism and a condition known as fructose intolerance arises.

GALACTOSE

Galactose from lactose is only utilised after conversion to glycogen and other glucose derivatives. If the enzymes for the conversion are not present, the patient, usually a child, suffers from galactose intolerance.

Physiological effects of dietary fibre

Food components go through phases when hypotheses are propounded about their biological role, there is public enthusiasm and then an increase of research. This sequence happened with dietary fibre in the 1970s. The laxative action of wholemeal compared with white bread has been known since classical Roman times (McCance and Widdowson, 1956). But in the early 1970s Dr Denis Burkitt, who had worked out the cause of Burkitt's lymphoma, and Dr Hugh Trowell, who had written the first textbook on kwashiorkor (Trowell et al., 1954), both back in England after medical service in East Africa, started discussing the possibility that diseases common in industrial countries but rare in Africa might be due partly to insufficient fibre in European and North American diets. They stimulated others to consider fibre. Reasoned hypotheses, based mainly on epidemiological data, linked low fibre intakes with a series of diseases: diverticular disease (Painter and Burkitt, 1971), cancer of the colon and rectum (Burkitt,

1971a), appendicitis (Burkitt, 1971b), varicose veins and haemorrhoids (Burkitt, 1972), coronary heart disease (Trowell, 1972), gallstones (Heaton, 1973) and diabetes mellitus (Trowell, 1973). The evidence and ideas about these and other diseases were put together in a book (Burkitt and Trowell, 1975).

Physiological and biochemical experiments are showing that different types of dietary fibre have different effects in the body. The early hypotheses concentrated on cereal fibre, particularly of wheat. Experiments show that wheat fibre increases faecal weight and shortens transit time more than most other types of dietary fibre (Cummings et al., 1978). This may be related to the high capacity of bran to bind water (Eastwood and Mitchell, 1976) and also its arabinoxylans are fermented in the large intestine (Meyer and Calloway, 1977). These effects relieve constipation overnight and by reducing colonic pressure during defaecation may well be preventive factors for haemorrhoids and diverticular disease (Gear, 1978). Wheat fibre does not, however, lower plasma cholesterol (Truswell and Kay, 1976).

Other types of dietary fibre have more effect in the stomach and small intestine, and some have little effect on faecal weight and transit time. Pectin in moderate and large amounts lowers the plasma cholesterol (Kay and Truswell, 1977) and relieves the symptoms of the dumping syndrome (Leeds et al., 1978). Guar gum also lowers plasma cholesterol and reduced blood sugar in diabetic patients (Jenkins et al., 1977). These substances appear to delay gastric emptying and by their viscosity slow the absorption of sugars and lipid micelles. Some types of dietary fibre may also act as ion exchangers (Eastwood and Mitchell, 1976). Lignin, for example, binds bile acids (Story and Kritcheusky, 1976). This may lead to a negative cholesterol balance and reduce the toxicity of some ingested foreign compounds.

On the other hand, the ion exchange property tends to increase faecal excretion of divalent cations, iron, zinc and calcium (Ismail-Beigi et al., 1977). This can contribute to mineral deficiency where high intakes of unleavened high extraction bread are combined with low intakes of zinc and iron as in parts of the Middle East (p. 105). The effect of fibre has not yet been disentangled from that of phytate. Large intakes of dietary fibre are followed by abdominal discomfort, flatus and frequency of defaecation. There is a wide individual variation in the amount that can be comfortably eaten.

5. Proteins

The contribution made by proteins to the energy value of most well-balanced diets is usually between 10 and 15 per cent of the total and seldom exceeds 20 per cent. Their importance lies in the fact that every cell in the body is partly composed of proteins which are subject to continuous wear and replacement. Carbohydrates and fats contain no nitrogen or sulphur, two essential elements in all proteins. Whereas the fat in the body can be derived from dietary carbohydrates and the carbohydrates from proteins, the proteins of the body are inevitably dependent for their formation and maintenance on the proteins in food. A four-volume monograph edited by Munro and Allison (1964) gives an admirable account of the metabolism of proteins. This is strongly recommended for further reading.

SOURCES AND CHEMICAL NATURE

Animal proteins can be divided into two kinds, fibrous and globular. Plant proteins are not so easily classified but, broadly speaking, most are glutelins or prolamines.

Fibrous proteins

These consist of long coiled or folded chains of amino acids bound together by peptide linkages. They are found in the protective and supportive tissues of animals such as skin, hair, feathers, tendons and the fins and scales of fish. The fibrous proteins in such tissues are very insoluble in water and for the most part indigestible. Nevertheless they are a valuable byproduct of the food industry since gelatin and other nitrogenous substances can be extracted from them. **Keratin,** the chief protein of hair, has been much studied by the wool industry. It is interesting chemically because it contains 11 per cent of the sulphur-containing amino acid, cystine. Its practical importance lies in its resistance to solution and its elasticity. The latter property is common to all the fibrous proteins. Their contracted molecules can be stretched out straight and, under suitable conditions, will remain stretched; this is the secret of a 'permanent wave' in the hair. Other fibrous proteins include the **collagen** of connective tissue, the **fibrin** of a blood clot and the **myosin** of muscle. The latter is an intracellular protein. All of these consist of long, elastic, molecular chains and although insoluble in water are more digestible than keratin. The Chinese have long known how to extract nourishment out of shark fins and other unpromising sources of fibrous proteins. The prudent housewife with a good stock pot, and particularly with the aid of a pressure-cooker, can do the same.

Globular proteins

These are found in the tissue fluids of animals and plants, in which they readily disperse either in true solution or colloidal suspension. Important from the standpoint of nutrition are **caseinogen** in milk, **albumin** in egg white, and **albumins** and **globulins** of blood. The exact configuration of their rounded molecules is a challenge to molecular biologists. For the nutritionist it is enough to know that they are not only easily digestible but also contain in their structure a good proportion of the essential amino acids (see below).

Glutelins and prolamines

These are the chief plant proteins. Glutelins, which are insoluble in neutral solutions, but soluble in weak acids and alkali, are present in cereals. They include glutenin from wheat, hordenin from barley and oryzenin from rice. These are probably not homogeneous substances. Prolamines are insoluble in water but dissolve in alcoholic solution. On hydrolysis they give large quantities of proline and ammonia. Typical prolamines are gliadin from wheat and zein from maize.

Wheat occupies a unique position in food because of its gluten content. Gluten is a mixture of two proteins, gliadin and glutenin; these two, when mixed with water, give the characteristic stickiness which enables the molecules, present in wheat flour, to be bound together by moderate heat with the production of dough, from which bread is baked. Rye has a small content of gluten and so (with difficulty) can be made into a loaf. Oats, barley, maize, millets and rice cannot be made into bread. The grains may be eaten after boiling or their flour made into porridge, bannocks, tortillas, etc.

Protamines and histones

These are basic proteins of low molecular weight. They are usually associated or combined with nucleic acids. Large amounts of protamine are found in male fish roes and also in cellular nucleoproteins. Protamines have a practical use in the commercial production of delayed-action insulins.

Coagulation and denaturation

Many water-soluble proteins when subjected to heat at about 100° C or above, as in the normal process of cooking, coagulate. The change of the white of an egg on boiling is a familiar example. Once a protein has undergone this change its properties are permanently altered; it can never be brought back into simple solution in water and its specific properties, e.g. enzymic, hormonal or immunological, are permanently destroyed. Proteins also undergo a lesser change, known as denaturation, in which they become less soluble in water. This occurs when they are exposed to a variety of agents such as moderate heat, ultraviolet light or alcohol and mild acids or alkalis. The exact nature of the denaturation process is obscure; it apparently involves some disorganisation of the specific arrangement of the component amino acids. To a certain extent it is reversible, once normal conditions are restored; but most enzymes and allergens lose their specific properties when once denatured. Proteins are most easily denatured at their isoelectric point, i.e. the particular pH at which the electric charges on their NH_2 and COOH groups precisely balance; this varies from one protein to another. It seems probable that many of the finer arts of cooking, such as simmering, the addition of vinegar, lye or wine, depend for their success on securing the proper degree of denaturation in preparation for the final coagulation.

AMINO ACIDS

Proteins consist of large molecules with molecular weights ranging from 1000 to over 1 000 000. In their native state some are soluble and some insoluble in water. They can be broken down by hydrolysis into simple units — the amino acids. These are all characterised by the presence of a carboxyl (COOH) group with acidic properties and an amino (NH_2) group with basic properties, attached to the same carbon atom; the rest of the molecule varies with the particular amino acid. The structure of an amino acid may be represented by the formula

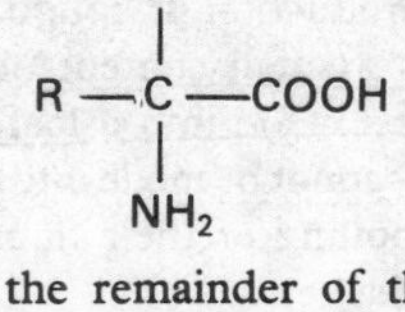

$$R - \underset{\underset{NH_2}{|}}{\overset{\overset{H}{|}}{C}} - COOH$$

where R represents the remainder of the molecule. It would be reasonable to expect that an infinite variety of compounds of this composition might exist in nature; but in fact only some 20 amino acids are commonly found in biological materials.

The amino acids are linked together in the protein molecule by the peptide linkage in which the basic (amino) group of one amino acid is linked to the carboxyl group of another, with the elimination of a molecule of water. Any two amino acids can be joined by this linkage to form part of a peptide chain and every amino acid may occur in varying amounts in different positions in the chain. Figure 5.1 lists 20 amino acids in the animal and plant kingdoms which resemble the 26 letters of the alphabet since each can be arranged in sequences to form an infinite number of proteins and sentences respectively. Every species of animal has its characteristic proteins — the proteins of beef muscle, for instance, differ from those of pork muscle. It is the sequence of amino acids in proteins that give each species its specific immunological characters and uniqueness.

Plants can synthesise all the amino acids they need from simple inorganic chemical compounds, but animals are unable to do this because they cannot synthesise the amino (NH_2) group; so in order to obtain the amino acids necessary for building protein they must eat plants, or other animals which have in their turn lived on plants.

The human body has certain limited powers of converting one amino acid into another. This is achieved in the liver, at least partly by the process of **transamination**, whereby an amino group is shifted from one molecule across to another under the influence of aminotransferases,

Name		Standard abbreviation	R
Glycine		Gly	H—
Alanine		Ala	CH_3
Valine	E	Val	$(CH_3)_2CH—$
Leucine	E	Leu	$(CH_3)_2CH—CH_2—$
Isoleucine	E	Ile	$C_2H_5—CH(CH_3)—$
Serine	E	Ser	$CH_2OH—$
Threonine	E	Thr	$CH_3—CHOH—$
Aspartic acid		Asp	$HOOC—CH_2—$
Glutamic acid		Glu	$HOOC—CH_2—CH_2—$
Lysine	E	Lys	$H_2N(CH_2)_4—$
Ornithine		Orn	$H_2N(CH_2)_3—$
Arginine		Arg	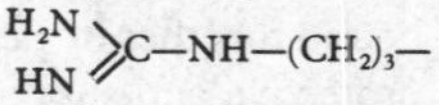
Histidine		His	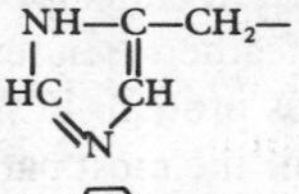
Phenylalanine	E	Phe	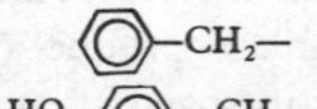
Tyrosine		Tyr	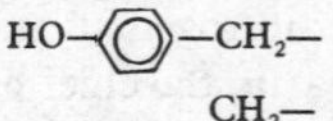
Tryptophan	E	Trp	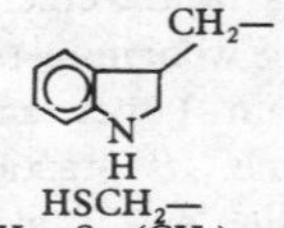
Cysteine		Cys	$HSCH_2—$
Methionine	E	Met	$CH_3—S—(CH_2)_2—$
Proline		Pro	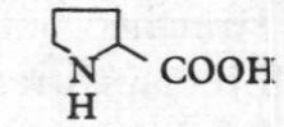
Hydroxyproline		Hyp	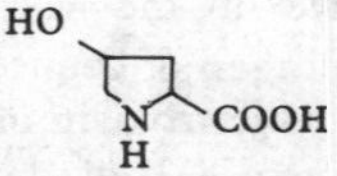

Fig. 5.1. The principal amino acids. Those marked E cannot be synthesised by man and are essential constituents of the diet.

the coenzyme of which is pyridoxal phosphate (p. 148). However, the ability of the body to convert one amino acid into another is restricted. There are several amino acids which the body cannot make for itself and so must obtain from the diet. These are termed **essential amino acids.**

Essential amino acids

The adult human body can maintain nitrogenous equilibrium on a mixture of eight pure amino acids as its sole source of nitrogen. These eight are: isoleucine, leucine, lysine, methionine, phenylalanine, threonine, tryptophan and valine. For growth in infants, histidine is also needed. In adults the essential nature of histidine was not clearly shown until 1975 (Kopple and Swerseid, 1975); when this amino acid is absent from the diet nitrogen balance may take two or three weeks before it becomes negative.

Characteristics of individual amino acids

Glycine. It is the simplest amino acid. During periods of rapid growth the demand for glycine may be enormous. For the young chick, glycine is an essential amino acid since its supply becomes, for a time, a limiting factor to growth. It is an important precursor in many syntheses in the body, such as those of the purine bases, porphyrins, creatine and the conjugated bile acids. Many aromatic substances, whether produced endogenously or consumed as drugs or food additives, are conjugated in the liver with glycine. The conjugate is then excreted in the bile or urine.

Glutamic acid. This dicarboxylic acid easily loses its amino group to keto acids such as pyruvic acid in this way giving rise to other amino acids in the body. Glutamic acid is the predominant amino acid in wheat protein (gliadin). The strong, meaty flavour of monosodium glutamate gives it commercial value as a flavouring agent for cooking. Glutamic acid also plays an important role in the metabolism of ammonia. It picks up an extra amino group in muscles to form glutamine, which is the source of urinary ammonia. Glutamic acid is the precursor of the neurotransmitter, γ-aminobutyric acid in the brain.

Arginine. This participates in the formation of urea in the liver, by the process known as the ornithine-arginine cycle, first described by Krebs. The reader is referred to textbooks of biochemistry for details.

Lysine. As most cereals contain very little lysine, it is the amino acid likely to be deficient in poor vegetarian diets. It is the parent substance of carnitine, which transports fatty acids within the cell.

Cysteine and methionine. These are the principal sources of sulphur in the diet of man. The body can make cysteine from methionine but not vice versa, so that methionine is the dietary essential. Cystine is formed when two molecules of cysteine are reduced and linked by an S—S bond. It is present in the keratin of hair and in insulin, in each of which it forms about 12 per cent of the whole protein molecule.

Methionine is also concerned with the important process of **transmethylation.** The chief dietary sources of labile methyl groups are methionine and betaine, $(CH_3)_3.N.CH_2.COOH$, which accordingly are called **methyl donors.** Methionine gives up the terminal CH_3 group attached to its sulphur atom. Dietary deficiency of methionine in rats results in a fatty liver which can be cured by restoring this amino acid to the diet, or alternatively by giving the choline which the body would normally form from it. Taurine, which like glycine is conjugated with the bile acids, is derived from the metabolism of cysteine.

Phenylalanine and tyrosine. These two amino acids which contain a benzene ring in their molecules provide the raw material from which the body makes the hormones adrenaline and thyroxine. They are also the origin of the pigment melanin which occurs in the hair, the choroid lining of the eye and in the skin. The body can convert phenylalanine to tyrosine, but not vice versa, so that the former is the dietary essential.

Histidine. This amino acid contains an imidazole ring, and the body's ability to synthesise it is limited. Histidine is an essential amino acid in childhood, when large amounts are needed for growth, and possibly in some circumstances in adult life. It is readily converted to histamine by an enzyme histidine decarboxylase present in many tissues, notably in the intestinal tract. Histamine is a stimulus for acid secretion in the stomach. It is also stored in granules in mast cells, from which it is released in many allergic reactions. In the skin this gives rise to urticaria or nettle rash, and in the lungs to constriction of the bronchi causing the symptoms of asthma.

Tryptophan. This is the raw material from which synthesis of some nicotinic acid takes place in the body. It is the precursor of 5-hydroxytryptamine (5-HT), also known as serotonin, a physiological substance which causes vasoconstriction and is present in many tissues, especially the argentaffin cells of the intestinal mucosa, and in the blood platelets. When the platelets break up in the formation of a blood clot, they release 5-HT which appears to prevent bleeding by causing vasoconstriction of the neighbouring blood vessels. 5-HT is also a neurotransmitter in parts of the central nervous system.

Proline and hydroxyproline. These consist essentially of a pyrrole ring. This same ring structure is found in the porphyrins which go to make haemoglobin and the cytochromes. These amino acids are prevalent in the collagen of connective tissue.

Amino acid sequences and protein structure

The order and arrangement of the amino acids in a protein can be determined by splitting off fragments of the chain by partial digestion with proteolytic enzymes or acid hydrolysis. Insulin was the first protein to have its amino acid sequence determined. This was done in 1951 by Sanger at Cambridge. Since then, the number of proteins whose amino acid sequence has been reported rose and is now over 1000. Insulin (Fig. 5.2) is composed of two chains containing 21 and 30 amino acids. The chains are held together in two places by S—S bonds of cysteine. The smaller chain has a loop in it. The three amino acids in the loop differ in samples of insulin obtained from different species of animals. The specificity of the order of the amino acids in proteins is remarkable. This is shown by the fact that the protein in the haemoglobin of patients with sickle-cell anaemia differs from normal haemoglobin by only one amino acid; valine replaces glutamine in a sequence of 580 amino acids.

DIGESTION

Proteins undergo hydrolysis by proteolytic enzymes in the gastrointestinal tract, resulting in the release of peptides and amino acids.

amount of faecal organic nitrogen. At the same time the stools and flatus are foul-smelling, due to the action of bacteria in the large intestine on undigested protein, producing hydrogen sulphide and other products of putrefaction.

The digestion of proteins may be continued until they are completely broken down to amino acids which are then absorbed. Van Slyke and Meyer (1912) first demonstrated the rise in amino nitrogen in the blood during protein absorption.

Yet there are quantitative difficulties in accounting for protein digestion and absorption entirely in the form of amino acids (Fisher, 1954). There is now good evidence that small peptides containing two to six amino acid residues are absorbed from the gut lumen at least as rapidly as free amino acids Matthews (1975) and by an independent transport mechanism in the cell.

Measurements of the net absorption of amino acids after a meal containing 15 g of milk protein show that it is 70 to

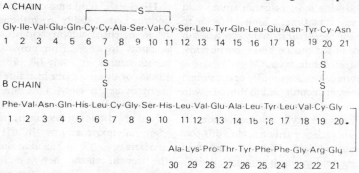

Fig. 5.2. Sequences of amino acids in the insulin molecule (Sanger, 1964).

Pepsin. This enzyme is secreted by the peptic cells of the mucosa of the stomach. It works best in an acid medium (optimum pH about 1.2) which is normally provided by the hydrochloric acid secreted by the oxyntic cells of the gastric mucosa. Pepsin breaks down proteins to smaller units, polypeptides, also composed of amino acids. The initial partial digestion of proteins in the stomach is not essential.

Rennin. This is another proteolytic enzyme secreted by the stomach of newborn mammals. It clots the protein of milk (caseinogen) and is the active principle of rennet, an extract from the stomach of animals or from certain plants used to curdle milk. There is no evidence, however, that rennin plays any part in protein digestion in the adult.

Trypsin. This is the chief proteolytic enzyme of the pancreatic juice. It acts best in an alkaline medium (optimum pH about 8) and converts proteins into polypeptides. The pancreatic juice is the principal means whereby proteins are normally digested. When disease of the pancreas obstructs or prevents the flow of the juice, failure of protein digestion is shown by the presence of undigested fibres of meat in the stools and by an increase in the

80 per cent complete in three hours (Mawer and Nixon, 1969). Patients with the genetic defect known as cystinuria are unable to absorb cysteine, arginine and lysine fully, owing to a failure of a transport system common to these amino acids.

In the first few days of life and in certain disease states traces of undigested protein may be absorbed. For instance a dietary protein occasionally exerts a general allergic response, such as urticaria, in people sensitive to it. Some part of the protein must have passed unchanged through the intestinal mucosa. Simple peptides and amino acids, being common to all species of animals, have no allergic or immunological properties.

It seems likely that, in general, proteins from animal sources are more easily and rapidly absorbed than vegetable proteins, perhaps because vegetable proteins are often enclosed in a cellulose covering. Phansalkar and Patwardhan (1955) have shown that the immediate urinary excretion of protein waste products is larger after a meal containing animal protein than when the same amount of protein is provided by vegetables.

Faecal nitrogen. The alimentary canal carries out the

digestion and absorption of protein effectively. Less than 10 per cent of the dietary protein usually appears as nitrogen in the faeces. Part of the faecal nitrogen comes from incompletely digested and absorbed foods. Large amounts of protein enter the alimentary canal also from the intestinal secretions and shed epithelial cells, and most of this is digested and absorbed. The metabolic faecal nitrogen can be measured by collecting the faeces during an experimental period on a diet containing no protein.

As stated in Chapter 3, Atwater concluded from his experiments that 92 per cent of the dietary protein was digested and absorbed. Subsequent experience has shown that among healthy persons eating the usual 'civilised' diets there is little variation from this figure. If the diet consists of unrefined cereals and contains much dietary fibre, digestion may be less complete and faecal losses of nitrogen higher.

Protein synthesis and turnover

The discovery of the general nature of the mechanisms of protein synthesis is one of the great achievements of modern science, comparable with the exploration of outer space. It has established biology alongside physics as a subject which attracts the best intellects in schools and universities. The discovery has been well publicised. Numerous articles in popular journals describe how deoxyribonucleic acids and ribonucleic acids carry codes, which sort a mixture of amino acids into the order appropriate for insertion into a specific protein molecule under construction.

For information on how proteins are synthesised from a mixture of amino acids a textbook on biochemistry (e.g. Lehninger, 1975) should be consulted. In nutritional practice, deficient synthesis is nearly always due to inadequacy of the amino acid mixture rather than to a failure of synthetic mechanisms; amino acid requirements are discussed later in this chapter.

The amount of protein synthesised daily depends on the requirements for growth, for the manufacture of digestive and other enzymes and for replacement of proteins broken down in the cells of the various tissues. The tissues of the body are under continuous repair. The rates at which they are broken down and replaced vary greatly. The mucosa of the small intestine is probably renewed every one to two days. The red blood cells have each a life of about 120 days. The skin is also being shed and replaced continuously. Isotope studies indicate that in the human body plasma albumin is being synthesised at the rate of about 10 g/day and fibrinogen at about 2 g/day. On the other hand collagen persists for a very long time and that laid down in the bones of infant rats has been shown to be still present after 300 days (half the life span).

As the rates of turnover of protein in cells is not easily measured, it is difficult to get an accurate estimate of the daily rate of protein synthesis. It is certainly greater than

Table 5.1. Total body protein synthesis rate in humans at various ages

Age group	No. of studies	Body weight (kg)	Age (range)	Total body protein synthesis (g kg^{-1}d^{-1})
Newborn (premature)	10	1.94	1–46 d	17.46
Infant	4	9.0	10–20 mths	6.9
Young adult	4	71	20–23 yr	3.0
Elderly	4	56	69–91 yr	1.9

the daily intake of protein in the diet, and amino acid liberated by the breakdown of old protein can be utilised again for synthesis.

The possibility of using amino acids labelled with ^{15}N as tools for measuring rates of protein turnover and synthesis was suggested by experiments carried out about 40 years ago (Schoenheimer et al., 1939). This approach has been much used but is beset with both methodological and technical difficulties. Two papers in Nature (Waterlow, 1975; Young et al., 1975) review the position, and Table 5.1 prepared by the latter authors gives estimates of synthesis rates at various ages. For an adult man synthesis amounts to over 200 g daily, or about five times the minimum dietary requirement. The rate of synthesis appears to be related to the basal metabolic rate.

Protein as a source of energy

A most important process in the metabolism of all amino acids is the removal of the amino group and its replacement by oxygen with the formation of a keto acid which is then available as a source of energy. The amino group is taken into the ornithine–arginine cycle in the liver and subsequently built up into urea. Most of the oxoacids formed by oxidative deamination are converted into pyruvic acid and so pass into the citric acid cycle. Alanine is the principal amino acid released from the muscle, and is used for gluconeogenesis when energy intake is insufficient. There are, however, other routes. For example, glutamic acid after deamination yields 2-oxoglutaric acid. This acid is one of the intermediary stages between citric acid and oxaloacetic acid in the cycle.

Glucose may be formed from many amino acids. Over 50 years ago Dakin (1913) fed single amino acids to diabetic dogs and in many instances was able to collect corresponding amounts of glucose in the urine. However, leucine, lysine, methionine and tryptophan do not form glucose in these circumstances; nor generally do cystine, isoleucine, phenylalanine and tyrosine. These amino acids may, however, give rise to acetoacetic acid. For this reason they have been called ketogenic amino acids, whereas the other amino acids are glucogenic. Acetoacetate and glucose formed from amino acids are important primary fuels of the tissues (Chap. 8).

An excellent account of the intermediary metabolism of amino acids is given by Krebs (1964). Before reading this, it might be advisable to study the chapter on protein metabolism in Lusk (1928). Some young biochemists appear to think that their subject only started when preparations of mitochondria first became available. There was much excellent biochemical work of direct application to nutrition carried out in the first 25 years of this century and for the study of this Lusk is the best guide.

Protein reserves

The amount of protein in the body is not constant, but depends to some extent on the protein content of the diet. If a person on a high protein diet is put on a low protein diet overnight, the daily output of nitrogen (N) in the urine does not drop immediately. It falls slowly and after four to six days reaches a level roughly similar to the amount of N in the diet. If a transfer back to a high protein diet is made the urinary N output rises slowly and after a few days approximates to the high intake (Martin and Robison, 1922). The excess N excreted or the N retained on changing from a high protein to a low protein diet and back is equivalent to between 175 and 350 g of protein in an adult man. This is called the **labile body protein.** In young children studied in Jamaica (Chan, 1968) the labile body protein represented less than 1 per cent of total body protein and such a small amount can hardly be considered as a store.

Addis and his colleagues (1936) were the first to show that when rats were given a diet deficient in protein, the protein content of the liver fell by 40 per cent and of the alimentary tract and pancreas by 30 per cent; the muscles and skin lost 8 per cent and the brain only 5 per cent of their original protein contents. Studies with ^{15}N-glycine show that endogenous amino acids from tissue breakdown are more efficiently utilised for resynthesis after adjustment to a low protein intake (Steffee et al., 1976).

There has been much argument as to whether a man or animal benefits from having this labile store full (p. 43).

A well fed human adult contains about 11 kg of protein, of which he can lose about 3 kg without serious loss of function or threat to life. Most of this loss is due to destruction of cell substance and cannot be regarded as a withdrawal from stores.

NITROGEN BALANCE

Nearly all the nitrogen in the diet and in the excreta is present in the form of amino groups ($-NH_2$). Amino N is readily determined by the Kjeldahl method. The material is first digested by heating with concentrated sulphuric acid and a catalyst. This converts the N into ammonium sulphate. After cooling, excess sodium hydroxide is added. The ammonia is then expelled by steam distillation into acid and estimated by titration. When nutritionists talk about urinary N or N balance, they are referring to amino N, not total N.

A subject is said to be in the N balance when the N intake (I) in the diet equals the N output in the urine (U), faeces (F) and by the skin (S):

$$I = U + F + S$$

Table 5.2 shows two examples: in the first the diet was low in protein and the balance is negative, which is interpreted as a loss of tissue protein; in the second the protein content of the diet was high, the balance positive and the subject can be presumed to be laying down tissue protein.

The N balance technique is used by physiologists to determine the minimum protein requirements of man. It is also used in the metabolic wards of hospitals to find out whether a patient is gaining or losing tissue protein on a particular therapeutic regime. A reliable estimate of the N balance can only be made if material is collected over a period of days on a constant regime. Five days is usually adequate but some preliminary days should be allowed for adjustment if the N intake on the test diet differs from that on the previous diet. If an accurate balance is required, it is necessary to determine analytically the N in an aliquot of the subject's diet. U can be determined precisely from an analysis of 24-hour samples of urine. Accurate collection of a 24-hour sample is an important task of the nursing staff in a hospital metabolic unit. The interval between the ingestion of food and the passage of the corresponding faeces is usually about 24 hours, but may vary greatly. For accurate work, it is necessary to mark the food at the beginning and end of the collection period with a dye or other readily detectable marker and to analyse the faecal material collected between the two marks. The output of N in the faeces is normally only a small fraction of the dietary intake. In some circumstances useful estimates of the N balance can be made without collecting faeces and assuming a small figure for faecal N.

It is difficult to measure the cutaneous N loss. Darke

Table 5.2 Nitrogen balances of an obese young woman after several days on diets containing 24 and 80 g protein/day (Passmore et al., 1958)

	g N/day	
Intake		
Food	3.9	12.7
Output		
Urine	5.3	9.3
Faeces	0.7	0.6
Skin	(0.2)	(0.2)
	6.2	10.1
Balance	−2.3	+2.6

(1960) measured the total cutaneous loss in 12 African subjects and obtained values between 188 and 480 mg N/day. Six medical students taking heavy physical exercise for about seven hours daily in Jamaica lost 3 to 4 kg of sweat, containing from 190 to 700 mg N (Ashworth and Harrower, 1967). In careful laboratory studies (Calloway and Margen, 1971) the total skin loss of N by subjects in a comfortable environment varied from 90 to 190 mg/day.

FACTORS AFFECTING N BALANCE

Growth

A 12-year old boy who gains 5 kg in weight in a year adds nearly 1 kg of protein to his body. To do this he must retain 160 g of N and be in positive N balance to the extent of about 0.4 g/day throughout the year. This N retention is controlled by growth hormone secreted by the anterior pituitary gland. Injections of growth hormone produce positive nitrogen balances both in man and in experimental animals. Other hormones which may promote nitrogen retention include insulin and the male sex hormones. The spurt in growth which occurs at puberty, so marked in boys, is associated with the development of the testes.

Injury and stress

After any injury or surgical operation there is an increased urinary excretion of N and a negative N balance (Chap. 51). It is part of a general catabolic response to injury, caused by increased secretion of adrenal cortical hormones, in response to the stimulus of trauma.

Physical exercise

It is common opinion, that those who do hard physical work require plenty of meat in their diets. In many families the working men are given an undue share of a limited supply of meat and eggs at the expense of the young children and mother. To justify this scientifically, it would be necessary to show that muscular activity increased protein metabolism and so would cause a negative N balance unless extra protein was given.

In 1889 two physiologists, Fick and Wislicenus, climbed a Swiss mountain, the Faulhorn, 1956 metres high. On the climb and during a recovery period they excreted in their urine 5.7 and 5.5 g of N/13 hours respectively. This represents a breakdown of protein no greater than would be expected during a day spent in light activities. Since then, several other investigators have failed to demonstrate a rise in urinary N during and following muscular activity. No support is available to justify the view that working men should get an undue proportion of protein from the family ration.

However, an athlete who goes into training may gain weight due to hypertrophy of muscle; this is brought about by synthesis of new protein and necessitates a positive N balance. The dietary needs of athletes are discussed in Chapter 63.

Intestinal bacterial flora

There is some evidence that in patients with renal failure on diets very low in protein, bacteria in the gut utilise ammonia to synthesise non-essential amino acids, which subsequently may be used for protein synthesis (Richards et al., 1967). In natives of New Guinea living on a diet very low in protein Oomen (1972) suggested that, intestinal bacteria may fix gaseous N and so make it available. The nitrogen-fixing organisms that have been identified in human faeces (Bergeson and Hipsley, 1970) use organic or ammonia N for preference and would only use trivial amounts of gaseous N under normal circumstances.

PHYSIOLOGICAL NEEDS

Proteins in the diet supply the amino acids required for the growth of young animals, infants and children and also those needed for the maintenance of the tissues in adults. The amounts needed for growth are much greater than those for maintenance. The newborn human infant probably needs about five times as much protein as the adult per unit of weight. As the child develops the rate of growth slows down and so the need for protein is progressively reduced, but until after puberty it remains larger than the adult's. Protein deficiency in children is widespread in Africa, Asia and Latin America as kwashiorkor (Chap. 29) but in adults is much less frequently found.

If the energy content of the diet is inadequate, protein is used to supply energy. In consequence protein deficiency is much more likely to occur if a diet is lacking in energy.

Obligatory N loss

This is total N loss on a N-free diet providing sufficient energy to meet requirements; it is also known as the endogenous N loss. Estimates (Young and Scrimshaw, 1968; Calloway and Margen, 1971) indicate that a representative figure for a 65 kg man is 3.5 g N/day (2.4 g in the urine, 0.8 g in the faeces, 0.2 g from the skin and 0.1 g miscellaneous). This is equivalent to 22 g of protein. This is the minimum need for protein under any circumstance.

Protein requirement for N balance

There is much individual variation in the minimum amount of protein that must be fed in order to maintain N equilibrium. Sherman (1920) reviewing all the evidence from European and American sources, concluded that the range of variation lay between 21 and 65 g/70 kg body weight/day. In many subsequent studies, the values have fallen within this range. A daily protein intake of 45 g or about 0.7 g/kg, provided it is of good quality (NPU at least 70, see below), is sufficient to keep most adults in N balance for a period of many weeks. This amount is less than adults normally eat. Whether consumption of higher amounts is necessary for health is discussed on page 43.

Protein requirement for growth

The infant grows fastest in the first three months of life and then the daily requirement of protein is 2.4 g/kg. As growth slows down, the need for protein declines, being 1.85, 1.62 and 1.44 g/kg daily at ages of 3 to 6, 6 to 9 and 9 to 12 months respectively. Thereafter protein requirements continue to decline slowly until growth stops. Growing children need more protein of better quality than do adults. However even if the protein intake appears adequate for a child, it cannot be utilised for growth unless the energy intake also meets requirements.

The subject of protein requirements has stimulated many writers. A review by Irvin and Hegsted (1971) has a bibliography of 373 papers.

Dietary sources

The protein content of almost every food used by man has been determined by measuring the total nitrogen by the Kjeldahl method and multiplying the value found by 6.25 or other appropriate factor (p. 14). The protein content is expressed as g/100 g of food in all well-known food tables. This does not relate the protein to the energy content of the food. Table 5.3 gives the protein content of some common foods expressed as the proportion of the energy in the foods provided by protein. Most satisfactory human diets provide from 10 to 15 per cent of the energy in the form of protein. The table enables one to distinguish at a glance foods which are poor, adequate and good as sources of protein in relation to their energy content. The low protein content of cassava and bananas is important. In those

Table 5.3 Protein content of various foods, expressed as their contribution (per cent) to the energy provided by each food

Value of food as a source of protein	Proportion of energy from protein (%)
Poor	
Cassava	3.3
Cooked bananas (plantains)	4.0
Sweet potatoes (*Ipomoea batatas*)	4.4
Taros	6.8
Adequate	
Potatoes	7.6
Rice (home-pounded)	8.0
Maize (wholemeal)	10.4
Millet (*Setaria italica*)	11.6
Sorghum (*Sorghum vulgare*)	11.6
Wheat flour (medium extraction)	13.2
Millet (*Pennisetum glaucum*)	13.6
Good	
Groundnuts (peanuts)	18.8
Cow's milk (3.5 % fat)	21.6
Beans and peas	25.6
Beef (lean)	38.4
Cow's milk, skimmed	40.0
Soya bean	45.2
Fish, fatty	45.6
Fish, dried	61.6

countries where these foods are the main source of energy, protein deficiency is widespread.

The quantity of protein in a food, however, may be misleading as a measure of its value for growth or maintenance of tissue. The quality of the protein is also important and is now discussed.

QUALITY OF PROTEINS

The nutritive value of a protein depends to an important degree on the relation of the amino acids in its molecule to those required for building new tissues. If the protein of the diet is seriously deficient in one or more of the essential amino acids, N equilibrium cannot be sustained, no matter how complete and excellent the diet may be in all other respects. If, however, another protein containing the missing amino acid in adequate amounts is added to the diet, N equilibrium and normal nutrition can be established. This capacity of proteins to make good one another's deficiencies is known as their **supplementary value.**

It has been known for a long time that proteins differ in quality. As long ago as 1915 the great American nutritionist Mendel, in a Harvey Society lecture, divided proteins into two classes: those which when fed to rats 'allowed growth' and those with which there was 'failure of growth'. Soon afterwards proteins were divided into animal and vegetable proteins. Formerly these were known as first and second class proteins respectively. However, many vegetable proteins, e.g. those from rice and soya bean, are little inferior to animal proteins and merit more than a second class label. Much more important is the fact that suitable mixtures of vegetable proteins are 'first-class' and promote growth in both laboratory rats and in children nearly as well as milk proteins. This is due to the proteins of different foods having different proportions of amino acids in their make-up. A relative lack of a particular amino acid in one protein can be made good in a mixture of proteins, provided such a mixture contains a protein which has an adequate amount of that particular amino acid. In any protein the amino acid which is furthest below the standard (see below) is known as the **limiting amino acid.** Tryptophan is the limiting amino acid in maize protein, lysine in wheat protein and the sulphur-containing amino acids (methionine and cysteine) in beef protein.

Many attempts have been made to give a numerical value to the quality of both individual dietary proteins and mixtures of proteins present in various human diets. It cannot be said that these have been entirely successful. Three international expert committees have examined on the subject (FAO, 1957; FAO/WHO, 1965; FAO-/WHO, 1973), but their reports have not escaped criticism. A succinct and critical account of the work of these Committees was given by Scrimshaw (1976) in a Shattuck lecture to the Massachusetts Medical Society. The reader who only requires sufficient knowledge of the quality of different proteins to enable him to advise individual patients can be content with the preceding paragraphs. Anyone responsible for planning diet schedules for hospitals, schools or the armed forces, especially in the tropics, should read on.

BIOLOGICAL TESTS

The protein to be tested can be fed to animals and its capacity to maintain the N balance or to promote growth measured. The methods used are not fully standardised and there is not complete agreement about the best ways in which to express the findings. Anyone who contemplates undertaking biological tests should first read accounts given by two masters of the subject, Platt (1964) and Allison (1964).

The tests are mostly based on estimations of the N balance. The **biological value** (BV) of a protein is defined as:

$$\frac{\text{Retained N}}{\text{Absorbed N}} \times 100$$

The protein to be tested is fed to the animal as the sole source of N in the diet and below the level needed for maintenance. The measured urinary and faecal N is corrected by subtracting the quantities lost on a protein-free diet. Then

$$BV = \frac{I-(F-F_m)-(U-U_e)}{I-(F-F_m)} \times 100$$

where I, F and U are the intake and faecal and urinary output of N on the test diet, and F_m and U_e are the faecal and urinary output on a protein-free diet.

The biological value (BV) makes no allowance for losses of N in digestion. This is included in the **net protein utilisation** (NPU) which is defined as:

$$\frac{\text{Retained N}}{\text{Intake of N}} \times 100$$

This is equal to BV × availability. NPU is normally measured with the protein intake at or below maintenance levels. It can be calculated from N balance data in man. In animals, gain of carcass N in weanling rats is more often used (Pellett, 1973). Values determined under other conditions have been termed 'operative' (NPU$_{op}$).

For a combined measure of both the quantity and quality of the protein in a diet, the net dietary protein value (ND$_p$V) is used. This is defined as:

$$\text{Intake of N} \times 6.25 \times \text{NPU}_{op}$$

As already described, it is often convenient to express the protein content of a food in terms of the percentage of the energy content provided by protein (Table 5.3). The protein content of a diet can be similarly expressed and an additional factor given for the quality of the mixed proteins. The **net dietary protein energy ratio** is defined as:

$$\frac{\text{Protein energy}}{\text{Net dietary intake}} \times \text{NPU}_{op}$$

The use of these indices has assisted in the testing of the qualities of many different types of diets.

Standard BV and NPU measurements, which consider only one intake level and zero, tend to overestimate the nutritional quality of some proteins, especially those limiting in lysine, because of the body's ability to adapt to partial deficiency. The best biological estimates of protein quality are provided by the slope of the intake–response line from several points in the range of intakes where the line is linear; it should not include zero protein intake. If carcass N retentions in animals are used in this way, the index is the **relative nutritive value** (Hegsted et al., 1968) and the line of the test protein is related to a standard (egg or lactalbumin). The ways in which this approach can be used in man, with N balances at several intake levels are considered by Rand et al. (1977).

Many nutritionists find this complex terminology, and indeed all modern literature on the biological testing of protein, difficult to follow. Fortunately a full understanding is not necessary for the dietitian either in the home or in the hospital. She should be able to understand the principles on which the chemical score is based and to apply chemical scores to diets which may be recommended.

CHEMICAL TESTING

Whereas biological methods for testing the quality of proteins have been available for over 50 years, chromatographic and microbiological methods for estimating the amino acid content of proteins only began to be used some 25 years ago. Orr and Watt (1968) and FAO (1970) have

Table 5.4 Content of essential amino acids in proteins (mg amino acid/g protein)

	Hen's egg	Cow's milk	Beef muscle	Wheat flour
Isoleucine	54	47	53	42
Leucine	86	95	82	71
Lysine	70	78	87	20
Methionine and cystine	57	33	38	31
Phenylalanine and tyrosine	93	102	75	79
Threonine	47	44	43	28
Tryptophan	17	14	12	11
Valine	66	64	55	42

published summaries of available results. Paul and Southgate (1978) give values for proteins in some foods consumed in Britain. Table 5.4 gives the amino acid content of the protein in hen's eggs, cow's milk, beef muscle and wheat flour.

AMINO ACID REQUIREMENTS

It is possible to feed human beings on artificial diets in which a mixture of amino acids is the sole source of nitrogen. If then one of the essential amino acids is omitted from the mixture, an adult subject goes into negative nitrogen balance, and an infant or young child ceases to grow. The missing amino acid can then be replaced in gradually increasing amounts, until the subject is again in nitrogen balance or until normal growth is resumed. In this way an estimate of the human requirements for each of the amino acids can be made.

Such experiments are difficult and tedious, and require much care and patience from both the investigators and their subjects. In the USA estimates of human requirements of amino acids have been made for adult men (Rose *et al.*, 1955), for adult women (Leverton *et al.*, 1956) and for infants (Holt *et al.*, 1960). Table 5.5 gives a summary of the findings. Comparison of the two right-hand columns of Table 5.5 shows that infants require more of their total protein to be supplied in the form of essential amino acids.

Table 5.5 Amino acids required to maintain N balance in adults and growth in infants under 6 months (FAO/WHO, 1973)

	Man (mg d^{-1})	Woman	Combined adult values (mg kg^{-1} d^{-1})	Infant
Histidine	—	—	—	28
Isoleucine	700	550	10	70
Leucine	1100	730	14	161
Lysine	800	545	12	103
Methionine and cystine	1100	700	13	58
Phenylalanine and tyrosine	1100	700	14	125
Threonine	500	375	7	87
Tryptophan	250	168	3.5	17
Valine	800	622	10	93

Amino acid scores

A chemical grading of the quality of a protein can be made by comparing its amino acid content with that of a reference protein and for this purpose hen's egg protein is recommended (Table 5.4).

Amino acid score =

$$\frac{\text{mg of amino acid in 1 g test protein}}{\text{mg of amino acid in 1 g reference pattern}} \times 100$$

The score should, in theory, be calculated for all the essential amino acids and the lowest score taken. In practice the scores need be calculated only for lysine, the sulphur-containing amino acids and tryptophan, as one or other of these is the limiting amino acid in common foods.

Table 5.6 compares the chemical scores and NPU values of proteins from single foodstuffs. It is difficult to obtain NPU values using man as the test animal, but relatively easy using the rat. The Table indicates that the results obtained with the two species agree sufficiently well to justify applying values obtained with rats to human diets. The chemical scores also agree with NPU values.

Table 5.6 The chemical score and net protein utilisation (NPU) of some common foods (FAO/WHO, 1973)

Protein	Chemical score	NPU determined on children	NPU determined on rats
Maize	49	36	52
Millet	63	43	44
Rice	67	63	59
Wheat	53	49	48
Soya	74	67	65
Whole egg	100	87	94
Human milk	100	94	87
Cow's milk	95	81	82

Most good mixed diets have a NPU value of around 70, and this figure is little affected by the amount of protein of animal origin in the diet. When 70 per cent or more of the dietary proteins come from a single staple food, e.g. maize, cassava or wheat, the NPU value of the food becomes of great importance and may determine whether or not protein requirements are met.

RECOMMENDED INTAKES

In nearly all communities adults eat more protein than is necessary to maintain N balance. Psychological and social factors as well as physiological needs determine intake. Much study has been devoted to three questions:

1. What is the minimum amount of dietary protein on which normal human life and activity can be sustained?
2. What is the desirable or optimal intake of protein for a man who has a free choice of food?
3. Is a high-protein diet beneficial or harmful?

These questions are important, since they raise the practical issue as to whether our present dietary habits provide the right amount of protein for our needs and, were we to increase our protein intake considerably, how would it affect our health?

The American physiologist Chittenden (1909) attempted to answer the second question by keeping healthy adult males, including himself, on diets containing as little as 40 g of protein daily for periods of up to one year. Chittenden asserted that this regime not only maintained, but often increased physical and mental vigour. He argued that reduction of the protein intake to the low levels used in his experiments is actually beneficial, claiming that the extra work in excreting the nitrogen from higher intakes of protein throws a strain on the kidneys and tends to cause renal and vascular disease.

However, there is good evidence that the kidneys can normally excrete the N end-products from large protein intakes without suffering damage. The Australian range-rider, the gaucho of the South American plains and the

Masai warrior of Central Africa all build up and maintain their good physique on diets which contain anything up to 250 or even 300 g of protein daily. A high protein intake seems to be tolerated throughout a lifetime without ill-effects. Nevertheless Chittenden's observation that adults can maintain good health on protein intakes far below current Western European and North American standards still remains true, and is a valuable contribution to knowledge.

In the opposite camp to Chittenden was Carl Voit, the great German pioneer in the scientific study of human nutrition. As early as 1881 he suggested 145 g as a suitable daily allowance of protein. But the chief exponent of the view that a high protein intake promoted the vigour and physical efficiency of 'superior' men was the physiologist Rubner. In the Germany of 1914 he was a man of influence, and probably did more than any army general to lose the war that then began; for on his advice German agriculture was continued on the old policy of rearing large herds of cattle and sheep. No additional pastures were ploughed. His failure to realise that cereals can yield up to six times more dietary energy per acre than cattle contributed importantly to the defeats which followed in 1917. When food became short in Central Europe as a result of the Allied blockade, it was too late to increase cereal production effectively. This mistake was avoided in Britain during World War II when Drummond was Scientific Adviser to the Ministry of Food.

A study of the diets of different races throughout the world shows that there is a great variation in the amount of protein on which man can subsist. A few, as already mentioned, may provide over 200 g protein. By contrast the diet of many millions of poor people in Asia, Africa and Latin America provides less than 50 g of protein per day. Attempts to relate racial constitution to dietary habits have often tended to support the view that generous intakes of protein are desirable — as for example McCarrison's (1936) comparison between the poor physique of rice-eating Bengalis and the good physique of milk-drinking Sikhs.

Animal experiments reviewed by Holt *et al.* (1962) do not support the view that a high level of labile body protein (p. 38) confers any biological advantage. They present good evidence to show that laboratory rats kept on low protein diets, which would allow no reserve of protein to accumulate, stand up to stresses such as exercise, unfavourable environmental temperatures, physical and chemical agents, injuries, infections, parasitic infestations and dietary deprivations as well as rats provided with a surplus of protein. It is naturally impossible to test these points experimentally in human subjects.

However some standard of requirements of protein is needed by government planners responsible for agricultural trade policies directed to ensuring a suitable diet for a country. It is also needed by those responsible for drawing up ration scales for institutions and members of various services, and by doctors responsible for the care of individual patients. Any recommendations must bear some relation to possible supplies. In this respect the countries of the world can be divided fairly sharply into two groups. Table 5.7 shows that the rich countries have 50 per cent more protein available than the poor countries. This table was prepared from data now 20 years old, but the differences remain today. In the poor countries many children die from lack of sufficient dietary protein and many more suffer serious ill health, grow slowly and fail to develop their full physical potential (Chap. 29). In these countries diseases due directly to lack of dietary protein are not common among adults. To what extent insufficient protein lowers resistance to other diseases or reduces physical capacity for work is a matter of opinion. In our judgment the majority of adults in these countries get sufficient protein for health.

However, when a family diet is barely adequate, the distribution of the food within the family is all important. There is ample evidence that if the children do not receive shares of the diet richer in protein than that given to the adults, they fail to develop normally and become liable to protein–energy malnutrition. This is perhaps the most important lesson which the nutritionist has to teach.

League of Nations Standards

The League of Nations Technical Committee on Nutrition (1936) was the first authoritative body to attempt to lay down a standard. Their recommendation that adults should have daily at least 1 g of protein/kg body weight was empirical. The figure has passed into textbooks of physiology and medicine and is still known widely. It remains a useful guide for administrators and doctors.

FAO/WHO Standards

Expert committees in 1957, 1965 and 1973 have each attempted to draw up standards based on a physiological approach, the requirement being derived from data for the obligatory N loss or the requirement to maintain N balance. The figures for adults have always been less than the League of Nations Standards. Their most recent figures for an adult man's daily requirement of protein are 53 g or 0.57 g/kg or 7.0 per cent of the energy intake. These are based on mixed dietary protein with NPU 70.

It has been traditional to use N balance for estimation of

Table 5.7 Daily consumption of livestock products (g/head). (FAO, 1962)

	Milk	Meat	Egg	Fish	Protein Animal	Total
The rich countries	573	152	30	34	44	90
The poor countries	79	30	4	24	9	58

human protein requirements and to give the subjects generous energy intakes. But other measurements are available which reflect body protein mass. When total body potassium and urinary creatinine are used, the study continued for several weeks and the energy intake adjusted precisely to maintain body weight. Scrimshaw (1976) finds that the 1973 FAO/WHO safe level of protein is insufficient for some healthy students.

British Standards

The Department of Health and Social Security (1969) recommended protein intakes equivalent to at least 10 per cent of the intake energy. This figure rests on no physiological basis. It is a little lower than the intake provided by good British diets of today. It was considered that diets containing less protein, although probably meeting physiological requirements, might be unsatisfactory in other respects and in particular might not meet requirements for some of the micronutrients.

The FAO/WHO figure for the adult requirement is certainly sufficient to maintain N balance, and there is evidence from the experiments of Chittenden that a few people have maintained health on such an intake for long periods. However, it is far below the level of intake freely chosen, especially by men engaged in active occupations, for whom a daily consumption of about 1.5 g/kg would be usual. It is possible that Rubner may be right and that this choice is the result of a hidden 'wisdom of the body', to use the words of Cannon, the great American physiologist. There may be long-term needs for protein in the synthesis of substances turning over slowly, which are not detected in balance studies of short duration. For this reason and also because of the difficulty of obtaining good diets using low protein food, the use of the FAO/WHO figures appears unsound for practical recommendations. A food supply in which 10 per cent of the energy is provided by protein is a safer target for food administrators in all countries and nowhere should it be beyond reach.

PROTEIN DEFICIENCY

If the supply of dietary protein is insufficient, the cells lack amino acids for their synthetic activities. The first effect of this on a young child is that growth slows down or stops. The effect on the organs and tissues is related to the speed of turnover of proteins (p. 37). This is fastest in the mucosa of the intestines and in the glands which secrete the digestive enzymes. In consequence a failure to digest and absorb the food, leading to diarrhoea and loss of water and electrolytes, is an early feature of protein deficiency. There is also a failure of the liver to maintain its normal structure and function. Fat accumulates in the liver cells. The liver also fails to synthesise plasma albumin and this is liable to lead to oedema. Later, protein deficiency leads to a failure

to maintain the structure of skeletal muscle and the production of red blood cells. Muscle wasting and anaemia result. The clinical consequences of these failures in protein synthesis are described in the chapter on protein-energy malnutrition (p. 256). Since the physiological turnover of collagen is slow, connective tissue is well maintained, as also is the protein in the central nervous system. Disturbances of mental function may follow severe protein deficiency occurring in early life.

As plasma is the tissue which is most easily sampled, analyses of plasma proteins are frequently used as an index of protein deficiency. Normal concentrations are given in Table 5.8. A plasma albumin concentration below 35 g/l suggests strongly protein deficiency, and in severe deficiency states the level often falls to 15 and sometimes lower. The concentration of immunoglobulins is often raised owing to the presence of infections. A low plasma albumin and a high plasma globulin are frequently found together where the people are poor with inadequate diet and an unhygienic environment. In marasmus the deficit of protein may be as great or greater than in kwashiorkor, but hypoalbuminaemia and fatty liver are not characteristic. When energy deficit predominates, the responses described above are modified.

Secondary or 'conditioned' protein deficiency may arise as a result of pathological processes. The following are examples.

1. Utilisation of protein as a source of energy, owing to an inadequate supply of carbohydrate.
2. Loss of protein in the urine as a result of disease of the kidneys.
3. Loss of protein (albumin and globulin) from the body by other routes such as haemorrhage and serous exudates from wounds.
4. Failure to absorb protein in various disorders of the intestines.
5. Failure by a damaged liver to synthesise proteins (particularly albumin) from the amino acids absorbed from the intestines.
6. Damage to tissues (trauma). Injuries such as burns, fractured bones or surgical operations are followed by a period of negative nitrogen balance. More tissue protein is catabolised than the diet can immediately replace. The breakdown is not confined to the immediate site of the trauma but is a general reaction to injury (p. 440).

Adaptions to low protein intakes

The health of most adults would probably be unaffected if they were put on diets providing either 50 or 150 g protein daily. Clearly the tissues of the body can adapt to widely different levels of protein intake. This is in sharp contrast to the effect of varying intakes of energy. The need for energy is fixed by the rate of energy expenditure. If the intake falls below or exceeds this need, then inevitably the

Table 5.8 Plasma proteins (g/litre)

	Mean	Range
Total protein	68	58–78
Albumin	43	35–56
Globulins	22	16–31
Fibrinogen	3	2–4

subject wastes or becomes obese. The problem of the nature of the adaptions to varying protein intakes have been much studied by Waterlow and his colleagues in the Tropical Metabolism Research Unit in Jamaica (Waterlow, 1968). The liver has a key role in the adaptive processes, for it is only in the liver that nitrogen can be transformed from amino acids into urea. The state of the liver must determine what proportion of the nitrogen in the amino acids entering it via the circulation is converted into urea, and what proportion is retained within the amino acid pool and used for synthetic processes in the protein turnover of the tissues. Studies with labelled amino acids indicate that in rats on a low protein diet the turnover of protein is maintained in the liver, but reduced in the muscles and skin. This is probably effected by changes in the activity of liver enzymes. In protein deficiency levels of amino acid activating enzymes are high and levels of argininosuccinase, the enzyme responsible for the formation of urea, are low. Table 5.9 (Stephen and Waterlow, 1968) shows the levels of activity of these enzymes in samples of liver obtained by biopsy from Jamaican children a few days after admission to hospital with severe malnutrition and one to two months later when they had

recovered well. Many experiments in rats (Stephen, 1968) confirmed by a few observations in man, have established that quantitative aspects of amino acid metabolism in the liver are determined by the dietary protein intake and directed to maintaining protein synthesis.

Alterations of hormone balance play an important part in the different responses of the body to protein deficiency, which may be acute or chronic and accompanied by varying degrees of energy deficit and by different infections. Energy balance determines whether insulin or cortisol predominate (Coward et al., 1977). When there is adequate carbohydrate this stimulates insulin secretion, which favours deposition of amino acids in muscle at the expense of the liver. If starvation predominates, insulin secretion is low but cortisol increased. Cortisol produces muscle wasting but deposition of protein in the liver.

Table 5.9 Enzymic activity of the livers of children with malnutrition

	Amino acid activating enzymes	Arginino-succinase
Soon after admission	1.44	1.06
One to two months later	0.91	1.46

The figures for the amino acid activating enzymes are the mean of 18 measurements and expressed in μmol P exchanged/mg protein hourly; for argininosuccinase the figures are the mean of 11 measurements and expressed in μmol urea/mg protein hourly. The changes on recovery are statistically significant.

6. Fats

Fats provide a convenient and concentrated source of energy. Unfortunately there is some confusion in terms. The housewife, when she goes to buy butter, margarine or lard, has a clear idea of what she means by fat. Biochemists, in an effort to be more precise, invented a new word—lipid which covers all the chemical substances included in the housewife's fat—triglycerides, phospholipids, sterols, etc. Lipids have been defined as substances which are insoluble in water but soluble in organic solvents such as ether, chloroform and benzene. They are actual or potential esters of fatty acids. But these criteria cannot be applied too rigidly or exclusively. The chemist uses the term 'fat' in a restricted sense to mean the 'neutral fats' which are mixtures of esters of fatty acids. The term 'oil' is applied indiscriminately both to liquid, digestible triglycerides (such as olive oil) and to indigestible mineral hydrocarbons (such as liquid paraffin). Hereafter we shall use the word 'fat' in the housewife's sense when referring to the fat content of foods and diets, but shall follow the more precise chemical nomenclature when considering the metabolism of lipids in the body.

In practical dietetics it is useful to refer to **visible fats**, meaning butter and margarine, lard and vegetable oils. This is convenient as visible fat can be accurately measured and therefore accurately prescribed. In contrast, many other foods contain different proportions of fat, which are closely associated with the other constituents in an emulsion or as part of the tissue. Hence the **total fat** in a diet is hard to measure, because different samples of the same food may vary widely in fat content, especially in the case of meat. Only approximate figures for total fat content are provided by food tables or nutrition labelling. Accurate assessments of the total fat in a diet require a chemical analysis of samples in the diet as actually consumed.

The fats in the body were divided by Terroine, the distinguished French physiologist, into *l'élément variable* and *l'élément constant*. The first is the fuel store of the body which can be expended; the second is part of the essential structure of the cells. This is still a useful distinction.

CHEMICAL CONSTITUTION AND NATURAL DISTRIBUTION

Triglyceride is the form in which fats chiefly occur both in foodstuffs and in the fat depots of most animals. Triglycer-ides are esters of glycerol and fatty acids and have the general composition:

$$CH_2.O.COR^1$$
$$CHO.O.COR^2$$
$$CH_2.O.COR^3$$

where R^1COOH, R^2COOH and R^3COOH are long-chain fatty acids with even numbers of carbon atoms

FATTY ACIDS

There are over 40 fatty acids found in nature. These give a diversity and chemical specificity to the natural fats similar to that given to the proteins by the amino acids. Characteristically fats are mixtures of triglycerides; no fat found in nature consists of a single triglyceride.

In any one fat, fatty acids are distributed amongst the glycerol molecules according to the 'principle of even distribution' (Hilditch and Williams, 1964). Thus in a mixture of triglycerides, molecules of a single fatty acid (say palmitic acid) are attached first to every molecule of glycerol. Triglycerides containing two molecules of palmitic acid are not found unless palmitic acid comprises more than a third of the total fatty acids present. Any fatty acid forming appreciably less than one-third of the total fatty acid never occurs more than once in any one triglyceride. Thus the composition of individual triglycerides is determined by biological order and is not the result of chemical chance.

Fatty acids have the basic formula $CH_3[CH_2]_nCOOH$, where n can be any number from 2 to 24, usually an even number. Those occurring in nature can be classified into three types. First, there are the saturated fatty acids; secondly, there are unsaturated fatty acids with one double bond (the monoenoic acids); thirdly, there are polyunsaturated fatty acids, sometimes abbreviated as PUFA, with two or more double bonds (the dienoic and polyenoic acids). The degree of unsaturation in any fat plays an important part in determining its physical nature. Fats consisting predominantly of saturated fatty acids are solid at room temperatures, while those with a high proportion of unsaturated acids are usually liquid (e.g. whale oil, cod-liver oil and olive oil). The extent to which a fat contains unsaturated fatty acids can be assessed from its ability to take up iodine (the iodine number). Vegetable and marine oils can be hardened and turned into solid fats by the action of hydrogen in the presence of a catalyst. This has enabled vegetable oils from all over the world to be used in the various processes of making margarine and other artificial butters such as *vanaspathis* in India. This hydrogenation converts most of the unsaturated fatty acids into saturated fatty acids.

Nomenclature

The carbon atoms in the fatty acids are referred to either by number or Greek letters; thus palmitic acid is

$$\overset{16}{CH_3}[CH_2]_{11}.\overset{4}{CH_2}.\overset{3}{CH_2}.\overset{2}{CH_2}.\overset{1}{COOH}$$
$$\underset{\omega}{} \quad \underset{\gamma}{} \quad \underset{\beta}{} \quad \underset{\alpha}{}$$

A shorthand designation for each acid gives the number of carbon atoms present and also the number of double bonds. Thus palmitic acid is written $C_{16:0}$ and oleic acid which has 18 carbon atoms and one double bond is $C_{18:1}$.

The more important fatty acids in nature are as follows:

Saturated acids

Butyric acid	$C_{4:0}$
Caproic acid	$C_{6:0}$
Caprylic acid	$C_{8:0}$
Capric acid	$C_{10:0}$
Lauric acid	$C_{12:0}$
Myristic acid	$C_{14:0}$
Palmitic acid	$C_{16:0}$
Stearic acid	$C_{18:0}$
Arachidic acid	$C_{20:0}$
Behenic acid	$C_{22:0}$

Monounsaturated acids

Palmitoleic acid	$C_{16:1}$
Oleic acid	$C_{18:1}$
Erucic acid	$C_{22:1}$

Polyunsaturated acids (PUFA)

Linoleic acid	$C_{18:2}$
Linolenic acid	$C_{18:3}$
Arachidonic acid	$C_{20:4}$

Palmitic acid is widely distributed in nature and may contribute from 10 to 50 per cent of total fatty acids in any fat. Of the other saturated fatty acids only myristic and stearic acid (the latter is present in up to 25 per cent of beef fat) are comparable in distribution to palmitic acid, though they are not invariably present in every fat.

Oleic acid is the most widely distributed fatty acid in nature. In most fats it forms 30 per cent or more of the total fatty acids.

The polyunsaturated fatty acids are of special interest. Linoleic and linolenic acids cannot be synthesised in the body and are known as 'essential fatty acids' (EFA). Arachidonic acid can be formed by conversion from linoleic acid. As long ago as 1929, Burr and Burr showed that these acids were essential for the growth and well-being of rats. Probably all species of animals, including man, require a small amount in their diet (p. 55). Essential fatty acids are present in large amounts in many vegetable oils. Polyunsaturated fatty acids have a major role in the synthesis of the prostaglandins, which are important hormones.

The ratio of dietary polyunsaturated to saturated fatty acids is often abbreviated to the P/S ratio. This has an influence on the plasma cholesterol and so is of interest in relation to coronary heart disease (p. 327).

Position of double bonds

Unsaturated fatty acids exist in different isomeric forms depending on the position of the double bonds. Two isomers of octadecadienoic acid, $C_{18:2}$, may be present in an edible oil, one of which functions as an essential fatty acid and the other does not. Chemists usually number the sites of double bonds by counting the carbon atoms from the carboxyl end. The active isomer of $C_{18:2}$ is designated $C_{18:2 \Delta 9,12}$ and the inactive one $C_{18:2 \Delta 6,9}$. An alternative system of numbering the sites counts from the methyl end, or ω carbon atom. In this system linoleic acid is $C_{18:2 \omega 6,9}$ and the inactive isomer is $C_{18:2 \omega 9,12}$. Biochemists often prefer the ω system because desaturase enzymes can only insert double bonds on the carboxylic side of an existing double bond. Thus the biologically important substance arachidonic acid, $C_{20:4 \omega 6,9,12,15}$ with four double bonds can be formed from linoleic acid $C_{18:2 \omega 6,9}$ but not from its isomer $C_{18:2 \omega 9,12}$. The ω system thus shows the potential of linoleic acid for conversion to arachidonic acid. All unsaturated fatty acids with their first or only double bond in the ω 6 position are grouped as *n*-6 acids, and linoleic and arachidonic are examples. Those with their first double bond at ω 9 are *n*-9 acids and these include oleic acid. The biologically active linolenic acid $C_{18:3 \omega 3,6,9}$ belongs to the *n*-3 group. This nomenclature is useful in understanding the role of essential fatty acids (p. 55).

Cis and trans isomerism. Any fatty acid which contains a double carbon bond (ethylene linkage) can exist in either of two geometrically isomeric forms. This is known as *cis* and *trans* isomerism. When two carbon atoms are held together by the double bond, there is no freedom of rotation for these groups about the axis of the bond and the molecule can be angled in one of two forms at each double bond. Thus oleic acid, a *cis* form, has a *trans* isomer elaidic acid.

$$\begin{array}{ll} H—C—[CH_2]_7CH_3 & CH_3—[CH_2]_7—CH \\ \quad \| & \qquad\qquad\qquad \| \\ H—C—[CH_2]_7COOH & H—C—[CH_2]_7COOH \end{array}$$

Oleic acid (*cis*)   Elaidic acid (*trans*)

The natural unsaturated fatty acids exist in the *cis* form, with their molecules bent back at each double bond. They cannot be packed together closely like the long straight chains of the saturated acids and the *trans* forms. *Trans* isomers of polyunsaturated acids do not have essential fatty acid activity and lack the ability possessed by *cis* isomers of lowering the level of lipoproteins in plasma (p. 326).

Distribution of fatty acids in animal and plant life

The chemical composition of the natural fats is related to the biological species from which they are derived. Organisms which have been classed together by biologists on morphological grounds have been found by chemists to share in general the same fatty acids in approximately similar proportions. Hilditch was a pioneer in finding out the biological distributions of the fatty acids. His book is the classic reference work on the subject (Hilditch and Williams, 1964).

In fats from all freshwater life, whether plant or animal, the unsaturated C_{16}, C_{18}, C_{20}, and C_{22} fatty acids predominate. They are present in varying proportions and in different states of unsaturation. The only important saturated acid is palmitic acid, which is usually present as 10 to 18 per cent of total acids.

In the marine world polyunsaturated C_{20} and C_{22} fatty acids, containing up to six double bonds, are most numerous. In highly developed fish and aquatic mammals the fatty acids form esters with other higher alcohols as well as with glycerol. The fats present in salmon and sea-trout, fish which live both in fresh and salt water, have fatty acids which conform to the general picture of other marine animals.

In land animals, and particularly in mammals, the unsaturated oleic acid and the saturated palmitic acid predominate. Palmitic acid forms about 25 to 30 per cent of the fatty acids in the depot fat of all the common mammals and this accounts for their hardness and low iodine value relative to marine oils. Stearic acid is found principally in the fat of ruminants, where it in part replaces oleic acid.

Milk fats, such as butter, differ from other animal fats in containing small amounts of short-chain C_4 to C_{12} fatty acids.

In plant seeds the fatty acids are less varied than in aquatic life. As in land animals, oleic acid and palmitic acid are prominent, but a third acid, linoleic acid (EFA), provides a large component. Linoleic and linolenic acids are amongst the most familiar constituents of the numerous seed oils. Coconut oil is an exception in that it is mostly made up of short-chain saturated fatty acids, with very little oleic and linoleic acid. Olive oil is very rich in oleic acid but contains little linoleic acid. The elucidation of the relationship of the different fatty acid components of the fats with the morphology and natural history of plants and animals from which they come is a fascinating biological problem.

Table 6.1 gives the relative amounts of the different fatty acids in some common foods and vegetable oils.

A diet rich in linoleic and linolenic acid can be obtained by eating plenty of vegetable seed oils. Arachidonic acid seldom occurs in vegetable oils, but animals have no difficulty in synthesising it from linoleic acid.

The proportion of essential fatty acids that remains in vegetable and marine oils after hardening by commercial hydrogenation is important. Completely hydrogenated fats of course contain none. Formerly most margarines contained little or no EFA. With the steady increase in the consumption of margarine during the first 50 years of the present century, national intakes of linoleic acid probably declined. Recently, owing to the interest in the physiological action of these acids, manufacturers have been at great pains to produce margarines containing linoleic acid. Products are now available in which 50 per cent or more of the fatty acids are polyunsaturated. This is achieved by skilful blending of vegetable oils that have not been hydrogenated.

WAXES

As defined chemically, waxes are fatty acid esters of higher alcohols. They occur widely in the cuticle of leaves and fruit and in the secretions of insects and may be mixed with very long-chain hydrocarbons (C_{21-35}). They replace the triglycerides to some extent in the tissues of aquatic animals (e.g. crustaceans). In some whales, wax esters form the major component of the depot fat. So far waxes have not been shown to be an important constituent of any of the higher land animals, nor do they contribute importantly to normal human diets.

PHOSPHOLIPIDS

After the triglycerides, the next largest lipid class in the body is the phospholipids. A great variety of these substances in present in the body.

Glycerophospholipids are an important group of phospholipids, found mainly in tissues and blood, and to a much lesser extent in depot fat. They form part of the structure of cell membranes and are concerned in the transport of fat about the body. They are derived from 2-glycerophosphate, by esterification with two fatty acid molecules and attachment to the phosphate radical of a nitrogen-containing alcohol, usually choline, ethanolamine or serine.

Phosphatidylcholine or **lecithin,** originally prepared from egg yolk, is the main phospholipid in plasma.

The constituent fatty acids in the phospholipids vary widely. Like the triglycerides, lecithin and related substances are not individual compounds, but each is a mixture. The distribution of the fatty acids does not follow the even pattern characteristic of the triglycerides. Nor is there evidence of so close an association between the

Table 6.1 Pattern of fatty acids in fats and oils (approximate percentage of total fatty acids)

	C_{4-12} saturated	$C_{14:0}$	$C_{16:0}$	$C_{18:0}$	$C_{16:1}$ + $C_{18:1}$	$C_{18:2}$	Other PUFA	Other FAs
Butter, cream and milk	13	11	26	11	30	2	1[b]	2
Beef	—	3	29	16	48	2	1	—
Bacon and pork	—	2	26	14	50	7	1	—
Chicken	—	1	26	7	45	18	2	—
Fish oil	—	5	15	3	27	7	43[a]	—
Coconut oil	58	18	10	3	8	2	—	—
Palm oil	—	1	40	4	45	9	—	—
Cocoa butter	—	—	26	35	36	3	—	—
Rapeseed oil	—	—	3	1	24	15	10[b]	40[c]
Olive oil	—	—	12	2	73	11	1	—
Groundnut oil	—	—	12	3	53	30	1	—
Sesame oil	—	—	9	5	40	43	—	—
Cottonseed oil	—	1	24	2	20	50	1	—
Corn (maize) oil	—	—	12	2	31	53	2	—
Soya bean oil	—	—	10	4	24	53	7[b]	—
Sunflower seed oil	—	—	6	6	33	58	—	—
Safflower seed oil	—	—	7	2	13	74	—	—
Margarine	3	5	23	9	33	12	1	5
Margarine, polyunsaturated	2	1	12	8	22	52	1	—

[a] Long-chain polyunsaturated fatty acids (C_{20} and C_{22}).
[b] $C_{18:3}$ (linolenic);   [c] $C_{22:1}$ (erucic).
Note. The composition of all these fats and oils varies depending on methods of animal husbandry and crop production. In margarines the proportion of fats and oils for the blend are adjusted to world market prices.

chemical constitution of the phosphatidyl esters and the biological species of their origin, as in the case of the triglycerides. Most animal phospholipids are characterised by a large proportion of highly unsaturated fatty acids including arachidonic acid

The **sphingomyelins** found in myelin in the nervous system are phospholipids in which phosphorylcholine is esterified with sphingosine, a complex base, structurally similar to a monoglyceride. **Glycolipids** (cerebrosides and gangliosides) contain sphingosine attached to hexoses and complex carbohydrates; they do not contain phosphorus. Glycolipids are important components of cell membranes. Little is known about their nutritional significance.

STEROLS

These comprise an important and widely distributed class of biological substances, all of which have the same basic ring structure. Sterols are solid alcohols and, like all alcohols, can form esters with fatty acids.

Cholesterol

Cholesterol is found in all animal tissues, so that some is present in all foods of animal origin, but eggs are the only common food rich in cholesterol. It is virtually absent from foods of plant origin.

Cholesterol metabolism. The cholesterol content of most Western diets is around 500 mg/day. In addition cholesterol is synthesised in the body from acetate via mevalonate and squalene, mainly in the liver but also in the intestinal wall.

Cholesterol is lost from the body in two main ways. Part is excreted unchanged in the bile, in which it is in solution as micelles formed with bile salts and lecithin. In the small bowel the biliary and dietary cholesterol mix and are partly absorbed. The remainder passes to the colon where much of it undergoes minor chemical transformation by the bacterial flora to coprostanol. Faecal coprostanol, cholesterol and related compounds constitute the faecal neutral steroids.

The other way in which cholesterol is lost is by oxidation in the liver to the primary bile acids, cholic and chenodeoxycholic acids (Fig. 6.1). These are then conjugated with glycine or taurine and excreted in the bile. In the small intestine the bile acids form the micelles which play an important role in absorption of the dietary fats (see below). Most of the bile acids are then reabsorbed from the lower ileum and recycle several times after each large meal. A small amount of the bile salts escape absorption during each enterohepatic cycle. They pass to the large bowel where the resident bacteria remove the glycine or taurine and the 7-hydroxyl group, thus forming the secondary bile acids, deoxycholic and lithocholic acids which are excreted as the faecal bile acids. About 0.5 g of faecal bile acids are excreted daily.

Cholesterol in the liver is in equilibrium with cholesterol in the plasma. Turnover studies can be interpreted as showing three body pools with fast, slow and very slow turnover rates.

Cholesterol metabolism is subject to feedback control. When dietary cholesterol increases, endogenous synthesis is suppressed and catabolism of cholesterol may be increased. The quantitative aspects of regulation of cholesterol metabolism vary between different species. In rats a high cholesterol intake is well absorbed but catabolism of cholesterol to bile acids is greatly increased so that body cholesterol increases only moderately. Rabbits cannot compensate in this way; when fed with cholesterol, they develop massive hypercholesterolaemia. In man cholesterol absorption is limited, but an increase is compensated by reduced endogenous synthesis; then a new steady state ensues in which the body pools of cholesterol are only a little enlarged. Nevertheless, plasma cholesterol generally falls when human subjects take a diet very low in cholesterol (Chap. 40). The regulation of cholesterol metabolism has been reviewed by Dietschy and Wilson (1970) and Lewis (1976).

DIGESTION AND ABSORPTION

The presence of fat in the food delays the emptying of the stomach. This may contribute to the feeling of satiety after a meal rich in fat. The mechanism of the delay has been attributed to the inhibitory action on the movement of the stomach of a hormone (enterogastrone) liberated when fat enters the duodenum, but this hormone has not been identified.

EMULSIFICATION AND HYDROLYSIS

Fats have to be reduced to small particles before digestion and absorption are possible. Conditions first become suitable for emulsification in the duodenum, below the point where the pancreatic juice and bile enter. Bile salts, and small quantities of fatty acids and monoglycerides liberated by pancreatic lipase, are then able to emulsify fat

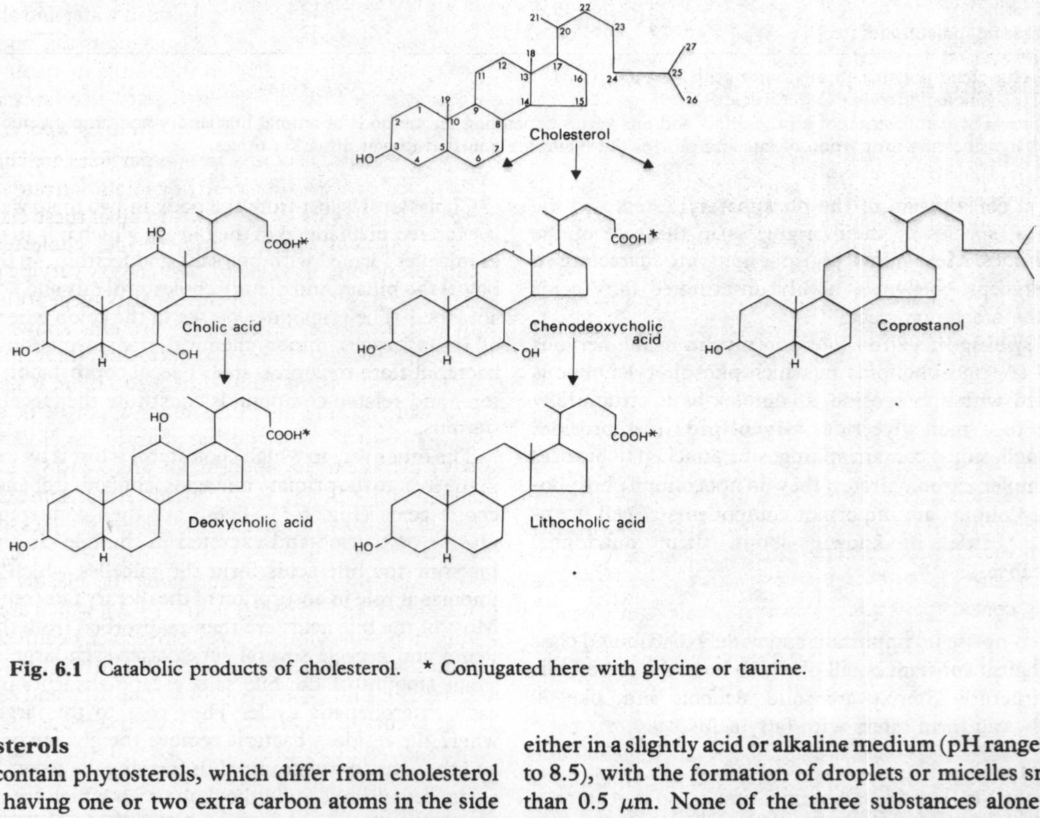

Fig. 6.1 Catabolic products of cholesterol.   * Conjugated here with glycine or taurine.

Plant sterols

Plants contain phytosterols, which differ from cholesterol only in having one or two extra carbon atoms in the side chain (Itoh *et al.,* 1973). A common one is ß-sitosterol which is 24-ethyl cholesterol. The plant sterols are poorly absorbed. They also interfere with absorption of cholesterol, and ß-sitosterol has been used to lower plasma cholesterol.

One of the plant sterols, **ergosterol,** is found in yeasts and fungi. Under the influence of ultraviolet light it is converted into vitamin D_2, ergocalciferol.

either in a slightly acid or alkaline medium (pH range of 6.0 to 8.5), with the formation of droplets or micelles smaller than 0.5 μm. None of the three substances alone is an effective emulsifier under the conditions found in the intestine and the combination of the three is necessary for the digestion of fat.

Pancreatic lipase splits triglycerides into fatty acids, diglycerides, monoglycerides and glycerol. Hydrolysis is slow at the 2-monoglyceride stage. Pancreatic juice also contains phospholipase and cholesterol esterase. The contents of the small intestine are not sufficiently alkaline to allow the fatty acids liberated by hydrolysis to form soaps with alkalis under normal conditions.

The final result is a clear microemulsion of lipids, which is then presented to the microvilli of the mucous membrane of the small intestine.

ABSORPTION

Fatty acids and monoglycerides pass into the cells of the mucous membrane as very small particles or micelles which can be demonstrated by the electron microscope. Within the cells further hydrolysis may take place under the influence of intracellular monoglyceride lipase and then the long-chain fatty acids are re-esterified into new triglycerides. In the processes of digestion and absorption, the fatty acids are mixed, so that the triglycerides of the food lose their identity and new triglycerides partly characteristic of the animal species are formed. After resynthesis the triglycerides enter the lacteals of the small intestine as small particles from 0.1 to 0.6 μm in diameter, known as chylomicrons (see below). These pass into the lacteals and the mesenteric lymph vessels, enter the thoracic duct and thence join the systemic circulation via the right subclavian vein. In experimental animals it is not difficult to make a fistula in the thoracic duct and collect the chyle therefrom. In clinical medicine an occasional opportunity to study the formation of chyle arises; if, as a result of injury, a leak occurs in the thoracic duct in the course of its passage through the thorax, the chyle escapes into the pleural cavity (chylothorax) and can be aspirated through the chest wall.

The major part of the fat absorbed enters the circulation via the thoracic duct, except for most short- and medium-chain fatty acids which pass to the liver via the portal vein.

COMPLETENESS OF DIGESTION AND ABSORPTION

Most fats, when fed to adult subjects in quantities up to 100 g/day, are digested and absorbed to the extent of at least 95 per cent. Much larger quantities, up to 250 g/day or even more, can sometimes be absorbed if the body is short of energy. Arctic explorers and lumberjacks frequently consume and digest such large amounts (Butson, 1950). In constitutionally thin people there is no evidence of a failure to digest or absorb fats. Normally, fats never form more than 10 per cent of the dry weight of the stools and the amount present is largely independent of the dietary intake. With a fat intake of 100 g/day or less, the presence of more than 7 g of fat daily in the faeces (taken as an average over a period of at least five days) constitutes evidence of some failure of fat absorption and justifies a diagnosis of steatorrhoea. Steatorrhoea is found whenever there is a failure of secretion either of the bile salts or the pancreatic juice, It also occurs in the malabsorption syndrome (Chap. 46).

LIPID TRANSPORT

After absorption from the alimentary canal nutrients are carried in the blood either to storage depots or to the muscles and other tissues where they serve as a source of energy. They are also taken from the storage depots to the active tissues when alimentary absorption is not taking place. In addition, nutrients pass to and from the liver and other tissues where synthetic processes and chemical transformation take place. For the transport of carbohydrate glucose serves as a convenient currency, for it is a simple chemical and readily soluble in water and almost all the carriage of carbohydrate throughout the body takes place in this form. Lipids are insoluble in water and for them no simple form of currency exists. They are carried in the blood attached to protein, as complex lipoproteins.

Four main classes of lipoprotein particles are characterised by their density, ultracentrifuge flotation rate and electrophoretic mobility (Table 6.2). In all of these classes the lipid component includes triglyceride, cholesterol and phospholipid but these are present in very varying proportions. The protein component consists of peptide chains known as apoproteins. Three apoproteins known as A, B and C are the main constituents, but their molecular structure is as yet not fully known and there is no agreed terminology. There are other minor apoproteins and also forms of A and C which differ slightly. In chylomicrons and VLDL the major apoproteins are B and C, LDL has predominantly B, and HDL mainly A but some C. Much fuller information is given in a review by Jackson et al. (1976).

In addition to these lipoproteins the plasma contains non-esterified, or free fatty acids (FFA), which are carried bound to plasma albumin; also present in health are small amounts of acetoacetic acid and β-hydroxybutyric acid derived from lipid metabolism in the liver and known as ketone bodies. FFA and ketone bodies serve as fuel for the tissues and are discussed in Chapter 8.

Table 6.2 The plasma lipoproteins (from Lewis, 1976)

Lipoprotein	Abbreviation	Density	S *	Electrophoretic mobility	Percentage composition			
					Protein	Triglyceride	Cholesterol	Phospholipid
Chylomicrons	—	0.96	>400	none	2	85	4	9
Very low density	VLDL	0.96–1.006	20–400	pre-β	10	50	22	18
Low density	LDL	1.006–1.063	0–12	β	25	10	45	20
High density	HDL	>1.063	—	α	55	4	17	24

*Lipoprotein flotation rate in Svedberg units in the ultracentrifuge.

Figure 6.2 is a simplified scheme illustrating the main features of lipid transport in plasma.

CHYLOMICRONS

Chylomicrons are the chief vehicle for the carriage of lipids from the alimentary canal. Chemically they are chiefly triglycerides and contain only about 2 per cent protein. A small amount of phospholipid is present, which probably provides a covering layer giving stability to the particles. They also contain a little cholesterol, both free and esterified.

Alimentary lipaemia

After a meal containing fat, a large number of chylomicrons appear in the blood. These are removed from the blood rapidly and, if only small amounts of fat (30 g or less) are taken at a meal, it is difficult to detect any increase in the plasma lipids. The clearing of chylomicrons from the plasma keeps pace with their formation in the intestinal wall. If a meal containing a large amount of fat is eaten, the plasma becomes milky. Alimentary lipaemia can be followed quantitatively by counting the chylomicrons, but this is difficult and it is simpler to measure the rise in either total serum lipids or in serum triglycerides. Man and Gildea (1932) found that three hours after a meal containing 60 g of fat, the total fatty acids in the sera of nine subjects increased by an average of 21 per cent. With a higher fat intake, large rises were found. The rise is usually at a maximum two to four hours after taking the fat. As chylomicrons contain only small amounts of phospholipid and cholesterol, the plasma concentration of these lipids is raised only slightly by a fatty meal. The triglycerides are removed from chylomicrons in a matter of minutes. This is effected by lipoprotein lipases, mainly in adipose tissue and muscle. Injection of heparin causes these lipases to appear in the blood, which then has 'clearing activity' but whether endogenous heparin plays any part in the removal of chylomicrons after a fatty meal is uncertain. After removal of the triglycerides, the remnants of the chylomicrons are taken up by the liver (Redgrave, 1970).

Lipid transformation in the liver

Triglycerides are synthesised in the liver partly from carbohydrate entering from the intestine, partly from fatty acid mobilised from adipose tissue (see below) as well as that derived from chylomicron remnants. Each of these sources is dominant under different metabolic conditions. Glucose is the main source when the diet is rich in carbohydrate; fatty acids from adipose tissue between meals and in starvation; chylomicrons after a fatty meal. Fat leaves the liver in very low density lipoproteins (VLDL) which, like the chylomicrons, are rich in triglycerides and have a high rate of turnover. The cholesterol-rich β or low density lipoproteins (LDL) in plasma appear to be derived in part, if not completely, from intravascular degradation of VLDL. The liver normally contains only 5 to 7 per cent of fat (wet weight) which cannot be seen under the microscope. In various dietary circumstances and as a result of toxins or disease, the amount of fat in the liver may increase greatly. As much as 50 per cent of its weight may be fat and in extreme cases the histological appearance may at first glance resemble adipose tissue. The two most important dietary causes of fatty liver in man are an excessive intake of ethyl alcohol and kwashiorkor. In the first of these there is increased hepatic synthesis of fatty acids, while insufficient amino acids for lipoprotein synthesis is probably the major abnormality in kwashiorkor.

Lipotropic factors

Before the discovery of insulin, patients with diabetes frequently had large fatty livers. Soon afterwards the Toronto School discovered that fatty livers developed in pancreatectomised dogs maintained on insulin for a long time. Best and his colleagues showed that dietary factors

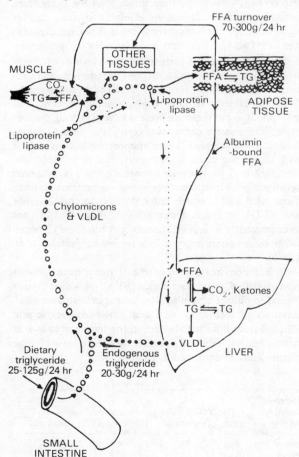

Fig. 6.2 Lipid transport in plasma. Key: O, chylomicrons; o, VLDL;..., remnants. (Modified from Lewis, 1976.)

play a part in controlling the fat content of the liver (Best and Taylor, 1961). Several substances were capable of preventing this accumulation of fat. Of these the most important was the base, choline, which forms part of phosphatidylcholine, the principal phospholipid in the plasma lipoproteins. However, choline is not an essential dietary substance and can be synthesised in the body. For this methyl (CH_3) radicals are necessary and these can be supplied by the amino acid methionine. Most foods of animal origin are good sources of choline and most animal proteins contain useful amounts of methionine. Moreover, there is no good evidence that a dietary deficiency of choline is responsible for any liver or other disorder in man.

PLASMA LIPOPROTEINS

As described above, the fat absorbed after a meal is carried in chylomicrons. After these have been cleared and in the fasting state there remain four classes of lipids in the blood—cholesterol, triglycerides, phospholipids and fatty acids. The first three come from the liver and are completely insoluble in the aqueous saline solution of plasma; plasma can only carry these lipids and remain clear because they are incorporated into the three types of lipoprotein summarised in Table 6.2. Most of the triglyceride originating in the liver is carried by VLDL or pre-β-lipoprotein. Within a few hours most of this triglyceride is taken up by the periphery by the same lipoprotein lipases that act on chylomicrons. This leaves LDL or β-lipoprotein, the main carrier of cholesterol. LDL is removed more slowly, over 2 to 5 days, probably mostly by the liver. The third type of lipoprotein, high density (HDL) or α-lipoprotein is not involved in triglyceride transport but some lipid and protein transfers readily back and forth between VLDL and HDL.

Fatty acids are carried in plasma attached to albumin. Unlike the other classes of lipid they are the form in which lipids are carried to the muscles and liver from the stores of triglyceride in the adipose tissue. How and when they are released is described below in the section on Adipose Tissue.

Although the plasma lipids are carried on proteins, in practice they are more often measured in the plasma after extracting them from protein. The concentration of cholesterol in healthy people can range between 3.6 and 7.8 mmol/1 (140 to 300 mg/100 ml). Measuring plasma cholesterol gives a good idea of the LDL concentration since most of the cholesterol is carried in LDL (Table 6.2); concentrations of the subsidiary carrier, HDL, usually vary much less than those of LDL. Most of the cholesterol in plasma is esterified at the 3 position (Fig. 6.1), chiefly in the form of linoleate. Plasma cholesterol concentration is influenced by dietary and other factors, which are described in Chapter 40.

Plasma triglyceride concentration reflects the concen-

tration of VLDL except when the subject has had a meal containing fat in the last few hours. Endogenous triglycerides come from the liver and are carried on VLDL; they are measured after an overnight fast, normal values ranging from 0.28 to 1.69 mmol/1 (25 to 150 mg/100 ml). After a meal there are in addition exogenous or alimentary triglycerides, carried on chylomicrons.

Plasma phospholipids are not usually measured in clinical or epidemiological laboratories. Depending on the metabolic conditions they may correlate with cholesterol or with triglycerides, as might be expected from their proportions in the lipoproteins.

ADIPOSE TISSUE

Dietary fat is brought to the adipose tissues direct from the intestine in the form of chylomicrons and from the liver as VLDL or pre-β-lipoproteins. Dietary glucose is also transported to adipose tissue and there converted into triglycerides.

It was once thought that adipose tissue was an inert store in which the surplus energy of the diet was kept in the form of fat until needed. Two Israeli scientists, Wertheimer and Shapiro (1948), in a classical review, were mainly responsible for dispelling this idea and demonstrating that adipose tissue has considerable metabolic activities. A major portion of the dietary energy, both as fat and carbohydrate is taken to adipose tissue and deposited as triglycerides. The fatty acid pattern of these triglycerides partly reflects that of the individual's customary dietary fat, notably in the proportion of linoleic acid which cannot be synthesised in the body. Between meals, when the adipose tissue reserves are drawn upon to provide fuel for the muscles and other tissue, the triglycerides are subsequently broken down to free fatty acids (FFA), which enter the blood and supply the tissues with energy. The deposition and mobilisation of fat in adipose tissue proceeds at rates which are ever varying, depending upon the supply of energy at the last meal and the immediate needs of the tissues, particularly those determined by muscular activity. These rates are controlled by endocrine factors and the autonomic nervous systèm. Insulin stimulates the synthesis of adipose tissue triglycerides from glucose and the uptake of plasma triglycerides into adipose tissue by the agency of lipoprotein lipase. Most other hormones, such as catecholamines and glucagon which appear in plasma in increased amounts during fasting, have the opposite effect and favour lipolysis.

ANATOMICAL CONSIDERATIONS

Adipose tissue is a large organ and very variable in size. In a healthy man it may amount to some 8 to 15 kg and in a healthy woman from 10 to 20 kg. In a very emaciated patient it is reduced to about 1 kg, and some very obese people carry around over 100 kg. Its distribution in the body is also uneven.

Distribution of adipose tissue.

Male connoisseurs of the female form are reputed to start their visual inspection at the ankle and work upwards. This traditional guide is generally reliable, but sometimes the amount of subcutaneous fat over the ankles and legs bears little relation to the amount of fat elsewhere. This is perhaps a relatively common but minor manifestation of the process responsible for the rare disease lipodystrophy, in which the fat disappears from the face, arms and legs and accumulates around the hips and thighs. As middle-age advances, especially in the male, many people acquire a greatly increased layer of fat over the abdomen and at the same time their limbs become thin.

The internal adipose tissue has an important role in providing protective cushions for the various viscera. The external fat acts as an insulator, conserving body heat.

Adipose tissue consists of mesenchymal connective tissue cells (adipocytes). Triglyceride is stored within these, usually as a single large droplet. The cells are supplied by a capillary network. Adipose tissue also receives nerves from the autonomic nervous system, the fibres of which appear to terminate in close relation to both cells and blood vessels.

CHEMICAL COMPOSITION

Punch biopsy through the skin, a minor procedure, provides samples of adipose tissue for analysis. Most contain about 80 to 85 per cent fat, the remainder being cell material and supporting tissue. Protein and water form about 2 and 10 per cent respectively. The results of analyses vary widely, even of samples taken from one individual, but at different sites. In obese subjects the fat content is seldom more than 90 per cent. Increased fat storage is associated with increases in both the size and number of adipocytes, but it is difficult to quantitate the changes.

The amount of cellular material in adipose tissue is not generally appreciated. Thus if a healthy man carries 10 kg of adipose tissue, of which 85 per cent is fat, he has 1.5 kg of fat-free adipose tissue. This is about the weight of his liver and contains about 200 g of protein.

Table 6.3 shows the fatty acid pattern (measured by gas–liquid chromatography) of adipose tissue obtained by needle biopsy from the buttocks of healthy men and women in London (Heffernan, 1964). Oleic acid was the major fatty acid and there were slightly more monounsaturated acids and less palmitic acid in women than men, making their fat softer. Patterns like these have been reported from different parts of the world. In general the human species has a characteristic pattern of fatty acids in adipose tissue, but it may be modified by diet. $C_{12:0}$ and $C_{14:0}$ fatty acids are 11 and 16 per cent respectively in

Table 6.3 Mean percentage of fatty acids in subcutaneous samples of adipose tissue from healthy adults (Heffernan, 1964)

Fatty acid	Men (8)	Women (8)
12:0	0.9	0.7
14:0	4.2	3.5
14:1	1.1	1.1
15:0	0.6	0.6
16:0	23.3	20.0
16:1	10.1	10.7
18:0	4.4	3.4
18:1	48.4	53.0
18:2	7.2	7.1

Polynesians who consume much of their fat as coconuts (Shortland et al., 1969) while $C_{18:2}$ fatty acid may be as high as 35 per cent in patients taking diets high in corn oil to reduce their plasma cholesterol (Albutt and Chance, 1969).

DEPOSITION OF FAT IN THE STORES

Triglycerides reaching adipose tissue in the form of chylomicrons and VLDL are hydrolysed by lipoprotein lipase at the luminal surface of the capillary endothelial cell; the free fatty acids liberated then pass across the endothelial cell into the adipose tissue cells. Endogenous heparin may have a role in this clearing of fat from the blood. Within the cells the fatty acids are again resynthesised into triglycerides. For this process to be complete an additional source of glycerol is needed. This provided by the breakdown of carbohydrate within the cell. The deposition of fat within the cell is thus determined in part by the available carbohydrate.

Fat is also formed in adipose tissue from glucose in the blood. When fat is being laid down rapidly there is always an increase in the small amount of glycogen present in adipose tissue cells. The control of fat formation by adipose tissue is determined largely by the available supply of insulin (Renold and Cahill, 1965). Insulin markedly increases the uptake of glucose by adipose tissue incubated in vitro. A failure to form fat from glucose is a characteristic feature of insulin deficiency.

Fat formation is of course dependent on the supply of nutrients provided by the diet. Under certain circumstances fat formation is greatly increased; for instance, during pregnancy it is normal for a woman to increase her fat stores by about 4 kg (Hytten and Leitch, 1971), presumably as an insurance to meet the future demands of lactation. Other animals, notably marine mammals, lay down much bigger stores. When suckling her young the mother seal cannot feed. Lactation only lasts about two weeks and the mother is reputed to lose 90 kg of weight, mostly fat, in the process. This fat has to be deposited by the mother in advance during pregnancy. The seal is born weighing about 14 kg and after two weeks weighs about 40 kg. Spawning salmon, migratory birds, hedgehogs and other hibernating animals lay down large stores of fat, which are accurately adjusted to meet future needs for energy. More knowledge about how this extra deposition of fat is controlled to meet physiological requirements might elucidate the problem of obesity in man.

ADIPOSE TISSUE AS AN ELECTRIC BLANKET

Starving people frequently complain of feeling cold. It is easy to appreciate that the subcutaneous adipose tissue acts like a good blanket and prevents heat loss. Under certain circumstances adipose tissue may also generate heat and thus act in the manner of an electric blanket.

Brown fat is present in limited amounts at various sites in many species of animals, including common laboratory animals such as the rat, the rabbit and the monkey. It is present in much larger amounts in all species which hibernate. This fat is easily visible lying between the shoulder blades in laboratory rats. The lipids present in brown fat undergo a series of cyclic changes, with hydrolysis of triglyceride and subsequent re-esterification of the fatty acids with glycerol derived from the blood. These reactions require ATP, and energy is utilised producing heat in the brown fat itself. This process is an essential part of the warming up of animals on arousal from hibernation. In many species of animals exposure to cold increases the amount of brown fat; however, the amount always remains a small proportion of the total adipose tissue and its capabilities as a heat producer are correspondingly limited.

Adult men and women have little brown fat. When they are cold, heat production can only be increased by shivering or muscular exercise. The newborn baby is unable to shiver, the necessary neuromuscular mechanisms having not yet developed. Although the newborn infant possesses no fat that is actually brown, some of the adipose tissue on the back, over the shoulder-blades and round the neck resembles brown fat. This adipose tissue is found in a loculated form: the cells contain many small vacuoles of fat and around these there are many large mitochondria. After the first few days, these cells have been found to be largely depleted of fat (Aherne and Hull, 1964). The newborn baby responds to cold by generating heat; this heat is probably produced by oxidation of the lipid contents of these fat cells. This at least is what the newborn rabbit does. Hull and Segall (1965) have demonstrated local heat production in the brown fat of infant rabbits exposed to cold. It is dependent on the sympathetic nervous system and is mediated by noradrenaline. This is an important part of the mechanism of temperature control in the first few weeks of life in many species, including man. On some cold winter mornings we regret having grown out of our electric blankets.

EFFECTS OF PARTICULAR FATTY ACIDS
ESSENTIAL FATTY ACIDS

Burr and Burr (1929) first showed that certain fatty acids (EFA) were essential in the diet for the health and survival of rats. When young rats are put on a fat-free diet immediately after weaning, they continue to grow normally for 2 or 3 weeks. The rate of growth then declines and usually stops within 8 to 10 weeks. During this period an eczematous scaliness of the skin develops, which is most marked over the tail. Animals also show decreased growth, increased permeability of the skin to water and on microscopical examination of the tissues there is swelling of the mitochondria (Wilson and Leduc, 1963). It can be prevented by giving vegetable oils, most of which are rich in linoleic acid, $C_{18:2}$ (n-6). Administration of linoleic acid alone can prevent the deficiency and linoleic acid is the widespread dietary EFA, but a number of other long-chain unsaturated fatty acids, both natural and synthetic, are also effective (Gurr and James, 1975). Arachidonic acid is the physiologically active form, but linoleic is readily converted to it in the body so that it can prevent the signs of deficiency. If hydrogenated coconut oil is added to the diet, the eczema develops sooner and growth ceases earlier. The need for EFA may thus be directly related to the amount of saturated fatty acids in the diet. The male rat needs about four or five times as much as the female for rapid growth.

A deficiency, similar to that found in rats, has been produced in mice and dogs and also in calves, pigs and poultry, although these species are not so susceptible. A variety of insects have been shown to require essential fatty acids. There is thus good reason to suppose that they are needed by all animal tissues.

Linoleic acid cannot be synthesised by animals. Dietary sources are readily converted in the tissues to arachidonic acid, $C_{20:4}$ (n-6). These two acids form an important proportion of the fatty acids in cell membranes and in the white matter of the central nervous system. Linoleic acid is also a precursor of prostaglandins, local hormones which have many and diverse effects in the tissues. One of these is to influence the sensitivity of the mechanism for blood clotting.

EFA deficiency in man

It was a long time before EFA deficiency was demonstrated in man. One adult volunteer lived on a very low fat diet for six months without developing any skin disorder (Brown et al., 1938). His diet contained about 2 g/day of butterfat; he lost weight and his serum linoleic and arachidonic acids fell. Other biochemical measurements such as trienoic fatty acids were not available at that time. A report by Hansen et al. (1958) that some cases of infantile eczema benefited from EFA therapy led to large numbers of luckless infants with this disease being dosed with vegetable oil preparation rich in EFA without any apparent benefit. Not until it was possible to keep a patient alive for a long period by intravenous feeding was the first unequivocal case of human EFA deficiency described. Collins *et al.* (1971) reported that a man of 44 had all but 60 cm of his small bowel removed surgically. Then he was given only intravenous feeding with preparations containing no fat, and after 100 days he developed a scaly dermatitis. When EFAs are deficient, attempts to replace them are made by elongating oleic acid, $C_{18:1}$ (*n*–9). Then large amounts of eicosatrienoic acid, $C_{20:3}$ (*n*–9) which lacks EFA activity, appear in the phospholipids of the plasma. This is accepted as evidence of EFA deficiency in animals. The ratio of $C_{20:3}$ (*n*–9) to arachidonic acid $C_{20:4}$ (*n*–6) in plasma lipids, the triene/tetraene ratio, rises in EFA deficiency and 0.4 is the upper limit of normal. Since then other cases have been reported from North America in adults and in children receiving intravenous feeding with no fat (Paulsrud *et al.*, 1973) and in patients with malabsorption whose dietary fats have been restricted to control diarrhoea (Press *et al.*, 1974). Clinical features include poor wound healing, anaemia, thrombocytopenia and centrilobular fatty infiltration of the liver. Intralipid, a preparation of soya oil (p. 447), contains 56 g/l of linoleic acid and its use in intravenous feeding prevents and cures EFA deficiencies. Intralipid was banned in the United States but, after many years of trouble-free use in Europe, has been approved by the FDA. EFA deficiency should become a rarity in patients on long-term parenteral feeding.

It is easy to visualise the need for EFA in the first two and a half years after conception, when new cell membranes are forming and myelin is being laid down in the brain. Linoleic acid provides 4 per cent of energy in breast milk but less in cow's milk. An adult man of 65 kg with 9 kg of body fat in which linoleic acid is 7 per cent of the fatty acids (Table 6.3), has a store of about 600 g. The experience of Brown *et al.* (1938) is not surprising, and EFA deficiency would not be expected in previously well-nourished individuals during a short period of negative energy balance. They draw upon their adipose tissue reserves of EFA as well as of energy. But if total parenteral nutrition is required and the fluid given is 80 per cent glucose and 20 per cent amino acids, fatty acid mobilisation is suppressed, the viscera and peripheral tissues are starved of EFA and biochemical signs appear rapidly (Wene *et al.*, 1975). Some types of injury such as extensive burns may increase the need (Helmkamp *et al.*, 1973).

Linoleic acid as a precursor of prostaglandins

Linoleic acid is the precursor of prostaglandins, substances first isolated from semen and thought to be secreted by the prostate gland. They are now known to be produced in most tissues and appear to have many and varied roles in both physiological and pathological processes. They are not stored in the body and on entering the circulation are rapidly converted, mainly in the lungs, into inactive metabolites which are excreted in the urine. Daily urinary excretion of metabolites of the main prostaglandins (PGE) is of the order of 300 nmol. Daily dietary intake of linoleic acid is of the order of 25 mmol. Thus only about one hundred thousandth of the linoleic acid in the diet is converted prostaglandins. Yet this appears as an essential role of linoleic acid and only fatty acids which can be converted into prostaglandins have EFA activity.

Figure 6.3 shows the stages in the conversion of linoleic acid into prostaglandins in the tissues. The most plentiful are PGE_2 and $PGF_2\alpha$. All prostaglandins are formed by ring closure and oxidation of an essential fatty acid, such as arachidonic acid (Fig. 6.4).

Linoleic acid and thrombosis

There are indications that the type of fat in the diet influences the tendency to thrombosis. This is not easy to measure because thrombosis is an uncommon event in

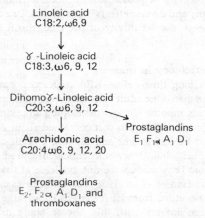

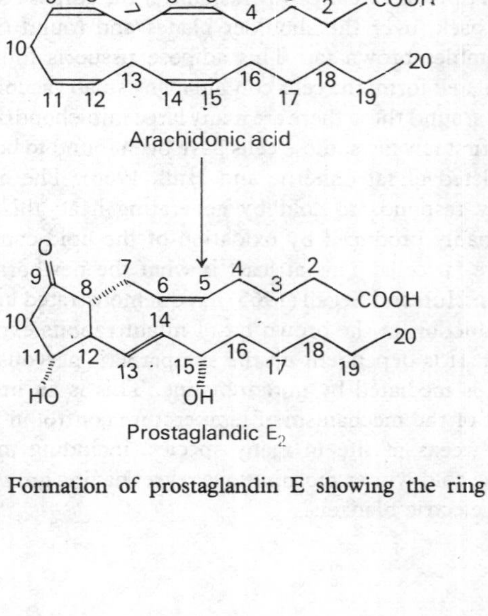

Linoleic acid
C18:2,ω6,9

↓

γ -Linoleic acid
C18:3,ω6, 9, 12

↓

Dihomoγ-Linoleic acid
C20:3,ω6, 9, 12 → Prostaglandins E₁ F₁α A₁ D₁

↓

Arachidonic acid
C20:4ω6, 9, 12, 20

↓

Prostaglandins
E₂, F₂α A₁ D₁ and
thromboxanes

Fig. 6.3 Formation of prostaglandins from linoleic acid.

Fig. 6.4 Formation of prostaglandin E showing the ring closure.

animals and healthy people, and not easy to visualise. In animals, it is possible to inflict a local injury to a blood vessel so that thrombosis is likely. Then thrombosis occurs more frequently in groups of animals given saturated fat in their diet than in those given polyunsaturated fats (Nordøy, 1976). Hornstra (1971) introduced a polythene loop-shaped cannula into the aorta of anaesthetised rats below the renal arteries. After a few days the transparent cannula became occluded by thrombus. It remained patent for only 4 days on average with a fat-free diet and for 7 days with 20 per cent sunflower oil in the diet. Using the same model and a range of oils in the diet, Hornstra (1975) found that occlusion time was positively related to the percentage of linoleic acid in the diet and negatively related to dietary palmitic and stearic acids.

In man, an increased intake of polyunsaturated fats is accompanied by changes in *in vitro* tests of platelet function which indicate that the platelets would be less likely to promote thrombosis *in vivo* (Kapp et al., 1971; Hornstra et al., 1973; O'Brien et al., 1976). It is suggested that high intakes of linoleic acid, via dihomo-γ-linolenic acid, lead to increased local formation of prostaglandin E_1, which is a potent inhibitor of platelet aggregation.

Other effects of polyunsaturated fat

While saturated fats, especially $C_{14:0}$ and $C_{16:0}$ raise plasma cholesterol, polyunsaturated fats, both EFA and others, tend to lower it. These effects are considered in more detail in Chapter 40.

Polyunsaturated fats appear to be absorbed more efficiently from the gut than saturated fats of the same chain length (Pinter et al., 1964). This property may be of some help in the dietetic management of steatorrhoea.

Recommended intakes

Official committees recommend that 1 to 2 per cent of dietary energy should be provided as EFA, i.e. about 2 to 5 g/day of linoleic acid in an adult.

As with some other nutrients, there are a few scientists with deep knowledge of fatty acid metabolism who consider that the optimum intake should be higher than the amount that prevents deficiency disease. Sinclair (1956) postulated that EFA intake is too low in industrial communities and contributes to endemic atherosclerotic diseases. Plasma cholesterol is lowered by diets high in polyunsaturated fat but with increasing severity of atherosclerosis there is, surprisingly, an increased percentage of linoleate in cholesterol ester in the lesions (Böttcher et al., 1960). But thrombosis plays a role in atherosclerotic disease (Chapter 41) and, as described above, polyunsaturated fats seem to reduce the tendency to thrombosis. Vergroesen et al. (1975) in reviewing the physiological role of EFA recommend that people should eat about 10 per cent of dietary energy as polyunsaturated fat, and so does the McGovern Committee (Select Committee of Nutrition and Human Needs, 1977). These views are not yet generally accepted.

Medium chain triglycerides (MCT)

These are fractionated from coconut oil (Table 6.1) and consist mostly of $C_{8:0}$ and $C_{10:0}$ They have been introduced into dietetics because they are hydrolysed by pancreatic lipase more easily than other triglycerides and because, once absorbed, they go direct to the liver in the portal vein in the form of fatty acids. Patients with steatorrhoea often absorb MCT much better than other fats so MCT is a valuable source of energy for such patients.

Erucic acid ($C_{22:1}$)

This very long chain monounsaturated acid is the principal fatty acid in rapeseed oil (see Table 6.1), one of the few vegetable oils that is easily grown in temperate areas of the world such as northern Europe and Canada. It has been found that when large amounts of rapeseed oil (50 per cent of total energy) are fed to experimental animals fatty change occurs in heart muscle. This is because erucic acid enters the myocardial cells but is oxidised more slowly than other fatty acids and so accumulates intracellularly in triglycerides (Abdellatif and Vles, 1973). Geneticists have now produced a variety of rapeseed, Canbra, that contains only 2 per cent of erucic acid.

A regulation in the UK and EEC now limits the erucic acid in edible oils and fats and in foods containing them to 5 per cent of the fat component.

DIETARY NEEDS FOR FAT

The amount of fat in diets varies greatly. In most prosperous countries fat usually contributes 35 to 45 per cent of the total energy. In some poor countries the figure is 15 per cent or even lower. It is very difficult to state what represents too much or too little fat for health. However, in all civilisations, Eastern or Western, old or new, fat has always been a necessity for the preparation of good meals. There is almost no country where a housewife can prepare the meals which she would like for her family without materials in which fat supplies at least 20 per cent of the energy. That the average figure in several countries is far below this reflects the wide prevalence of poverty. Many people cannot enjoy their traditional diet through lack of fat. In Britain in 1934–38 fat provided 38 per cent of the total energy in the diet. As a result of wartime rationing and restrictions on food this figure fell gradually and reached a minimum of 33 per cent in 1947. Thereafter it has risen steadily and in 1977 was 42 per cent. This small wartime restriction of the fat intake caused much publicly voiced discontent. Many of the ailments of the time were ascribed to a shortage of fat in the diet, not only by harrassed housewives but also by some physicians.

A national diet containing 33 per cent of fat certainly supplies far more fat than is necessary to meet physiological needs. Hence no conceivable physical harm could have arisen from this restriction. Nevertheless, there was much discontent. In retrospect it seems clear that the true explanation of this discontent was that many articles of food cooked with inadequate amounts of fat are insipid and unpalatable to traditional British tastes. In any country social requirements of fat for good living are far higher than physiological requirements for physical health. In the present state of knowledge it is difficult to state a minimum fat requirement for man. Human diets low in fat are almost always also low in protein and other nutrients necessary for the maintenance of health. It is thus very difficult to ascribe any disease arising in these conditions specifically to a deficiency of fat.

Minimal requirements for fat may indeed be very low. Mitra (1942) made a study of the dietary habits of the Hos, an aboriginal tribe in Bihar, India. He investigated 250 families and found that 200 made no use of any kind of fat in their cooking. This was not due to poverty, for many of the Hos had acquired some money by collecting forest products and they visited bazaars in nearby towns where they could have purchased fats had they so wished. They did not do so because they were ignorant of the use of fats and oils in cooking; their culinary practices were limited to boiling and—very occasionally—baking. The Hos possessed cattle but used them only as beasts of burden; they drank no milk and ate no meat. The total daily fat intake of different families was estimated as varying from 2.4 to 3.8 g/head, which would provide at most 2 per cent of the total energy, but might contain 1 g or so of EFA. Although the health and nutrition of these aborigines were by no means ideal, they presented no signs or symptoms which could be attributed to fat deficiency, their general level of nutrition and physique being no worse than that of neighbouring villagers who regularly consumed vegetable oils.

High fat diets are almost always also high in energy so—except in those physically active—lead to obesity. High fat diets are also usually associated with high plasma cholesterol and β-lipoprotein concentrations and this may be a factor contributing to a variety of diseases, but this effect may be due to a low P/S ratio in the fatty acids of the diet rather than to the total amount of fat.

PRACTICAL RECOMMENDATIONS

Although scientific precision is lacking for making such recommendations, two seem sensible. First any community which wishes to feed well and in a civilised tradition (either Eastern or Western) should obtain at least 20 per cent of its energy from fat. Secondly, individuals in prosperous communities who lead sedentary lives and have reached middle age would be well advised to limit their fat intake to 25 to 30 per cent of their total energy. The possible value of reducing intakes of animal fats and the use of vegetable oils in the prevention and treatment of atherosclerosis are discussed in Chapter 41.

A high fat intake is essential for very active people spending over 17 MJ(4000 kcal/day). Lumberjacks in the sub-Arctic and workers on polar expeditions often require this amount of energy and would have to spend much of their working day eating to obtain such a high energy intake solely from bulky carbohydrate sources. Fats give them the necessary energy quickly, so that they can get on with their job in the short time allotted to them.

7. Alcohol

Ethyl alcohol (ethanol, C_2H_5OH) is formed in nature by the fermentation of sugar and used by man for several purposes. It may serve as a disfectant, a drug, a food or a preservative. In classical experiments with a human calorimeter Atwater and Benedict (1902) showed that the energy liberated by oxidation of ethanol can be utilised by the body and that its use replaces similar amounts of energy derived from carbohydrate and fat. As a source of fuel for the body ethanol differs from carbohydrate and fat in two important respects. First, ethanol cannot be utilised by muscle; indeed it is almost entirely metabolised in the liver. Secondly, ethanol is metabolised at a fixed rate which is unaffected by its concentration in the blood.

ABSORPTION, DISTRIBUTION AND DISPOSAL

Ethanol being soluble in both water and lipids diffuses rapidly through cell membranes and into cells. Hence an oral dose is soon absorbed from the alimentary canal, part of it from the stomach, and distributed throughout the total body water. Indeed it can be used as a measure of total body water. Thus in a 65 kg man with a total body water of 40 litres a dose of 30 g (about 4 fl. oz of whisky), given on an empty stomach, quickly raises the ethanol concentrations in all body fluids, including the blood, to about 750 mg/1; such a concentration certainly impairs judgment and may or may not lead to symptoms of intoxication. Most people are drunk at blood levels over 1500 mg/1. Absorption is delayed if alcohol is taken slowly throughout the course of a meal. Some Russians are said to prepare themselves for a drinking session of vodka with a litre of milk. Most people would have difficulty taking so much and in a study in New Zealand blood alcohol rose only marginally less when 240 ml of milk was taken before 90 ml of whisky. There were considerable individual variations (Janus and Sharman, 1972).

After absorption ethanol appears in both expired air and in urine in concentrations related directly to the blood concentration, since ethanol is not actively secreted by either of these organs, but simply diffuses out from them. The amounts of ethanol disposed of in these ways is small and over 90 per cent of an ingested dose is metabolised in the liver. The rate of metabolism varies widely in individuals and ranges from 60 to 200 mg/kg an hour. The hourly rate is usually about 100 mg/kg and this means that a 65 kg man after a 30 g dose of ethanol clears his blood in about $(30 \times 1000)/(65 \times 100) = 4.6$ hours.

Metabolism in the liver

Ethanol is metabolised almost entirely in the liver. The first step is oxidation to acetaldehyde. There are two enzyme systems that may carry out this reaction.

Alcohol dehydrogenase is a non-specific enzyme present in the liver of all mammals. Its natural substrates are alcohols produced in intermediary metabolism, for example in steroid and bile acid metabolism. It also oxidises ethanol and methanol when these are ingested. The enzyme is present in the cell cytoplasm. Its co-factor is NAD; NADH is produced, and the oxidation is linked to the formation of high energy bonds in ATP.

$$CH_3CH_2OH + NAD^+ \longrightarrow CH_3CHO + NADH + H^+$$
alcohol dehydrogenase

The microsomal ethanol-oxidising system (MEOS) is not present normally in liver, but may be induced by repeated ingestion of ethanol. It is included in the mixed function oxidase system which is induced by many drugs. The system is dependent on NADPH and cytochrome P-450, and catalyses the direct utilisation of molecular oxygen without formation of ATP.

$$CH_3CH_2OH + NADPH + H + O_2 \longrightarrow CH_3CHO + NADP + 2H_2O$$
MEOS

Acetaldehyde formed by these enzymes is converted into acetyl CoA by aldehyde dehydrogenase. The acetyl CoA may then be used as a source of energy in the citric acid cycle or enter a synthetic pathway, e.g. for fatty acids or cholesterol. As the acetyl CoA can pass into the blood stream and be metabolised elsewhere, ethanol may serve as source of energy for other tissues, including muscle. However, as the rate-limiting reaction is the formation of acetaldehyde which occurs only in the liver, the rate of clearance of ethanol alcohol from the blood cannot be increased by muscular exercise.

When, as in normal persons, ethanol is disposed of by alcohol dehydrogenase and acetaldehyde dehydrogenase, all the energy is utilised in the tissues; ethanol then spares isoenergetically the metabolism of carbohydrate and fat. When ethanol is first converted to acetaldehyde by MEOS, part of the energy liberated cannot be utilised and is dissipated directly as heat. It is not known how much ethanol has to be taken or for how long before MEOS activity is induced in man. However it is certain that part of the energy in the ethanol taken in by some heavy drinkers is not available for utilisation in the tissues.

When ethanol is oxidised by alcohol dehydrogenase, NAD is converted to NADH. The NAD may be reformed in a reaction which is coupled with the formation of lactic acid from pyruvic acid and subsequent lactic acid acidosis.

Many substances, both nutrients and drugs, e.g. caffeine, have been tested to see if they accelerate the removal of ethanol from the blood. Positive results have been obtained only with fructose. In patients with a blood ethanol over 1500 mg/1 who received an intravenous infusion of 200g of fructose (500 ml of a 40 per cent solution), the rate of ethanol clearance was 23 per cent higher than in untreated controls (Brown *et al.*, 1972). This effect may be due to more rapid reoxidation of $NADH_2$ by glycerate derived from fructose. If fructose is used to treat anyone in an alcoholic coma, the risk of inducing a dangerous lactic acid acidosis should be appreciated.

Two therapeutic points arise from the nature of the enzymic mechanisms for the removal of ethanol. First, methanol is far more dangerous than ethanol because the formaldehyde formed by its oxidation damages the retina irreversibly and a single dose may cause permanent blindness. As ethanol and methanol are oxidised by the same enzyme and compete for it, ethanol slows down the oxidation of methanol and the production of its toxic product. Hence ethanol should be administered to a patient who has ingested methanol. Secondly, acetaldehyde does not normally accumulate in the tissues after taking ethanol, because it is removed by acetaldehyde dehydrogenase as fast as it is formed. This enzyme can be inhibited by a drug, disulfiram (Antabusè). If after the administration of this drug a patient takes a drink he rapidly develops unpleasant symptoms, nausea, giddiness and headache, due to the accumulation of acetaldehyde in the blood. This may help a chronic alcoholic to give up drinking.

For a fuller account of the enzymic mechanisms which are responsible for the metabolism of ethanol, papers by Pirola and Lieber (1976) and a symposium edited by Lieber (1977) should be consulted.

INTAKE

The amount of ethanol and energy value in various alcohol beverages is given in Table 21.1. Beers, wines, fortified wines and spirits contain about 30, 100, 150 and 300 g/1, respectively. Assuming an hourly clearance rate of 100 mg/kg, a 65 kg man could in 24 hours dispose of 156 g, i.e. the ethanol in 9 pints (5.2 litres) of beer, 1.5 litres of table wine or half a bottle (0.5 litre) of whisky. This calculation provides one basis for the poster that appeared in the Paris Metro, 'Les prescriptions de l'Académie de Médecine; Jamais plus qu'un litre de vin par jour!' Another is the steep rise in the incidence of cirrhosis seen when daily consumption of alcohol regularly exceeds 80 g in men (less in women) in a French wine-drinking community (Thaler, 1977).

The energy content of ethanol is normally 29.7 kJ (7.1 kcal)/g. Its density is 0.794 g/ml. Allowing for a small loss, excreted directly in the urine, the energy provided by alcoholic drinks can be quickly calculated by a formula derived from Gastineau (1976):

6.7 (or 1.6) x percentage of alcohol drink (by volume) x fluid ounces drunk
= energy provided in kJ (or kcal)

Two 4-oz glasses of wine with an alcohol content of 12 per cent would supply

6.7 (or 1.6) x 12 x 8 = 540 kJ (or 155 kcal)

A litre of wine, containing about 100 g ethanol, provides nearly 3 MJ or 710 kcal, about half the basal metabolism for 24 hours.

Ethanol can be given in small divided doses up to this total amount to patients, if liver function is not impaired. It provides a source of energy which is readily absorbed and utilised; it is also suitable for intravenous nutrition (p. 448). Given in repeated small doses ethanol usually has a pleasant sedative effect and is not intoxicating.

Data provided by Customs and Excise indicate that in 1975 consumption of alcoholic beverages per head of population in the UK was 206 pints of beer, 11.3 pints of wine and 4.8 pints of spirits. The ethanol in these beverages accounted for 5.6 per cent of the total energy available in the national food supply. This figure has been increasing steadily and was only 3.0 per cent in 1950.

Nevertheless the United Kingdom is a relatively small consumer of alcohol. The *Encyclopaedia Britannica* gives an international league table of alcohol consumption for 1970. The data are expressed in litres of ethanol consumed each year per head of population over 15 years of age. France tops the list with 22.6 litres, followed by Italy 15.0, Austria 14.4, West Germany 13.5, Portugal 13.4, Switzerland 13.0, Spain 12.8, Australia 11.8, Hungary 11.1, Belgium 10.9, New Zealand 10.8, Czechoslovakia 10.5, USA 10.1, Denmark 8.7, Canada 8.4 and the UK and Sweden 7.2. Other countries are relatively sober, but no figure is given for the USSR. There is very little data about individual consumption in any of these countries, but in all of them there must be many people who get far more dietary energy from ethanol than from protein. One individual dietary survey of the crew of a British oil tanker sailing to the Persian Gulf showed that they took on average 13 per cent of their energy as ethanol (Eddy *et al.*, 1971). Clearly it is important to record intakes of alcoholic beverages in any dietary survey. If this is not done energy intake is likely to be underestimated, perhaps by a large amount. However, in individuals with a high intake of ethanol, part of it is likely to be oxidised by MEOS and then the energy is not all physiologically available. For such persons a figures of 22 to 25 kJ (5 to 6 kcal)/g may be appropriate for calculating the energy value of ethanol consumed.

The increasing consumption of alcohol in Britain in the 1970s has been put in historical perspective by Spring and Buss (1977), who analysed the unique records of HM Customs and Excise, which go back to 1684. Then ethanol consumption, almost all as beer, was more than double what it is today. The trend of consumption after 300 years has in general been downwards, except for a peak in the prosperous late Victorian era and a more recent but still relatively small increase in the 1970s (Fig. 7.1). Spring and Buss describe how beer has been partly replaced by spirits and wine as well as by tea and coffee and how economic and social factors and taxes have affected the consumption of different alcoholic beverages.

OTHER CONSTITUENTS

There is more to beers, wines and spirits than ethanol and sugar. They contain negligible protein or vitamins except for a little nicotinic acid and less riboflavin in beer; thus they provide 'empty calories'. Some wines contain appreciable amounts of iron; 13 mg/1 is an average figure for Medoc wines, and haemosiderosis can occur in people who habitually consume large quantities of certain wines or kaffir beer (see p. 103).

Associated with ethyl alcohol are congeners—higher alcohols, fused oil, etc—which are present in larger amounts in some drinks than others. Much of the discomfort of a hangover is due to the congeners rather than to ethanol itself. Pawan (1973) gave the same dose of ethanol in eight different drinks at weekly intervals to healthy volunteers. Hangovers were most distressing after brandy, then came red wine, rum, whisky, white wine and gin in descending order, while after vodka and pure ethyl alcohol the subjects only suffered a little tiredness and thirst.

EXCESSIVE INTAKES

Many of us take alcoholic drinks when with friends on convivial occasions or to reduce feelings of shyness, stress or fatigue. Such **social drinking** in moderation has no adverse effect on physical health, and most social drinkers consider it a psychological benefit. However, a social drinker is exposed to two hazards. First, he may go on binges and, secondly, he can become dependent on alcohol, having to take large amounts every day. He has then become an alcoholic.

A binge may last several hours and involve very large intakes of ethanol, up to 500 g, with very little food. The blood concentration rises to a high figure and there are gross signs of intoxication, the liver removes the ethanol at the usual slow hourly rate of about 100 mg/kg, and it may take two or more days after drinking has ceased to clear the blood. Then, provided the binger has not driven a car or got otherwise involved with the police, or developed acute gastric erosion or hypoglycaemia, he may be little the worse for the episode. If the binges are not repeated too frequently, general health and nutrition remain good. Regular weekend bingers run a risk of developing pancreatitis.

Alcoholism

An alcoholic is a person who cannot stop drinking when there is good reason for doing so. He may need a shot in the morning to start the day. Tolerance of the drug increases and consumption may rise to two to three bottles of wine or more than one bottle of spirits a day; thus the daily intake of ethanol is more than a normal liver can metabolise. In regular heavy drinkers the liver clears ethanol from the blood more rapidly than normal and the brain is more tolerant of its effects.

Such persons may seldom show signs of intoxication, but may never be completely sober.

In almost all alcoholics, family life and personal relationships are disturbed. Though they may retain their job, their competence is greatly reduced. Many, especially in the professional and managerial classes, keep up their position because they have the support of long-suffering wives or colleagues.

Some alcoholics retain their physical health surprisingly well for many years and may appear well nourished. Others become malnourished. Because of their social and financial problems, feeding arrangements are usually unsatisfactory. Appetite is poor, sometimes as a result of a chronic gastritis induced by their drug. As a result they may be in a state of partial starvation or develop signs of deficiency of one or more nutrients.

The types of malnutrition which are most characteristically associated with alcoholism are deficiencies of thiamin, nicotinic acid, vitamin B_6, folic acid, protein, magnesium, potassium and zinc. The effects of these are all described in other chapters. Impairment of judgment and coordination from intoxication make alcoholics liable to trauma; their poor nutritional and social status increase

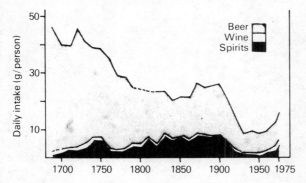

Fig. 7.1 Average daily intakes of alcohol from beer, wine and spirits in Britain from 1684 to 1975. Calculated from the records of HM Customs and Excise (Spring and Buss, 1977).

their susceptibility to infections. Any of these illnesses may necessitate admission to hospital. Removal of the supply of alcohol may precipitate in about two days **delirium tremens**, characterised by mania, hallucinations and tremor. This acute withdrawal syndrome occurs when blood alcohol approaches zero in a person who has become habituated to having alcohol constantly in his blood.

Alcoholics are at greater risk than other persons of developing cirrhosis of the liver (p. 413), peripheral neuropathy (p. 287), Wernicke's encephalopathy (p. 288), carcinoma of the oesophagus and stomach (p. 511), pancreatitis (p. 420) and cardiomyopathy (p. 343). To what extent each of these conditions is directly due to the toxic action of ethanol or the indirect effect of deficiencies of nutrients in a poor diet is discussed in the appropriate section of the book. Alcoholics also have higher death rates from several non-nutritional diseases, especially suicide and pneumonia.

There are no reliable figures for the prevalence of alcoholism in any country. Various indices like hospital admission rates for alcoholism and death rates from cirrhosis of the liver vary disproportionately between different countries (Walsh and Walsh, 1973) and only show the tip of the iceberg. Although the physical aspects of the disease are usually easily recognised, its social and economic manifestations are often overlooked. Many alcoholics do not recognise that they are ill. In Britain and the USA the abuse of alcohol by middle-aged persons is a much more serious problem than the use of marihuana, LSD or heroin by young people, but it receives less publicity.

The outlook for an alcoholic who continues drinking is inevitably progressive social, psychological and physical deterioration. If he gives up the use of the drug and becomes a total abstainer, in a large proportion of cases there is a marked improvement in health and often a return to normal life. Total abstinence is essential and no ex-alcoholic can afford to risk social drinking. It can seldom be achieved by the patient's unaided effort and expert professional care and supervision is needed, often at first in an institution.

There are no specific nutritional measures during rehabilitation. All patients need a good mixed diet and may require vitamin supplements for a period to build up depleted reserves.

8. Fuels of the Tissues

The energy supplied in the diet is mostly in the form of complex macromolecules of carbohydrate, protein and fat. This energy cannot be utilised by the tissues until these have been broken down into smaller molecules, monosaccharides, free fatty acids (FFA) and amino acids (AA). An account of the energy present in foods and of the small losses that occur in making it available to the tissues has been given in Chapter 3. Chapters 4, 5 and 6 describe how the digestive processes break down the large molecules into smaller ones which can be transported in the blood and may be utilised by the tissues. The tissues are not dependent on a continuous supply of energy from the digestive tract. Much of the energy that is absorbed, often the greater part, is not used directly but only after the smaller molecules have been converted back into macromolecules, glycogen, triglycerides and proteins. These then form stores or reserves that can be mobilised to meet the continuing but varying needs of the tissues for energy. Ethyl alcohol is an additional source of energy, as described in Chapter 7. In the present chapter the fuels of the tissues are discussed. Table 8.1 lists substances that circulate in the blood stream and which the tissues can utilise directly. These fuels are utilised in varying proportions dependent on the dietary supply and the needs of individual tissues. The metabolic mixture is regulated by feedback mechanisms dependent on concentrations of the fuels in the blood and is controlled mainly by endocrine secretions.

The immediate sources of energy for metabolism in cell tissues are compounds with high energy phosphate bonds. Of these, adenosine triphosphate (ATP) is the most important. It is formed in cells from adenosine diphosphate (ADP) and inorganic phosphate (P_i), and the energy needed for its formation comes from the fuels in oxidative reactions which are coupled with phosphorylation. The hydrolysis of ATP to ADP and P_i provides the cells with the energy required for mechanical work, organic syntheses and for the ionic pumps which maintain the gradient of electrolytes between intracellular and extracellular fluids.

High-energy phosphate compounds

ATP is not the only phosphorylated intermediate involved in the transfer of energy. Phosphocreatine, which serves as an energy-rich store in muscle, can be used to regenerate ATP. Guanosine triphosphate (GTP) is generated in the citric acid cycle at the stage where succinate is formed from succinyl-CoA; it then readily donates a phosphate group to ADP to form ATP. GTP is involved in gluconeogenesis by phosphorylating malate and in the synthesis of DNA and RNA. Glycerol phosphate is required in its phosphorylated form both for the conversion of fatty acids to triglycerides and for the shuttle of electrons across mitochondrial membranes. There are a range of energy-rich phosphorylated intermediates in the flow of energy within a cell, but ATP forms a link between them and, for simplicity, we can think of food energy as being converted into ATP energy.

The standard free energy liberated in the complete oxidation of glucose to CO_2 and water is 2870 kJ mol^{-1} (686 kcal mol^{-1}). In the process, 38 moles of ATP are formed (see below). The standard free energy of ATP is 30.5 kJ mol^{-1} (7.3 kcal mol^{-1}). The thermodynamic efficiency of conversion is therefore 38 x 30.5/2870, or about 40 per cent. Some 60 per cent of the energy in the glucose molecule is liberated as heat and dissipated and 40 per cent is stored in the ATP molecules. When the ATP is hydrolysed to ADP, this energy is utilised either for work or for

Table 8.1 Substances which circulate in the blood and are utilised by tissues as a source of energy

Fuel	Source
Prime fuels	
Glucose	Dietary carbohydrate
	Glycogen stores
	Gluconeogenesis in the liver from certain amino acids and glycerol
Free fatty acids	Triglycerides in adipose tissue
Secondary fuels	
Ketones*	Free fatty acids and certain amino acids; formed in the liver
Lactic acid	Formed in tissues from glucose when the supply of oxygen is inadequate
Glycerol	Triglycerides
Additional fuels	
Ethyl alcohol	Dietary
Fructose	Dietary carbohydrate
Galactose	Dietary carbohydrate

* Ketones is a collective term for acetoacetic acid and its derivatives ß-hydroxybutyric acid and acetone.

synthesis of new materials and ultimately dissipated as heat. A small fraction may be incorporated in the synthesised glycogen and only appear as heat when this is broken down.

Production of ATP

Figure 8.1 shows the various stages in the breakdown of glucose at which ATP is produced. Detailed descriptions of these metabolic pathways and those for fatty acid and amino acid oxidation can be obtained from textbooks of biochemistry, e.g. Lehninger (1975). Glucose is first broken down to pyruvate by glycolysis and this occurs in the cytoplasm of cells; pyruvate undergoes oxidative decarboxylation to form acetyl-CoA, which is then oxidised in the citric acid cycle by enzymes present in mitochondria. The greater part of the transduction of energy in glucose to ATP occurs in the citric acid cycle, but some occurs during glycolysis and this is important because it does not depend on oxygen.

Glycolysis

The first stage in glycolysis is the conversion of one molecule of glucose to two molecules of glyceraldehyde-

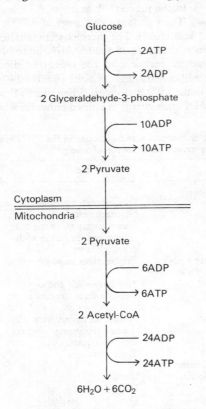

Fig. 8.1 Transfer of energy from glucose to ATP under aerobic condition. Net production of ATP is 38 mol from 1 mol of glucose.

3-phosphate (GAP). This requires two molecules of ATP. Under aerobic condition the conversion of 2 GAP to two pyruvate molecules produces 10 ATP molecules, so that there is a net yield of 8 ATP from the conversion of glucose to pyruvate. Anaerobic glycolysis is the only source of energy for the ionic pumps in red blood corpuscles which do not contain mitochondria and is also a main source in cells of the renal tubules. Cells of malignant tumours also get most of their energy by aerobic glycolysis.

Anaerobic glycolysis. Under anaerobic conditions pyruvate is reduced to lactate, and this utilises six molecules of ATP for two molecules of pyruvate. Hence when one molecule of glucose is converted to lactate, the net yield of ATP is only two molecules. For this reason much more glucose has to be utilised to provide a given amount of energy to a tissue under anaerobic conditions than when it is supplied with oxygen. Lactate diffuses out of anaerobic tissues into the blood stream whence it is taken up by the liver and converted back into glucose (**the Cori cycle**). It may also be taken up by other tissues and serve as a fuel for them. In health, anaerobic conditions occur only in muscle during moderately severe exercise (p. 74). In a fit person lactate begins to appear in the blood when oxygen consumption rises above 1.5 l/min, i.e. brisk walking at 4.5 miles/hour or over. In heavy exercise blood lactate rises rapidly because production in muscle greatly exceeds the liver's capacity for uptake and gluconeogenesis in the Cori cycle. Unless we are physically very active, only a very small part of our daily energy is utilised anaerobically.

In pathological conditions where the supply of oxygen to a tissue is reduced, anaerobic glycolysis is an important additional source of energy. In this respect it is unique, as metabolism of both free fatty acids (FFA) and amino acids (AA) is dependent on oxidations. Disorders of the circulation, either local or generalised, reduce the supply of oxygenated blood to a tissue and so may make it dependent on anaerobic glycolysis. Lactate then diffuses into the blood stream and may cause a metabolic acidosis. This commonly accompanies acute circulatory failure, e.g. in shock after a severe haemorrhage or a coronary thrombosis. Severe burns are a special case because regenerating cells, which form the granulomatous mass in a healing wound, have a high need for energy and, as the blood supply has inevitably been damaged by the burn, they depend on anaerobic glycolysis. The glucose for this has to be provided from the liver by gluconeogenesis from either lactate (the Cori cycle) or amino acids. These considerations help to explain the rapid weight loss that often occurs in patients with severe burns.

Oxidations

Of the 38 molecules of ATP that may be formed from the breakdown of one molecule of glucose, 24 arise from the oxidation of two molecules of acetyl-CoA in the citric acid cycle. Most of the energy in FFA is also transduced in the cycle. Thus one molecule of palmitic acid can yield 129 molecules of ATP, of which 96 arise in the oxidation of eight molecules of acetyl-CoA; the corresponding figures for other fatty acids differ slightly (see Table 8.2) and depend on the chain length and degree of unsaturation of each acid. Amino acids after deamination are also oxidised in the cycle, but the intermediary metabolism and the point of entry into the cycle (Fig. 8.2) of individual acids varies greatly.

OVERALL PRODUCTION OF ATP IN THE HUMAN BODY

Table 8.2 shows how the carbohydrate, fat, protein and ethanol in a diet which provides 10.7 MJ might generate 145 moles of ATP. The energy equivalence of ATP under the conditions found in the body is uncertain and not quite the same as the standard free energy but may be taken as 33 kJ (7.8 kcal) mol^{-1}. On this basis a man who is in energy balance on a diet providing 10.7 MJ converts about 4.5 MJ, or 44 per cent of the dietary energy into ATP energy, the remainder appearing directly as heat. The ATP produced varies a little with the exact fatty acid composition of the diet and the nature of the carbohydrate also affects the yield. The energy conversion of protein hydrolysis and oxidation depends on the AA composition of the protein and about 30 per cent of the protein energy is excreted as urea without being converted to either ATP or heat.

The production of ATP does not proceed at a constant rate but varies in response to the demand for energy by the cells. The concentration of ATP, [ATP], in the cell fluid is small, amounting to about 1 mmol kg^{-1} in tissues such as

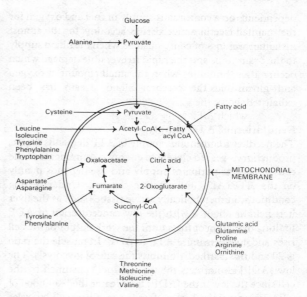

Fig. 8.2 Points of entry of derivatives of dietary carbohydrate, fat and protein into the enzyme systems of the citric acid cycle situated in the mitochondria of cells.

the liver or brain, but can be as high as 6 mmol kg^{-1} in skeletal muscle. Hence an adult may have only 200 millimoles of ATP in the body, despite a production of about 140 moles each day. The ATP pool is turning over extremely rapidly and for the whole body would only last about a minute; rapidly metabolising tissues such as the brain may only have enough ATP for 2 to 3 seconds. This

Table 8.2 Estimated daily production of ATP from the energy ingested by a subject on a Western diet

Food eaten	Amount g	mmol	Energy kJ/g	content total kJ	ATP generated in moles per mol substrate		total
Carbohydrate as glucose (mol wt 180)	300	1667	15.6	4 680	38		63.3
Fat as triglyceride (mol wt av. 861.5) yielding on hydrolysis	100	116	37	3 700			
Glycerol (mol wt 92)	10.7	116			20	2.3	
Fatty acids saturated, e.g. palmitic acid (mol wt 254)	22.1	87			129	11.2	
monounsaturated, e.g. oleic acid (mol wt 282)	49.1	174			144	25.1	
polyunsaturated, e.g. linoleic acid (mol wt 280)	24.4	87			142	12.4	51.0
Protein as amino acid (mol wt av. 110)	80	727	16	1 280			
Oxidation in deamination to urea						1.4	
as glucose		288				10.4	
as 3-hydroxybutyric acid		145				3.7	
as acetoacetate		61				1.4	16.9
Alcohol as ethyl alcohol (mol wt 46)	35	761	29	1 020	18		13.7
				10 680			144.9

dependence on a continuous supply of fuel and oxygen for the maintenance of active tissues accounts for the almost instantaneous loss of consciousness when the blood supply to the brain stops and the rapid irreversible damage which occurs after 2 minutes when the small amount of oxygen and glucose in the cerebral blood stream has been exhausted.

Regulation of ATP supply

The need for a continuous supply of ATP demands that its production is geared closely to energy requirements of the cells. This integration of supply and use depends mainly on the ATP/ADP ratio within the cell. Under resting conditions, in metabolically active tissues such as the liver it is held at about 2 with the low concentration of ADP limiting oxidation of fuels until the work output of the cell rises and converts more ATP to ADP. In muscle the ratio is 20 and this markedly inhibits the rate of glycolysis. The low [ADP] also affects the type of fuel consumed by the cell since the lower the [ADP] the greater the likelihood of FFA being oxidised in preference to glucose. This relationship holds in part because oxidation of NADH in mitochondria depends on three steps requiring ADP; as [ADP] falls NADH oxidation is reduced, [NADH] rises and therefore [NAD$^+$] falls. This fall limits glycolysis at the step from glyceraldehyde-3-phosphate to diphosphoglycerate (the first intermediary en route to pyruvate) and also conversion of pyruvate to acetyl-CoA. During the oxidation of FFA to acetyl-CoA half the electrons bypass the NADH step and are transferred to flavoproteins, which are more powerful reducing agents than NAD$^+$ and less affected by ADP. Thus resting muscles consume predominantly FFA and no glucose; [ATP] is high, [ADP] low and [NADH] high. Most other tissues at rest also consume FFA since the ATP/ADP ratio is sufficiently high to limit glycolysis.

Organs and tissues increase their demand for glucose as energy output increases. This is readily seen in exercising muscle which, despite continued oxidation of FFA, increases its consumption of glucose as [ATP] falls. In unusual circumstances, when the demand for glucose cannot be met, e.g. in patients with burns, life is threatened. Then not only is Cori cycle activity high but, as [ADP] falls, glucose oxidation is increased and thereby reduces [NADH] as much as is compatible with the supply of oxygen. Thus the balance of ADP and ATP has a key role in determining not only the rate of oxidation of fuels by cells but even the type of fuel used. Inorganic phosphate (P$_i$) does not exert a regulatory role since [P$_i$] is about 10 mmol l^{-1} (20 times that of ADP) and so does not usually limit rephosphorylation of ADP. But in patients fed intravenously without phosphate for prolonged periods, [P$_i$] can fall markedly and lead to a fall in cellular [ATP] and a reduced rate of glycolysis (Travis *et al.*, 1971).

ENERGETICS OF FUEL ASSIMILATION AND STORAGE

Assimilation

Energy is needed for the digestion and absorption of nutrients. Carbohydrates, fats and protein are broken down by hydrolytic reactions that do not require energy, but energy is needed to synthesise the enzymes present in the secretions of the alimentary tract. Sugars and amino acids need to be actively transported across the intestinal mucosa; the cost of transport for sugars is about 2.5 per cent of their energy content, but for amino acids may be more expensive if the γ-glutamyl cycle is involved; absorption of lipids does not require energy. Gastric and pancreatic digestion are unlikely to utilise more than 5 per cent of ingested energy, since the rise in energy expenditure in response to a meal varies from 10 to 20 per cent of the energy ingested, and this includes metabolic costs involved in the distribution and storage of the fuels.

Storage

Glucose

Glucose is stored as glycogen in the liver at a small cost since only 1 mole of ATP is needed for 1 mole of glucose. When liver glycogen is used as a reserve to provide glucose for the rest of the body, the energy cost doubles since glucose must then be reformed for transport to the tissues. When glucose is stored as fat the energy cost is much greater since the fatty acids have to be synthesised and then esterified with glycerol phosphate derived from glucose. The overall equation for the synthesis of glyceryl tripalmitate from glucose is

$$14\ C_6H_{12}O_6 + 18\ ADP + 12\ O_2 + 2H^+$$
$$= C_{51}H_{98}O_6 + 18\ ATP + 33\ CO_2 + 36\ H_2O$$

It is an oxidation with a very high respiratory quotient and in the tissues is coupled with the net formation of about 18 moles of ATP. Subsequent oxidation of the glyceryl tripalmitate produces only 407 moles of ATP compared with 504 which can be derived from the 14 moles of glucose by direct oxidation. Thus the storage of glucose as fat involves the loss of 16 per cent of the ATP equivalents of glucose. The intermediary steps in the synthesis of palmitate from glucose are numerous and details of their complex energetics are given by Lehninger (1975). Table 8.3 summarises the differences in the energy derived from glucose when it is metabolised in different ways.

Triglyceride

The storage of dietary fat as triglyceride (TG) is much less costly than that of dietary carbohydrate since the energy cost of the repeated hydrolysis and re-esterification is small. For re-esterification a fatty acid has to be converted to its coenzyme-A derivative at the cost of two high-energy phosphate bonds. Thus in the epithelium of the small intestine the recombination of two fatty acids with a

Table 8.3 Net ATP production from glucose metabolised by different pathways

Route	mol ATP yield/ mol glucose
1. Direct oxidation	38.0
2. Oxidation after preliminary glycogen storage	37.0
3. (a) Conversion to palmitic acid	2.0
(b) Storage as glyceryltripalmitate	1.3
(c) Indirect oxidation after preliminary storage as tripalmitate	30.4

Note the yield of ATP is about 16 per cent less if the glucose is first stored as fat. These calculations ignore the energy cost of substrate transport, hormone synthesis and cyclic AMP activation of triglyceride.

monoglyceride requires 4 ATP. In adipose tissue 2 ATP are needed to form glycerol phosphate from glucose and 6 ATP to esterify it with three fatty acids. Thus a total of only 12 ATP are required for the esterifications needed to convert a dietary into a storage triglyceride. A total of 437 ATP can be provided by the oxidation of the triglyceride. The additional energy needed for the synthesis of lipoprotein carriers is minute so that the overall cost of fat storage is only about 3 per cent of the total energy ingested as fat.

Amino acids

The energy cost of storing amino acids is greater than that of dietary fat since approximately four energy-rich phosphate bonds are needed for each peptide bond synthesised. The cost of this depends on the source of the ATP used but, if it comes from direct oxidation of glucose with the generation of 38 mol ATP/mol glucose, then the storage of 1 gram of tissue protein would cost 2.9 kJ, approximately 17 per cent of the protein's metabolisable energy. This cost does not include the energy involved in the synthesis of the nucleotides needed for synthesis of the peptide bonds and this may require an additional 10 per cent of energy (Buttery and Annison, 1973). The energy needed for AA transport into cells may be much higher but the cost is uncertain since only some amino acids are actively transported into cells. Nevertheless the cost of storing AA as protein is substantially higher than that of storing carbohydrate as glycogen or fat as TG.

ENERGETIC DIFFERENCES IN SUBSTRATE OXIDATION

The loss of energy available from glucose when it is first stored as fat has already been explained, but the route of substrate oxidation may also affect the yield of ATP. This is illustrated by comparing the energy derived from FFA oxidised via ketone body production rather than directly in the citric acid cycle.

Energetics of fatty acid and ketone body metabolism

Fatty acid oxidation starts with successive cleavages from the chain of two carbon units of acetyl-CoA. In the liver a small part of the acetyl-CoA is normally converted to acetoacetic acid. Acetoacetic acid together with its derivatives ß-hydroxybutyric acid and acetone, collectively known as ketone bodies, enter the blood and serve as fuel for other tissues.

Table 8.2 gives a figure of 51 mol ATP generated from 100 g of dietary fat. This was calculated on the assumption that all of the fatty acids underwent cleavage into two carbon units. If the fatty acids were broken down into acetoacetate before oxidation, net production of ATP would be 49 mol. Taking the energy equivalence of ATP as 33 kJ mol⁻¹ and the total energy of the triglyceride as 3700 kJ, the efficiencies of conversion in direct oxidation of fatty acids and in oxidation via ketones are 45 and 43 per cent respectively. The corresponding figure in the utilisation of glucose given in Table 8.2 is 43 per cent. All of these calculations are too uncertain to allow precise comparisons, but they do show that the thermodynamic efficiency of the formation of ATP is high and substantially the same whether glucose, FFA or acetoacetate is the primary fuel.

The state of metabolism may affect the distribution of different fuels between tissues. Thus in starvation peripheral utilisation of fuels changes and ketone body production plays a crucial role in providing energy to the brain. The mechanisms and control of ketone body production are set out later.

If the liver generates ß-hydroxybutyrate from acetoacetate, this deprives it of a NAD-linked step for energy production; but energy becomes available in the peripheral tissues from the oxidation of ß-hydroxybutyrate back to acetoacetate. Hence there is some advantage in the transfer of additional energy from the liver to the peripheral tissues in the form of ß-hydroxybutyrate rather than acetoacetate. If 80 per cent of the ketones produced are ß-hydroxybutyrate (i.e. a ß-hydroxybutyrate/acetoacetate ratio of 4 : 1), then there is a shift in energy distribution; less becomes available to the liver during the preliminary oxidation to ketone bodies and more is available from the ketone bodies going to peripheral tissues. This extra energy more than compensates for a 3 per cent loss of energy in regenerating acetyl-CoA from ketone bodies in the periphery. This loss is, as we shall see, a small price to pay for the chance of producing for the brain a fuel which is derived from fat rather than from protein.

Substrate cycling

The body expends energy not only on the distribution and storage of fuels but also in making these fuels readily available for use by different tissues. The main fuel of the body is FFA, which is continually released into the blood stream from the fat depots and circulates at concentrations which permit rapid uptake by the tissues. Not all the fatty acid entering the circulation is removed for immediate oxidation; most is recycled by the liver and returned as TG in very low density lipoproteins to the adipose tissue for release once more as FFA and glycerol. This process provides in the blood a continuous supply of fatty acids which can be boosted by increasing lipolysis when the demand for energy increases. The continuous recycling of fuel, however, imposes an additional energy cost, of about 40–50 kJ/day (Table 8.4). A rather higher cost of about 65 kJ may be involved in the Cori cycle where approximately 36 g glucose recycles from lactate in those tissues which have to rely on glycolysis for their fuel supply. These two substrate cycles are inexpensive but they play a crucial role in the distribution of fuel to the tissues.

A more expensive process is the turnover of about 275 g protein which is synthesised and degraded each day throughout the day. This turnover is crucial since the continuous release of amino acids allows cells in the liver and other tissues to respond to sudden metabolic demands by synthesising enzymes in amounts appropriate for the new requirements. Thus an inflow of excess AA leads to the rapid induction of enzyme responsible for catabolising AA. An inflow of carbohydrate also leads to rapid induction of enzymes for glycogen storage and glucose oxidation. The presence of an infection may cause reprogramming of protein synthesis in the liver with the secretion of fibrinogen, transferrin and many glycoproteins but a fall in synthesis of albumin. Turnover of muscle protein is also essential to allow the body to respond to fasting and to maintain prolonged exercise, since muscle protein is a source of AA for gluconeogenesis in the liver. In severe exercise the rate of efflux of AA from muscle corresponds to the rate of protein breakdown and matches the large increase in the hepatic requirements for glucose (see below).

Turnover of protein is an integral part of the body's capacity to adjust its fuel supply to needs imposed by the environment, and the cost of protein turnover is substantial. Table 8.4 includes only the cost of synthesising the peptide bonds of 275 g protein a day and excludes any cost associated with protein breakdown, ribosomal synthesis or AA transport and recycling. If the cost of AA recycling is

high, then the cost of protein turnover rises and may account for over 25 per cent of the resting metabolic rate.

Energy has to be provided at varying rates for many different metabolic processes; of these, the most expensive is probably the maintenance of the electrochemical gradients across cell membranes by the energy-demanding sodium pumps. The cost of sodium pumping is difficult to estimate but it may be as much as 50 per cent of the resting metabolic rate.

Two cycles are present in the early stages of glucose metabolism. The conversion of glucose to glucose 6-phosphate by hexose kinase utilises ATP and it is reversed by glucose 6-phosphatase. Similarly the conversion of fructose 6-phosphate to fructose 1,6-diphosphate utilises ATP and is reversed by hexose diphosphatase. Both these cycles appear to accomplish nothing and all the energy from the breakdown of ATP is dissipated as heat. Hence they have been called **futile cycles.** They may be present either as a flaw in biological design or as a subtle form of control of metabolic processes. Hexose kinase is inhibited by some substances lower down on the glycolytic pathway; a fall in concentration of one of these might increase the rate of cycling and so lower ATP/ADP ratio in the cell. In this way the activity of the cycle could be a factor in controlling the rate of oxidation of glucose.

The amount of energy expended in these continuously operating substrate cycles is uncertain and difficult to measure. They are ways in which the body can change its rate of fuel combustion without changing its work output. How much any of these cycles contributes to the variability in the resting metabolic rate of different individuals and of one individual from day to day is unknown.

FLOW OF ENERGY BETWEEN ORGANS
Quantitative estimates of the utilisation of different fuels by the different organs of man and of the flux of fuels between organs depend on measurements of blood flow and of differences in arterial and venous concentrations of the fuels. Until techniques were available for catheterising the veins draining the principal organs of the human body

Table 8.4 The energetic significance of substrate cycling

Cycle	ATP used (mol/ mol substrate)	Substrate ATP energy lost (per cent)	Estimated substrate turnover (mmol/day)	Energy used in turnover (kJ/day)
Glucose-lactate (Cori cycle)	4	11.1	200	65
Triglyceride-adipose tissue re-esterification	8	1.8	150	45
Protein turnover	4	17.2	2500	804
Glucose 6-phosphate-glycogen	1	2.8	2000	161

and so obtaining repeated samples of venous blood, conclusions had to be drawn from animal experiments. Although the same fuels are used by all higher animals there are marked species differences in the mixtures used under differing circumstances. Catheterisation of large veins requires a meticulous technique, experience and, for physiological studies, a supply of willing volunteers. Much of what follows is derived from catheterisation studies carried out since 1970.

Glucose absorption and distribution

Glucose is rapidly absorbed from the upper small intestine and enters the blood stream, from which most of it is extracted by the liver. When starchy foods are eaten gastric emptying, digestion and absorption is slower and a meal containing 100 g starch is absorbed over a 2–3 hour period. During this time the liver extracts about 50 g of the glucose, having quickly shut down its own production of glucose from AA. Insulin concentration rises in the portal vein in response to rises in blood glucose and amino acids and secretion of gut hormones. The liver stores a large part of the glucose as glycogen, uses the glucose as its own fuel and allows additional glucose to pass into the main circulation where it supplies both the brain and muscle with energy and restocks the muscle with glycogen. Glucose uptake by the liver differs from that in peripheral tissues in that the liver has both a specific transport system for glucose with a large capacity and a kinase for phosphorylating glucose with a low affinity for glucose. This ensures that phosphorylation responds to the concentration of glucose without the need for insulin. Thus the rate of glucose extraction by the liver responds to the concentration of glucose in the portal blood without the need for insulin or other hormonal controls. In contrast, muscle and adipose tissue have a rate-limiting step at the transport stage of uptake and this is insulin-sensitive; once uptake has occurred the hexokinase has a very high affinity for glucose so it is rapidly stored as glycogen or metabolised. The peripheral distribution of glucose is thus finely controlled by the plasma insulin.

Storage of glucose as fat

Most of the glucose stored after a starchy meal may be converted at first to glycogen rather than fat. Glycogen is, however, a temporary store whereas fat is a long-term store of energy. Some glucose is converted to fat in both the liver and adipose tissue. The relative importance of these two organs for fat synthesis in man is uncertain, but the liver is probably the dominant site. Glucose contributes to TG synthesis both by providing the glycerol for the esterification of FFA and by being converted into FFA. The three-carbon unit glycerol phosphate needed for the re-esterification is generated in both the liver and fat cells during glycolysis, but in the liver glycerol phosphate can also be synthesised from glycerol itself. The glycerokinase

needed for this conversion is absent or of low activity in fat cells. Glucose generates FFA via the two-carbon unit, acetyl-CoA. When [ATP] is high, activity of the citric acid cycle is limited and so accumulating acetyl-CoA is then used for synthesising FFA rather than for oxidation. After a meal glucose flowing directly to the fat cells is used mainly for synthesis of glycerol phosphate rather than FFA, but in the liver it is used for synthesis of FFA and subsequent conversion to TG.

Triglyceride distribution after a meal

Digestion and absorption of fat is much slower than that of starch and protein because fat delays gastric emptying and enters the circulation mainly through lymphatic channels as chylomicrons (p. 52). After a meal containing fat, chylomicrons may enter the blood faster than they are removed and the plasma is then opalescent. Chylomicrons are droplets of fat about 1 μm in diameter with a large central core of TG and small amounts of phospholipid, cholesterol and protein (p. 51). Lymphatic absorption delays the influx of fat into the blood and channels it past the liver to peripheral tissues. Chylomicron TG is broken down in adipose tissue, muscle and liver, where FFA and glycerol are released by lipoprotein lipase. The FFA is re-esterified with newly formed glycerol phosphate and then stored as TG. Thus there are two hydrolyses with re-esterification before dietary fatty acids are stored, but this is accomplished with little loss of energy.

Most of the ingested fat is probably taken up from the blood by adipose tissue but some is removed by the liver and muscle. This distribution depends on lipoprotein lipase activity in the tissues. Activity varies during the day, and after a meal rises in adipose tissue and falls in muscle. Between meals this is reversed so that muscle then becomes the preferential site of storage of TG. Control of this cyclical variation directs the energy flow from one organ to another. The maximum clearance rate of TG in a 70 kg man is about 15.5 g h^{-1} (Kissebah et al., 1974). Thus after a meal containing 50 g of fat it takes more than three hours to clear the blood. Clearance is rarely at a maximum since the rate is proportional to plasma [TG]. At the normal fasting value of 1 mmol l^{-1} clearance is 7 g h^{-1} and reaches the maximum rate when the concentration exceeds 5 mmol l^{-1}. Hence after a meal clearance of fat from the blood proceeds slowly and it is necessary for a patient to fast for 12 hours before his basal plasma [TG] can be measured.

The daily turnover of TG in the fat depots is about 140 g, or 6 g h^{-1} (Kissebah et al., 1974), and greater than the normal dietary intake. Hence the fatty acid composition of adipose tissue TG is only slowly affected by the type of fat in the diet. But when American subjects were given diets in which corn oil or linseed oil was the only source of fat, after a year or more the proportion of polyunsaturated fatty acids in their adipose tissue fatty acids rose markedly

(Hirsch, 1965). When coconut oil is the major source of dietary fat, medium chain fatty acids never reach the fat stores since being water-soluble they pass in the portal blood to the liver, where they are oxidised.

Amino acid absorption and distribution

Proteins like starch are rapidly digested in the duodenum and jejunum and after a meal concentrations of amino acids and glucose rise in the blood at about the same time. Once absorbed, AAs pass to the liver in both plasma and red blood cells. About 25 per cent of the alanine and an appreciable proportion of serine, threonine, methionine, leucine, isoleucine and tyrosine are carried from one tissue to another in red blood cells.

After a meal concentrations of all amino acids rise in the systemic circulation but the greatest increases are in leucine, isoleucine and valine. The liver extracts from the portal blood most of the excess AA, but relatively less of those with branched chains, valine, leucine and isoleucine; these, which contribute 20 per cent of the weight of non-collagen proteins, account for 50 per cent of the increased output of AA from the liver. Within 30 min of ingesting a protein-rich meal there is an appreciable increase in the uptake of valine, leucine and isoleucine by muscles and a smaller increase of other AAs.

Glutamate and aspartate form about 20 per cent of ingested protein but do not appear in appreciable quantity in the portal blood because they are rapidly converted to alanine in the intestine. Alanine has a key role in integrating protein and carbohydrate metabolism since it is readily extracted by the liver, provides the carbon skeleton for gluconeogenesis and carries nitrogen for excretion as urea.

Wahren et al. (1976) studied protein absorption and AAs distribution in normal man. They showed that the greater part of the branched chain AAs reach the systemic circulation and are not oxidised in the liver. After a meal of 47 g of beef protein containing about 10 g of branched chain AAs, only 1 g of these passed each hour into the systemic circulation, but plasma [AA] was raised by 50–100 per cent for up to 8 hours. This prolonged output into the systemic circulation is not due to slow digestion of proteins; the intestines and to a lesser extent the liver moderate the flow of AAs to the rest of the body by temporarily increasing their own protein mass. As the AA supply to the liver increases there is a surge in the synthesis of export proteins, including albumin, and breakdown of hepatic cell proteins is slowed. The result is an increase in the mass of hepatic protein. Subsequent rapid turnover of both gut and liver proteins maintains the outflow of AAs to the periphery for several hours.

Dietary amino acids mix in the blood with those recycling from the tissues; the total daily turnover of AA is about 350 g, i.e. about 15 g h^{-1}. Entry of AA from the intestine may double their flow in the portal blood for 3 hours following a meal. After entry into liver and muscle cells a proportion of the AAs is metabolised to provide either substrate for gluconeogenesis or energy in the citric acid cycle (Fig. 8.2). Over 24 hours the rate of oxidation of AA by the tissues approximately matches the amount ingested but there is a surge in oxidation after each meal. The liver is the major site for oxidation and the only site for generating urea.

Although the liver acts as a temporary store of AAs in the form of protein, the main long-term store is in muscle. Muscle protein increases during the day, as AAs flow from the gut, and AAs are released when there is a need for gluconeogenesis. This cyclical net movement of AA does not involve alanine, which passes to the liver from muscle even in the postprandial phase. Alanine is then serving as a nitrogen carrier, the alanine carbon coming from blood glucose and muscle glycogen, and the nitrogen from the oxidation of other AA especially the branched chain ones. The alanine carbon is used once more for glucose synthesis in the liver. In this way a **glucose–alanine cycle** transfers nitrogen from muscles to the liver.

Plasma alanine concentrations remain unchanged after a meal despite the large inflow of alanine from three sources, ingested alanine, intestinal metabolism of glutamate and aspartate, and the glucose–alanine cycle. Therefore net synthesis of glucose from alanine is unlikely after a meal. Muscle nitrogen can be transferred to 2-oxoglutarate to form glutamate and to pyruvate to form alanine, but the latter is the major carrier. Glutamine serves as a nitrogen source for AA production in the kidneys, particularly when ketosis develops during starvation (see below) and there is a need for ammonium production to balance the ketones excreted in the urine. Blood glutamine concentrations after a meal may actually fall, especially in red blood cells (Aoki et al., 1976), reflecting the dominance of the pyruvate–alanine transamination systems in muscle.

The sequence of changes in AA metabolism after a meal is closely regulated by hormones. There is an increase in both plasma insulin and glucagon concentrations. Insulin stimulates the uptake of AA by peripheral tissues and glucagon ensures that the liver continues to put out the glucose needed by the brain. Without glucagon the insulin-stimulated liver would immediately inhibit glucose output and this would be a serious problem after a low carbohydrate meal. An increase in both glucagon and insulin secretion is therefore necessary after ingesting protein (Felig et al., 1976).

With the inflow of dietary protein there is an increase in metabolism, the specific dynamic action or thermic effect of food (p. 19) which was originally considered to be specific to protein ingestion. This increase, which usually amounts to a rise of 10 per cent, persists for many hours, up to half of the increase may be accounted for by the increased metabolic activity in the splanchnic bed. This includes the energy cost of the digestive processes and the increase in protein turnover in the gut and hepatic tissues.

The increase in AA oxidation after a meal was once considered a main cause of the specific dynamic action of proteins, but this now seems unlikely since the oxidation would necessarily involve generating additional ATP. This energy could be dissipated in futile cycles or used for biological work; however, additional ATP from AA oxidation need not automatically increase total energy expenditure since the increased ATP from AA oxidation could be balanced by a fall in ATP produced by oxidation of either glucose or FFA. The metabolic rate would then remain unchanged.

A more acceptable explanation for the increased metabolism after a protein meal is the cost of synthesising extra protein. In the experiments of Wahren et al. (1976) the energy cost of resynthesising the 47 g of amino acids into gut and hepatic proteins includes that needed for syntheses of peptide bonds, each synthesis requiring four energy-high phosphate bonds. If this energy is provided by the oxidation of glucose then the cost of synthesising 1 g of protein amounts to 2.9 kJ for the 47 g of ingested amino acids. This, spread over a 6 hour period, would increase the resting O_2 uptake of the 70 kg man studied by half the total increase actually observed. Thus the increase in metabolic rate after a protein meal is most simply explained as the result of the energy cost of the digestion, distribution of the protein meal and the increased protein turnover which results.

FUEL RESERVES IN MAN

When food is unavailable the body has to rely on its own stores of fuel; these are summarised in Table 8.5, modified from an article on starvation by Cahill (1976). The store of carbohydrate is small and mostly as glycogen in muscle and liver. Muscle glycogen is usually considered to be available for energy production in the muscle only. In muscle it plays a key role in maintaining a subject's capacity to remain active (see below). When fasting, the crucial provision of glucose for the brain depends initially on liver glycogen and, after 12 to 18 hours, on synthesis of

glucose by both the liver and kidneys. The glucose is derived at first mainly from AA coming from muscle protein. The total mass of body protein amounts to about 12 kg in a 65 kg man and of this about 50 per cent is in muscle. Not all of this protein is available, however, since studies in Jamaica have shown that collagen proteins, constituting 25 per cent of muscle and total body proteins, are not depleted in severe malnutrition (Picou et al., 1966). The non-collagen protein in muscle, in the form of myofibrillar proteins and the enzymes of the muscle sarcoplasm, can provide under extreme condition up to 4 kg of protein for gluconeogenesis (see also p. 68). Other tissues, including the liver, intestine, skin, brain and adipose tissue, lose protein as starvation develops and contribute about another 1 kg of amino acids. However, simple starvation, unaccompanied by infection or the provision of a protein-deficient diet, seems to deplete muscle protein selectively, and muscles bear the brunt of a poor energy intake. In time, other tissues contribute their amino acids for glucose production, but this is clinically less obvious in patients with marasmus.

Triglycerides are stored without water, unlike protein or glycogen, which are deposited within cells with five times their weight of water. TG have a lower specific gravity, but twice the energy value of protein and carbohydrate. This high energy density makes fat a highly economical fuel for storing for use in times when food is scarce. On the other hand, when excess fat is deposited in obesity, large energy stores accumulate for only a moderate increase in weight.

The transition in fuel supplies from the fed to fasted state

As glucose absorption slows after a carbohydrate meal, plasma insulin falls and plasma glucagon rises. This altered glucagon/insulin ratio ensures continued hepatic glucose output of glucose for the brain and other glycolytic tissues. Glucagon stimulates gluconeogenesis as well as hepatic glucose output but insulin also has an important role; as plasma insulin falls, glycogen synthesis declines and

Table 8.5 Available fuel reserves in an adult man (modified from Cahill, 1976, and Halliday 1967.)

Tissue	Glucose and glycogen		Mobilisable proteins		Triglycerides	
(weight in kg)	g	kJ	g	kJ	g	kJ
Blood (10)	15	255	100	1 700	5	185
Liver (1)	100	1 700	100	1 700	50	1 850
Intestines (1)	0	0	100	1 020	0	0
Brain (1.4)	2	34	40	680	0	0
Muscle (30)	300	5 100	4 000	68 000	600	22 200
Adipose tissue (15)	20	340	300	5 100	12 000	444 000
Skin, lung, spleen (4)	13	220	240	4 080	40	1 480
Total	450	7 649	5 000	82 280	12 695	469 715

glycogenolysis increases, and when blood glucose also falls muscle and adipose tissue reduce their uptake of glucose. At the same time the hormone-sensitive lipase in adipocytes is activated and increases FFA output rapidly, so providing fuel for most of the body's tissues. If the interval between a meal is longer than 12 hours, e.g. in those who do not eat breakfast, then liver glycogen reserves become depleted and additional glucose has to be produced, mainly from AA.

Muscle glycogen falls progressively during the first five days of starvation, and may contribute 140 g of glucose to the brain during this crucial period when hepatic glycogen reserves are exhausted and circulating blood ketones are still at too low a concentration to supply the brain (Ruderman, 1975). Muscle glycogen could yield 25–30 g glucose for the brain each day during early starvation by generating pyruvate which enters the Cori cycle. If fasting continues, blood glucose falls slightly, plasma insulin falls markedly and plasma glucagon rises. The lower insulin leads to decreased uptake of AA by muscle, but a lower rate of protein synthesis increases their concentration within muscle. Then there is an efflux of AA from muscle to the liver. In starvation, muscle changes from a state of net synthesis to one of net catabolism of protein.

Muscle is the major reserve of AA in the body but the amounts of each AA released from muscle do not reflect their proportions in the muscle proteins. Catabolism releases mainly alanine and glutamine (Table 8.6). Alanine is the preferred substrate for gluconeogenesis in the liver, and glutamine contributes to gluconeogenesis in the kidneys as starvation progresses. The carbon skeletons of the alanine and glutamine effluxing from muscle are derived from several sources: some pyruvate and 2-oxoglutarate is derived from AA metabolism and can then be transaminated to alanine and glutamate. Additional glutamate is taken up by muscle from blood and used for glutamine synthesis.

In prolonged starvation the flow of alanine from muscle falls and this is reflected in a steady decline in urea synthesis and excretion. Glutamine output tends to persist

since, after 10 days of fasting, ammonia becomes the main nitrogen product in the urine.

Ketone body production

The increases in plasma FFA and glucagon during fasting both promote synthesis of ketone bodies from fatty acids in the liver. These are used by most tissues, including the brain, as fuels and reduce the need for glucose. Initially production of ketones is small, but, as fasting continues, it rises progressively until they become the substrate with the highest concentration in the blood (Fig. 8.3). After comparing the concentration of the different circulating fuels, it is not surprising that ketones come to dominate the fuel economy of some tissues during starvation. The change from glucose oxidation to FFA oxidation with the addition of ketone body metabolism occurs within a matter of three days of fasting and subsequently further changes occur until ketone bodies become the major fuel for the brain (Table 8.7).

For many years the state of ketosis was considered undesirable because severe ketosis develops rapidly in a poorly controlled diabetic and may cause a fatal acidosis. Yet the development of ketosis in a normal subject is a beneficial physiological response to both starvation and a low carbohydrate diet. In these circumstances ketogenesis is controlled and does not become excessive. The advantages of switching to metabolise ketones rather than free fatty acids are many. First, the transformation of FFA into ketone bodies produces a fuel which can be used by·the brain; without this source of energy the brain would need 120 g of glucose daily and this would have to be provided by tissue proteins. The demand for glucose would soon put an intolerable strain on the tissues and the survival time in

Table 8.6 The pattern of release of some amino acids from the human forearm and their contribution to muscle protein (data from Ruderman, 1975)

Amino acid	Percentage of all amino acids released	Percentage of muscle protein
Alanine	28.0	6.4
Glutamine	23.0	6.6
Lysine	8.7	12.6
Glycine	7.9	4.0
Histidine	2.8	3.1
Valine	2.8	3.5
Leucine	2.0	6.2
Isoleucine	2.0	3.9
Aspartate	0	7.0
Glutamate	− 7.9 (net uptake)	11.7

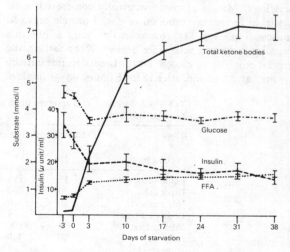

Fig. 8.3 Concentrations of blood total ketone bodies and glucose, serum insulin and plasma free fatty acids (FFA) in 37 obese subjects during prolonged starvation. Values are means ± SE. (Owen and Reichard, 1975.)

Table 8.7 Fuel supplies and utilisation during a short fast and prolonged starvation (adapted from Cahill, 1976)

Tissue	Fuel	Fasting 3 days (g/day)	Starvation 6 weeks (g/day)
Energy supplies from			
Adipose tissue	FFA	180	180
Liver	Ketones	150	150
	Glucose	150	80
	Glycerol	20	20
	Lactate + pyruvate	40	40
	Amino acids	70	20
Muscle	Glycogen	20	0
	Amino acids	75	20
Energy utilised by			
Brain	Glucose	100	40
	Ketones	50	100
Liver	Amino acids	70	20
Muscle	Amino acids	75	20
Other tissues	Glucose	50	40
	FFA	30	30
	Ketones	100	50

starvation would be severely limited. Another advantage of ketones is that they readily pass across cell membranes without the need for specific transport systems or binding proteins, as required for glucose and FFA. Being water-soluble the ketones readily reach a concentration where they are oxidised in preference to glucose without the need for additional regulatory mechanisms at the cell level. Ketones also reduce the rate of oxidation of branched chain AA in muscle and thereby reduce the efflux and loss of AA from muscle.

Ketone body synthesis

The three ketone bodies acetoacetate, β-hydroxybutyrate and acetone are generated from acetyl- CoA only in the liver, but the reactions are readily reversible in all tissues, where the acetyl-CoA can be oxidised in the citric acid cycle. The generation of NADH during fatty acid oxidation also favours the conversion of acetoacetate to β-hydroxybutyrate. The reverse of these reactions predominates in the peripheral tissues because of the continuous use of acetyl-CoA by the citric acid cycle.

Normally only acetoacetate and β-hydroxybutyrate are measured in blood; acetone is readily formed by decarboxylation of acetoacetate and is excreted in the breath where it is responsible for the characteristically sweet odour of a ketotic subject. The ratio of β-hydroxybutyrate to acetoacetate varies in part because of changes in the ratio of NAD/NADH in the liver. In the blood the ratio may rise from 2 up to 5 or even 10 under conditions of rapid fatty acid oxidation. The reduction of acetoacetate to β-hydroxybutyrate has the advantage of transferring reducing equivalents from the liver to the peripheral tissues where they yield an additional three molecules of ATP for each molecule of β-hydroxybutyrate oxidised.

Two major events seem to determine the development of ketosis. First there is a rise in the plasma [FFA]. This occurs when plasma insulin falls and provides the liver with the substrate for ketogenesis. An acute rise in plasma [FFA], however, produces only a small increase in ketone body production (Grey *et al.*, 1975) in well-fed individuals, so that a further major change in liver metabolism must occur to ensure that FFA is converted to ketone bodies rather than re-esterified to TG as occurs in some patients with hypertriglyceridaemia (Chapter 40). Ketogenesis is activated by an increase in the ratio of plasma glucagon to insulin but the relative importance of glucagon and insulin is uncertain. The control of ketogenesis seems to be exerted at the carnitine acyltranferase step and may depend on the availability of carnitine. This step is reponsible for the movement of FFA from the cytoplasm into the mitochondria and, if this is blocked, the FFA are re-esterified in the cytoplasm and do not enter the mitochondria for oxidation to acetyl-CoA (McGarry and Foster, 1977). Subsequent conversion of acetyl-CoA to acetoacetate appears to be increased if liver glycogen stores are low, as would be expected during starvation, but the mechanism accounting for this effect is uncertain. Once the liver has been primed for ketogenesis then the availability of FFA determines the rate of ketone body production; a fall in plasma [FFA] in response to a glucose-induced release of insulin leads to a very rapid fall in the concentration of ketone bodies in blood.

Changes in ketone body metabolism during starvation

The concentration of ketone bodies in the blood reflects the balance between their rate of production in the liver and their rate of oxidation in the three principal tissues metabolising ketones, brain, kidneys and muscles. The rate of oxidation is proportional to blood concentrations during the first few days of starvation as ketone body concentrations rise from the normal value of 0.5 to 1 up to 3 mmol l^{-1}. At this stage they are oxidised at near maximal rates and provide 30–40 per cent of total energy requirements. Ketones contribute about 10 per cent of the energy for muscle after an overnight fast but this proportion rises to 50–80 per cent after 3–7 days of starvation (Owen and Reichard, 1975).

The increase in plasma ketones during prolonged fasting results from a reversal in the progressive changeover in muscle from FFA to ketone body oxidation. After 6 weeks of fasting perhaps only 10 per cent of the muscle's fuel comes from ketone bodies but the brain and kidneys are now almost totally dependent on ketones. Muscle continues to take up acetoacetate but releases β-hydroxybutyrate, this reductive step signifying the increased consumption of fatty acids and the ready availability of NADH within muscle. Thus the late switch in fuel consumption by muscle boosts the supply of ketones for the brain and so reduces the need for muscle protein to be used for gluconeogenesis. This extraordinary survival mechanism is further helped by the effect of both ketones and FFA in reducing oxidation of branched chain AA in muscle (Aoki *et al.*, 1975; Cahill, 1976). Conservation of these, particularly leucine, enhances synthesis of muscle proteins and tends to limit the rate of muscle protein breakdown.

Normally from 1–3 mmol of ketones are excreted in the urine daily, about 1 per cent of the amount produced. At low plasma concentrations the greater part of the urinary ketones is acetoacetate, but when plasma β-hydroxybutyrate rises to about 2 mmol l^{-1} its urinary output begins to increase exponentially (Johnson and Passmore, 1961). When in starvation plasma ketones reach 5 mmol l^{-1} the predominant urinary ketone is β-hydroxybutyrate. The ability of the kidneys to conserve ketones is nutritionally significant, since an equimolar amount of amino acids is needed to generate ammonia to balance the excretion of acid; β-hydroxybutyric acid is a weaker acid than acetoacetic acid. During starvation this action of the kidneys protects the body from being depleted of up to 8 g of nitrogen daily.

Fuel supply during exercise

At rest the overall uptake of glucose by the muscles is very small, about 20–25/min and 10 to 15 per cent of the total body glucose turnover, and the RQ of muscles at rest is close to 0.7, reflecting the dominance of fat as a fuel (Andres *et al.*, 1956). Most of this is in the form of FFA and is derived from endogenous triglyceride within the muscles. When exercise starts, the immediate source of additional energy is ATP but, as we have seen, the supplies are very small; they can be generated rapidly from the small store of phosphocreatine which provides enough energy for ι man to run for about 100–200 metres. This supply is also soon exhausted and then glycolysis of muscle glycogen provides energy anaerobically but only in small amounts. If work is to continue, the muscles must soon shift to oxidation of a mixture of carbohydrate and fat.

Glucose is the major fuel at first during muscular work and as exercise proceeds there is a greater proportion of fat in the mixture. Yet carbohydrate still provides 40 per cent of the fuel, even if heavy exercise is continued for nearly 3 hours (Table 8.8). Studies of samples of blood obtained from the femoral artery and vein confirm this finding and show also the proportions of the fuel provided by blood glucose and muscle glycogen (Fig. 8.4). More details of the fuels used by muscles are given in a report of a seminar at Yale University (Felig and Wahren, 1975).

During continued exercise exogenous glucose for the muscles has to come from glycogen stores in the liver and, once these are depleted, from AA catabolism and gluconeogenesis. Alanine output from muscle increases rapidly in response to exercise and in proportion to the intensity of the work. At the same time branched chain AA pass into the muscles for oxidation and their concentration in blood falls. With the increased need for glucose production the hepatic extraction of alanine goes up progressively from 40 to 90 per cent. During the exercise the brain continues to demand its usual supply of glucose so the additional demand for glucose by the muscle must be met at the cost of muscle proteins. All these changes are associated with a fall in plasma insulin.

A failure of carbohydrate supply may in some circumstances be a limiting factor in exercise. For example, in a study of the effect of prolonged exercise and starvation on secretion of growth hormone (Fonseka *et al.*, 1965), two medical students offered to walk 28 miles in 7 hours with no breakfast. One of them after 23 miles collapsed suddenly; he was given oral glucose and after 30 min he had recovered fully. Measurements of his respiratory exchanges indicated that he had utilised 150 g of carbohydrate during the walk and the proportion of carbohydrate in his metabolic mixture had fallen from 65 to 35 per cent. The other student, who completed the walk without apparent difficulty, was estimated to have utilised only 125 g of carbohydrate and at the end of the walk only 10 per cent of his metabolic mixture was carbohydrate. The three highly trained Scandinavian athletes who provided the

Table 8.8 Relative proportions of carbohydrate and fat in the fuel mixture during prolonged heavy work with energy expenditure at 900–1000 W (Christensen and Hansen, 1939)

Time (min)	Respiratory quotient	Percentage of energy from Carbohydrate	Fat
0–30	0.910	69	31
30–60	0.890	63	37
60–90	0.875	57	43
90–120	0.855	50	50
120–150	0.840	45	55
150–162	0.825	40	60

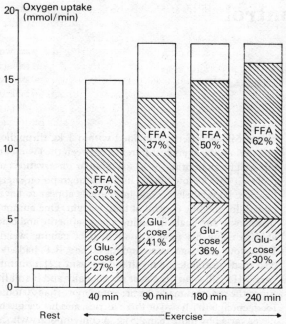

Fig. 8.4 Uptake of oxygen and substrates by the legs during prolonged exercise. Hatched areas represent the proportion of total oxygen uptake contributed by oxidation of FFA and blood glucose. Open portions indicate oxidation of non-bloodborne fuels (muscle glycogen and intramuscular lipids). (From Ahlborg *et al.*, 1974.)

data for Table 8.8 may be calculated to have used on average 325 g of carbohydrate during their prolonged period of heavy exercise, but they had probably eaten breakfast.

These estimates of the amounts of carbohydrates used in prolonged physical work indicate a need for a large store of muscle glycogen before taking part in any athletic event requiring a high or prolonged expenditure of energy. The dietary means to ensure such a store are described in Chapter 64.

Recovery from exercise

Once exercise has stopped, muscles continue to extract circulating glucose at three to four times the resting rate for some time, and this presumably helps to restore their stock of glycogen. However, the rate is far less than during severe exercise, and so gluconeogenesis in the liver drops to about twice the pre-exercise rate. Much of this glucose comes via the Cori cycle from circulating lactate which increases to concentrations of 10 mmol l^{-1} towards the end of exhausting exercise.

At the end of exercise insulin concentrations rapidly increase, particularly in the portal blood. This increase may depend on a fall in catecholamine output as well as a tendency for blood glucose to rise as glucose extraction by muscle falls. Despite the rise in plasma insulin, plasma glucagon remains high for some time and this may help to replenish hepatic glycogen stores.

The changes in amino acid metabolism are equally rapid after exercise. During the exercise period muscle is in negative nitrogen balance and urea production rates may rise by 60 per cent in trained athletes. After exercise, however, the increasing insulin aids uptake of amino acids from protein supplied in the next meal and athletes usually remain in nitrogen balance on the day of an event. In this way the well-known absence of a marked negative nitrogen balance during heavy and prolonged exercise is explained.

9. Energy Balance and Control of Body Weight

Body weight does not remain constant throughout the 24 hours. Weight increases during the day as food is ingested and is then lost between meals both as fuel is oxidised for energy with the exhalation of carbon dioxide and as water evaporates from the skin and lungs. Some subjects have marked weight gains during the day because water is being retained and gravitates into the legs; when the weight increase exceeds 2 kg between morning to evening, then an abnormality of electrolyte and water balance is likely (Edwards, 1977). Anyone who weighs himself each morning after emptying the bladder, but before breakfast, also finds significant variations from day to day. A careful study of these has been made on young women in New Zealand by Robinson and Watson (1965). A gain or loss of more than 0.5 kg each day was found in 13 per cent of the daily weighings and of more than 1.0 kg in nearly 2 per cent. A gain or loss of as much as 2 kg is unusual except in association with the cyclical changes in a woman's water balance during the menstrual cycle. The daily changes are not cumulative; they compensate one another and reflect primarily changes in water balance from day to day and week to week with a day-to-day standard deviation of about 0.5 per cent of body weight (Garrow, 1978).

If weight is measured at monthly or yearly intervals, then the results may be very different since in addition to short-term fluctuation in body fluids there may be slower changes in both the body's fat content and in the mass of lean tissue. The Metropolitan Life Insurance Company (1960) report that in the United States women of height 172 cm (5 ft 8 in) weighed on average 62 kg when aged 20 to 40 years and 73 kg when aged to 60 to 69 years. Thus there was a gain of 11 kg in four decades. These are average figures: in many women the gain was much greater whereas others retained their weight unchanged. In some people weight increase is rapid. Thus many women become obese because of a failure to lose the weight which it is normal to put on during pregnancy. For the majority it is a gradual process. The data show that USA men and women on average gained weight steadily throughout adult life. There was no middle-age spread and the gain between the ages 20 to 24 and 25 to 29 was as great as in any other period.

Long-term changes in weight vary greatly from person to person. Gordon and Kannel (1973) found that very few of the individuals weighed at yearly intervals for 18 years as part of the famous prospective study of health in Framingham, Massachusetts, remained within 1 kg throughout this period, the average difference between the lowest and top weight amounting to 10 kg. Similar observations are reported by Garrow (1978) in his monograph on energy balance. Nevertheless some individuals appear to have a system for the fine control of body weight. One author of this book is fortunate in having a good appetite and being able to enjoy his food without fear of gaining weight. Forty-four years ago, as an undergraduate, R.P. had a tail-coat made to enable him to attend a cousin's 21st birthday party. He still wears the coat occasionally and it still fits. Since the coat was made, he has eaten more than 20 tons of food, enough to fill two or three lorries, and his weight has never varied by more than 2.5 kg. A contemporary who has slowly acquired by middle-age a modest spread amounting to some 10 kg has not been a glutton. The energy equivalent of tissue gained is about 26 kJ/g so his total dietary excess has been some 260 MJ. Spread over 20 years this amounts to an average daily excess of only about 35 kJ or 8 kcal. This figure is important because it shows how little excess energy is needed on a daily basis to accumulate a large reservoir of energy over a period of years. Even a rapid weight gain of 10 kg over a year, amounting to 26 MJ, would imply an average net imbalance of only 80 kJ/day.

Slower adjustments in weight may indicate changes in lean tissue as well as in fat. With ageing, the amount of lean tissue declines even when body weight stays the same. Conversely, a footballer training for a new season may lose weight as his body fat content falls, but this decrease is minimised by an increase in muscle mass as training progresses. Overeating, however, leads to an increase in weight as both lean tissue and fat are deposited.

Short-term control of food intake

The physiological and psychological factors involved in the short-term regulation of food intake in man are complex and difficult to disentangle one from another. Adult men fed a liquid diet tended to compensate for any pre-meal drink by reducing the volume of feed consumed, but this adjustment is imperfect (Jordan 1973). Compensation occurred if the drink was taken as long as one hour before the meal and depended both on the subject seeing the volume of the pre-meal drink and on his assessment of this volume from oral stimuli; if the drink was pumped into his stomach, then compensation was poor. Similarly, the short-term control of energy intake is inadequate since it is possible to disguise the energy content of the drink and double the energy ingested with little effect on the next meal. When student volunteers were maintained for weeks on a liquid feed without knowing either the volume or energy content of the fluid being drunk, then many students begin to eat more 2–5 days after the feed had been diluted and thereby maintained weight. Others, however, failed to adjust and were unaware of losing 5 kg in weight. Whether these individual differences in the capacity to adjust are related to the likelihood of developing obesity is unknown. Obese and non-obese people are unable to distinguish high and low energy liquid meals which taste and look alike and which are of equal volume.

Nan Taggart (1962), of Aberdeen, has provided a good example of how appetite can regulate food intake to maintain the body weight accurately over a week, but not on a day-to-day basis. For 11 consecutive weeks she weighed every item of food that she ate. During this period she also weighed herself accurately under standard conditions each morning, except on Sundays when she did not go to the laboratory. She did not analyse her results until all the figures were collected. She was surprised to find that her average intake of food on Monday to Friday provided 9.6 MJ/day; whereas on Saturdays it provided 10.8 MJ/day and on Sundays 12.8 MJ/day. During the weekdays she lost on average 480 g which she regained at the weekend. Until the results had been analysed she did not realise that she ate more at the weekends, and at no time was she conscious of undue hunger or repletion. It would appear that during the first five days of the week she was about 2.9 MJ deficient and this was responsible for the loss of weight. Yet she was not hungry on Friday night, nor was she aware that she ate much more on Sundays than on other days.

A deficit of 2.9 MJ is the equivalent of one meal. An examination of daily records of energy intake and expenditure (Durnin, 1961) suggests that some people may be either in energy excess or deficit by as much as three good meals before an adjustment of food intake is made.

Measurements of the food intake of a group of students who undertook a period of five days of hard exercise between two periods of artificially restricted sedentary life, showed that in none of the students did the food intake change abruptly with the changes in energy expenditure (Passmore et al., 1952). During this experiment one of the subjects developed mumps, which restricted his food intake for four days. Figure 9.1 shows that for this subject over a period of 13 days, energy intake equalled energy expenditure despite large daily fluctuations in the energy balance.

CONTROL MECHANISMS

The body weight depends on a balance between energy intake and energy output. The balance is regulated by a mechanism situated within the central nervous system. This receives an input of information which may come from within the body, i.e. chemical and nervous stimuli, or from the outside world, i.e. the sight and smell of food and the social milieu. The output may be behavioural, i.e. feeding or changes in physical activity, or metabolic adaptations.

CENTRAL REGULATION

Feeding is a motor activity dependent on the hypothalamus, a structure at the base of the brain which also regulates the production of many hormones and, through the automatic nervous system, many of the vegetative functions of the body including the temperature. Destruction of the ventral hypothalamic nuclei in experimental animals or, as happens very occasionally in man, damage to the hypothalamus following a head injury, leads to excessive feeding (hyperphagia). Destruction of the lateral nuclei suppresses feeding (aphagia). These nuclei have been considered to operate as satiety and feeding centres respectively, but this is oversimplification. The effect of damage to these centres may be slight unless adjacent axons in nerve pathways from lower parts of the brain are also damaged.

The nature of these pathways is now being studied in rats by observing the effect on feeding behaviour of injecting through cannulas permanently implanted into specific areas in the hypothalamic region chemical neurotransmitters (Leibowitz, 1976). These pharmacological experiments indicate that there are both α- and ß-adrenoreceptors and also dopamine receptors on neurones in the hypothalamus which are activated by nerve impulses in

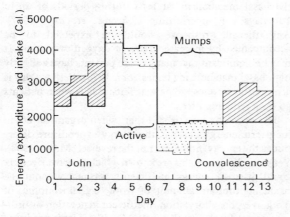

Fig. 9.1 Energy balance in a young man during four periods: (a) 3 days—sedentary life; (b) 3 days—activity; (c) 4 days—mumps; (d) 3 days—convalescence. Thin line = daily energy intake; thick line = daily energy expenditure. Cross-hatched areas show excess intake over expenditure; stippled areas show excess expenditure over intake.

pathways from the midbrain and medulla. Thus the neuronal regulatory mechanism is probably widespread in the brain and not confined to small discrete areas, as earlier experiments had suggested. New techniques in neurobiochemistry and neuropharmacology are leading to fresh understanding of neuroanatomy and neurophysiology. However, the functions of newly discovered pathways in the brain are as yet far from completely worked out.

OUTPUTS FROM THE CONTROL CENTRES

Feeding behaviour

This is a motor activity initiated or suppressed by sensations or perceptual states arising from incoming stimuli. Feeding may be initiated by hunger, which is a complex sensation arising from physiological changes in the state of the body's store of energy, and inhibited by fullness, a sensation arising in the alimentary canal. Feeding behaviour is also markedly influenced by appetite and satiety. These depend on the nature and quality of the food and the immediate physical environment of the eater and they are also influenced by his habits, family customs and indeed by his education and cultural background. One man's food may appear as another man's poison.

Physical activity

Hunger causes wild animals to go and search for food and may stimulate civilised men and women to activity needed to prepare a meal at home or go out to a restaurant. In circumstances when food is not available continuous hunger suppresses spontaneous activity. This occurs in experimental animals and in man. Thus when only about half the normal food supply is provided, as in prisoner of war camps in the Far East (Smith and Woodruff, 1951) and in the famous Minnesota experiment (Keys et al., 1950), all unnecessary movements are curtailed and in this way energy expenditure is so reduced that survival is possible. This is an important adaptive change.

To what extent satiety promotes a drive to exercise in affluent societies is uncertain and has been little studied. On more than one occasion the authors after a long session preparing this book and a good lunch have gone out and climbed to the top of Arthur's Seat in Edinburgh before returning to work and a good evening meal. Is this an example of a physiological drive to exercise initiated by a high food intake in those whose work is sedentary? Such a drive may be an important control on body weight in some persons.

Metabolic changes

When food intake is reduced, the resting metabolic rate falls slowly. This can be attributed in part to wasting of tissues and a reduction of cell mass. This is one of the factors that permits survival when the food supply is reduced greatly.

Is there a metabolic mechanism which protects some people from the usual consequence of continuing dietary excesses? It is a common observation that some people eat heartily, never worry about their diet and yet remain thin, while others gain weight readily unless they are continuously watching their diet. Nearly 70 years ago it was suggested (Grafe and Graham, 1911) that normal individuals can dispose of a dietary excess by increasing their metabolic rate and so burning it off. Obese individuals are said to lack this physiological control. Grafe called it a **luxus consumption** mechanism; interest in it has revived and it is now usually referred to as the thermic response or thermogenesis. Two critical reviews (Sims, 1976; Garrow, 1978) agree that the hypothesis of a difference in dietary-induced thermogenesis as a cause of obesity has been neither proved or disproved.

The hypothesis was put forward by Grafe to account for observations that dogs who were overfed did not gain the anticipated amount of weight. A failure to gain weight equivalent to the excess dietary energy has now been reported in several overfeeding experiments; of these the most carefully carried out over a long period was that by Sims et al. (1968) on volunteers among the prisoners in Vermont State Gaol. There are many difficulties in such experiments. Subjects soon tire of even the best food and find a long-continuing surfeit unpleasant. Strict discipline is needed. Accurate bookkeeping of daily dietary energy and of energy expenditure in physical activity is not easy, and any systematic error is cumulative. Furthermore the weight gain is not all fat: normally in overfed subjects it is about 63 per cent fat, 14 per cent extracellular fluid and 23 per cent cell mass. For these reasons some claims that excess dietary energy cannot be all accounted for as fat laid down are unconvincing.

There is good evidence that overfeeding does not raise the basal metabolism, at least during periods of up to 14 days of overfeeding (Strong et al., 1967). Any thermic response would be expected to be accompanied by increased rates of oxygen utilisation. It may be significant that many obese patients have a slightly high basal metabolism (James et al. 1978). Perhaps this is acquired in response to past surfeits; it falls when patients go on a reducing diet.

The orthodox view is still that 'when organisms are in long-term energy balance, the energy expenditure determines the energy intake and not the reverse' (Miller, 1968). Yet several mechanisms are known which after overfeeding could dissipate energy inefficiently as heat without the usual appropriate amount of work, e.g. uncoupling of oxidative phosphorylation, inefficient generation or utilisation of ATP and 'futile cycles' (p. 68). Heat is produced in these ways in brown fat as part of the mechanism of temperature regulation in all newborn and many adult mammals. In man brown fat atrophies early in life. A thermic response to surfeit may or may not exist; if it does, it has yet to be identified at the molecular level.

There is no control of absorption of energy in the gut, and faecal losses remain at about 5 per cent of dietary intake during overfeeding (Strong et al., 1967).

INPUTS TO THE CONTROL CENTRES

Nervous stimuli
A hungry man can sometimes feel his stomach contracting. If a small balloon attached to a catheter is swallowed and attached to a manometer, contractions of the stomach can be recorded in most of us just before a meal and cease when food is taken. These contractions may be presumed to signal that the stomach is empty and probably play a role in initiating feeding. However, this signal is not essential and a dog whose stomach has been completely denervated feeds normally. In man the gastric nerves are cut extensively in many operations on the stomach and the vagus nerve is often cut to reduce acid secretion in patients with peptic ulcer. Usually, none of these procedures affect food intake.

Chemical stimuli
A fall in blood glucose, as after a small dose of insulin, causes hunger and the cessation of eating after a meal is associated with a rise in blood glucose. However, since a diabetic may be ravenously hungry when his blood sugar is high, this cannot be a direct cause of satiety. Mayer (1953, 1972) showed that hunger and satiety were associated with small and high differences between glucose concentrations in arterial and venous blood respectively, and suggested that satiety was due to a high insulin-dependent rate of transport of glucose into cells in the hypothalamus. An analogue of glucose, 2-deoxyglucose, which enters the cells but is not metabolised, promotes feeding. It is presumed that it blocks intracellular glucose receptors which otherwise would be signaling satiety. As the inhibitory effect of the analogue is increased when it is injected into the portal vein, glucose receptors may also be present in the liver (Van der Weele and Sanderson, 1976). The effect on the liver is abolished by vagotomy. Glucose receptors may therefore pass information via the vagus to the brain about a fall in the glucose supply to the liver arising from a fall in blood glucose concentration or in liver blood flow or perhaps in hepatic glycogen. How important these peripheral receptors are in comparison with central receptors is uncertain.

After a meal a rise in blood glucose is associated with a fall in free fatty acids (FFA) in the blood and during starvation concentration of FFA rises. Sensations of hunger and satiety are closely associated with blood FFA which may well be a signal determining feeding behaviour.

Amino acids may also affect feeding behaviour. Animals fed a very low or a very high protein diet or an imbalanced amino acid mixture reduce their food intake. Amino acids compete for specific transport systems to enable them to cross the blood–brain barrier. Hence excess or deficiency of any one amino acid in the blood may alter the amino acid mixture which becomes available to neurones. It has been suggested (Harper, 1976) that intracerebral histidine may determine food intake and that other amino acids act only by competing with histidine for a transport system. Histidine can be converted in the brain to histamine and it is now known that there are some neuronal pathways in which histamine is the chemical transmitter. However, other and more important transmitter substances, e.g. catecholamines and 5-hydroxytryptamine (5-HT) are formed in the brain and depend on an available supply of tyrosine and tryptophan; the inhibitory neurotransmitters, γ-aminobutyric acid and glycine, are also formed in the brain from amino acids. These may all be competing for places in the transport system and their rates of synthesis may depend on nutritional factors. Anderson (1977) contends that animals have distinct appetites for energy and protein; the one for energy is dependent on pathways in which a catecholamine (noradrenaline) is the transmitter and the one for protein is dependent on a 5-HT pathway.

Thermal stimuli
When we are cold we often feel hungry and on a very hot day appetite may be markedly depressed. Central mechanisms for regulation of body temperature are situated in the hypothalamus close to the feeding and satiety centres. Brobeck (1957) showed that the amount of food eaten by rats was closely related to the temperature at which the animal house was maintained, and suggested that we eat to keep warm. Civilised man protects himself against changes in temperature in the environment by means of clothing, heating and air conditioning. Obese tissue provides extra insulation against cold and thin people feel cold more intensely than others.

Stimuli from adipose tissue
The neural, chemical and thermal stimuli described above may all have an important role in determining feeding behaviour of wild animals and sometimes of man. Each can initiate feeding. But each acts on a short time scale and as has been shown food intake by man is not adjusted rapidly to changes in energy expenditure. Several days may elapse before appropriate changes in behaviour restore the energy balance and so maintain body weight. There must be a long-term regulating mechanism which presumably depends on information on the size of the fats stores (Kennedy, 1953; Hervey, 1969). The nature of the signal is not known, but a natural steroid with a high fat : water partition coefficient could monitor the amount of fat in the body by the dilution principle. Administration of progesterone to rats increases food intake and in certain circumstances decreases energy expenditure and leads to gain in weight and fat (Hervey, 1971).

Habit and pleasure

The affluent seldom eat primarily because they are hungry. Meals are prepared at certain times by custom in our homes, canteens and restaurants and we eat when we know that they are ready. The initiating of feeding is therefore in our society more in response to custom and habit than to physiological stimuli. For most people the variable that determines energy balance is not the times when we start eating but what makes us stop. What determines whether we have one or two pieces of toast at breakfast? Why on some occasions are we unable to eat a whole helping of potatoes, which is normally enjoyed? There is no easy answer to these questions. Often we have finished eating before products of digestion can have entered the blood in significant amounts; though we may feel full the stomach is seldom distended to its capacity. Eating is associated with pleasure and we stop when it ceases to be pleasant. Cabanac (1971) pointed out that a feeling of pleasure in response to a sensory input depends on the state of the body as well as the nature of the stimulus. Thus putting the hand into water at 20°C is very pleasant when immersed in a hot bath, but very unpleasant when in a cold bath. Similarly he found that a sweet-tasting and an orange-smelling stimulus were rated as very pleasant when fasting, but unpleasant and neutral respectively one hour after ingesting 50 g of glucose. The regulating system may be reset at different levels in different individuals and this may account for the great difficulty in preventing a relapse in obesity.

GENERAL CONSIDERATIONS

Mammals and other higher animals evolved in an environment where food was usually scarce. They had to work for it and to get enough to meet their energy needs and to maintain a store of energy in the form of fat for when food was not available easily. This store had the additional use of providing insulation against heat losses in a cold environment, but it had to be kept within limits so as not to impede movements or by its weight increase their energy cost. The size of the store that migratory birds build up before their departure is a critical factor for the success of their journey (Weis-Fogh, 1967). Seals and other aquatic mammals build up a large store during pregnancy to meet energy needs during lactation when they are on land and cannot get their normal food. How the sizes of these stores are monitored so that they are just sufficient to meet the specific energy requirements of migration and lactation is unknown. They are examples of how physiological adaptations have evolved to meet special circumstances with precision. For most of the three million years of his existence *Homo sapiens* has lived in an environment where food is scarce. He is adapted to be able to withstand long periods of a restricted energy supply.

Eating is a pleasure which all higher animals appear to enjoy. Overindulgence, except for brief occasions, was impossible until a continued assured food supply from the cultivation of cereals became available about 7000 years ago. Because of the uncertainties of agriculture the great majority of the population worked hard in the field and only a minority of people, mostly the wealthy, could overeat regularly. Only since the beginning of the nineteenth century has there been large industrial communities with assured food supplies and at first the cost of food in relation to wages acted as a brake on consumption. Only since 1945 have there been large communities with an abundant and varied food supply which most of the members could afford to purchase. There has been so short an experience of abundant food that the processes of evolution have not had time to produce effective physiological adaption. Attitudes to food change slowly, not always for the better. Ancient religions lay down occasions for feasting and fasting. Contemporary man is good at feasting but seldom fasts. It is not surprising that the energy balance is often upset or that the physiological, psychological and social factors that determine it in each individual are poorly understood. Of all the regulatory mechanisms in the brain, that which determines and fixes the reserve of energy as body fat is perhaps the most complicated. Figure 9.2 indicates relations of the inputs and outputs already discussed, but it is no more than a sketch of possibilities. Neither the exact nature nor the relative quantitative importance of the various components of the diagram can be stated.

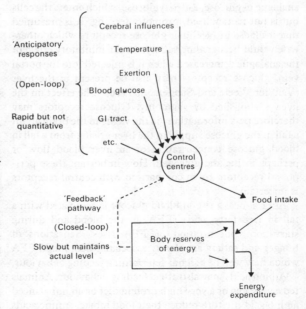

Fig. 9.2 Hypothetical organisation of the regulation of energy balance. GI = Gastrointestinal. (From Hervey, 1971.)

10. Water and Electrolytes

The body of a 65 kg man contains approximately 40 litres of water: of this about 25 litres are within the cells and about 15 litres in the extracellular fluids. The principal cation in the cell water is K and in the extracellular fluids Na. The maintenance of the different concentrations of ions on each side of the cell membrane is one of the most fundamental processes in biology. These ionic gradients can only be preserved by the expenditure of energy. Whenever a muscle or nerve is active, there is a change in the electrolyte equilibrium at the cell membrane and Na enters the cell and K leaves. During the recovery processes—both of muscle and nerve—this sodium is pumped out of the cell and the original equilibrium restored.

The normal concentration of ions, both in the intracellular and extracellular fluids, is preserved by a balance between the intake of water and electrolytes in the diet and the output in the excretions. Disturbances of this balance are of great importance in clinical practice. Present knowledge of electrolyte disturbances in disease followed the development of rapid methods of analysis using flame photometry and, more recently, atomic absorption spectrometry. By these means Na, K, Ca and Mg concentrations in small quantities of biological materials can be measured quickly and accurately. Older chemical methods involved much time and analytical skill. Radioactive tracer techniques have also facilitated studies of electrolyte distribution. These are examples of an important sequence—advance in analytical technique → new physiological knowledge → fresh clinical understanding.

WATER BALANCE

The water intake comprises the fluid drunk and the water in the food eaten. The water formed by the oxidation of carbohydrate, protein and fat is also available (metabolic water). The output consists of the urine, the water in the faeces and the water evaporated from the skin and lungs. Table 10.1 shows a normal water balance in a young man leading a sedentary life.

The data in Table 10.1 can only be obtained if the facilities of a metabolic ward are available; details of the method are given by Consolazio et al. (1963). The table shows that the liquid drunk is roughly equal to the urine output. These are easily measured and form the basis of a fluid balance chart which can be kept by the nursing staff in any ward. It is a useful guide to the water balance provided that there are not large losses from the alimentary tract or from sweating caused by fever or a hot environment.

Measurement

For research purposes, if the facilities of a metabolic ward are available, the complete water balance can be determined. Details of the method are given in Consolazio et al., (1963).

In brief, the fluid consumed is easily measured and the water in the solid components of the diet can be estimated by homogenising and drying a duplicate sample of the whole day's food.

The metabolic water can be calculated, since the oxidation of the proximate principles yields water in the following amounts:

1 g starch	0.60 g water
1 g protein	0.41 g water
1 g fat	1.07 g water

If the subject is neither losing or gaining weight, the composition of the diet provides a measure of the nutrients actually oxidised. If the subject is losing weight, an addition must be made for the water produced by the oxidation of protein and tissue fat; conversely, if the

Table 10.1 The daily water balance of a young man leading a sedentary life on a diet providing 8.8 MJ (2110 kcal)/day (Passmore et al., 1955a)

(Mean of five daily measurements)	Water ml/day
Intake:	
Water content of solid food	1115
Liquid drunk	1180
Metabolic water	279
	2574
Output:	
Urine	1295
Faecal water	56
Evaporative water loss	1214
	2565
Water balance	+9

subject is gaining weight the excess nutrients laid down do not yield water. The metabolic water is usually small in proportion to the total intake of water and any error is of little significance in calculating the water balance.

The urine volume is easily measured, as is the faecal water by weighing the faeces before and after drying. The evaporative water loss is determined from the invisible weight loss.

The invisible weight loss = weight of food and liquid consumed ± any change in body weight – the weight of urine and faeces.

These are all simple measurements.

The evaporative water loss = the invisible weight loss – weight of CO_2 expired + weight of O_2 absorbed.

Under normal circumstances the evaporative water loss is about 93 per cent of the invisible weight loss. The exact figure depends on the RQ and may vary from 90 to 102 per cent.

Fluid intake

In normal life the intake of fluids is largely determined by social custom and habit. The kidney is the principal organ regulating the amount of water in the body. Thirst is normally an additional physiological regulating mechanism. It was at one time thought that thirst was produced by dryness of the mouth and throat. More probably the sensation of thirst arises as a result of the concentration of sodium in the blood. An increase of 1 per cent in the osmolality of the blood causes thirst. The sensory receptors for thirst are in the hypothalamus and the thirst centre is closely connected with the feeding centres. Thirst is predominantly associated with water depletion, but not with salt depletion. Indeed if there is an associated salt depletion such as may occur in the tropics as a result of losses in the sweat, the thirst mechanism may not operate adequately. For this reason men doing heavy manual work, and also febrile patients, may easily become dehydrated and salt depleted without complaining of thirst. Such people may have to be persuaded to drink sufficient water, to which salt has been added. Fitzsimmons (1972) has reviewed the physiological mechanisms involved in thirst.

In medical practice fluids can be given in other ways than by mouth—into the veins, subcutaneously or into the peritoneal cavity.

Fluid output

Output from the skin. Water is commonly lost from the skin by sweating. Rates as high as 2500 ml/hr have been recorded in hot climates, both in the tropics and in hot industrial occupations. A loss of 500 ml/hr is not uncommon. Unless this water is replaced by increased intake, the body becomes dehydrated. Severe symptoms result from dehydration when about 10 per cent of the total body water has been lost.

Output from the lungs. The expired air is saturated with water vapour at 37°C. Under normal conditions only about 300 ml/day are lost in this way. When the inspired air is very dry, losses may be considerable. On the slopes of Mount Everest, for instance, the cold dry air draws off much more moisture from the lungs than is lost in a temperate climate. The losses are exaggerated by the increased ventilation of the lungs necessitated by the low oxygen content of the inspired air. It is probable that earlier Everest climbers became dehydrated from this cause which impaired their fitness for the final assault. In Sir John Hunt's first successful expedition this was appreciated and special attention was paid to the water intake of every member of the expedition. Each was made to drink 5 to 7 pints (3 to 4 litres) daily (Pugh and Ward, 1953). This apparently small point in physiology probably preserved the fitness of the climbers and may have made the difference between success and failure in the final assault on the summit.

Output from the gastrointestinal tract. The small loss of water in the faeces is the balance of large exchanges which take place in the intestines. The saliva, the gastric secretions, the bile and the secretions of the pancreas and glands of the small intestine may together add up to 8 litres or more fluid daily. All but a small proportion of this is normally reabsorbed in the gut. If, however, there is diarrhoea, vomiting or an intestinal fistula, fluid losses may be large and cause dehydration. In infants and small children particularly, gastroenteritis with diarrhoea and vomiting may cause a rapid and dangerous reduction in the total body water.

Output from the kidneys. The volume of the urine is very variable and in general reflects the fluid intake but the minimum volume is determined by the nature of the diet.

The urine is normally more concentrated than the blood and to achieve this concentration the kidneys must do work. The concentrating power of the kidneys can be assessed from simple measurements of its specific gravity. A more precise assessment is obtained from measurements of osmolality, usually obtained by determining the effect of the urinary solutes in lowering the freezing point. Osmolality is expressed in terms of osmoles. One gram molecule in 1 kg of water of any un-ionised substance is equal to 1 osmol. When a substance is ionised forming cations and anions, both exert an osmotic effect. For monovalent ions 1 equivalent weight has an osmolality of 1 osmol, but for divalent ions one equivalent weight is equal to only 0.5 osmol. The fluids of the body are dilute and it is convenient to express their concentration in terms of milliosmoles (mosmol).

The osmolality of the blood is normally just under 300 mosmol and the healthy human kidney can produce urine with an osmolality of 1200 mosmol, i.e. it can concentrate the blood plasma four times. The concentrating power of the kidneys of many animals is much higher than this, particularly those who live in deserts and have to survive on a very limited water intake. The relation between the specific gravity and osmolality of the urine varies slightly, depending on the constituents of the urine. For a healthy subject on a good mixed diet the relationship is approximately as follows.

Sp. gr.	1.007	1.015	1.020	1.025	1.030	1.035
mosmol	400	600	800	1080	1200	1400

The main constituents of the urine are nitrogenous end products, of which over 80 per cent is usually urea, and sodium chloride. Although there are over 100 other substances present in urine, the amounts are normally so small that they contribute no more than about 15 per cent of the osmolality. As the amounts of urea and sodium chloride in the urine depend on the dietary intake of protein and salt, the osmolar load on the kidneys depends mainly on the dietary intake. Thus the diet determines the amount of work that the kidneys have to do.

Consider a diet providing 100 g of protein and 10 g of salt. The protein contains 16 g of nitrogen which must be excreted, mostly as urea. The molecular weight of urea is 60 of which 28 comes from its two atoms of nitrogen. Thus every gram of dietary nitrogen leads to the formation of just under 2 g of urea and the urine of the subject eating 100 g/day of protein contains about 30 g of urea. As the mol. wt of urea is 60, this is equivalent to 0.5 osmol or 500 mosmol. The 10 g of salt yield Na^+ and Cl^-, both in amounts of $(10 \times 1000)/58.5 = 170$ mmol, and their combined osmolar load is 340 mosmol. Thus the protein and salt in the diet produce an osmolar load of 840 mosmol. This figure may be arbitrarily raised to 1000 to take in the other urinary constituents. As the kidneys cannot concentrate urine normally to more than 1200 mosmol/litre, the subject must pass $1000/1200 = 830$ ml of urinary water. This is known as the **obligatory water** and is required to enable the kidneys to clear the dietary osmolar load. All people normally drink far more water than is essential for renal function. If the daily water intake of a person on the above diet was 1500 ml, then 670 ml of this can be described as **free water**. The conception of the division of the urinary water into obligatory and free portions, the obligatory being determined by the osmolar load of the diet, is useful under two circumstances. The first is when disease of the kidneys reduces their power of concentration. The second is when the supply of water is limited, as it may be to survivors of shipwreck in a lifeboat and to other castaways.

The normal control of the urine volume depends on a regulatory mechanism, elucidated mainly by Verney (1957), which involves a nerve centre in the hypothalamus and the antidiuretic hormone (ADH) secreted by the posterior pituitary gland, regulating fluid absorption in the renal tubules. The hypothalamus contains cells—osmoreceptors—which are sensitive to changes in concentration of the solutes in the plasma. A dilution of the plasma (as after drinking a glass of water) is sensed by the receptor cells which are connected by nerve fibres with the posterior pituitary gland. The secretion of ADH by the gland is inhibited, and a diuresis sets in. Conversely, if the plasma becomes concentrated, the osmoreceptors are stimulated and signal the posterior pituitary to increase the secretion of ADH and a diminished urine flow results. If the hypothalamus or posterior pituitary gland is injured by disease, secretion of the hormone may be impaired or stopped. Very large volumes of dilute urine are passed. This condition is known as diabetes insipidus.

Water balance in infancy
At birth the full function of the kidneys is not developed, and for the first two or three days of life the daily urinary volume is only about 20 ml. The volume of the colostrum may be little more than this. Kidney function improves simultaneously with the development of lactation. At 2 weeks the urinary volume is usually about 200 ml and the volume of milk ingested about 500 ml. At 3 months the volume of milk may be 800 to 900 ml and the urine volume about 300 ml daily. The excess water is eliminated by evaporation, at a higher rate than is usual in adults. Naturally there are great variations. Infants are particularly liable to lose large quantities of fluid by diarrhoea and vomiting. Indeed dehydration is a common and dangerous feature of many febrile illnesses in infancy and early childhood.

Water retention and depletion
Oedema. This is the condition when excess fluid in the body causes the subcutaneous tissues to swell and pit when pressure is applied with the finger. It is important to remember, however, that this simple clinical test is not very sensitive; oedema is not usually apparent until the limb volume is increased by 10 per cent or more (Drury and Jones, 1927). Overhydration sometimes results in oedema of the lungs which causes difficulty in breathing.

Dehydration. This can be suspected from the sunken features, particularly the eyes which recede into the orbits. The skin and tongue are dry. The skin becomes loose and lacks elasticity. On pinching it stands up, away from the subcutaneous tissue. The patient is usually, but not always, thirsty.

SALT

Man's need for sodium chloride has been a subject of dispute since the beginnings of medical practice. The first known salt mines have been found in the Austrian Tyrol and date from the late Bronze Age, about 1000 B C. In a scholarly review Kaunitz (1956) pointed out that it is not known accurately when man first began to use salt. Sanskrit and its daughter languages have no common root for salt, so perhaps the Indo-Europeans at the time of their first migrations did not know of its use. However, salt was certainly available in the early civilisations and Homer called it 'divine'. For at least 3000 years sodium chloride has played 'an amazingly important part in the lives of men. Wars have been fought over its sources, and for centuries its trade was more important than that of any other material' (Kaunitz). The salaries which we draw are in lineal descent from the salt money paid to the Roman soldiers. Imperial governments, such as those in the Roman provinces and in British India, have found a salt tax a convenient source of revenue; everyone paid it. This was because salt was the best food preservative available. Salted meat and fish were an important part of the diet in early times, yet a separate supply of salt in addition to that present in the food is not essential for man. There are good records of primitive people who do not use it (Glieber-mann, 1973).

Most people suffering from congestive cardiac failure or hypertension benefit if the sodium in their diet is restricted. The hormones of the adrenal cortex—and in particular aldosterone—are responsible for conserving the body's sodium and regulating the excretion of any excess. This is brought about by a direct effect on the renal tubules. It has been argued that the salting of food is a bad habit deleterious to health, in that it is liable to strain the regulating mechanisms of the adrenal cortex. The possible role of high salt intakes on the production of hypertension is discussed on page 341.

From these considerations it must be clear that to make recommendations of human needs for salt is very difficult. It is certainly true that the physiological processes of the body can go on without the deliberate addition of salt to food: yet many people have become accustomed to add salt at the table to food cooked with salt. Their taste buds would not accept only 5 g/day of salt as recommended by the Select Committee on Nutrition and Human Needs of the US Senate (1977).

SODIUM AND POTASSIUM IN THE BODY

The body of a healthy 65 kg man contains about 4000 mmol of Na, equivalent to 256 g NaCl. of this the major part, just over half, is in the extracellular fluid, about 1500 mmol is in bone and less than 500 mmol in the cells. When ^{24}Na is injected, it equilibrates rapidly with all the Na in the intra- and extracellular fluid, but only with a small part of that in bone. Total exchangeable sodium is about 2800 mmol or 40 mmol/kg. Most of the Na in bone forms part of the structure of the crystals of bone minerals and is not available as an immediate reserve.

By contrast, the potassium content of the extracellular fluids is only about 80 mmol, whereas the tissues contain about 3500 mmol. Four-fifths of this amount is in the skeletal muscles. The total potassium, measured with ^{42}K or ^{40}K, is a measure of the cell mass. ^{42}K is injected and its dilution after 24 hours is the total exchangeable potassium. ^{40}K is a natural isotope and is present as a small fraction (0.00119 per cent) of the potassium throughout nature; it emits gamma rays which may be measured in a whole body counter. The store of potassium in the bones is negligible.

SODIUM AND POTASSIUM BALANCES

Table 10.2 shows the sodium and potassium exchanges in a healthy young man. Intake is from the food only, as this subject took no table salt. Output is in the urine and faeces; occasionally significant amounts of sodium are lost in the sweat.

Table 10.2 The daily sodium and potassium balance of a young man leading a sedentary life on a normal diet (Passmore et al., 1955b)

	Sodium (mmol/day)	Potassium (mmol/day)
Intake:		
Food	135	60
Condiments	0	0
	135	60
Output:		
Urine	130	55
Faeces	5	10
Skin	negligible	negligible
Total	135	65
Balance	0	-5

Intake of sodium
Most normal people ingest 5 to 18 g NaCl/day, corresponding to 70 to 300 mmol Na. The food as served seldom contains more than 200 mmol Na/day; the remainder is taken as table salt.

Table 10.3 gives the sodium content of a selection of foods. In general, natural foods contain relatively little sodium, but large amounts may be added in cooking, either as NaCl or as sodium bicarbonate in baking powder. Also in most forms of processing and preserving, salt is added. Most bakers add salt to bread in a concentration of about 1 per cent; wheat flours contain less than one-hundredth of this amount in the natural state. Similarly butter, bacon and many other foods are commonly salted in preparation. Low sodium diets must therefore be prepared mainly from unprocessed vegetable foods. Foods of animal origin usually contain more sodium.

Diets low in sodium
The terms **restricted sodium regime** and **low sodium diet** are clearly defined in this section to avoid repetition and duplication; they are used with the same exact meaning in other chapters of this book.

Table 10.3 Sodium content of some common foods

Food	Description	Sodium mmol/100g	Sodium mg/100g
Rich sources			
Salami		78	1800
Fish	Smoked or kipper	43–78	1000–1800
Bacon	Raw, lean	83	1900
Beef	Corned	39	910
Ham	Boiled, lean	48	1100
Sausage	Raw	34	780
Bovril			
Marmite		200	460
Cornflakes		52	1200
Shellfish	Fresh, tinned	9–24	210–550
Bread	All extractions	24	560
Tomato juice	Canned	10	230
Worcester sauce		48–61	1100–1400
Tomato ketchup		48	1100
Butter	Fresh, salt	38	870
Vegetables	Tinned	10–14	230–330
Margarine		35	800
Biscuits	Savoury	26–52	610–1200
Cheese	Hard (Cheddar, etc.)	26	610
Moderate sources			
Milk	Fresh, whole	2	50
Fish	Fresh	4	100
Biscuits	Sweet	9–22	200–500
Beef, lamb & pork	Raw	3–4	60–90
Eggs	Fresh, whole	6	140
Cheese	Cream	13	300
Vegetables	Root, raw*	3–6	60–140
Flour	Self-raising	15	350
Wines		0.2–1.0	4–28
Beers		0.2–1.0	4–23
Pulses		1.3–2.6	30–60
Oatmeal	Raw	1.3	30
Cornflour		2.2	50
Cream	35% fat	1.3	30
Fruits	Dried, uncooked	1.3	30
Poor sources			
Fruit	Fresh	0.4–1.3	1–30
Prunes	Dried	0.52	12
Fruit juices	Fresh, canned	0.04–0.2	1–4
Vegetables	Other	0.09–0.6	2–13
Rice	Raw	0.3	6
Shredded wheat		0.3	8
Sago	Raw	0.1	3
Lard		0.09	2
Flour	Wheat, various	0.09–0.2	2–4
Nuts	Various, without shells unsalted	0.04–0.9	1–20
Sugar		0	0

* Beetroot, carrots, celery, radish, turnips, watercress.

Table 10.4 gives the sodium content of the regimes expressed in three different ways. Unfortunately each has been used indiscriminately by writers of textbooks, physicians, dietitians and laboratory workers. It is therefore important to make certain that in any discussion of the sodium content of a diet or article of food the unit is clearly stated.

The sodium content of all foods is subject to wide variations, and calculations of the content of diets based on tables are liable to an error of up to ±50 per cent.

Restricted salt regime. It is possible to reduce the dietary sodium intake to about a third of normal by eliminating the use of all table salt, reducing cooking salt to a minimum and by suitable selection of foods. A restricted salt regime

Table 10.4 Approximate daily intake of sodium on different regimes (1 mmol Na = 23 mg Na or 58.5 mg NaCl)

| | Sodium expressed as | | |
	mmol	g Na	g NaCl
A normal diet	150	3.5	9.0
Restricted salt regime	100	2.3	6.0
Low sodium diet, moderate	50	1.2	3.0
Low sodium diet, strict	25	0.6	1.5

allows the diet to be chosen from normal foods, but the foods which are rich sources of sodium should be excluded as far as possible or reduced to a minimum.

For most patients a restricted salt regime is a hardship, but one which can be undertaken for weeks or months with self-discipline. The regime does not exclude the sharing of meals with one's family or friends, but it does involve the selection of suitable articles of food.

The following points must be firmly impressed on patients and may be given to them as a printed list.
1. No table salt is permitted.
2. Salt used in cooking and baking powder must be reduced to a minimum.
3. Sodium-rich foods, such as ham and bacon, sausages, all tinned meats and fish, shellfish, cheese, all sauces (except special home-made ones) and all biscuits, scones and shop cakes must be avoided.
4. The maximum amount of ordinary bread allowed is five thin slices daily and the maximum amount of butter is 30 g daily.
5. Helpings of fresh meat and fish, should be small, and some vegetables naturally contain moderate amounts of sodium, e.g. beetroot, carrots, celery, radish, turnip and watercress. Potatoes are low in sodium if cooked without added salt, e.g. in their skins.
6. One egg and 250 ml (½ pint) of milk daily are allowed.
7. All fruits and nuts are permitted.
8. Sugar and jams, rice and sago are freely allowed.

Low sodium diets. With the use of special foods and dietary measures, the daily sodium intake can be greatly reduced (Diets No. 12 and No. 13). Strict adherence to such diets is necessary if these low intakes are to be achieved; the use of special salt-free bread and butter is essential. The provision of a low sodium diet is usually only possible for patients in hospital. If taken at home, expert dietary supervision and instruction are necessary. Salt-free bread and butter are not easy to obtain in many places.

By restricting the diet to washed rice, fruit and fruit juices, as first advocated by Kempner (1945), it is possible to reduce the sodium intake to below 10 mmol/day. Patients find this diet monotonous and unappetising. Hence it is seldom recommended.

Uraemia may develop in a patient with cardiac or renal disease who is on a low sodium diet. The doctor must keep this danger in mind.

Intake of potassium

The potassium content of foodstuffs is very variable; natural diets provide from 50 to 150 mmol K/day. The usual figure is about 65 mmol/day, equivalent to 5 g of potassium chloride. Potassium deficiency or excess (p. 88) rarely arise primarily as a result of dietary deficiency or excess: nor is the treatment of such conditions confined to simple dietary corrections.

Table 10.5 shows that most of the common foods contain moderate amounts. Cereals (including rice and wheat), cheese, eggs, fats and almost all fresh fruits contain less than 8 mmol/100 g and have been used in constructing low potassium diets. There are certainly great variations in the potassium content of different samples of the same food. The figures in the table are really only of illustrative value and in accurate metabolic balance studies it is essential to determine the potassium content of the diet by analysis of a sample.

Output in the urine

Output of sodium. Most of the daily output of sodium is in the urine which usually contains 100 to 200 mmol/24 hours, and reflects the dietary intake. Concentrations range from 40 to 100 mmol/litre. In most subjects studied a well-marked diurnal variation in sodium excretion has been found. The highest excretion is usually at

Table 10.5 Potassium content of foods—rich and moderate sources (ranked in descending order of potassium per usual serving)

| Food | Potassium | |
	mmol/100g	mg/100g
Potatoes (chips)	25	1020
Treacle (molasses)	37	1470
Milk, fresh, whole	4	150
Beef, lamb, poultry	7–9	300–350
All Bran	27	1070
Fish, various types	6–9	230–360
Chocolate, drinking	10	410
Soya flour	41–51	1660–2030
Dried fruits, various, raw	18–47	710–1880
Fruit, fresh	2–11	65–430
Fruit juices, pure, canned	3–7	110–260
Vegetables, raw, salad	4–27	140–1080
Vegetables, boiled	1–10	50–400
Breakfast cereals	2–15	100–600
Coffee, instant	100	4000
Nuts	9–23	350–940
Rice, polished, raw	3	110
Bread, white and brown	2–5	100–220
Syrup, golden	6	240
Eggs, fresh, whole	4	140
Biscuits, savoury	4–12	140–500
Biscuits, sweet	2–6	90–230
Cheese, full fat	3–5	110–190
Jam	2	100

Foods low in potassium are honey, cream, butter, margarine, brown and white sugar, corn starch, cooking oils, beer and tea.

about midday and the lowest at night. The kidney tubules can conserve sodium by reabsorbing most of the sodium reaching them in the glomerular filtrate. This regulatory mechanism is controlled by aldosterone. If the body sodium is depleted as by excessive sweating, reabsorption may be almost complete and sodium chloride can no longer be detected in the urine by the test of adding silver nitrate, which yields a white precipitate of silver chloride. This test is useful in clinical practice in the tropics as an indication of the extent of a primary salt deficiency arising as a result of excessive sweating. In temperate climates difficulties of interpretation, arising from other factors, make the test of little value.

The efficiency of the aldosterone-renal tubule mechanism for conserving sodium is of great biological value. When the adrenal cortex is destroyed in Addison's disease this mechanism is upset and large amounts of sodium are lost in the urine. Many of the clinical features of Addison's disease—notably the muscular weakness and low blood-pressure—result from lack of sodium in the body and can be relieved by giving sufficient salt. In chronic renal failure the kidneys' ability to conserve sodium is often impaired and patients may become markedly depleted of sodium.

Healthy kidneys have no difficulty in excreting any quantity of salt that may be taken in the diet, provided there is a sufficient excretion of water. As already stated, the kidneys cannot concentrate the urine above a specific gravity of about 1.035. This limit to the kidneys' capacity to excrete salt is of practical importance for survival in deserts or after shipwreck, when fresh water may not be available.

Sodium accumulates in the body in congestive heart failure and in certain types of kidney disease. Therapeutic doses of cortisone or other adrenal cortical hormones also inhibit sodium excretion and so may lead to sodium excess in the tissues.

Output of potassium. This reflects closely the dietary potassium intake. In healthy people on a normal diet it is around 60 mmol/24 hours. Increased amounts of potassium are found in the urine whenever the tissues are losing potassium. Perhaps the most important cause is a breakdown of cellular proteins such as occurs in diabetes, in underfeeding and after injury. In most tissues 1 g of nitrogen is associated with about 2.7 mmol of potassium. By means of metabolic studies it is possible to determine from the nitrogen and potassium balance the K/N ratio of the cellular material lost or gained; this may be a useful guide to changes in the cells. Some potassium can be displaced from the cells by an excess of other cations, especially H^+. Any condition giving rise to acidosis is liable to cause cellular depletion of potassium.

In patients given diuretics, e.g. the thiazide group, to increase the output of sodium and water in the urine an important side-effect is a concomitant increase of potassium excretion. This can lead to potassium depletion if the intake is not supplemented. In severe renal failure, either in acute anuria or in the late stages of chronic renal disease, the normal intake of potassium is not excreted in the urine and a state of potassium excess occurs.

Output in the gastrointestinal tract
In health the faeces contain very small amounts of sodium (about 5 mmol/day) and only a little more potassium. The digestive juices contain large amounts of both, but these are normally reabsorbed in the gut. However, diarrhoea may cause large losses in the stools; in this way the body may be depleted in amounts up to 90 mmol/24 hours of both sodium and potassium. When severe diarrhoea is present in infants suffering from protein–energy malnutrition, potassium deficiency frequently develops and as much as 10 to 30 per cent of the total body potassium may be lost; this may be responsible for sudden cardiac failure. Similar losses can also occur in adults with diarrhoea, either acute or chronic, and from intestinal fistulae.

Output through the skin. Unless there is active sweating, the loss of sodium through the skin is small and usually neglected in balance studies. When there is active sweating the situation is very different. The sodium content of sweat varies greatly from one individual to another, but generally lies within the range 20 to 80 mmol/l. People acclimatised to heat usually conserve some of their body sodium by secreting a dilute sweat containing only about 30 mmol/l. As the daily volume of sweat may be several litres (14 litres is the measured record) sodium losses from this source may be very large and much greater than the urinary loss. In such circumstances, unless there is a corresponding increase in salt intake, sodium depletion soon follows.

Sweat contains about 9 mmol/l of potassium, range 5 to 16 (Ahlman *et al.*, 1952) and losses from the skin are usually negligible.

Sodium depletion
Sodium depletion is characteristically associated with dehydration, as for instance in heat exhaustion. The essential chemical pathology is a reduction in the extracellular fluid. The blood volume is also reduced and the red cells form a higher proportion of the blood volume, shown by a high haematocrit value. As a result of the low blood volume the veins are collapsed, blood-pressure is low and the pulse is rapid. Sodium chloride usually cannot be detected in the urine. Thirst may be absent, although the mouth is dry. Mental apathy is usually noticeable. Loss of appetite and vomiting may also be present. In pure sodium deficiency, muscular cramps occur and are well known to miners who work in hot pits. A full account of the symptoms and signs of salt deficiency is given by McCance (1936), based on observations made on himself and his

students after experimental depletion. A guide to the extent of the deficiency of both sodium and water is provided by the concentration of serum sodium and the haematocrit reading (normal values, 135 to 145 mmol Na/l and 38 to 47 per cent). Although sodium and water deficiency can usually be detected easily enough from the history and clinical examination, the extent of the deficiency cannot be so easily judged.

It is now well recognised that sodium depletion may be present without water depletion—a condition which has been called **water intoxication.** This is fully described and discussed by Black (1968). The condition occurs when thirst provoked by heavy sweating is quenched by water to which no salt has been added. It may also arise in the treatment of water or sodium deficiency if too much water is given either intravenously or by mouth. In addition to anorexia, weakness and mental apathy, there may be muscular twitchings, convulsions and even coma from oedema of the brain which may be difficult to distinguish from uraemia.

Sodium excess
Any excess of sodium in the body accumulates principally in the extracellular fluids. The increased concentration of sodium is partially offset by an increase in these fluids. Sodium excess may result in oedema. Rats fed on diets containing a large excess of salt develop enlarged hearts with high blood pressure and abnormal electrocardiograms. In some the kidneys are also enlarged and glomerulonephritis may occur. Experimental chronic salt toxicity was described by Youmans (1957), but he is properly cautious in applying these results to man. Dahl (1972) gives epidemiological evidence associating the high incidence of raised blood pressure in certain countries with an habitual high salt intake.

The ideal sodium intake for infants is that of breast milk. In the first 3 months of life unmodified cow's milk with its higher sodium carries a risk of hypernatraemia. Weanling rats are more susceptible to the hypertensive effect of a high sodium intake. Both the Committee on Nutrition of the American Academy of Pediatrics (1974) and the Department of Health and Social Security (1974) advise that salt should not be added during processing or preparation of infant foods.

Potassium deficiency
The chief features of potassium deficiency are muscular weakness and mental confusion. The weakness is well illustrated by a rare disease, familial periodic paralysis. The patient is subject to recurrent attacks of muscular weakness and paralysis which last for several hours. The attacks are associated with low levels of plasma potassium. They are probably caused by a periodic oversecretion of aldosterone by the adrenal cortex.

The absence of characteristic symptoms makes it diffi-

cult to recognise potassium deficiency clinically. The concentration of potassium in the plasma may bear little relation to the amount in the tissues. When tissues are breaking down and losing potassium, plasma concentrations may actually be higher than normal.

The cardiac muscle is involved in the general muscular weakness. The electrocardiogram commonly shows S–T depression and a broad low T wave. Sudden death is a possible consequence.

The smooth muscle of the small intestine may become paralysed (**paralytic ileus**); this leads to abdominal distension, which may be an important early sign of potassium deficiency, especially in children.

Patients with chronic diarrhoea or a chronic wasting disease or those on long-term diuretic therapy nearly always need an oral supplement of about 50 to 100 mmol of potassium daily, best given as slow-release potassium tablets. Intravenous potassium is always needed in diabetic ketoacidosis and in severe acute diarrhoea. Infants and young children are especially at risk of potassium deficiency, because of the small reserves in their tissues.

Potassium excess
The toxic effects of potassium fall first on skeletal and cardiac muscle and so broadly resemble the effects of depletion (hyperkalaemia). Muscular weakness and mental apathy are generally marked. The electrocardiogram may show tall peaked T waves. Concentrations of potassium in the blood are above the normal range of 3.8 to 5.0 mmol/l. Causes of potassium excess include renal failure, adrenal insufficiency or shock after injury, in which condition the potassium can leak out into the blood from the damaged cells. An excessive dose of potassium given by vein may cause death by stopping the heart. The need to supplement with potassium by mouth the diet of patients receiving diuretics of the chlorothiazide class has brought to light a new hazard. Ulceration of the small bowel may occur, needing surgical treatment. The probable cause is the presence of localised high concentrations of potassium in the intestinal fluids (Ashby et al., 1965).

CHLORIDE

Chloride is taken into the body largely as sodium chloride and excretion of Cl^- in the urine, sweat and gastrointestinal tract usually follows closely the excretion of Na. Plasma Cl lies between 98 and 106 mmol/l. However, Cl^- may be lost to the body in urine in association with NH_4^-, or in vomit in association with H^+. This leads to the subject of acid–base equilibrium.

ACID–BASE BALANCE

Human life is possible only if the blood is kept within a

narrow range of alkalinity. In health the blood is maintained between pH 7.35 and 7.45. This precise equilibrium is maintained by two mechanisms. First, the rate of excretion of carbonic acid (a weak acid) through the lungs acts as a very fine adjustment. Secondly, the kidneys are able to excrete urine with either an acid or an alkaline reaction. In disease of the lungs or of the kidneys, these controlling mechanisms may no longer work normally and an acidosis or alkalosis results. Such effects are of great interest to the physiologist and of much practical importance to the physician, but are outside the scope of this book. Here we shall be concerned only with the dietary aspect of acid–base balance which, compared with the renal and respiratory aspects, is very minor.

It has long been known that the urine of the rabbit is normally alkaline and the urine of the dog acid. This is related to the nature of their diets. The fresh urine of an omnivorous animal is usually slightly acid, but in vegetarians it is often neutral, and in large meat-eaters more strongly acid. This is chiefly because sulphuric acid is produced by metabolic oxidation of the sulphur amino acids in protein, and phosphoric acid is formed from the oxidation of nucleoproteins and phospholipids. The hydrogen ion produced in this way on a mixed diet is around 70 mmol/day (Black, 1968). Except when kidney function is seriously impaired (Chap. 44) the pH of the blood is easily maintained by the kidneys excreting a correspondingly more or less acid urine.

Fruits and vegetables are alkali-producing foods, but they may taste acidic and are often thought to be 'acid' foods. Many food faddists and some physicians (who should know better) have made much of the 'acidity' of fruits and vegetables. This acidity is due to the presence in plant tissues of a variety of organic acids—citric acid (citrus fruits, pineapple, tomato and most summer fruits), malic acid (apples, plums and tomatoes), benzoic acid (cranberry and bilberry), tartaric acid (grapes), oxalic acid (strawberries, unripe tomatoes, rhubarb and spinach). Sinclair and Hollingsworth (1969) give some details of the amount of acid present in fruits and vegetables. They state that very few foods are ever as acid as gastric juice. Further, the body can easily oxidise malic and citric acid. Benzoic acid is excreted by the kidney as hippuric acid. Tartaric acid is hardly absorbed at all. Oxalic acid forms insoluble calcium salts and so is not easily absorbed from the intestines; nevertheless it can also be oxidised and excreted. Figures given by Sinclair and Hollingsworth indicate that the intake of these acids, even from large quantities of fruits and vegetables, is well within the capacity of the body to deal with them. They do not cause acidosis. The digestive disturbances from which young gentlemen are known to suffer after an illicit visit to an orchard are attributable to sudden intake of large quantities of indigestible dietary fibre.

However, there are two organic acids produced within the body which can give rise to acidosis. These are lactic and acetoacetic acid. Large quantities of lactic acid may accumulate in the blood after severe muscular exercise (up to 10 mmol/l). The rapid breathing during recovery from exercise helps to restore the acid–base balance by blowing off carbonic acid.

In many pathological states the tissues are inadequately oxygenated and then lactic acid accumulates, e.g. in heart failure. A serious form of **lactic acid acidosis** arises as a medical emergency in some patients with diabetes and liver disorders in the absence of tissue hypoxia. It is precipitated by drugs, especially biguanides, and by intravenous infusion of fructose.

Acetoacetic acid (and its derivative β-hydroxybutyric acid) are produced in excess in diabetes that has been inadequately treated and in other conditions in which fat metabolism predominates (p. 358). These acids accumulate in the blood and as both are stronger acids than carbonic acid, they displace the bicarbonate in the blood. As a result the dangerous condition of acidosis develops. Ketone bodies are excreted in and present in blood plasma in fasting and starvation but acidosis is rare unless renal function becomes impaired.

11. Minerals

Man's food, whether of vegetable or animal origin, is derived from the soil or the sea. The chemical composition of both depends on the rocks that lie beneath them. These are composed of complex mineral salts which contain many elements. The classification of these from a nutritional point of view presents difficulties, and no classification is altogether satisfactory. Salts of sodium and potassium are for the most part readily soluble in water. They are easily absorbed from the alimentary canal and, as they form the main cations of the body fluids, are usually considered along with water (Chapter 10). Most of the other elements, but not iodine and fluorine, are present in salts which are relatively insoluble. Consequently they are not easily absorbed from the gut. Further, they are for the most part present in the plasma bound to one of the proteins. Hence they are only excreted in the urine in small amounts, and the major proportion of the dietary intake appears in the faeces. The amounts present in the tissues are regulated by the control of absorption in the small intestine, in which the epithelial cells play a major role.

Deficiency of an element in the tissues is less likely to arise from deficiency in dietary intake than from factors in the diet reducing absorption or from a disorder of the absorbing epithelium.

An excessive concentration of any of these elements in the tissues has adverse effects. This may arise if there is so large an amount in the diet that the controlling mechanism in the small intestine is overwhelmed. It may also arise if the element enters the tissues by other route; excess iron may accumulate as a result of repeated blood transfusions, and excess lead from atmospheric pollution and absorption through the lungs.

Calcium, magnesium, phosphorus and sulphur are important components of bone and other supporting tissues. They are considered first, together with strontium. The latter is always associated in small amounts with calcium in bone. It is only of importance because of the hazards that may arise from the presence of the isotope ^{90}Sr from the fall-out from atomic explosions which may contaminate food.

This chapter concludes with iron and zinc. Other elements are considered in the next chapter, starting with iodine and fluorine. Fe, Zn, I and F all have important physiological roles. Others present in biological material in very small amounts and known as **trace elements** are components of enzyme systems and are therefore essential nutrients. A final set of elements, of which strontium has already been mentioned, appear to have no role in metabolism and their presence in foods and tissues seems to be adventitious. Some are known only by their toxic effects. Metallic elements may enter the body through contamination of foods and drinking water by the atmosphere as a result of the use of these elements in industry.

Knowledge of the amounts of trace elements in foods and tissues and of their effects on health was rudimentary until a few years ago owing to the difficulties of analysis by orthodox chemical methods. The development of atomic absorption spectrometry has revolutionised analytical procedure and is leading to rapid advances in understanding of their nutritional roles. The account given in Chapter 12 is partly based on the report of a WHO Expert Committee (1973). A useful account of a human metabolic study of the dietary intake and urinary and faecal excretion of six trace elements is also available (Robinson *et al.*, 1973). The textbook by Underwood (1977) is recommended for reference.

A bewildering variety of units have been used to express results. To clarify the exposition and allow better comparisons between different elements, much of the quantitative data is given in molar units. The atomic weight of each element is given which enables the reader to convert data in the literature into these units.

CALCIUM
Ca (at. wt 40)

The body of an adult normally contains about 1200 g of calcium. At least 99 per cent of this amount is present in the skeleton, where calcium salts (chiefly phosphate) held in a cellular matrix provide the hard structure of the bones and teeth. Obviously all of this calcium comes from the diet. Among common foods, milk is much the richest source, which is one reason why milk and cheese are especially valuable for growing children. Half a litre (just under a pint) of cow's milk contains about 0.6 g of calcium. Most other foods contribute much smaller amounts. The calcium retained in the normal human skeleton has therefore been extracted from a very large volume of food, even when the diet has contained abundant milk and cheese. For reviews of calcium metabolism with special reference to nutrition the reader is referred to reviews by Leitch (1964), Fourman and Royer (1968) and Nordin (1976).

CALCIUM IN THE SKELETON

In life the skeleton is not made up of dry bones, as seen in a museum. Bone contains a living cellular matrix on which the minerals are deposited. Its chemical composition is approximately water 25 per cent, protein 20 per cent, fat 5 per cent, small amounts of glycosaminoglycans and nearly 50 per cent mineral. Most of the mineral is the calcium salt, hydroxapatite $Ca_{10}(PO_4)_6(OH)_2$, but there are small and variable amounts of magnesium, sodium carbonate and citrate.

About 200 years ago John Hunter showed that the architecture of the bones is completely reorganised during the process of growth; no single strut or brace of bone remains fixed and permanent in any part of the body. Two different kinds of cells are constantly altering the structure of the bones, even in adult life. While the osteoblasts lay down fresh calcium salts, especially where new stresses have developed, osteoclasts are constantly eroding redundant calcium deposits. A well-adjusted equilibrium exists between the calcium coming and going from the bones and the calcium present in small but normally constant amounts in the fluids of the body. In an adult man about 700 mg of calcium enter and leave the bones daily (Whedon, 1964). Thus the bones not only provide physcial support to the body but also a large reserve of two essential elements—calcium and phosphorus—on which the body can draw in case of need.

Effects of age

In a young child the skeleton is replaced completely in between one and two years. In an adult its metabolism is slower and the turnover probably takes 10 to 12 years. After the bones have stopped growing in length at about the age of 18 or earlier in a girl, they may continue to get slightly more dense for a few years, but by the age of 40

years or earlier they begin to atrophy (Exton-Smith *et al.*, 1969). There is no change in the quality of older bones which have the same histological structure and chemical composition, but their substance is slowly reduced. This atrophy, known as **osteoporosis,** is part of the ageing process like greying of the hair and hardening of the lenses of the eyes. Like these processes, osteoporosis with advancing age cannot be prevented, but it proceeds at varying rates in individuals and there are possibilities that it may be slowed down. Osteoporosis in itself causes no disability, except that the bones are more liable to break. When the condition is advanced, trivial injuries may cause a fracture. An old lady may break the neck of her femur when she falls after tripping up on a carpet. Such fractures in the old are common and not only cause much suffering and disability, but are also an economic problem to the community owing to the number of hospital beds and staff required for their care.

Measurements of bone mass

The volume of a bone changes with age, but as it atrophies, its mass is reduced and its density falls. The shadow of a bone on a radiograph can give a measure of its density. Owing to variations in the amount of soft tissue around the bones and in the times of exposure and development, routine radiographs are an insensitive index of bone density. Probably about 40 per cent of the bone mass has to be lost before a diagnosis of osteoporosis can be made. However, these technical difficulties can be overcome and radiographic measurements of bone density have been made for research purposes. Figure 11.1 shows the ageing of bone in the two sexes. The data are derived from radiographs of the first metacarpal bone of the wrist under standardised conditions, from which an estimate of the area of dense cortical bone is made and the ratio of this to

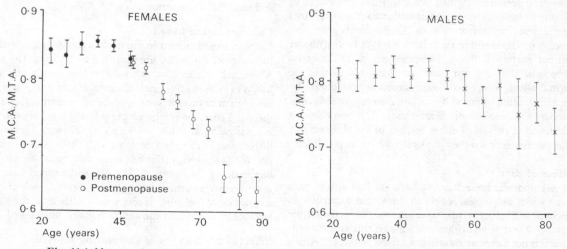

Fig. 11.1 Metacarpal cortical/total area ratios in normal men and women (mean ± S.D.) (redrawn from Nordin, 1971).

the total bone area on the film is an index of the bone density. Similar data from the USA are presented by Garn (1972).

Information about both the chemical composition and histological structure of bone can also be obtained by examination of a bone biopsy. For this purpose a small plug of bone, usually from the crest of the iliums is taken with a special trephine; the procedure is done under local anaesthesia and is simple. Inevitably the sample taken is a very small fraction of the skeleton and the value of the method is limited by the finding of large differences in samples from the same subjects taken close together.

Effects of hormones

Figure 11.1 shows a sharp decline in the density of bone in women following the menopause. Clinically this appears as a great increase in the incidence of fractures, especially fractures of the wrist after a fall, at this period of life. It is attributed to the loss of oestrogens secreted by the ovary. Osteoporosis is also a feature of several endocrine disorders, e.g. Cushing's disease, hyperparathyroidism and hyperthyroidism, and it follows the prolonged use of corticosteroid hormones for therapeutic purposes. There is thus no doubt that the maintenance of bone throughout life is dependent on the correct balance between the various endocrine secretions. Oestrogens have been given to large numbers of women and androgens to men with the aim of reversing or delaying the progress of osteoporosis. Unfortunately there is no clear evidence that either hormone has had any such effect. However, in women who had had bilateral oophorectomy the oestrogen, mestranol, significantly delayed bone mineral loss provided treatment was started soon after the operation (Aitken et al., 1973).

Effect of immobilisation

If a young person is confined to bed by illness the output of calcium in the urine goes up and well marked osteoporosis may develop in a few months. Osteoporosis may also develop in a limb still more quickly if it is put into a plaster and not exercised. Bones, like other organs of the body, atrophy if they are not used. In many old people the normal ageing process of osteoporosis is accelerated by inactivity, often imposed by various chronic diseases, e.g. osteoarthritis and chronic heart disease. The best chance a middle-aged person of either sex has of avoiding serious osteoporosis is to keep as physically active as possible.

Effect of diet

An osteoporotic bone has lost both calcium and protein and so it is not unreasonable to think that a diet low in calcium and protein might accelerate the osteoporotic process. There is no evidence to support this view. Osteoporosis is not more common in those parts of Asia and Africa where diets are low in these nutrients than in the well fed countries of Europe and North America (Nordin, 1966).

Indeed in the USA osteoporosis is probably more common in the white than in the Negro population, who in general eat poorer diets. Similarly in South Africa osteoporosis is more common in Blacks than Whites (Walker et al., 1971). This difference might be due to a genetic factor or more probably to differences in physical activity. Garn (1972) found no correlation between dietary calcium and density of bone in middle-aged subjects.

If patients with severe osteoporosis are given large amounts of calcium either in the diet or as a calcium salt, some of this is retained in the body and they go into positive calcium balance at least for a short time. Yet there is no clinical or radiographic evidence that this slows down or reverses the osteoporotic process.

Calcium deficiency alone has produced rickets in an infant (Kooh et al., 1977). A 10 month infant developed all the clinical, radiological and biochemical signs of rickets after receiving a diet based on lamb with no milk because of disaccharide intolerance; calcium intake was estimated at 180 mg/day, but a multivitamin preparation had provided 10 μg of vitamin D every day. His rickets responded to the addition of an unfortified skimmed milk formula to the diet while his vitamin D was temporarily withdrawn.

CALCIUM OUTWITH THE SKELETON

The amount of calcium in the extracellular fluids and soft tissues of a normal adult does not exceed 10 g. Calcium has an important role in determining the excitability of peripheral nerves and muscle including the heart. It is essential for the clotting of blood. Sodium oxalate is often added to samples of blood drawn for chemical analysis to precipitate the calcium and so prevent clotting. The enzyme rennin is dependent on calcium for its activity. This enzyme is secreted by the stomach of young mammals and causes the curdling of milk (i.e. clotting of caseinogen) as a preliminary to digestion. Calcium activates a number of enzymes and moderates the action of cyclic AMP.

Calcium in the blood

Calcium concentration in the plasma normally lies within the range of 2.1 to 2.6 mmol/1 (8.5 to 10.5 mg/100 ml). About half this amount is bound to plasma albumin and half is in ionised solution. If the level of albumin plasma is lower than normal in consequence of protein deficiency, there is a corresponding reduction in the level of protein-bound calcium. This produces no obvious metabolic disturbance, in marked contrast to the effects of a reduction in the ionised portion of plasma calcium as sometimes happens, e.g. in rickets. If the pH of the blood rises (as after excessive vomiting with loss of chloride anions) the ionisation of calcium is depressed although the total amount of calcium in the serum remains unchanged.

Effects of reduction in circulating ionised calcium

The motor nerves become over-susceptible to stimuli.

This particularly affects the face, hands and feet, producing the twitching known clinically as **tetany**. Muscles lose tone and become flaccid, so that infants with rickets are late in sitting, standing and walking. The isolated animal heart ceases to beat when transfused with fluid lacking calcium; however, there is no good evidence that calcium deficiency in the myocardium is ever a cause of heart failure in man.

CALCIUM INTAKE

Before birth and during lactation. For the fetus the supply is assured, since the mother's body always yields all the calcium that it requires. If she is short of calcium herself she may develop osteomalacia in consequence. In this sense, the fetus is a true parasite. After birth the infant becomes dependent for the first time on a dietary source to supply the calcium necessary for the development of his bones. The natural source is his mother's milk, which provides about 30 mg Ca/100 ml, no matter how malnourished she may be. Nevertheless intestinal absorption of calcium is probably enhanced both in pregnancy and during lactation. Malnutrition is more important in influencing the volume of milk that the mother can yield, though this varies very much, even in apparent health. Test-weighings of infants before and after breast feeds show that a good mother produces on average 500 ml milk/day after a few weeks and at 6 months 1 litre or more, providing at least 300 mg/day of calcium. Cow's milk contains about four times more calcium (roughly 120 mg/100 ml). This is not surprising since a calf calcifies its skeleton much faster than a human infant. There is no evidence that infants fed cow's milk, and therefore having a higher calcium intake than breast-fed infants, suffer any disability from the excess. Indeed in the first few days of life, a failure of calcium absorption in infants on preparations of cow's milk may lead to tetany.

In childhood and later life. Table 11.1 shows the calcium content of some common foods. Milk and cheese are the most valuable sources. However, pulses, other vegetables and particularly cereal grains contribute. In diets where cereals provide more than 50 per cent of the energy, they also provide a major part of the calcium.

Drinking water can provide significant amounts. In Britain the average intake from this source is about 75 mg Ca/day; but the variations are large: from almost nil in water from peaty hill lochs in Scotland to 200 mg or more in London water drawn from chalk or limestone areas.

Absorption

The calcium content of a diet is no direct index of the amount actually utilised since absorption in the gut is always far from complete. Normally between 70 and 80 per cent is excreted in the faeces. Absorption is an active process which depends on an adequate supply of oxygen and of glucose or other source of energy. The many factors that influence the extent of calcium absorption are still not fully understood, though some at least are known, as described in the following paragraphs. The subject has

Table 11.1 Calcium content of some common foods (Selected values from various food tables)

Food	Description	Range (mg/100 g or 100 ml)
Cheese	Hard—from whole or skimmed milk	400–1200
Cheese	Soft—from whole or skimmed milk, and processed	60–725
Milk	Cow's—fresh whole	120
Milk	Human	35
Nuts	Various—without shells	13–250
Pulses	Raw—dried	40–150
Herring	Raw—edible parts	33
Roots, gourds and stems	Raw—various, except potato	20–80
Vegetables★	Raw—green, leafy	25–250
Eggs	Fresh, whole	50–60
Oatmeal	Raw, 65 per cent extraction	55–60
Whole wheat	100 per cent extraction	30–40
Wheat flour †	70 per cent extraction	13–20
Millets	Most varieties	20–50
Fruits	Various—raw, fresh	3–60
Fish ‡	Fresh	17–32
Beef, mutton, pork and poultry	Raw—edible portions	3–24
Maize	Various millings	5–18
Rice	Raw, polished	4
Potatoes	Raw—all seasons	7–10

★Green vegetables most commonly used in temperate climates all fall in the lower part of the range and therefore contribute little to the calcium content of the diet.
† In Britain this is fortified and Ca is 140 mg/100 g.
‡ Sardines and other small fish eaten whole provide anything up to 400 mg Ca/100 g and may therefore be important sources of calcium.

been reviewed by Malm (1958) and by Kodicek (1967).

Substances assisting absorption

Vitamin D. This vitamin is essential for absorption of calcium. The active derivative 1,25 dihydroxy vitamin D acts by promoting the synthesis of a carrier protein (p. 123).

Proteins. Absorption of calcium from the small intestine is influenced by the nature of other nutrients undergoing absorption at the same time. McCance and his colleagues (1942) demonstrated the importance of proteins in facilitating calcium absorption. The probable explanation is that amino acids liberated in the course of protein digestion form soluble calcium salts which are easily absorbed. Any advantage from increased absorption is likely to be more than counterbalanced by the increased urinary loss of calcium on high protein diets.

Lactose. This enhances the absorption of calcium in animals. In man this action appears to depend on the hydrolysis of lactose. This has prompted the suggestion that persistence of small intestinal lactase beyond infancy in people of northern European stock has developed by natural selection because it would reduce the risk of rickets (Flatz and Rotthauwe, 1973).

Substances interfering with absorption

Phytic acid. Mellanby (1925) showed that puppies developed rickets when fed a diet poor in vitamin D and calcium, and containing large amounts of bread. The puppies that ate the most bread grew fastest and developed the most severe rickets. Mellanby at first attributed this to the growth-promoting properties of the bread, which allowed the puppies to grow at a rate faster than their bones could lay down calcium. He soon found, however, that the effect was not due solely to the quantity of bread eaten; there were also qualitative differences. Whole wheat flour was more rachitogenic than white flour, and oatmeal worse than either. The fascinating story of the elucidation of the nature of this anticalcifying factor in cereals was well told by Mellanby (1950). In brief, it was eventually proved that the factor is phytic acid (inositol phosphoric acid).

McCance and Widdowson (1942) published the first human experiments on the dietary influence of phytic acid.

1. Less calcium is absorbed from diets consisting largely of brown bread than from those consisting largely of white.
2. The amount of calcium absorbed from diets containing brown bread could be raised by adding calcium to the bread.
3. The absorption of calcium from white bread could be prevented by adding sodium phytate.
4. The absorption of calcium from brown bread diets could be improved by removing phytic acid from the bread. The latter point is illustrated in Table 11.2 taken from their data.

These experimental results become available at a crucial time in the World War II when the outcome of the Battle of the Atlantic still lay in the balance. Food from North America was vital, but there were not enough ships to transport it; consequently a change from white bread to bread containing more of the whole grain became essential. The advice given by the Medical Research Council was that calcium carbonate should be added to the new 'National Loaf' in amounts sufficient to offset its increased content of phytic acid.

Since that time of crisis there have been some second thoughts. In the first place many cereals contain an enzyme—phytase—which splits phytic acid so that it no longer binds calcium and makes it unavailable for absorption. Rye in particular and also wheat contain enough phytase to destroy much of the phytic acid during the leavening of bread when conditions for enzymic action are good. Thus although 50 per cent or more of the phosphorus in the original whole grain may be in the form of phytic acid, the amount in the bread may be much less. However, oats contain little phytase and what there is may be destroyed by commercial kiln heating. This perhaps accounts for their tendency to produce rickets in puppies. Mellanby's animal experiments suggest that rickets would be especially common among porridge-eating Highlanders in Scotland. In fact the disease was never prevalent in Scotland except in the cities. Mellanby himself suggested that the amount of milk taken with porridge might provide enough calcium to offset the rachitogenic properties of oatmeal, but perhaps there is a better explanation. Cruickshank and his colleagues (1945) struck a blow in defence of the honour of Scotland's traditional cereal when they showed in four Aberdonian volunteers that the phytate phosphorus present in oatmeal was hydrolysed in the gut and so caused little interference with the absorption of calcium. Perhaps the important point is that in those who eat oatmeal regularly the digestive juices acquire the ability to split calcium phytate. For puppies, on the other hand, oatmeal is an unfamiliar food.

Most nutritionists agree with Walker (1951), who in a scholarly review of the subject concluded that 'the importance of phytic acid as an anticalcifying factor in human nutrition has not been established'. His chief argument against the interpretation of the experiments of McCance and Widdowson is that they were not continued long enough for the subjects to become adapted to the change in diet. However, Indian children in Britain, when their diet is based on chapattis, may develop rickets and it is possible that this may be due in part to impaired absorption of calcium, caused by a high intake of phytic acid (Ford *et al.*, 1972).

Dietary fibre. Dietary fibre from plants low in phytate binds calcium in proportion to its uronic acid content. Uronic acids can be digested by bacteria in the colon and this may be part of the process whereby calcium absorp-

Table 11.2 Intake and absorption of calcium on diets largely composed of bread

Bread	Subject 1			Subject 2		
	Intake	Absorption		Intake	Absorption	
			%			%
	mg/day	mg/day	of intake	mg/day	mg/day	of intake
Brown	550	89	16	522	57	11
Dephytinised brown	590	231	39	566	169	30
White	488	250	51	478	219	46

tion is increased slowly after a change to a high fibre diet (James *et al.*, 1978).

Phosphate. Before the discovery of phytic acid it was generally believed that phosphate intake had a crucial influence on calcium absorption. This belief originated from experiments showing that a high dietary Ca/P ratio caused rickets in rats.

Subsequent human experiments show that phosphate intake has little or no influence on calcium absorption, at least within the range within which these normally occur in foodstuffs. Malm (1953) for instance, showed that six Norwegian men given excess phosphate by mouth in amounts sufficient to provide an extra 250 to 1000 mg P/day for four to eight weeks, maintained their normal calcium balance. In breast-fed babies, a supplement of phosphates did not hinder absorption of calcium (Widdowson *et al.*, 1963).

Ca/P ratios in food can therefore be forgotten, along with other once popular but now outmoded scientific fashions. This firm dictum appeared in the first edition. We see no reason to modify it, as regards normal diets, and it is supported by a later study (Spencer *et al.*, 1975). However, the absorption of calcium in the first few weeks of life from artificial milks presents special problems. (Widdowson, 1965). In such preparations the Ca/P ratio may be important.

Fats. Fatty acids form insoluble soaps with calcium. Thus fatty acids, and particularly those that are saturated, may carry into the faeces significant amounts of calcium. They may also carry with them fat-soluble vitamin D. Hence it is understandable how patients with chronic intestinal disorders leading to increased fat in the faeces (steatorrhoea) may develop osteomalacia after a time.

Oxalic acid. This can inhibit the absorption of calcium because calcium oxalate is insoluble. Soluble oxalates are present in certain fruits and vegetables, but the amounts of these consumed are seldom sufficient to have any practical influence on calcium absorption.

CALCIUM OUTPUT

Lactation

A lactating mother commonly loses 150 to 300 mg of calcium daily in her milk. The mammary glands withdraw this amount from the blood, which is simultaneously replenished from the calcium pool, and so the plasma concentration is maintained, though at a somewhat lower level probably because of the reduced plasma albumin concentration. If the diet is grossly deficient in calcium, the bones must provide the calcium for the milk. However, in the whole period of lactation the total amount of calcium secreted would never exceed 100 g, which is small by comparison with the total amount normally present in the bones. Furthermore, there is evidence that calcium absorption is enhanced in late pregnancy and during lactation. Prolactin increases the rate at which vitamin D is converted to the active 1,25 dihydroxy form (Boass *et al.*, 1977). It is understandable, therefore, why there is usually no radiographic evidence of loss of calcium salts from the bones during lactation, although in women previously seriously depleted of calcium, breast-feeding may precipitate the clinical features of osteomalacia.

Excretion

In the faeces. Most of the calcium found in the stools is that part of the dietary intake which, for one reason or another, never gets absorbed. The remainder comes from shed epithelial cells and the digestive juices daily poured into the intestinal tract. Assuming this quantity to be about 8 litres and also that these juices have the same content of ionised calcium as the blood serum, 400 mg Ca/day is likely to be secreted into the lumen of the bowel. The amount ultimately reabsorbed depends on the various factors mentioned above which influence calcium absorption.

In the urine. The urine normally contains 100 to 350 mg Ca/day. The amount varies greatly from person to person (Davis *et al.*, 1970) and is higher in the summer (Robertson *et al.*, 1974). In women the fasting overnight level of calcium excretion increases after the menopause (Nordin, 1971). This may provide an explanation for postmenopausal osteoporosis. A milk drink before going to bed might reduce nocturnal bone loss. Urinary excretion of calcium falls when dietary protein is reduced and rises when it is increased (Chu *et al.*, 1975; Linkswiler, 1976). The calcium loss is usually greater than any increased absorption on moderate and high protein intakes. This phenomenon helps to explain how people in developing countries have no more osteoporosis—possibly

Table 11.3 Examples of calcium balances in healthy individuals (All figures in mg/day)

Sources	Subject	Diet	Intake	Urine	Faeces	Total excretion	Balance
1	South African male	Normal mixed European	1008	135	858	993	+15
2	Bengali male	Rice and fish	536	80	395	475	+61
3	German boy aged 11	Orphanage diet: wholemeal bread and vegetables	944	43	509	552	+392
4	South Indian children	Orphanage diet: wheat, pulses and vegetables	204	26	101	127	+77

Sources: 1. Walker *et al.* (1948). 2. Basu (1946). 3. Widdowson and Thrussell (1951). 4. Begum and Pereira (1969).

less than in Europe and North America, despite lower calcium intakes.

In the sweat. Men working in extreme heat may lose over 100 mg/hr of calcium in the sweat (Consolazio *et al.*, 1962). Under these conditions the sweat may contribute 30 per cent of the total calcium output. Normally this loss is about 15 mg/day and insignificant (Whedon, 1964).

CALCIUM BALANCE

An adult on a normal mixed diet is usually in a state of calcium equilibrium, i.e. the amount lost in the faeces and urine is approximately equal to the amount present in the food. Table 11.3 gives the data of the measured calcium exchanges of healthy individuals living on very different diets.

In growing children the body is normally in positive balance, with calcium being steadily retained for the formation of new bone. As the table clearly shows, when the need of the bones is great, net absorption of dietary calcium via the intestinal mucosa can be much greater than normal. This appears to be due to a mechanism regulating supply to requirements.

Adaption to low calcium intakes

Nicholls and Nimalasuriya (1939) showed that growing children in Sri Lanka often maintained a positive calcium balance on intakes of about 200 mg Ca/day. Their observations have since been amply supported by observations made on citizens of such diverse places as Johannesburg (Walker and Arvidsson, 1954), Mysore (Murthy *et al.*, 1955) and Peru (Hegsted *et al.*, 1952). The adult Bantu, receiving no more than 300 mg Ca/day, have a normal plasma calcium concentration and, more important, normal amounts in their bones, as determined by chemical analyses of samples obtained both at operation and in the postmortem room

Malm (1958) made a thorough study of the adaptation of 26 Norwegian prisoners to diets low in calcium. The subjects were healthy men aged 20 to 69 years, some of whom were investigated continuously for a year or longer. Table 11.4 illustrates a metabolic study of a man in whom, after several months on a low calcium diet, the faecal loss was so reduced that he was virtually in balance.

Of the 26 subjects, 22 adapted satisfactorily, 10 rapidly and 12 slowly as in the example. One man made a slight adaptation, but in three there was no adaptation. These studies have been cited as examples of 'adaptation' to a low calcium intake. Adults who have grown accustomed over a long period to a calcium intake greatly in excess of their true needs, may no longer absorb enough calcium to keep themselves in equilibrium when their dietary intake is reduced.

Calcium regulation

Figure 11.2 summarises the main features of the calcium exchanges. The calcium in the blood and tissues form a miscible pool containing 4 to 7 g. The concentration of calcium in the plasma is regulated accurately. Intake and output is also regulated, so that the store in the bones remains constant. Control is possible at three sites, the alimentary canal, the bones and the kidneys. Parathyroid hormone, calcitonin and vitamin D have regulatory roles.

A slight fall in plasma calcium stimulates secretion of parathyroid hormone, which increases calcium absorption from the intestine and resorption from bones and also conserves renal excretion of calcium. These effects are partly due to increased rate of formation of 1,25-dihydroxy

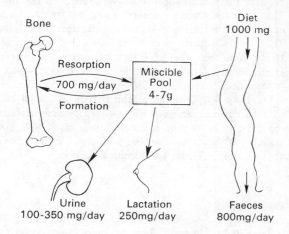

Fig. 11.2 Calcium exchanges in the body.

Table 11.4 An example of adaptation by a Norwegian to a low calcium diet (Case No. 502, Malm, 1958)
(All figures in mg/day)

Days observed	Intake	Urine	Faeces	Balance	Total gain or loss
210	942	238	605	+ 100	+ 21 g
210	436	200	323	− 88	− 18.5 g
196	454	209	252	− 7	− 1.3 g

vitamin D (Kodicek, 1974). A rise in plasma calcium triggers secretion of calcitonin and decreases secretion of parathyroid hormone; production of 1,25-dihydroxy vitamin D declines, reducing intestinal calcium absorption and inhibiting osteoclasts.

Recommended intake

Numerous experiments have been performed to determine the amount of calcium which the diet must provide in order to maintain calcium balance. Most inevitably have been carried out over short periods. Sherman (1920) estimated the average intake necessary for balance in such circumstances at 450 mg/day. Sherman (1941) indeed believed that the ordinary mixed diet of Americans and Europeans was 'more often deficient in calcium than in any other chemical element'. His views no doubt weighed heavily with the Food and Nutrition Board of the National Research Council in the USA when, in 1941, it first recommended 0.8 g as a suitable daily allowance for an adult, with larger amounts for adolescents and mothers with infants. Nutritionists and dietitians in the USA in attempting to raise calcium intakes to these high levels induced a widespread milk-drinking neurosis. The associated high intakes of saturated fatty acids may have contributed to atherosclerosis. The British Medical Association (1950) also recommended similar high calcium intakes.

These recommendations were based partly on the results of experiments conducted on individuals accustomed to a good Western diet (rich in calcium and protein) and partly on informed guesswork. In many parts of Africa and Asia children develop healthy bones and adults remain in calcium balance despite much lower calcium intakes. They are nearly always well supplied with vitamin D from strong sunlight, and their protein intakes are often lower than in northern industrial countries. The FAO/WHO (1962) Committee on Calcium Requirements suggested that a practical allowance for adults should be between 400 and 500 mg/day. They add: 'The usefulness of exceeding this has not been proved. In a number of countries the average daily intake is considerably higher, in some cases as high as 1500 mg a day. There is no evidence that such a high intake is undesirable, but neither is there any indication that raising calcium intake above 1 g will serve any useful purpose.' The Committee recommended the following allowances for children and adolescents:

Age	Practical allowance (mg daily)
0–12 months (not breast fed	500–600
1–9 years	400–500
10–15 years	600–700
16–19 years	500–600

During pregnancy and lactation it was recommended that the allowance should be between 1000 and 1200 mg a day. These recommendations appear realistic and the British Department of Health and Social Security (1969) adopted them with minor modifications.

There are, however, those who consider that higher intakes of calcium are desirable. This is because calcium balance in normal British subjects receiving less than 600 mg/day is often negative (Marshall et al., 1976) and because they are not convinced that a high intake may not retard the progress of osteoporosis.

Calcium is a good example of a nutrient whose requirements cannot be decided on their own; intakes of vitamin D, protein and sometimes phosphorus must be taken into account.

Hypercalcaemia

In infants

Idiopathic hypercalcaemia of infants was first described by Lightwood (1952) of St Mary's Hospital, London. Soon after, it was reported in many other parts of Britain and in Northern Europe, though infrequently in the USA. These reports are reviewed by Forfar and Tompsett (1959) and by Mitchell (1967). It is now rare.

The disease usually starts between the ages of 5 and 8 months. Infants affected suffer from loss of appetite, vomiting, wasting, constipation, flabby muscles and a characteristic facial appearance. The concentration of calcium in the plasma is raised, as may be that of urea and cholesterol, and also the blood pressure. Calcification may occur in the heart and kidneys. Mental retardation may be marked and the damage to brain and other organs irreparable. The infants not infrequently die. Speculation about the aetiology is summarised by Leitch (1964). Excessive absorption of calcium results from overdosage with cholecalciferol, and many of the infants had received excessive amounts of vitamin D preparations. In others there was no evidence of such overdosage. It is to this latter group of cases that the name idiopathic hypercalcaemia should be restricted. Perhaps these infants had some idiosyncrasy or hypersensitivity to the vitamin.

Treatment consists in providing a diet as low as possible in calcium, and free from vitamin D. The commercial product, Locasol (Trufood Ltd), is satisfactory since on reconstitution with water to a 12.5 per cent (1 in 8) solution, it provides a fluid which is similar to breast milk except that it contains rather less calcium and no vitamin D. It can be used as a beverage suitably flavoured and also in preparing soups, puddings and dishes permitted in the low calcium diet. After being on this diet for some months additional calcium may be allowed provided its effect on plasma calcium and on growth is carefully controlled.

In adults

Hypercalcaemia occurs in adults as a result of hyperparathyroidism or excessive doses of vitamin D. It has also been reported in patients with peptic ulcer with impaired renal function treated with a milk diet and large doses of alkali—the milk-alkali syndrome. It can be reduced by treatment with calcitonin (West *et al.*, 1971).

For a healthy man there is no danger of excessive calcium intake, since the homoeostatic mechanisms of the body ensure that the amount of calcium retained from the food does not exceed the amount needed to replace the wear and tear of the bones and soft tissues.

THERAPEUTIC USES OF CALCIUM

In tetany and when the bones are decalcified due to poor calcium absorption, as in rickets, osteomalacia and the malabsorption syndrome, or when excessive calcium has been lost from the body, as in hyperparathyroidism or chronic renal disease, calcium lactate or gluconate should be given by mouth. A level teaspoonful of calcium lactate weighs about 2 g and provides 400 mg of absorbable calcium. An effective therapeutic dose is three teaspoonfuls given three times a day in water before meals (providing about 3.6 g of calcium). Proprietary effervescent tablets are available. Calcium gluconate can be given intravenously in aqueous solution for the immediate relief of tetany.

PHOSPHORUS
P (at. wt 31)

As phosphate is a major constituent of all plant and animal cells, phosphorus is present in all natural foods. Food manufacturers also use it as a food additive for various reasons. Total food supplies in the United Kingdom provide 1.5 g P/head daily of which about 10 per cent is added artificially.

Primary dietary deficiency of phosphorus is not known to occur in man, though it may arise in cattle grazing on land lacking in phosphates. In people taking large quantities of aluminium hydroxide antacids, dietary phosphate is bound and not absorbed. This can lead to secondary phosphate depletion. Occasional cases have been reported. There is muscle weakness and bone pains. Plasma inorganic phosphate is very low and urinary phosphorus only about 15 mg/day (Dent and Winter, 1974).

Most of the phosphate in the body is present in bones which contain from 600 to 900 g P. Bone ash was a component of many ancient and mediaeval remedies and later glycerophosphates have had a great vogue as a tonic. Now with all other tonics it is in disrepute.

Phosphate metabolism may be disturbed in many types of disease, notably those involving the kidneys and bone. The plasma concentration of phosphate is controlled mainly by renal excretion, and normally falls within the range 0.8 to 1.4 mmol/1 (2.5 to 4.5 mg P/100 ml) in the fasting state. Foods rich in calcium and protein are generally rich in phosphorus, and dietitians are seldom asked to provide diets with a specified content. There is no recommended intake in Britain. The US recommended intake (p. 155) of P is equal to that for calcium except in infancy: 800 mg/day for adults is a generous allowance for most circumstances (Marshall *et al.*, 1976).

The effects on young infants fed on preparations of cow's milk with a much higher phosphate content than human milk are discussed on page 525.

MAGNESIUM
Mg (at. wt 24)

All human tissues contain small amounts of magnesium. The whole adult body contains about 25 g or 1 mol of the metal. The greater part of this amount is present in bones in combination with phosphate and bicarbonate. Bone ashes contain rather less than 1 per cent magnesium. It seems likely that the bones provide a reserve supply of magnesium, as of calcium and sodium, which is available when there is a shortage elsewhere in the body.

About one-fifth of the total magnesium in the body is present in the soft tissues, where it is apparently mainly bound to protein. The plasma normally contains 0.6 to 1.0 mmol/1 (1.4 to 2.4 mg/100 ml). Next to potassium, magnesium is the predominant metallic cation in living cells. The concentration in cell water is about 10 mmol/1 and so there is a large gradient across the cell membranes. Inside the cells the metal is concentrated within the mitochondria where it is a co-factor for cocarboxylase and co-enzyme A and concerned with energy transfer.

Fortunately, from the standpoint of the nutritionist, most foods contain useful amounts, particularly those of vegetable origin, because magnesium is an essential component of chlorophyll. A typical British diet contains 200 to 400 mg or 8 to 17 mmol/day (Marshall *et al.*, 1976), which should be ample to maintain normal reserves. Cereals and vegetables between them normally contribute more than two-thirds of the daily magnesium intake. The

US recommended intake for adults is 350 mg (15 mmol)/day. Vitamin D appears to increase Mg absorption from the intestine.

It is unlikely therefore that magnesium deficiency would arise in man from simple lack of foods containing it.

Magnesium deficiency

Excessive losses of magnesium in the faeces or urine occur in many diseases and the resulting magnesium deficiency leads to apathy and muscular weakness and sometimes to tetany and convulsions. These features are not characteristic and diagnosis is made by finding a low plasma Mg.

Diarrhoea even for a few days in young children may cause magnesium deficiency which is commonly found in children admitted to hospital with protein-energy malnutrition. In adults it may arise in patients with prolonged diarrhoea from any cause, with intestinal fistulae or with the malabsorption syndrome.

Increased urinary losses occur in various renal disorders, in diabetic ketoacidosis, where it follows osmotic diuresis and muscle wasting, in hyperparathyoidism and sometimes in hyperthyroidism and in hyperaldosteronism. Many alcoholics have a low plasma Mg.

Magnesium salts given by mouth are poorly absorbed and tend to cause diarrhoea. For patients with diarrhoea receiving intravenous fluids a daily addition of 20–30 mmol of Mg to the infusion prevents deficiency. The dose for children is 10 mmol/kg. To replace established depletion larger doses are needed, but plasma Mg should be repeatedly checked to avoid hypermagnesaemia.

STRONTIUM
Sr (at. wt 88)

At the end of the eighteenth century, a mineral was found in the ore from the lead mines of Strontian in Argyllshire by Hope (1798). He wrote: 'Considering it a peculiar earth, I thought it necessary to give it a name. I have called it strontites from the place where it was found, a mode of derivation, in my opinion, fully as proper as any quality it may possess.'

Although widely distributed in nature and present in foods and in the skeleton, strontium is probably not an element essential for human life and aroused little medical interest until the start of atomic explosions. These produce the radioactive isotope of the element ^{90}Sr which is widely dispersed in the fallout. The isotope subsequently may become incorporated into plants and animals and so into human food.

Strontium, like calcium and magnesium, is a divalent metal and its biological behaviour is in many ways similar to that of calcium. In general strontium is present in those foods which are rich in calcium, especially milk and to a lesser extent fresh vegetables; it is also stored in bone.

Concentrations of strontium in biological material tend to be about one thousand times less than those of calcium.

Widdowson et al. (1963) reported balance studies on babies and discussed some aspects of strontium metabolism in adults. Cow's milk is richer than human milk in strontium as it is in calcium. The intake of strontium was four to eight times greater in bottle-fed babies than in breast-fed babies, and the amount of strontium retained was dependent on the quantity of milk ingested. Breast-fed babies excreted more strontium than they were receiving, due to a large urinary output. The urinary output of strontium was slightly reduced, when supplementary phosphate was given. In all infants, the ratio strontium : calcium was higher in the urine and faeces than in the bones. The body thus appears to discriminate against strontium in favour of calcium, especially in the breast-fed infant.

SULPHUR
S (at. wt 32)

All living matter contains proteins and all proteins contain some sulphur; this element is therefore essential for life. The greater part of the sulphur in the human body is present in the two sulphur-containing amino acids, methionine and cysteine, or in the double form of the latter, cystine. Several enzyme systems, for example those containing co-enzyme A and glutathione, depend for their activity on free sulphydryl (SH) groups. Sulphate ions are present in the cells and sulphate also occurs bound to various organic molecules. Of these the best known are heparin and chondroitin sulphate.

Two known vitamins, thiamin and biotin, contain sulphur. Sulphate esters of fatty acids are said to occur in the body, although practically nothing is known of their significance. Much of the vitamin D in milk is present as the water-soluble sulphate. The prefix thio (Greek: theion = sulphur) is used to denote certain compounds containing sulphur. Thiosulphate and thiocyanate have been detected in body fluids; the latter occurs in saliva, especially of tobacco smokers.

A review of the intermediary metabolism of sulphur-containing substances by Dziewiatkowski (1962) showed how little was known about the origin of the sulphur in these compounds and of the amounts formed and broken down daily. No reliable metabolic balances of total sulphur intake and output in man have been reported due to the difficulty in estimating small amounts of sulphur in biological material.

Most of the sulphur in the diet is provided by the sulphur-containing amino acids, but there is always some inorganic sulphate. In the urine most of the sulphur is present as sulphate. Metabolic studies on obese women, given diets with varying amounts of protein and energy, showed that urinary excretion of sulphate and nitrogen were closely correlated (Jourdan *et al.*, 1979). Provided the supply of sulphur-containing amino acids is adequate, sulphur deficiency does not occur. The old nostrum of 'brimstone and treacle' cannot have been of any nutritional value.

IRON
Fe (at. wt 56)

The amount of iron in the body of a healthy adult is about 4 g (74 mmol), distributed in the body roughly as follows: in haemoglobin 2.5 g (45 mmol), in tissue iron 0.3 g (5 mmol) and in iron stores 1.0 g (18 mmol). Tissue iron is present in myoglobin and the cytochromes.

Iron is thus an essential component of three different processes involved in the transfer of oxygen, and hence is of great importance in human nutrition. A deficient supply of iron is a very common cause of **anaemia** which is usually mild or moderate in degree. If the supply is deficient for a long period severe anaemia may develop which could lead to a fatal result. Fortunately this is rare, for three reasons. First, the body conserves iron well; normal losses in the bile, faeces and sweat are small and the urinary excretion is only 52 to 138 μg/day or 0.4 to 1.4 per cent of intake (Man and Wadsworth, 1969). Secondly, in health a store of iron is maintained in the

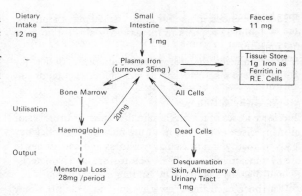

Fig. 11.3 Summary of daily iron metabolism in man (adapted from Moore, 1961).

tissues, bound to protein, in a form known as ferritin. Thirdly iron-deficient persons absorb iron more efficiently.

During the reproductive period of a woman's life additional losses of iron are inevitable. These occur at the menstrual periods and in the transfer of iron to the infant, when in the uterus and at the breast. There may also be a large loss of haemoglobin due to haemorrhage at labour. Thus, a woman during her reproductive life has a loss of iron at least double that of a man or of a woman after the menopause. If there are gynaecological disorders, the loss

Table 11.5 Iron content of some common foods

Food	Description	Range (mg/100 g)
Black (blood) sausage		20
Liver	Raw	6.0–14.0
Corned beef	Tinned	3.0–11.0
Beef, mutton	Raw, fresh	2.0–4.3
Fish	Raw	0.5–1.0
Eggs	Whole, fresh	2.0–3.0
Pulses	Various	1.9–14.0
Millets*	Various, raw	4.0–5.4
Oatmeal	Raw	3.8–5.1
Wheat flour	High extraction	3.0–7.0
Wheat flour	Low extraction	0.7–1.5
Cocoa	Powder	2.7–14.3
Chocolate	Plain	2.8–4.4
Treacle		9.2–11.3
Dried fruit	Various	2.0–10.6
Greens, leafy vegetables †	Raw	0.4–18.0
Potatoes and other root vegetables	Raw	0.3–2.0
Fruits	Tinned and fresh	0.2–4.0
Nuts	Various, without shells	1.0–5.0
Milk	Cow's, fresh whole	·0.1–0.4

* Cereals, other than milled rice, may contain up to 9 mg Fe/100 g. However, the associated high phytic acid content may reduce their value as sources of iron.

† Green vegetables commonly used in the tropics all fall in the upper part of the range and may therefore be useful sources of iron, while the vegetables (less green) most commonly used in temperate climates are generally from the lower part of the range and are consequently less important in their contribution to the iron content of the diet.

may be much greater. The intake of iron in the diet is often not able to meet this increased demand; hence anaemia is very common in women in all countries of the world. It causes much ill-health and domestic unhappiness. It is also very common in infants and young children whose intake of iron is unable to meet the demands for rapid growth.

The chief features of iron metabolism in man are set out in Fig. 11.3. Books on the subject are edited by Hallberg *et al.* (1970) and by Jacobs and Worwood (1974).

INTAKE

The mean daily intake of iron in the diet of households in Britain in 1975 was 11.6 mg/head. Table 11.5 shows the iron content of some common foods. It can be seen that there is a wide range of values for each food. This depends in part on the soil and other conditions under which the foods were raised.

As, however, only a small proportion of the dietary iron requires to be absorbed to balance the daily losses, the factors determining absorption are in general more important than the total intake of iron.

Absorption

Since the iron content of the body remains remarkably constant in health and only a small part of the dietary iron is absorbed, it follows that there is a fine regulatory mechanism controlling absorption of iron.

The study of the absorption of iron has been greatly assisted by the use of ^{59}Fe, which can be identified subsequently in the blood and excreta. The results of this experimental method have been summarised by Moore (1973) of the Washington School of Medicine, St Louis, a pioneer in this field. Besides using ferrous sulphate labelled with ^{59}Fe, Moore (1961) obtained foods containing radioactive iron by growing vegetables in nutrient solutions to which the isotope was added or by injecting iron into hens, chickens or rabbits so that eggs, liver and muscle contained the labelled iron. Absorption from ^{59}Fe-labelled foods fed singly exceeded 10 per cent from animal foods (haem iron), except for egg. Of vegetable foods absorption of the non-haem iron was poor from rice and spinach and tended to be better from soya beans. There is great variability between subjects for some foods and absorption is higher in iron-deficient subjects. Data are still limited for iron absorption from foods fed as a single test meal (Fig. 11.4) and are only starting to be collected for ordinary mixed meals; for this purpose extrinsic radioactive iron is being used, mixed with the food (Hallberg *et*

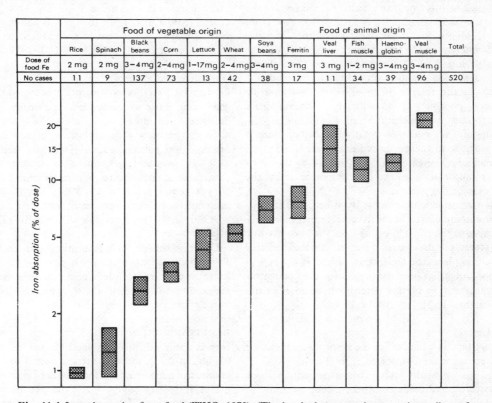

Fig. 11.4 Iron absorption from food (WHO, 1972). (The hatched areas are between the antilogs of the log standard error on each side of the geometric mean. Scatter of individual cases is considerably greater.)

al., 1977). By feeding a vegetable food labelled with ^{55}Fe and an animal food labelled with ^{59}Fe, Martinez-Torres and Layrisse (1971) have shown that vegetable foods slightly reduce absorption of meat iron while meat in the meal doubles absorption of iron from maize or beans.

Iron absorption occurs in the duodenum and jejunum, after ferric iron present in foods has been reduced. Iron is absorbed via the brush border of the intestinal mucosa. In the mucosa cells, it can be either bound to the plasma globulin, **transferrin,** and absorbed into the blood stream or combined with another protein, apoferritin. The ferritin so formed remains within the cells and is excreted when mucosal cells are shed into the lumen. Control of iron absorption depends on the amount of iron deposited in this **ferritin curtain.**

Systemic regulation

The two most important conditions determining iron absorption are (1) the state of the iron stores in the body and (2) the state of activity of the bone marrow. When the stores are low and new red cells are being rapidly produced iron absorption is increased. This has been demonstrated in growing children and in pregnant women. Absorption is also increased both in man and in experimental animals when anaemia results from haemorrhage. In averaging the overall results of 58 experiments in adult patients with iron deficiency, Moore found 20 per cent of the ^{59}Fe was absorbed, whereas in 133 experiments on control subjects considerably less than 10 per cent was absorbed. These averages cover wide variations in individual experiments.

Patients in the relapse stage of pernicious anaemia absorb iron poorly, but immediately a haemopoietic response results from the administration of vitamin B_{12} the absorption of iron becomes greatly increased. Here it seems reasonable to assume that when the rate of red blood cell formation is increased, a signal is sent to the small intestine to allow more iron to be transported across the mucosal cells to the plasma.

Another factor which undoubtedly affects iron absorption is the amount of iron in the tissues. Neither the nature of the signals to the small intestine from the bone marrow and iron stores, nor the control system within the intestinal wall which regulates the absorption of iron is as yet well understood but it has been suggested that the concentration of transferrin in plasma determines whether or not iron passes through the mucosal cell.

Dietary factors

The dietary factors which affect the absorption of iron are quite different for the two forms of food iron.

Non-haem or ionic iron. This is present in foods mainly as ferric hydroxide complexes, directly bound to organic molecules such as proteins, amino acids and organic acids. Before such iron can be absorbed, it has to be split from the complex and reduced to the divalent state. A number of dietary factors may affect this process, rendering the iron available or unavailable. For example, iron forms insoluble salts with the phytates and phosphates in coarse vegetable foods. Hence cereals are poor sources of available iron. In Jamaica Ashworth *et al.* (1973) showed that less than 5 per cent of ^{59}Fe incorporated into maize was absorbed by young children. The phosphates in egg yolk may make the iron unavailable. Tea also decreases iron absorption (Dister *et al.*, 1975).

Reducing substances, such as ascorbic acid, favour the absorption of ionic iron. Ascorbic acid not only promotes reduction of trivalent to divalent iron but, in addition, combines with iron to form a soluble chelate in the presence of a low pH. Meat increases the absorption of iron from other sources. This has been attributed to cysteine.

Haem iron. This is the iron bound to porphyrin in haemoglobin and myoglobin. Unlike ionic iron, the absorption of haem iron is not affected by phosphates and phytates, nor by ascorbic acid. The haem complex is absorbed intact into the intestinal epithelial cell and only then is the iron split off. Its absorption is therefore more efficient than that of ionic iron.

The above account may help to explain the gradation of efficiency of absorption of iron through vegetable to animal-origin foods when given singly (Fig. 11.4). Absorption of iron from a mixed Western diet is about 6 per cent in normal males, 14 per cent in normal females and 20 per cent in iron-deficient subjects (WHO, 1972).

Gastrointestinal factors

Gastric HCl facilitates absorption of non-haem iron by converting ferric to ferrous iron. Achlorhydria and iron deficiency anaemia are epidemiologically associated although patients with achlorhydria may have normal haemoglobin concentrations (Davidson and Fullerton, 1938). It has been demonstrated that achlorhydria reduces absorption of ferric iron administered with food by about 50 per cent (Jacobs *et al.*, 1964). On the other hand prolonged iron deficiency may lead to gastric atrophy which is sometimes reversible with iron therapy in young adults.

Other gastrointestinal conditions can influence iron absorption. Patients who have had partial gastrectomy are liable to develop iron deficiency anaemia. Any cause of malabsorption or intestinal hurry is usually associated with iron deficiency.

IRON TRANSPORT

Iron is absorbed into the blood stream and not into the lymph. In the blood it is carried bound to a β-globulin known as transferrin. Normal plasma contains about 2.5 g/l of transferrin. This gives the plasma a total iron binding capacity (TIBC) of from 45 to 72 μmol/1 of iron (250 to 400 μg/dl). TIBC is increased when the need for iron is increased as in the later stages of pregnancy, in iron deficiency anaemias and in siderosis. Decreased values are found in infections, uraemia and kwashiorkor and in haemorrhagic anaemias. Normally the TIBC is not fully saturated, and in health the plasma contains about 100 to 150 μg of iron/dl. In iron deficiency the concentration is much lower and the degree of unsaturation very much greater.

By their mobility in an electrophoretic field a number of genetic variants of transferrin have been identified. These are useful as genetic markers but each appears to have the same functional capacity.

The transport system has to deal with some 360 μmol (20 mg) of iron daily liberated from broken-down red cells and also absorbed iron going to and from the cells and the storage depots. The daily turnover of plasma iron is about 630 μmol (35 mg). Only a very small proportion of this originates from the diet, even when iron absorption is at a maximum.

UTILISATION

Most of the iron utilised by the body is needed by the bone marrow to make haemoglobin for new red blood corpuscles. The life of a red blood corpuscle is about 120 days. It is then destroyed, the haemoglobin broken down, stored in the reticuloendothelial system and then the iron liberated. For this reason 1/120 of the total haemoglobin in the body has to be replaced daily in the bone marrow.

The intracellular iron present in all cells is also being continuously turned over. The amount of this **tissue iron** is only about 5.3 mmol (300 mg), but a significant part of must be replaced daily to make good losses in dead or desquamated cells.

STORAGE

Iron combines with a protein to form a complex compound, ferritin, which is normally stored in the fixed phagocytic cells of the reticuloendothelial system, chiefly in the liver, spleen and bone marrow. The normal amount of iron in this store is about 1 g. It is only turned over slowly and hence is not immediately available for increased haemoglobin synthesis if this is needed urgently, as after a severe haemorrhage.

The storage iron may be greatly increased; if this occurs the ferritin molecules become conglomerated and form a substance, haemosiderin. This can be readily detected in tissues because on addition of ferricyanide a blue colour (Prussian blue) is formed which can be seen easily with the naked eye. The first stage of iron deficiency is a reduction of storage iron without anaemia. The amount of storage iron can be estimated by examination of bone marrow which has been stained with Prussian blue. It is now more conveniently assessed by measuring the small amount of ferritin in the plasma. This is possible with a radio-immunoassay, and the normal value is 35-70 ng/ml (Jacobs *et al.*, 1972).

SIDEROSIS

This term is used to describe the presence of excess iron in the body, as demonstrated by the presence of haemosiderin in the tissues. This may occur under several circumstances (1) an excessive iron intake, (2) excessive destruction of red cells in haemolytic conditions and after multiple blood transfusions, and (3) a failure to regulate absorption.

Nutritional siderosis

An excessive intake of iron is common among the Bantu who cook their maize and other cereals in iron pots. Some of the iron gets into the food and as much as 100 mg or more may be ingested daily. The home-brewed kaffir beer is very rich in iron and a gallon (4 litres) or more may be drunk daily. Bothwell and Bradlow (1960) measured the iron content of 147 livers from Bantu who had died from accidents. In all but 16 the normal maximum (1 g/kg) was exceeded.

Wines, especially cheap wines, are rich in iron. Although most contain less than 10 mg/l, some have been reported to contain over 30 mg/1 and one sample 350 mg/1. Siderosis is common amongst chronic alcoholics in Boston, many of whom may regularly drink over a litre of cheap wine daily. MacDonald (1964) has given an interesting account of the habits of these people and of their pathology. He found a similar state of affairs in Normandy when large amounts of cider were drunk of which the iron content was as high as 16 mg/1.

Haemolytic conditions

Excess iron accumulates in the tissues of patients with all types of haemolytic anaemia. In these disorders red blood corpuscles are broken down more rapidly than normal. Severe anaemia may result. Repeated blood transfusions for any disorder may lead to siderosis. Since iron liberated from destroyed cells is not excreted and since 500 ml of blood transfused contains over 200 mg of iron, a considerable accumulation may occur.

Hereditary haemochromatosis. In this rare disease excessive amounts of iron are deposited chiefly in the liver and spleen, but also in the pancreas, skin and many other organs. It is associated with various disorders including cirrhosis of the liver, diabetes mellitus, and sometimes a bronze discoloration of the skin. There is a failure of the control mechanism for iron absorption in the alimentary canal. The disease was attributed to a genetic defect by Sheldon (1927), who first described it.

Treatment is by phlebotomy, which is the only satisfactory way of reducing the great amount of iron in the body (up to 50 g). A venesection of 500 ml removes about 250 mg of iron and this must be carried out weekly for approximately two years, by which time the haemoglobin and plasma iron concentration should have fallen and the patient be greatly improved. Thereafter the removal of one litre of blood once or twice a year is needed.

Siblings with significant iron deposits in the liver should also be treated by phlebotomy. The iron-chelating agent desferrioxamine produces such a small excretion of iron that it is not recommended and a low iron diet is of no value.

Pathological effects of siderosis

It is not clear whether a minor degree of siderosis affects health. It is certainly very common amongst Bantu with no apparent clinical manifestations. Bothwell and Bradlow (1960) found that with a slight overload all the iron was present in the parenchymal cells of the liver, but with increasing concentrations it also appeared in the Kupffer cells and in the portal tracts. Here the excess iron may set up fibrosis. Siderosis is certainly one of the numerous factors discussed on page 413, which appear to cause cirrhosis of liver.

OUTPUT

The crucial fact that the iron liberated by the continuous breakdown of red blood corpuscles is not excreted but conserved and utilised was first demonstrated by McCance and Widdowson (1937). Neither the kidneys nor the cells of the intestinal and sweat glands appear to have the power to concentrate iron. In consequence the iron content of their cell-free secretions is not higher than that of plasma and the total loss in this way is very small (0.5–1 mg daily).

It has often been postulated that large quantities of iron may be lost in the sweat and that in hot countries this contributes to iron deficiency. However, it is difficult to collect samples of sweat for analysis which do not contain desquamated skin cells, rich in iron. In Dar es Salaam Wheeler et al. (1973) found that losses of iron in the sweat in six male students ranged from 0.25 to 0.52 mg/day and were slightly greater than those in the urine; they concluded that such losses could be important when iron was not being properly absorbed.

Most of the iron in the faeces has, of course, never been absorbed into the body. Losses in menstruation and during pregnancy and lactation are further discussed on page 424.

RECOMMENDED INTAKES

As all the iron present in many diets is not readily digested and absorbed, a recommended figure for dietary iron intake may be misleading. Most authorities recommend 10 mg per day for men and post-menopausal women. This is based on an estimated requirement of absorbed iron of 0.5 to 1 mg per day and absorption of 10 per cent of the intake. Women during the reproductive period need more iron, and usually absorb it more efficiently. Hallberg et al. (1966) measured menstrual losses in a large sample of 476 Swedish women. The distribution was markedly skewed. Blood losses were equivalent to less than 1.4 mg Fe each day of the month in 90 per cent of women but were over 2

mg Fe/day in the top 5 per cent of the distribution. The Department of Health and Social Security (1969) recommended 12 mg daily for women during their reproductive life. This meets the requirements of most menstruating women but not of some 10 per cent who have excessive menstrual losses. Their higher requirements can seldom be met from the diet and most of them require medicinal iron. The FAO/WHO and USA recommendations (Tables 15.1 and 15.2) are much higher and provide a greater margin of safety. However, they are unrealistic because they cannot be met by natural diets and satisfactory means of fortifying foods with iron are not as yet available. Iron is added to bread and other foods in some countries, but this is not absorbed from bread in amounts effective in preventing anaemia.

Therapeutic uses

Fortunately the treatment and even the prevention of iron deficiency anaemia is not dependent on dietary means. Ferrous salts by mouth are cheap and effective, as discussed on page 425. In certain conditions (e.g. the malabsorption syndrome) ferrous salts taken by mouth may be ineffective. In such cases iron-sorbitol may be given intramuscularly or dextriferron by slow intravenous infusion.

Toxic effects

Accidental poisoning with ferrous sulphate occurs usually in children who have taken medicinal tablets, mistaking them for sweets. Within an hour there is nausea and vomiting, soon followed by diarrhoea and gastrointestinal bleeding. Circulatory collapse and death may follow.

Up to 20 per cent of patients taking oral preparations of iron complain of epigastric pain, colic and constipation. Ferrous sulphate is widely believed to cause more adverse reactions than organic preparations, such as ferrous gluconate and ferrous succinate, but this is not borne out by trials carried out by Kerr and Davidson (1958) on antenatal patients and on healthy non-pregnant young women. Pills containing various preparations of iron with identical coating and the same iron content, and similar control pills without iron were given to matched groups of patients in a double blind trial. No significant difference in the incidence of adverse symptoms between the different preparations of iron tested or between the iron pills and the control pills containing lactose was found. Hence it was concluded that intolerance to iron preparations is largely psychological in origin.

ZINC
Zn (at. wt 65)

The total body content of zinc in an adult is over 2.0 g (30 mmol). This is half the body content of iron and much higher than the corresponding figures for any other trace element (Widdowson *et al.*, 1951; Schroeder, 1965). Zinc is part of or necessary for over 20 enzymes, including carbonic anhydrase, alcohol dehydrogenase, alkaline phosphatase, lactic dehydrogenase, superoxide dismutase and pancreatic carboxypeptidase. The tissues that contain the highest concentrations of zinc are the choroid of the eye and the prostrate. Semen has 100 times the concentration of blood plasma. Relatively high concentrations are present in the skin but most of the body zinc is in the bones, where the concentration is 3 μmol/g (200 μg/g), compared with an average of 0.5 μmol/g (30 μg/g) in fat-free tissues of the body.

Normal plasma concentrations range from 12 to 17 μmol/l (80-110 μg/dl); red cells contain 200 μmol/l (13 μg/ml); hair contains 2–4 μmol/g (125–250 μg/g) in newborns and adults. Urinary excretion ranges from 6–9 μmol/d (0.4–0.6 mg/d) and sweat may reach 15 μmol/l (1 mg/l). The main route of excretion is in the faeces, which contain both endogenously zinc excreted in pancreatic and intestinal juices and unabsorbed zinc from the diet.

Deficiency states
Zinc deficiency has been demonstrated in man in several circumstances.

A clinical syndrome characterised by small stature, hypogonadism, mild anaemia and low plasma Zn occurs in older children and adolescents in poor peasant communities in Iran and elsewhere in the Middle East where the staple diet is unleavened bread, *tanok* (Prasad *et al.*, 1963). After giving supplements of 120 mg zinc sulphate (410 μmol or 27 mg Zn) daily for several months, puberty developed and growth rates were accelerated (Halsted *et al.*, 1972). The zinc intake is low and its absorption is impaired by phytate in the unleavened bread (Reinhold *et al.*, 1973). This syndrome occurs in girls as well as youths.

Zinc responsive growth failure has also been reported in young children from middle-class homes in the USA, in Denver, Colorado. The children had hypogeusia (impaired taste acuity), poor appetite and hair zinc under 1.1 μmol/g (70 μg/g). Dietary histories showed that they had been eating little meat. The children improved markedly with daily supplements of 0.4–0.8 mg zinc/kg (Hambidge *et al.*, 1972).

Indolent venous leg ulcers healed more rapidly when patients where given oral zinc sulphate in a double-blind trial. (Hallbrook and Lanner, 1972). Control patients with low initial plasma zinc showed the slowest wound healing. A similar benefit from oral zinc sulphate was found in the healing of excised pilonidal sinus in apparently well-nourished US airmen (Pories *et al.*, 1967). Zinc appears to be one of the nutrients required for optimal wound healing.

Evidence of zinc deficiency has been found in chronic alcoholics, in patients with malabsorption (Solomons *et al.*, 1976) and in children with protein–energy malnutrition (Hansen and Lehmann, 1969). Conditions which can lead to increased urinary loss of zinc are the nephrotic syndrome, diabetes, chronic febrile illness and stress from surgery or burns; urinary zinc rises in response to injury (Fell *et al.*, 1973; WHO, 1973). Plasma zinc is low in Down's syndrome (Halsted and Smith, 1970) and often in patients on long-term haemodialysis. Affected men may suffer from impotence. Antoniou *et al.* (1977) studied eight such men; they added zinc chloride to the dialysis bath for four of them. After a few weeks not only was plasma zinc normal, but sexual potency was restored, with plasma testosterone increased and FSH back to normal levels. None of these gratifying changes took place in the control patients.

A syndrome of acute zinc deficiency has been reported in patients receiving prolonged intravenous alimentation. In four post-operative surgical patients in Auckland, for example, there was diarrhoea, mental apathy, a moist eczema especially round the mouth, loss of hair and a very low plasma zinc (Kay and Tasman-Jones, 1975). All the features responded well when zinc sulphate was added to the intravenous fluids. Zinc should be one of the nutrients included in the fluids given for total intravenous feeding.

Acrodermatitis enteropathica, a rare disease due to an autosomal recessive gene, was usually fatal early in infancy until Moynahan (1974) in London showed that good results followed treatment with small doses of 35 to 150 mg zinc sulphate daily. Others have confirmed this, and the disease appears to be due to failure of zinc absorption leading to low concentrations in plasma. The clinical features are loss of hair, a pustalar dermatitis and diarrhoea.

DIETARY INTAKE
Good dietary sources of zinc are meats (3–5 mg/100g), whole grains and legumes (2–3 mg/100g). Oysters (70 mg/100g) are outstandingly rich in zinc. White bread, fats and sugar are poor sources. Human milk at first contains about 1 mg/100 ml but the concentration later falls. Provisional tables of the zinc content of American foods have been prepared by Murphy *et al.* (1975). Phytate interferes with the absorption of zinc (Rheingold *et al.*, 1973) but when phytate is extracted, lignin and some of the hemicelluloses in whole wheat also show zinc binding *in vitro* (Ismail-Beigi *et al.*, 1977).

There are several indications that zinc could be important in the nutrition of mother and infant. Human maternal plasma zinc falls in pregnancy. In pregnant rats mild zinc deficiency leads to reduced learning ability of the offspring (Underwood, 1977). Cavell and Widdowson (1964) found negative zinc balances in the newborn and the zinc concentration in hair declines sharply in the first few months of life.

Requirements for zinc have been calculated from the known losses in faeces, urine and sweat and the amounts accumulated during growth. The USA included zinc in the main table of recommended dietary allowances for the first time in 1974 (p. 155). These are based on an assumed absorption of 20 per cent of dietary zinc (WHO, 1973).

The gap between nutritional requirement and toxic dose seems wide. Patients have been given 200 mg of elemental zinc daily in divided daily doses therapeutically for impaired wound healing over long periods without apparent toxic effects (WHO, 1973). Acute toxicity with nausea, vomiting and fever has been reported after home dialysis using water stored in a galvanised tank (Gallery et al., 1972).

12. Trace Elements

IODINE

I (at. wt 127)

The adult body contains 20 to 50 mg (160 to 400 μmol) of iodine; about 8 mg of this amount is concentrated in the thyroid gland. Since the thyroid normally weighs only 0.05 per cent of the whole body it is evident that this concentration is intense. Iodine is contained in the hormones stored and secreted by the gland.

HISTORY

Iodine was discovered in 1811 by Courtois, who was working in Paris to keep Napoleon supplied with gunpowder. He used kelp (dried seaweed) as a source of lye for the manufacture of nitre and found the iodine in it. The chemical properties of the new element were investigated by Gay-Lussac and by Humphry Davy who—by the personal permission of Napoleon—was passing through Paris on his way to Italy at the time. Andrew Fyfe of Edinburgh in 1819 was apparently the first to demonstrate its presence in the animal body. In 1820 the Geneva physician, Coindet, successfully treated goitrous patients with tincture of iodine. This was enthusiastically pursued by several French and Swiss investigators, notably by Chatin of Paris. Chatin carried out extensive and surprisingly accurate analyses of iodine in foodstuffs and drinking waters and came to the conclusion that although the element is universally distributed in nature, it is relatively deficient in areas where goitre is endemic. He provided the first sound scientific backing for the belief that goitre is due to deficiency of iodine. In 1860 Boussingault instigated an experiment on the use of iodine in the prevention of goitre among school children in three areas of France. Unfortunately the dose given was far too large and toxic effects were observed. This brought discredit on the whole idea. Soon afterwards the mounting enthusiasm for bacteriology, engendered by Pasteur, sent the medical profession on a false trail in pursuit of an infective cause for goitre. Nevertheless many humble people suffering from goitre continued to take iodine as a secret nostrum.

Interest in iodine was revived when Baumann (1895), of Freiburg in the Black Forest (a goitre area), discovered that the thyroid gland contains iodine. Thereafter the Americans began to take up the trail. Marine and Lenhart (1911) found that goitre in trout could be prevented with iodine; Marine and Kimball (1920) published the results of their classic experiment in school children in Akron, Ohio, which succeeded in proving what the French had failed to show a generation before—that sodium iodide in suitable doses reduces the incidence of goitre in children. Their results were confirmed and enthusiastically supported by numerous doctors in Switzerland.

Meanwhile Kendall and Osterberg (1919) in America, after much painstaking work in the laboratory, succeeded in isolating from thyroid glands a crystalline iodine-containing compound which they called 'thyroxin'. Harington (1926) determined its chemical structure and in the following year successfully accomplished its synthesis in collaboration with Barger of Edinburgh (Harington and Barger, 1927). Gross and Pitt-Rivers (1952) demonstrated the presence of another hormone, triiodothyronine, in the thyroid gland.

PHYSIOLOGY

All vertebrate animals require iodine and they all possess thyroid tissue in some part of the body. This tissue has the specific property of taking up iodine, storing it, and subsequently releasing it in controlled amounts in the form of thyroid hormones. Iodine is unique among the necessary mineral elements in that it is an essential component of specific hormones.

The iodine in food and water is quickly absorbed from the alimentary canal, mostly as inorganic iodide; a proportion of this is taken up by the thyroid gland, the amount depending on the activity of the gland. In the gland the iodide is oxidised to iodine, which is immediately bound to tyrosine with the formation of mono- and diiodotyrosines. These substances are subsequently converted into the hormones triodothyronine (T_3) and thyroxine (T_4). This takes place in the epithelial cells of the gland. Thyroxine is then bound to a globulin to form thyroglobulin in which form it is stored in the vesicles of the gland. From the gland it is released, as required, into the blood stream loosely bound to an α-globulin. With a normally active gland plasma concentrations of T_4 range from 75–150 nmol/l and of T_3 from 1.1–2.2 nmol/l. The output of thyroid hormones is controlled from the pituitary gland by means of the thyrotropic hormone.

The thyroid secretions determine the level of metabolism in many cells. If the secretion is deficient, basal metabolism falls, the circulation is reduced and the whole tempo of the patient's life is slowed down.

The secretions also control in some way the state of the connective tissues. A lack of the hormone causes accumulation of mucinous material under the skin and in other organs. This coarsens the features and gives the patient suffering from thyroid deficiency a characteristic appearance (myxoedema).

The part played by lack of iodine and other dietary factors in causing enlargement of the thyroid gland (goitre) is discussed in Chapter 30.

SOURCES

The iodide content of plants and animals is determined by the environment in which they grow. As most soils contain little iodide, most foodstuffs are poor sources. Fruits, vegetables, cereals, meat and meat products may contain up to 100 μg/kg, but the amount varies greatly in different samples and is usually between 20 and 50 μg/kg. The only rich source of iodide is sea food. The following analyses were obtained on fish in Glasgow by Wayne et al. (1964): haddock 6590, whiting 650 to 3610, and herring 210 to 270 μg/kg. It was estimated that diets in Glasgow provided from 40 to 1000 μg/day. If sea-fish is eaten at one or two meals in a week, this provides an intake of about 150 μg/day which is sufficient to prevent goitre in normal circumstances.

Much attention has been directed in the past to the iodide content of drinking waters in areas where goitre occurs, as compared with the waters in goitre-free districts. As a result there has been a tendency to regard drinking water as an important source of iodide. But fresh water usually contains only small amounts of iodide, e.g. 1 to 50 μg/1 in Britain (Murray et al., 1948), so that it contributes little to the needs of the body. The iodide content of the water in a locality is more important as an index of the amount of iodide that is likely to be provided by the cereals and vegetables that grow in the soil which the water irrigates. Among people who do not live largely on home grown food it is a matter of little consequence. Contrary to usual belief, sea water is a relatively poor source of iodide, containing less than 20 μg/1.

RECOMMENDED INTAKES

Various figures, ranging from 50 to 300 μg/day, have been proposed for the requirements of an adult. The Department of Health and Social Security (1969) recommend 150 μg/day. All such figures are based on scant evidence; moreover they may be unrealistic, since the physiological need for iodine is influenced by many dietary and environmental factors such as the amount of cabbage and other brassicae eaten, the hardness of the drinking water, the climate, the age and sex of the people and their exposure to infections or other stresses. These factors are discussed in connection with goitre in Chapter 30.

PROPHYLACTIC AND THERAPEUTIC USES

Small doses of iodine are of great value in the prevention of goitre in areas where it is endemic, and are of value in treatment, at least in the early stages. Larger doses have a temporary value in the preparation of patients with hyperthyroidism for surgical operation.

FLUORINE
Fl (at. wt 19)

In 1805 Gay-Lussac first detected fluorine in the animal body. Traces of this element are regularly present in human tissues, notably in the bones, teeth, thyroid gland and skin. There is now no doubt that traces of fluorine in the teeth help to protect them against decay, and traces of fluorine have been shown to be needed for normal growth in rats (Schwartz and Milne, 1972). West Germany now includes fluoride among the nutrients with an official recommended intake: this is 1 mg/day in adults and smaller amounts below the age of 10 years (Deutsche Gesellschaft für Ernährung, 1975).

SOURCES

The chief source is usually drinking water, which, if it contains 1 mg/1 or 1 part per million (p.p.m.) of fluoride, supplies 1 to 2 mg/day. Soft waters may contain no fluorine, whilst very hard waters may contain over 10 p.p.m. Compared with this source, the fluoride in foodstuffs is of little importance. Very few foods contain more than 1 p.p.m. The exception is sea-fish which may contain relatively large amounts of the order of 5 to 10 p.p.m. Another significant source is tea, particularly China tea, which in the dry state may contain as much as 100 p.p.m. In Britain and Australia, where people are addicted to tea, the adult intake from this source may be as 1 mg daily.

METABOLISM

Ingested fluorides are completely ionised and rapidly absorbed and distributed throughout the extracellular fluid, in a manner similar to chloride. Levels in the blood and tissues are so low that it has been difficult to make reliable analyses. Fluoride is rapidly excreted in the urine, even by those with severe kidney disease. The relation of urinary output to the total intake is complicated and related to the state of the bones. Fluoride is a bone seeker. In rats, 60 per cent of a dose of radiofluoride can be found in the skeleton after two hours. It is also deposited in dental enamel. The study of both storage and mobilisation of fluoride is technically difficult. Reports by WHO (1970) and the Royal College of Physicians, London (1976) give good accounts of available knowledge.

Prevention of dental caries
Epidemiological studies in many parts of the world have established that where the water supply contains fluorine in amounts of 1 p.p.m. or more, the incidence of dental

caries is much lower than in comparable areas where the water contains only traces of the element. Fluorides become deposited in the enamel surface of the developing teeth of children. Such fluorotic teeth are usually resistant to caries for reasons not yet fully understood. Fluoride may strengthen the structure of the tooth and reduce the solubility of tooth minerals (Hodge, 1964); alternatively it may be that traces of fluoride discourage the growth of acid-forming bacteria. Fluoride is not deposited in fully developed adult teeth, so that no benefit to adults' teeth can be expected when they begin for the first time to drink water containing traces of fluoride.

The deliberate addition of traces of fluoride to those public water supplies which are deficient in fluoride is now a widespread practice throughout North America where about 100 million people are drinking water artificially fluoridated. In at least 17 other countries similar projects have been started.

fluoride up to 1 p.p.m. to the water supplies of those areas where it is lacking, is strongly supported by these trials.

Fluorosis in animals

This may occur in cattle and sheep whenever the vegetation on which they graze is contaminated by fluoride-containing dust. A notable outbreak was caused by the eruption of Mount Hekla in Iceland in 1845 (Roholm, 1937). Smoke from brick kilns in England and from the aluminium works at Fort William in Scotland (Agate *et al.*, 1949) have likewise caused fluorosis in livestock. The first sign is usually seen in the teeth of young growing animals, which are mottled with white patches and present a rough enamel surface. In adult animals the first effect is generally the development of bony changes. The surfaces of the long bones and lower jaw become thickened and densely calcified, often with bony outgrowths (exostoses). The animals become weak and their milk yield is reduced.

Table 12.1 Average number of carious teeth per child

Children's ages	Control areas		Areas with water to which fluoride was added		Percentage reduction
	1956	1961	1956	1961	
3 years*	3.53	3.32	3.80	1.29	66
4 years*	5.18	4.83	5.39	2.31	57
5 years †	5.66	5.39	5.81	2.91	50
6 years †	6.32	6.22	6.49	4.81	26
7 years †	7.08	6.89	7.06	6.05	14

* Full dentition.
† Deciduous canines and molars only.

In the United Kingdom fluoridation of the water supply up to 1 p.p.m. was begun in three experimental areas, Anglesey, Kilmarnock and Watford, in 1956. Three neighbouring areas in which the water was unchanged served as controls. A dental survey of the children was carried out then and again in 1961 (Ministry of Health, Scottish Office, 1962). Large numbers of children were involved in this very careful study. Table 12.1 summarises the results. There can be no doubt that in the three areas where fluoride was added to the water, a substantial reduction in caries followed. Similar findings have been recorded from all over the world. Furthermore, in the Scottish burgh of Kilmarnock fluoridation which was started in 1956 was discontinued 6½ years later because of a reversal of opinion of the Burgh Council. Careful studies of the children's teeth showed not only a substantial reduction of caries in 1961 and 1963 but an increase of caries was quite apparent by 1968 (Department of Health and Social Security, 1969b).

In view of the widespread incidence of caries throughout the United Kingdom, the case for the addition of

Fluorosis in man

In many parts of the world where the fluoride content of the water is high (over 3 to 5 parts per million) mottling of the teeth is common. The enamel loses its lustre and becomes rough. Bands of brown pigmentation separate patches as white as chalk. Small pits may be present on the surface (Fig. 12.1). All the teeth may be affected, but

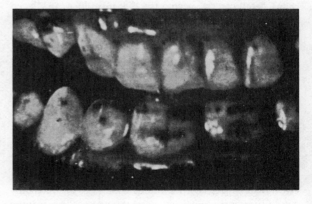

Fig. 12.1 Fluorosis in a Sudanese man. (By courtesy of Professor D.A. Smith.)

mottling is usually best seen on the incisors of the upper jaw. Dental fluorosis is not usually associated with any evidence of skeleton fluorosis or indeed with any impairment of health.

Severe fluoride poisoning has been reported in several localities in India, China, Argentina and the Transvaal, where the water supply contains over 10 p.p.m. fluoride. Fluoride poisoning has also occurred as an industrial hazard among workers handling fluoride-containing minerals such as cryolite, used in smelting aluminium. The effects are much the same as in animals; there is a loss of appetite and an increased density (sclerosis) of the bones of the spine, pelvis and limbs. In addition the ligaments of the spine become calcified, producing a 'poker back', resembling the condition called ankylosing spondylitis. There may also be ossification of the tendinous insertions of muscles, producing characteristic 'rose-thorn' shadows in the radiograph (Hunter, 1955). Neurological disturbances secondary to the changes in the vertebral column can occur. Jolly *et al.* (1969) give a full account of the clinical features of fluorosis in North India where, in localised areas, the water may contain 14 p.p.m. of flouride.

Fluoride and osteoporosis

As osteosclerosis is a consequence of excess fluoride, it is reasonable to speculate that osteoporosis might be promoted by a deficiency of fluoride. Lack of knowledge of the factors that determine the progress of the osteoporosis, which occurs in all of us when middle age is reached, and the uncertainties of measuring its rate of progress, make attempts to verify this hypothesis extremely difficult. Such evidence as has been produced (*British Medical Journal* 1972) is conflicting. However, Jowsey *et al.* (1972) at the Mayo Clinic, who did bone biopsies on 11 patients with osteoporosis, found in all of them an increase in new bone formation after giving sodium fluoride (45 mg/day).

OPPOSITION TO FLUORIDATION OF WATER
The fluoridation of public water supplies is opposed by many people on two accounts: (1) it introduces an alleged hazard, and (2) as it is generally impractical to provide an alternative water supply, to which fluoride has not been added, it is impossible for an individual to opt out of a fluoridation scheme. The compulsion to drink the treated water is considered as an interference with a fundamental right of an individual to a choice in what he consumes.

Health statistics

The health of two communities comparable in every way except that one has a high and the other a low fluoride water supply has been studied on several occasions. For instance there is a striking contrast in the water supply of two towns in Texas. In Bartlett, which has an unusually high fluoride content in its drinking water (8 p.p.m.) the incidence of general disease was no different from that in Cameron with a water content of 0.4 p.p.m. except that there was a slightly lower incidence of cardiovascular abnormalities in the former (Leone *et al.*, 1955). In the United Kingdom trials the organisers kept in constant touch with the 89 general practitioners and the public health authorities in the districts concerned. Neither there nor elsewhere has there been any evidence to suggest that the addition of fluoride to the drinking water increased the incidence of any disease or indeed had any effect on the health of the people, except for the benefit to the children's teeth. All proposals for fluoridation are limited to raising the level to 1 p.p.m. Fluoride poisoning does not occur unless the level is 10 p.p.m. There is thus a 10-fold margin of safety.

This conclusion was tested in Dublin High Court in 1963. Eminent scientific medical and dental workers from many countries gave evidence in a case arising from a challenge to the position of fluoridation in the Irish Constitution. The hearing lasted 65 days. In his judgment the Hon. Mr Justice Kenny commented on the passionate conviction, even fanaticism, of the witnesses opposing fluoridation, but stated that in his opinion fluoridation, as proposed, did not involve any element of risk to health.

The opposition to fluoridation comes from those who react emotionally to any suggestion of an enforced alteration in the natural quality of their food and drink. But it is surely reasonable that people unfortunate enough to have a defective water supply should sanction the efforts of public health experts to improve it to the level enjoyed by others more fortunate.

The citizen of today should be provided with a supply of water that is safe, clean and pleasant to taste. In many localities it is inevitable that the water may need to be treated in various ways. Bacteria must be killed and bad-tasting organic material precipitated. If the water contains unnaturally small amounts of fluoride—insufficient to confer protection against dental decay—it seems reasonable that fluoride should be added to the extent necessary to bring its concentration to a satisfactory level.

There are still many people in Britain vigorously opposing fluoridation schemes at local government Councils. If any of them read this section we hope that they will turn to Chapter 56 where they may find a creative outlet for their crusading zeal.

Those who have to argue the case for fluoridation in local health councils can brief themselves accurately by reading one of four reports (Department of Health and Social Security, 1969b; British Dental Association, 1969; WHO, 1970; Royal College of Physicians, London, 1976).

COPPER
Cu (at. wt 64)

DIETARY INTAKES
Some pastures lack copper, so cattle grazing on the her-

bage may develop anaemia due to Cu deficiency. In other species osteoporosis or ataxia (swayback) can occur. However, primary Cu deficiency has never been reported in adult man, presumably because his diet usually comes from a variety of lands. Normal adult diets provide 15–45 μmol (1–3 mg)/day and the estimated daily requirement for children is 0.8 μmol/kg. Green vegetables, many species of fish, oysters and liver are good sources, providing 4 μmol/MJ or more, whereas most other foods, e.g. milk, meats, bread, provide less than 2 μmol/MJ. As milk is a poor source, some infants are at risk of Cu deficiency, which has been reported when feeds contain less than 1.6 μmol/MJ (42 μg/100 kcal). All medicinal iron preparations contain traces of Cu.

EXCRETION AND METABOLISM

The major portion of the dietary Cu appears in the faeces and very little in the urine. The low urinary output is due to almost all the Cu in plasma being bound to a specific protein, caeruloplasmin, which is not excreted; the remainder is loosely bound to albumin. The total body Cu in an adult is about 2 mmol (100 to 150 mg). There is a higher concentration in the liver than in other tissues; in the later months of pregnancy Cu is transferred from the maternal to the fetal liver, where a reserve is built up for use when the infant is on a milk diet. Lack of this reserve makes premature infants more prone to Cu deficiency.

Copper is a component of many enzyme systems, e.g. cytochrome oxidase, dopamine hydroxylase, superoxide dismutase and lysyl oxidase. Cu depletion in experimental animals leads to a failure to use ferritin iron, which accumulates in the liver. This may be due to a decline in caeruloplasmin activity. Iron metabolism is closely dependent on Cu, and in animals it is difficult to distinguish between the anaemias arising from deficiencies of the two elements.

Deficiency states

Anaemia due to Cu deficiency has not been reported in adults, except after prolonged intravenous feeding following extensive bowel surgery (Dunlap *et al.*, 1974). Infants, especially those who are premature, may develop Cu deficiency, which usually presents as chronic diarrhoea. Plasma Cu and caeruloplasmin concentrations are low; neutropenia and later anaemia develop and do not respond to iron (Al-Rashid and Spangler, 1971). Cu deficiency has been reported in protein-energy malnutrition (Graham and Cordano, 1969).

Menkes' syndrome is a rare genetically determined failure of Cu absorption, leading to progressive mental retardation, failure to keratinise hair, which becomes kinky, hypothermia, low concentrations of Cu in plasma and liver, skeletal changes and degenerative changes in aortic elastica (Danks *et al.*, 1972). Formerly the children always died within three years of birth, but there is now hope that with adequate Cu therapy they may thrive.

Toxicity

Copper sulphate is widely used for killing algae and bacteria in swimming baths and is potentially dangerous to man and animals. Concentrations should not be allowed to exceed 12 μmol/1 in drinking water.

Excess Cu accumulates in the tissues in a rare genetically determined condition, **Wilson's disease** or hepatolenticular degeneration. Deficient synthesis of caeruloplasmin in the liver leads to Cu being transported in plasma loosely bound to albumin. There appears to be a positive Cu balance throughout life, and the excess Cu is deposited in the tissues, mainly in the liver and basal nuclei of the brain. This leads to cirrhosis of the liver and brain disturbances, e.g. coarse tremor and personality changes. The outlook was hopeless until the discovery that the chelating agent, D-penicillamine, promotes Cu excretion. Now, provided that the diagnosis is made early and treatment continued for life, the outlook is fairly good.

COBALT
Co (at. wt 59)

Cobalt is a constituent of vitamin B_{12}, an essential nutrient for man and many other animals (p. 142). No other role for the element in human nutrition has been identified. Vitamin B_{12} is the only compound of cobalt that is nutritionally effective in man and other monogastric animals. In cattle and sheep, bacteria in the rumen are able to use metallic Co to synthesise vitamin B_{12} and are thus the ultimate source of the vitamin in human diets.

When Co salts have been used as a non-specific bone marrow stimulus in the treatment of certain refractory anaemias, doses of 500 μmol/day produced serious toxic effects including goitre, hypothyroidism and heart failure. An outbreak of severe cardiomyopathy with a high mortality affecting heavy beer-drinkers in Quebec, the USA and Belgium was traced to Co deliberately added to the beer to improve its head (Morin *et al.*, 1967). The beer contained up to 25 μmol/1 of Co, and some of the men were said to be drinking 12 litres daily.

CHROMIUM
Cr (at. wt. 52)

Chromium is present in all organic matter and appears to be an essential nutrient. Only the trivalent form is biologically active, and it cannot be oxidised to the hexavalent form in the tissues. Analytical methods are still difficult and uncertain, and this makes interpretation of the literature hazardous. Dietary intakes in the USA vary from 0.1 to 2 μmol (5 to 100 μg)/day; most of this is not absorbed and urinary excretion is low. Plasma concentrations are usually between 0.4 and 1.0 μmol/1 and a lower figure may suggest a deficient intake. The total body content in adults is 100 to 200 μmol (5 to 10 mg). The concentration of Cr in hair ranges from 3 to 6 μmol/kg and low values may be an index of deficiency (Hambidge, 1974).

In experimental animals, Cr deficiency leads to a reduced rate of removal of ingested glucose, due to a low sensitivity of peripheral tissues to insulin. An organic compound of Cr, termed 'glucose tolerance factor' (GTF) is much more active than inorganic chromium salts. The richest source of GTF is brewer's yeast; black pepper, liver, wholemeal bread, even beer appear to be moderate sources (Toepfer et al., 1973). Its chemical composition has still to be elucidated but it contains nicotinic acid in combination with trivalent Cr.

Jeejeboy et al. (1977) reported the case of a woman who was maintained on long-term parenteral nutrition for 3½ years after complete removal of the small intestine for mesenteric thrombosis. She then lost weight, her glucose tolerance was impaired and she had to be given insulin. Cr concentrations in her blood and hair were one-tenth and one-quarter of normal respectively. When 250 μg CrC1$_3$ was added daily to the intravenous fluid, glucose tolerance returned to normal, insulin was stopped and she remained well for another 1½ years. In some patients with impaired glucose tolerance, especially children with protein-energy malnutrition, tolerance has improved after giving a Cr supplement. In some areas protein-energy malnutrition appears to be associated with Cr deficiency.

A review, *Chromium in Biological Systems* (Mertz. 1969), runs to 70 pages and 265 references. Yet there appears to be little hard knowledge and no certainty about the role of chromium in human nutrition.

MANGANESE
Mn (at. wt 55)

Manganese deficiency has not been described in man but can be produced in many laboratory animals and in poultry has been of commercial importance. The features in all species are deformities of bone, poor growth and ataxia of the newborn, from abnormal formation of otoliths in the inner ear. Manganese is a co-factor in phosphohydrolases and phosphotransferases involved in the synthesis of proteoglycans in cartilage.

Human diets provide from 20–150 μmol (1–8 mg)/day (Guthrie and Robinson, 1977). The average British diet is calculated to contain 4.6 mg/day, half coming from tea (Wenlock et al., 1979). Unrefined vegetarian diets can provide more. About 5 per cent is absorbed. The body of an adult man contains 12–20 mg with higher concentrations in bones, liver and kidneys. Excretion is via the bile. Foods rich in Mn are whole cereals, legumes and leafy vegetables; tea is very rich. Meat, milk and refined cereals are poor sources. Infants before weaning may have a low intake.

Manganese is relatively non-toxic to laboratory animals and poisoning of man due to food contamination is unknown. Mineworkers in Chile have developed 'manganese madness' with severe psychotic symptoms and Parkinsonism.

SELENIUM
Se (at. wt 79)

This element is irregularly distributed in soils; some contain too much and some too little. In North America, soil concentrations are too high in parts of Wyoming and the Dakotas. Certain plants, Grey's vetch and locoweed, thrive on such soils and accumulate Se in their leaves and seeds. Two diseases of the livestock grazing on these plants, 'blind staggers' and 'alkali disease', were shown in 1935 to be caused by acute and chronic selenium intoxication respectively (Krehl, 1970). In alkali disease animals' hooves become deformed and they loose hair.

That selenium is an essential nutrient was discovered later. Schwarz was investigating dietary causes of liver necrosis in rats. This could be produced by a diet in which the source of protein was Torula yeast. Brewer's yeast would prevent the necrosis and Schwarz recognised three nutritional components with this activity—cystine, vitamin E and a third factor. This was found to be an organic derivative of selenium, factor 3 (Schwarz and Folz, 1957); the effect of the cystine was later shown to be due to contamination of its sulphur with selenium. Soon after this it was discovered that white muscle disease of lambs in New Zealand could be prevented by selenium treatment.

There is an overlap between selenium deficiency and vitamin E deficiency in different animal species. Most of the deficiency syndromes can be prevented or cured by either Se or vitamin E, e.g. liver necrosis in rats and white muscle disease of lambs. But fetal resorption in rats responds only to vitamin E and pancreatic atrophy in chicks responds only to Se. The reason for the interchangeability of vitamin E and Se is that Se is an integral part of glutathione peroxidase (Hoekstra, 1975), which destroys lipid hydroperoxides and guards against oxidative damage to lipid membranes.

The soil contains very little selenium in the South Island of New Zealand, and residents of Dunedin have a mean blood concentration of 0.86 μmol/l compared with 1.3 to 4.3 μmol/l in the USA and Britain, and up to 10 μmol/l in parts of Venezuela with high Se levels in soil. Robinson (1976) and her colleagues have carried out metabolic experiments in Otago and are trying to establish whether any disease is associated with low blood concentrations of Se. There is no excess of human liver or muscle disease in New Zealand.

Analyses of the Se content of some foods in the British diet is given by Thorn et al. (1978), together with references to reports from other countries. Most of Se comes from cereals and meat (mean content 110 and 120 $\mu g/kg$), but fish is richer (mean content 320 $\mu g/kg$). Milk, vegetables and fruit contain little. The estimated daily intake of Se is about 60 μg, less than estimates in North America and other European countries but more than in New Zealand.

MOLYBDENUM
Mo (at. wt 96)

There is no evidence that deficiency of Mo is responsible for any disorder of man. However, it is an essential nutrient. Animals on a low Mo diet do not grow normally and the element forms an essential part of several enzyme systems, e.g. xanthine oxidase.

The amount of Mo present in plants varies greatly depending on the soil, being relatively high in those grown on neutral or alkaline soils with a high content of organic matter and low in those grown on acid sandy soils. Consequently dietary intakes vary, but are usually within the range 0.5 to 2.0 mg/day. Concentrations in human whole blood ranging from 30 to 700 nmol/1 have been reported in different geographical areas, but concentrations in the liver are less variable (30 to 50 $\mu mol/kg$). The output in the urine may be up to half the total daily intake.

A very high incidence of gout in some areas of Armenia, USSR, has been attributed to very high intakes of Mo (10–15mg/day) from local plants growing on the Mo-rich soil. Another effect of high Mo intakes reported from India is an increased urinary loss of copper (Deosthale and Gopalan, 1974). On the other hand Mo has a cariostatic effect in animals, and it has been reported that dental caries rates are lower than average in children brought up in areas where the soil has a high Mo content.

VANADIUM
V (at. wt 51)

Vanadium deficiency has been produced in chicks and rats. High concentrations of V in the liver decrease synthesis of cholesterol, and in the aorta lead to mobilisation of cholesterol. Animal experiments have led to conflicting claims that V can prevent or promote dental caries. Analyses of the V contents of samples of the same food vary widely and it is difficult to measure the small amounts present in diets, but daily intakes may range from 0.1 to 1 mg. Radish is the richest known food source. There is no evidence that man ever suffers from either deficiency or excess of dietary V, but industrial exposure may be a hazard. This negative picture may be changed when the biological effects of the element have been studied more intensively.

NICKEL
Ni (at. wt 59)

Traces of Ni are present in human tissue and there is evidence that it is an essential nutrient for rats, chicks and swine. However it is difficult to produce Ni deficiency in animals and there is no evidence of its existence in man. Nickel alloys are widely used for lining cooking vessels and pasteurisation equipment, and in the food industry but this has not led to poisoning, as far as is known. In animals the toxic dose is high relative to normal intakes.

SILICON
Si (at. wt 28)

Silica is second only to oxygen in abundance in the biosphere. The element and its salts are poorly soluble in water and only trace amounts are present in tissues. It is an essential nutrient for the growing chick and rat; abnormalities occur in the bones of deficient animals. Silicon may be an integral part of proteoglycans of cartilage and of the ground substance of connective tissue (Carlisle, 1976).

LITHIUM
Li (at. wt 7)

Lithium is not an essential element for animals or man, as far as is known. It is present in drinking water and also in vegetables and its concentration in the former appears to be inversely related to the prevalence of coronary heart disease (Voors, 1969). Lithium has a place in psychiatry and is used in the prevention of recurrent attacks of mania and depression. These effects are regarded as pharmacological. The dose is regulated so that the plasma concentration lies close to 1.0 mmol/1, which does not alter concentrations of sodium and potassium; adverse effects are liable to arise if the concentration rises above 2 mmol/1.

BORON
B (at. wt 11)

Boron was shown to be an essential nutrient for plants as long ago as 1910, but there is no evidence that the element plays a role in any aspect of animal metabolism. Human diets provide about 2 mg/day; most of this is absorbed from the gut and appears in the urine. The dose producing toxic symptoms in man is about 50 times this amount and it is not likely that boron presents a problem in human nutrition. Boric acid was formerly used as a food preservative, but has been declared unsafe as a food additive by an FAO/WHO Expert Committee.

TIN
Sn (at. wt 119)

Rats raised in an all-plastic isolator system with a highly purified diet did not grow normally until they received a supplement of stannic sulphate, 1 p.p.m. of diet. This suggests that tin is an essential nutrient, but the experiments await confirmation. Naturally occurring Sn deficiency is unknown either in animals or man.

The widespread use of tin and tinfoil in cans and in packages of food presents potential hazards to man. Although in most countries cans are now coated with lacquer, which greatly reduces food contamination by tin, many canned foods contain higher concentrations of tin than unprocessed food. Human diets have been reported as containing from 30 to 140 μmol (3.5 to 17 mg)/day, more than would be present in unprocessed food. Such intakes have a high safety margin, as the toxic dose for man is about 40 to 60 μmol/kg of body weight. Ingested tin is poorly absorbed and is mainly excreted in the faeces. Apart from rare reports of gastrointestinal symptoms, there is no good evidence of human toxicity from inorganic tin in foods. The upper limit permissible in a canned food is usually taken as 2.1 mmol (250 mg)/kg. As 1 kg of such a food would constitute a toxic dose for a 65 kg man, this limit seems to allow too small a safety margin.

ALUMINIUM
Al (at. wt 27)

Aluminium is the third most abundant element in the earth's crust and its compounds are widespread in soils. Although present in trace amounts in biological material it does not appear to be an essential element. Al cooking vessels are much used, but the metal is too insoluble for these to be a hazard. Aluminium hydroxide is used therapeutically as an antacid. It is also given to patients with chronic renal failure to reduce phosphate absorption and in these circumstances the small amounts of Al that are absorbed may accumulate in the body (Berlyne et al., 1972; Clarkson et al., 1972). It is responsible for an encephalopathy that can occur in uraemic patients on long-term dialysis (p. 382).

LEAD
Pb (at. wt 207)

As far as is known, lead has no essential role or beneficial effect on the tissues. Ever since lead was first mined and smelted, people have been at risk of absorbing toxic amounts in their drinking water, in their food and in the air. Lead poisoning may lead to anaemia, a peripheral neuropathy or an encephalopathy. It is now mainly an industrial hazard of lead workers, but there are still homes where the water supply comes through lead pipes, people who make home-made wines using pewter vessels, and lead toys and paints which children suck. Children are more susceptible than adults to comparable degrees of exposure to lead. The atmosphere may be a danger in the vicinity of an industrial plant, and in a town where there is much traffic pouring out lead in exhaust fumes.

A blood concentration above 2 μmol/l suggests undue exposure, and higher concentrations are associated with the risk of developing lead poisoning. In industrial societies from 1 to 2 μmol (200 to 400 μg) are ingested in the food daily; 90 per cent of this is unabsorbed and appears in the faeces, most of the remainder being excreted in the urine. Thus a faecal specimen containing more than 4 μmol or a urine specimen containing more than 400 nmol/l suggests excess contamination of the food. The concentration of lead in the atmosphere of Los Angeles in 1969 was found to be 22 nmol (4.5 μg)/m^3. This indicates that citizens would be inhaling about 400 nmol/day, a significant additional lead load. In spite of an increase in atmospheric lead, Weiss et al. (1972) have found that the lead content of contemporary hair in the USA is lower than that of locks of hair preserved from 50 to 100 years ago.

Although the amounts of lead of concern to biologists are measured in micromoles and nanomoles, industry in the United States processes over one million tons per year. Continuing surveillance of the lead hazard is necessary in all industrial communities.

ARSENIC
As (at. wt 75)

Minute amounts of arsenic may have an essential role in animals (Nielsen et al., 1975), but the element is better known to all readers of detective stories as a poison. It is present in soil and water and in many plant and animal foods. The diet of an adult man contains normally from 6 to 50 μmol (0.4 to 3.9 mg)/day, and 43 μmol/day has been suggested as an acceptable upper limit. Shellfish contain much more arsenic than other foods. Organic arsenicals are sometimes added to poultry and pig diets, in the belief that they stimulate growth, possibly by modifying intestinal flora. This may raise As concentrations in muscle and liver to 6.5 and 26 μmol/kg. However, the As in such foods is organically bound and appears to be rapidly excreted without significant retention of elemental As.

MERCURY
Hg (at. wt 201)

Mercury is not known to have any essential role in the metabolism of living tissues. However, Hg compounds have a number of important uses in industry and elsewhere. Most of the Hg that may contaminate the environment is in metallic or inorganic form. Mercury poisoning produces tremors and stomatitis, but the symptoms are reversible when the patient is removed from further exposure to Hg. Nearly all of us have mercury in our mouth in the form of dental amalgam but this is a stable alloy; the Hg is not absorbed and causes no trouble.

The dangerous forms of Hg are the alkyl derivatives, methylmercury and ethylmercury which are much more toxic than the other compounds and produce an encephalopathy which appears to be irreversible. Alkyl mercury derivatives are taken into the body in the food and poisoning has occured after eating carnivorous fish from polluted waters and seed grain previously treated with mercurial fungicide.

When waters are contaminated with inorganic Hg, microorganisms in the water convert it into methylmercury which then moves up the food chain, becoming more concentrated as it passes through plant-eating small fish to carnivorous large fish like tuna, swordfish and pike. Severe cases of poisoning occurred in fishermen and their families round Minimata Bay in Japan when it was polluted by effluent from a factory. In Sweden and parts of North America it was subsequently discovered that fish in inland lakes contained amounts of mercury up to 25 μmol/kg and the sale of fish from these lakes was banned. Even some deep-sea tuna have contained appreciable amounts of mercury. The dangers were taken up by the world press, and the governments have now made arrangements to monitor the amounts of mercury in fish. In Britain the Working Party on the Monitoring of Foodstuffs for Mercury and other Heavy Metals (1971) found that the mercury in canned tuna ranged from 0.5 to 4 μmol/kg, about half as methylmercury. Most of the deep-sea fish landed in Britain contain very small amounts, e.g. cod average 400 nmol/kg, while in coastal fish from a few estuaries receiving effluents from large chemical plants the content averaged 2.5 μmol/kg. WHO (1973) considers that the provisional tolerable weekly intake of mercury is 1.5 μmol (300 μg), of which no more than 1.0 μmol should be methylmercury. Hg poisoning from fish thus appears at present to be a potential rather than a real hazard. However, a case has been reported in New York: the patient was a lady who ate 0.5 kg of swordfish daily (Korns, 1972).

Tragic outbreaks of a different method of poisoning have occurred in Pakistan, Guatemala and Iraq after illiterate peasant families have eaten seed grains dressed with an alkyl mercury compound to prevent fungal disease, despite a red dye on the grain and warnings on the sacks. After a latent period of 2 to 5 weeks ataxia and visual disturbances develop and may lead to permanent paralysis or death. In the 1972 Iraq epidemic 6500 cases were admitted to hospital and there were 459 deaths (Bakir *et al.*, 1973).

In surveillance of populations for evidence of mercury ingestion, blood or hair can be examined. Concentrations below 100 nmol (20 μg)/1 of whole blood are satisfactory.

CADMIUM
Cd (at. wt 112)

Cadmium does not appear to be an essential nutrient. It is virtually absent from the body at birth, but accumulates in it slowly; by the age of 50 years there may be 200 to 300 μmol (20 to 30 mg). Cd is poorly absorbed from food and water. The highest concentration is in the renal cortex, and when this reaches 2 mmol/kg it may damage the kidneys.

Cd is present naturally in the geosphere, but various industrial processes increase exposure. Cd poisoning is a recognised industrial hazard. Superphosphates used as fertilisers may contain 130 to 180 μmol (15 to 21 mg)/kg, and the element is present in some plastics used for pipes and containers in the food industry. In Japan cadmium has been incriminated in Itai-itai disease, a severe and often fatal osteomalacia with aminoaciduria which affected over 200 people living on rice grown on land irrigated by waste water from a mine upstream from the area (*Lancet*, 1971). Municipal drinking waters contain about 10 nmol/1; soft waters are liable to contain more, especially after standing in galvanised pipes. Rats given drinking water containing 50 μmol/1 develop hypertension and this can be reversed if Zn is given. The cadmium content of human kidneys gradually increases throughout life; and in some centres, but not others, plasma cadmium has been higher in people with hypertension than in controls (*Lancet*, 1976). Toxicity tests on animals show complex relations between Cd and Zn, and Cu and Se, perhaps due to competition for binding sites on protein. The only British food known to contain more than negligible amounts of Cd is shellfish collected from the Bristol Channel, near a zinc smelter. However, in a Somerset village, near a long-disused zinc and lead mine, the cadmium content of vegetables from the gardens and of the villagers' blood is being investigated in 1979.

COMMENT

Because until recently accurate analysis of trace elements in biological material was either impossible or extremely difficult, precise knowledge of the ranges of concentrations in tissues that may be essential for health or be toxic is available in very few cases. Now that better analytical methods are available there has been an upsurge of research in the biological role of these elements. Though it would be unwise to predict what this will reveal and what practical effects will follow in the prevention and treatment of disease, there are several fields in which valuable results may be obtained.

The first is infant feeding. Infants have a less varied diet than adults and their main food, milk, is a poor source of some of the trace elements. There are reports of low concentrations of some elements in children suffering from various forms of protein-energy malnutrition. There is now a good case for studying in detail intake and tissue concentrations of trace elements in relation to the growth and development of children. It is not known to what extent manufacturing processes either add to or reduce the amounts present in foods for infants and young children. These are not normally analysed for trace elements, nor are they subject to any statutory controls in this respect. Research might show that both upper and lower limits for the concentration of certain elements in infant foods are desirable.

In some countries, an association has been demonstrated between the softness of the drinking water and an increased mortality from cardiovascular diseases. Research may show that a deficiency of one element or an excess of another, or the combination of the two, has an adverse effect on the myocardium or other tissues. There are other diseases in which trace elements could well be involved: dental caries (Rothman *et al.*, 1972), gallstones (Burnett *et al.*, 1976) and other calculi, degenerative diseases of various tissues and cancer.

There are also the continuing hazards of pollution of the environment by industrial processes. It has long been known that traces of lead and mercury can enter the body after contamination of the food, the drinking water or the air, and have severe toxic effects. The ways in which inorganic mercury can be converted to the more dangerous alkyl mercury and contaminate foods have been worked out in the last 10 years. Cadmium is now under suspicion in this respect. Clearly there is a need to keep a close watch on the environment to ensure that it is not contaminated by dangerous amounts of any of these elements.

Agricultural scientists know well that there are many antagonisms and synergisms between the different trace elements and with other nutrients. In plant nutrition they cannot be considered in isolation, nor can they in human nutrition, as a story from India told by Krishnamachari and Krishnaswamy (1973) and Agarwal (1975) shows. There are living near the Nagarjunasagar dam in Andhra Pradesh men whose spines have become stiff early in life and their legs bent at the knees with the deformity known as genu valgum. The fluorine content of the water in the area is high and this accounts for the osteosclerosis of the spine; it also probably increases the effects of a mild copper deficiency to induce osteoporosis in the legs. The copper deficiency arises because their main supply dietary source is their staple cereal, sorghum. The lack of copper in the cereal arises from increased molybdenum in soil, due to increased alkalinity, following a rise in subsoil water.

Wordsworth provides a fitting final comment to this chapter:

'Dust as we are, the immortal spirit grows
Like harmony in music; there is a dark
Inscrutable workmanship that reconciles
Discordant elements.'

13. Fat-soluble Vitamins

The vitamins are organic substances which the body requires in small amounts for its metabolism, yet cannot make for itself at least in sufficient quantity. They are not related chemically and differ in their physiological actions.

As the vitamins were discovered, each was first labelled with a letter, but once a vitamin had been isolated and its chemical structure identified, it was given a specific name. It is entirely correct to use this specific name provided it is applied only to a single chemical substance. However, there are advantages in certain circumstances for retaining some of the original letters as labels for the following reasons.

1. Many of the vitamins, such as vitamins A, D, K, E and B_{12}, each consist of several closely related compounds with similar physiological properties.

2. It is useful still to talk about the 'vitamin B complex' because the vitamins concerned in it (though unrelated chemically) often occur together in the same foodstuffs.

FACTORS INFLUENCING UTILISATION

Availability. Not all of the vitamin may be in absorbable form. For instance most of the nicotinic acid in cereals is bound in such a way that it is not absorbed from the gut. Fat-soluble vitamins may fail to be absorbed if the digestion of fat is impaired.

Antivitamins. These are present in some natural foods (Chap. 25). Several synthetic analogues of vitamins have proved to be highly poisonous (e.g. aminopterin, desoxypyridoxine), because they block the true vitamins at their site of action in enzyme systems. Some drugs antagonise a particular vitamin. Examples are given under individual vitamins.

Provitamins. Substances occur in foods which are not themselves vitamins but are capable of conversion into vitamins in the body. Thus the carotenes are provitamins of vitamin A and to some extent at least the amino acid tryptophan can be converted to nicotinic acid. Vitamin D is synthesised in the skin by the action of sunlight on a derivative of cholesterol (p. 121).

Biosynthesis in the gut. The normal bacterial flora of the gut is capable of synthesising significant amounts of certain vitamins (e.g. vitamin K, nicotinic acid, riboflavin, vitamin B_{12}, folic acid). Bacteria may also extract vitamins from the ingested food and retain them until excreted in the faeces. In health the small intestine of man is for the most part sterile. The large intestine carries a heavy load of bacteria, but usually absorption from the large intestine is limited to water and salts. It is unlikely that bacterial activity significantly affects the amounts of vitamins available to a healthy human body. When intestinal disease is present, and particularly if there is diarrhoea (a common concomitant of nutritional disorders), the small intestine may harbour large numbers of bacteria. These are more likely to reduce than to increase the amounts of available vitamins as is clearly demonstrated in the blind loop syndrome.

Interactions of nutrients. If the diet is rich in carbohydrates or alcohol more thiamin is needed for metabolism. The requirement for vitamin E is increased when the intake of polyunsaturated fats is high. There are several other interactions of nutrients like this. For this reason the nutritive value of a diet in respect of a given vitamin may differ from the chemical analysis of its vitamin content.

VITAMIN A OR RETINOL

HISTORY

In experiments carried out between 1906 and 1912 Hopkins showed that young rats fed on a diet of casein, starch, sugar, lard and inorganic salts failed to grow and finally died. The addition to the diet of only 3 ml of milk daily, supplying not more than 4 per cent of the total energy, enabled the rats to thrive. He thus demonstrated the existence of an 'accessory food factor' in milk. In 1913 two groups of American workers extracted this growth factor with ether, thus showing that it was fat-soluble. Osborne and Mendel (1913) extracted it from butter, and McCollum and Davis (1913) from butter, egg yolk and cod-liver oil. Two years later the latter workers proposed the name 'fat-soluble A' to distinguish it from 'water-soluble B' which they had detected in whey, yeast and rice polishings. Vitamin A, as it came to be called, was further distinguished from fat-soluble vitamin D following the demonstration that it was ineffective in the cure of rickets produced experimentally in puppies by Mellanby in 1918.

The relationship of vitamin A to the plant pigment carotene was first demonstrated by Rosenheim and Drummond (1920). They showed that the vitamin A potency of vegetable foods was closely related to their content of carotene—a pigment that had been isolated from carrots nearly a century before. The final proof that carotene is the precursor of vitamin A was largely due to the subsequent work of Moore (1957) at Cambridge, who has written an admirable monograph on the vitamin.

CHEMISTRY OF RETINOL

The retinol molecule consists of a hydrocarbon chain with a β-ionone ring at one end and an alcohol group at the other (Fig. 13.1). It is the main form of vitamin A in foods and was formerly known as vitamin A_1. Pure crystalline retinol is the reference standard for vitamin A activity. The usual form is the *all-trans* stereoisomer. Isomers with *cis* configuration at the 11 or 13 position occur less commonly and have somewhat lower biological activity. Vitamin A_2 is 3-dehydroretinol; it has about half the biological activity of retinol but is of little biological importance, only occurring in the livers of some Indian fish.

The terminal alcohol group can be oxidised in the body to an aldehyde, retinal, or a carboxylic acid group, retinoic acid. In foodstuffs the alcohol is usually esterified with fatty acids (retinyl esters).

Retinol itself is a pale yellow, almost colourless compound, soluble in fats and fat solvents but not in water. It is stable to heat at ordinary cooking temperatures but liable to oxidation and destruction if the fats that contain it turn rancid. Vitamin E, if present, protects it from oxidation. Retinol is also destroyed by exposure to sunlight.

CONVERSION OF β-CAROTENE INTO RETINOL

There are about 100 naturally occurring pigments, the carotenoids, which are chemically similar in structure to β-carotene (Fig. 13.1). They are responsible for most of the yellow-red colour of vegetables and some fruits (Goodwin, 1954). The most important, β-carotene, has a widespread distribution in association with chlorophyll, the green pigment necessary for photosynthesis; it can be split in the middle of its long hydrocarbon chain by an enzyme in the small intestinal mucosa, β-carotene-15,15'-oxygenase, to yield two molecules of retinol. β-Carotene is therefore a provitamin A. It is the only carotenoid which has a structure identical with retinol in both halves of the molecule. A few other carotenoids, e.g. α-carotene, γ-carotene, cryptoxanthin and β-zeacarotene, on cleavage yield one molecule of retinol (Olson and Lakshmanan, 1970). Most of the other carotenoids, such as xanthophyll, the other yellow pigment associated with chlorophyll, and lycopene, the red pigment of tomatoes, have no provitamin A activity.

Dark-green leaves are a good source of β-carotene, carrots are an excellent source, and red palm oil is very rich in α-carotene. In many parts of the world where animal foods are seldom eaten almost all the vitamin A intake comes from such vegetable sources. Even in Europe and North America about half the vitamin A comes from β-carotene.

Absorption of β-carotene from the diet is very variable and depends on the quantity and quality of the dietary fat. The conversion of β-carotene to retinol takes place mainly in the intestinal mucosa in man and most animals, but the liver and probably other tissues are alternative sites. Many studies have shown that 6 μg of β-carotene has the biological activity of 1 μg of retinol. Most of this difference is due to the poor absorption of carotene. The vitamin A activity of a diet is usually expressed in retinol equivalents. This is calculated by adding to the retinol content one-sixth of the β-carotene content.

Formerly vitamin A activity was expressed in terms of international units (iu). Carotene was available in pure form before vitamin A and by definition 1 iu of vitamin A was made equal to 0.6 μg of β-carotene and all values of vitamin A were expressed in this unit. Since crystalline retinol became available there is no longer a need for an international unit; the term 'retinol' should be used to mean vitamin A alcohol, while the term 'vitamin A' should be used to include all compounds with vitamin A activity (FAO/WHO, 1965). All values for vitamin A expressed as international units in the old literature may be converted into the equivalent value of retinol using the factor 1 iu = 0.3 μg of retinol.

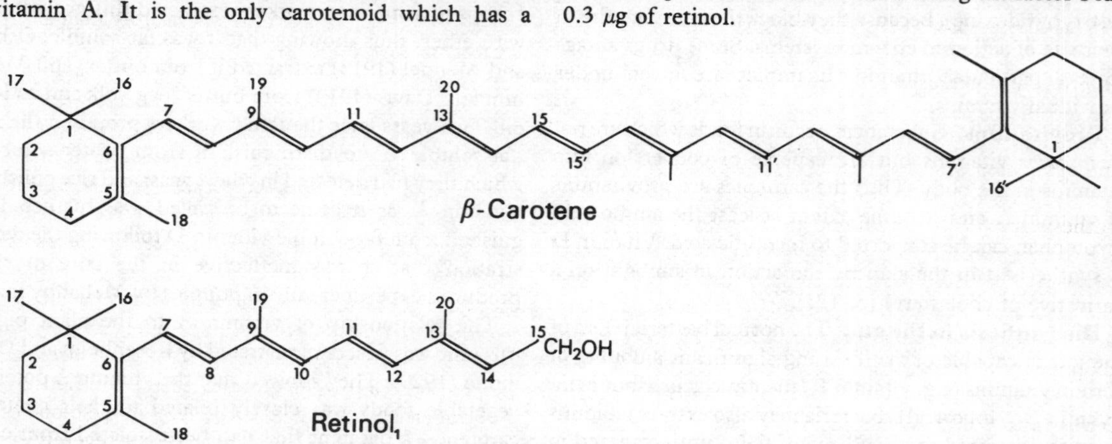

Fig. 13.1 Formulae for β-carotene and retinol.

PHYSIOLOGICAL ACTION

In night vision

Retinol is essential for vision in dim light. The ability of the eye to see in dim light is dependent on the presence of the retinal pigment rhodopsin (visual purple), which is bleached in the presence of light and in the process acts as a stimulus to the rods of the retina (Wald, 1968). The bleaching of visual purple is the means whereby the human eye can see at night. The aldehyde formed from retinol is an essential component of visual purple. Patients suffering from vitamin A deficiency are often troubled with night blindness (p. 274).

In epithelial surfaces

Vitamin A deficiency results in a morphological change, first described by Wolbach and Howe (1952). Cells undergo squamous metaplasia whereby they become flattened and heaped one upon another. The heaping up of dry epithelium on the scleral conjunctiva produces the condition of xerophthalmia (Chap. 31). If the deficiency of vitamin A continues and is severe, softening of the cornea will result (keratomalacia) with subsequent necrosis, and blindness follows.

The peak incidence of xerophthalmia occurs among children 3 to 4 years of age (Oomen, 1969) and it is usually found in association with protein-energy malnutrition. Diets lacking in protein are often low in vitamin A activity, and in protein-energy malnutrition both absorption of retinol and its transport in the blood are impaired. In the skin the condition of follicular keratosis develops. The sebaceous glands become blocked with horny plugs of keratin so that their secretions diminish. In animals at least, similar changes occur in the epithelial lining of the bronchial tree, with loss of cilia, the accumulation of bacteria and fatal bronchopneumonia. Squamous metaplasia in the urinary tract of dogs results in the formation of urinary calculi, but there is no good evidence that vitamin A deficiency is a cause of renal stones in man.

Biochemical action

The role of retinol in the formation of visual purple is well established, but the part it plays in the metabolism of epithelial cells, bone and other tissues is far from certain. In rats deficient in vitamin A there is a decrease in synthesis of a fucose-containing glycopeptide in the goblet cells of the small intestine (De Luca et al., 1971) and also in synthesis of a glycolipid containing mannose in the liver (De Luca et al., 1973). It is possible that retinol acts as a carrier for carbohydrates necessary for the manufacture of components of intracellular membranes.

Transport

Retinol is carried from the intestines as retinyl palmitate in chylomicrons and is taken up by the liver. It is released from the liver as retinol and circulates in the blood bound to a specific transport protein, retinol-binding protein (RBP), which forms a complex with plasma prealbumin (PA). Both RBP and PA can be measured by immunoassay and concentrations of both are low in children with kwashiorkor (Smith et al., 1973). After ingestion of retinol, 80 per cent is absorbed. Usually 30 to 50 per cent is stored in the liver, 20 to 60 per cent is conjugated and excreted in bile as the glucuronide. The remaining 10 to 20 per cent of a radioactively labelled dose appears in the urine as metabolites such as methylated derivatives of retinoic acid (Rietz et al., 1974; Hanni et al., 1976).

Storage

The livers of people killed accidentally in Britain contain on average 270 μg/g of retinol, or about 400 mg in the whole liver (Huque and Truswell, 1979). This is sufficient to meet requirements for many months or years with no dietary intake. Liver stores are not inexhaustible and in postmortem surveys in Canada and the USA it has been found that some 20 to 30 per cent of people have had liver vitamin A in the low range of 0 to 40 μg/g by the time of death (Hoppner et al., 1968; Raica et al., 1972). In Bangladesh 78 per cent of people had low concentrations ($<$ 40 μg/g) in the liver (Abedin et al., 1976).

HUMAN DEFICIENCY

Vitamin A deficiency was induced in 16 human volunteers in an experiment carried out in Sheffield from 1942 to 1944. Anyone with a special interest in vitamin A should study the account of this investigation (Hume and Krebs, 1949). It is noteworthy that although night blindness and some follicular keratosis resulted, there was no xerophthalmia. The clinical effects of vitamin A deficiency are usually seen only in people whose diet has been deficient for a long time both in dairy produce and vegetables. Deficiency of vitamin A occasionally develops from faulty absorption, caused by a variety of diseases of the alimentary tract. Owing to the large store of the vitamin this is very rare and could only occur in a previously healthy man after many months of severe illness.

Diagnosis

The Sheffield experiment showed that the most sensitive test of retinol deficiency is the measurement of ability to see in dim light ('dark adaptation'). For this purpose Wald's method of measuring 'final rod threshold' as modified by Dow and Steven (1941) is perhaps the most reliable.

Retinol can be measured in the blood by means of the blue colour that it develops in the presence of antimony trichloride or trifluoracetic acid (Carr-Price reaction). There is also a fluorimetric procedure. Methods are given by Sauberlich et al. (1974). The level in the blood does not begin to fall until the body's reserves are severely depleted. Mean values for the plasma concentrations of retinol and carotenoids are given in Table 13.1. The lower limits which can be considered satisfactory are 200 and 800 μg/1 ml for retinol and carotenoids respectively. The concentration of carotenoids reflects the recent dietary intake of the precursor.

When an individual regularly consumes very large amounts of foods rich in carotenoids, the plasma can become distinctly orange-yellow and the skin can become tinged with the same colour. This is called **hypercarotenaemia.** Unlike jaundice, in which bile pigments accumulate in the body, the eyes do not become yellow. Hypercarotenaemia is a benign condition; vitamin A is not formed in toxic amounts and the skin reverts to its normal colour on changing to an ordinary diet.

DIETARY SOURCES
Retinol is chiefly found in milk, butter, cheese, egg yolk, liver and some of the fatty fish. The liver oils of fish are the richest natural sources of vitamin A, but these are used as nutritional supplements rather than foods.

Carotenes are found chiefly in green vegetables in association with chlorophyll, so that the green outer leaves of vegetables are good sources of carotene, while the white inner leaves contain little. Other useful sources are yellow and red fruits and vegetables, particularly carrots (Table 13.2). All vegetable oils are devoid of vitamin A activity, with the exception of red palm oil which is extensively produced in West Africa and Malaysia. In Great Britain and some other countries vitamin A is added artificially to margarine to provide the same concentration as that of good summer butter.

The yellow colour usually present in dairy products, cheese, butter and eggs, is due to carotenoids, but gives no indication of the amount of vitamin A present.

Losses in the preparation and handling of food
Both retinol and carotene are stable to ordinary cooking methods, though some loss may occur at temperatures above 100° C as when butter or palm oil is used for frying. Fruits and other foods that are dried in the sun lose much of their vitamin A potency. Considerable losses of retinol

Table 13.2 Dietary sources of vitamin A activity

Source	Range (μg retinol equivalent/ 100g edible portion)
Supplying preformed retinol	
Fatty fish and their oils	
Halibut–liver oil	600 000–10 800 000
Cod–liver oil	18 000–27 000
Shark–liver oil	13 500–180 000
Herring and salmon, fresh and tinned	45–90
Sardine	trace
Dairy produce	
Butter	830
Margarine, vitaminised	900
Eggs, fresh, whole	140
Milk, fresh, whole	40
Cheese, whole, fatty type	320
Meats	
Liver, sheep and ox	15 000–18 000
Beef, mutton, pork	0–4
Supplying carotene	
Fruit and vegetables	
Red palm oil	4000–10 000
Carrots	2000
Leafy vegetables	685
Tomatoes	100
Apricots, fresh	250
Bananas	30
Sweet potatoes, white	50
Sweet potatoes, red and yellow	670
Orange and juice	8

Negligible sources
Lard and vegetable oils, white fish, cereals (except maize), potatoes, sugar, jams and syrups

may occur in fish-liver oils bottled in colourless glass and displayed in shop windows before being sold to the public. The stability of carotene in tinned foods was dramatically shown by Drummond (1939) who found that cooked carrots that had been sealed in air-tight containers in 1824 for the Arctic voyage of *HMS Hecla* had much the same carotene content as fresh carrots when the containers were finally opened in 1939.

Table 13.1 Plasma concentrations of retinol and carotenoids (μg/1) and retinol-binding protein and prealbumin (mg/1)

Country	Retinol	Carotenoids	RBP	PA	Reference
Britain					
Adults	450 (150–900)	1330 (150–3700)	–	–	Leitner *et al.* (1952)
Canada					
Adults	650	1130	–	–	Philips *et al.* (1970)
South India					
Healthy children	240	500	–	–	Chandra *et al.* (1960)
Children with vitamin A deficiency	100	180	–	–	
Cairo					
Healthy children	224	–	23.7	143	Smith *et al.* (1973)
Children with kwashiorkor	101	–	15.2	75	

RECOMMENDED INTAKES

Hume and Krebs (1949) showed that an intake of 440 μg/day given to depleted human volunteers slowly restored dark adaptation to normal, and concluded that the minimum protective intake was no greater than this. They also showed that volunteers receiving 880 μg/day maintained normal dark adaptation for a year. The FAO/WHO (1967) recommended intake for adults of 750 μg/day is based mainly on these findings. Rodriguez and Irwin (1972) have prepared a 'conspectus' of research on vitamin A requirements of man. British diets on average provide about 1300 μg retinol equivalents/day, of which about two-thirds comes from carotenes.

The recommended intake for infants is based on measurements of intake of retinol by breast-fed infants. As vitamin A is essential for growth, children might be expected to need more than adults per weight of body weight. There is no experimental or field data from which requirements of children and adolescents can be calculated and the recommendations in Table 15.1 are based on interpolation from infant and adult requirements.

THERAPEUTIC USES

Retinol is invaluable in the treatment of xerophthalmia and of night blindness—when this is due to dietary failure. It should also be given to patients with the malabsorption syndrome or obstructive jaundice, and to malnourished people who show Bitôt's spots (p. 305) or follicular keratosis.

Where vitamin A deficiency is prevalent, minor disorders of the eyes and skin often improve more rapidly if children are given prophylactic doses of the vitamin. A total dosage of 7.5 mg of retinol given in capsules over a period of one week should achieve the maximum therapeutic benefit. There is also the clinical impression that this often improves their growth and well-being.

Pharmaceutical preparations of vitamin A and their dosage for prevention and treatment of xerophthalmia are described on page 274. The prescription of vitamin A or its sale over the counter for trivial conditions like sunburn is not justified by any reliable clinical trial (*Drug and Therapeutics Bulletin*, 1975).

TOXICITY

The early explorers of the Arctic learnt from the Eskimos that it is unwise to eat the liver of the polar bear; it causes drowsiness, headache with increased cerebrospinal fluid pressure, vomiting and extensive peeling of the skin. Analysis has shown that polar bear liver may contain nearly 600 mg retinol/100 g (Rodahl and Moore, 1943). Husky dogs' livers contain half this amount; death and disease have occurred in Antarctic explorers who were forced to eat their dogs (Shearman, 1978).

About 20 cases of children under 3 years old with retinol poisoning have been described in the USA. Usually they have been the victims of misguided maternal enthusiasm, receiving a daily dose between 30 to 150 mg for several months. Some concentrated preparation has usually been given in large doses, in the mistaken belief that if a little does good, more should do better. The characteristic changes observed were anorexia, irritability, a dry itching skin, coarse, sparse hair and swellings over the long bones due to bony exostoses. The liver was sometimes enlarged. Plasma retinol concentrations were about 900 μg/1. Rapid recovery followed withdrawal of the vitamin.

In adults 17 cases have been reviewed by Muenter *et al.* (1971). Most of them were women who had taken 14 to 90 mg/day of retinol for over 8 years for chronic skin diseases. The clinical features were skin changes, headache, muscular stiffness and enlarged liver. Plasma retinol concentrations were from 0.8 to 20 mg/1. At least one death has occurred in a food faddist.

VITAMIN D OR CHOLECALCIFEROL (Fig 13.2)

HISTORY

Cod-liver oil was used in Scotland as a traditional folk remedy at least as early as the eighteenth century. Its nutritional value was recognised by Professor Hughes Bennet (1812–75) of Edinburgh. The famous French physician Trousseau began to use it in the treatment of rickets about 100 years ago. Mellanby (1918) first clearly showed by his classical studies on puppies that rickets is a nutritional disease responding to a fat-soluble vitamin present in cod-liver oil. The vitamin was prepared in pure form in 1931 simultaneously in Britain and Germany.

CHEMISTRY

A number of distinct but closely related compounds possess rickets-preventing (antirachitic) properties. These are all sterols. Certain sterols on exposure to ultraviolet irradiation undergo a small structural change which makes them antirachitic. Only two 'activated' sterols are of importance in nutrition and therapeutics. These were first described as vitamin D_2 and D_3 and are still known by these labels. The material originally described as vitamin D_1 was subsequently shown to be an impure mixture of sterols.

Cholecalciferol, vitamin D_3

This substance is the natural form of vitamin D. It is produced by the ultraviolet irradiation of 7-dehydrocholesterol, a sterol widely distributed in animal fats, such as the oily secretions in mammalian skin and the oil of the preen glands of birds.

Ergocalciferol, vitamin D_2

Ergocalciferol is manufactured by exposing ergosterol, a sterol found in fungi and yeasts, to the action of ultraviolet light. Irradiation of egosterol gives rise to several related substances—some toxic—of which only ergocalciferol has marked antirachitic properties. The irradiation has to be carefully controlled so that toxic substances are not present, except in traces, in the final product.

Although ergocalciferol is widely used in therapeutics, it occurs very rarely in nature. It is absent in almost all plant and animal tissues. Ergocalciferol differs from cholecalciferol only in an extra methyl group at C-24 and a double bond between and C-22 and C-23, and undergoes the same hydroxylations in the body.

SOURCES

Only a very few foods provide the vitamin (Table 13.3). The only rich sources are the liver oils of fish, which obtain the vitamin by ingesting plankton living near the surface of

the sea and so exposed to sunlight. Many people obtain little or no vitamin from their diet and get their supply by synthesis from 7-dehydrocholesterol, which takes place in the stratum granulosum of the skin through the action of ultraviolet light. ,

Since in man cholecalciferol is formed in one organ of the body (the skin) and it acts on distant target organs (the gut and the bones), it could be classified as a hormone rather than a vitamin, as suggested by Loomis (1967). The rate of synthesis in the skin is determined by the degree of exposure to ultraviolet light and probably by the amount of pigment. Loomis points out that *Homo sapiens* evolved in a tropical environment where he was exposed heavily to sunlight. His skin was probably brown, containing large amounts of melanin which protects against solar damage. When such early men migrated north, the sunlight was less intense and they were also less exposed to it, owing to the necessity to clothe themselves in furs against the cold. A heavily pigmented child is probably more susceptible to rickets because the melanin reduces penetration of u.v. light and less 7-dehydrocholesterol is irradiated, and natural selection would have favoured the evolution of a people with fair skins. This attractive hypothesis for the evolution of the white races is by no means proven.

Loomis has estimated that the pink cheeks of a European infant (area about 20 cm²) can synthesise daily about 10 μg of vitamin D if adequately exposed; this is enough to prevent rickets. The 25–hydroxycholecalciferol (25–OH–D$_3$) and 25–hydroxyergocalciferol (25–OH–D$_2$) in plasma can be distinguished by immunoassay (Preece *et al.*, 1975). This makes it possible to see how much of the circulating form of the vitamin comes from sunlight and

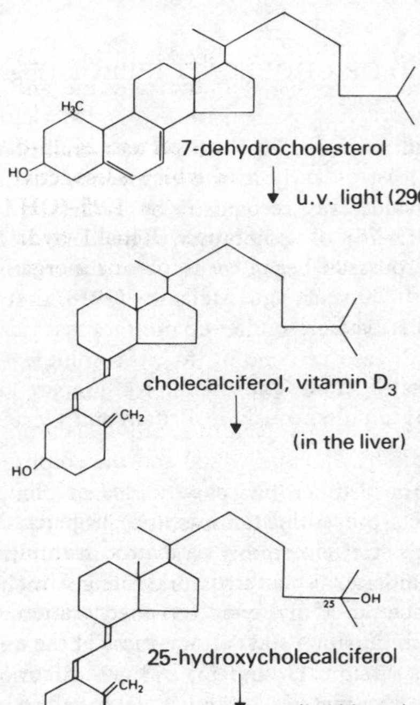

Fig. 13.2 The metabolism of vitamin D. Ergocalciferol undergoes the same 25- and 1- hydroxylations.

Table 13.3 Vitamin D in foods (1μg is equal to 40 of the old international units)

Food	Mean vitamin D (μg/100g)
Naturally containing the vitamin	
Cod liver oil	213.0
Herrings, kippers	22.0
Salmon (canned)	12.5
Sardines, pilchards (canned)	7.5
Tuna (canned)	6.0
Eggs	1.75
Butter	0.75
Liver	0.75
Cheese (cheddar)	0.25
Cream (double)	0.25
Milk, unfortified (summer)	0.03
Fortified with vitamin D	
Margarine	8.0
Infant milks (after dilution)	about 1.0
Some yogurts	about 2.0
Milk in USA, Canada	1.1

Cereals, vegetables and fruit contain no vitamin D. Meat and white fish contribute insignificant amounts.

fish oils as 25–OH–D$_3$, and how much as 25–OH–D$_2$ from pharmaceutical preparations and fortified milk. In the USA, where milk is fortified, five times as much 25–OH–D$_3$ was found in normal adults in St Louis, Missouri, which shows that sunlight is the principal source of their vitamin D (Haddad and Hahn, 1973).

Breast milk contains 0.5–1.3 μg/dl, mostly as the water-soluble vitamin D sulphate (Lakdawala and Widdowson, 1977) and this is enough to prevent rickets. Cow's milk contains much less.

PHYSIOLOGY (Fig. 13.3)

Vitamin D in food is absorbed in the small intestine only when fat digestion and absorption are normal. It is carried in chylomicrons to the liver. Here vitamin D of cutaneous or dietary origin is converted in the microsomes to 25–hydroxy vitamin D (25–OH–D), the circulating form of the vitamin which is carried on a special α_2–globulin that corresponds to the Gc system of plasma proteins (Mourant et al., 1976). The plasma 25–OH–D concentration is normally above 5 μg/l (12 nmol/l). The amount of vitamin D stored in the human body is not as large as that of vitamin A. More is stored in the adipose tissue than the liver (Mawes et al., 1972). It is excreted in the bile as more polar hydroxylated metabolites, some in the form of glucuronides.

The active form of vitamin D is 1,25–dihydroxy vitamin D (1,25–(OH)$_2$D), which is formed only in the kidney by the action of a specific mitochondrial 1–hydroxylase on 25–OH–D. The dihydroxy metabolite is about 10 times more active than vitamin D$_3$ itself on the target tissues and acts more quickly. It was the 10 to 12 hour delay before vitamin D stimulated intestinal calcium absorption that prompted the search for active intermediates. These were discovered in the laboratories of de Luca (1976) in Wisconsin and Kodicek (1974) in Cambridge, England, whose accounts are recommended for further reading.

1,25–(OH)$_2$D functions as a hormone which, along with parathyroid hormone and calcitonin, regulates calcium and phosphate metabolism. Three effects of 1,25–(OH)$_2$D are now well established. (1) It promotes calcium absorption in the upper small intestine by inducing the synthesis of a specific calcium-binding protein in the epithelial cell. It appears to pass to the nucleus of the cell and there stimulate production of a specific messenger RNA. (2) It acts on bone to mobilise calcium into the circulation. This effect requires the presence of parathyroid hormone. (3) It facilitates phosphate absorption by stimulating a separate phosphate transport mechanism in intestinal epithelial cells. This is independent of the calcium transport system and is easiest to demonstrate in the distal small intestine where little calcium is absorbed.

A fall in plasma calcium is monitored by the parathyroid glands which then secrete more parathyroid hormone. Parathyroid hormone stimulates the 1–hydroxylase in

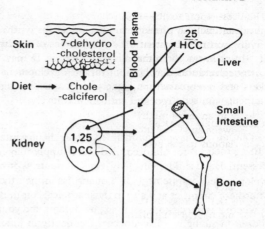

Fig. 13.3 Intermediary metabolism of vitamin D (modified from Fraser and Kodicek, 1970).

kidney mitochondria and secretion of 1,25–(HO)$_2$D increases. By its actions on the intestine and bone it increases plasma calcium. But if plasma calcium rises synthesis of 1,25–(OH)$_2$D shuts off and 24,25–dihydroxy vitamin D is produced instead, which is less active. Rats on a low calcium diet produce more 1,25–(OH)$_2$D than animals given high calcium rations. Renal 1–hydroxylation of 25–OH–D is also sensitive to plasma inorganic phosphate concentration.

PATHOLOGY

Vitamin D deficiency alters the processes involved in the growth of bones. Growth in length of the long bones normally occurs at the band of epiphyseal cartilage lying between the shaft (or diaphysis) and the epiphysis. New cartilage is continuously formed at the epiphyseal end, while at the diaphyseal end the cartilage degenerates and is invaded by capillaries and osteoblasts, forming osteoid tissue in which calcium salts are deposited. The formation of new cartilage keeps pace with its degeneration and with the simultaneous formation of new bone at the end of the diaphysis, so that the bone grows in length. Growth ceases when no further new cartilage is formed and the diaphyseal bone meets and fuses with the epiphysis.

Experiments on animals have shown that in vitamin D deficiency the epiphyseal cartilage grows, but the normal degeneration of this cartilage becomes defective, so that there is widening of the zone between diaphysis and epiphysis. At the diaphyseal end the cartilage is irregularly invaded by excessive osteoid tissue in which little calcification takes place. Calcification is also reduced beneath the periosteum which covers the outer surface of the bones; there is an overgrowth of osteoid tissue below the periosteum and delay in the normal outward thickening.

These anatomical lesions in animals deprived of vitamin D are accompanied by the biochemical effects of calcium depletion and the general manifestations of rickets (p. 277).

INTERACTION WITH DRUGS

Some drugs, notably phenobarbitone, induce the synthesis of hydroxylating enzymes in the microsomes of the liver cells. In this way the metabolism of vitamin D may be accelerated and this may account for the development of rickets and osteomalacia in some patients on prolonged treatment with sedatives and anticonvulsants.

RECOMMENDED INTAKES

Most authorities have recommended a daily dietary intake of 10 μg (400 iu) for children. A dietary supply may not be essential, and children in many tropical countries do not develop rickets despite negligible quantities in their food. In northern countries and also in those tropical communities where it is the custom not to expose infants and young children to sunlight, rickets occurs frequently in infants unless the vitamin is available in the diet. Experience has shown that 10 μg daily is sufficient to protect a child against rickets and this intake involves no risk of hypervitaminosis. The vitamins should also be provided, about 2.5 μg/day, for older children and adults who are deprived of sunlight for long periods for any reason. Intakes above the recommended levels are potentially dangerous and should be avoided.

PROPHYLACTIC AND THERAPEUTIC USES

The uses of vitamin D in the prevention and treatment of rickets and of osteomalacia are discussed in Chapter 32.

Synthetic 1,25(OH)$_2$D and analogues such as 1,α-hydroxy vitamin D are effective in the treatment of hypocalcaemic states caused by disease, such as hypoparathyroidism and vitamin D-resistant rickets (Chap. 44). Their use in renal disease is described in Chapter 44.

TOXICITY

An important characteristic of vitamin D is the narrow gap between the nutrient requirement and the toxic dose. As little as five times the recommended intakes, i.e. 50 μg/day, over prolonged periods, has led to hypercalcaemia in infants and nephrocalcinosis in adults. Furthermore, some individuals are sensitive, either constitutionally or because of disease. Toxicity from excessive vitamin D may arise when the mother of an infant mistakes her instructions and gives some concentrated calciferol preparation by the teaspoonful—in the mistaken belief that it is similar to cod-liver oil—without realising that it may be 50 times more potent. It may also occur when the vitamin is given in massive doses for the treatment of bone disease due to malabsorption or chronic renal disease.

The earliest toxic symptom in children is usually loss of appetite. Nausea and vomiting are frequently associated. Thirst and corresponding polyuria soon follow. Constipation may alternate with bouts of diarrhoea. Pains in the head and elsewhere are frequent but inconstant features. The child becomes thin, irritable and depressed, gradually falling into a stuporose condition which may suggest

meningitis. Fatal cases have been reported in which metastatic calcification was found at autopsy in the arteries, renal tubules, heart, lungs and elsewhere.

Plasma calcium may be 3 mmol (120 mg)/1 or even higher. Plasma inorganic phosphorus shows no regular change and the alkaline phosphatase is unaffected. The erythrocyte sedimentation rate is often increased. Radiography shows an increase in density at the growing points of the bones, but elsewhere the bones may be less well calcified than usual. Metastatic calcification may be seen. The prevention of calciferol poisoning depends on detecting the early symptoms and reducing the dose accordingly.

VITAMIN K AND RELATED SUBSTANCES

HISTORY

The Danish workers Dam and Schönheyder (1934) described a nutritional disease of chickens characterised by bleeding which was not due to vitamin C deficiency. Bleeding could be prevented by giving a variety of foodstuffs: lucerne (alfalfa) and decayed fish meal were particularly effective. The active principle in these materials could be extracted with ether and thus a new fat-soluble vitamin was discovered. Dam (1935) named it vitamin K (Koagulations-vitamin). With the aid of the Swiss chemist Karrer and his colleagues, Dam finally isolated the vitamin in 1939. In the same year, and only a few months later, the successful synthesis of vitamin K was announced from three different laboratories in the USA.

CHEMISTRY

The vitamin, a naphthoquinone, was found to exist in nature in two forms. Vitamin K$_1$, originally isolated from lucerne, is the only form that occurs in plants. It is called phytylmenaquinone or phylloquinone by nutritionists but in the British and US pharmacopoeias its name is phytomenadione. It has a 20-carbon phytyl side-chain attached to 2-methyl-1,4-naphthoquinone (menadione or menaquinone). It is a yellow oil, soluble in fat solvents, but only slightly soluble in water.

Vitamin K$_2$ was originally isolated from putrid fish meal but it was subsequently found that it is one of a family of vitamin K$_2$ homologues produced by bacteria, with 4 to 13 isoprenyl units (20 to 65 carbons) in the side-chain attached to the basic 2-methyl-1,4-naphthoquinone. They are called menaquinone–4 to menaquinone–13, according to the number of isoprenyl units. These are sometimes abbreviated as MK–4 to MK–13. The whole group are called multiprenyl-menaquinones (Fig. 13.4).

PHYSIOLOGICAL ACTIVITY

Absorption of vitamin K$_1$ requires bile and pancreatic juice. It is transported from the intestine in chylomicrons and in the blood on β-lipoproteins.

The only known function of vitamin K is as a co-factor for the synthesis in the liver of four proteins which participate in the coagulation cascade—prothrombin or factor II, and factors, VII, IX and X. Vitamin K acts after the constituent amino acids of these proteins have been strung together on the ribosomes. It allows several glutamic acid residues in the molecules to be carboxylated, as

Phylloquinone k_1

Menaquinones (MK-n)

Menadione (synthetic)

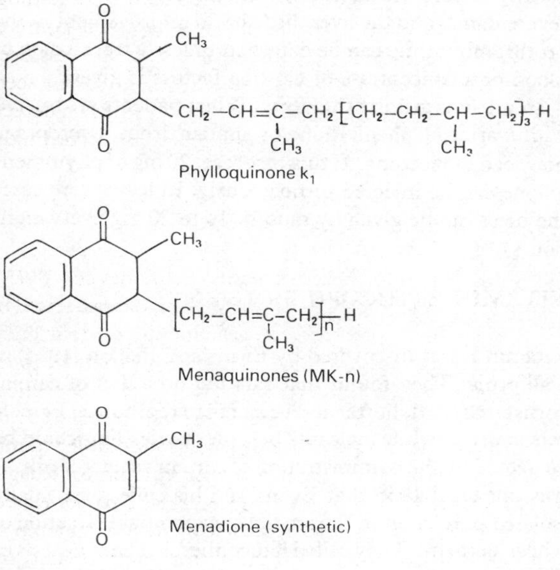

Fig. 13.4 Structures of vitamin K.

many as 10 at one end of the prothombin molecule; the residues can then bind calcium, a step required before prothrombin can be attached to phospholipid during its activation to thrombin. In vitamin K deficiency the clotting time is prolonged and so is the prothrombin time; activities of factors VII, IX and X, but not of other coagulation factors, are much reduced (Ansell *et al.*, 1977).

Vitamin K_1 normally comes into the body in the diet. Vitamins K_2 are synthesised by bacteria in the lumen of the large intestine. There is uncertainty about how well this fat-soluble vitamin can be absorbed from this low level of the gastrointestinal tract. Rats deprived of the vitamin in their diet only develop deficiency if coprophagy is prevented. Udall (1965) instilled vitamin K_1 into the caecum of patients receiving anticoagulants but this did not raise their depressed coagulation factors in plasma. Rietz *et al.* (1970) analysed the different types of vitamin in human liver: about 50 per cent was vitamin K_1 and the rest a mixture of menaquinones with 7 to 11 isoprenyl units. This indicates that about half of the vitamin normally derives from gut bacteria, a deduction supported by the occurence of vitamin K deficiency in patients given antibiotics that reduce the intestinal bacterial flora (Ansell *et al.*, 1977). How or at what level the K_2 vitamins are absorbed is not known. Body stores of vitamin K are not large but there are modest amounts in the liver.

HUMAN DEFICIENCY

Primary deficiencies
Primary deficiency has only once been clearly demonstrated in adults (Colvin and Lloyd, 1977) but has been seen in infants. Newborn babies have a sterile intestinal tract and are fed on foods relatively free from bacterial contamination. Cow's milk contains small amounts of vitamin K but breast milk is a very poor source. Infants in the first week of life have less prothrombin in their blood than normal adults and sometimes have a prolonged prothrombin time. There is usually spontaneous improvement within a few days. At one time bleeding in the newborn was attributed solely to hypoprothrombinaemia due to lack of vitamin K but even if the vitamin has been provided an immature liver may be slow in starting synthesis of prothrombin, and there are other causes of haemorrhage in the newborn which do not involve prothrombin.

Conditioned deficiences
Defects in absorption
As vitamin K is fat-soluble, it is not surprising that any defect in absorption of fats may result in vitamin K deficiency.

Biliary obstruction. The secretion of bile salts is as necessary for the normal absorption of vitamin K as for other fat-soluble substances. Severe bleeding during or, more frequently, a day or two after an operation for the relief of jaundice due to obstruction of the common bile duct was a complication much feared by surgeons. Today this danger can be reduced by giving vitamin K by injection before operation.

Malabsorption. In coeliac disease and other conditions in which fats are not effectively absorbed, bleeding due to deficiency of vitamin K may occur.

Intestinal antibiotics. If antibiotics which reduce colonic flora are given for more than a week to a patient who has been eating poorly, vitamin K deficiency, hypoprothrombinaemia and bleeding can occur, especially in those who are ill with other diseases (Ansell *et al.*, 1977).

Liver disease
In severe disease of the liver synthesis of prothrombin may fail and bleeding result even if an ample supply of vitamin K is given.

Antagonists: anticoagulants
It has been known for some time that cattle develop a tendency to bleed if they are fed on spoilt sweet clover. The substance responsible for this effect was isolated and synthesised as dicoumarol by Stahmann, Huebner and Link (1941) in Wisconsin. Dicoumarol prolongs the prothrombin time of the blood; this discovery opened up a new field in the treatment of thrombosis.

Dicoumarol itself has now been replaced in clinical use by other synthetic analogues such as warfarin and phenindione. They antagonise the actions of vitamin K and inhibit synthesis of prothrombin and factors VII, IX and X in the liver. Overdosage with these drugs can be overcome by adequate dosage of phytomenadione (vitamin K_1).

LABORATORY DIAGNOSIS

The effects of vitamin K deficiency can be detected by determining the 'prothrombin time'. The essential basis of this test is as follows: freshly drawn blood that has been prevented from clotting by the addition of oxalate (which precipitates calcium) is centrifuged. To the separated plasma, an excess of calcium salts is then added to overcome the effect of the oxalate, and also a source of thromboplastin (generally derived from brain tissue). The time it then takes for the plasma to clot is taken as an inverse measure of its prothrombin content.

DIETARY SOURCES

Vitamin K is present in fresh green leafy vegetables, such as broccoli, lettuce, cabbage and spinach. Beef liver is a good source but most other animal foods, cereals and fruits are poor sources unless they have undergone extensive bacterial putrefaction. Testing the response of prothrombin time to intravenous vitamin K_1 in a patient not absorbing the vitamin because of obstrucive jaundice showed that the adult dietary requirement is about 40 μg/day (Barkhan and Shearer, 1977).

THERAPEUTIC USES

In haemorrhagic disease of the newborn. In about 1 of every 800 infants born, bleeding occurs between the second and fifth days of life somewhere in the body either into the skin, nervous system, peritoneal cavity or alimentary tract (melaena neonatorum). Vitamin K deficiency is not always the cause and trauma at birth is undoubtedly responsible in some cases. Because of the low incidence of bleeding in the newborn and the improved efficacy of vitamin K in its treatment, most obstetric units in Britain no longer give vitamin K as a routine prophylactic measure either to infants or expectant mothers shortly before delivery. They confine its use to the prevention of bleeding in newborn infants who have suffered from trauma at birth or who show signs of bleeding. Water-soluble analogues of vitamin K should not be used in the newborn, especially if premature, because they may cause hyperbillirubinaemia and kernicterus. In some underdeveloped countries haemorrhagic disease of the newborn is more common. Then there may be a case for giving every baby a prophylactic dose of 1 mg of vitamin K_1 intramuscularly. This preventive measure rarely has an adverse effect but may be a significant addition to the budget of the health service.

In biliary obstruction and fistula, and in malabsorption. Vitamin K preparations are invaluable in cases where its absorption has been impaired by lack of bile salts, pancreatic secretion or by other causes of malabsorption. This is an essential preoperative measure if surgery is contemplated in such cases. Phytomenadione should be given preoperatively for three days in a dose of 10 to 20 mg daily intramuscularly. The plasma prothrombin time is usually restored to normal within a week. When there is severe damage to the liver, little or no improvement in the prothrombin time can be expected unless a transfusion of blood or a concentrate of clotting factors is given.

In anticoagulant therapy. When patients are treated with warfarin, phenindione or similar drugs, overdosage may lead to bleeding. If this is severe, 20 mg of phytomenadione can be injected intravenously. In less severe cases the drug can be given by mouth (10 to 20 mg every eight hours).

VITAMIN E (TOCOPHEROLS)

Vitamin E was discovered by Evans and Bishop (1923) in California. They found that rats fed on a diet of casein, cornstarch, lard, butter and yeast fail to reproduce. Female rats aborted, while male rats became sterile. This could be corrected by the administration of certain vegetable oils. It was not until 1936 that Evans and his colleagues finally isolated pure vitamin E from the unsaponifiable fraction of wheat-germ oil. They called it tocopherol. The synthesis of α-tocopherol was accomplished in 1938 by Karrer in Switzerland and by Smith in the USA.

CHEMISTRY

Eight tocopherols and tocotrienols with vitamin E activity have been identified, differing from each other in the number and position of the methyl groups round the ring of the molecule (Figs. 13.5 and 13.6). All have the same physiological properties; α-tocopherol, which is synthesised commercially, is the most potent. Relative to it the

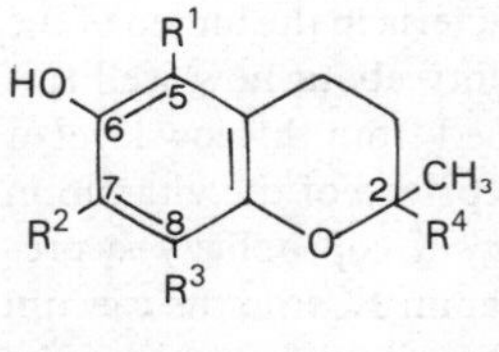

Tocols
$R4 = CH_2(CH_2CH_2\overset{CH_3}{\underset{|}{CH}}CH_2)_3H$

Tocotrienols
$R4 = CH_2(CH_2CH = \overset{CH_3}{\underset{|}{C}}CH_2)_3H$

Naturally occurring tocopherols

Tocol	Tocotrienol	Methyl Positions
α -(alpha)	ζ -(zeta)	5, 7, 8
β -(beta)	ϵ -(epsilon)	5, 8
γ -(gamma)	η -(eta)	7, 8
δ -(delta)	8 -(methyl-tocotrienol)	8

Fig. 13.5 The tocotrienols are now designated in accordance with methyl positions corresponding to the tocopherols. In descending order they are now called α-, β-, γ-, and δ-tocotrienols respectively

Fig. 13.6 *d*-α-Tocopherol.

biological activities of *ß*–and γ–tocopherol and α–tocotrienol are 40, 8 and 20 per cent. Other forms have little activity. The tocopherols are yellow, oily liquids, freely soluble in fat solvents and remarkably stable to heat, even at temperatures above 100°C. The term vitamin E is useful as a name for any mixture of biologically active tocopherols.

BIOCHEMICAL ROLE
Being fat-soluble, vitamin E is found in all cell membranes. Here it may prevent the destructive non-enzymic oxidation of polyunsaturated fatty acids by molecular oxygen. This action is similar to that of antioxidants used in the food industry to prevent fats going rancid (p. 209). The products of oxidative deterioration of fat may appear in the tissues as pigments, which can be estimated by fluorimetric methods, and are associated with cell damage. They are likely to be found in the tissues of old animals and of those on diets lacking vitamin E. Hence it seems sensible to guess that the vitamin may have a role in preventing a large number of degenerative disorders. Yet there is no evidence to support this view (see below). Tappel (1973), who gives a good account of the cellular action of the vitamin, states that: 'The more research is done on the substance, the more intriguing it appears. Thus there is a nagging suspicion that there is a very important use for the vitamin and we are just not smart enough to see it.'

Deficiency in animals
In animals a bewildering array of different diseases are produced on regimes deficient in vitamin E. Fetal resorption occurs in female rats and other rodents; degeneration of the seminiferous epithelium of the testis occurs in rabbits, dogs and some monkeys; muscular dystrophy occurs in herbivores, affecting voluntary, cardiac and smooth muscle; nutritional encephalomalacia occurs in chicks; haemorrhages and exudative diathesis in turkeys; liver cell necrosis can occur in rats and pigs if the diet is also deficient in selenium. In monkeys a haemolytic anaemia occurs and the red cells show increased sensitivity to peroxide *in vitro*. In general, high intakes of polyunsaturated fat make animals more susceptible to deficiency and non-toxic intakes of selenium are protective, though there are exceptions (p. 112).

Human deficiency
The vitamin is certainly present in human tissues and there is good circumstantial evidence that it is necessary for their normal metabolism. But in view of its wide distribution in foods primary dietary deficiency of the vitamin is most unlikely. However, premature infants are born with an inadequate reserve of the vitamin; they have subnormal plasma vitamin E and, if given a formula rich in polyunsaturated fat or iron medication, they may develop haemolytic anaemia. Prophylactic vitamin E is advisable in such cases (Graeber *et al.*, 1977).

Apart from premature babies, firm evidence of vitamin E deficiency has only been found in patients with malabsorption of fat, due to cystic fibrosis (Farrel *et al.*, 1977), abetalipoproteinaemia (Muller *et al.*, 1977) and other diseases (Leonard and Losowsky, 1971). Plasma vitamin E concentration is reduced; the red cell survival, measured with ^{51}Cr tagged cells, is shortened; *in vitro* red cells show haemolysis in the presence of hydrogen peroxide, but anaemia and clinical manifestations attributable to vitamin E deficiency are unusual. Experimental depletion over three years likewise produced low plasma levels, some shortening of the life span of red cells but no symptoms or anaemia (Horwitt, 1960).

The normal plasma concentration of vitamin E is 5 to 10 mg/l α-tocopherol. Since it is carried on low density lipoproteins the concentration is correlated with that of plasma lipids and a correction should be made if plasma lipids are abnormal. About 1 μg α-tocopherol/mg total lipid in plasma is normal (Farrel *et al.*, 1977).

DIETARY SOURCES
The richest sources are vegetable oils, in descending order wheat germ, sunflower seed, cotton seed, safflower, palm, rapeseed and other oils (Slover, 1971). In consequence margarine and shortening are major sources in the diet. Eggs, butter, wholemeal cereals and broccoli are moderately good sources. Meats, fruits and vegetables provide small amounts, and white bread and sugars negligible amounts of vitamin E (Thompson *et al.*, 1973). Breast milk contains four times as much as natural cow's milk. Mixed Western diets have been found to provide 5 to 10 mg α–tocopherol equivalents per day (Smith *et al.*, 1971; Thompson *et al.*, 1973). Some people appear to be in good health on diets containing less than this.

In the USA recommended intakes were set too high in 1968. They were halved in 1974 to 15 mg in adults (p. 154). In Canada about half of this again is recommended, 9 mg α–tocopherol in men and 6 mg in women, and we think these are better figures (Health and Welfare, Canada, 1975). Vitamin E requirements increase with the polyunsaturated fat content of the diet but not in a linear fashion and probably not in the range of polyunsaturated fat intakes between 2 and 10 per cent of energy (Jager, 1975).

THERAPEUTIC USES AND TOXICITY
Vitamin E is one of those embarrassing vitamins that has been identified, isolated and synthesised by physiologists and biochemists and then handed to the medical profes-

sion with the suggestion that a use should be found for it, before there was any evidence of human deficiency. Although vitamin E has been recommended in the treatment of such conditions as habitual abortion, sterility, muscular dystrophies, diabetes, coronary heart disease, skin disorders, and to delay ageing and to improve sexual performance, there is no satisfactory evidence from controlled trials that it is useful in any human ailment, except the anaemia of premature infants and in the malabsorption syndrome. Some athletes are dosed with the vitamin by their coaches. This is modern black magic. In a controlled trial, a daily dose of vitamin E given as part of a training programme had no effect on either physiological functions or athletic performance (Sharman *et al.*, 1971).

So far there is no clear evidence that vitamin E is poisonous, even in doses much above physiological levels. However, Briggs (1974) has raised some doubts about its safety.

14. Water-soluble Vitamins

VITAMIN C

Deficiency of vitamin C, now known as ascorbic acid, is the cause of scurvy. As ascorbic acid is widely distributed in the tissues of all plants and animals, with the notable exception of the dried seeds of cereals and pulses, scurvy is not a disease that occurs in people on natural diets containing fresh foods. Scurvy was classically a disease of sailors and, as it frequently incapacitated the crews of sailing ships, it had a profound effect on the history of the colonisation of the world by seafaring Europeans. When in 1497 Vasco da Gama sailed round the Cape of Good Hope and established the first European trading colony on the coast of Malabar in India, 100 out of his crew of 160 men died of scurvy on the voyage. Although many sea captains, notably Jacques Cartier on a voyage in 1535 to Newfoundland, discovered the value of fresh fruits in the treatment and prevention of scurvy, it was not until about 1850 that scurvy ceased to occur in the merchant navies of the world. Scurvy has also determined the fate of many besieged cities.

Nowadays scurvy is uncommon but still an important disease. It is seen occasionally in socially deprived people, mostly either old people living alone or persons addicted to alcohol or other drugs, who live on unsatisfactory diets containing no fresh foods. Outbreaks also occur in times of scarcity or famine in the populations of semidesert areas in Africa and Asia.

A daily intake of 10 mg of ascorbic acid is more than sufficient to prevent scurvy. Most people in Europe and North America get in their daily diet from three to ten times this amount. There are many nutritionists who consider that high intakes of ascorbic acid are of benefit to health and would reduce the prevalence of various diseases. Nevertheless there have been, and are, many examples of apparently healthy populations and individual people whose habitual intake of ascorbic acid is only a little above that known to be sufficient to prevent scurvy.

ASCORBIC ACID

Attempts to isolate and identify the antiscorbutic factor became practical when in 1907 Holst and Frölich found that guinea-pigs, like man and monkeys, were susceptible to scurvy. Funk in 1912 in a paper entitled 'The Etiology of Deficiency Diseases' introduced the term Vitamine for the first time and the antiscorbutic factor was soon termed vitamin C. Ascorbic acid was identified as vitamin C 20 years later in 1932 by Glen King, who had started his work as a postgraduate student in Sherman's laboratory in Columbia University and completed it in Hopkins' laboratory at Cambridge. Previously, in 1928, Szent-György, also working in Hopkins' laboratory, had been studying natural reducing substances and isolated ascorbic acid from the adrenal glands, oranges and cabbage leaves, but had not recognised its properties as a vitamin.

Chemistry

Ascorbic acid (AA) is a simple sugar with molecular weight 176. It is a white crystalline substance which is stable when dry but easily oxidised when in solution in water, especially in an alkaline medium and on exposure to heat, light and traces of metals especially copper. In a cold acid solution it is fairly stable. The first stage of oxidation to dehydro-ascorbic acid (DHA) is readily reversible (Fig. 14.1), but subsequent oxidation to dioxogulonic acid cannot be reversed.

Ascorbic acid is a powerful reducing agent and this is its main role in the tissues of both plants and animals. However, unlike the other water-soluble vitamins of the B group it has not been shown to act as a specific coenzyme in any biological oxidation-reduction system. Its main function in cells appears to be balancing or setting the redox potential. The oxidised form (DHA) is readily reduced by the tripeptide glutathione (GSH), and its main biological role may be to maintain glutathione in the tissues in its oxidised form (GSSG).

Two aspects of failure of electron transport which occur in ascorbic acid deficiency are important in clinical medi-

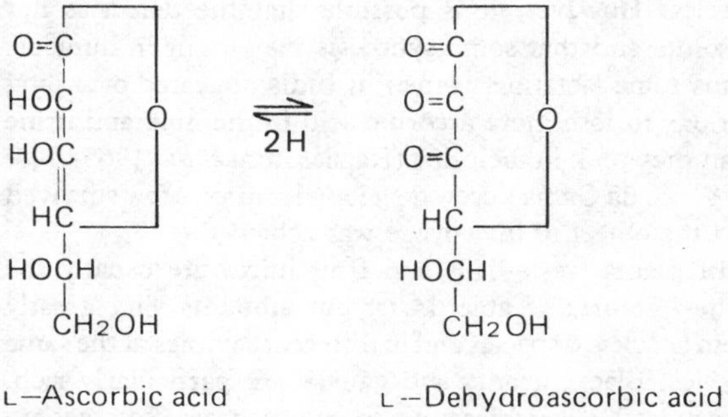

Fig. 14.1 Reversible oxidation of ascorbic acid.

129

cine. The first is a failure to synthesise hydroxyproline from proline. An inadequate supply of hydroxyproline for the synthesis of the protein collagen in connective tissues is the biochemical disorder mainly responsible for the features of scurvy and is discussed later.

Secondly, the enzyme *p*-hydroxyphenylpyruvic acid (pHPPA) oxidase, a key enzyme in the metabolism of tyrosine, is dependent on ascorbic acid. The activity of pHPPA oxidase is low in about 30 per cent of preterm infants and may not reach adult levels until three months in up to five per cent of full-term infants. In these infants there is an abnormally high concentration of tyrosine in the blood. Fortunately such hypertyrosinaemia is usually without effect on the development of the child but if it is persistent and severe, brain damage may result. pHPPA oxidase deficiency can be relieved by giving ascorbic acid and a milk formula diet low in tyrosine.

Ascorbic acid in the lumen of the gut helps in the reduction of ferric to ferrous iron, a necessary stage before iron is absorbed. The physiological importance of this reaction of ascorbic acid is uncertain. Although an iron-deficiency anaemia is common in natural scurvy, it has not been found in volunteers in whom the disease was produced experimentally.

Ascorbic acid is utilised during the production or release of steroid hormones by the adrenal glands in response to stress. The importance of this action is discussed later.

Sources of ascorbic acid

All plant and animal tissues appear to contain ascorbic acid, although no systematic survey has been made. It is synthesised from glucose via L-gulonic acid and L-gulonolactone. This takes place in the liver of all higher animals except primates, the guinea-pig, an Indian fruit-eating bat, the red-vented bulbul and some other birds. In these animals a mutation has probably been responsible for the loss of an enzyme on the synthetic pathway for ascorbic acid; this may be similar to the mutations responsible for the group of diseases known as Inborn Errors of Metabolism. Scurvy differs from these diseases only in that the defect appears to be present in all members of an affected species. However, it is possible that the defect is not absolute and that some synthesis may occur in humans. Thus some lactating women in India appeared over long periods to lose more ascorbic acid in the milk and urine than they took in their diet (Rajalakshmi *et al.*, 1965). Not all Vasco da Gama's crew developed scurvy; a few survived and the object of his voyage was achieved.

In plants fresh fruit and fruit juices are usually the richest sources (Table 14.1), but amounts vary greatly from species to species and in different samples of the same species. Blackcurrants and gauvas are particularly rich. Green leafy vegetables are also good sources. Potatoes are not a rich source, but as large amounts may be eaten they provide the major intake of ascorbic acid in some countries, e.g. Scotland.

Losses of ascorbic acid due to oxidation are inevitable during cooking. They can be kept to less than 50 per cent if the fresh food is put straight into boiling water from which the oxygen has been driven off and, when frying potatoes, by rapid immersion in hot deep fat. As traces of copper and an alkaline medium facilitate oxidation, copper pots and baking soda should not be used. Losses continue when vegetables are kept warm on hot plates, so vegetables should be served as soon after cooking as possible.

Losses also occur on storage, especially if the fruit or vegetables are damaged. Manufacturers of canned and frozen fruits and vegetables take good care to use only material of high quality which is processed quickly: Such foods may contain more ascorbic acid than reputedly fresh foods which have been lying in markets or shops for some days before being sold.

Fresh early potatoes contain about 30 mg/100 g of ascorbic acid before cooking and over 75 per cent of this may be lost after 9 months storage. This and the additional losses on cooking probably account for the occasional cases of scurvy seen in old people in Edinburgh. These usually occur in April and May and never in the months immediately after the fresh crop has become available.

Liver is a good source of ascorbic acid and fresh milk contains some. Fresh meat provides only traces but with offal supplies sufficient to prevent scurvy, as many Arctic explorers know. A classical example of the protective role of meat was when the Indian Third Cavalry division was besieged by the Turks in Kut-el-Amara in Mesopotamia in December 1915 (Hehir, 1922). When the garrison surrendered in April 1916, scurvy had broken out in the Indian sepoys, but not in the British soldiers who had eaten their horses.

Distribution, utilisation and excretion in the human body

Ascorbic acid is readily and rapidly absorbed in the small intestine and little or none is lost in the faeces with a normal diet, but absorption of large pharmacological doses may be incomplete.

After absorption it is distributed in the blood but taken up unevenly by the tissues. The classical studies of Hodges and his colleagues (Hodges *et al.*, 1971: Baker *et al.*, 1971) on nine volunteers in the Iowa State Penitentiary using isotopically labelled ^{14}C ascorbic acid showed that when the subjects received 75 mg of ascorbic acid daily, the average size of the pool in which this was distributed was 1500 mg. The pool fell to 300 mg after 55 days on an ascorbic acid-free diet (Fig. 14.1). It was calculated that on a diet providing 30 mg daily the size of the pool would be 1000 mg.

Plasma concentrations. This is related to the dietary intake and is about 12 mg/l (68 μmol/l) on a diet contain-

Table 14.1 Sources of ascorbic acid

Food	Ascorbic acid (mg/100g edible)	
	Raw	Cooked *
Fruits		
Blackcurrants	200	140
Guavas (canned)	—	180
Strawberries	60	—
Citrus fruits—orange, grapefruit, lemon juice	40–50	—
Redcurrants and gooseberries	40	28
Raspberries, loganberries and blackberries	20–25	14–26
Melons and pineapple	25	—
Bananas	10	—
Cooking apples	—	12
Peaches and apricots	7–8	—
Dessert apples, pears, plums, grapes, figs, cherries	2–5	—
Salads		
Green peppers	100	—
Watercress, mustard and cress	40–60	—
Radish, lettuce, tomato	15–25	—
Onions	10	—
Carrots	6	—
Celery	7	—
Parsley	150	—
Vegetables		
Broccoli tops and brussels sprouts	(100)	35
Cauliflower, cabbage and spinach	50–60	15–25
Asparagus, leeks	—	18–20
Peas	25	14
Parsnips and turnips	—	10–17
New early potatoes	—	18
Main grop potatoes	—	9
Sweetcorn	—	9
Runner beans	—	5
Lentils	0	0
Animal foods		
Liver	(23)	15
Milk	2	1

* Usually stewed fruit and boiled vegetables.

ing about 100 mg. It falls to 1 mg/1 (5.7 μmol/l) after about four weeks on diets containing less than 10 mg of ascorbic acid. Depletion studies have shown that a plasma concentration below 1 mg/l indicates that the subject is at high risk of developing scurvy and that between 1 and 2 mg/l he is at moderate risk. Values above 2 mg/l are acceptable White blood cells normally contain over 150 mg/l and a value below 70 mg/l indicates a high risk of developing scurvy. The amount in the white blood cells provides a better index of depletion of ascorbic acid than does the amount in the plasma, but the estimation is technically more difficult.

Concentration in organs. All organs and tissues have a higher concentration than plasma. Concentrations are high in glandular organs, especially the adrenal glands where it may be 50 times more than the concentration in plasma. There is much data about the ascorbic acid content of guinea-pig organs but relatively little in man. Table 14.2 gives data obtained from autopsies in Pittsburgh in 1934.

The figures are averages and there were wide individual variations, but it was not possible to relate the finding to dietary intakes or plasma concentrations in life. The figures show very high concentrations in early life and a steady fall with increasing age. As the weights of the glandular organs are small, the brain and liver—each of which weighs about 1.5 kg—contain the major amount of ascorbic acid and presumably provide a store which is available when the dietary intake is reduced. The total ascorbic acid in all the organs listed in Table 14.2 falls some way short of the 1500 mg found in the ascorbic acid pool. There must also be some in muscle. In guinea-pig muscle concentrations are usually between 30 and 40 mg/kg. Values for human muscle are certainly lower. If a figure of 20 mg/kg is taken, then a 70 kg man with 30 kg of muscle would have 600 mg of ascorbic acid in his muscles. This would be the largest store of the vitamin in his body.

The aqueous humour of the eye also has a much higher concentration than the plasma. Kinsey (1947) found values

Table 14.2 Average values (mg/kg) for the ascorbic acid content of human organs obtained at autopsy (from Yavorsky *et al.*, 1934)

| | Age group | | | |
Organ	1–30 days (11)	1–10 years (11)	11–45 years (17)	46–77 years (19)
Adrenal gland	581	550	393	230
Brain	460	433	n.m.	110
Pancreas	365	225	152	95
Thymus	304	190	n.m.	46
Spleen	153	157	127	81
Kidney	153	98	98	47
Liver	149	163	135	64
Lung	126	58	65	45
Heart	76	42	42	21

Number of subjects are shown in parenthesis. n.m. = not measured.

of from 200–250 mg/l in rabbits whose plasma concentration ranged from 5 to 20 mg/l. The concentration in aqueous humour rose to over 500 mg/l one hour after an injection of ascorbic acid. The aqueous humour supplies the nutrition of the lens which is also rich in ascorbic acid.

The ascorbic acid content of human connective tissue has been measured by Crandon *et al.* (1953) in samples of the anterior rectus sheath obtained during abdominal operations. Amounts between 30 and 60 mg/kg were found in patients with plasma concentrations ranging from 4 to 13 mg/l whose dietary intake may be presumed to have been satisfactory. Values from 0 to 15 mg/kg were found in 12 patients with plasma concentrations below 1 mg/l.

Urinary excretion. How the kidneys deal with ascorbic acid was worked out by Friedman, Sherry and Ralli (1943). Ascorbic acid passes into the glomerular filtrate in the same concentration as in the plasma but, provided the plasma concentration is below 14 mg/l, almost all is reabsorbed in the renal tubules. Thus the kidneys conserve the vitamin well and very little appears in the urine with normal dietary intakes. Estimations of the urinary output of ascorbic acid are of no value in assessing the risk of scurvy for this reason. If, however, the plasma concentration is raised above 14 mg/l by giving preparations of ascorbic acid, the renal tubules fail to absorb this. With increasing plasma concentrations the renal clearance of ascorbic acid rapidly rises and soon approaches that of inulin. Then almost all the dose is lost in the urine. Studies with ^{14}C ascorbic acid have shown that intermediary metabolites, not yet all identified, are present in the urine in significant amounts (Baker *et. al.*, 1975).

Rate of utilisation. In the Iowa studies the urine, faeces and expired air were analysed for their content of labelled carbon after injection of ^{14}C ascorbic acid. Less than 2 per cent of the label was found in the faeces, showing the completeness of absorption, and only about 2 per cent in the carbon dioxide of the expired air. Nearly all was present in the urine and most of it not in ascorbic acid itself or in the first two products of its oxidation, dehydroascorbic acid and dioxogulonic acid, but in unidentified

metabolic products. From the output of the label the rate of utilisation of the vitamin was calculated. This was 45 mg/day when the body pool was at a maximum of 1500 mg. When after depletion the body pool fell to 300 mg and signs of scurvy began to appear, the catabolic rate was below 9 mg/day (Fig. 14.2). The rate of utilisation thus appears to be determined by the size of the pool and so is related to the dietary intake and not to any specific physiological need.

Ascorbic acid and extracellular connective tissue
Although ascorbic acid is ubiquitous in the cells of the body and is a powerful biological reducing agent, manifestations of its deficiency are obvious only in extracellular structures. The characteristic feature of scurvy, both the natural disease in man and the experimental disease in guinea-pigs is an 'inability of the supporting tissues to produce and maintain intercellular substances' (Wolback and Howe, 1926).

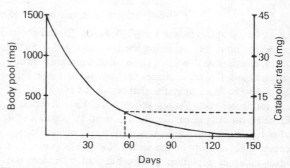

Fig. 14.2 Curve of ascorbate pool derived from data of nine men whose body pool of ascorbate was labelled with ^{14}C L-ascorbic acid. They were then fed on a diet devoid of vitamin C. Initially the body pool averaged 1500 mg. The average daily rate of catabolism was 3 per cent of the existing body pool. Thus the maximal rate approximated to 45 mg/day. When the body pool fell below 300 mg total and the catabolic rate below 9 mg/day, signs of scurvy began to appear (about 55 days). From this curve one can estimate the approximate body pool size from the dose. Thus with a daily intake of 30 mg the pool size should be about 1000 mg. (From Hodges, 1973.)

Burt Wolback was a Boston pathologist who studied the histological lesions in scurvy for many years and summarised it in a beautifully illustrated paper presented at the Lind bicentenary symposium in Edinburgh (Wolbach, 1953). The capillary haemorrhages are due to a defect in the basement membrane that lines the capillaries and the intracellular cement that joins the endothelial cells together. The failure of wounds to heal is due to a defect in the formation of scar tissue. In children and young guinea-pigs the failure of cartilage, bone and dentine to develop normally is due to a defect in the extracellular matrix in which the cells of the tissues, respectively the chondroblasts, the osteoblasts and the ondontoblasts, lay down the hard minerals. This matrix is composed of the protein collagen which forms about one-fifth of the wet weight of both bone and cartilage. Changes in the matrix prevent the osteoblasts laying down new bone and lead to demineralization. This is responsible for the breakdown of old fractures as was graphically described by Walter (1748) in his account of Anson's voyage round the world.

But a most extraordinary circumstance, and what could be scarcely credible upon any single evidence, is that the scars of wounds which had been for many years healed were forced open again by this virulent distemper. Of this there was a remarkable example in one of the invalids on board the *Centurion*, who had been wounded about fifty years before at the Battle of the Boyne, for though he was cured soon after, and had continued well for a great number of years past, yet on his being attacked by the scurvy, his wounds, in the progress of the disease, broke out afresh and appeared as if they had never healed: nay, what is still more astonishing, the callus of a broken bone which had been completely formed for a long time, was found to be hereby dissolved, and the fracture seemed as if it had never been consolidated.

The biochemical lesion. This is in the formation of defective collagen, the protein forming the basement membrane of capillaries, the fibrous tissue in scars and the matrix of the hard tissues. The collagen molecule, which is very large, is assembled outside the cells from smaller units of procollagen which are synthesised by connective tissue cells and secreted into the extracellular spaces. Not all collagens are identical in their molecular structure, but all are characterised by a unique combination of amino acids in their makeup. Glycine provides about one-quarter and proline and hydroxyproline, in approximately equal proportions, about one-third of the constituent amino acids. The procollagen chain is a coil which has many repeating units of —glycine—hydroxyproline—proline—. Hydroxyproline is not found in proteins other than collagen and it is formed from proline by the action of an enzyme system, proline hydroxylase, present in fibroblasts (Fig. 14.3). In scorbutic animals this reaction is defective and, although

collagen is formed, it lacks hydroxyproline and the cross-links between the chains in the molecule are unstable.

The proline hydroxylase enzyme system has been studied both *in vitro* and in fibroblasts growing in tissue culture (Leven and Bates, 1975). Ascorbic acid appears to have two roles. Production of hydroxyproline by the isolated system *in vitro* is negligible in its absence; nevertheless other reducing substances, e.g. thiol compounds and even inorganic reducing agents such as sulphite, can replace it. Therefore, ascorbic acid is not a specific oxygen receptor for the enzyme system. In living cells the addition of ascorbic acid to the culture medium rapidly increased activity of the enzyme but a similar effect can be produced by a low partial pressure of oxygen and in other ways (Barnes, 1975). The precise role of ascorbic acid in collagen synthesis therefore remains uncertain.

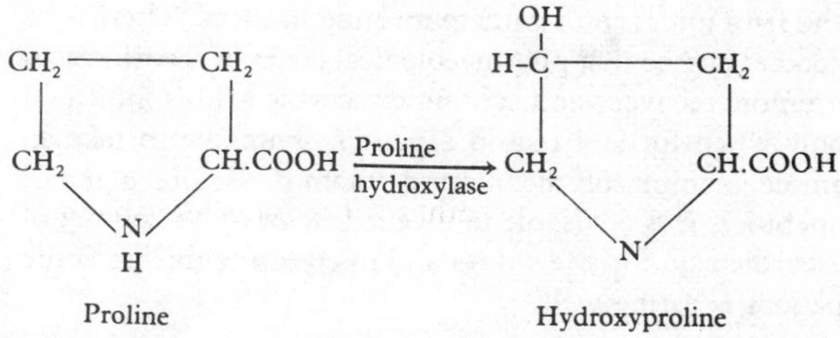

Fig. 14.3 Action of proline hydroxylase.

Ascorbic acid, the adrenal cortex and stress

In the eighteenth century Lind (1753) and many others reported that scurvy was more likely to break out in ships when the crews were exposed to cold, damp and rough seas, fatigued by hard work or debilitated by other diseases. Non-specific stresses clearly predisposed the men to the disease. The first association of vitamin C with the adrenal glands was the observation of McCarrison (1919) that they were hypertrophied in scorbutic guinea-pigs. The high concentration of ascorbic acid in adrenal glands was shown to be depleted by fatigue (Van Eekelen and Kooy, 1933) and by infections (Harris *et al.*, 1937). Soon after the discovery of the role of the pituitary hormone, ACTH, in promoting secretion of adrenocortical hormones in conditions of stress, injections of ACTH were shown to deplete the adrenal cortex of ascorbic acid and to increase the concentration of ascorbic acid in the adrenal veins. These findings lead to the view that a major physiological role of ascorbic acid was in the synthesis of steroid hormones in the adrenal cortex in response to stresses of various kinds. However, this attractive theory failed to explain the fact that, when the adrenal glands are destroyed, as in Addison's disease, the patient's signs and symptoms, mainly extreme muscular weakness, in no way resemble those found in scurvy. It has been disproved by the finding that isolated adrenal cells, in which almost all the ascorbic acid had been removed during preparation, were still able to synthesise adrenocortical hormones in response to stimulation by ACTH (Kitabchi and West, 1975). Adrenal function tests, e.g. plasma cortisol before and after ACTH, are normal in scurvy (Kitabchi and Duckworth, 1970).

It is difficult to believe that the high concentrations of ascorbic acid in the adrenal glands serve no biological purpose. A new theory is that ascorbic acid has a continuous inhibitory effect either on the synthesis of adrenocortical hormones or on their release from the gland into the blood stream. The role of ACTH would then be to reverse this inhibition by releasing ascorbic acid from the cells which could then secrete the hormones.

On the practical side injuries of any sort, especially burns and including surgical operations, increase utilisation of ascorbic acid. Such a patient needs a good supply of the vitamin. Visitors to the hospital who bring fresh fruit and fruit juices contribute to meeting his need. There is no good evidence that pharmacological doses of ascorbic acid promote recovery and synthetic ascorbic acid is indicated only when for any reason a patient is unable to take an ample amount of the natural vitamin. Before a major operation it is advisable to give a dose of up to 250 mg of ascorbic acid for a few days and to continue this until the patient is eating well.

Toxicity

Ascorbic acid appears to be one of the safest substances in the pharmacopoeia. Many people have now taken 2 g or more daily for long periods without untoward effect; this is 200 times the dose needed to cure scurvy and 20 to 40 times the usual dietary intake. It would seem that no adverse effect could arise from taking large amounts of the natural vitamin present in foods. There are, however, doubts about the safety of taking pharmacological doses for long periods. Nausea and diarrhoea occasionally occur, but as these gastrointestinal symptoms are likely to lead the subject to stop taking the drug, they are not likely to be dangerous. More important is a possible increased risk of renal stones. Oxalic acid is one of the metabolites of ascorbic acid that appears in the urine and increased excretion might lead to stone formation, especially in subjects with hypercalciuria. A rise in plasma cholesterol and destruction of vitamin B_{12} have also been reported. These and other possible hazards are reviewed by Barnes (1975), who points out that they are most likely to be significant in patients with inborn errors of metabolism; he rightly cautions against the use of high doses in infants and rapidly growing children

Ascorbic acid as a drug

Ascorbic acid is a cheap and safe drug. There have been many claims that it is useful in the treatment of a large number of diseases. Its most enthusiastic advocate is Linus Pauling (1976), whose book *Vitamin C and the Common*

Cold and the Flu has had a great influence. Pauling became interested in ascorbic acid in 1966 when he received a letter from Irwin Stone, the successful novelist, advising him to take large doses of it daily. He and his wife then began to take 1 g or more daily and at once 'noticed an increased feeling of wellbeing, and especially a striking decrease in the number of colds that we caught and in their severity.' He then began to study the literature on ascorbic acid and the first edition of his book appeared in 1970 and soon had large numbers of readers.

Pauling was greatly respected by scientists for his work as a chemist on the structure of large molecules and especially by biologists for his explanation of how a small change in the chemical composition of haemoglobin was responsible for the sickle cell phenomenon in red blood corpuscles. He was also well known to the general public for his work to promote peace and had the rare distinction of receiving two Nobel prizes, one for science and one for peace. Furthermore, his book on vitamin C was beautifully written and easily read by the general public despite the fact that it contained complicated scientific argument and many references to the literature. As a result of his advocacy, very large numbers of the public in America and other countries began to take tablets of ascorbic acid regularly.

Pauling's hypothesis was based on a study of the evolution of the diet of primates. He calculated the average content of ascorbic acid in 110 natural plant foods, as might be eaten by a gorilla, and showed that a human adult eating a diet made up of these foods would obtain 2.3 g of the vitamin, some 50 times the USA recommended intake. Furthermore, he showed that the potential rate of synthesis of ascorbic acid, as reported in several species of animals, if extrapolated to man, indicated a human daily requirement of up to 10 g.

Three studies of the effect of ascorbic acid on the common cold were available to him, one from Minnesota, USA (Cowan *et al.*, 1942), one from Scotland (Glazebrook and Thomson, 1942) and one from Switzerland. The authors of the first two reports both considered that the vitamin had no effect on the prevalence and severity of respiratory infections but Pauling concluded that they had misinterpreted their data and that it indicated a beneficial effect. The Swiss report (Ritzel, 1961) claimed benefit, but the trial was on a small scale, 31 out of 140 subjects receiving a placebo developing colds as against 17 out of 139 of these receiving 1 g of ascorbic acid daily. The difficulties of organising controlled clinical trials are now much better appreciated; they are especially great for the common cold and influenza, which are infections caused by a variety of pathogenic organisms, and investigators are usually dependent on their subjects for the diagnosis of an attack and judgment of its severity. Pauling's book has stimulated at least 15 such trials, not all of which have been technically good. The largest and best designed was carried out in Toronto (Anderson *et al.*, 1974), in which 2349 subjects out of 3520 who enrolled completed the three months of study. The subjects were divided into eight groups who received a placebo or a dose of ascorbic acid both prophylactically throughout the trial and during episodes of infection. Table 14.3 shows the treatment schedules and an abstract of their results. One of the placebo groups had fewer episodes and of less severity than any of the other groups. None of the groups receiving ascorbic acid had a sickness experience that was statistically different from the placebo groups. However, the authors state that their 'results were compatible with an effect of small magnitude from both the prophylactic and therapeutic regimens'. Other experimenters (Coulehan *et al.*, 1974; Wilson *et al.*, 1976) have also presented data indicating a possible small benefit.

This small benefit has to be offset against any possible hazard. Ascorbic acid in large doses has been taken by many thousands of persons for long periods without untoward effect. Nevertheless it is known to increase the urinary output of oxalic acid and of uric acid, and intestinal absorption of iron. Large doses are therefore dangerous to those with a liability to urinary stones or to iron-storage disease. The Canadian workers found that after an abrupt withdrawal of a high dose, blood concentrations of ascorbic acid were abnormally low, and this might be dangerous. For these reasons we cannot recommend that large doses should be taken for long periods for prophylactic purposes. The risk of taking up to 4 g daily for a few days for therapeutic purposes should be acceptable.

There is no satisfactory evidence from *in vitro* studies that ascorbic acid is an antiviral agent effective against any of the virus responsible for infections of the upper respiratory tract. There is, however, a good study (Zuskin *et al.*, 1973) showing that a dose of 500 mg inhibits the bronchospasm induced by inhaling a histamine aerosol. Ascorbic acid is thus an antihistamine and, if any of the effects of respiratory infections can be attributed to the liberation of histamine as a result of immunity reaction or injury to tissue, it might be beneficial in this way.

Orthomolecular medicine. Pauling claims in his book that large doses of ascorbic acid may be beneficial in cancer, heart disease, schizophrenia and other diseases. This view is derived from his concept of orthomolecular medicine which '...is the preservation of good health and the treatment of disease by varying the concentrations in the human body of substances that are normally present in the body and are required for health.... To achieve the best of health, the rate of intake of essential foods should be such as to establish and maintain optimum concentrations of essential molecules, such as those of ascorbic acid. There is no doubt that a high concentration of ascorbic acid is needed to provide the maximum protection against infection, and to permit the rapid healing of wounds. I believe that in general the treatment of disease by the use of substances such as ascorbic acid, that are normally present in the human body and are required for life is to be preferred to the treatment by the use of powerful synthetic substances or plant products, which may, and usually do, have undesirable side effects.'

Orthomolecular medicine is an attractive idea, and the principle can sometimes work in practice. Thus large doses of vitamin D, 100 times the daily requirement, were used effectively to treat tuberculosis of the skin; such dosage carried a grave risk of hypervitaminosis D and the treatment was given up soon after the introduction of relatively safe antituberculous drugs. There may well be other pathological processes sensitive to large doses of vitamins or be individuals whose defence and repair mechanisms requiring abnormally high concentrations of a vitamin or other natural substance to operate effectively. Pauling has not demonstrated this—at least not to the satisfaction of the medical establishment.

THIAMIN—VITAMIN B$_1$

History

In 1890 the Dutch physician Eijkman (1897), working in a military hospital in Java, fed some domestic fowls on the food provided for his patients suffering from beriberi. He noticed that they developed weakness of the legs and head retraction. Their food consisted mainly of polished rice; a

Table 14.3 Ascorbic acid in the prophylaxis and treatment of the common cold (from Anderson *et al.*, 1974)

Treatment (g ascorbic acid/day) Prophylactic	Therapeutic	Mean number of episodes	Mean days of symptoms	Mean days off work
Placebo	Placebo	1.53	5.40	1.18
Placebo	Placebo	1.47	4.16	0.94
0.25	Placebo	1.53	4.77	1.11
1.0	Placebo	1.51	5.04	1.09
2.0	Placebo	1.51	4.87	1.29
Placebo	4	1.52	4.82	0.97
Placebo	8	1.58	4.52	1.05
1	4	1.57	5.38	1.13

new head cook at the hospital discontinued this supply of 'military' rice, so that thereafter the birds had to be fed on whole-grain 'civilian' rice, with the result that they recovered. Many great advances in science have started from such chance observations pursued by men of inspiration. Eijkman deservedly won the Nobel Prize many years later for showing that there was something existing in very small amounts in the germ and pericarp of rice that protected fowls from a disease resembling beriberi, and for recognising the fact that it was an unknown nutrient. He extracted it from rice polishings with water and alcohol.

Thirty years later Jansen and Donath (1926), working in the same laboratory, succeeded in isolating this factor (thiamin) in crystalline form. They used small rice birds (*Munia maja*) instead of fowls for testing the activity of the different fractions which they prepared in the course of isolating the vitamin. Thiamin deficiency, they found, could readily be produced in this bird; it was also produced in pigeons, rats and mice by numerous other workers who were seeking in the 1920s to identify and isolate the vitamin.

The crystalline vitamin was found to contain a sulphur atom united in a hitherto unknown (thiazole) ring. The structure of the vitamin was finally elucidated and its synthesis accomplished by R. R. Williams and Cline (1936). Williams began his search for the vitamin in 1913 in the Philippines, under the guidance of E. B. Vedder, a pioneer in the clinical study of beriberi. R. R. Williams patented the synthesis in North America. All the proceeds went to the Williams-Waterman Fund which supported nutrition research in many countries between 1935 and 1955.

Thiamin deficiency in birds

The condition produced in birds by acute thiamin deficiency is characterised by head retraction and convulsions indicating a disorder of the nervous system. These features are due to an acute biochemical lesion in the brain, not necessarily associated with any anatomical lesion of the brain or peripheral nerves. The giving of pure synthetic thiamin rapidly relieves this biochemical lesion.

Chemistry

Thiamin hydrochloride is a white crystalline substance. The molecule consists of a pyrimidine ring joined to a sulphur-containing thiazole ring. It is readily soluble in water, but not in most fat solvents nor in fats. It is rapidly destroyed by heat in neutral or alkaline solutions; in acid solution, however, it is resistant to heat up to 120°C. Thiamin can be converted by controlled oxidation into an inactive product, thiochrome, which is strongly fluorescent in ultraviolet light. This property is used for the chemical estimation of the vitamin in biological materials. It is also measured microbiologically with *Lactobacillus viridescens*.

Physiological activity

Thiamin was the first vitamin whose precise activity in the body was stated in biochemical terms. This was achieved at Oxford between 1928 and 1935. Peters (1963) has written an historical account of the work. It was first demonstrated that lactic acid accumulates in the brains of thiamin-deficient pigeons. It was then found that minced brain tissue from such birds took up less oxygen than brain tissue from normal birds in the presence of added glucose or lactic acid *in vitro*. This failure of oxidation could be corrected by adding thiamin in catalytic amounts to the brain tissue. It was thus established for the first time that a vitamin could be an essential part of an enzyme system. At the start it seemed likely that thiamin was specifically concerned with lactic acid, but it was found that pyruvic acid also accumulated in the brain and blood of such birds and that thiamin is specifically concerned with its removal. It is now known that thiamin pyrophosphate (TPP) is the coenzyme of carboxylase, the enzyme concerned with the oxidative decarboxylation of pyruvic acid.

The fact that thiamin is concerned with a stage in the breakdown of carbohydrate explains how signs of deficiency of the vitamin develop most rapidly in animals fed diets rich in carbohydrates. The onset of deficiency is delayed by a diet rich in fat. There is evidence from dietary surveys that the same may also be true in man.

The brain and nerves have a respiratory quotient of unity, which shows that their energy is derived mostly from the oxidation of carbohydrate. The role of thiamin in the breakdown of carbohydrate explains how deficiency in animals leads rapidly to a biochemical lesion in the brain. TPP is also required for the decarboxylation of 2-oxoglutarate in the citric acid cycle and of the keto acids formed after deamination of the branched chain amino acids, leucine, isoleucine and valine; it is also needed in the transketolase reaction in the hexose monophosphate pathway. Thiamin is present in the body mostly as TPP but about 10 per cent is thiamin triphosphate.

Thiamin is absorbed from the small intestine by an active process which is impaired in alcoholics with folate deficiency (Thomson *et al.*, 1971).

The total amount of thiamin in the well-nourished human body is small, amounting in all to about 25–30 mg. The highest concentration is found in the heart, brain, liver, kidneys and skeletal muscles. The body has no means of storing any excess so that no benefit derives from taking large doses; the excess is lost in the urine.

Experimental deficiency in man

Human volunteers have been fed on diets deficient in thiamin but adequate in other respects (Williams *et al.*, 1942; Keys *et al.*, 1945). The first reported symptoms have usually been loss of appetite (anorexia) and mental changes resembling anxiety states, with irritability and easy exhaustion. To what extent these are specific effects of the deficiency is open to question. They may be the non-specific result of an unaccustomed regime and a distasteful diet.

Laboratory diagnosis

The amount of thiamin in the urine reflects recent intake but is no reliable test of deficiency, since it falls to low levels before the tissues are depleted. Several metabolites are excreted in the urine as well as unchanged thiamin.

A satisfactory laboratory test must show whether a patient's symptoms can reasonably be attributed to lack of thiamin. The point at which a dietary deficiency of the vitamin becomes important is when it is sufficiently severe to cause a biochemical lesion. The rise in the level of pyruvic acid in the blood of patients with beriberi was first shown in 1936 by Platt and Lu (1936). This test is made more sensitive by measuring the accumulation of pyruvic acid in the blood following exercise or an oral dose of glucose (Thompson and Cumings, 1970). However, thiamin deficiency is by no means the sole cause of an elevated blood pyruvic acid: the test is not specific unless accom-

panied by a therapeutic trial, demonstrating improvement following the administration of thiamin.

A more specific test is the measurement of the transketolase activity in the red blood corpuscles with and without the addition of TPP *in vitro*. If TPP increases activity by more than 25 per cent, this indicated thiamin deficiency (Brin, 1962). An assessment of the thiamin status of rice eaters in Malaya by Chong and Ho (1970) used this test.

Dietary sources

All animal and plant tissues contain thiamin and it is therefore present in all whole natural foods; but the only important stores in the biological world are in the seeds of plants. The germ of cereals, nuts, peas, beans and other pulses and in addition yeast are the only rich sources. All green vegetables, roots, fruits, flesh foods and dairy produce (except butter) contain significant amounts of the vitamin, but none are rich sources. As the vitamin is not soluble in fats, it is not found in butter or in any separated vegetable or animal oil. Pork resembles human flesh in having a higher content of thiamin than beef or mutton. In

Table 14.4 Sources of thiamin

Source	Description	Thiamin		
		µg/MJ	mg/1000 kcal	mg/100 g
Satisfactory or rich sources not usually associated with beriberi				
Whole wheat	—	290	1.2	0.4
Pulses	Various	290	1.2	0.4
Millets	Sorghum	290	1.2	0.4
Rice	Home pounded	84*	0.35*	0.08–0.14*
Rice	Parboiled and milled	76*	0.32*	0.11*
Poor sources associated with beriberi				
White bread †	70 per cent extraction flour	48	0.20	0.05–0.07
Rice	Raw, milled	36	0.15*	0.02–0.04*
Sugars and jams	—	0	0	—
Alcoholic beverages	—	0	0	—
Moderate sources protective against beriberi if consumed in large amounts				
Fruits and vegetables	Fresh	120–290	0.5–1.2	0.02–0.20
Pork	Fresh	240–360	1.0–1.5	0.72–1.04
Beef	Fresh	70–120	0.3–0.5	0.07–0.30
Mutton	Fresh	120	0.5	0.16–0.20
Fish	Fresh	70–240	0.3–1.0	0.01–0.10
Milk	Cow's	170	0.7	0.04
Eggs	Whole	150	0.6	0.09
Rich sources used in the treatment of beriberi				
Yeast ‡	Brewers', dried	—		6–24
Bran	Rice or wheat	—		2–4
Marmite	Yeast extract	—		2.4–3.0

Note. Butter, vegetable oils and other fats contain no thiamin, but as the vitamin is not needed for their metabolism they are not beriberi-producing.

* Assuming losses of 50 per cent in washing and cooking.
† Unfortified.
‡ Bakers' yeasts have much less thiamin than brewers' yeast and are unreliable for therapeutic purposes.

the refining of sugar and many cereal products all the naturally occurring vitamin may be removed: there is also none in distilled spirits. The labile thiaminase present in certain uncooked fish may also decrease the thiamin content of rice diets in the Far East. The distribution of the vitamin within cereal grains and the effect of milling and other food processing are discussed on page 213. The thiamin content of some common foods is given in Table 14.4.

As thiamin is readily soluble in water, considerable amounts may be lost when vegetables are cooked in an excess of water which is afterwards discarded. It is relatively stable to temperatures up to boiling point, provided that the medium is slightly acid, as in baking with yeast. But if baking powder is used, or if soda is added in the cooking of vegetables, almost all the vitamin may be destroyed. The loss of thiamin in the cooking of an ordinary mixed diet is usually about 25 per cent. Modern processes for freezing, canning and dehydrating food result in only small losses.

Recommended intakes

While there is a relationship between the utilisation of thiamin and the amount of carbohydrate in the diet, it is more practical to relate thiamin intake to total dietary energy. Williams and Spies (1938) calculated the thiamin/energy ratio of 100 diets, of which 66 were associated with beriberi. Beriberi did not occur when the ratio was greater than 62 $\mu g/MJ$. This can be taken as the minimum protective intake. FAO/WHO (1967) recommended a daily intake of 96 $\mu g/MJ$ (0.4 mg/1000 kcal) for all classes of consumers, including nursing mothers. This provides a sufficient margin of safety.

THIAMIN-ENERGY RELATIONSHIPS IN FOODS

It should be emphasised that beriberi is not a disease of famines. Indeed cardiovascular beriberi may occur among people with good supplies of polished rice and good appetites to eat it. It results from a poorly balanced diet. The thiamin/energy ratio of foods indicates those which protect against beriberi and those which are liable to produce the disease, if consumed in excessive amounts. Thus pulses and most whole cereals have a ratio of about 290 $\mu g/MJ$ (1.2 mg/1000 kcal) and are actively protective against beriberi. Raw polished rice has a value of about 36 $\mu g/MJ$ (0.15 mg/1000 kcal) and is beriberi-producing. Most fruits, vegetables and flesh foods have a ratio just above a critical level of about 60 and are weakly effective in preventing beriberi.

Therapeutic uses

Thiamin is life-saving in the treatment of cardiovascular and infantile beriberi (p. 286) in Wernicke's encephalopathy (p. 288) and in some forms of cardiomyopathy (p. 287). It may be given, though without expectation of dramatic results, in cases of nutritional neuropathy. There is no reliable evidence that it is useful in any other disorder of the nervous system. The prescription of synthetic thiamin, either alone or in combination with other vitamins, as a general tonic or appetiser, is supported by no scientific evidence and is now discredited.

In prescribing thiamin it should be remembered that the healthy human body contains only about 25 mg of the vitamin. Furthermore, it has no means of storing any excess taken in the diet; the excess is lost rapidly in the urine. The human body is certainly an effective machine for dissolving thiamin pills and transferring the solution to the urinal.

NICOTINIC ACID (NIACIN) AND NICOTINAMIDE

History

Nicotinic acid has been known to organic chemists since 1867. As early as 1913 Funk isolated it from yeast and rice polishings in the course of an attempt to identify the water-soluble anti-beriberi vitamin. But interest in the acid was lost when it was found ineffective in curing pigeons of beriberi and did not arise again until 1935, when its amide was found to be a component of the respiratory coenzyme NAD.

Nicotinic acid was shown to be the 'pellagra-preventing' (P-P) vitamin in the following manner. In the 1920s Goldberger and his colleagues in the US Public Health Service recognised that human pellagra responded not only to treatment with animal protein but also to boiled extracts of yeast almost devoid of protein (Goldberger et al., 1928). This naturally led to the supposition the the P-P factor was identical with 'heat-stable vitamin B₂' present in yeast. An important step towards the isolation of this factor was the discovery of a suitable laboratory animal for testing its potency in various concentrated preparations derived from natural sources; it was found that a pellagra-like disease could be produced in dogs and pigs (Chick et al., 1938). Following the discovery by Ruffin and Smith (1934) that a crude extract of liver was effective in human pellagra, and therefore a source of the P-P factor, Elvehjem and his colleagues (1937) finally isolated nicotinamide from liver as the factor that would cure black-tongue in dogs. Reports of the dramatic therapeutic effects of nicotinic acid in human pellagra quickly followed from several clinics.

Chemistry

Nicotinic acid is a simple derivative of pyridine. Although related chemically to nicotine, it possesses very different physiological properties. It is a white crystalline substance readily soluble in water and resistant to heat, oxidation and alkalis: it is in fact one of the most stable of the vitamins.

Nicotinic acid is easily synthesised commercially. It occurs naturally in the body in the form of the amide, nicotinamide (niacinamide).

Physiological activity

Nicotinamide is a component of the respiratory coenzymes NAD and NADP, concerned with tissue oxidation. The lack of NAD in pellagra may account for the inflammatory changes that occur in the skin and gastrointestinal tract, though the precise mechanism involved is still obscure. In pharmacological doses nicotinic acid inhibits lipolysis in adipose tissue, but this is probably not a physiological action. A full account of the metabolic effects of nicotinic acid is given by Gey and Carlson (1971).

Laboratory diagnosis of deficiency

Nicotinic acid can be estimated in blood and other biological material by a chemical technique (Swaminathan, 1938), based on a reaction with cyanogen bromide and aniline leading to the formation of a yellow colour. A microbiological method (Snell and Wright, 1941), in which the amount of lactic acid produced by *Lactobacillus arabinosis* grown on synthetic medium is also reliable.

Attempts to diagnose deficiency by measuring nicotinic acid itself in body fluids have proved disappointing. Blood normally contains about 5 mg/l mainly as NAD, but in states of manifest deficiency the amount is not greatly reduced.

The urinary excretion of the nicotinic acid metabolite, N'-methylnicotinamide, is used as a measure of reserves of nutritional status (p.468). For methodology see Pelletier and Brassard (1977). The other major metabolite is the 2-pyridone of N'-methylnicotinamide.

Dietary sources

The human body is not entirely dependent on dietary sources of nicotinic acid, as it may also be synthesised from trytophan (Fig. 14.4). Observations on a large group of patients (Horwitt *et al.*, 1956) suggest that on average about 60 mg of tryptophan are needed to replace 1 mg of dietary nicotinic acid. The nicotinic acid equivalent (the nicotinic acid content plus one-sixtieth of the tryptophan content) of a food or diet is a better measure than the nicotinic acid content alone. Its use removes one anomaly: milk and eggs are poor sources of nicotinic acid, although they have long been recognised as beneficial to patients with pellagra; each of these foods has a high nicotinic acid equivalent.

Nicotinic acid is widely distributed in plant and animal foods, but only in relatively small amounts, except in meat (especially the organs), fish, wholemeal cereals and pulses (Table 14.5). Table 14.6 gives the nicotinic acid equivalent of some foods and shows the important contribution that may come from tryptophan. In many cereals, especially maize, and perhaps also in potatoes, the greater part may

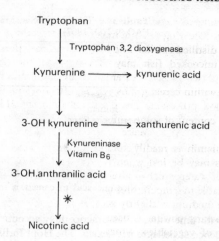

Fig. 14.4 The conversion of tryptophan to nicotinic acid. In deficiency of vitamin B_6, kynurenic acid and xanthurenic acid appear in the urine in increased amounts.
*Several intermediary steps.

be in a bound unabsorbable form (Kodicek, 1962; Mason *et al.*, 1973). Nicotinic acid can be liberated from the bound form, niacytin, by treatment with alkali. For a long time in Mexico *tortillas* have been made from maize

Table 14.5 Nicotinic acid and nicotinamide in foods

Food	mg/100g edible part
High content	
Liver and kidney	7.0–17.0
Beef, mutton, pork	3.0–6.0
Fish	2.0–6.0
Brewers' yeast	30–100
'Bovril'	82
'Marmite'	60
Groundnuts	16
Coffee (instant)	30
Wheat bran (outer only)	25–46*
Wheatgerm meal	3.0–7.0*
Rice (lightly milled)	2.0–4.5*
Wheat, wholemeal flour	4.0–5.5*
Sorghum	2.5–3.5*
Millets (various)	1.3–3.2*
Moderate content	
Pulses	1.5–3.0
Nuts	1.0–2.0
Dried fruit	0.5–5.0
Oatmeal	1.0*
Rice (highly milled) raw	1.5*
Wheat flour 70 percent extraction †	0.7*
Low content	
Maize meal, potato, vegetables, fresh fruits, eggs, milk and cheese	

* Much of the nicotinic acid in some, possibly all, cereals is in bound form, not biologically available. † Unfortified.

Table 14.6 The nicotinic acid equivalents in some common foods (data from FAO/WHO, 1967)

Food	Nicotinic acid	Tryptophan	Nicotinic acid equivalent
	(all values in mg/MJ)		
Milk—cow's	0.3	162	3.0
human	0.6	106	2.4
Wheat, white flour	0.6*	71	1.8
Maize	1.2*	25	1.6
Maize grits	0.4*	17	0.7
Beef	5.9	306	11.0
Eggs	0.1	275	4.8

* Nicotinic acid in cereals is mostly unavailable.

treated with lime water. This practice may account for a low incidence of pellagra in Mexico. The Hopi Indians of Arizona roast sweetcorn in hot ashes: this is another traditional practice that liberates the nicotinic acid (Kodicek et al., 1974), but the ways of food preparation used in Africa and Asia do not have this fortunate effect. In a normal European diet about half the nicotinic acid equivalent is provided by meat and fish.

Cooking causes little actual destruction of nicotinic acid but considerable amounts may be lost in the cooking water and 'drippings' from cooked meat if these are discarded. In a mixed diet, from 15 to 25 per cent of the nicotinic acid of the cooked foodstuffs may be lost in this way. Commercial processing and storage of foodstuffs cause little loss.

Recommended intakes

The Joint Committee of FAO/WHO (1967) recommended an intake of 1.6 mg/MJ (6.6 mg/1000 kcal) nicotinic acid equivalents in the diet. Most authorities base their recommendations on this figure.

In pregnancy larger than normal amounts of nicotinamide metabolites are excreted in the urine, whether comparison is made on ordinary diets or after a load of 2 g L-tryptophan. Administration of oestrogens and of oral contraceptives containing oestrogens likewise increase nicotinamide metabolites in urine (Wolf, 1971; Horwitt et al., 1975). The first enzyme on the kynurenine pathway, tryptophan dioxygenase, is induced by oestrogens. This suggests that more tryptophan is converted to NAD during pregnancy so 60 mg tryptophan in the diet may then be equivalent to more than 1 mg nicotinic acid. On the other hand, if the protein intake is low it would be unwise to assume that the usual proportion of tryptophan is converted to nicotinic acid.

Therapeutic uses

Nicotinic acid and nicotinamide have specific and dramatic effects in pellagra and Hartnup disease (Chap. 34). The acid, though not the amide, causes transient vasodilation when taken by mouth, resulting in flushing, burning and tingling, especially round the neck, face and hands. Nevertheless nicotinic acid has been widely used as a vasodilator drug in chilblains and other vascular disorders and also in a variety of diseases, quite unconnected with nutritional failure.

Pharmacological doses (1 g thrice daily) of nicotinic acid are sometimes used to lower plasma lipids in patients with hyperlipidaemia.

RIBOFLAVIN

History

Riboflavin was discovered in the course of the search for the hypothetical 'heat-stable vitamin B_2'. Identifying this vitamin by means of its growth-promoting properties in rats, Kuhn and his colleagues (1933) finally isolated the factor from milk; from 5400 litres of whey they extracted 1 g of crystalline riboflavin. However, riboflavin did not have all the properties previously ascribed to vitamin B_2, e.g. it did not cure black-tongue in dogs. Evidently, therefore, riboflavin was only one of several factors present in the heat-stable fraction of the vitamin B complex.

An important clue to the nature of Kuhn's crystals was that they were yellow. One year previously Warburg and Christian (1932) had described their 'yellow enzyme', a respiratory catalyst. They obtained it from extracts of yeast and went on to show that it consisted of a protein component combined with a yellow pigment, neither of which alone was enzymically active, though effective in combination. It was an inspired guess that the yellow pigment of Warburg's enzyme was identical with the new vitamin, for so it proved to be. In 1935 riboflavin was synthesised by two independent groups of workers under Kuhn in Heidelberg and Karrer in Basle.

Chemistry

Riboflavin is a yellow-green fluorescent compound, soluble in water but not in fats, composed of an alloxazine ring linked to an alcohol derived from the pentose sugar ribose. Though stable to boiling in acid solution, in alkaline solution it is readily decomposed by heat. It is also destroyed by exposure to light.

In plant and animal tissues riboflavin is linked with phosphoric acid to form flavin mononucleotide (FMN). This with adenosine monophosphate forms flavin adenine dinucleotide (FAD). FMN and FAD are the prosthetic groups of the flavoproteins enzymes involved in oxidation-reduction reactions.

For further reading there is a monograph on riboflavin edited by Rivlin (1975).

Dietary sources

The best sources of riboflavin are liver, milk, eggs and green vegetables. Riboflavin differs from other components of the vitamin B complex in that it occurs in good amounts in dairy produce, but is relatively lacking in cereal grains. It is also present in beer. Ordinary methods of cooking do not destroy the vitamin apart from losses that occur when the water in which green vegetables have been boiled is discarded. If foods, especially milk, are left exposed to sunshine, large losses may occur. Especially good sources of the natural vitamin are yeast extract (e.g. Marmite) and meat extract (e.g. Bovril). Table 14.7 gives the riboflavin content of some common foods.

Effects of deficiency in animals

Riboflavin deficiency in animals always results in a failure to grow. A great variety of lesions have been reported in animals; these include dermatitis, loss of hair, conjunctivitis, corneal vascularisation and opacities, impaired reproduction with congenital malformations in the offspring, anaemia with hypoplastic bone marrow, neuropathy and fatty liver.

Effects of deficiency in man

Sebrell and Butler (1938) described the clinical effects of feeding human subjects for four months on a diet

Table 14.7 Natural sources of riboflavin

Food	Range (mg/100 g edible portion)
Good and moderate sources	
Wheat bran	0.5
Wheat and barley (whole grain)	0.12–0.25
Wheat germ	0.25
Pulses (fresh)	0.1–0.3
Fish (various)	0.2–0.4
Beef, mutton and pork	0.10–0.3
Liver and kidney	2.0–3.3
Eggs	0.3–0.5
Cheese	0.3–0.5
Cocoa powder	0.3–0.4
Chocolate (plain)	0.2
Brewers' yeast	1.3–4.0
Yeast extract, e.g. Marmite	5.0–6.0
Wheat germ, e.g. Bemax	0.67
Meat extract, e.g. Bovril, Oxo	1.8–2.6
Milk (fresh cow's)	0.15
Green leafy vegetables*	0.05–0.30
Maize (whole)	0.1
Oatmeal	0.15
Millets	0.10–0.15
Wheat flour (wholemeal)	0.10–0.15
Nuts	0.2
Dried fruit	0.1
Beers	0.05–0.10
Poor sources	
Maize (meal)	0.02–0.1
Rice (lightly milled)	0.05–0.1
Rice (highly milled)	0.03–0.05
Wheat flour (70 per cent extraction)	0.03–0.05
Fruits (fresh, tropical and temperate)	0.01–0.1
Potato	0.05
Vegetables	0.09

* Green vegetables and fruits in tropical countries are, in general, richer in riboflavin than those in temperate regions.

providing about 0.5 mg/day of riboflavin. Their subjects developed angular stomatitis, cheilosis and nasolabial seborrhoea (p. 303) which responded to the administration of riboflavin. Two years later Sydenstricker and his colleagues (1940) first described among pellagrous patients in southern USA an invasion of the cornea by capillary blood vessels similar to that seen in rats suffering from riboflavin deficiency. This ocular lesion, accompanied by lachrymation and photophobia, was often associated with angular stomatitis and other features of the orogenital syndrome (p. 304). These lesions responded to the administration of riboflavin. However, other factors besides riboflavin deficiency can cause angular stomatitis, and circumcorneal vascularisation was not seen in human subjects with experimental riboflavin deficiency by Hills *et al.* (1951).

In view of the importance of riboflavin in cell respiration it seems surprising that the clinical changes attributed to its deficiency are minor and do not by themselves threaten life. Even though riboflavin has a wide distribution in the foodstuffs used by man there are still many people who live for long periods on a very low intake and consequently minor signs of deficiency are common in many parts of the world. Why these conditions do not progress and lead to serious illness remains a mystery.

Laboratory diagnosis

In the presence of ultraviolet light riboflavin has a brilliant greenish-yellow fluorescence which provides a means of detecting and estimating small quantities in extracts of biological materials. It can also be estimated by microbiological assay. These methods have been of value in measuring the riboflavin in foodstuffs, in human urine and faeces, and in the tissues of animals.

Urinary riboflavin reflects the recent intake. It tends to increase when the nitrogen balance is negative. The most promising test for quantifying any functional effect of deficiency in the tissues is the measurement of activity in erythrocytes, glutathione reductase, with and without added FAD *in vitro*. An activation coefficient of over 1.30 with added FAD indicates inadequate riboflavin in the tissues (Tillotson and Baker, 1972; Thurnham *et al.*, 1972).

Recommended intakes

The Joint Committee of FAO/WHO (1967) recommended an intake of 130 μg/MJ (0.55 mg/1000 kcal) in the diet, and this is the basis of most other recommendations.

Therapeutic uses and toxic effects

Synthetic riboflavin, both for oral and parenteral administration, is readily available, but its therapeutic uses are not well supported by objective clinical evidence. It may be tried empirically in cases of angular stomatitis and the other lesions that sometimes co-exist, especially if they occur in cases of the malabsorption syndrome, in which the absorption of riboflavin may be impaired. Those who wish to prescribe this vitamin may give it by mouth in doses of 5 mg three times daily. There is no evidence that larger doses produce any further benefit.

Thus far, no one seems to have been adversely affected by treatment with synthetic riboflavin.

THE ANAEMIA-PREVENTING VITAMINS

History

Pernicious anaemia, described by Addison in 1849, occurs sporadically in most human races, apparently without relation to dietary habits. A constitutional or genetic predisposition to the disease was early recognised and in many cases it has now been shown to be the result of autoimmune reactions. As its name implies, the disease was fatal and feared until Minot and Murphy (1926) demonstrated the value of whole liver by mouth in its treatment. This was followed by the classic experiments of Castle (1929), who showed that beef muscle mixed with normal gastric juice caused new blood formation in patients with pernicious anaemia, though neither was effective alone. He called the unknown factor in gastric juice 'intrinsic factor' and that in beef 'extrinsic factor', suggesting at the same time that the two interact to produce the remedial substance present in liver. Later it was found that the need for intrinsic factor could be circumvented, not only by giving large amounts of liver by mouth but also by injecting extracts of liver intramuscularly. Thereafter the search for the hypothetical 'anti-PA' vitamin was directed towards its isolation from extracts of liver. Each new concentrate of liver could only be tested by therapeutic trials on human patients with Addisonian anaemia. The lack of a suitable animal to assist in laboratory trials delayed the discovery of vitamin B_{12}. The history of the early work on Addisonian anaemia is given by Davidson and Gulland (1930).

Then, as happened repeatedly in the history of the vitamins, a new and unexpected development came from an unrelated field of biochemistry. Folic acid had been isolated as a factor necessary for the growth of certain microorganisms (p. 145). In Addisonian anaemia folic acid resulted in dramatic therapeutic responses. It soon became apparent, however, that although folic acid corrects (at least temporarily) the defect in the formation of red cells it did not prevent or cure the degenerative changes in the nervous system which are often a serious feature of pernicious anaemia. The 'anti-PA' vitamin of liver extract, vitamin B_{12}, was finally isolated in 1948.

VITAMIN B_{12}—CYANOCOBALAMIN AND RELATED SUBSTANCES

The discovery that protein-free extracts of liver, given by injection, were effective in pernicious anaemia, led to many attempts over a period of 20 years to isolate from liver the active principle concerned. Progress was necessarily slow through lack of any easy means of detecting the vitamin until Mary Shorb discovered that liver extracts effective in pernicious anaemia had growth-promoting properties for the micro-organism *Lactobacillus lactis dorner*. The search for the growth factor proceeded rapidly and, aided by the fact that it was found to have a red colour, the isolation of crystalline vitamin B$_{12}$ was achieved almost simultaneously in Britain (Smith and Parker, 1948) and the USA (Rickes *et al.*, 1948). Proof soon followed of its effectiveness in the treatment of both the haematological and neurological manifestations of pernicious anaemia.

Chemistry

About 1 ton of fresh liver was needed for the isolation of 20 mg of the red crystals. These were found to have a molecular weight of about 1350 and to contain, surprisingly, 4 per cent of the mineral element cobalt, which previously was known to be an essential nutrient for sheep and cattle. The crystalline material was named cyanocobalamin. It is freely soluble in water and resistant to boiling in neutral solution though unstable in the presence of alkalis. It was subsequently found that the cyano-group in the molecule was an artefact of the extraction procedure.

The chemical nature of the vitamin was elucidated by two teams working in cooperation under Dorothy Hodgkin at Oxford (Hodgkin *et al.*, 1955) and Todd at Cambridge (Bonnett *et al.*, 1955). The cobalt is contained in a porphyrin-like ring which is linked to a nucleotide containing a base, ribose and phosphoric acid. In nature, vitamin B$_{12}$ usually occurs in combination with protein.

Vitamin B$_{12}$ is present in the body in several forms, including 5'-deoxyadenosylcobalamin, the major coenzyme form, methylcobalamin and hydroxocobalamin. The last is available commercially and is even more effective therapeutically than cyanocobalamin. The vitamin is produced commercially as a cheap by-product of the cultivation of *Streptomyces griseus* used in the preparation of the antibiotic streptomycin.

Physiological action

Deficiency of vitamin B$_{12}$ probably affects every cell in the body but is most severely felt in tissues where the cells are normally dividing rapidly, e.g. in the blood-forming tissues of the bone marrow and in the gastrointestinal tract. The nervous system is also affected and this may lead to degeneration of nerve fibres in the spinal cord and peripheral nerves.

The effect of the deficiency can be detected by examination of biopsies of bone marrow. Abnormal cells—megaloblasts—are seen. These are larger than the nucleated cells that give rise to normal red blood corpuscles and have characteristic large reticulated nuclei. When megaloblasts are present in the bone marrow the circulating red cells derived from them are bigger than normal (macrocytic) though usually carrying a normal concentration of haemoglobin (normochromic).

Megaloblastosis occurs because DNA formation is limited but that of RNA is not. As the cells develop they synthesise RNA normally but DNA synthesis does not keep pace. The consequence is slower replication of cells which have more nuclear chromatin than normal, but not enough for division, and a larger cytoplasm than nucleus. In vitamin B$_{12}$ deficiency there is impaired synthesis of thymidylate, the nucleotide of thymine and the characteristic base of DNA—the other bases of DNA occur in RNA as well. Deoxythymidylic acid (dTMP) is formed by methylation of deoxyuridylic acid (dUMP) with the participation of a folate coenzyme, N^{10}-methylene tetrahydrofolate (p. 146). Vitamin B$_{12}$ plays a supporting role in regenerating this active form of folate from its end product, methyl folate, the most abundant form of folate in the body. This occurs during the methylation of homocysteine to form methionine. The entry of methyl folate into red cells also requires vitamin B$_{12}$ (Herbert, 1976). Consequently, the megaloblastic anaemia of folate deficiency is morphologically the same as that seen in vitamin B$_{12}$ deficiency and red cell folate is subnormal in both. However, in vitamin B$_{12}$ deficiency plasma vitamin B$_{12}$ is subnormal but plasma folate normal.

Vitamin B$_{12}$ plays a separate biochemical role, unrelated to folate, in the maintenance of myelin in the nervous system. This is probably due to dependence of propionate catabolism on vitamin B$_{12}$. The normal sequence is from propionyl coenzyme A via methylmalonyl coenzyme A to succinyl coenzyme A, which is metabolised in the citric acid cycle. Deoxyadenosyl vitamin B$_{12}$ is essential for the last step. In vitamin B$_{12}$ deficiency 15- and 17-carbon fatty acids and branched fatty acids appear in nervous tissue. It is likely that the odd-numbered fatty acids are formed when propionyl coenzyme A is used instead of acetyl coenzyme A for fatty acid synthesis and that branched chain fatty acids result when methylmalonyl coenzyme A substitutes for malonyl coenzyme A. Patients with vitamin B$_{12}$ deficiency usually excrete methylmalonic acid in their urine. This has been used as a test for deficiency; it does not occur in folate deficiency. An animal model for subacute combined degeneration of the spinal cord (p. 300) has been found, the fruit bat *Rousettus aegypticus*. Coprophagy has not been observed in these animals; their usual sources of vitamin B$_{12}$ are presumed to be from stagnant water and insect pests on fruit. When kept in cages and given fruit and distilled water, after 200 days their plasma B$_{12}$ fell and their pattern of flying was disturbed, presumably because they had become ataxic due to demyelination of the spinal cord (Green *et al.*, 1975).

Hydroxocobalamin has an affinity for cyanide; this appears to be a detoxication mechanism in people exposed to repeated small amounts of cyanide in food or in tobacco smoke.

Dietary intake

Vitamin B_{12} is unique amongst vitamins in that it is not found in any plants. The dietary intake varies according to the amount of animal products consumed. High cost, low cost and poor American diets have been estimated to provide 32, 16 and 3 μg/day respectively and a poor Asian diet 0.5 μg/day (Bozian *et al.*, 1963). Vitamin B_{12} is present in several forms in foods. The main ones are adenosyl- and hydroxocobalamin, of which 34 and 55 per cent are absorbed. Methylcobalamin is found in egg yolk and cheese, and sulphitocobalamin in some canned foods. Little or no cyanocobalamin occurs in foods. Cooking may affect the forms and they may interchange in the intestine before absorption (Farquharson and Adams, 1976). Vitamin B_{12} activity is usually stable during food preparation but boiling in an alkaline medium can lead to moderate losses. Most vegetarians will drink milk and so get a modest supply. Cow's milk contains about 0.3 μg/100 g. How strict vegetarians, who eat no animal product, get the vitamin remains a mystery. There may be traces in microorganisms and moulds which contaminate their food.

Alimentary absorption

There is now no doubt that vitamin B_{12} is the 'extrinsic factor' originally postulated by Castle, but it still remains to be explained exactly why a normal gastric secretion is needed for its proper utilisation. As Castle himself (1955) has said: 'It can be stated with assurance that pernicious anaemia is usually an example of a highly specific isolation of the affected person from his alimentary environment. Thus his disease would not develop if the patient could effect daily the transfer of a millionth of a gram of vitamin B_{12} the distance of a small fraction of a millimetre across the intestinal mucosa and into the blood stream. This he cannot do, principally as a result of failure of his stomach to secrete into its lumen some essential but still unknown substance.' We now know that intrinsic factor is a glycoprotein secreted by the parietal cells of the stomach. Vitamin B_{12} is absorbed in the distal part of the ileum and not in the jejunum.

The normal requirements of an adult to prevent signs of deficiency are probably about 1 μg/day. When micrograms of vitamin B_{12} are given to patients with pernicious anaemia by mouth, little absorption, if any, occurs. When milligrams are given, a very small percentage of the dose is absorbed but probably a sufficient quantity to prevent deficiency. This may be due to simple diffusion. For the absorption of physiological doses and also of the vitamin present in foods, intrinsic factor is essential. Neither the nature nor the mode of action of intrinsic factor is as yet established. The failure to produce it in pernicious anaemia arises from an autoimmune reaction, which destroys the secreting glands in the stomach. This may arise from a genetically determined defect in immunological tolerance.

The tapeworm *Diphyllobothrium latum* infects many species of freshwater fish. Human infection occurs round the world wherever raw or insufficiently cooked fish is eaten. The adult worms which may reach a length of 15 metres assimilate the vitamin from the food and make it unavailable to the host (p. 428). In a variety of intestinal diseases, e.g. the malabsorption syndrome, especially the blind loop syndrome, an increased bacterial flora may affect absorption of vitamin B_{12}, because the bacteria assimilate it from the food. In ileal disease vitamin B_{12} cannot be absorbed and after total gastrectomy intrinsic factor is lost. Some drugs, e.g. *p*-aminosalicylic acid, biguanides, slow-release potassium and colchicine, interfere specifically with the absorption of vitamin B_{12}. In each of the above ways anaemia due to secondary vitamin B_{12} deficiency may arise.

Excretion and storage

Normal persons living on American diets excrete in their urine about 1.3 μg/day (Reizenstein *et al.*, 1964). Cobalamin is attached to three proteins in the blood, transcobalamins I, II and III, which are α-, β- and γ- globins respectively. II is the functionally important carrier because it gives up its vitamin B_{12} to the tissues. The other two transcobalamins bind the vitamin more permanently. Some vitamin B_{12} is excreted in the bile but this is partly reabsorbed in normal people, with fresh intrinsic factor, in an enterohepatic cycle. Loss of endogenous, as well as exogenous, vitamin explains why deficiency develops more rapidly in malabsorption than on an inadequate diet. Excess intake is stored, mostly in the liver. Total body cobalamin in normal adults is 2 to 5 mg of which half or more is in the liver. This is about 1000 times the estimated daily utilisation and losses.

Primary deficiency in man

A completely vegetarian diet, containing no milk, eggs or other foods of animal origin, is practically devoid of cobalamins, provided that all its components are fresh and free from fermentation by microorganisms. People who follow such a diet have occasionally developed megaloblastic anaemia or more commonly developed neurological manifestation of vitamin B_{12} deficiency (p. 300).

Laboratory diagnosis

The plasma concentration in healthy persons normally lies between 200 and 960 pg/ml. A value below 80 is diagnostic of vitamin B_{12} deficiency. Values between 80 and 200 are equivocal. The capacity of the bowel to absorb vitamin B_{12} is a valuable test used in the investigation of complex cases of megaloblastic anaemia. If a 1 μg dose of radioactive B_{12} is given to healthy persons, only about 30 per cent is recovered in the faeces, whereas over 70 per cent is recovered in patients with pernicious anaemia and in malabsorbtion The two may be differentiated by giving another dose of radioactive B_{12}, this time with intrinisc factor which corrects absorption in pernicious anaemia. The measurement of the urinary excretion of the isotope (Schilling test) is now in general use as a test. To ensure prompt urinary excretion of the absorbed radioactive B_{12} a 'flushing' dose of 1000 μg 'cold' vitamin B_{12} is often given.

Recommended intakes
It is impossible to state accurately any figure for a desirable daily intake of vitamin B_{12}. Two things, however, are certain: a remission can be brought about in pernicious anaemia by the daily injection of 1 μg of vitamin B_{12}; people in apparent health may get only 0.5 μg/day in their diet. Faecal and urinary excretion is normally between 1 and 2 μg/day. Only the effects of gross deficiency of the vitamin are known and it is possible that a minor degree of deficiency operating over several years might have pathological consequences. For these reasons, a daily intake of 3 to 4 μg seems desirable.

Therapeutic uses
Vitamin B_{12}, given by injection, provides complete and satisfactory treatment in cases of pernicious anaemia. The general practice is to give 1000 μg of hydroxocobalamin by injection twice weekly until the haemoglobin is normal. Subsequently an injection of 1000 μg every six weeks is all that is needed to keep the patient in health. The blood should be examined every six months. These doses may appear excessive as much of the vitamin is excreted in the urine. Nevertheless, it is not unreasonable to give large doses at first to refill the depleted reserves. A similar dose schedule is required in subacute combined degeneration of the cord and in vitamin B_{12} deficiency due to other causes.

FOLATE (FOLIC ACID, FOLACIN)

History
The classical studies of Dr Lucy Wills (1931) in Bombay drew attention to the importance of nutritional megaloblastic anaemia in pregnant women (Chap. 48). She reproduced this anaemia in monkeys by means of a diet composed chiefly of polished rice and white bread, similar to that eaten by her patients. This anaemia did not respond to any vitamin known at that time, nor to purified liver extract (presumably containing vitamin B_{12}). Yet good clinical responses were obtained with an autolysed yeast preparation (Wills, 1933) which was generally ineffective in pernicious anaemia. Therefore yeast contained an antianaemic principle (the 'Wills' factor') that was different from the factor present in purified liver extract.

Then an unexpected clue came from an unrelated field

of biochemistry; Mitchell *et al*. (1941) obtained from spinach a preparation, called by them 'folic acid', that was a growth factor for *Lactobacillus casei*. This preparation would cure a dietary anaemia in chicks. The isolation of a crystalline active principle was announced in 1945 by a large team of American industrial chemists, who soon accomplished its synthesis. The pure synthetic substance was pteroylglutamic acid (PGA). The most complex part of the molecule was a pterin. This group of biological compounds was known from the pioneer work of Gowland Hopkins. In 1885 he had begun to investigate the pigments present in the wings of butterflies. Many years later he summarised (Hopkins, 1942) the chemical properties of the pterins extracted from them; he recognised their chemical similarity to the purines of nucleic acid and suggested that one at least was physiologically important for mammals.

It was soon found that synthetic folic acid would cure dietary anaemia in chicks and also in monkeys. Hence it was reasonable to try it empirically in pernicious anaemia; dramatic responses occurred comparable to that produced by liver extract. However, the neurological lesions were not improved and were often made worse (Davidson and Girdwood, 1947). Some time was to elapse before it was shown that the real therapeutic role of folic acid lay in the treatment of the megaloblastic anaemias of malnutrition, pregnancy and malabsorption (Chap. 48). Thus Lucy Wills' original observation that there are at least two different dietary factors concerned with megaloblastosis was shown to be correct.

Chemistry
Folic acid, often referred to as folacin in the USA, consists of a pterin ring attached to *p*-aminobenzoic acid and conjugated with one molecule of glutamic acid. It is a yellow crystalline substance, sparingly soluble in water and stable in acid solution. When heated in neutral or alkaline media, however, it undergoes fairly rapid destruction, so it may be destroyed by some methods of cooking (see below). Several closely allied compounds have been identified in living matter:

1. Up to six additional molecules of glutamic acid may be attached through the γ-carboxyl group to pteroylmonoglutamic acid. The test organism, *Lactobacillus casei* can utilise pteroyltriglutamic acid but not compounds with more than three glutamic acid residues, the pteroylpolyglutamates.

2. Two reduced forms of folate, 7,8-dihydrofolate and 5,6,7,8-tetrahydrofolate (THF), may be present in the tissues.

3. In the course of its numerous metabolic functions folate, usually in the tetrahydroform, may have active one-carbon groups on the N-5 or N-10 positions or bridging the two. The most important of these are 5-methyl-THF, 5,10-methylene-THF, 5,10-methenyl-THF, 5-formyl-

THF and 10-formyl-THF and 5-formimino-THF. The structural relation between folic acid and THF is shown in Fig. 14.5.

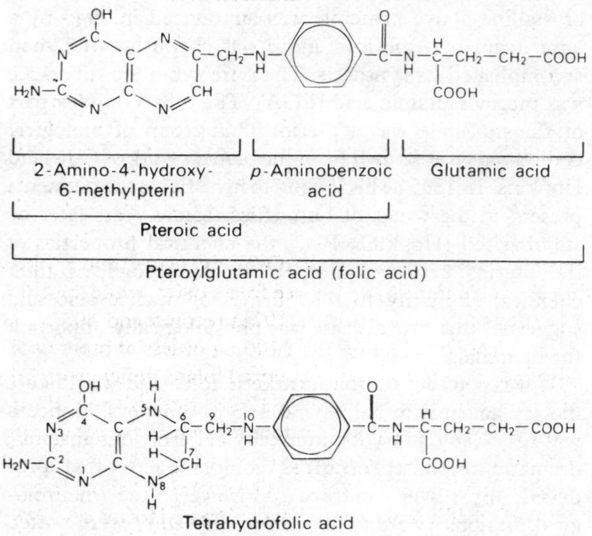

2-Amino-4-hydroxy-6-methylpterin   p-Aminobenzoic acid   Glutamic acid

Pteroic acid

Pteroylglutamic acid (folic acid)

Tetrahydrofolic acid

Fig. 14.5 The structure of folic acid and THF. The N-5 and N-10 nitrogen atoms participate in the transfer of one-carbon groups.

Metabolic roles

Folic acid in its tetrahydro form has an essential role in one-carbon transfers in the body. It receives one-carbon radicals from, for example, serine, glycine, histidine and tryptophan, and donates them at two steps in purine synthesis and one important step in pyrimidine synthesis—insertion of the methyl group in deoxyuridylic acid to form thymidylic acid, the characteristic nucleotide of DNA.

It is failure of this synthetic step that explains the megaloblastosis seen in folate deficiency and in vitamin B_{12} deficiency. The interdependence of the two vitamins can be explained as follows. The form of folate needed for synthesis of thymidylate is 5,10-methylene-THF, which has to be made from THF. The principal way in which THF is generated from methyl-THF, the dominant form of folate in human liver and plasma, is in the homocysteine → methionine reaction for which vitamin B_{12} is the cofactor. When vitamin B_{12} is deficient, most of the folate is trapped in the methyl-THF form which cannot be used in synthetic reactions, of which the most important for the body is the formation of thymidylate for DNA synthesis (Herbert and Zalusky, 1962).

Absorption, excretion and storage

About three-quarters of the folate in foods is in polyglutamyl forms. These are normally hydrolysed to free folate by a conjugase (a γ-L-glutamyl carboxypeptidase) present in small intestinal epithelium. Free folate is actively absorbed from the upper small intestine (Hempner et al., 1968). At some stage during absorption it appears to be reduced and methylated to methyl-THF. Plasma folate activity for L. casei, but not for Streptococcus faecalis (Table 14.8) reaches a peak about one hour after feeding various forms of folate (Chanarin and Perry, 1969). Methyl-THF is the principal form of folate present in the liver as well as in plasma.

Folic acid is stored mainly in the liver which normally contains 5 to 15 mg/kg. Small amounts are excreted in faeces and urine, but additional amounts are presumed to be metabolised and some is lost by desquamation of cells from body surfaces.

Deficiency

Megaloblastic anaemia due to a simple dietary deficiency of the vitamin is common and sometimes severe amongst poor people in the tropics. It is unusual in prosperous countries, except in pregnancy when the need for the vitamin is increased. Absorption from the small intestine is reduced by many gastrointestinal diseases. Secondary folic acid deficiency is therefore not uncommon.

Almost all the antiepileptic drugs used in the treatment of epilepsy reduce plasma folate concentrations (Reynolds, 1973), but megaloblastic anaemia is only a rare complication of antiepileptic therapy. In addition to antiepileptics other drugs may impair folate metabolism, e.g. oral contraceptives, pyrimethamine, co-trimoxazole and ethanol.

Laboratory diagnosis

Folate may be estimated in fluids by microbiological assay. The normal plasma concentration is between 6 and 20 μg/l. Folate deficiency is possible if the plasma concentration is below 6 and certain if below 3. Erythrocytes contain much more (160–650 μg/l) and provide a means of measuring tissues stores, which is now used in diagnosis. Various folate absorption tests are in use. A dose of folate is given by mouth and plasma concentrations determined at intervals thereafter. These are of special value in doubtful cases of the malabsorption syndrome.

Another test depends on the breakdown of a loading dose of histidine. This is normally converted first to formiminoglutamic acid, FIGLU, and the formimino group transferred to THF, and then to glutamic acid. In the absence of adequate amounts of folic acid in the tissues, the second stage does not take place; FIGLU accumulates and is excreted in the urine. However, this test is not specific. FIGLU excretion is increased in vitamin B_{12} deficiency.

Dietary sources

Folic acid is present in foods in several different forms. The methods used for analysis of foodstuffs and body

Table 14.8 Responses of assay organisms to different forms of folate

	Streptococcus faecalis	*Lactobacillus casei*	*Pediococcus cerevisiae*
Folic acid	+	+	−
Pteroyldiglutamic acid	+	+	−
Pteroyltriglutamic acid	−	+	−
Pteroylheptaglutamic acid	−	+	−
THF	+	+	−
5-Formyl-THF (folinic acid)	+	+	+
5-Methyl-THF	−	+	−

fluids are microbiological. Three organisms are commonly used (Table 14.8). *Lactobacillus casei* responds to all forms of folic acid with up to three glutamic acid residues: this is free folate. To demonstrate the pteroylpolyglutamates, foods are treated with a conjugase obtained from chicken liver and again microbiologically analysed for folate: this is total folate. Absorption of polyglutamates is not as complete as that of free folate.

Some indications of the relative folic acid content of foods is given in Table 14.9. The richest source is liver, in which most of the folate is 5-methyl-THF and well absorbed. Other foods contain most of the folate as polyglutamates and are less reliable as dietary sources (FAO/WHO, 1970). Table 14.9 shows free and total folate in a selection of uncooked foods. Fruits are poor sources, except orange juice, cantaloupes and avocados (Dong and Oace, 1973). There are no complete tables of folate activity in foods, measured by modern methods. The best available are given by Hoppner *et al.* (1972), who report on 178 foods, mostly before cooking, and by Paul and Southgate (1978). More data about the amounts of the various forms present in different foods are needed.

When different forms of folate, labelled with isotopes, were given to patients with leukaemia (Butterworth *et al.*, 1969) and to healthy volunteers (Godwin and Rosenberg, 1975), the heptaglutamate was shown to be split to monoglutamate during digestion and about 55 per cent of it was absorbed. The availability of five pure forms of folate including THF and pteroylheptaglumate, and of the folate in 12 natural foods was assessed by measuring urinary folate with an assay of *Lactobacillus casei* (Tamura and Stokstad, 1973). Availability appeared to be low, 25 to 50 per cent, from lettuce, egg, orange and wheat germ, but 50 to 96 per cent for lima beans, liver, brewers' yeast and bananas. This suggests that factors in foods as well as the forms of folate may influence absorption.

Food preparation can cause serious losses of folic acid—in canning, in prolonged heating, when cooking water is discarded, and from reheating. Reducing agents in food tend to protect the folic acid. Herbert (1973) suggests that if everyone were to eat one helping of fresh vegetables or fresh fruit each day nutritional folate deficiency would be wiped from the face of the earth.

Recommended intakes

For non-pregnant adults, FAO/WHO (1974) and Canada (1975) recommend 200 μg free folate daily, while the USA (1974) and West Germany (1975) recommend 400 μg as total folate. In normal adults 100 μg or less of pteroylglutamic acid have prevented or cured folate-deficient megaloblastic anaemia (Herbert, 1968) but is not always sufficient to maintain or restore plasma folate concentration. The safe requirement appears to be 200 μg/day as available folate. This would correspond to 300 μg/day as total folate if it is assumed that conjugated forms are 50 per cent utilised and make up 50 per cent of the total. Canadian diets provide, on average, 240 μg total folate of which

Table 14.9 Folate in foods (data mostly from Hoppner *et al.*, 1972)

Food	Folate (mg/100g)	
	Free	Total
Good sources		
Liver (ox)	−	140
Spinach	175	204
Broccoli tops	90	105
Kidney (ox)	63	80
Lima beans	25	113
Peanuts	28	106
Asparagus	58	64
Beets	68	92
Cabbage	25	30
Lettuce	24	24
Avocados	31	36
Fair sources		
Bread (wholemeal)	17	54
Bread (white)	8	35
Oranges	13	24
Bananas	11	20
Egg	12	21
Rice	15	29
Cod (frozen)	6	19
Milk (human)	−	5
Poor sources		
Beef	4	7
Chicken, lamb, pork	1–3	3–7
Milk (cow's)	4	5
Potatoes (fresh)	10	13
Apples, grapes	3	6

Values are for fresh (uncooked) foods: cooking losses can be considerable.

140μg are free (Hoppner, 1972). Further analyses are needed. For infants, human milk provides 5 μg folate/100 ml, and 5 μg folate/kg body weight has been estimated as the daily requirement (Sullivan *et al.*, 1966). In pregnancy there is an additional requirement of about 100 μg of available folate (Chanarin and Perry, 1977). Many doctors in the UK prescribe a daily supplement containing 400 μg during pregnancy. We recommend 50 μg/day in infancy, 300 μg/day in adults and 500 μg/day in pregnancy, all expressed as total folate.

Therapeutic uses and toxicity

Folic acid is required for the treatment of nutritional megaloblastic anaemia, the megaloblastic anaemias of pregnancy and infancy, and in some cases of the malabsorption syndrome. A daily dose of 5 to 10 mg by mouth is usually sufficient. It should never be used in Addisonian anaemia because it may make the neurological features of the disease worse. A small daily dose (400μg) is recommended during pregnancy.

Folic acid normally has no adverse effects. However, when it is used to treat megaloblastic anaemia secondary to the use of antiepileptic drugs, the epilepsy may be aggravated (Reynolds, 1973). Certain synthetic analogues are highly poisonous, notably methotrexate which is used as an antimetabolite in the treatment of leukaemia.

VITAMIN B₆—PYRIDOXINE AND RELATED COMPOUNDS

The vitamin was first identified as the factor in the vitamin B complex, distinct from thiamin and riboflavin, that would cure a specific nutritional dermatitis in rats. Birch and György (1936) concentrated the vitamin in 1936; soon after, it was isolated and synthesised. György (1971) has recalled the history.

Biochemical action

The three forms of vitamin B_6 found in foods are shown in Fig. 14.6. Pyridoxine is the commonest in vegetable foods, and the corresponding aldehyde (pyridoxal) and amine (pyridoxamine) are the usual forms in animal foods. The three are interconvertible in tissues and have equal biological activity in rats. Pyridoxine hydrochloride is the commonly available synthetic preparation. Pyridoxal 5'-phosphate and pyridoxamine 5'-phosphate are two coenzymes found in animal tissues. The vitamin can occur partly in these coenzyme forms in foods but the phosphate is split off during digestion. Vitamin B_6 is a generic term for the whole group of compounds; pyridoxine is sometimes used incorrectly in this way. An enzyme, pyridoxal kinase, in the cells converts pyridoxine and related compounds to pyridoxal (or pyridoxamine) 5'-phosphate (PLP).

PLP is the coenzyme for over 60 different enzymes. Most of them are on the pathways of amino acid and protein metabolism and include aminotransferases and decarboxylases. In one way or another PLP is involved in the metabolism of all the amino acids. Two aminotransferases present in red blood cells are used to assess nutritional status in respect of vitamin B_6. They are aspartate aminotransferase and alanine aminotransferase and catalyse respectively:

Aspartate + 2-oxoglutarate $\rightleftharpoons$ oxaloacetate + glutamate
Alanine + 2-oxoglutarate $\rightleftharpoons$ pyruvate + glutamate

Other important enzymes dependent on PLP are (1) the decarboxylases which produce amines and also γ-aminobutryic acid in brain, (2) ALA synthetase which produces δ-aminolaevulinic acid, the first stage in the synthesis of porphyrins and haem compounds, and (3) kynureninase, an enzyme on the pathway from tryptophan to nicotinic acid (Fig. 14.4). If the tissues contain insufficient vitamin B_6 the kynurenine is converted into xanthurenic acid, which then appears in the urine where it can be measured.

Vitamin B_6 deficiency has been produced by dietary means in monkeys, dogs, pigs, rats and chickens. Pigs develop a microcytic hypochromic anaemia and a peripheral neuropathy; dogs developed epileptiform convulsions, whereas monkeys were found to have atheromatous changes in the arteries.

Human deficiency

Primary dietary deficiency is rare because of the wide distribution of the vitamin in foods. A minor epidemic of convulsions in infants in the USA was traced to a milk formula which provided little vitamin B_6 because of a manufacturing error (Coursin, 1954). Biochemical evidence suggesting pyridoxine deficiency has been found in patients with malabsorption and in protein-energy malnutrition. Several drugs antagonise pyridoxine, notably isoniazid, hydralazine, penicillamine and oestrogens. Peripheral neuropathy is an adverse effect of doses of isoniazid above 300 mg/day, which may sometimes be required in the treatment of tuberculosis. It can be prevented by giving 10 mg/day of pyridoxine.

In adequately nourished infants, convulsions sometimes respond to the administration of pyridoxine. This is **pyridoxine dependency** (as opposed to deficiency) and appears to be an inborn error of metabolism (Scriver, 1967). In adults hypochromic anaemia is occasionally encountered with normal or increased iron reserves, i.e. hypochromic sideroblastic anaemia. Some such cases respond to pyridoxine but the dose has to be large, usually 20 to 100 mg/day by mouth and even intramuscular PLP may be required (Mason and Emerson, 1973). Plasma PLP is subnormal in patients with rheumatoid arthritis; large doses of pyridoxine bring the PLP concentration to normal but unfortunately do nothing for the arthritis (Schumacher *et al.*, 1975).

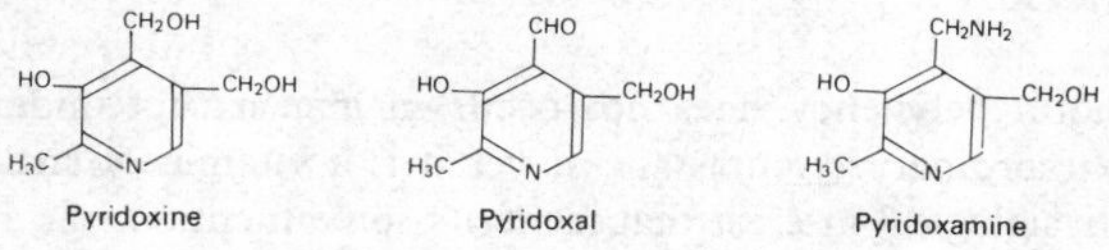

Fig. 14.6 The three forms of vitamin B$_6$

Some women taking oral oestrogen-containing contraceptives become pyridoxine-deficient judged by biochemical criteria. This may be because oestrogens induce increased activity of the enzyme system in the liver which converts tryptophan to nicotinic acid, and this may increase requirements of pyridoxine. Such women may become depressed, and in some cases the depression disappears when pyridoxine (20 mg twice daily) is given (Adams *et al.*, 1973). There is now evidence that depression is sometimes associated with disturbance of amine metabolism in the brain, particularly of 5-hydroxytryptamine which is a product of tryptophan metabolism. However, Nobbs (1974) found biochemical features of pyridoxine deficiency in only one out of 23 patients with depression who were not taking oral contraceptives.

Laboratory diagnosis
Plasma PLP can now be measured and normal adult values in the USA are available (Rose *et al.*, 1976). The principal urinary metabolite is 4-pyridoxic acid but methods for its assay are tedious. Much use has been made of the tryptophan load test. In this, 2 g L-tryptophan is given and urinary excretion of xanthurenic acid measured. The method is straightforward, but factors other than vitamin B$_6$ may influence the test, e.g. the state of protein metabolism and oestrogens. Aminotransferase activity in red blood cells (see above) can be assayed with and without added PLP *in vitro*; the greater the percentage stimulation by PLP the more the likelihood of vitamin B$_6$ deficiency. Laboratory tests for vitamin B$_6$ are reviewed by Sauberlich *et al.* (1974).

Dietary sources and recommended intakes
Vitamin B$_6$ can be measured in foodstuffs by microbiological assay. The vitamin is widely distributed both in plant and animal tissues. Liver, whole grain cereals, peanuts and bananas are good sources (around 0.5 mg/100 g). Most foods are moderate sources, but fats, oils, sugar, cornflour and alcoholic spirits contain none.

For infants 0.3 mg/day is recommended in the USA (Chap. 15) but breast milk alone would not provide so much, as it contains 0.01 mg/100 ml or less. Adult diets provide 1.5–2 mg/day, which is sufficient to meet most people's requirements. The need for vitamin B$_6$ appears to be increased by high protein diets. In pregnancy xanthurenic acid excretion is increased after a tryptophan load. It

may be a consequence of induction of tryptophan oxygenase (Fig. 14.4) by a physiological rise in circulating oestrogens. There is also a fall in plasma PLP which may be prevented by a daily dose of 4 mg pyridoxine (Lumeng *et al.*, 1976). No clinical benefit has followed a supplement of 2 mg/day (Hillman *et al.*, 1963) but gestational diabetes has sometimes responded to large doses of pyridoxine (Coelingh *et al.*, 1975). In the USA 2.5 mg/day are recommended in pregnancy (Chap. 15), 0.5 mg above the non-pregnant recommendation; the Deutsche Gesellschaft für Ernährung (1975), however, recommends 3.6 mg/day in pregnancy, 2.0 mg above the normal requirement of 1.6 mg for women. It would not be easy to obtain so much from ordinary diets.

The toxicity of pyridoxine is very low. The pharmacological dose is up to 100–150 mg/day. It is used with moderate success as an antiemetic, e.g. in radiation sickness. In even larger dosage it appears to be a good antidote to poisoning with the rocket fuel hydrazine (Kirklin *et al.*, 1976).

PANTOTHENIC ACID

Pantothenic acid is a constituent of coenzyme A and present in all living matter; its distribution in natural foodstuffs is so widespread that deficiency of the vitamin is unlikely to occur in man except perhaps when processed foods form a large proportion of the diet.

After the discovery of riboflavin, nicotinic acid and pyridoxine it was soon realised that there was still at least one other factor left in materials containing the hypothetical 'vitamin B$_2$'. This 'filtrate factor' was first recognised by its ability to prevent a specific type of dermatitis that develops round the eyes and beak of chicks fed on a diet deficient in it, and by its ability to prevent grey hair in black rats similarly fed. Attempts to isolate this factor were proceeding along orthodox lines using rats and chicks as the test animals when, as in the case of folic acid, the microbiological approach unexpectedly revealed the vitamin. R. J. Williams (1939) first isolated the vitamin, using the growth of yeast at a test of its presence, and later achieved its synthesis. He called it pantothenic acid because of its apparently universal distribution in living matter.

Chemistry
Pantothenic acid consists of a dimethyl derivative of butyric acid joined by a peptide linkage to the amino acid β-alanine. The vitamin itself is a pale yellow oily liquid that has never yet been crystallised, but its calcium salt crystallises readily and this is the form in which it is generally available. Though stable in neutral solution, it is easily destroyed by heat, both on the acid and alkaline side of neutrality.

Biochemical function

Pantothenic acid is the characteristic part of coenzyme A, the rest of the coenzyme being adenosine diphosphate. Coenzyme A participates in numerous reactions as donor or acceptor of acetyl and acyl groups, e.g. in pyruvate and fatty acid oxidation, in acetylation of choline and sulphonamide drugs, in synthesis of fatty acids, cholesterols, steroids and porphyrins. Pantothenic acid is also part of the prosthetic group of acyl carrier proteins which functions in fatty acid synthesis.

Deficiency in animals

Lack of pantothenic acid in the diet of rats produces failure of growth, greying of the hair, an accumulation of porphyrin on the whiskers round the nose and haemorrhage and necrosis in the adrenal glands. Some rats develop a fatal aplasia of the bone marrow, with anaemia and leucopenia. Deficiency leads to a typical dermatitis and a neuropathy characterised by myelin degeneration of the tracts in the spinal cord in chicks, a fatty liver in dogs and a peripheral neuropathy affecting the sensory nerves in pigs.

Human deficiency

Spontaneous deficiency has never been described. Experimental depletion was produced by feeding a deficient diet (Hodges et al., 1958). The subjects complained of malaise, vomiting and abdominal discomfort, perhaps due to a diet of sugar, corn starch, vitamin-free casein, corn oil and water. They also had insomnia, fatigue and tenderness in the heels. The more definite effects were only obtained by giving the antagonist ω-methyl pantothenic acid as well. For biochemical assessment pantothenic acid has been measured microbiologically in urine; reported experience is summarised by Sauberlich et al. (1974). Most adults excrete 3 mg/day or more, and less than 1 mg/day is provisionally considered abnormally low.

Dietary sources and therapeutic uses

Pantothenic acid is found universally in all living matter. The best sources are liver, kidney, yeast, egg yolk, wheat germ or bran, peanuts and some vegetables. On the other hand, there is no pantothenic acid in sugar, confectionery, butter, margarine, shortening, lard, sago, spaghetti, tapioca, corn starch, alcoholic spirits or Coca Cola. In most cooking and baking procedures there is little loss of the vitamin, but temperatures above boiling point may cause considerable loss. Frozen meat may lose much of its original content in the drip that occurs with thawing.

So far there is no clearly defined use for synthetic pantothenic acid, though it may be tried, in doses of 10 mg daily of the calcium salt by intramuscular injection, in patients suffering from the burning feet syndrome. It will not prevent the development of grey hair in man.

BIOTIN

Biotin deficiency does not occur in man except under extraordinary circumstances; yet it is a vitamin of such physiological interest that it merits some mention.

Rats fed on the raw whites of eggs as their sole source of animal protein develop a dermatitis and become emaciated. Raw egg-white contains a particular protein (avidin) which combines with biotin rendering it unavailable to the rat. By cooking the eggs the avidin is denatured and the biotin liberated. The vitamin was synthesised in 1943. Billings (1970, 1975) has prepared annotated bibliographies on biotin.

Biotin is one of the most active biological substances known; extremely small amounts have marked effects on the growth of yeast and certain bacteria. This provides the means by which it can be measured in foodstuffs. It forms part of several enzyme systems, notably one that fixes CO_2 derived from bicarbonate ions and then incorporates the CO_2 into the pathway of fatty acid synthesis. It also participates in the pyruvate carboxylase system where a N atom in the biotin ring combines with CO_2. This CO_2 is subsequently transferred to pyruvate with the formation of oxaloacetate. This reaction is important in the formation of glucose from pyruvate.

Deficiency in man

Sydenstricker and his colleagues (1942) produced biotin deficiency by feeding four volunteers a diet very poor in all the vitamins of the B group. This diet was composed largely of dried egg-white which supplied 30 per cent of the energy in the diet. Other known components of the B complex except biotin were added in synthetic form. After 10 weeks on the diet the subjects were fatigued, depressed and sleepy, with nausea and loss of appetite. Muscular pains, hyperaesthesiae and paraesthesiae developed, without reflex changes or other objective signs of neuropathy. As the authors point out, these features could not be distinguished from those previously attributed to thiamin deficiency. The tongue became pale with loss of papillae. The skin became dry, 'crackled', with fine branny desquamation (p. 303) and anaemia and hypercholesterolaemia developed. All of these signs and symptoms were relieved by the injection of a concentrated preparation containing 150 to 300 μg of biotin daily. The authors concluded: 'The phenomena observed were similar to some of those observed in spontaneous avitaminoses.'

Biotin deficiency has been described in an eccentric man who lived on a diet consisting mainly of six dozen raw eggs weekly, washed down with 4 quarts of red wine daily (Williams, 1943). He had a severe dermatitis which responded to injections of the methyl ester of biotin. A second spontaneous human case of biotin deficiency was reported by Scott (1958) in a boy with bulbar poliomyelitis who had received six raw eggs daily by gastric tube for 18 months. He developed scaly dermatitis and loss of hair. A third case of biotin deficiency was reported in a man with cirrhosis of the liver who consumed raw eggs (Baugh et al., 1968).

Human milk contains 0.7 μg/100 ml of biotin, only a third of the content of cow's milk. If the mother is malnourished, the intake can become critical and cases of seborrhoeic dermatitis have been reported in breast-fed infants which responded to biotin (Nisenson, 1964).

Dietary sources and therapeutic uses

Yeasts and bacteria of many species either make or retain biotin; it seems probable that man, if indeed he cannot make the vitamin in his tissues, can obtain all he needs from the numerous microorganisms that are present in his food or inhabit his large intestine. Moreover, biotin is present in a variety of bacteria-free foods. Liver, kidney and yeast extract are very rich sources. Pulses, nuts, chocolate and some vegetables (e.g. cauliflower) are fair sources. Other meats, dairy produce and cereals are relatively poor.

The human body probably utilises a few micrograms of biotin daily. It is doubtful whether this needs to be provided in the diet.

15. Dietary Standards

Circumstances when food supplies and diets have had to be planned have been described since history was first written. The Bible relates that Joseph advised Pharoah on the stores needed as a precaution against famine. The Greeks had to victual their ships for voyages across the Mediterranean Sea, and Hippocrates prescribed therapeutic diets. Requirements had to be based on observations of the amounts of food eaten by healthy persons. The Roman unit of weight, the librum, became the European pound which varied slightly from region to region. A pound of wheat flour or other cereal provides the energy needed to meet the basal metabolic rate of an adult man and is a practical unit for planning food supplies when a cereal provides a greater part of the dietary energy.

In the nineteenth century, when knowledge of the chemical constituents of foods was first available, it became possible to state dietary requirements in terms of nutrients rather than foods. Since about 1925, when quantitative knowledge of requirements for vitamins began to be accumulated, it has become possible to give estimates of human dietary requirements for an increasing number of nutrients. Many committees have given much time to this task, and their reports give recommended intakes or allowances of nutrients and are used as dietary standards.

RECOMMENDED DIETARY INTAKES OR ALLOWANCES

Tables giving recommended dietary intakes (RDI) or allowances (RDA) have now been prepared in most of the larger countries. The terms RDI and RDA are not distinguishable. The tables are now used in five different ways: the first three are well established in practical nutrition, the other two were introduced only recently.

Assessment of dietary surveys

RDI provide a standard against which the nutrients in the food eaten by different sections of the community or a whole country can be assessed. In the annual reports of the British National Food Survey the diets of samples of different sections of the population are compared against the recommended intakes of the Department of Health and Social Security (1969). In this way it is possible to detect any group with a low intake of one or more nutrients. Any such group may then be investigated and, if clinical or biochemical evidence of deficiency (Chap. 55) is found, steps are taken to improve their diet or provide a supplement of nutrients.

Planning diets

Authorities planning diets of ordinary food for institutions, e.g. boarding schools, old people's homes and prisons, and for the armed services and special therapeutic diets for individuals, should ensure that the diet meets the RDI. Caterers in institutions usually derive their menus from traditional wisdom, but if a complaint about underfeeding arose RDIs would be used in the enquiry.

Planning food supplies

International agencies use RDIs in planning long-term aid for underdeveloped regions and for calculating food supplies needed for famine relief. All national governments should, in forming agricultural policies, use RDIs as the common ground between economic planners and nutritionists. However, it is not possible to diagnose the nutritional deficiencies present in a country by comparing average food available per head against the RDI, because the distribution of available foods in various sections of the population is often very uneven.

Nutritional labelling

For canned and packed foods the amounts of important nutrients in an average serving may be given on the label, expressed as a proportion of the recommended intake for the intended consumer (Chap. 26).

Nutrient density

The nutrient value of any food may be expressed in terms of its content of nutrients and of energy, each related to RDI. This is the nutrient density (Hansen, 1973) and for any one nutrient in a food is

$$\frac{\text{(Nutrient in 100 g)/(energy in 100g)}}{\text{(RDI of nutrient)/(RDI of energy)}}$$

This concept is especially useful for new types of manufactured foods and foods enriched with synthetic foods. Thus the nutrient density of thiamin in bread made from 70 per cent extraction white flour (thiamin 0.08 mg and energy 1.43 MJ/100 g) in the diet of a sedentary man (RDI, thiamin 1.1 mg and energy 11.3 MJ/day) is

$$\frac{0.08}{1.43} \times \frac{11.3}{1.1} = 0.57$$

As the value is far below 1.0, the bread is a poor source of

Table 15.1 World Health Organization Recommended Intakes (Passmore et al., 1974)

Age	Body weight (kg)	Energy a (MJ)	Energy a (kcal)	Protein a,b (g)	Vitamin A d (μg)	Vitamin D e,f (μg)	Thiamin c (mg)	Riboflavin c (mg)	Niacin c (mg)	Folic acid e (μg)	Vitamin B$_{12}$ e (μg)	Ascorbic acid e (mg)	Calcium g (g)	Iron e,h (mg)
Children														
<1	7.3	3.4	820	14	300	10.0	0.3	0.5	5.4	60	0.3	20	0.5-0.6	5-10
1-3	13.4	5.7	1360	16	250	10.0	0.5	0.8	9.0	100	0.9	20	0.4-0.5	5-10
4-6	20.2	7.6	1830	20	300	10.0	0.7	1.1	12.1	100	1.5	20	0.4-0.5	5-10
7-9	28.1	9.2	2190	25	400	2.5	0.9	1.3	14.5	100	1.5	20	0.4-0.5	5-10
Male adolescents														
10-12	36.9	10.9	2600	30	575	2.5	1.0	1.6	17.2	100	2.0	20	0.6-0.7	5-10
13-15	51.3	12.1	2900	37	725	2.5	1.2	1.7	19.1	200	2.0	30	0.6-0.7	9-18
16-19	62.9	12.8	3070	38	750	2.5	1.2	1.8	20.3	200	2.0	30	0.5-0.6	5-9
Female adolescents														
10-12	38.0	9.8	2350	29	575	2.5	0.9	1.4	15.5	100	2.0	20	0.6-0.7	5-10
13-15	49.9	10.4	2490	31	725	2.5	1.0	1.5	16.4	200	2.0	30	0.6-0.7	12-24
16-19	54.4	9.7	2310	30	750	2.5	0.9	1.4	15.2	200	2.0	30	0.5-0.6	14-28
Adult man (moderately active)	65.0	12.6	3000	37	750	2.5	1.2	1.8	19.8	200	2.0	30	0.4-0.5	5-9
Adult woman (moderately active)	55.0	9.2	2200	29	750	2.5	0.9	1.3	14.5	200	2.0	30	0.4-0.5	14-28
Pregnancy (later half)		+1.5	+350	38	750	10.0	+0.1	+0.2	+2.3	400	3.0	50	1.0-1.2	i
Lactation (first 6 months)		+2.3	+550	46	1200	10.0	+0.2	+0.4	+3.7	300	2.5	50	1.0-1.2	i

a Energy and Protein Requirements: Report of a Joint FAO/WHO Expert Group, FAO, Rome, 1972.

b As egg or milk protein.

c Requirements of Vitamin A, Thiamin, Riboflavin and Niacin: Report of a joint FAO/WHO Expert Group, FAO, Rome, 1965.

d As retinol.

e Requirements of Ascorbic Acid, Vitamin D, Vitamin B$_{12}$, Folate and Iron: Report of a Joint FAO/WHO Expert Group, FAO, Rome, 1970.

f As cholecalciferol.

g Calcium Requirements: Report of a FAO/WHO Expert Group, FAO, Rome, 1961.

h On each line the lower value applies when over 25 per cent of calories in the diet come from animal foods, and the higher value when animal foods represent less than 10 per cent of calories.

i For women whose iron intake throughout life has been at the level recommended in this table, the daily intake of iron during pregnancy and lactation should be the same as that recommended for non-pregnant, non-lactating women of childbearing age. For women whose iron status is not satisfactory at the beginning of pregnancy, the requirement is increased; and in the extreme situation of women with no iron stores, the requirement can probably not be met without supplementation.

Table 15.2 Food and Nutrition Board, National Academy of Sciences–National Research Council: *Recommended Daily Dietary Allowances*, Revised 1974. Designed for the maintenance of good nutrition of practically all healthy people in the USA

	Age (years)	Weight (kg)	Weight (lb)	Height (cm)	Height (in)	Energy [b] (kcal)	Protein (g)	Vitamin A Activity (RE) [c]	Vitamin A Activity (IU)	Vitamin D (IU)	Vitamin E activity [e] (IU)
Infants	0.0–0.5	6	14	60	24	kg×117	kg×2.2	420 [d]	1400	400	4
	0.5–1.0	9	20	71	28	kg×108	kg×2.0	400	2000	400	5
Children	1–3	13	28	86	34	1300	23	400	2000	400	7
	4–6	20	44	110	44	1800	30	500	2500	400	9
	7–10	30	66	135	54	2400	36	700	3300	400	10
Males	11–14	44	97	158	63	2800	44	1000	5000	400	12
	15–18	61	134	172	69	3000	54	1000	5000	400	15
	19–22	67	147	172	69	3000	54	1000	5000	400	15
	23–50	70	154	172	69	2700	56	1000	5000	–	15
	51+	70	154	172	69	2400	56	1000	5000	–	15
Females	11–14	44	97	155	62	2400	44	800	4000	400	12
	15–18	54	119	162	65	2100	48	800	4000	400	12
	19–22	58	128	162	65	2100	46	800	4000	400	12
	23–50	58	128	162	65	2000	46	800	4000	–	12
	51+	58	128	162	65	1800	46	800	4000	–	12
Pregnant	–	–		–		+300	+30	1000	5000	400	15
Lactating	–	–		–		+500	+20	1200	6000	400	15

a The allowances are intended to provide for individual variations among most normal persons as they live in the United States under usual environmental stresses. Diets should be based on a variety of common foods in order to provide other nutrients for which human requirements have been less well defined.

b Kilojoules (KJ) = 4.2 × kcal.

c Retinol equivalents.

d Assumed to be all as retinol in milk during the first six months of life. All subsequent intakes are assumed to be one-half as retinol and one-half as β-carotene when calculated from international units. As retinol equivalents, three-fourths are as retinol and one-fourth as β-carotene.

thiamin and other richer sources are needed in the diet to meet the RDI. If the flour is enriched with thiamin so as to contain 0.24 mg/100 g, as is the law in the UK, then its nutrient density is 1.7 Bread made from such flour is a good source of thiamin. Even if eaten with a thick covering of butter or jam, providing extra energy but little or no thiamin, the nutrient density would be above 1.0 and thus satisfactory.

How recommended dietary intakes are derived

Committees produce RDIs. Their first step is to decide whether a compound is an essential nutrient for man. If an organic compound, it must cure a deficiency disease. If an inorganic element, it must be found regularly in the body and shown to have a function. The next decisions are how low the intake of the nutrient can fall before disease occurs and how much of it prevents or cures the deficiency disease. For most nutrients the minimum requirement needed to prevent deficiency disease can be stated with some precision.

Persons who show no evidence of deficiency disease may not be in full health. Amounts of a nutrient greater than the minimum requirement may be utilised physiologically and this may promote health. Some biochemical studies are aimed at defining criteria of optimal nutrition and here there are possibilities for different opinions. Thus the US Food and Nutrition Board was formerly concerned that the tissues should be saturated with vitamin C while in Britain the Department of Health and Social Security (1969) considered that 'in the UK few of us are saturated with the vitamin but we do not appear to suffer any ill effects as a result.' In the 1960s the RDA for ascorbic acid for adults was 70 mg in the USA and only 30 mg in the UK. The USA no longer uses tissue saturation as a criterion and the difference between the recommendations in the two countries has narrowed.

Safety factors have to be added to average minimum requirements to deal with three variables. The first is the range of physiological requirements, which is very wide for some nutrients; the safety factor covers the majority (about

Water-soluble vitamins							Minerals					
Ascorbic acid (mg)	Folacin f (µg)	Niacin g (mg)	Ribo-flavin (mg)	Thia-min (mg)	Vitamin B_6 (mg)	Vitamin B_{12} (µg)	Cal-cium (mg)	Phos-phorus (mg)	Iodine (µg)	Iron (mg)	Mag-nesium (mg)	Zinc (mg)
35	50	5	0.4	0.3	0.3	0.3	360	240	35	10	60	3
35	50	8	0.6	0.5	0.4	0.3	540	400	45	15	70	5
40	100	9	0.8	0.7	0.6	1.0	800	800	60	15	150	10
40	200	12	1.1	0.9	0.9	1.5	800	800	80	10	200	10
40	300	16	1.2	1.2	1.2	2.0	800	800	110	10	250	10
45	400	18	1.5	1.4	1.6	3.0	1200	1200	130	18	350	15
45	400	20	1.8	1.5	2.0	3.0	1200	1200	150	18	400	15
45	400	20	1.8	1.5	2.0	3.0	800	800	140	10	350	15
45	400	18	1.6	1.4	2.0	3.0	800	800	130	10	350	15
45	400	16	1.5	1.2	2.0	3.0	800	800	110	10	350	15
45	400	16	1.3	1.2	1.6	3.0	1200	1200	115	18	300	15
45	400	14	1.4	1.1	2.0	3.0	1200	1200	115	18	300	15
45	400	14	1.4	1.1	2.0	3.0	800	800	100	18	300	15
45	400	13	1.2	1.0	2.0	3.0	800	800	100	18	300	15
45	400	12	1.1	1.0	2.0	3.0	800	800	80	10	300	15
60	800	+2	+0.3	+0.3	2.5	4.0	1200	1200	125	18+ h	450	20
60	600	+4	+0.5	+0.3	2.5	4.0	1200	1200	150	18	450	25

e Total vitamin E activity, estimated to be 80 per cent as α-tocopherol and 20 per cent other tocopherols.

f The folacin allowances refer to dietary sources as determined by *Lactobacillus casei* assay. Pure forms of folacin may be effective in doses less than one-fourth of the RDA.

g Although allowances are expressed as niacin, it is recognised that on the average 1 mg of niacin is derived from each 60 mg of dietary tryptophan.

h This increased requirement cannot be met by ordinary diets; therefore, the use of supplemental iron is recommended.

95 per cent) of individuals. The second is the possible increase in the requirements caused by the minor stresses of everyday life; however, RDIs do not allow for infections, injuries and other illnesses. A third variable sometimes considered is the different availability of a nutrient in various foods. For example FAO/WHO recommendations for iron (Table 15.1) are adjusted for the proportion of animal food in the diet, because haem iron is more readily absorbed than iron in vegetable foods (Chap. 11).

RDIs for energy contrasted with those for nutrients

There is a fundamental difference between energy and other nutrients. It is not possible to recommend exactly how much energy an individual requires to get from his food. It depends on how physically active he is at work and at leisure, and varies from time to time. If all of a class of 100 students were to eat exactly their RDI of energy for two weeks, about half would lose and half would gain weight. If the students were forced to continue this experiment for a year, then a few of them would be seriously undernourished and some would have become obese. RDIs for energy are a catering average; individuals take more or less according to appetite which follows their energy expenditure. On the other hand, RDIs for protein, vitamins and minerals supply the needs of the great majority of people and without causing adverse effects from overdosage in any.

RDIs in different countries

In some countries figures for the RDI of some nutrients, e.g. protein, ascorbic acid, calcium and iron, have changed over the years. For these nutrients there is uncertainty how to define both adequate and optimal nutritional status. Foods rich in good quality protein or ascorbic acid or calcium or iron are usually expensive, and it is impractical to set RDIs for these nutrients as high as they are in some richer countries. When the American RDAs were first published in 1943, a practical Indian nutritionist remarked to R.P., 'They are a beautiful dream.' For other nutrients which are less controversial or have not attracted as much research interest by nutritional scientists, the dietary standards change little with time or place. Examples are thiamin and nicotinamide.

The Committee on International Dietary Allowances of the International Union of Nutritional Sciences (1975) published a report which compares RDIs in 20 countries; the changes from the 1930s to the present in some central countries have been summarised by Truswell (1976). All the RDIs for European countries are assembled in the report of the Second European Nutrition Conference (Zöllner, et al., 1977). There are 15 tables; some countries, including France, do not have their own dietary standards.

There are big differences in the number of nutrients given in the main tables. The British Department of Health and Social Security (1969) gives 10, the FAO/WHO handbook (Table 15.1) 12 and the US report (Table 15.2) 18. In West Germany the Deutsche Gesellschaft für Ernährung (1975) has 24 nutrients, including water and fluoride. Countries which have a short list of nutrients in the main table may discuss the range of requirements or of usual intakes of other nutrients in the text. There are differences, too, in the number of groups in the population for which separate RDIs are given; figures are often interpolations from measurements on other groups. West Germany has a total of 14 groups for females and the USSR has no fewer then 49, all with different RDIs for protein (Truswell, 1978).

Two of the better known tables are given as examples. Table 15.1 is from the FAO/WHO Handbook on Human Nutritional Requirements (Passmore et al., 1974). This condenses judgments on energy and nutrient requirements by a series of expert committees convened in the 1960s or early 1970s. The values given provide a basis for assessment of nutrient intakes but in some cases they would be unacceptably low for prescription of diets in affluent populations. Table 15.2 gives the US recommended dietary allowances drawn up by the Committee on Dietary Allowances, Food and Nutrition Board (1974). These are the best-known recommendations from an

Table 15.3 Tentatively recommended daily allowances of energy and nutrients for patients on complete intravenous nutrition. The allowances cover resting metabolism, some physical activity and specific dynamic action, but no increased need resulting from trauma, burns, or other conditions (Wretlind, 1975)

Nutrient	Allowance/kg body-weight	
	Adults	Neonates and infants
Water (ml)	30	120–150
Energy (MJ (kcal))	0.13 (30)	0.38–0.50 (90–120)
Amino acid–nitrogen (mg)	90 (0.7 g amino acids)	330 (2.5 g amino acids)
Glucose (g)	2	12–18
Fat (g)	2	4
Sodium (mmol)	1–1.4	1–2.5
Potassium (mmol)	0.7–0.9	2
Calcium (mmol)	0.11	0.5–1
Phosphorus (mmol)	0.15	0.4–0.8
Magnesium (mmol)	0.04	0.15
Iron (μmol)	1	2
Manganese (μmol)	0.6	1
Zinc (μmol)	0.3	0.6
Copper (μmol)	0.07	0.3
Chloride (mmol)	1.3–1.9	1.8–4.3
Fluoride (μmol)	0.7	3
Iodine (μmol)	0.015	0.04
Thiamin (mg)	0.02	0.05
Riboflavin (mg)	0.03	0.1
Nicotinamide (mg)	0.2	1
Pyridoxine (mg)	0.03	0.1
Folic acid (μg)	3	20
Vitamin B_{12} (μg)	0.03	0.2
Panothernic acid (mg)	0.2	1
Biotin (μg)	5	30
Ascorbic acid (mg)	0.5	3
Retinol (μg)	10	100
Ergocalciferol or chole-calciferol (μg)	0.04	2.5
Phytylmenaquinone (μg)	2	50
α-Tocopherol (mg)	1.5	3

industrial country. The report explains how the recommendations have been derived and how they are meant to be used.

Recommendations for parenteral feeding

When a patient who is comatose or has severe gastrointestinal disease has to be fed entirely by intravenous fluids for more than a few days, it is necessary to ensure that he is given all the essential nutrients. The list of nutrients for which recommendations are made in most tables is not long enough for this purpose, since they do not include some nutrients that are required in small amounts and are widespread in foods. Disorders attributable to deficiencies of essential fatty acids, zinc, chromium and other nutrients have occurred in patients on prolonged parenteral feeding and are described in other chapters. Table 15.3 gives recommendations for water, energy and 28 nutrients, and is based on experience in Stockholm. All patients who depend only on intravenous fluids for their supply of nutrients should be given this formula.

THE FUTURE: A NEED FOR TWO DIETARY STANDARDS

Committees have long been aware that their recommendations are used both for assessment and planning, and aware also of the difficulties in providing figures suitable for both purposes. The chief difficulty is that diets customary in many countries, and accepted as good, often provide far more of some nutrients, especially protein, calcium and vitamin A, than appears to be needed to meet physiological requirements. This difficulty and others are considered by Hegsted (1975) in a critical review. He suggested the need for two standards. The first, based on estimates of nutrient needs, would be for use in assessment or evaluation of diets. The second, for which food supplies, food habits and the aims of nutrition education would be considered, would be for use in planning.

This approach was used at the Round Table Discussion on Recommended Intakes at the Second European Nutrition Conference in Munich in 1976. Two levels of dietary standards were suggested. 'The **group physiological requirement,** or "safe level", is useful for evaluating diets or diagnosing an unsatisfactorily low intake of one or more nutrients. The **recommended intake,** or **desirable range,** is intended for teaching, for menu planning by housewives, dietitians, caterers, and ultimately for agricultural economic planning. These prescriptive values are higher than the requirements and may be expressed in foods.... Where a country's recommended intake for protein is generous—say 65 g for an adult—this cannot be used as a criterion for assessing if a diet is adequate; a low standard has to be found such as the FAO/WHO value of 37 g or the British "minimum" of 45 g/day' (Wretlind *et al.*, 1977.)

The second of these approaches indicates that recommended intakes might be more useful and practical if based on available food supplies, rather than on estimates of physiological needs. Passmore *et al.* (1979) have made an estimate of what foods constitute an average British diet, based on data in reports of the National Food Survey. The diet is expressed in terms of 12 classes of foods. They suggest that the health of the population might be improved if consumption of oils and fats, sugar and alcoholic beverages were reduced. Economic factors might reduce consumption of meat but this would have no adverse effect on health. The loss of energy from decreased consumption of these foods could be made good by increased consumption of grain products, potatoes, fruit and vegetables. Figures are suggested for the amounts of these changes which might be practical over 10 years. None of the changes is revolutionary but most of them reverse trends in consumption in recent years. This suggestion for an improved national diet could be used as a basis for recommended intakes for purposes of planning, as indicated at the Munich discussion.

PART II

Food

16. Foods and Food Composition Tables

The physiological roles of the essential nutrients, carbohydrates, fats, proteins, minerals and vitamins have now been considered. Next it is necessary to describe the principal foods of man in terms of these nutrients. Foods are conveniently classified in ten categories: (1) cereals, (2) starchy roots, (3) sugars and syrups, (4) pulses, nuts and seeds, (5) vegetables, (6) fruits, (7) meat, fish, eggs and novel proteins, (8) milk and milk products, (9) oils and fats, and (10) beverages. First a brief account is given of food tables, which describe individual foods in terms of their content of nutrients.

It is now 100 years since the first food composition tables were published, in 1878, by König in Germany (Somogyi, 1974). These were followed by the classic American tables compiled by Atwater and Woods (1896). Some of the many tables now available are listed in Table 16.1. Every dietitian and nutritionist should be in possession of one of these or some other suitable table of food values, for it is these tables that enable dietetics to be a science as well as an art.

Widdowson and McCance (1943) have aptly stated: 'There are two schools of thought about food tables. One tends to regard the figures in them as having the accuracy of atomic weight determinations; the other dismisses them as valueless on the grounds that a foodstuff may be so modified by the soil, the season or its rate of growth that no figure can be a reliable guide to its composition. The truth, of course, lies somewhere between these points of view.' To understand the information that tables provide, and to assess their reliability and accuracy it is necessary to read the introductions which describe how they have been compiled. If this is not done the tables may be abused by improper application.

Applications

Clinical practice

Accurate prescribing of diets containing known amounts of some of the important nutrients is essential for the treatment of certain diseases. Diets low in energy for obese patients, diets containing known amounts of carbohydrate and fat for diabetics, diets rich in protein for the nephrotic syndrome, and diets with a low sodium content for patients with congestive heart failure are well-known examples.

Accurate interpretation of a dietary history may be a value aid to diagnosis. For example, an estimate of the amount of ascorbic acid in a patient's previous diet may assist in deciding whether a purpuric rash is a manifestation of scurvy or of some blood disease. Many problems of this nature arise in clinical medicine.

Community health

In a dietary survey after intakes of the different foods have been measured, tables have to be used to calculate intakes of the various nutrients; then comparisons with recommended intakes (Chap. 15) allow judgments to be made as to whether these intakes are or are not sufficient to maintain the group in good health. From statistics of national agricultural production and of imports and exports of food and census data, food tables are used to calculate the amounts of nutrients per head of population in a country. In this way Ministries of Agriculture make use of food tables in planning national diets. The food industry also uses food tables in planning and promoting the use of new foods.

In prescribing diets for closed communities such as the armed services, boarding schools, old people's homes, prisons, etc, it is important to make sure that any recommended ration scale is compared with acceptable standards and that its use is not likely to cause deficiency disease.

The large number of calculations required, even for an individual patient, let alone a community sample, make the use of a computer very helpful. Food tables are now available as input material for computers. These can save the dietitian's time but are more cumbersome to modify or correct than printed tables.

Clinical research

Tables are useful as a guide in the planning stages, but they rarely provide information about intake of nutrients which is precise enough to allow an accurate balance to be drawn up.

Limitations

How far can food tables help to provide answers to the practical problems discussed above? There is the drawback that each figure in the table can only be an average of the analyses of a limited number of samples of each food. Laboratory errors are small for most methods and can be minimised by replication. Sampling error is very important, especially when whole dishes or meals are analysed. For any single plant or animal foodstuff there are small individual genetic variations; there are large possibilities of differences in composition due to the variety or strain, and equally large effects from conditions of culture or husbandry and maturity or freshness. The effect of cooking is considered in Chapter 23. For this reason it is best to use tables based on analyses of local foods. A few principles can be set out which indicate the significance of these variations and so allow an intelligent use of the tables.

Water

Variation in the water content of foods is the main cause of variation in the content of other nutrients. Thus figures for the composition of foods containing large amounts of water are always uncertain. Cereal grains contain relatively little water and, although there are variations in the nutrient content of different varieties of the same cereal, these are relatively small. Cereals have been extensively analysed and tables give reliable figures for most of them. Diets with a high cereal content are usually eaten by poor people. Thus the error involved in calculating the nutrients consumed by a farm worker in Kenya, living mainly on maize and sorghum, is much less than the error in making a similar calculation for a business executive in Chicago with his varied diet.

Proximate principles

Perhaps the least variable of the chemical constituents of foods is protein. On numerous occasions when the protein content of a diet has been calculated from tables and simultaneously determined by analyses of aliquot portions of the diet, there has been very good agreement. The error in using tables to calculate the protein content of a diet is not likely to be more than 7 per cent.

The error in estimating carbohydrate and fat from the tables is also not very great—with one important exception. This is the calculation for meat. There are large variations in the fat content of different helpings of beef, mutton or pork and people vary greatly in the amount of fat on meat they eat or reject. These greatly affect the calculated energy value.

Energy

The energy value of a diet can usually be calculated with an accuracy sufficient for practical purposes. However, it is necessary to know the way in which the energy values given in a table have been calculated in order not to make invalid comparisons with other data. The error introduced by the use of tables should not be more than 10 per cent unless the diet contains large quantities of meat. Thus estimates can be made with the help of the tables, which s   for most clinical and public health purposes. The   ve sufficient accuracy for use in prescrib-   e and diabetic patients. The error will be   sing simple diets based on cereals and at a   h mixed diets. Errors of up to 10 per

cent are too great for most metabolic studies, and tables of food analyses are of little use to clinical scientists and physiologists, who must make their own analyses on aliquot samples of their subjects' diets.

Vitamins

The variations in the vitamin content of foods is very much greater than the variations in proximate principles. They are especially large in all classes of vegetables and fruits and particularly for vitamin A activity and ascorbic acid content. These variations are so great that the use of tables to give a quantitative assessment of the vitamin content of a diet may produce a set of figures that have no factual basis. With poor diets containing only small amounts of foods rich in vitamins, the errors are less. For instance food tables should enable a statement to be made as to whether a diet contains less or more than 5 mg of ascorbic acid, i.e. whether or not it is likely to be associated with scurvy. Similar assessments can be made for vitamin A activity and the principal vitamins of the B group.

Minerals

For minerals the tables are of limited value. There are enormous variations in the iron content of different samples of the same food. Different tables can give very different values for the iron content of a diet. This is due mainly to the fact that foods are readily contaminated with iron during preparation. For calcium and trace elements, the value of the figures is limited by uncertainty as to how much of the element is available for absorption.

Sampling and other problems

Those who prepare food tables have difficulty in ensuring that the foods actually analysed are a representative sample of the foods eaten. Their difficulty arises with simple agricultural products, such as cereals, fresh meat and vegetables, but is much greater with manufactured foods. Representative sampling of foods such as cakes, ice cream, meat pies and other made-up dishes is impossible. The more these foods contribute to a diet, the less accurate is an estimate of intake of nutrients based on tables. Stock and Wheeler (1972) and Kaser et al. (1947) have compared the nutrient content of diets determined by chemical analysis and calculated from tables.

The preparation of each of the tables listed opposite was a major task, and inevitably they soon become out of date. For example the 1978 British tables give figures for energy and some 33 nutrients for all common foods together with appendices showing 18 amino acids, 16 fatty acids, cholesterol, etc. for selected foodstuffs. New foods appear in every country, and nutritionists become interested in new components of diets. Thus most tables at present available provide inadequate information about amounts of fibre and trace elements in foods—subjects of great current interest. Those who use food tables should not grumble too much about their inadequacies; rather they should be grateful to those who prepare the tables for their immense efforts which provide so much useful information.

The Group of European Nutritionists set up a working party to study the general principles which have to be considered in the preparation of national food composition tables. The report (Southgate, 1974) considers the selection of food items and of nutrients, sampling procedure, statistical expression and the best chemical methods.

Table 16.1 A selected list of food tables

Food tables	Source
AFRICA *Food Composition Table for Use in Africa* Woot-Tsuen Wu Leung *et al.* (1968)	Obtainable from FAO *or* Nutrition Program, National Center for Chronic Disease Control, Public Health Service, US Department of Health, Education and Welfare, 9000 Rockville Pike, Bethesda, Md
WEST AFRICA *Aliments de l'ouest Africain—Tables de Composition* Toury, J., Giorgi, R., Favier, J.C. and Savina, J.F. (1965)	Organisation de Coordination et de Cooperation pour la lutte contre les grandes Endemies-Organisme de Recherches sur l'Alimentation et la Nutrition Africaines, Dakar, Senegal
ETHIOPIA *Food Composition Table for Use in Ethiopia* Ågren, G. and Gibson, R. (1968)	Obtainable from Children's Nutrition Unit, Addis Ababa, PO Box 1768
GHANA *Food Composition Table* (1969)	Food Research Institute—Food Research and Development Unit, Accra
SOUTH AFRICA *Studies on the Chemical Composition of Foods Commonly Used in Southern Africa* Fox, F.W. (1966)	South African Institute for Medical Research, Johannesburg
ASIA EAST ASIA *Food Composition Table for Use in East Asia* (1972)	US Department of Health, Education and Welfare (National Institute of Arthritis, Metabolism and Digestive Diseases, National Institutes of Health, Maryland 20014) *or* FAO, Food Policy and Nutrition Division, Rome
INDIA *Nutritive Value of Indian Foods* Gopalan, C., Rama Sastri, B. V. and Balasubramanian, S.C. (1974)	National Institute of Nutrition, Indian Council of Medical Research, Hyderabad 7
JAPAN *Standard Tables of Food Composition in Japan* (1963) *The Amino Acid Composition of Foods in Japan* Tamura, E. (1966)	Resources Bureau, Science and Technology Agency, Tokyo Resources Bureau, Science and Technology Agency, Tokyo
PAKISTAN *Nutritive Value of Foodstuffs and Planning of Satisfactory Diets in Pakistan. Part I, Composition of Raw Foodstuffs* Chughtai, M.I.D. and Waheed Khan, A. (1960)	Division of Biochemistry, Institute of Chemistry, Punjab University, Lahore
PHILLIPPINES *Food Composition Table Recommended for Use in the Philippines. Handbook I,* 3rd revision (1964)	The Food and Nutrition Research Center, National Science Development Board, Manila
AUSTRALIA *Tables of Composition of Australian Foods,* revised edition Thomas, S. and Corden, M. (1977)	Australian Commonwealth Department of Health, Nutrition Section, Canberra
EUROPE DENMARK *Fodevare-og ernaeringstabeller* Rich Ege-Nyt. (1969)	Nordish Forlag, Arnold Busck ......agen

Food tables	Source
FINLAND *Ruoka-Aine-Taulukko* Turpeinen, O. and Roine, P. (1967)	Department of Biochemistry, College of Veterinary Medicine, Hameentie 57, Helsinki
FRANCE *Tables de Composition des Aliments* Randoin, L., Legallic, P., Dupuis, Y. and Beradin, A. (1961)	Institut Scientific d'Hygiene Alimentaire, Centre National de la Recherche Scientifique, Paris
HUNGARY *Food Composition Tables*, 7th edition Tarján, R. and Lindner, K. (1972)	Medicinakonyvkiado, Budapest
ITALY *Composizione in alcuni principi nutritivi e valore calorico degli alimenti comunemente in Italia* (1968)	National Institute of Nutrition, Rome (for internal use of the Institute, not published)
NETHERLANDS *Nederlandse Voedingsmiddeln Tabel*, 30th edition (1977) (revised regularly)	Voorlichtingsbureau voor de Voeding, Laan Copes van Cattenburch 44, Den Haag-2011
NORWAY *Naerings Middel Tabell*, 3rd edition (1966)	Pub. Landsforeningen for Kosthold of Helse, Oslo
POLAND *Tabele skladu I wartosci odzywczych produktow spozywczych* Szczygla, A. (ed.) (1972)	Panstwowy Zaklad Wydawrietw Lekarskich, Warsaw
SWEDEN *Fadoämnes-Tabeller* Abramson, E. (1971)	Svenska Bokförlaget, Bonniers, Stockholm
WEST GERMANY *Die Zusammensetzung der Lebensmittel: Nährwerttabellen* Souci, S.W., Fachmann, W. and Kraut, H. (1973)	Wissenschaftliche Verlagsgesellschaft MBH, Stuttgart
UNITED KINGDOM *McCance and Widdowson's The Composition of Foods,* 4th revised edition Paul, A.A. and Southgate, D.A.T. (1978)	H.M. Stationery Office, London
USSR *Tabulky Kalorickych a biologickych Kudnor potravin,* 2nd edition Muller, S. (1969)	SPN, Bratislava, Czechoslovakia
MIDDLE EAST *Food Composition Tables for Use in the Middle East* Publication No. 20 (1963)	Division of Food Technology and Nutrition, Faculty of Agricultural Sciences, American University of Beirut, Lebanon
IRAN *Food Composition Tables* Hedayat, H., Mermillod, M.J. and Hormazdyary, H. (1965)	Ministry of Health, Food and Nutrition Institute, Teheran
ISRAEL *Tablaoth Herkev Hamsonoth* Guggenheim, K. (1964)	College of Nutrition and Home Economics, Ministry of Education and Culture, Jersualem
TURKEY *Gida Komposizyon Cetvelleri* Koksal, O. and Baysal, A. (1966)	School of Public Health, Ankara
AMERICA USA *Amino Acid Content of Foods* US Department of Agriculture, Home Economics Report No. 4 Orr, M.L. and Watt, B.K. (1957, reviewed 1968)	Obtainable from Superintendent of Documents, U.S. Government Printing Office, Washington, DC 20402
Composition of Foods. Raw, Processed, Prepared Agriculture Handbook No. 8. Watt, B~~ ~~ and Merrill, A.L. (1963) Revision Posati, L.P. and Orr, ~~Dairy and Egg Products~~ Revision 8-2: *Species and Herbs* Marsh, A.C., Moss, M.K. and Murph~~y,~~	Obtainable from Superintendent of Documents, US Government Printing Office, Washington, DC 20402

Food tables	Source
CANADA *Nutrient Value of Some Common Foods* Health and Welfare, Canada (1971)	Nutrition Division, Department of National Health and Welfare, Ottawa
LATIN AMERICA *INCAP-ICNND Food Consumption Table for Use in Latin America* Woot-Tsuen Wu Leung and Flores, M. (1961)	Obtainable from INCAP, Apartado Postal No. 11-88, Guatemala City, Guatemala, C.A.
CARIBBEAN *Food Composition Tables for Use in the English Speaking Caribbean* (1974)	Caribbean Food and Nutrition Institute, Kingston, Jamaica

OTHERS

Food tables	Source
SOUTH PACIFIC *Some Tropical South Pacific Island Foods* Muaj, M., Pen, F. and Miller, C.D. (1958)	University of Hawaii Press, Honolulu, Hawaii
TROPICAL COUNTRIES *Tables of Representative Values of Foods Commonly Used in Tropical Countries* (MRC Special Report Series No. 302) Platt, B.S. (1962)	HM Stationery Office, London

FAO Updated Annotated Bibliography of Food Composition Tables (Food Composition Section, Food Consumption and Planning Branch, Nutrition Division, Rome, 1975) lists food tables from 72 countries.

17. Cereals

Cereal grains are the seeds of domesticated grasses. Stable civilisations have arisen only when primitive hunting communities have learned how to raise successive cereal crops from cultivated land. Without the use of cereals man is reduced to an uncertain and unsettled nomadic life. They have been modified and improved by centuries of cultivation and selective breeding.

In many rural areas, including large parts of Asia and Africa, cereals provide more than 70 per cent of the energy in the common diet. As a country becomes more prosperous this proportion falls, but cereals remain the most important single food. In the national diet of the UK bread and flour products provide about 29 per cent of the energy, about 15 per cent coming from bread. Only isolated people, such as the Eskimos and a few pastoral tribes, are almost entirely carnivorous and do not cultivate cereals or root crops.

The principal cereals are wheat, rice, maize, millets, barley, oats and rye. The amounts of cereals produced in the different regions of the world are given in Table 17.1, but this does not distinguish between that eaten by man and that fed to animals. Wheat is the cereal of choice in temperate or dry climates in most parts of the world.

Rice is the cereal of choice in most damp tropical climates. It grows best in the deltas of the great rivers since it is essentially a mud plant requiring an abundant water supply.

Maize is a poor man's food, being hardy, easily cultivated and relatively immune from the predation of birds. In North America it is grown mainly for cattle fodder.

Millets grow in hot climates, on poor soil with limited water supply. They are the principal crops in many dry areas in the tropics.

Barley is grown mainly for cattle fodder and for brewing. Oats are a hardy crop and at one time the staple food of the people of Scotland, but now are grown chiefly for cattle fodder. Rye grows in poor soil in cold climates. In the last five hundred years it has been progressively replaced by wheat.

The name 'corn' is generally used in the English-speaking world to mean the most familiar local cereal—whatever the species. Thus 'corn' in Scotland means oats, in England, wheat, and in the USA, maize. The choice depends largely on climate and economic factors, but custom and precedent are also important. All cereals can be ground into flour for cakes or porridge, but only wheat and rye bake into bread.

The whole grains of all cereals have a similar chemical constitution and nutritive value. They provide energy and protein, which is usually of good quality. They contain appreciable amounts of calcium and iron, but the value of these minerals is partly discounted by the presence of phytic acid which may interfere with their absorption. Cereals are totally devoid of ascorbic acid and practically devoid of vitamin A activity. Yellow maize is the only cereal containing significant amounts of carotene. Whole cereal grains also contain useful amounts of the water-soluble B group of vitamins.

Table 17.2 shows how similar are the nutritive values of the whole grains of all the principal cereals, although their limiting amino acids differ. To make a balanced diet, cereals should be supplemented by animal proteins, minerals and vitamins A and C. These are provided by meat, milk and fresh green vegetables. When cereal grains are consumed in their entirety an adequate supply of the B group of vitamins is ensured except in the case of maize, in

Table 17.1 Cereal production in the world in 1975 (data from FAO, 1977)

	Wheat	Rice	Maize	Millets	Barley	Oats	Rye
			(millions of metric tons)				
Western Europe	55		27		45	12	4
Eastern Europe and USSR	91				49	17	18
North America	75	4	150	19	18	14	
Latin America	15	9	39				
China	41	81	35	26			
Far East	33	111	16	21			
Near East	28	3	4		8		
Africa	4		14	16	3		
Oceania	12						

Table 17.2 Nutritive value of the main whole cereal grains (values per 100 g)

	Energy		Pro-tein (g)	Limiting amino acid	Fat (g)	Cal-cium (mg)	Iron (mg)	Thia-min (mg)	Nicotinic acid (mg)	Ribo-flavin (mg)	Carotene (μg)	Ascorbic acid (mg)
	MJ	kcal										
Wheat (whole meal)	1.40	334	12.2	Lysine	2.3	30	3.5	0.40	5.0	0.17	Trace	0
Rice (husked)	1.49	357	7.5	Lysine (threonine)	1.8	15	2.8	0.25	4.0	0.12	Trace	0
Maize (whole meal)	1.19	356	9.5	Tryptophan (lysine)	4.3	12	5.0	0.33	1.5	0.13	Up to 800	0
Millet (sorghum)	1.44	343	10.1	Lysine	3.3	30	6.2	0.40	3.5	0.12	Trace	
Oats (rolled)	1.61	385	13.0	Lysine	7.5	60	3.8	0.50	1.3	0.14	Trace	0
Rye	1.34	319	11.0	Lysine	1.9	50	3.5	0.27	1.2	0.10	Trace	0

which the nicotinic acid is not biologically available. If, however, the grains are first milled and outer portions of the seed, including the germ and scutellum, discarded, there is a grave risk that there will be an insufficiency of the B group of vitamins. Fortunately oats, barley, millets and rye are usually only lightly husked and most of the whole grain is eaten. Wheat and rice, however, are invariably subjected to some degree of milling. The extent to which the milling process removes the vitamins is of importance. For a proper understanding of the nutritive value of the cereals and of the changes they undergo in preparing them as food for man it is necessary to consider the structure of the cereal grain and the composition of its parts.

WHEAT

Wheat is the most important crop in the world. There are 14 species, wild or cultivated, of the genus *Triticum*. *Triticum aestivum* or *vulgare*, the common bread wheat, contains three sets of chromosomes, i.e. 21 in its reproductive cells. Archaeological evidence indicates that it originated from relatives of einkorn (seven chromosomes) and emmer (14 chromosomes) around 8000 BC in western Asia. The genetics of wheat is a highly specialised and an important branch of science. New varieties of wheat are being developed in the main wheat-growing countries.

Anatomy of the grain. A readable monograph on *Wheat in Human Nutrition* by Aykroyd and Doughty (1970) elaborates many of the points mentioned below. The grain is a seed with the structure shown in Fig. 17.1. The outer coverings are the pericarp and testa which are hard, and contain much indigestible fibre. Beneath them is the aleurone layer, which is an envelope of cells rich in protein. These outer layers form about 12 per cent of the weight of the grain. Inside is the endosperm, comprising about 85 per cent of the weight of the grain, and consisting of an inner and outer portion. The germ (or embryo)—

situated at the lower end of the grain—consists of the shoot and root. The embryo is attached to the grain by a special structure, the scutellum. The embryo and scutellum are only just visible to the naked eye and form about 3 per cent of the total weight of the grain.

Distribution of nutrients in the grain. This is not uniform. The germ is relatively rich in protein, fat and several of the B vitamins. So also is the scutellum, which contains about 50 times more thiamin than the whole grain. Thus an important part, perhaps as much as half of the total thiamin in the grain, may be present in the scutellum. The outer layers of the endosperm and the aleurone layer contain a higher concentration of protein, vitamins (especially nicotinic acid) and phytic acid than the inner endosperm. The inner endosperm contains most of the starch and protein in the grain, though the protein is at a slightly lower concentration than in the outer layers and germ.

Wheat is usually ground into flour before being prepared as food. Flour containing the whole grain may be used but usually the germ and a varying proportion of the outer layers are separated from the central portion of the grain and discarded as bran. The proportion of the whole grain that is utilised to make flour is known as the **extraction rate.** Thus an 85 per cent extraction rate flour contains 85 per cent by weight of the whole grain and 15 per cent is discarded as bran. It is important to remember that the extraction rate refers to the proportion of the original grain in the flour and not in the bran. Thus flour of a 'high extraction rate' has lost little of the aleurone layer and outer endosperm.

Nutritive value of flour
Tables 17.3 and 4 show the effects of milling at different extraction rates on the composition of the resulting flours. The nutritional significance of these changes have to be considered against the background of the diet. Whole wheat is devoid of vitamins A, D and C and contains very

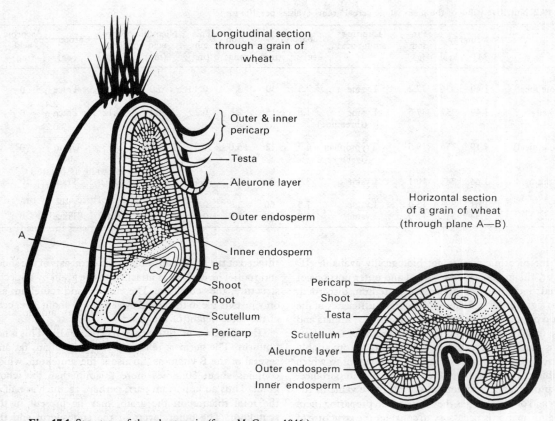

Longitudinal section through a grain of wheat

Outer & inner pericarp

Testa

Aleurone layer

Outer endosperm

A

Inner endosperm

B

Shoot

Root

Scutellum

Pericarp

Horizontal section of a grain of wheat (through plane A—B)

Pericarp

Shoot

Testa

Scutellum

Aleurone layer

Outer endosperm

Inner endosperm

Fig. 17.1 Structure of the wheat grain (from McCance 1946.)

little fat and these have to supplied by other items in the diet. There are many records of healthy communities who get up to 70 per cent of their dietary energy from wheat. In an experiment which is now a classic Widdowson and McCance (1954) showed that children in orphanages in Germany were healthy and grew well on diets in which 75 per cent of the energy was provided by wheat, about 20 per cent by vegetables and only about 5 per cent by foods of animal origin. Furthermore there was no difference between groups of children whose bread was made from flour of 100, 85 and 70 per cent extraction. This experiment confirmed common observation that bread made from flour was a nutritious food, even if the extraction rate was as low as 70 per cent as in most white bread.

Significance of milling losses for health

Protein. In the sample of 72 per cent extraction for which the data is given in Table 17.3, protein provides about 13 per cent of the energy. This proportion in the whole diet is more than enough to meet the needs of growth and maintain N balance provided the quality of the protein is satisfactory. Weanling rats whose sole source of protein was 75 per cent extraction flour did not gain weight as fast as those fed whole wheat flour (Chick, 1942) but did so when lysine was added to their white flour (Hutchinson *et al.*, 1956). Lysine is the first limiting amino acid in wheat protein. However, in older rats, who grow more slowly, and also in children wheat protein contains sufficient lysine for growth provided the energy need is met, and

Table 17.3 Nutritive value of some unfortified wheat flours (values per 100g). (Paul and Southgate, 1978)

Percentage extraction	Energy MJ	Energy kcal	Protein (g)	Fat (g)	Dietary fibre (g)	Calcium (mg)	Total phosphorus (mg)	Phytate P (mg)
100	1.35	318	13.2	2.0	9.6	35	340	240
85	1.39	327	12.8	2.0	7.5	20	270	100
72	1.43	337	11.3	1.2	3.0	15	130	30
40	1.48	347	10.8	1.3	3.0	11	90	15

Table 17.4 Some micronutrients in whole wheat flour and in flours of different extraction rate (values per 100 g) (Paul and Southgate, 1978)

Percentage extraction	Thiamin (mg)	Riboflavin (mg)	Niacin (mg)	Pyridoxine (mg)	Total folate (μg)	Vitamin E (mg)	Iron (mg)	Zinc (mg)
100	0.46	0.08	5.6	0.50	57	1.0	4.0	3.0
85	0.30*	0.06	1.7*	0.30	51	trace	2.5	2.4
72	0.10*	0.03	0.7*	0.15	31	trace	1.5	0.9
40	0.10*	0.02	0.7*	0.10	10	trace	1.5	0.7

* Before fortification

there is no need for supplementation with lysine in ordinary circumstances. Contrary to much old-fashioned teaching bread is a good source of protein no matter what kind of flour it is made from.

Water-soluble vitamins. In low extraction flours large losses of these occur during milling, as Table 17.4 shows. When white bread made from 70 per cent extraction flour provides no more than 30 per cent of the dietary energy and the other foods are varied and of good quality, requirements of all the known vitamins in this group are likely to be met. This is the situation in prosperous industrial countries where primary dietary deficiencies due to lack of any known vitamin are uncommon. Yet the loss of the vitamins in milling increases the risk of deficiency in individuals whose diets are otherwise poor and lacking in these vitamins. For this reason white flours are often fortified with thiamin and nicotinic acid and sometimes with riboflavin. Thus in Britain without such fortification the average diets in households with low incomes would only just meet thiamin requirements. Hence there is a good reason for fortifying all low extraction flours with thiamin. Average intakes of other vitamins in this group are satisfactory without fortification. There is no evidence at present that losses of vitamins in milling cause a significant hazard to health in prosperous communities. Yet under exceptional circumstances they may be dangerous and outbreaks of beriberi have occurred in communities living mainly on white bread, e.g. in British troops beseiged in Kut, Mesopotamia, in 1915 (Hehir, 1922) and in isolated fishing communities in Newfoundland (Aykroyd, 1930).

Nearly all the vitamin E present in whole wheat is removed by milling but other dietary sources usually produce adequate amounts.

Dietary fibre Whole wheat flour contains three times as much dietary fibre as white flour (Table 17.3). It has been known since the time of Galen to have a mild laxative effect, which a few people find disagreeable. The fibre is chiefly in the form of arabinoxylans, which have a high capacity for absorbing water (McConnell et al., 1974). This increased faecal bulk decreases transit time and so prevents constipation. Wheat fibre, unlike some other forms of dietary fibre, does not lower plasma cholesterol (Kay and Truswell, 1977). In one small British study a high intake of wheat fibre appeared to be associated with a low incidence of coronary heart disease (Morris et al., 1977). Phytic acid is associated with fibre and by binding minerals, especially divalent cations, may make them unavailable. There are thus both advantages and disadvantages from a high intake of wheat fibre. The role of dietary fibre and its effects on health are now the subject of much discussion and research. Many nutritionists consider that moderate amounts of fibre are beneficial and wheat fibre has impressive effects on colonic function.

Minerals. Whole wheat flour contains amounts of calcium, iron and zinc which would be nutritionally valuable if they were absorbed, but this is greatly impeded by binding to dietary phytate. Low extraction flours have lost much of these minerals (Tables 17.3 and 17.4) but what remains may be better absorbed because of the loss of phytate. All wheat flours are thus an unreliable source of minerals. White flour is often fortified with iron preparations, but it is uncertain whether significant amounts of these are absorbed and no benefit to health has been demonstrated (Ministry of Health, 1968; Callender and Warner, 1968; Elwood et al., 1971). Calcium was added to flour in Britain in 1942 (p. 94), but after nearly 40 years there is no evidence that our bones are any stronger as a result of the addition. The impairment of zinc absorption by unleavened wholemeal bread is described in Chapter 11.

Selection of flour

In poor rural communities in which over 60 per cent of dietary energy comes from wheat flour, the extraction rate should be low to ensure an adequate supply of B vitamins. Such flour is usually made into unleavened bread.

Increasing prosperity always leads to a more varied diet and a decreasing consumption of cereals. A great variety of breads and flour products (cakes, pastries and biscuits or cookies) are made by bakers who have to suit their customers' choices and their purses. In exercising their craft skills bakers have to select their raw material from an enormous variety of flours whose baking qualities depend on the strain of wheat, its condition of growth and the extraction rate during milling. Plant geneticists and agronomists contribute greatly to the efficiency of production of wheat and much to the baking properties of its flour (Spicer,

1975) but relatively little to its nutritive value. The protein content of the wheat grain may be a little below 10 g/100 g or, in a few selected strains, as high as 20 g/100 g, but all wheats are satisfactory sources of protein. It is the millers who most affect the nutritive value of the final product.

Milling

In prehistoric times wheat was crushed and ground with a large stone in a stone quern. Drawings indicate that this was usually a woman's job in Egypt, where the first mention of millers was about 1500 BC (Darby *et al.*, 1976). Most of the flour consumed was whole meal but white flour, perhaps 80 per cent extraction, could be obtained by using sieves made from papyrus, rushes, flax or horsehair. To use white bread in a household was a sign of prestige amongst the wealthy in Athens and Rome. For some classical writers, e.g. Plato and Cato, wholemeal flour appeared to have an appeal as a symbol of the simple and good life of the countryside (McCance and Widdowson, 1956); this view has been held by some people throughout history and persists today. Throughout the Middle Ages in Europe wheat was ground between large stones frequently in watermills. The flour was mostly of high extraction but white flour could be produced and was used by the rich. Thus Chaucer's prioress ate white loaves, but the poor widow in The Nun's Tale could afford only brown.

In the eighteenth century new sources of power and new machinery began to improve milling techniques. The price of white flour fell, and by the beginning of the nineteenth century it was the accepted food of the poor in Europe and North America. Millstones were replaced by steel rollers in about 1870, when there were also great improvements in techniques for sieving and bolting flour.

At this time various chemicals began to be added as flour improvers and preservatives (p. 209). The former are needed to give flours good baking qualities. Since pure vitamins became commercially available in about 1940 some of these have been added as has iron, and in Britain, calcium.

The quality of flours is regulated by laws. In Britain there are the Bread and Flour Regulations. In drawing up these the Government is advised by the Food Standards Committee, whose report (1974) on *Bread and Flour* gives a full account of the considerations on which the law is based. There is a list of permitted additives and limits are set to the amounts allowed in flours. Low extraction flours must have nutrients added to bring the content of thiamin, nicotinic acid and iron up to 0.24, 1.60 and 1.65 mg/100 g respectively. Calcium in the form of *creta preparata* must be added (7 to 14 oz to 280 lb of flour). It is now recommended that the additions of nicotinic acid and calcium be discontinued, but the necessary legislation has not yet been passed.

In the United States most low extraction flours are enriched with thiamin, riboflavin, nicotinamide and iron up to 0.44, 0.26, 3.5 and 2.9 mg/100 g respectively.

Calcium and vitamin D may also be added. The law varies in different states and the additions are not usually compulsory but are needed to satisfy labelling regulations for enriched bread.

Millers have to produce the flour which their customers, whether they be commercial or home bakers, demand. Two other factors have influenced the production of white flour. First, because most of the fat in the whole grain is removed, white flour is much less likely than whole meal to go rancid and so is a better commercial product. Secondly, in the Middle Ages millers kept the bran as payment for the milling and sold it as cattle fodder. The amount of bran retained could not be controlled by the customer, and both of Chaucer's millers were rogues:

A theef he was for sothe of corn and mele,
And that a sly and usaunt for to stele.

The lower the extraction rate, the more the bran that the miller can sell. We would not presume to say to what extent, if any, these factors influence the commercial policy of millers today.

Baking

This is one of the most ancient of human crafts. Early in classical times there were large numbers of professional bakers in Rome, and in most cities bread-making has always been carried out by bakers; but it is also a domestic art and before modern means of transport were available much of the bread eaten by country folk was baked in the home. Nowadays in Great Britain there are only a few housewives—and an occasional man—who like to bake their own bread but the number may be increasing.

Wheaten flour has the property that, after being mixed with water and made into dough, it rises if gas is liberated in the dough either by natural yeast fermentation or from the addition of artificial baking powder. Other flours and even potatoes can be used to dilute wheaten flour. However, this is not a common practice, except when there is a lack of wheat.

Cultivated yeasts are generally used for the fermentation process. Young growing yeast is first mixed with sugar and a little flour. Fermentation soon begins and the yeast culture is then added to the dough and kneaded thoroughly. Fermentation is then allowed to proceed until the carbon dioxide has blown the dough up to one and a half times its original size. This may take from one to four hours, depending on the nature of the yeast culture added. The dough is then kneaded again, shaped into loaves and baked in ovens at about 230°C. The Chorleywood Bread Process, introduced in 1961, is a mechanical process which eliminates the need for the traditional and lengthy bulk fermentation of dough. High-speed mixers develop the dough in less than five minutes. As they have a high cost and high consumption of power, they can be used only by large bakeries. About 200 plants belonging to the major milling groups now produce about 70 per cent of British bread by this process. The nutritive value of the flour is not altered (Knight *et al.*, 1973).

Activated Dough Development is another process introduced in 1962 in the USA. In this the changes in the physical properties of the dough brought about by fermentation or mechanical mixing are achieved by chemical reducing agents. Of these the most used is L-cysteine, now a permitted additive in the United Kingdom. This confers some of the advantages of the Chorleywood process without the need for expensive equipment.

The protein complex gluten (a mixture of gliadin and glutelin) present only in wheat and rye gives the dough the viscid property which keeps it together and so lets it rise when distended by gas. Good bread has a firm, strong texture and the loaf stands up well. Flours made from hard wheats such as those grown in the USA and Canada have this property of 'strength' and make good bread. British wheat is 'weak' and not good for bread-making though ideal for biscuits or crackers.

Bread

Bread has the same nutritive properties as the flour from which it was baked, but the nutrients are diluted by the water added to make the dough. In the final product the water content should not be outside the range of 35 to 40 per cent. The energy content of breads lies within the range 0.9 to 1.05 MJ (215 to 250 kcal)/100 g and the content of other nutrients is correspondingly reduced from the figures given for flours in Tables 17.3 and 4.

The flour used in bread-making is nearly always solely wheat flour, but sometimes other cereal flours and soya bean flour may be added in small amounts. Bread made from mixtures of wheat and rye are well known. There are also many speciality breads which may contain milk and milk products. There are three main types of bread.

White bread. This is made from low extraction flours which may contain additives and additional nutrients as already described.

Brown bread. By law in Britain this has to contain crude fibre in amounts of not less than 0.6 g/100 g. It is usually made from a mixture of whole wheat and white flours with a minimum of about 50 per cent whole wheat, which corresponds to an extraction rate of 85 per cent. Caramel may be added for colouring.

Wholemeal bread. This has to be made from whole wheat flour. Bleaching and improving agents are not permitted, but preservatives are.

These three breads provide respectively about 90, 8 and 2 per cent of the market in Britain. Consumption of brown bread has been rising slowly and steadily for over 20 years. Consumption of wholemeal bread was falling but is now rising. These proportions reflect consumers' choices, but may be partly determined by availability. There are 8000

bakeries, but 200 large plants owned by national milling groups account for 70 per cent of bread production and their breads are delivered everywhere. Wholemeal bread is made mostly by small bakers and is less widely available, though shops selling a variety of wholemeal bread can be found easily in most towns.

There is no doubt that white bread is a good commercial product. It is the bread that is best suited for making sandwiches, which are now so commonly taken to work. Yet those of us who appreciate the taste of wholemeal and brown breads, as well as their additional nutritive properties, wonder why we are in such a small minority. To eat good wholemeal bread is one of the pleasures of living which many seem not to know about. The bigger millers appear to be content to manufacture a second-rate product and to make no attempt to promote their goods of quality.

High protein breads. Persons wishing to lose weight have to reduce their intake of carbohydrate, but still require protein. For such people bread with more than the normal amount of protein, 13.0 to 13.5 g/100 g of dry matter, may be useful. Such breads are made by adding protein to flour, and this protein may be wheat gluten, skimmed milk or soya flour. The law now permits the terms 'protein bread' and 'high protein bread' to apply to breads containing 16 and 22 per cent of protein respectively. Such breads have been described as 'starch reduced', but this may be misleading and it is recommended that this term should not be permissible.

As lysine is the limiting amino acid in wheat flour, the addition of this amino acid has been suggested. However, lysine is not the limiting amino acid in British diets, which usually provide sufficient lysine from other foods.

Biscuits. These are made from flours which are baked with very little water. Sometimes a small amount of baking powder is added. In the days of sailing ships, biscuits were consumed in large quantities at sea. In making modern fancy biscuits, sugar, fat, chocolate and flavouring agents may be added. Some biscuits such as Scottish shortbread contain up to 30 per cent fat. British wheats are very well suited for biscuit manufacture. Biscuits made in Edinburgh, Reading and other towns have acquired an international reputation for quality, and large quantities are exported. In the USA British biscuits are called 'crackers'.

Cakes and confectionery. These are made by baking wheaten flour with sugar and fat, to which eggs are sometimes added. Fruit and nuts may also be incorporated. Until sugar became regularly available and cheap, cakes were a luxury and, in the Middle Ages, were usually made only for feasts and festivals. Flour of high-extraction rate is not suitable for cake-making. Rich cakes may contain large amounts of fat and sugar and so are of high energy value.

Breakfast cereals. These only became popular in the twentieth century. Collins (1976) records the history of this development. They are prepared from a number of cereals, including wheat, maize and rice and are not usually eaten in large amounts, but people appreciate their palatability, their ready cooked state and the attractive packages. Their chief nutritive value is that they are always eaten with milk. Some products are fortified (voluntarily) with B vitamins and even iron. A comparative evaluation of the nutrients provided by breakfast cereals available in Britain was reported in *Which?* (1976). There are many children who do not like milk as a drink, but consume a good amount with their daily breakfast cereal.

Other products

Toast. Toast is made by applying dry heat to bread This drives off some of the moisture. There are also changes in the starch grain and a little caramel is formed, which gives the colour. As water is driven off, the content of nutrients—expressed as a proportion of weight—rises. Patients on accurately prescribed diets should weigh their bread before toasting.

Macaroni, spaghetti and vermicelli. These and other forms of Italian 'pasta' are made from a very hard variety of wheat (*Triticum durum*) which flourishes in the warm, dry Italian climate. Only the endosperm is used for making flour for 'pasta'; consequently it is not rich in the B group of vitamins. Their very high gluten content enables the characteristic mouldings to be made.

Thus far we have described European methods of preparing wheat. In Asia and North Africa wheat is often eaten as unleavened bread. The flour used is usually of high extraction, often milled in the home.

Chapattis. These are the common form in which wheat is eaten in India, Pakistan and Iran. They are made from wholemeal flour (atta). Coarse sieves remove some of the fibre and bran. This may amount to 5 to 7 per cent of the total weight so Indians usually eat 93 to 95 per cent extraction flour. One method of making a chapatti is as follows: the dough is first prepared by mixing the atta with water and kneading. Usually salt and a little oil are added. A portion of the dough is rolled on a wooden board until it is flat, thin and circular. It is then placed on a flat iron pan over an open fire and slowly cooked. When one side is done, the chapatti is turned over and the other side cooked. There are many minor variations in technique and chapatti-making is a subtle art. Those made by an expert are soft and tasty with the delicious flavour of whole wheat.

RICE

Rice is second to wheat in global importance as a staple food for man. It gives a higher yield per hectare but requires warm conditions. There are two cultivated species, *Oryza sativa*, Asian rice, is the major one; *O. glaberrima*, African rice, is grown in parts of West Africa. The earliest archaeological remains of rice from around 3000 BC

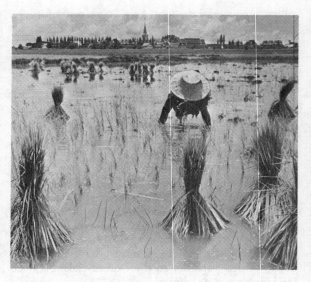

Fig. 17.2 Thailand. Replanting the rice (FAO photo by Eric Schwab.)

were found in China. Most rice is grown under semi-aquatic conditions in paddy fields, but there are varieties which grow on dry land. The International Rice Research Institute (IRRI), set up in 1962 in the Philippines, has bred high yielding, semidwarf varieties, starting with IR8. Two crops of rice a year of this and other varieties can be grown under favourable conditions. A picture of rice cultivation is shown in Fig. 17.2.

The rice grain has a botanical structure similar to the wheat grain. Hinton (1948) has made micro-dissections and gives analyses of the thiamin content of the components of individual grains (Table 17.5). Pericarp, aleurone and the scutellum together contain 79 per cent of the total thiamin present in the grain, although constituting only 6.2 per cent of the weight. By contrast the endosperm, which represents 92 per cent of the grain by weight, contains only 8.8 per cent of the thiamin.

Changes similar to those already described for wheat occur when rice is milled. These changes are important because rice so often forms such a large proportion of the total food of rice-eaters. The chemical properties of rice in relation to the nutritive value of rice diets are given in two monographs (Aykroyd *et al.*, 1940; FAO, 1954a).

From time immemorial a variety of methods have been used by men for husking 'paddy'—the rice grain in the husk. The domestic labour of preparing rice by hand-pounding is still undertaken in most parts of the East. The paddy is placed in a stone or wooden mortar, about 6 inches in diameter and 8 inches deep, and pounded with wooden pestles about 6 foot long. Usually two or more people pound together. The pounding breaks the outer husk and allows it to be separated by winnowing. Some of the germ and part of the pericarp is removed, the amount

Table 17.5 Thiamin content of fractions of the rice grain

Part of grain	Proportion of grain (per cent)	Thiamin content ($\mu g/g$)	Proportion of the total thiamin of the grain (per cent)
Pericarp and aleurone	5.95	31· ⎫	32.5
Covering to germ	0.20	12 ⎭	
Epiblast	0.27	78	3.9
Coleorhiza	0.20	94	3.5
Plumule	0.31	46	2.7
Radicle	0.17	62	2.0
Scutellum	1.25	189	43.9
Outer endosperm	18.80	1.3 ⎫	8.8
Inner endosperm	73.10	0.3 ⎭	

depending on the vigour and duration of the pounding. It is possible to produce a refined white rice almost totally devoid of vitamins by home-pounding. Yet home-pounded rice normally retains over half of the outer layers of the grain, thus conserving the greater part of the vitamins. It is essentially a high-extraction cereal grain and a satisfactory source of B vitamins. However, pounding is a wearisome domestic drudgery even if, as in many parts of Bengal and Thailand, a simple mechanical device enabling the mortar to be worked by the feet is used. It is therefore not surprising that mechanical rice mills have spread among the rice-eating people. The housewife is relieved of domestic labour, at no financial cost, since many mills are content to retain as their fee the bran removed, which is sold as cattle fodder. Mills can produce a highly refined rice, almost devoid of vitamins as·Table 17.6 shows.

Parboiling. There is, however, one process which is widely applied both in the home and the mill in the preparation of rice, which has a profound effect upon the content of the B group of vitamins in the final product. Parboiling is the steaming or boiling of unhusked rice after preliminary soaking. This splits the woody outer husk and renders its subsequent removal easier. Small quantities of paddy may be parboiled in domestic vessels before pounding. In the bigger mills it is steamed under pressure in large cylinders. The parboiling either drives the vitamin into the interior of the grain or may fix the scutellum so that it is less readily removed in the milling process (Hinton, 1948b). This fixes the vitamins so that they are not removed with the bran and remain behind in the milled grain. Figure 17.3 shows the effect of varying degrees of

Table 17.6 Thiamin content of rice at different stages of milling

	$\mu g/g$ of rice
Husked only	4.0
Once polished	1.8
Twice polished	1.0
Thrice polished (ready for market)	0.7

milling upon the two samples of the same paddy, one parboiled and one raw; even in very highly milled samples of parboiled rice the major portion of the thiamin is still present. Similar results are obtained for nicotinic acid.

This is important for in all parts of the world where rice forms the staple article of diet, beriberi has been liable to break out, except where it was the custom to parboil the rice. The parboiling of rice is the simplest preventive measure against beriberi. There is a manual on the technology of rice parboiling (Gariboldi, 1974). Probably one-fifth of the world's rice is parboiled.

In addition to milling, the rice grain is subject to another severe loss of vitamins in the washing and cooking of the cereal. Rice, purchased in the bazaar, must be washed in the home before cooking, which itself involves the use of water. Much of the water is often subsequently discarded. The B group of vitamins are all very soluble in water and heavy losses may thus result in the home. Experiments conducted under cooking conditions common in South India showed that half the thiamin and nicotinic acid that escaped the mills might be thrown away as domestic waste. Even higher losses may occur. Such losses can be reduced,

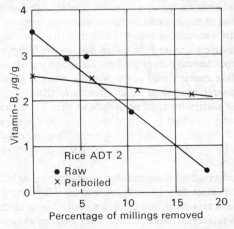

Fig. 17.3 The effect of milling in the raw and parboiled states on thiamin content of rice (Aykroyd *et al.*, 1940).

first by seeing that rice reaches the home as clean as possible; this requires clean and good storage conditions in shops and bazaars. Secondly, within the home a minimum of water should be used for cooking, and all surplus should not be discarded but taken as the drink known as 'congie'.

ENRICHMENT OF RICE

A field trial in the Philippines (Salcedo *et al.*, 1948) indicated that rice enriched with thiamin and other nutrients could prevent beriberi. An enrichment programme presents many technical difficulties, especially the problem of enforcement (FAO, 1954b), and has seldom been undertaken.

Protein content

Most samples of milled rice contain 6.5 to 8.0 g/100 g of protein, providing 7.0 to 8.5 per cent of the energy. This is less than in other cereals, but no other cereal protein is of such good quality. Lysine is the limiting amino acid. A variety has been bred with 14 g/100 g of protein which was well utilised in nitrogen balance experiments on man (Clark *et al.*, 1971)

MAIZE

Maize (*Zea mays*) is second to wheat in world food production. Most of this is used as feed for livestock but maize is the staple food of man in Central America and in many parts of Africa, South America and elsewhere. It is also used in the food industry in the manufacture of corn starch, glucose and some whiskies.

Maize originated in Central America and cobs have been found in archaeological material dated 5000 BC. It was the staple food of Mayan and Aztec civilisations but pellagra and protein-energy malnutrition, common in maize-eating communities in the nineteenth and twentieth centuries, did not arise. The reasons for this are fascinating and are discussed by Béhar (1969).

Columbus found maize growing in Cuba in 1492 and brought some to Europe where it quickly became established in Mediterranean countries and later in other parts of Africa and also in some places in Asia. The Pilgrim Fathers were given seeds of Indian corn by the Indians and corn was a central part of the first Thanksgiving dinner in 1621. Today nearly half of the world's maize is grown in the belt stretching from South Dakota to Ohio.

Maize differs from other cereals in that its numerous kernels are attached to a rigid stem and the entire ear is enclosed by the modified leaf sheath. This impedes the dispersal of grain and maize is dependent on man for its propagation.

Maize is in general much more resistant to drought than either wheat or rice. In addition it gives a high yield per acre and is relatively free from the predation of birds. It matures rapidly so that a good crop can be grown in a short season. For these reasons maize has acquired a well-deserved reputation as a poor man's cereal.

The maize grain has the same general structure as that of rice and wheat. The following preparations are used as human food.

Sweetcorn ('corn on the cob') is a type with short maturing season. It is eaten before the sugar in the endosperm has been converted to starch.

Whole maize grain. This is the whole grain which is removed from the cob after drying, usually in the sun.

Whole maize meal. Whole maize grain is ground to meal fineness either by hand-pounding or by modern techniques. The meal is not subjected to any 'bolting' and contains 97 to 100 per cent of the original grain.

Decorticated maize meal. This is the wholemeal with most of the pericarp, but none of the germ, removed by sieving or simple fanning. It usually contains 90 to 96 per cent of the original grain.

Degerminated maize meal. The wholemeal is passed through finer sieves, which remove most of the pericarp and germ. It usually contains about 85 per cent of the original grain.

Hominy or samp. This is the starchy portion of the endosperm, left after the whole grain has been softened by steaming, the pericarp removed and the germ loosened by a handling machine. In the USA hominy has acquired culinary prestige and its nutritive deficiencies are made up by other foods. In southern Africa where it may contribute a large part of the dietary energy among the poor, samp contributes to protein-energy malnutrition.

Maize may be boiled and made into a porridge. This is the usual method in Europe and Africa. Maize may also be made into flat bread. Maize itself will not make leavened bread, but it can be mixed with wheat flour and baked into good loaves.

The nutrient value of maize resembles that of other cereals in general, but differs in some important respects. Yellow maize contains a mixture of carotenoids some of which, β-carotene, cryptoxanthin and β-zeacarotene, have provitamin A activity. Values range from 100 to 800 μg/100 g (expressed as β-carotene) (Quackenbush *et al.*, 1961). The principal protein in maize is zein, which forms about half the total protein in the whole grain. Zein is an imperfect protein, lacking lysine and tryptophan. This defect is important in the relation of maize to pellagra (Chap. 34). Truswell and Brock (1962) measured the nutritive value of maize protein in human adults. The biological value is about 57—not so low as was once thought. A supplement for maize protein should contain both lysine and tryptophan and possibly isoleucine. Opaque-2 is a strain of maize, homozygous for a recessive gene, which is relatively rich in lysine and tryptophan. This quality of its protein allowed the nitrogen balance to be maintained in adult men, with no other significant source of protein in their diet (Clark *et al.*, 1967). The soft kernels of Opaque-2 maize limit its acceptability and yields were poor in the original strain. Cereal geneticists are now working to solve these problems (CIMMYT-Purdue. 1975).

The nicotinic acid present in maize is in a bound form and does not become available. For this and other reasons pellagra is associated with maize eating (see p. 289). In preparing Mexican *tortillas*, the grains are softened by heating in lime-water and then ground directly into a dough and cooked on a hot iron plate. The treatment with lime-water makes the nicotinic acid biologically available (Laguna and Carpenter, 1951), and the lime may provide an important contribution to calcium intake.

MILLETS

Millets are cereals very resistant to drought and so have been extensively cultivated in arid regions. They are the staple food of many people in Africa and also in some areas of Asia and Latin America. With the spread of irrigation and the introduction of drought-resistant varieties of wheat, millet cultivation is tending to decline, notably in India. Ripening millets need to be watched to protect them from birds. Millets have always been regarded as a poor man's food and there are social prejudices against their use. Although this is understandable (they are much less tasty than wheat or rice) it is unfortunate, for they have good nutritive value and their protein is a valuable addition to rice protein in predominantly rice diets.

There are a variety of different millets which have an even greater variety of names. Common millets are: (1) *Sorghum vulgare*, often known as the large millet, or sorghum. In India, where it is widely grown, it is known as *juar* in the north and *cholam* in the south. (2) *Eleusine coracana* is known as *finger millet* in Africa and as *ragi* in South India. (3) *Pennisetum typhoideum* is widely grown in India and known as *bajra* in the north and *cambu* in the south. There are a variety of names for it in use in Africa; it is often referred to in scientific literature simply as 'millet'. These are the three most important millets in Africa and Asia. In South America *quinoa* (*Chenopodium quinoa*) is a hardy millet which is widely grown in the cold arid countryside on the altiplano. Many other species of millets are grown locally.

Millets, like all other cereals, have to be husked. The grains may then be soaked and boiled and made into a porridge or ground into a meal. These processes are usually carried out in the home since millet-eaters are mostly simple peasants. Refined millet products have not yet appeared on any international market on an appreciable scale.

OATS

In Scotland oats became the staple food of the people in the seventeenth and eighteenth centuries, gradually replacing barley and rye. In the nineteenth century oats were in turn gradually replaced by wheat. Oatcakes and brose (uncooked oatmeal treated with water, milk or whisky) ceased to be common daily foods, while porridge survived chiefly as a breakfast dish. In the twentieth century oats have been largely ousted even from this limited position by the ubiquitous breakfast cereals; few Edinburgh people today eat porridge for breakfast.

In the milling of oats only the fibrous pericarp is usually removed and the germ is retained. Most forms of oatmeal are thus not highly refined. Oatmeal contains more protein (12 g/100 g) and more oil (8.5 g/100 g) than other common cereals. Frequently nowadays the grains are not ground, but crushed flat between rollers. Heat is applied during the process and the grains are thus partially cooked. The resulting 'rolled oats' are the basis of several convenient breakfast preparations.

The decline in the consumption of oatmeal is probably attributable in the main to a change in cooking habits. Porridge as traditionally cooked in Scotland is prepared the night before and left to warm on the hob of the kitchen fire overnight, or in the haybox. The introduction of gas and electric cookers has abolished this traditional practice, and although proprietary brands of rolled oats can be made into porridge in a few minutes before breakfast, a ready-cooked breakfast cereal or a loaf of wheaten bread is less trouble for the housewife working with one eye on the clock. Oatmeal is making a small come-back in the form of 'muesli' a nutritious breakfast dish of Swiss origin in which it is mixed with fruit and sometimes honey and taken with milk.

BARLEY

Barley is widely grown in almost all parts of the world. It was once much used as a human food. It produces the most satisfactory malt for brewers and is the basis of the best beers and much whisky in many countries. It is widely used as a cattle food.

RYE

Rye (*Secale cercele*) was once a common crop all over Europe and is still grown extensively in the north and east. The crops are resistant to cold. Many people like rye bread, which is tasty, rich in the B group of vitamins and also contains roughage.

TRITICALE

Triticale is a new cereal, the result of crossing two genera, *Triticum* (wheat) and *Secale* (rye). The aim is to combine the winter hardiness of rye with the properties of wheat that are commercially valuable. Some promising varieties are being developed by geneticists in Canada and Mexico.

18. Starchy Roots; Sugars and Syrups; Pulses, Nuts and Seeds; Vegetables; Fruits

STARCHY ROOTS

The potato is the most important food of this class in temperate climates. In the tropics cassava (also known as manioca, yuca and tapioca), the yams, the sweet potato and taro are all important foods. Sago, as it is very rich in starch, is usually classified with these foods, though in fact it is derived from the pith of a palm. Arrowroot and a large number of other roots are also eaten in small quantities in the tropics. Such roots all contain large quantities of starch and so are good sources of energy. For the most part they are poor in protein, minerals and vitamins.

Table 18.1 gives values for the principal nutrients in starchy roots. They are easily cultivated, often giving high yields even on poor soil, and so have been widely used by peasants in many parts of the world. The common garden root vegetables contain much less starch and are discussed on page 182 under Vegetables. Figure 18.1 shows a typical cassava plantation in the tropics and Fig. 18.2 a market.

COMMON POTATO (*Solanum tuberosum*)

This is a native of the New World. It flourished and continues to flourish on the *altiplano* in the Andes and was the staple food of the peasants under the Inca civilisation. It was introduced into Europe by the early explorers, at first as a curiosity. Cultivation spread rapidly throughout the European continent in the second half of the seventeenth century and in the eighteenth century. The intro-

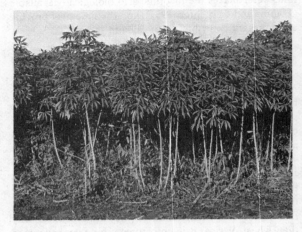

Fig. 18.1 Plantation of yuca (cassava or marioca).

duction of the potato was initially a great blessing since it provided the peasants with a cheap alternative crop to cereals. Until the eighteenth century the history of all European countries was marked by famines due to failure of the main cereal crops as a result of drought or disease. Potato cultivation provided a second crop which allowed a population to survive despite a failure of the cereal harvests. The last serious famines in Scotland were during the 'six dear years' of William III's reign at the end of the seventeenth century, prior to the extensive cultivation of

Table 18.1 Starchy roots (potato, sweet potato, yams, taro). Composition in terms of 100 g of the retail weight, as purchased

	Range	Selected value	Notes
Moisture, per cent	65–85	—	—
Energy { kJ	210–520	330	—
Energy { kcal	50–125	80	—
Carbohydrate, g	10–25	18	—
Protein, g	1.5–2.5	2.0	Tapioca and sago as sold in Europe, 0.3–0.4
Fat, g	Trace	0	—
Calcium, mg	10–30	20	—
Iron, mg	0.5–2.0	0.8	—
Carotene, μg	0	0	Sweet potato: most varieties 300; deep yellow and red up to 4500
Ascorbic acid, mg	5–25	15	—
Thiamin, mg	0.05–0.10	0.075	—
Ribofalvin, mg	0.03–0.08	0.05	—
Nicotinic acid, mg	0.5–1.5	1.0	—

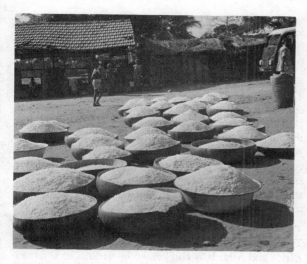

Fig. 18.2 Cassava market in French Togoland.

potatoes. In Ireland the potato flourished exceedingly well and completely ousted cereal crops. The peasants became entirely dependent on one food crop again, and they paid the inevitable penalty. The potatoes were attacked by the blight (*Phytophthora infestans*); the harvest failed for three years from 1845 to 1847 and the people suffered one of the most disastrous famines in history. The population fell from 8.2 million in 1841 to 6.6 million in 1851. Probably over one million died and many were forced to emigrate. Ireland has not yet recovered her former population and Boston, Glasgow and many other cities owe a large part of their present population to the direct effect of the potato blight.

The potato has two remarkable properties. First, it is the cheap food that can best support life when fed as the sole article of diet. Hinhede (1913) describes a man who lived on a diet of 2 to 4 kg of potatoes daily with a little margarine as the only other source of food for 300 days. Secondly, potatoes yield more energy per acre than any cereal crop. The importance of this fact to an eighteenth-century

peasant can be illustrated by some calculations from data collected by Young (1771) of yields on English farms (Table 18.2).

The first column gives Young's data in bushels, a measure of volume. The second column gives the weight of the crops and the third their approximate energy value. The last column gives the amount of land required to provide the total energy needs of a family of a man and wife with three young children (estimated at 42 MJ or 10 000 kcal/day). Thus the peasant needs less than half as much land to feed his family if he grows potatoes in place of cereals as his main crop. He also needs less land for his subsidiary crops to provide protective foods. These conditions are ideal for the landlord. Salaman (1948) in his classic book on the history of the potato has pointed out that in 'potato civilisations' the peasants have been at the mercy of their landlords. Probably at no time in history has man been reduced to more misery and abject poverty than the South American peasants under their Inca rulers and the Irish under their English landlords.

Potatoes contain 75 to 80 per cent of water and yield from 290 to 380 kJ (70 to 90 kcal)/100 g. Of the energy, 7.6 per cent comes from protein, a negligible amount from fat and most from starch. The protein content is low, about 2 g/100 g, but it has a high biological value, when fed to man (Kofrányi *et al.*, 1970). Potatoes are a useful source of protein, especially if large amounts are eaten, and of dietary fibre (Flynn *et al.*, 1977).

Potatoes contain small but not very important amounts of minerals and the B group of vitamins. They are a good source of potassium. Potatoes are not rich in ascorbic acid, but when they are eaten in large quantities they often provide a considerable proportion of the ascorbic acid in the diet. However, their ascorbic acid content is very variable; figures ranging from 4 to 50 mg/100 g are given in the literature. This wide variation is due, in part at least, to losses in storage. A figure of 30 or over is only found in freshly dug potatoes, whereas from March in the northern hemisphere until the new harvest values are usually below 10 mg. This seasonal variation can be important. In Edinburgh for instance, where patients with scurvy are occasionally seen, they appear usually in the spring and early summer. They are almost always old men living alone. The disease is seldom found after the new potatoes arrive in the shops; they probably serve to prevent scurvy throughout the autumn and winter.

The effect of cooking on the ascorbic acid content of potatoes is discussed in Chapter 22.

Potatoes are easily digested and well absorbed and are thus a good food for invalids. They are a valuable and useful food with an important place in the British diet. Their reputation for being fattening is undeserved. They do, of course, form fat if eaten in amounts sufficient to make the energy value of the diet greater than the daily energy expenditure. But so do all other foods. The energy

Table 18.2 Average yields from English farms in the eighteenth century

	Average annual yield per acre		Energy value of crop	Acres required to provide 42 MJ daily for a year
	Bushels*	kg	MJ	
Wheat	23	650	8900	1.7
Barley	32	820	11400	1.4
Oats	38	690	9300	1.6
Potatoes	427	10900	31900	0.5

* Young's figures for 1711. With modern agricultural techniques all yields per acre are higher, but the difference between potatoes and cereals still holds.

density of potatoes is 26 per cent that of beef steak, for example, and 10 per cent that of butter.

From consideration of epidemiological data Renwick (1972) put forward the hypothesis that the geographical and temporal distribution of the congenital abnormalities anencephaly and spina bifida might be explained by a teratogenic effect of eating potatoes affected with potato blight during early pregnancy. Even when first presented there were statistical details which did not fit the hypothesis, and subsequently some dozen reports from all over the world have each presented further evidence against the hypothesis.

CASSAVA (Manihot esculenta)

These shrubs, of which there are several species, are native to South America, but are now widely grown in tropical Africa and some parts of Asia. Cultivation is easy, new trees being propagated from stem cuttings. When they have grown to a height of 6 to 12 feet they are dug up and the tubers or thickened roots cooked.

Cassava is the principal food of many people in the tropics. The fresh root contains 50 to 75 per cent of water, less than 1 per cent of protein and the remainder mostly starch. Only about 3 per cent of the energy is derived from protein: this is less than half of the proportion of energy derived from protein in potatoes, yams and taro. This low-protein content places cassava in a different nutritional class from the other starchy roots. Kwashiorkor is common in all communities dependent on cassava. As an easily cultivated food providing energy it is a valuable crop for many people; but it should only be cultivated along with other crops which can provide additional protein.

The leaves and outer parts of the roots contain a glyceride, linamarin, from which hydrogen cyanide is released by enzymic action. This is removed by grating the roots and then drying them in the sun. There is in West Africa a close association between the consumption of cassava and the prevalence of neuropathies (p. 300) and the patients often have a raised plasma concentration of thiocyanate, to which cyanide is converted by a detoxicating mechanism (Osuntokun et al., 1969). It is likely that the consumption of cassava contributes to the aetiology of these neuropathies through its cyanide. However, this can only be a subsidiary factor since they also occur in patients who have never eaten cassava. Cassava also appears to contain a goitrogen.

Tapioca as sold in western countries is a preparation of cassava from which most of the protein is removed: in fact it is almost pure starch.

YAMS

The two most important cultivated varieties are the greater yam (Dioscorea alata) and the lesser yam (D. esculenta). Both are climbing tropical plants. The tubers take 4 to 12 months to develop. Those of the larger species are big and may be as large as a football. The lesser yam has clusters of smaller tubers. Several wild yams may also serve as a source of food.

Like potatoes, yam tubers are rich in starch, but also contain significant amounts of protein.

SWEET POTATO (Ipomoea batatas)

This herbaceous plant with starchy tubers is extensively cultivated in the southern states of the USA and other hot climates. The crop is propagated from stem cuttings, and the tubers weigh up to 0.5 kg each. They have the same general properties as the potato and when fresh may contain up to 30 mg/100 g of ascorbic acid. Many varieties are coloured yellow or red. The pigments are carotenoids and anthocyanins and the sweet potato can be a useful source of vitamin A activity in the diet.

TARO (Colocasia esculenta)

This is widely grown in the Pacific Islands and in parts of Africa and Asia. It is also known by various local names such as dasheen, eddo, keladi and cocoyam. The Colocasia plant is a herbaceous perennial with tubers 15 to 30 cm long, which are used for propagation. They have the same general nutritive properties as yams and potatoes. The young leaves and stalks are also eaten as fresh vegetables.

SAGO

This is obtained from the pith of the sago palm (Metroxylon sagu) which is widely grown in Malaya, Indonesia and other parts of the Far East. The tree has to be felled and split before the starch is washed out. The commercial preparations ('pearl sago') are almost devoid of protein.

INVALID FOODS

Sago, tapioca, arrowroot and ground rice have each some reputation as 'invalid foods'. The commercial preparations on sale in temperate countries are almost pure starch. Provided it is realised that these foods are almost devoid of proteins, minerals and vitamins, they are useful as easily assimilated sources of energy. Taken with a suitable source of protein, as in milk puddings, they are valuable foods for the sick and also for young growing children.

SUGARS AND SYRUPS

Sugar consumption in the UK was 35 g/head daily in 1855 and rose steadily, interrupted only by rationing in the two world wars, to 138 g/head daily in 1958. Since then it has fallen slightly and the figure for 1971 was 123 g (Fig. 18.3). Thus although sugar was cheap, consumption rose with increasing affluence, but there appears to be a maximum which has now been reached in some countries.

During the Middle Ages cane sugar was part of the spice trade that came from the East to Venice and so into Europe. In the thirteenth and fourteenth centuries the price of sugar lay between one to two shillings a pound—more than a week's wages for a servant. It was much in

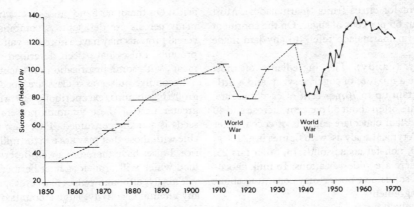

Fig. 18.3 Total amount of refined sugar available for daily consumption in the UK (g/head) (Department of Health and Social Security, 1974*a*). From 1971 to 1976 the figure has varied from 111 to 125g and has been related to difficulties in the supply.

demand by apothecaries for making their confections. The supply increased with the development of the sugar colonies—the West Indies and the Atlantic Islands. The cultivation of sugar was closely associated with the growth of slavery. The history of both is well told by Aykroyd (1967) in a book entitled *Sweet Malefactor*, which can be recommended to anyone interested in the background of West Indians.

In the middle of the seventeenth century the presence of cane sugar in beetroot was discovered by the German chemist Nargraf, and during the Napoleonic Wars much sugar beet was planted in France with a view to achieving independence from outside sources. During the nineteenth century sugar beet cultivation was greatly extended in Germany and France and more recently in Great Britain. There was also a great increase in imports of sugar from cane grown in the colonies.

Sugar is readily preserved and so is very suitable as an article of trade. This, together with its cheapness and its usefulness as a flavouring agent, made it popular with the new industrial urban populations. As a cheap and easily digested form of energy, sugar is a valuable food; but as it lacks every nutrient save carbohydrate, its very attractiveness is a danger in that it tends to displace other more nutritious foods from the diet. With the increase in sugar consumption there has been an increase in the incidence of dental disease.

Chemists have devoted much technical ingenuity to removing the last traces of 'impurities' from commercial sucrose, even employing animal charcoal as a clearing agent to precipitate the minute amounts of coloured matter that are naturally associated with it. Crystalline table sugar is thus one of the purest chemicals regularly produced in large quantities by modern industry. It is practically 100 per cent sucrose and contains no other nutrients, such as minerals or vitamins. 'Brown sugar' is less highly refined sucrose containing traces of other sugars and minerals, and

colouring matter; perhaps for this reason it has a better flavour and is esteemed for use in coffee. Public demand for brown sugar has sometimes tempted the manufacturers to produce a spurious imitation of it by simply adding a synthetic brown dye. The raw sugar cane that is chewed in considerable quantities—especially by children—in the sugar-growing areas of the tropics contains only traces of protein, vitamins and minerals.

Syrups are highly concentrated solutions in which the sugar is unable to crystallise out owing to the presence of small quantities of other substances. They include molasses, treacles and golden syrup which are by-products of the manufacture of crystalline cane sugar. These contain 20 to 30 per cent of water in addition to sugar. They may also contain nutritionally significant amounts of calcium and iron, some of which probably comes from the vessels in which they have been processed. Molasses are popular remedies for the treatment of several diseases; there is no scientific support for their use.

Various natural syrups exist of which perhaps the most famous is the maple syrup obtained from the sap of the maple in Canada and New England. It contains about 20 per cent of water and the remainder carbohydrate.

Honey is a pleasant attractive food. At many times and places it has acquired a special reputation either as a medicine or as a nutritious food. Unfortunately this reputation is undeserved. Most honeys consist of about 20 per cent water and about 75 per cent of sugars, mostly fructose and glucose, with only traces of other nutrients. However, despite these dismal chemical analyses, honey and maple syrup continue to be appreciated by all who enjoy pleasant and attractive food.

Jams are made by boiling either fresh fruit or a pulp preserved with SO_2 (sulphited pulp) with sugar. Pectin may or may not be added, dependent on the amount present in the raw material. The minimum fruit content in Britain varies from 30 to 40 per cent for different fruits, but is only 20 per cent for citrus fruits (marmalades). Most jams contain about 65 per cent of sugar. On the continent of Europe the term marmalade refers to any jam made from a fruit purée.

Confectionery (candy). The ingredients of most toffees (candy) are a mixture of sugar, a syrup and a little fat; they may contain up to 70 per cent of carbohydrate. Boiled 'sweeties' are often about 50 per cent sucrose and 40 per cent glucose. Plain chocolate consists of cocoa, other fats and sucrose. A typical analysis, with figures in g/100 g, is cocoa butter 20, non-fat cocoa solids 15, other fats 25, sucrose 40, but there are wide variations. In milk chocolate, non-fat milk solids and butter may constitute about one-fifth of the ingredients.

PULSES, NUTS AND SEEDS

Pulses or legumes are the seeds of the *Fabaceae* or *Leguminosae* family—peas, beans and lentils. The English word *pulse* is taken from the Latin *puls*, meaning pottage or thick pap. The family is large and different species are capable of surviving in very different climates and soils. They are cultivated in almost all civilised parts of the world, so there are very few people to whose diet pulses do not make some regular contribution.

In the East, pulses make a much more important contribution to the diet of all classes of society than in the West. So it is proper to consider the role of pulses in Eastern diets first.

PULSES IN EASTERN DIETS
The nutritive properties of pulses resemble in many respects those of the whole cereal grains; but there are important differences, which enable pulses to be a valuable supplementary food to cereals and especially to rice.

First, all pulses have a higher protein content than cereals. Most contain about 20 g of protein/100 g dry weight. The biological value of pulse protein is not high owing to their low content of sulphur-containing amino acids. On the other hand pulses are rich in lysine in which many cereals are deficient. A combination of pulse and cereal proteins may have a nutritive value as good as animal proteins. Pulses have been described as 'the poor man's meat', with some justification on chemical grounds.

Secondly, pulses as a class are good sources of the B group of vitamins (except riboflavin). More important, the greater part of these vitamins present in the harvested seeds is actually consumed. There are no losses comparable with those that may arise in the milling and cooking of rice. Pulses have therefore a well-deserved reputation as a food which will protect against beriberi.

Thirdly, although pulses like cereal grains are devoid of any vitamin C activity, large amounts of ascorbic acid are formed on germination; sprouted pulses are an excellent preventive against scurvy (p. 298).

Hospitals dietitians in Asia and Africa find sprouted pulses a useful item for their menus, especially when fresh vegetables and fruits are scarce and expensive. The sophisticated may find them useful at cocktail parties—for guests like them; they are cheap, and supplement the nutritive value of the other refreshment.

Soya bean *(Glycine max)*
The soya bean has been eaten in China for several thousand years. The whole dry grain contains about 40 per cent of protein (twice as much as in most other pulses) and also up to 20 per cent of fat. Soya forms the basis of a great variety of the sauces and pastes with which Chinese cooks garnish their food. To the Chinese peasant subsisting on rice, the extra protein and fat, and incidentally B vitamins, provided by even a small amount of soya, can be of immense value in maintaining his physiological activities. For the Chinese gourmet, soya is one of the raw materials out of which the cooks create their delicious works of art.

No other people have acquired the Chinese taste for soya, but the bean has become an important raw material for the international food industry. Production in the USA rose between 1935 and 1973 from 2 to 45 million tons per year. Soya bean oil is a major raw material of modern

Table 18.3 Pulses (peas, beans and lentils). Nutrient in 100 g of dry weight

	Range	Selected value	Notes
Moisture, per cent	8–15	—	—
Energy { kJ	1340–1460	1400	—
{ kcal	320–350	340	—
Carbohydrate, g	55–65	60	Soya bean, 20
Protein, g	17–25	20	Soya bean, 38
Fat, g	1–5	4	Soya bean, 18
Calcium, mg	100–200	150	—
Iron, mg	2–8	6	—
Carotene, μg	12–120	60	—
Ascorbic acid, mg	0	0	When sprouted, 10–15
Thiamin, mg	0.2–0.6	0.4	—
Riboflavin, mg	0.1–0.3	0.2	Soya bean, 0.75
Nicotinic acid, mg	1.5–3.0	2.0	—

margarine. Soya bean cake is used in animal husbandry as a good source of protein, and is fed to cattle, pigs and poultry. Soya flour is being increasingly used in human foods. The lists of ingredients on the packs in a supermarket show that it is present in many sausages, biscuits, breakfast foods and other cereal products and in made-up dishes. Human consumption of soya protein is increasing with the development of textured vegetable proteins and other artifical meat (p. 191). Soya protein is an important constituent in some infant foods and milk substitutes.

Lentils

Lentils are the seeds of *Lens esculenta* of which many varieties are known. The plants are small, about 25 to 50 cm high, with small leaves and pale blue flowers. The plant originated in the Mediterranean countries and has been an important crop there for a long time. Esau sold his birthright to his brother Jacob 'for bread and pottage of lentils' (Genesis xxv, 34). Latterly lentils were introduced into India and large areas planted, especially in Bengal. There are several varieties: the Indian and Egyptian kinds are orange-red in colour and these are the lentils most commonly imported into Europe. A green variety also exists. Lentils may be made into soups or ground into a flour.

Dhals

In India, besides the lentils several other pulses (or dhals) are widely cultivated. The best known are Bengal gram (*Cicer arietinum*), black gram (*Vigna mungo*), green gram (*V. radiatus*) and red gram or pigeon pea (*Cajanus cajan*). A pulse, khesari dhal (*Lathyrus sativus*), was once sown widely in Central India. Its special value was that it was very resistant to drought. Even if the main cereal crop failed in a dry season, some khesari could be harvested. However, it was found that if large amounts of khesari dhal were eaten, paralysis of the lower limbs commonly followed. This condition, lathyrism, is discussed on page 301.

Groundnuts (*Arachis hypogaea*)

Also known as peanuts and monkey nuts, groundnuts are in fact the seeds of a leguminous plant. They are therefore properly pulses and not nuts. The plants originated in Brazil, but are now grown widely all over the tropics. After flowering, the ends of the flower stalk bend down and the young pods are forced into the ground by the direction of growth. They ripen underground and have to be dug up at harvest.

Groundnuts resemble other pulses in general nutritive value, except that they are rich in fat. The whole seed contains about 40 per cent of fat, twice the amount in soya beans.

As most children know, peanuts are good to eat, but few would care to eat a lot of them. The cultivation of groundnuts is seldom intended as a primary source of human food. The chief product is the oil, which can be used either as cooking oil or for making margarine and soap. The secondary product is the residue or cake left after the expression of the oil. Groundnut cake is excellent cattle food. It is also in theory an excellent protein-rich food for man. However, it is difficult to overcome the unpleasant taste. Experience has shown that as a diluent of flours from millets, wheat or other sources up to 10 per cent can be well tolerated; in higher proportions the mixture becomes nauseating and unpalatable.

Other pulses

The Lima bean (*Phaseolus lunatus*), a native of Peru, the cow pea (*Vigna unguiculata*) and the locust bean are other pulses which are widely grown in many parts of the tropics and in subtropical areas.

This list gives only a small selection of a large number of different pulses cultivated in various parts of the world. They all give remarkably similar chemical analyses and have the same general nutritive properties.

Physicians, nutritionists and dietitians should strongly recommend the increased cultivation of pulses in tropical areas and especially if there is evidence of protein deficiency or beriberi. The choice of which pulse to grow can be left to the tastes of the inhabitants and the judgment of agriculturalists.

PULSES IN WESTERN DIETS

Pulses are less important in the diets of people in North America and Western Europe than in the East and other tropical areas. This is because the greater variety of foods consumed much reduces the risk of protein deficiency or lack of vitamins of the B group. For most people, peas or beans are pleasant foods which can be enjoyed.

The popular garden pea (*Pisum sativum*) is best eaten picked fresh from one's own garden. It is now cultivated extensively on a large scale and mostly by mechanical means. Peas have become much more freely available at all times of the year as a result of canning or freezing. The best canned or frozen peas are now as good nutritionally as fresh peas from a garden and taste nearly as good.

The common garden bean is the kidney bean (*Phaseolus vulgaris*) or French bean. In France it is known as the haricot, and in North America as the green or snap bean. It is a native of Central America and so can be added to the list of foods acquired by the Old World from the New. There are many varieties. In Britain the beans are sometimes picked when still very immature, and the whole pod sliced and eaten (the *haricot vert* of the French). The popular scarlet runner bean (*Phaseolus coccineus*) which also originates from tropical America is always eaten sliced in the green pod. Other varieties are grown in which the beans are allowed to mature. They may then be dried. Haricot beans, navy beans and pea beans are names for different varieties. In recent years there has been a great increase in the canning of kidney beans; the tin (can) of baked beans has become a common article of diet. The broad bean (*Vicia faba*) has been cultivated in Europe for at least 2000 years and is probably a native of Asia.

DIGESTIBILITY OF PULSES

Pulses have a reputation for being indigestible. This was acquired at the time of Galen or even earlier. It is only partially deserved. In health, the digestion of pulses and the absorption of their principal nutrients is practically complete and about as effective as is the assimilation of cereals. However, even in minor gastrointestinal disorders their digestion may be incomplete. Flatulence may be assessed objectively by measuring flatus volume or breath hydrogen. It appears to be largely due to stachyose and verbascose (p. 28) and is more marked with *Phaseolus vulgaris* than with other legumes (Murphy, 1975).

TOXINS

Some pulses may sometimes contain toxic substances. The effects of those associated with the lathyrus pea are described on page 221, with groundnuts contaminated by a fungus on page 224 and favism from broad beans on page 430.

A monograph by Aykroyd and Doughty (1964) entitled *Legumes in Human Nutrition* gives an account of their history, lists the species grown as food for man and discusses their nutritive value.

NUTS

We know of no record of any people who regularly consumed large quantities of nuts, except for some bushmen in Botswana. In Great Britain during the last war it was possible to register as a vegetarian, surrender one's meat ration and receive in return up to 2 lb of nuts weekly. In 1941 there were only 16000 registered vegetarians, but the numbers rose to 70000 by 1947.

However, nuts are an occasional small luxury which everyone enjoys. As the different popular nuts grow in many parts of the world there is a small but flourishing international trade. Most of the imported nuts go direct to the manufacturers of confectionery and biscuits and to bakers.

Most nuts have a high content of fat and protein, but as they are eaten in such small amounts their nutritive value is generally insignificant, compared with their flavouring properties. A variety of different kinds of nuts are described in the Glossary.

Coconuts (*Cocos nucifera*)

This palm contributes to human needs in many ways. As its fruit is not botanically a nut but rather a stone-fruit or loupe, coconuts are a little out of place here. Coconut palms grow on low-lying land often near the sea, and their graceful leaves and the curves of their trunk give great

charm to many tropical landscapes. To the hot and thirsty traveller there is no more refreshing drink than the water inside a green coconut and it is also hygienic. However, coconut water is of little nutritive value; it is a minor luxury of the tropics and available to any small boy who can climb a palm unseen by the owner. The white flesh inside the nut, when dried, is known as 'copra'. It has a high content of oil, and coconut oil is the most valued product of the palm. It is widely used as a cooking oil in the tropics and is exported for soap making. The residual cake after the oil has been extracted is known as 'poonac' and is used as a cattle food. Copra itself is a good food and can be eaten either dried or fried. It is rich in fat (over 30 per cent). Dried coconut is imported into temperate countries and used by confectioners and cake makers, who value its flavour.

The fresh sap of the palm (sweet toddy) is a pleasant drink but it contains few nutrients. Sweet toddy is readily fermented by yeasts and this product has been the chief alcoholic drink in many parts of the tropics.

SEEDS

Many other miscellaneous seeds play a small part in various diets. On the music-hall stage no Russian peasant is complete unless he is chewing **sunflower seeds.** These have a composition similar to groundnuts and are cultivated widely in Russia and elsewhere as a source of oil. Chewing the seeds of these and similar plants no doubt provides an additional small source of nutrients to many peasants.

VEGETABLES

There are hundreds of 'common vegetables' eaten in different parts of the world. Everyone knows what 'vegetables' are and yet they defy exact classification or description. Some vegetables, like spinach, cabbage and lettuce are leaves; others—onions, turnips and radishes—are roots; egg-plants (brinjals or aubergines), gourds and marrows are fruits; celery is a stalk and cauliflower and globe artichokes are flowers. Clearly there is no biological structure common to 'vegetables' and largely determining their chemical composition, as in the case of cereal grains.

Nevertheless, despite the great variety of botanical structure, vegetables all possess the same general nutritive properties.

SOCIAL FACTORS

Before discussing the nutritive properties of vegetables it is proper to state that man should eat vegetables because he likes them; vegetables may also be good for him, as nutrition education posters proclaim, but this should be a secondary consideration. In the Middle Ages few people ate vegetables regularly. Only the religious houses kept vegetable gardens and these were very poorly stocked. An

Table 18.4 Vegetables: (a) Green, leafy (cabbage, brussels sprouts, lettuce, spinach, parsley, amaranth, coriander, fenugreek, neem, etc.) Composition in terms of 100 g of the retail weight, as purchased

	Range	Selected value	Notes
Moisture, per cent	75–80	—	—
Energy { kJ	40–200	80	—
Energy { kcal	10–50	20	—
Carbohydrate, g	1–12	3	—
Protein, g	1–4	2	—
Fat, g	Trace	0	—
Calcium, mg	25–500	100	In temperate zones, 75
			In tropical zones, 250
Iron, mg	1–25	5	—
Carotene, μg	600–6000	1800	In the higher range in the tropics
Ascorbic acid, mg	10–200	50	In temperate zones, 30
			In tropical zones, 180
Thiamin, mg	0.03–0.08	0.05	—
Riboflavin, mg	0.03–0.25	0.08	Kale and spinach up to 0.5
Nicotinic acid, mg	0.2–1.0	0.5	—
Folic acid, μg	20–100	50	—

interest in gardening arose at the time of the Reformation in Europe. It had spread to England in the seventeenth century and to Scotland in the eighteenth. Many new vegetables were introduced, not a few coming from the New World. Both landowners and merchants began to take pride in their vegetable gardens and the produce greatly improved the quality of the table which they kept. The poor followed their example. It was soon demonstrated that a small well cared for cottage garden could provide a varied supply of vegetables for a family. English cottage gardeners acquired a well deserved reputation for their skill as vegetable growers; any tourist in rural England today will see that this skill is still maintained. This is less true in Scotland.

With the industrial revolution many who moved from the country to the town were cut off from their supply of fresh vegetables. To meet the needs of the cities large commercial market gardens were started. These have been for the most part well run and they continue to produce a great number of excellent varieties of vegetables. Some delay in the passage of the vegetables from the market gardens to the greengrocers' shops in the cities is inevitable. This may be extended, sometimes to days, by a complicated trade with too many middlemen.

In industrial countries there is nowadays a satisfactory variety of canned and frozen vegetables. The keen gardener will claim that these do not taste quite so good as the produce he brings straight into his own kitchen. Nevertheless the quality and nutritional value are excellent. The food technologist has taken over from the housewife much of the drudgery of cleaning, preparing and even the cooking of vegetables. A regular supply of vegetables, either fresh, frozen or canned, should be an essential part of good living and good feeding. Vegetables add to the elegance and attractiveness of a meal. In many underdeveloped tropical countries the need for vegetables for health

reasons is particularly important. Modern methods both for growing and marketing require to be developed on a large scale. The picturesque vegetable market of small tropical towns cannot be adapted to meet the needs of big cities.

NUTRITIVE PROPERTIES OF VEGETABLES
These are shown in Tables 18.4 and 18.5.

The value of vegetables as a source of energy is very small. Most provide from 40 to 200 kJ (10–50 kcal)/100 g. To obtain 4.2 MJ (1000 kcal) it would be necessary to eat 2 to 3 kg of vegetables. The large bulk of vegetables helps to promote satiety and this, with their low-energy value, makes them useful in the prevention and treatment of obesity. Vegetables are also of little value as a source of proteins and essential amino acids. All vegetables contain dietary fibre. This increases the bulk of the faeces. In this way vegetables, by increasing the size of the stool, have a mild laxative effect.

Most vegetables contain amounts of calcium and iron that are probably physiologically significant. However, it is doubtful if the actual figures given for these minerals in food tables are of much value. The mineral content of different samples of the same vegetable may vary greatly. Oxalic acid in some leafy vegetables may interefere with calcium absorption. Workers at the Indian National Institute of Nutrition (1977) find the urinary calcium over 6 hours after eating amaranth (providing 450 mg calcium) did not increase; with the same amount of calcium in the form of milk urinary calcium increased by 33 mg.

Even though much of the iron present in vegetables may not be absorbed, the ascorbic acid which they also contain may aid its absorption (p. 130).

All vegetables contain small amounts of the B group of vitamins, but their contribution to the total intake is seldom great. Most leafy vegetables are fair sources of

Table 18.5 Vegetables: (b) Others (onions, turnips, cauliflower, leeks, egg plants, pumpkins, gourds, etc.). Composition in terms of 100 g of the retail weight, as purchased

	Range	Selected value
Moisture, per cent	70–90	—
Energy kJ	40–200	100
Energy kcal	10–50	25
Carbohydrate, g	2–10	5
Protein, g	0.5–2.5	1.5
Fat, g	0–0.4	0
Calcium, mg	20–100	65
Iron, mg	0.5–4.0	1.5
Carotene, μg	0–180	90
Ascorbic acid, mg	5–100	25
Thiamin, mg	0.05–0.20	0.07
Riboflavin, mg	0.01–0.20	0.05
Nicotinic acid, mg	0.1–1.0	0.5
Folic acid, μg	2–30	10

riboflavin. In the tropics a small supply of greens may reduce the incidence of angular stomatitis, often attributed to an insufficiency of riboflavin.

The chief nutritive value of vegetables is as a supply of β-carotene, ascorbic acid and folate. Cereals and pulses in general lack all these vitamins. So vegetables are able to make good deficiencies likely to arise on diets containing excessive amounts of cereals. It is in this way that vegetables balance a diet.

The β-carotene content of vegetables is very variable. The great majority have good vitamin A activity. There is a rough relation between colour and β-carotene content. All green leafy vegetables are rich and some, such as kale, very rich. Cucumber, cauliflower, some of the gourds and other pale vegetables may contain very little.

All vegetables contain valuable amounts of ascorbic acid, but the quantities are variable and losses in cooking and preparation may be great. However, a single helping of vegetables (3 oz: 90 g) daily, even if it has been badly treated by the cook, will usually provide at least 10 mg of ascorbic acid, an amount known to prevent scurvy. The losses of vitamins in cooking and preserving are discussed in more detail in Chapter 23.

In many tropical countries it is impossible to over-emphasise the improvement in health that is likely to arise from even a small increase in the vegetable supply. A poor woman with insufficient iron, vitamin A and ascorbic acid in her diet may find great improvement in her health as a result of taking one helping of good garden vegetables a day. In Africa and Asia there are few keen and competent gardeners; some are school-masters who set an excellent example to their pupils, but their numbers are few in relation to the need. A single enthusiast in a village or small town, by giving instruction and encouragement to his neighbours in the art of gardening, can carry out first-class

preventive medicine in his spare time. Oomen and Grubben (1977) have produced a beautifully illustrated book to encourage consumption of leafy vegetables in the tropics. Many grow wild and are not familiar to expatriate health educators.

Other types of 'vegetables' which may serve as food for man deserve brief mention.

Seaweed and marine algae have been used as a human food by the Chinese for many centuries and today seaweeds are eaten regularly in significant amounts by several Japanese communities. Carrageen 'moss' is a seaweed still eaten on the west coasts of Scotland, South Wales and Ireland. As already described (p. 29), agar and alginic acid are polysaccharides derived from seaweeds which are used by housewives and food technologists to alter the texture and consistency of foods, especially in making jellies.

The chief carbohydrates in seaweeds are mannitol and the polysaccharides alginic acid and laminarin. Seaweeds contain less than 1 per cent of fat, but appreciable amounts of protein, and a high content of minerals. An account of the nutritional properties of seaweed with a bibliography is given by Black (1953). There are several million tons of seaweed round the shores of the British islands that could be harvested. So far attempts to make a palatable food have met with little success.

FUNGI

Ramsbottom (1953) has given a good account of the use of mushrooms and toadstools as food. The British appear to be uniquely conservative in their fear of toadstools. Only certain species are poisonous, notably the Death Cap (*Amanita phalloides*) which has been responsible for nearly all the deaths. Many British toadstools are excellent eating. In other parts of the world a great variety of fungi are eaten. Fungi are for the most part delicious food and are eaten for their flavour. As they only contain up to 3 per cent protein, less than 1 per cent fat and about 2 per cent carbohydrate, their nutritive value is small. Mushrooms contain unusual amounts of trehalose (p. 28).

Fungi are valuable as one of the few luxury foods that are freely available to poor countrymen. With the increase in commercial cultivation they are also becoming available at cheaper prices in the cities. They are much appreciated by all who love good food and have good digestions.

FRUITS

Since the beginning of civilisation men of ingenuity who have had a little land to spare have used it to cultivate orchards and fruit gardens. In this art there has been a steady and progressive increase in skill and technical knowledge. The modern grower can provide fruit of great variety and excellent quality.

No other class of foods has such a variety of pleasant and attractive flavours. By delicacy of colouring, fruits attracts the eye as well as the palate. For thousands of years vintners have been preserving the best and most delicate flavours in wines and liqueurs. Housewives have been similarly engaged for about three hundred years in preserving and jam making. In the last hundred years they have been greatly assisted by food technologists. All these skills have contributed beyond measure to the pleasures of the table and the art of living.

The nutritive value of fruits is much less important. The only essential nutrient in which fruits are rich in ascorbic acid. Almost all fruits contain physiologically significant amounts of this vitamin and some are very rich. As fruits are often eaten raw, large intakes of the vitamin may be provided. Table 14.1 gives the ascorbic acid content of some fruits. How important fruit is in a national diet depends on one's opinion as to man's requirements of ascorbic acid.

Fruits, of course, like vegetables contain dietary fibre which is indigestible and so adds bulk to the stools; fruits are thus mild natural laxatives. For this reason a few people with sensitive colons can take fruit only in very small quantities; if larger amounts are taken diarrhoea follows. Prunes contain derivatives of hydroxyphenylisatin, which stimulates the smooth muscle of the colon. Pectin present in fruit assists in the formation of jellies and is of great value to jam-makers.

Most fruits contain small quantities of carotene and the B group of vitamins. The amounts present are not usually great enough to increase significantly the intake of these nutrients by people who are already living on a good mixed diet, but under certain circumstances they may be very valuable. In many parts of the tropics there is a sudden and obvious improvement in the health of the children coincident with the mango or jack-fruit season. Children may eat enormous quantities of these fruits which are rich in carotenoids with provitamin A activity.

Fruits contain little or no protein or fat. Most contain 5 to 20 per cent of carbohydrate. Ripe fruits contain no starch. Fructose and glucose are the chief sugars found. These two sugars are often present in equal proportions. Apples and pears contain much more fructose, while apricots and peaches contain sucrose.

Fruits contain a great variety of organic acids. These have already been referred to on page 89. They are responsible for the sourness of unripe fruit. During ripening the concentration of these acids falls and that of the sugars rises. As already described, the body readily disposes of these acids; most are easily oxidised, some excreted in the urine and a few are not absorbed from the gut. They do not give rise to acidosis.

Bananas are a fruit which requires special mention. They contain much larger amounts of carbohydrate than most fruits and so can act as a useful source of energy. There are about 50 varieties of bananas. They vary widely in composition, but may contain carbohydrate 20 g, protein 1 g, fat 0.2 g with an energy value of about 335 kJ (80 kcal)/100 g. In some parts of the tropics they may be the staple food of children and are often eaten together with large quantities of cassava. As a consequence the consumption of carbohydrate is high, while that of protein is low and kwashiorkor may occur.

The staple diet of many Africans is matoke (*Musa species*), a banana usually eaten green. This contains a high concentration of 5-hydroxytryptamine (5-HT), which has widespread actions on the circulatory and nervous systems. Crawford (1962) in East Africa and Foy and Parratt (1962) in West Africa have shown that matoke eaters may excrete 20-100 mg/day of 5-hydroxyindolyl acetic acid in their urine. 5-HIAA is derived from 5-HT by oxidation. It has been suggested that this might in part be responsible for endomyocardial fibrosis which is common in parts of Africa. However, there is little evidence to support such a view (Crawford et al., 1970).

In small quantities bananas are a pleasant and attractive

Table 18.6 Fruits fresh or canned* (apple, raspberry, orange, peach, mango, tomato, papaya, banana, etc.). Composition in terms of 100 g of retail weight as purchased

	Range	Selected value	Notes
Moisture per cent	75-90	—	—
Energy { kJ	80-300	200	—
Energy { kcal	20-80	50	—
Carbohydrate, g	2-20	10	—
Protein, g	0.2-2.0	0.5	—
Fat, g	0-1	0.5	Avocardo 20
Calcium, mg	5-40	20	—
Iron, mg	0.1-1.0	0.3	—
β-Carotene, μg	0-2000	240	Mango 600-1500 Tomato 600-1800 Orange 90-120
Ascorbic acid, mg	0-300	30	Very variable
Thiamin, mg	0-0.1	0.04	—
Riboflavin, mg	0-0.1	0.05	—
Nicotinic acid, mg	0.2-1.0	0.4	—

* Canned fruit often contains added sugar.

food and have acquired a well merited reputation in temperate climates. They are very easily digested. In ripe bananas 15 to 20 per cent of the pulp consists of sucrose, fructose or glucose and 1 to 2 per cent is starch (Palmer, 1971). It is important that bananas given to children be fully ripe. They can be digested by babies as early as the third month. Bananas contain no gluten hence their value in coeliac disease. They are also a food for convalescence.

19. Meat, Fish and Eggs; Novel Proteins

MEAT AND MEAT PRODUCTS

Meat was an important part of the hunter-gatherer's diet. Today the technically undeveloped agricuralists in many parts of the world have little or no meat to eat, along with the urban poor. By contrast annual consumption in the USA is about 200 lb/head; almost as much is eaten in several industrial countries and by a rich minority of people in other countries. Protein of animal origin is not essential for man as has been amply demonstrated by many vegetarians who have led full and active lives. Yet as soon as the income of a family or community rises, there is nearly always an increase in the amount of meat they consume. Although higher standards of living are often associated with better health, this is not necessarily attributable to a larger consumption of meat. Communities eating large amounts of meat and other animal products usually have high rates of coronary heart disease.

Much more land and energy is required for the production of meat than of grain. People concerned about food supplies for the poorest countries have joined with those anxious about atherosclerotic diseases in rich countries in calling for a reduction of high meat production.

MEAT PRODUCTION

The flesh of more than 100 species of animals is eaten by man. Production of beef and mutton is the responsibility of stockmen and butchers who over the generations have developed a *mystère* of what determines the quality of meat. To their traditional wisdom there is now added *meat science*. This is a growing subject and a systematic account of it is given in a short textbook by Lawrie (1974). Genetics and physiology are being applied to improve the live animal and biochemistry and electron microscopy to understand changes in the muscle tissues after slaughter.

We are now in the middle of a revolution in meat production and a significant proportion of our supply is no longer produced on a farm but in a factory. In western countries, this applies to nearly all of the poultry, much of the pork and a small but increasing proportion of beef cattle. Factory farming makes a more efficient use of animal foodstuffs and so appeals to economic man. There is, however, a natural concern that factory meat may be of poorer quality and of less nutritive value than farm meat.

So far there is little justification for such fears. Thus Harries *et al.* (1968) showed that there were no significant differences in the amounts of the important nutrients present in samples of 'barley beef' from stall-fed cattle and in beef from farm animals. The adipose tissue of lambs fed on large amounts of barley is noticeably softer than in lambs that grazed in the field. This is due to a larger proportion of odd-numbered and branched chain fatty acids, derived from increased generation of propionate in the rumen (Duncan *et al.*, 1974).

QUALITY OF MEAT

Meat is appreciated for its digestibility, tenderness and flavour.

Digestibility

The muscle proteins are more rapidly and easily digested than the connective tissue proteins, mostly collagen, and fat. As an animal ages there is relatively more connective and the meat of an old ewe is tougher than that of a young lamb. The collagen content varies with cut. Thus it may be as low as 2.5 per cent in a fillet of beef and as high as 23.6 per cent in skin meat (Bender and Zia, 1976).

Fat delays the emptying of the stomach and the proportion of fat in a helping of meat may vary from 8 to 50 per cent. Cuts of pork often contained large amounts of fat and this probably explains why pork acquired the reputation of being indigestible.

Tenderness

We like our meat to be tender and perceive its tenderness through three sensory components: first, the ease of initial penetration by the teeth; next, the ease with which the meat breaks into fragments; and, lastly, the amount of unchewable residue. The ultimate measurement must be semiquantitative rating of tenderness given by a reliable taste panel but several workers have devised tests to try and express this by physical laboratory methods. Tenderness varies with species, breed and age of the animal. Coarse muscle fibres are less tender and connective tissue, especially elastin, is associated with toughness. Marbled meat, with fat between the muscle fibres is usually more tender. After slaughter the proportions of these structures do not change but there can be large variations in tenderness, depending on how the meat is handled. Rigor mortis is the macroscopic expression of interdigitation of the actin and myosin filaments in the muscle fibres as the ATP is used up in anaerobic glycolysis. Conditions which retard or reduce the degree of muscle fibre shortening in rigor mortis give more tender meat. The tenderness of beef and venison improves if it is stored at temperatures just above freezing for 10 to 14 days, called 'conditioning'. Tenderness first decreases with the onset of rigor mortis and then slowly improves. The detailed biochemical explanation of this second phase is still being worked out. It appears to result from the local action of muscle proteases or cathepsins, with some weakening of the attachment of actin filaments and increased water-holding capacity of the non-fibrous, sarcoplasmic proteins.

Flavour

The flavour of meat is a complex sensation. Much of it is water-soluble due to substances such as inosinic acid, hypoxanthine derived from ATP, glycopeptides and amino acids such as glutamic acid. There is a gradual loss of flavour during storage, even frozen, due to evaporation of volatile substances. The flesh of full-grown male pigs contains traces of an unpleasant 'boar odour', which 92 per cent of women but only 56 per cent of men can smell. It has been identified chemically as 5, α-androst-16-ene-3-one. Substances in the animals' feed can sometimes give undesirable flavours in the meat and volatile taints can be absorbed during frozen storage.

NUTRITIVE PROPERTIES

The energy value of meat depends on its fat content, which as already stated varies greatly. For this reason, the use of food tables to calculate the energy content of diets containing much meat is subject to large errors. However, meat is a good source of energy as lean muscle contains about 20 per cent of protein and 5 per cent of fat.

The protein of meat is of high biological value, but this may be somewhat reduced when the proportion of connective tissue protein is high.

Meats are usually rich in iron and also in zinc, but contain little calcium. They are an important source of

nicotinic acid and riboflavin. Indeed in most British and American diets about half the total nicotinic acid and one-quarter of the total riboflavin come from meat. Meats also contain some thiamin; pork contains the most. There is very little vitamin A or ascorbic acid in muscle meats but they provide moderate amounts of vitamin B_{12}.

Meat would be more nutritious if the saturated fat content could be reduced (Munro, 1976) especially in beef and sheep which hydrogenate polyunsaturated fats in their rumens. Pig meat and chicken have a higher P:S ratio than beef and mutton. Some consumers are asking for meat with low amounts of fat both within and around the muscle bundles. By feeding encapsulated polyunsaturated oils a CSIRO team in Australia produced beef fat with 25 per cent linoleic acid. This can lower plasma cholesterol in man (Nestel et al., 1973) but has not been a commercial success.

Offal

This curious word—a corruption of off-fall—is defined by the Meat Inspection Regulations 1963 as 'any part of a dead animal removed from the carcase in the process of dressing it, but does not include the hide or skin'. Some offals, e.g. liver, kidney, heart and tongue, are foods of repute found on the menus of the best restaurants. Others, e.g. sweetbreads (pancreas and thymus), tripe (dressed stomach of ox or sheep), feet (pigs' and calves'), brains, chitterlings (pigs' intestines), maws (pigs' stomach), lambs' fries (testicles) and udders, are often regarded as local delicacies, but are more likely to be found in back street eating houses. Nevertheless all offal is of good nutritional value. Carnivorous animals in custody do not thrive on 'muscle meat' alone. Bone and offal contribute greatly to the nutritional value of their diet. Liver contains more vitamins and absorbable iron than muscle and so is a valuable food. At one time lightly cooked liver was the only means of saving the lives of patients with pernicious

Table 19.1 Meat and offal (composition in terms of 100 g of the retail weight, as purchased) based on Paul and Southgate, 1978

	Chicken	Beef (lean steak)	Lamb chop (inc. fat)	Liver	Notes
Moisture, per cent	74	67	49	67–70	
Energy { kJ	508	821	1558	567–748	
{ kcal	121	197	377	135–180	
Carbohydrate, g	0	0	0	0.6–2.2	
Protein, g	20	19	15	20	Duck 11
Fat, g	4*	14†	35	6.3–10.3	
Calcium, mg	14	6	7	7	Tongue and blood sausage 32–35
Iron, mg	0.7	2.3	1.2	7–21	Blood sausage 20; kidney 6; heart 4
Retinol equiv., µg	trace	trace	trace	9300–18 100	Kidney 100–150
Ascorbic acid, mg	0	0	0	10–23	Kidney 7–14; heart 6
Thiamin, mg	0.1	0.08	0.09	0.21–0.31	Pork 0.9; bacon 0.6
Riboflavin, mg	0.16	0.26	0.16	2.7–3.3	Kidney 2; heart 1
Nicotinic acid equiv., mg	11.6	8.2	7.1	14–19	Kidney 7–14

* Fat 18 g if skin eaten as well.
† More if visible fat included, e.g. beefburgers 20 g.

anaemia. Liver nowadays plays a very small part in hospital dietetics. Liver, kidneys and pancreas, being rich in cells, contain more nucleic acids than muscle. For this reason patients with gout have been advised to avoid them. Brain contains large amounts of lipids and especially phospholipids. In a pre-scientific age it acquired a spurious reputation as a food for the intellect.

Sausages

These have been used throughout historical times as a convenient form in which meat can be preserved and transported. Odysseus, waiting to revenge himself on the suitors, sat impatiently like 'a man before a great fire taking a sausage full of fat and blood, turning it this way and that and longing to have it roasted more speedily'. Cities like Oxford and Cambridge, Bologna and Hamburg have achieved fame from their sausages as well as from their universities. The basis of all sausages is a mixture of meat and bread and their quality depends on the proportion and quality of the meat. In Britain the best sausages contain pork and the cheaper varieties beef.

Germany has a great reputation for the variety of its sausages, many made from liver and offal. A variety of seasonings are used; chipolata sausages contain chives; saveloys, pigs' brains. With such varied recipes, any general statement of the nutritive value of sausages would be liable to a large error. In the absence of any precise knowledge of the composition, protein 12 g, fat 20 g, carbohydrate 12 g and energy 1.2 MJ (280 kcal)/100 g is a reasonable estimate.

Meat extractives, beef tea, soups, etc.

Meat extracts have been used for generations and some, like Liebig's extract are famous. Such extracts contain the freely water-soluble contents of muscle—potassium, phosphates, peptides, nucleotides, creatine, vitamin B_{12} and other vitamins. When reconstituted with hot water, 'beef teas' have a very low concentration of solids and do not supply significant amounts either of energy or protein, but they usually contain large amounts of sodium (Table 8.1). However, they stimulate appetite and hence may be useful in the feeding of convalescents.

'Slugs and snails and puppy-dogs' tails' or chacun a son goût

Those of us who have been brought up as members of one of the great religions of the world—particularly caste Hindus, but to a lesser extent all Mohammedans, Jews and Christians—seldom realise the extent to which our daily diet is artificially restricted. Religious taboos are partly responsible, but custom and tradition are much more important. There are many foods which would cause any 'civilised' man to revolt at the very thought of eating them; yet some of these foods are very palatable and many are nutritious. They can play an important part in the diet of

unsophisticated people. Nicol (1953) has recorded how the Isoko tribe in Nigeria may obtain up to 20 g of protein/head daily from mud-fish, monkeys, pangolin, porcupine, cane-rat, Gambian rat, snails, palm weevils and frogs. Without the addition of these luxuries to their diet, the Isoko would be very poorly off. Young boys show much ingenuity in hunting and trapping such animals.

Bristowe (1953) gives an interesting account of the insects that may be eaten in Vietnam and Thailand. Even wealthy and well-bred people consider the larvae of a coffee-boring moth (*Zeuzero coffeae*) delicious when roasted and eaten with rice and salt. Bristowe has made an impressive list of insects known to be appreciated by man. Properly cooked and served, locusts can be an attractive and nourishing food. Flying ants cooked in butter are considered to be a delicacy in certain parts of Africa.

Many South Americans rear guinea-pigs especially for the table, and they are reputed to be very tasty. Some Polynesians regard dog-flesh as a delicacy. These practices seem particularly distasteful to laboratory-trained nutritionists.

There are many records of the inhabitants of besieged cities in Europe eating cats, dogs and even rats with avidity. Man's range of foods is much wider than social conventions normally permit. Amongst primitive people these foods may contribute significantly to the total protein content of the diet and so improve health—particularly of small boys. A visiting nutritionist may well fail to be informed about these foods, unless special enquiries are made. Few of these foods have been analysed and little is known about their nutritive value.

It used to be thought that the inhabitants of certain parts of Africa would be better off nutritionally if the wild animals were exterminated and the grazing lands used for cattle, sheep and goats. This view is now being challenged. Pirie (1962) quotes figures showing that the yield of meat from game such as blesbok, eland, wildebeest and springbok, if properly protected and culled, is likely to be greater than that obtained from domestic animals grazed on the same land. He also discusses the possibility of hippopotamus farming in swamps. Talbot (1964) has provided a useful review of wild animals as a source of food.

FISH AND OTHER SEA FOODS

Fish are an important source of animal protein for some people. Lean fish contains less than 1 per cent of fat and about 10 per cent of protein with energy values ranging from 220 to 330 kJ (50 to 80 kcal)/100 g. The familiar lean fish on the British coast are cod, haddock, pollack, saithe, brill, ling, whiting, John Dory, sole, plaice and turbot. These fish have a reputation—for the most part well merited—as being a light and easily digested food, suitable for invalids. Fat fish contain 8 to 15 per cent of fish oil and so have a higher energy value than lean fish—330 to 660 kJ (80 to 160 kcal)/100 g. Fat fish eaten in Great Britain are herring (including the preserved forms, kippers and bloaters), pilchards, salmon, whitebait, eel, sardines and sprats. Intermediate species—usually with 2 to 7 per cent of fat—are hake, halibut, mackerel, mullet and trout.

Fish proteins have a high biological value similar to the proteins of land animals. Yet, although many fish are delicious, on the whole fish are less tasty than meat, and a fish diet tends to be monotonous. Good cooks have a great variety of sauces and garnishes by which they make fish more interesting and appetising. In the Middle Ages, housewives used the herb garden with skill to flavour the flesh of coarse fish such as carp, pike, perch, roach, dace and chub, which came out of the fishponds kept by the great manor houses. The monosyllabic names of these fish indicate that they were familiar to the earliest users of the English language. The art of cooking them is now all but lost. Too few anglers' wives have the skill to make these fish palatable.

The content of protein in fish is somewhat less than in meat and there is often a large waste in the scales and bones. This should be remembered in calculating the relative cost of proteins of different origin.

The only fish offal commonly eaten is the roe, both the hard roe and the soft roe or milts. Cod roe and herring roe contain 20 to 25 per cent of protein and are rich in nucleic acids. True caviare is the roe of the sturgeon; many imitations are produced by colouring other fish roes. This rich and tasty food contains about 30 per cent of protein and 20 per cent of fat.

Fish oils are rich sources of the fat-soluble vitamins A and D. Marine fish are the richest source of iodine in the diet and a good source of fluoride. Small fish—such as sprats and sardines—may be a useful source of calcium when eaten whole, together with the bones. In the great river deltas of the East, where there is extensive cultivation of rice (a cereal poor in calcium) and few or no dairy cattle, the general level of calcium intake is always low. This can be improved by proper use of the small fish which abound in the ditches, tributaries and irrigation canals that lead off from the big rivers.

Shellfish

Lobsters, crayfish, crabs, shrimps and other crustaceans have little fat and an energy value of about 200 kJ (50 kcal)/100 g. They are very tasty and have become an expensive 'prestige' food. As the demand for them is high, many natural breeding grounds are overfished and becoming exhausted. But the coarse, big muscle fibres of the larger species are not easily digested. Some people are sensitive to the proteins of these creatures and develop a variety of allergic reactions from eating them. Shellfish are not as rich in cholesterol as has been thought (Schulze and Truswell, 1977).

Oysters, mussels and other molluscs contain rather more protein (15 per cent) than most fish. They also contain about 5 per cent of the carbohydrate glycogen, but little fat. Oysters have acquired a reputation as an expensive luxury food, whereas the other molluscs are often regarded as poor man's fare; all can be attractive and useful foods. Oysters are the richest food source of zinc (containing up to 100 mg/100 g).

These shellfish live on seashores and are sometimes gathered near the output of urban sewage. Unfortunately they may harbour bacteria, particularly those of the Salmonella group. Proper supervision is necessary both of sewage disposal and the collection of shellfish, to prevent the danger of infection. Though shellfish such as mussels and winkles are safe if properly cooked, it is well to be sure that those eaten raw—such as oysters—come from a pure source. Mussels occasionally cause neurotoxic poisoning (p. 221).

Fish-meal and fish-flour

These two products of the fishing industry are used as feeds for dairy animals and poultry and so add to the world's supply of protein-rich foods. But they can be used with greater nutritional efficiency directly as food for man. They can be incorporated in stews and staple starches or scattered on cooked foods such as porridge. Prepared from small whole fish, they have excellent nutrient content. Objections have been raised on grounds of hygiene (the alimentary contents), flavour, keeping quality and simple fastidiousness. All of these objections can and should be overcome. Care must be taken that the processes for preparing fish-flour from fish-meal do not destroy any amino acids in the crude fish-meal.

An increase in the consumption of sea food requires improved methods of conservation. Many offshore waters—notably the North Sea and the waters around Iceland and the Faeroes—have been overfished. Very rich fishing grounds are available in deeper and less accessible waters, though in many parts of the world such as Africa, South America and South-east Asia the traditional methods of fishing—the nets and the boats—are ill-adapted for exploiting these fields. Recently modern methods of fishing with motor trawlers and drifters have been greatly extended in tropical seas. Previously unfamiliar species of deeper water fish will be exploited. They can be made acceptable by turning their unattractive shapes into fish fingers.

We are becoming aware that the living resources of the sea are not unlimited. The prospects of greatly increasing the world's catch of marine fish, some 60 million tons a year, do not seem very bright at present. Several species are threatened by overfishing. The catch of whales gets less each year and the Peruvian anchovy (Engraulis ringens) which had reached 20 per cent of the total world catch by

1970 completely failed in 1972, with disastrous effects on the price of fish-meal for animal feedstuffs. Landings of herring from British coastal waters have been falling steadily since 1963. Too many ships from several different countries have been fishing in the North Sea. It is hoped that new international agreements on the extent of fishing rights off the shores of maritime countries will allow better control of tonnage, size and species of fish caught. Then fish populations can be managed in a more rational and conservative way.

Instead of hunting haphazardly ocean fish whose population size and rates of replacement are little known, an alternative approach is fish farming. The supply of freshwater fish can be increased by systematic cultivation with proper stocking and the use of mineral and nitrogen fertilisers added to the fishponds. In the tropics much progress along these lines has been made, often stimulated by the Fisheries Divisions of FAO. In Europe the fish ponds which in medieval times supplied fish in winter to the monasteries and other great houses have long been in disuse. Nowadays trout served in restaurants is likely to have come from a fish farm. Experimental marine fish farms in the Scottish lochs for salmon (Young, 1977) and flat fish (Kerr, 1977) are now ready for commercial development.

EGGS

Since the egg forms a complete food for the embryo chick, it is naturally rich in essential nutrients. An average hen's egg, weighing about 2 oz or 60 g, contains 6 g of protein and 6 g of fat and yields about 330 kJ (80 kcal). The proteins—most of which are albumins in the white of the egg—have the highest biological value for human adults of all food proteins. The amino acid composition of whole hens' eggs is sometimes used as a standard against which the chemical score of other proteins is compared. Values of the amino acid pattern of egg proteins are given by Lunven et al. (1973). A hen's egg contains about 30 mg of calcium and 1.5 mg of iron; however, the iron is bound, possibly to the protein conalbumin, and poorly absorbed in man (Callender et al., 1970). The yolk is a fair source of vitamin A and also contains significant amounts of thiamin, nicotinic acid and riboflavin; most of the yellow colour of yolks is xanthophyll (lutein) which is a carotenoid but not a vitamin A precursor. There is little or no ascorbic acid. Tolan et al. (1974) compared the nutrients in eggs from free-range battery hens; eggs from free-range hens contained more folate and vitamin B_{12}.

Eggs have been described as nature's 'convenience food', since they come in an hygienic pack, are easily stored and readily opened and cooked. For this reason and also because of their nutritive value they are well suited to the needs of old people who usually like them. An egg contains about 250 mg of cholesterol and when eaten in large numbers may raise the plasma cholesterol. They should therefore be restricted in a dietary regime designed to lower plasma cholesterol.

The eggs of many other species of birds are eaten in various parts of the world and all have approximately the same nutritive value as eggs of domestic hens.

NOVEL PROTEIN FOODS

Attempts to find new foods rich in protein arise from two main motives. There is the need for new infant foods suitable for preventing protein-energy malnutrition, so prevalent in many countries, and also for a cheap alternative to meat. Everywhere prices of meat have been rising for many years and in some countries the supply has declined. A suitable alternative to meat might obtain an established place in our diets, just as 100 years ago the manufacture of margarine provided a valuable alternative to butter. There is also the fear that world population will outgrow its supply of conventional foods. The term 'novel protein' is used to describe several different types of product and no definition is generally acceptable. Defatted soya flour and fish protein concentrates are products of food technology which have been available for many years, and the former is widely used in the food industry. In as much as they are not conventional foods, they can be described as *novel*.

PLANKTON, ALGAE AND LEAVES

It is possible to extract and concentrate an edible material from biological sources which themselves cannot be used as human food because of their high content of indigestible material. The Japanese have been pioneers in preparing foods from plankton, the mass of small crustacea and coelenterates that abound on the surface waters of the sea, and from chlorella, the green alga which forms the scum on top of many pools. In England Pirie (1975) has devised a process on a small factory scale for extracting protein from green leaves and grasses. He has entertained his friends with the product which has the consistency of a friable cheese and only a slight taste which is not unpleasant. These are three potential sources of novel protein, which a hungry world may need some day, but for which no one shows much enthusiasm at present.

PROTEIN-RICH MATERIAL FROM MICROORGANISMS

Large industrial firms are using their resources to develop new foods from microorganisms. Thus British Petroleum have plants in France and in Scotland in which yeast is grown on petroleum oil, and in England Rank Hovis McDougall are growing a fungus, *Fusarium graminearum* on a hydrolysed bean starch. Imperial Chemical Industries are converting the methane and other hydrocarbons in natural gas into methanol, which is being used to grow bacteria for conversion into foods. The immediate aim, which has already been partially achieved, is to produce products which are suitable protein concentrates for animal feeding. However, it is the intention to go on to produce new human foods. Before such preparations could be accepted as human foods, they would have to undergo toxicity trials for the presence of possible carcinogens and mutagens. These trials should involve several generations of animals of different species, including primates. Some of these products may become important human foods in the future, but it is very unlikely that they will be on the market before 1980. For this reason they are not discussed further. For a review of single-cell protein for human food see Lovland et al. (1976).

PROTEINS FROM LEGUMES AND OIL SEEDS
There are available in the USA and Britain vegetable protein products which have been textured and flavoured to resemble meat. Textured vegetable protein (TVP) is a registered name in the USA. Stews, meat pies and goulashes have been prepared from these products and their resemblance to the real thing is as close as that of good margarine to butter. A TVP preparation from soya bean is in use in school meal programmes in the USA and is on sale in Britain. In as much as the raw materials of these products are conventional foods, and as there is no reason to think that the physical changes brought about in the texturing and spinning have harmful effects, there seem to be no new problems of toxicity.

Just as margarine is now enriched with vitamins A and D to give it a nutritive value similar to that of butter, it is sensible to make new foods as nutritious as meat. It has been suggested that they should contain in 100 g of dry matter a minimum of 50 g protein, 1.3 g methionine, 10 mg iron, 2 mg thiamin, 0.6 mg riboflavin and 5 μg vitamin B_{12}. The natural ingredients contain no vitamin B_{12} and this

would have to be added. Vegetable proteins in general have less methionine than animal proteins and most products would require enrichment with this amino acid to bring their biological value up to approximately that of most meat. Artificial additions of iron, thiamin and riboflavin might or might not be needed. With these safeguards there is no reason to think that the substitution of meat by such foods in a mixed diet would have any adverse affect on nutrition.

These new products should be welcomed as attractive and nutritious cheap alternatives to meat with an appeal to families, schools, homes for old people and others whose purchases of meat are restricted by small incomes. Yet it is important that no one should be deceived into thinking that they are eating meat when they are not. There are no special difficulties in ensuring that manufacturers of novel protein foods label their containers with the appropriate description of their contents. Caterers who buy these products and use them to prepare 'meat pies', 'meat stews', etc., either for consumption in restaurants and canteens or for outside sale, are under the same legal obligations as manufacturers to inform their customers by correct labelling of their products. Many articles of food are likely to be prepared from mixtures of meat and novel proteins, but as yet there are no regulations regarding the proportion of meat in the mixture necessary to ensure that the article can still be described as a meat product.

The introduction of novel protein foods thus poses many new problems. These have ben considered by the Food Standards Committee (1974), whose report contains much detailed information and amplification of the problems. It is a basis for discussion and subsequent legislation. The Protein Advisory Group (PAG) of the UN was concerned with international aspects of novel proteins and issued several statements on the subject (PAG, 1974).

20. Milk and Milk Products; Oils and Fats

MILK AND CHEESE

Milk is the sole natural food on the human infant for the first few months of life. After about 3 to 6 months it is desirable to give supplementary foods and gradually wean the infant on to a good mixed diet. In this process milk slowly loses its dominant place in the infant's diet, but for the first two years of life it is important that milk should remain the largest single item of food.

From the age of 2 years and until growth ceases, children grow more rapidly and reach maturity sooner if given ample quantities of milk. Increased growth rates are generally associated with improved health and vitality and with relative freedom from disease. All nutritionists agree that a regular intake of milk is beneficial to growing children. There are, however, many people who have doubts as to whether large quantities (more than 2 pints or 1 litre daily) are desirable. It is not proven that the unusually rapid growth promoted by such large intakes is beneficial. In many tropical countries little milk is available and older children may not be able to take large amounts because of lactase insufficiency (p. 407). Widdowson and McCance (1954) showed that children can grow well on a diet composed almost entirely of wheaten bread and vegetables, with no milk. The same has been found in Guatemala, India and other countries with well-balanced combinations of vegetable foods.

As a complete food easily given, readily digested and absorbed, milk is a good food for invalids, especially for patients with acute illnesses. There is no evidence, however, that milk is an indispensable food for adults. As a good source of the principal nutrients it can be recommended for those who like it. Kon (1972) has prepared a small handbook on milk and milk products especially useful for public health workers.

CHEMICAL COMPOSITION OF MILK

This chapter is concerned with milk as a food for adults and for children after weaning from the breast or bottle. Human breast milk is considered only incidentally and its composition and that of the various infant milk preparations are discussed in Chapter 61.

Typical values for the carbohydrate, protein, fat and energy content of milks consumed by man are given in Table 20.1. The values for human milk are taken from analyses of pooled samples in Britain (DHSS, 1977).

Protein

Cow's milk contains much more protein than human milk. About 80 per cent of this protein is casein. The rest, whey proteins, broadly resemble those found in plasma and include lactalbumin and various immunoglobulins which have a role in defence mechanisms in early life (p. 522).

Fat

The fat in freshly secreted milk is present in fine globules, many of which are as small as 0.5 μm in diameter. Fat in this form is easily digested. When milk is left to stand these globules run together to form cream. The fat content of both human and cow's milk varies greatly.

In some mammals the fat content of the milk is very high. The milk of whales and sea lions, for instance, contains over 40 g/dl of fat. In these animals lactation lasts for a very short period, during which the mothers cannot feed. The milk transfers an enormous quantity of fat from the mother to the young in the course of a few days. Elephant's milk contains 20 g of fat and reindeer milk 17 g/dl.

Carbohydrate

The carbohydrate in all milks is lactose. This sugar is much less sweet than sucrose. Human milk contains more lactose than cow's milk. Cow's milk is frequently 'humanised' by diluting and then adding sucrose or glucose. The young infant thus becomes accustomed to an unnaturally sweet food at an early age.

Minerals

Calcium is present in all milks in good quantities. Human milk usually contains between 25 and 35 mg/dl. Cow's milk contains about 120 mg/dl. The calcium is present chiefly in combination with caseinogen. For some unknown reason milk also contains significant amounts of citric acid—up to 0.23 mg/dl—which must reduce the ionisation of a small part of the calcium. Nevertheless the calcium in milk is generally more readily absorbed than that in other foods, probably because of its combination with amino acids. Milk is thus a most valuable food for the formation of bone.

Milk contains very little iron. All milks provide 0.1 to 0.2 mg/100 ml. Young mammals depend for their initial supply of iron on stores accumulated during intrauterine life. In the human infant these stores are sufficient for only

Table 20.1 Typical analyses of milk from various species

	Carbohydrate (g/dl)	Protein (g/dl)	Fat (g/dl)	Energy kJ/dl	Energy kcal/dl
Human	7.3 (7.1–7.8)	1.07 (0.95–1.20)	4.2 (3.7–4.8)	293 (272–314)	70 (65–75)
Cow	5.0 (4.2–6.8)	3.5 (2.5–4.0)	3.5 (3–6)	275	66
Buffalo	4.5	4.3	7.5	430	103
Goat	4.5	3.7	4.8	320	76
Ewe	4.9	6.5	6.9	450	109
Mare	5.7	1.3	1.2	160	29
Camel	4.1	3.7	4.2	290	69

four to six months, and if iron is not then provided in the diet anaemia is likely to follow. Infants born prematurely have smaller reserves of iron in the liver, and so are more liable to develop anaemia.

Vitamins

Table 20.2 gives normal values for the vitamin content of cow's whole milk and human milk. If the dietary intake of any vitamin is high some of the excess is likely to appear in the milk, especially vitamin A and riboflavin.

Cow's milk is a useful but not rich source of vitamins. Its riboflavin may be especially valuable to children on poor diets and its nicotinic acid may help to prevent pellagra in maize-eaters. Cow's milk contains little vitamin D mostly as the aqueous-soluble sulphate and unless enriched cannot be relied on to prevent rickets. The ascorbic acid content is also not high and it is destroyed by pasteurisation, boiling or allowing the milk to stand in sunlight.

DIGESTION OF MILK

Milk clots when it enters the stomach. This is due to the action of an enzyme—rennin. The clotting converts the caseinogen into insoluble casein. The casein clot contracts into a tough mass which is subsequently digested. Infants secrete little pepsin in the stomach; the clot is digested by trypsin and other proteolytic ensymes in the small intestine. The biological significance of this clotting is not known; it is reputed to make milk less easily digested. It can be partially prevented by diluting the milk with water,

Table 20.2 Normal values for the vitamin content of cow's milk (whole raw) and human milk (DHSS, 1977; Paul and Southgate, 1978)

	Cow's milk /dl	Human milk /dl
Vitamin A (μg) summer	43	50
winter	30	
Vitamin D (μg)	0.15	0.8
Thiamin (μg)	40	20
Riboflavin (μg)	190	30
Nicotinic acid (μg)	80	220
Ascorbic acid (μg)	1.5	3.8

thus reducing the concentration of calcium which is necessary for the formation of the clot. Clotting can also be prevented by the addition of sodium citrate. Both of these means have been much used, but whether they increase the digestibility of milk is doubtful. Milk is readily digested and absorbed by infants and growing children.

Cow's milk—owing to its high protein content and its content of phosphate and citrate—exerts a strong buffering action, thus lowering the acidity of the gastric juice. It is perhaps for this reason that milk is often so effective in reducing the discomfort caused by a peptic ulcer and the associated hyperacidity.

MILK PRODUCTS

Soured and fermented milks

In many countries, milk is drunk sour or curdled. Various bacteria are used for this purpose—*Lactobacillus acidophilus* found in man, *L. bifidus* found in the alimentary tract of infants and *L. bulgaricus* found in cows. All these bacteria cause a breakdown of the lactose in the milk with the formation of lactic acid (up to 3 per cent). The natural method of preparation is to boil the milk and somewhat reduce its volume. After cooling it is inoculated with a small portion of the previous day's milk as a starter. The souring takes about 24 hours. Condensed and reconstituted dried milk can be used for the purpose. Commercial preparations of the bacterial cultures are also available as starters. Sour milk (yogurt) contains all the protein, fat, calcium and vitamins of the original milk. It is a safe preparation in countries where standards of dairy hygiene are low, for the original milk is sterilised by boiling and the subsequent profuse growth of *L. acidophilus* overgrows any chance pathogenic contaminant. There are many traditional forms of sour milk which are appreciated as national drinks.

Yogurt originated in South-east Europe and Turkey. If the milk has been much concentrated by boiling, the yogurt is diluted with water for drinking and is then known as *doogh* in Afghanistan and Iran, or *eyran* in Turkey. If souring is allowed to take place when the milk is warm (about 55° C), a preparation known as *laban* is formed, which may contain a little alcohol from yeast fermentation. *Kefir* is a sour milk made in the Caucasus with lactobacilli and a lactose-fermenting yeast, which may have an alcohol content of 1 per cent. *Koumiss* is a popular Russian drink prepared from mares' milk, which is rich in lactose. It may contain up to 3 per cent alcohol.

Consumption of commercially produced yogurt has increased greatly and in Britain in 1975 was 23 ml/head weekly. Sales increased 450 per cent in the USA in the 10 years to 1974. The organisms most used for the processing are *L. bulgaricus* and *Streptococcus thermophilus*. Composition varies greatly and a draft prepared for the *Codex Alimentarius* suggests a minimum content of non-fat milk solids of 8.5 g/dl and of milk fat 3 g/dl. Skimmed yogurts are also popular and for these a maximum fat content of 0.5 g/dl is suggested.

The great Russian scientist Metchnikoff at the end of the nineteenth century conceived the idea that yogurt was an elixir of life. His theory was that the putrefactive bacteria present in the large intestine produce toxins that shorten life. He thought that by taking yogurt, the milk-souring bacilli would become dominant in the intestine and oust the usual putrefactive bacteria. He himself took yogurt regularly and established it as a fashion in many European cities. Metchnikoff was mistaken: *L. bulgaricus* cannot proliferate in the human bowel. But yogurt is a nutritious and convenient food. The modern consumer may derive extra satisfaction from knowing that it tends to lower plasma cholesterol (Mann, 1977).

Dahi is a sour milk preparation made in innumerable Indian homes. Whole milk brought to the boil and then allowed to cool to about body temperature and kept at this heat in an earthen vessel. A small amount of yesterday's dahi is added as a starter. When cool, dahi is a delicious drink, especially in the hot weather, although perhaps an acquired taste for Europeans. The butter fat may be removed from dahi by churning and used to make *ghee*. The remaining sour milk is known as *lassi* and is also a popular drink.

Curds (junket)
Curds are the clotted proteins formed when fresh milk is artificially inoculated with rennet (a commercial preparation of rennin, prepared either from calves' stomachs or vegetable sources). Sweetened and flavoured forms are junket.

Whey
Whey is the fluid that separates from the clot in making cheese. It contains most of the lactose in the original milk, and a little lactalbumin, but almost no casein or fat. Whey is often wasted and efforts are being made to find economic ways to concentrate the lactalbumin, a good quality protein, which could be a useful protein supplement.

Butter
This is discussed later in this chapter.

Cream
Cream contains all the fat and usually from one-third to half of the protein and lactose in milk. The standards for cream have varied in different countries and from time to time. In the UK it has been recommended by the Food Standards Committee that cream should contain 20 per cent of butterfat, double cream 48 per cent, whipping cream 35 per cent and half cream 12 per cent. The last is approximately the top of the milk and can be used for adding to coffee and fruit.

The famous Devonshire cream or clotted cream is prepared by heating the milk in special pans. This brings about a rapid and effective separation of the fat. Devonshire cream may contain 60 per cent of fat.

Evaporated and condensed milk
Evaporated milk is the liquid product obtained by the partial removal of water from milk or skimmed milk. Condensed milk is the product obtained in the same way, but with the addition of sugar. The first came into use to meet the needs of the people in the new industrial towns in Europe and North America in the nineteenth century, and both products are now finding new markets in the greatly increased urban populations of Asia, Africa and South America. Clearly, legal composition standards are needed and those in force in Britain are shown in Table 20.3. There are also important labelling requirements, including the statement, 'should not be used for babies except under medical advice', on partly skimmed milk products and 'unfit for babies' on skimmed milk products. In some countries infants fed on these products have become blind, due to the development of keratomalacia.

Skimmed milk
This is milk from which the fat has been removed in the making of butter or cream. It is a byproduct of the butter industry and since it is readily dried, large quantities of the

Table 20.3 Compositional standards laid down in Britain for evaporated and condensed milk

	Percentage of milk fat	Minimum percentage of milk solids including fat
Evaporated full cream milk	9.0*	31.0
Condensed full cream milk	9.0*	31.0
Evaporated partly skimmed milk	4.5*	26.5
Condensed partly skimmed milk	4.5*	26.5
Evaporated skimmed milk	0.5†	22.0
Condensed skimmed milk	0.5†	26.0

* *Minimum permitted.*
† *Maximum permitted.*

dried product are available on the world market. In Great Britain skimmed milk has been traditionally fed to pigs and is despised as a human food. This is unfortunate, since it contains most of the protein and nearly all the calcium in the original milk. It also contains the B group of vitamins. Skimmed milk is thus a good food. Largely through the good offices of the United Nations Children's Fund (UNICEF) many thousands of tons of dried skimmed milk have been distributed to children in countries which are short of dairy cattle. The improvement in health of children receiving this milk has been demonstrated in controlled experiments and vast numbers of children have benefited.

Dried skimmed milk from the USA has been enriched with vitamin A but milk donated by European countries has not. Because xerophthalmia is reported in at least 73 developing countries, WHO (1977) recommends that all dried skimmed milk used in aid programmes be enriched with vitamin A.

Consumption of low fat liquid milk (2 per cent fat) is increasing in the USA and Sweden. It is lower in energy and saturated fat than is full cream milk.

Casein

Various preparations of casein are on the market. Casilan, a calcium caseinate is one which is well known. These preparations have little taste and provide a most convenient and effective means of enriching diets with protein in dietetic practice, as in the treatment of burns, prolonged fevers and in convalescence from severe illnesses. They can be added to soups, puddings, milk drinks, cocoa, etc.

Cheese

Milk production is inevitably subject to large seasonal variations. In the summer months when pastures are good, cows yield more milk than in the winter; a surplus in summer is therefore common. Cheese-making is an effective method of preserving some of this surplus and has been a traditional occupation of European farmers' wives for generations. There are over 400 varieties.

The basic process in cheese-making is the clotting of the milk. The milk may or may not be soured first. Rennet is used to form the clot, usually at a temperature of about 30° C. The clot, which contains almost all the protein in the milk, also entangles the fat and many of the other nutrients. The clot is then gently separated from the whey and salted. It is pressed to remove moisture and a firm cake is made. The cheese is then put in cheese bags and kept in a cool room to ripen. During ripening bacterial fermentation takes place; the particular bacteria and moulds responsible give the cheese its characteristic texture and flavour. Many variations in the details of cheese-making exist. Cow's milk is usually employed, but Roquefort cheese comes from ewe's milk and some Norwegian cheeses from goat's milk. The blue colour characteristic of Stilton, Gorgonzola and

Roquefort is produced by moulds developing during the ripening process. The most famous English cheeses are Cheddar, Cheshire, Wensleydale and Stilton. France produces the greatest variety: Camembert, Brie, Livarot and Pont l'Eveque are famous French soft cheeses; Roquefort, Saint Paulin and Port-du-Salut are semi-soft cheeses. Italy produces the blue Gorgonzola, semi-soft Bel Paese and the hard Parmesan. Limburger is a soft, strongly flavoured Belgian cheese. Holland produces many notable Dutch cheeses—particularly the round red Edam—and Denmark the famous Danish blue. Gruyère, with its characteristic holes, comes from Switzerland. These and many other cheeses are described by Eekhof-Stork (1976). France has the highest cheese consumption of any country (daily average 40 g/head) followed by Israel.

Those who will not eat cheese forego a food which is not only tasty but also nutritious. Most cheeses contain 25 to 35 per cent of protein and this protein is of high biological value. The fat content usually varies from 16 to 40 per cent. Cheeses are also rich in calcium, vitamin A and riboflavin. There are also dietetic cheeses made from skimmed milk; cottage cheese contains 4 per cent fat.

The cheese reaction. Many cheeses contain tyramine, the amine of the amino acid tyrosine. The amounts vary greatly, but a portion of cheddar may contain 20 mg. Tyramine stimulates the sympathetic system and may cause a big rise in blood pressure. The tyramine naturally present in foods is normally destroyed very quickly in the tissues by monoamine oxidases (MAO). However, drugs such as phenelzine and tranylcypromine which are used for the treatment of depression, inhibit MAO. If patients on these drugs eat a large portion of cheese, the tyramine present is not destroyed and may produce alarming reactions. Headache, severe nausea and dizziness frequently occur, with severe hypertension, followed occasionally by cerebral haemorrhage or cardiac failure. Patients taking MAO inhibitors have to be careful with other food, drinks and medicines containing amines.

Khoa, rabri, churkom, dried reindeer milk and other delicacies

Cheese-making is characteristically a European art. There are, however, a number of ways in which surplus milk can be concentrated, sometimes into forms which may be preserved for a long time. In India, *khoa* or *mawa* is made by boiling milk briskly in an open pan until about two-thirds of the water has been evaporated and it has the consistency of dough; *rabri* is made by skimming off successive layers of cream from simmering milk and adding sugar when the liquid residue is greatly reduced; the skimmed-off clots are then blended back into the liquid residue to make a sweet concentrate. In the Himalayas the Sherpas heat any excess *lassi* and the clot formed, mainly casein, is strained through bamboo baskets and then dried before an open fire to make *churkom*. In Lapland reindeer milk is put in a reindeer stomach over an open smoking fire. As the water evaporates and the milk is 'cured', more is added and it may take two or three weeks before the stomach is filled with grains of dried milk. This quantity may last a Lapp family for the winter.

Nearly all indigenous soured milk products have the advantage that they are much less likely to be contaminated with pathogenic organisms than fresh milk. They can therefore be strongly recommended in places where the standards of dairy hygiene are low.

OILS AND FATS

These are valuable foods because they are (1) concentrated sources of energy, (2) essential to the art of good cooking, as practised in all civilised countries, and (3) important sources of fat-soluble vitamins. As discussed in Chapter 6, good cooking usually demands that at least 20 per cent of the energy in the food should come from fat. This applies to traditional methods of cooking both in the West and East. Fats and oils are expensive, so that this level is often not achieved by poor families. Amongst the well-to-do, fats and oils often provide 40 per cent of the energy; there is clear evidence that—in sedentary people at least—such a high intake disturbs the normal mechanisms for the transport of fat in the blood; this may lead in turn to atherosclerotic changes in the arteries and an increased tendency to thrombosis (p. 333).

Butter (milk fat) is generally the housewife's favourite: but the depot fat from the carcasses of many animals is also used for cooking. Vegetable oils used for cooking in many parts of the world include olive oil, cotton-seed oil, coconut oil, red-palm oil, soya-bean oil, groundnut oil, mustard oil, gingelly (sesame) oil, and sunflower seed oil. The

Table 20.4 World production and exports of fats and oils, 1972–73 (Lysons, 1975) (thousands of metric tons in terms of oil or fat)

	Production	Exports
Butter	5325	758
Lard	4075	354
Soya bean oil	7900	3352
Sunflower seed oil	3240	560
Groundnut oil	2860	810
Cottonseed oil	2785	340
Rapeseed oil	2240	869
Coconut oil	2335	1200
Palm oil	2060	1170
Palm kernel oil	430	312
Olive oil	1420	336
Fish oil	815	507
Sesame oil	690	114
Maize oil	305*	31*
Sunflower oil	195*	54*
Whale oil	45	44

* figures for 1970.

world production of edible fats and oils is shown in Table 20.4. In the last 50 years there has been an enormous increase in the manufacture of hardened fats—artificial butters—from vegetable and marine oils. Margarine manufacture is a major industry.

The principal constituents of all fats and oils are the triglycerides or neutral fats. Fats contain very little water; the energy value of all food fats and oils is high and lies between 3.3 and 3.8 MJ (800 and 900 kcal)/100 g. The natural fats vary greatly in the nature of the fatty acids which they contain (p. 49). These variations have little effect on the energy value of the fat or oil but determine the consistency of the fat. The proportion of polyunsaturated to saturated fatty acids (P/S ratio) determines whether at room temperature a fat is hard or liquid. Land animals have hard fat with a low P/S ratio. Marine animals and vegetable seeds usually contain oils with higher P/S ratios.

Margarine and butter

A French chemist, Mège-Mouries, made the first recognisable substitute for butter in 1869, stimulated by the shortage of the natural product during the Franco-Prussian War. He used suet (beef or sheep fat). At about the same time there was a growing need for a cheap substitute for butter for the industrial populations in the big towns of western Europe and the USA. At first animal fats were used; the meat-packing industry in Chicago rapidly produced these fats as a byproduct. But supplies were soon insufficient. At the end of the nineteenth century—largely as a result of Dutch enterprise—ways were found of hardening vegetable oils by hydrogenation. Margarines consist predominantly of fat; the aqueous part, up to 16 per cent, forms a water in oil emulsion and contains non-fat milk solids and salt for flavour. To celebrate the centenary of margarine an excellent account of its economic, social and scientific history was produced by van Stuyvenberg (1969).

The vitamin content of butter depends on the quality of the cow's diet. Good summer butter may contain up to 1300 μg of retinol/100 g, but winter butter as little as 500 μg. The vitamin D content of butter varies and at most is 2.5 μg/100 g. In Britain vitamins are artificially added to margarine: margarine sold by retail is required by law to contain on average the equivalent of 900 μg of retinol and 8 μg of vitamin D/100 g. The raw materials of margarine may have a high P/S ratio but this tends to be lowered by the hardening process in manufacture. However, some brands of margarine now have up to 50 per cent of *cis, cis* linoleic acid. The consumption of such margarine helps to lower the plasma cholesterol concentration and they are useful in diets for the treatment of hyperlipoproteinaemia (p. 327).

Whether butter, had any nutritional advantage over margarine enriched with vitamin A was an old issue. Much experimental work on rats and one good clinical trial with children (Leichenger *et al.*, 1948) produced no evidence that butter was more nutritious.

Ghee

In India and, in other parts of the East, butter fats are first clarified by heating and the resulting product is known as *ghee*. Ghee may be made either in the home or as an industrial product. Processes vary. Good ghee may contain almost all the vitamins present in the original milk fat, but losses may be up to 50 per cent.

Suet, lard and dripping

In Western countries various cooking fats besides butter and margarine are used. These include suet (perirenal fat of beef and sheep), lard (pig fat), beef dripping and several commercial preparations. All of these are of high energy value of 3.3 to 3.8 MJ (800 to 900 kcal)/100 g; the natural ones contain only traces of vitamins.

Vegetable oils

The large number of vegetable oils used originally in the tropics and Mediterranean countries are all of high energy value (about 3.8 MJ/100 g). With one exception all are devoid of any vitamin activity. This is one reason why many tropical diets are low in vitamin A activity. The one exception is red-palm oil (from the palm *Elaeis guineensis*), which contains 24 to 48 mg of carotene/100 g. The palm is a native of West Africa where is grows wild and also is extensively cultivated. There are plantations in Indonesia, Malaysia and other parts of Asia. In comparative studies in Nigeria, Nicol (1952) showed that children receiving red-palm oil were in better health than those that had none. The use of vegetable oils, particularly corn oil and sunflower seed oil, for lowering the plasma cholesterol concentration is discussed in Chapter 47.

Regulations in Britain and the EEC limit the level of erucic acid (p. 57) in edible oils and fats to 5 per cent.

21. Beverages; Herbs and Spices

BEVERAGES

The needs of the human body for water have already been discussed (p. 81). To meet them man must drink. *Homo sapiens* is not very fond of plain water and prefers flavoured fluids such as beer, wine, spirits, tea, coffee, cocoa, fruit juice, or even synthetic 'colas' and 'lemonades'. Americans encourage the consumption of plain water by serving it iced.

Beverages are appreciated for their flavour and for the pharmacological action of certain ingredients which many contain. Some are also a source of energy and a few provide small amounts of micronutrients.

Flavours are provided by the essential oils in the herbs, berries, and other fruit and grains which go to form the basic ingredients of many drinks. In tea and coffee gardens, in orchards, hop fields and vineyards, cultivators use the experience of generations to produce the best raw materials. Tea blenders, vintners, distillers, housewives and many others use traditional skills to refine and concentrate the basic ingredients. All humanity is grateful for the labours of such skilled craftsmen. To the epicure with a trained palate, the appreciation of well-made tea and coffee—of fine wines and spirits—is one of the privileges of living in a civilised society. Chemists are now moving into this field of knowledge, but they are not yet as reliable as wine tasters, tea tasters and other experts with long-standing traditions. The chemistry of 'Bouquet and Essence' was discussed in a learned editorial in the *Lancet* (1961) with references to appropriate French and German literature. The supreme qualities of 'Scotch' still remain a mystery, immune from science.

SOFT DRINKS

These include any fruit squash, crush and cordial (as distinct from fruit juice), colas, soda water, tonic water, sweetened artificially carbonated water that may or may not be flavoured, and ginger beer. They may be sold as concentrates or powders requiring dilution or ready to drink. Those that are sold at final volume for drinking are usually carbonated and thus fizzy. Cola drinks originated in 1886 in the United States and contained extracts from the kola nut, prepared by a pharmacist, John Pemberton. They are now manufactured throughout the world by many companies who use cola essences mostly provided by two American companies. The precise formulation of these essences is a closely guarded secret even within the companies. Large amounts of soft drinks are consumed, the total production in the UK in 1974 being 816 imperial gallons or 66 litres per head of population. The corresponding figure for the USA is just over 100 litres per head.

Soft drinks have little value in nutrition except that they encourage people to drink water. Some citrus squashes contain significant amounts of natural vitamin C or may be enriched with it, when claims are made on the label. Most soft drinks are sweetened. If sugar is used, this may contribute to obesity, especially in children, and the drink is unsuitable for diabetics. In one British product the content of glucose has been advertised as especially valuable for giving energy; but in fact glucose taken by mouth is no better than sucrose as a source of energy. Cola drinks usually contain caffeine in concentrations from 50 to 200 mg/l. In fruit-flavoured squashes, often to be seen standing next to the bed of patients in hospital, clinicians need to know that the potassium content may be quite low. Bateson and Lant (1973) measured this in 16 proprietary squashes found in a London hospital and the highest potassium concentration was 9 mmol/l.

Fruit juices

Fruit juices are obtained from fruit by mechanical processes. After removal of a portion of the water, they may be sold as a concentrated juice. Fruit juice has become an almost essential component of an American breakfast. This is a pleasant habit which is spreading slowly into Europe. Fruit juices contain approximately the same nutrients as whole fruit but have lost most of the pectin. The most important nutrient is vitamin C. This varies greatly depending on the fruit from which the juice was prepared. Citrus fruit juices may be expected to contain between 30 and 50 mg/dl and pineapple and tomato juices about half as much. Apple juices contain little of the vitamin. Fruit juices are also useful for patients on low sodium diets or receiving diuretic drugs for any reason, as their content of potassium is high and of sodium low. A reasonable assumption is that juice contains not more than 2.5 mmol/l of Na^+ and not less than 30 mmol/l of K^+ and that K^+/Na^+ ratio is at least 20:1.

Tea, coffee and cocoa

These beverages contain small amounts of three drugs, caffeine, theobromine and theophylline. These are methyl derivatives of xanthine. Caffeine is the most active; it is a stimulant to the nervous system and often prevents fatigue; many people find that caffeine appears to facilitate mental work. Most people in western countries are habituated to caffeine; they are accustomed to take it, but they do not become addicted to it. The British housewife, who is so frequently 'dying for a cup of tea', may feel tired and frustrated if she does not get it, but otherwise suffers no serious symptoms.

An excessive intake of caffeine can cause sleeplessness and so may aggravate emotional instability and mental illness. In some persons coffee appears to sensitise the heart and increase the incidence of extrasystoles and possibly other arrhythmias; otherwise it is doubtful if any ill effects arise from the use of tea and coffee. Both contain tannin, which is a weak protein precipitant and astringent. Tea and coffee do not impair digestion when taken in moderate amounts and not excessively strong, whether by healthy people or patients.

Caffeine is a weak diuretic. It is of little medicinal value for this purpose, nor are tea and coffee contraindicated for this reason.

Tea

Tea has been drunk in China for thousands of years. It was introduced into Europe in the seventeenth century and was at first a great luxury. After the discovery that tea could be grown easily on large estates in Sri Lanka and India, enormous quantities were imported into Great Britain, where for nearly a hundred years it has been a cheap and popular beverage.

Several varieties of the shrub are cultivated. Fertile soil, a warm climate and a good rainfall are necessary conditions for growth and these are found in Sri Lanka, Assam and the hill districts of South India. The shrubs are allowed to grow up to a height of about 4 ft and are pruned each year. The young and tender leaves, 'two leaves and a bud' of each shoot, are picked by hand, usually by women. After picking, the leaves are taken to a factory, usually on the estate, where they are withered, mashed or rolled and allowed to ferment. They are then dried. Most Indian and Ceylon tea sold in Great Britain is blended by mixing samples grown in different gardens.

Green teas commonly consumed by the Chinese are withered at high temperatures, so that the enzymes responsible for the fermentation are destroyed and this process in the manufacture is omitted.

The great variety of teas on the market are of interest to the connoisseur, but not to the physician or dietitian. They can be recommended as an attractive drink to all except a few unfortunates, in whom tea appears to cause indigestion, probably owing to the tannin present. Sinclair and Hollingsworth (1969) reported the analyses of many types of tea; they found the tannin content of a cup (150 ml) of infusion to vary from 60 to 280 mg. Caffeine contents varied from 50 to 80 mg. The mild stimulating effect of caffeine has already been described. Its pharmacopoeial dose is 60 to 300 mg, so that many cups have to be drunk before this maximum is exceeded. Tea contains up to 10 mg/100 g of fluoride in the dry leaves.

The usual British custom (though not practised by connoisseurs) is to add sugar and milk. In this way some people may obtain a significant addition to their intake of energy and protein.

Coffee

Coffee beans are the seeds of coffee trees that are widely cultivated in the tropics. They have been grown in Ethiopia and Arabia for hundreds of generations. There are large plantations in India, Indonesia, Africa and especially in Brazil.

A variety of trees are grown. Most are 10 to 15 ft high with evergreen leaves. Shade trees are necessary to protect them from excessive sun. They bear clusters of white flowers which develop into the beans. A tree provides the best crop when between 6 and 14 years old; it requires regular and skilful pruning.

The beans have to be roasted and ground before the infusion is made. Sir Robert Hutchison found about 100 mg of caffeine and 200 mg of tannin in a teacupful of coffee, made by infusing 2 oz (60 g) in a pint (450 ml) of water (Sinclair and Hollingsworth, 1969). Analyses of cups of coffee and tea by Al-Samarrae et al. (1975) showed that Londoners may get from 58 to 168 mg of caffeine in a cup of coffee and from 43 to 92 mg in a cup of tea. Coffee made at home was slightly weaker than that served in cafés (averages 92 and 99 mg/cup respectively), but homemade tea was stronger (averages 70 and 56 mg/cup).

Coffee rapidly loses some of its flavour after grinding; the best coffee is made from beans ground in the home. Preparations of dried ground coffee are convenient but lack bouquet. Instant coffee is a modern form of coffee that has been made into an infusion from coffee beans in the factory. This liquid is spray dried and the powder sold in airtight containers. In the home it is conveniently made into a drink by simply adding warm water. Instant coffees have overtaken the traditional ground beans in popularity in many industrial countries. They contain 20 to 40 mg of caffeine per gram of powder.

Coffee is a popular drink and in moderate amounts a mild cerebral stimulant and diuretic. People habituated to several cups of coffee during the day feel tired if this is stopped and may have headaches. But coffee is not inert. Too much can produce anxiety symptoms, cardiac arrhythmias, gastrointestinal discomfort or insomnia. Some people are more sensitive to the pharmacological actions of coffee or are allergic to it. Decaffeinated coffee has most of the taste without most of the pharmacological effects. Retrospective studies suggesting that a large intake of coffee is a factor in the development of coronary heart disease are not being confirmed (Chapter 41).

Roasted coffee beans and instant coffee powder made from it contain 10 to 40 mg nicotinic acid/100 g (Böddeker and Mishkin, 1963); the darker the roast the more nicotinic acid. One cup of coffee thus provides around 0.6 mg of the vitamin (Okungbowa et al., 1976).

Coffee may be adulterated and—especially in times of scarcity—a great variety of substances are used for this purpose. The most important is chicory which is frequently added to French coffee. Chicory is the root of a wild endive. It is dried, partly caramelised and then added to coffee in proportions varying from 10 to 80 per cent. Chicory's great attraction is its cheapness. There is no reason to think that it is in any way injurious to health.

Cocoa
Cocoa is made from the fruit of a tree indigenous in Central and South America. It is a small tree—about 20 ft high—and grows only in damp tropical lands. Cultivation has spread from tropical America to West Africa, Sri Lanka and other parts of Asia. West Africa now provides the greater part of the world's supplies. The fruit is a gourd in which the numerous seeds are embedded. The seeds are removed from the pulp, placed in heaps and allowed to dry in the sun for several days. During this process they lose their bitterness and acquire the pleasant taste characteristic of cocoa. The seeds are then roasted and ground.

The chief xanthine derivative in cocoa is theobromine, but it also contains some caffeine and tannin.

Natural waters
The most important quality of a natural water is that it should be free from pathogenic organisms. Cholera and typhoid are the classical water-borne diseases and there are many others. The constant vigilance of water engineers and public health authorities is necessary to protect civilised communities from these diseases. So accustomed have many of us become to the services of these experts that they are often too readily taken for granted. In countries where clean water is not available everywhere, much ill-health is attributable to water-borne diseases.

Natural waters may contain too little iodine and too little or too much fluoride with effects discussed on page 109 Soft waters contain little or no calcium, but very hard waters may contain 200 mg calcium per litre or more and so may provide a useful proportion of the daily intake of this mineral. Communities' drinking water can sometimes become accidentally contaminated by industrial effluents such as cadmium (p. 115) and mercury (p. 114) and where the water is collected off heavily fertilised agricultural land its content of nitrate needs to be monitored because of the possibility of methaemoglobinaemia (p. 528) in bottle-fed infants.

Mineral waters
Natural springs of water with a strong odour or taste have always excited the imagination of man. From time immemorial healing powers have been attributed to such mineral waters; and indeed in more credulous times many were accredited with miraculous properties. All over the world there are watering-places and spas whither many resort to drink the waters in search of health. There is no doubt that large numbers of patients have benefited from visits to spas. Such benefit, however, can usually be attributed to a change of regime and a new and more regular habit of life rather than to any special medicinal property of the water. Indeed the mineral salts present in many spa waters are in such low concentrations as to be virtually devoid of physiological or pharmacological action.

Mineral waters contain small quantities of sodium chloride, sodium carbonate and bicarbonate, also salts of calcium and magnesium and sometimes iron or hydrogen sulphide. They are usually mildly alkaline. The total mineral content is seldom as high as 8 g/1 and is often much less. Many of these waters are naturally aerated with carbon dioxide.

The best-known waters come from France and Germany. Perrier, Contrexéville, Vichy, Apollinaris and Evian waters are bottled on a large scale and have a worldwide sale. Their pleasant sharp taste makes them refreshing to drink and for this they can be recommended. Inasmuch as their use may restrict the intake of other less desirable beverages, they may promote health.

The popular modern taste for carbonated water as a diluent or 'mix' for alcoholic drinks or fruit juices no doubt derives from the earlier taste for naturally aerated waters. 'Soda water' in its traditional siphon is simply water from any wholesome source, with carbon dioxide forced into it under pressure. It has no medicinal properties.

ALCOHOLIC DRINKS
Alcohol is a drug which depresses the higher nerve centres. Its first effect is to reduce the sense of worry and so to promote a feeling of well-being. It also loosens the imagination. Men and women come out of themselves, are more sociable and generally less intolerant of their fellow beings. For these reasons alcohol promotes good fellowship. If not abused, it is a valuable social stimulant which has been appreciated by many civilised men.

Alcohol, even in small doses, impairs the judgment and inhibits the skills necessary for fine movements. Euphoria usually prevents the subject from appreciating this loss. It is in this way that alcohol is so specially dangerous for motorists, even in small amounts. The other dangers of the misuse of alcohol are discussed in Chapter 7.

For these reasons many thoughtful people are total abstainers and advocate total abstinence for others. Of the four men who have had the greatest influence on human thought, two—Jesus Christ and Socrates—are reputed to have been wine-drinkers. The other two, Gautama Buddha and Mohammed, are said to have been abstainers. Lesser men are similarly divided, though the divisions do not always follow religious lines. Whatever one's personal views, it is important to appreciate the sincere opinions of others. We ourselves believe that alcohol has a valuable role in promoting social intercourse and thereby health. In certain circumstances alcohol is a valuable drug in the treatment of disease; it can stimulate appetite, act as a useful bedtime sedative—especially for elderly or injured people—and is a good source of energy.

From the earliest times man has used yeasts to ferment carbohydrates and so to produce ethyl alcohol (ethanol). A great variety of carbohydrate sources have been used. The best alcoholic drinks are made from fruit or cereal grains. But there are many other sources, ranging from the sap of palm trees used in Africa to the fermented milk of mares of the Tartars.

Ethanol is seldom the only product of fermentation when microorganisms grow in a carbohydrate medium; given a good supply of oxygen they generally yield acetic acid instead, with the production of vinegar. The cellulose contained in wood pulp when fermented yields a high proportion of methyl alcohol which—in contrast to ethanol—is highly toxic for man and can cause permanent blindness. Many fermented liquors contain small amounts of congeners, higher alcohols (fusel oils), aldehydes, ethers and volatile acids which can have toxic effects; they are partly responsible for the 'hangover' (Pawan, 1973). By their traditional art, the brewer, vintner and distiller—aiming at a benign and beneficent drink—generally manage to exclude these toxic products.

Beer, ale and stout
The best brews are made from malted barley. The barley grains are moistened and allowed to sprout for a few days in a warm atmosphere. This activates the enzyme diastase which begins to split the starch in the grains. At the proper moment the activity of the enzyme is stopped by heating ('malting') the sprouting grain in kilns. The temperature at which the malting is carried out determines the final appearance of the brew. For dark beers and stout (also known as 'porter' in London), the heat is sufficiently intense to produce some caramel which gives the colour. The dried malt is ground and then mixed with water to produce the 'mash'. The quality of the water is most important; the waters of Edinburgh, Dublin and Burton-on-Trent have each been the foundation on which large brewing industries have been built. The fluid from the mash is called 'wort'. The wort is boiled with the result that all further enzymic action is stopped and intruding microorganisms are killed. Generally hops are added during the boiling to impart the distinctive bitter flavour to the brew. The chemical substances responsible in the essential oil of hops are now known and synthetic iso-humulones are increasingly used, to many people's regret.

The wort, once cooled, is piped off into vats where it is inoculated with a pure culture of yeast. The maintenance of a good yeast culture is one of the most carefully guarded and unpredictable secrets of good brewing. In the making of British-type ales, selected strains of *Saccharomyces cerevisiae* and a temperature of 15–20°C are used. Much of the multiplying yeast rises to the top. In the making of lager-type beers, a cooler temperature and selected strains of *Saccharomyces carlsbergensis (uvarum)* are used. Fermentation occurs at the bottom of the vessel so that carbon dioxide rises up through the wort. Prolonged cool storage follows. This type of beer originated in Munich and *lager* is the German word for a storage cellar. When the fermentation has reached the proper stage the wort is filtered off into casks where some further fermentation may take place. Various clearing agents are usually added, such as gelatin, isinglass or tannin—sometimes with additional hops.

Most beers, ale and stout contain from 3 to 7 g ethanol/100 ml, though some 'special brews' may contain much more. Their energy value is usually between 125 and 250 kJ (30 and 60 kcal)/100 ml—about the same as milk. But they differ from milk in that they contain no protein, fat or useful amounts of calcium. The only vitamins present in beer are small amounts of nicotinic acid and riboflavin. The Food Standards Committee (1977) *Report on Beer* is recommended for a readable introduction to the science of making beer.

Country beers and toddies
In many parts of the world country beers are made by fermenting cereals such as maize, millets or rice. Where palm trees grow, toddy can be made by fermenting the sweet sap. In Japan sake is made from rice, in Mexico pulque from the agave plant, and in Africa beers are usually made from sorghum. Wild yeasts are generally used for the fermentations. Such beers and toddies are usually produced for their intoxicating effects. Their alcohol content varies greatly, and they may contain as little as 1 g or as much as 7 g/100 ml. This alcohol is, of course, a source of energy, and country beers and toddies may also contain thiamin, riboflavin, nicotinic acid and ascorbic acid in amounts which are nutritionally significant. Thus these beverages are sometimes useful foods. Platt (1955) has given an interesting account of the alcoholic drinks traditional amongst indigenous Africans. In some villages, excessive amounts are drunk and this may be responsible for much poverty and ill-health. Elsewhere, the beer may be a valuable supplementary food and a useful 'cement' to the cultural life of the village. In Africa, as elsewhere, alcoholism is an old problem, but reformers should not condemn these country beers hastily, without a knowledge of the social circumstances and the amounts of alcohol and vitamins usually derived from them by the local people.

Mead, cider, country 'wines'

Mead made from honey was perhaps the first alcoholic drink. Homer and the writers of the Norse sagas were familiar with it. The Roman conquerors of Britain tried hard to introduce wine in its place; relics of their efforts remain in the terraced hillsides overlooking the Severn river. Wine-making continued on a small scale in the mediaeval monasteries in order to provide for the Eucharist. But in our cold and uncongenial climate, the only fruit that could be depended on to produce fermentable sugars was the apple. Cider made from fermented apple juice was the *vin ordinaire* of the British.

A few people in Britain still make their own home brews, such as elderberry, cowslip and dandelion 'wine'. The wild yeasts present in these materials, mixed with raisins or some other good source of sugar, generally produce a benign and sometimes potent brew.

Wines

The grape is unique among fruits in that no additional sugars need be added to enable wild yeasts present on the fruit to carry out a satisfactory fermentation. In the making of wine the French are pre-eminent; the great clarets, sauternes, burgundies and champagnes—Château Lafite, Châteu d'Yquem, Richebourg, Veuve Clicquot—are names to conjure with. Then there are the German wines of the Rhine and Moselle—the Schloss Johannisberg and Berncastler Doktor. All these are the proper delight and solace of civilised Europeans. Other countries also produce some fine wines and every gourmet has his favourite. Italian, Greek, Hungarian, South African, Australian, Chilean and Californian wines all have their special virtues. Taken with a meal they are excellent adjuvants to appetite.

An admirable account of the making of wines and of their individual qualities has been provided by Marrison (1957). *The World Atlas of Wine* (Johnson, 1971) gives maps and descriptions of the vineyards from which the world's wines are produced.

But there is also a dark side to the story of wine. In the grape-growing areas of the world *vin ordinaire* is the common drink of the people and is used to quench thirst. Two wine-growing countries, France and Italy, have the highest alcohol consumption in the world and also a high incidence of cirrhosis of the liver. Natural wines contain 8 to 13 g of ethanol/100 ml and some unfermented sugars, but no other nutrients in significant amounts. One bottle (650 ml) of *vin ordinaire* provides about 1.9 MJ (450 kcal). They may also contribute to iron overload (p. 103).

French wines contain very variable amounts of histamine—from 0.1 mg/l in the best champagnes to 30 mg/l in some burgundies. As little as 20 µg of histamine if injected intravenously produces headache and it is possible that histamine contributes to the after effects of too much cheap wine.

Fortified wines, such as sherry, port and madeira, have alcohol added to raise the concentration up to 20 g/100 ml.

Spirits

The art of concentrating ethanol by distillation from fermented liquors was probably discovered by one of the great Arabian physicians despite their traditional abstinence. The word 'alcohol' is derived from the Arabic—*al Kohl* (the powder). Most likely it was first prescribed solely as a drug.

The number and variety of distilled spirits used by modern man is legion. Only the most notable can be mentioned here.

Whisky. The name derives from the Gaelic *uisgebeatha* (water of life) and certainly much of life in the Scottish Highlands still revolves round it. In a similar way the French call brandy *eau-de-vie*, the Italians *acquavite*, whilst the Danes call their spirits *akvavit*.

Most Scotch whisky now on sale is 'blended' from a mixture of pot-stilled 'malt' whisky with 'patent-still' grain spirit. The unique flavour and aroma of pure malt whisky is probably due to the fact that the wort from which it is distilled is made from barley, malted over peat fires. The method of distillation in potstills—based on the principle of the alchemists' retort—also adds something to its quality. Potentially toxic substances present in the first distillate and those remaining in the pot are discarded. Pure malt whisky is the best way to 'treat' a Highlander.

Patent 'Coffey-still' whisky is produced by spraying wort into a tall wooden chamber into which superheated steam is introduced from below. The various alcohol-containing fractions are drawn off by pipes placed at different levels in the chamber. The alcohol so produced forms the body of most exported 'Scotch'.

The best Scotch is matured for at least seven years in oak casks which have previously contained sherry. From them it acquires the characteristic colour and loses its initial rawness by esterification of its higher alcohols.

The strength of a whisky is generally stated in terms of 'proof'. 'Proof' spirit is traditionally of such a strength that gunpowder will ignite when mixed with it in a teaspoon. Nowadays the meaning of 'proof' is more precisely defined. At 51° F proof spirit contains 57.07 per cent alcohol by volume or 48.24 per cent by weight. Whisky sold in Great Britain is almost uniformly 70 per cent proof, i.e. the alcoholic strength is approximately 30 per cent. A standard bottle of whisky containing 700 ml therefore provides about 230 g of ethanol, which at 30 kJ/g amounts to 6.9 MJ (1600 kcal). But apart from its energy value, whisky has no other purely nutritional virtues.

Other whiskies. *Irish.* Irish whiskey has much the same qualities as Scotch, though most is kept for home consumption and little is exported. 'Poteen' is the traditional name for the product of the illicit stills, at one time commonly hidden in the hills.

Bourbon. This is 'the water of life' for gentlemen of Scottish ancestry living in the Southern States of the USA. It was first produced in Bourbon County, Kentucky. The mash consists chiefly of maize ('corn') to which some malted barley or wheat is added. Originally it was matured in casks that had been used to import molasses. Nowadays the casks are deliberately burnt on the inside to reproduce the traditional flavour.

Rye. Rye whiskey is made in Canada and the USA. The brands are distilled from mashes of combinations of cereals, including rye.

Other distilled spirits. *Brandy.* 'Une fine champagne'—a brandy distilled from champagne grapes—is the perfect ending to a gourmet's meal. No other distilled spirit has such a fine aroma or is prepared with so much care. The names of Cognac and Armagnac, the two producing areas, are justly celebrated by *bon-viveurs* throughout the world.

Rum. Molasses provide the carbohydrate from which this distilled spirit is prepared. It was the crude drink of those who had traffic among the sugar-cane growing islands of the West Indies, such as British sailors and New England slavers. Nowadays some well-matured and gentle rums are produced.

Gin. This is essentially a Dutch drink. It arrived in Britain when William of Orange succeeded to the British throne at the end of the seventeenth century. Properly made, it is an almost pure aqueous solution of ethanol, derived from a variety of sources, but deliberately flavoured by the addition of various vegetable agents, of which juniper (*genièvre* in French—hence 'Geneva') is the principal ingredient. Gin thus differs from the spirits so far mentioned in that its flavour is due to additives rather than the materials from which it is made. In eighteenth-century Britain almost any crude distilled spirit was cheaply and freely sold as 'gin' with tragic consequences to the desperate inhabitants of the verminous city slums. Nowadays gin is a civilised drink and the heart of a good cocktail.

Vodka. This is another neutral spirit distilled from fermented rye or potatoes. Vodka is the nearest to pure aqueous ethanol of all these beverages, colourless and contains very little congeners. It is the standard liquor of the Russians, but has lately been adopted in the West. It may yet help to smooth out differences of opinion!

Calvados. This is the traditional liquor of the Celts in the westermost parts of France. It is made by distilling cider which in turn is made from apples. A similar liquor is called 'applejack' in the USA. Vermont farmers make it for their own use, not by distillation, but by leaving the cider barrels outside in the depth of winter. The unnecessary water in the barrels turns to ice, but the ethanol-containing fraction—having a lower freezing point—can be siphoned off into smaller barrels. This process is repeated at each

major frost. Thus a hard winter produces a real 'hard' liquor.

Slibovitz. This is a distinctive drink made in Yugoslavia by distilling fermented plums.

Ouzo. In Greece may be any kind of spirit with added flavourings.

Arak. Once out of Europe or North America the names of distilled liquors and their origins become confused. The word *arak* or *raki* applies throughout most of the East to any distilled spirit. It is usually made by distilling 'toddies' produced from fermented palm sap and can be very toxic.

Liqueurs. For centuries monks and other skilled people have worked to produce the perfect ending to a good meal. The best French brandy has obvious pride of place, but after it follow the great liqueurs, made by adding sugar to ethanol, with secret and subtle flavouring agents.

Table 21.1 gives the alcohol content and energy value of alcoholic beverages commonly taken in Britain today.

HERBS AND SPICES

In all parts of the world herbs and spices are used to flavour food and so make it more attractive and appetising. Large numbers of plants have been cultivated for this purpose. Their flavour resides in essential oils, or oleo resins, often in specialised parts of the plant. In Britain in the Middle Ages, mint, balm and basil, sage and thyme, chives, garlic and fennel, marjoram, horse radish, parsley and rosemary were grown in herb gardens. Rosengarten (1969) defines herbs as aromatic products from temperate regions and spices as the exotic products of tropical lands. Herbs are usually leafy and spices often seeds, fruit or flower parts, bark or roots. In tropical countries, chillies, turmeric, coriander seeds, pimento, cumin, pepper, capsicum, cinnamon, cloves, nutmeg, vanilla and ginger are grown and commonly used. From time immemorial there has been a profitable trade in spices between the East and Europe.

In any part of the world, even in the poorest homes, it is unusual to find neither condiments nor spices. They are essential to the culinary art and promote appetite, good feeding and thus health. In communities without refrigerators herbs and spices may have some preservative action on meat and certainly counteract the taste of spoiled or monotonous food. Several such as cardamon, dill, peppermint and anise have a carminative action, helping to bring up wind after a heavy meal. Nevertheless they have little direct nutritional value. Individual daily intakes in India may vary from 7 to 30 g. The energy value and protein content of this is negligible. Some condiments such as green chillies are rich in ascorbic acid (100 mg/100 g); they may contribute significantly to the ascorbic acid content of the diet. Most herbs and spices contain the B group of vitamins and minerals such as calcium and iron in appreci-

Table 21.1 Alcohol content, sugar and energy value of common alcoholic beverages (Paul and Southgate, 1978)

	Alcohol g/dl	Sugars g/dl	Energy kJ (kcal)/dl	
Beers				
Brown ale, bottled	2.2	3.0	117	(28)
Draught ale, mild	2.6	1.6	104	(25)
Draught ale, bitter	3.1	2.3	132	(32)
Lager, bottled	3.2	1.5	120	(29)
Strong ale	6.6	6.1	301	(72)
Ciders				
Dry	3.8	2.6	152	(36)
Sweet	3.7	4.3	176	(42)
Vintage	10.5	7.3	421	(101)
Wines				
Red	9.5	0.3	284	(68)
White, dry	9.1	0.6	275	(66)
White, sweet	10.2	5.9	394	(94)
Champagne	9.9	1.4	315	(76)
Fortified wines				
Sherry, dry	15.7	1.4	481	(116)
Sherry, sweet	15.6	6.9	568	(136)
Port	15.9	12.0	655	(157)
Spirits (70 per cent proof)				
Brandy, gin, rum, whisky	31.7	trace	919	(222)

able concentrations, but the quantities eaten are too small to be significant.

Some herbs contain substances which are poisonous to man. Most of these are well known locally and tradition assures that they are avoided. Toxic effects of nutmeg, wormwood oil and Worcester sauce are described on page 222. In Jamaica herbal teas may be responsible for liver disease (p. 413).

In industrial countries natural flavouring agents are being replaced to a considerable extent by artificial chemical ones. A variety of artificial sauces is a feature of the table in most cheap restaurants and indeed in many homes.

22. Food Processing

Many species of animals collect and store food, but only *Homo sapiens* processes it. He has acquired techniques for preserving and cooking his food and developed arts which give it taste and flavour. The techniques of food processing use both physical and chemical methods, the application of heat and the addition of salt being prototypes. Any chemical that is added to a food deliberately for any of the above purposes is known as a food additive. This chapter describes some of the benefits from food processing. The next three chapters describe how adverse effects may arise in the course of food processing; these are loss of nutritive value, and the introduction of pathogenic organisms and toxic substances. These chapters are followed by one entitled 'Consumer protection', which describes methods used to ensure that foods purchased in shops and markets are, as far as possible, both safe and nutritious.

DEVELOPMENT OF FOOD TECHNOLOGY

Apart from fruits and salads, man seldom eats food that is fresh and raw. The preservation, preparation and cooking of foods are domestic arts, which have been practised since before the time that man learnt to write and to record his history. The study of the utensils used for these purposes, which have been found at prehistoric sites of human habitations, is an important part of archaeology. Meat, fish and fruits were preserved by drying, vegetables by pickling, and many foods by salting. Excess milk was converted into cheese, and barley was malted and brewed into beer. The basic arts of cooking (boiling, roasting, baking and frying) have been practised since time immemorial. The use of herbs and spices as flavouring agents is also very ancient, and natural colouring agents, e.g. cochineal, have been used for a long time to make foods appear pleasing to the eye. In the traditional farmhouses of Europe, the farmer's wife processed and prepared a large variety of foods.

The industrial revolution drew large numbers of people into towns, away from the countryside where their food was grown. Women were increasingly employed in factories and offices and so were less available for their traditional roles of preparing food in the home. At the same time, many new chemicals and physical processes were introduced, e.g. refrigeration on a large scale. In industrialised countries between 1850 and 1950 a steadily increasing proportion of food was prepared in factories and after 1950 the food industry expanded rapidly. In the United Kingdom in 1970, it employed 8.1 per cent of the population in industry, a proportion exceeded only by the construction industry, mechanical engineering and electrical engineering. Supermarkets selling ready prepared foods and precooked meals increasingly continue to replace the shops of traditional grocers, greengrocers, butchers and fishmongers. In the USA in 1975, about 40 per cent of all meals, whether eaten in the home, in restaurants or in food service-stations, were prepared and cooked outside the home. This proportion is likely to increase. The preparation of food has become food technology, which is based on food sciences.

New foods have been developed which serve as substitutes for traditional foods that may have become scarce or too expensive. Margarine is the classical example. Margarines are an acceptable alternative to butter (p. 197); they are fortified with vitamins A and D, and some contain large amounts of polyunsaturated fatty acids, which are almost absent from butter. Meat substitutes, prepared from novel proteins of vegetable origin (p. 192), are rapidly becoming acceptable alternatives in many meat dishes. Many new food preparations play a big part in the diets of infants and young children.

The food industry is, however, not without its critics. There is a large and widespread demand for **health foods**, and there are advocates for compost-grown vegetables and free-range chickens. Such people believe that fresh foods and those grown without the use of artificial fertilisers have mysterious beneficial properties. If you are lucky enough to be asked to dinner by a friend in the country, you may be given chicken from his backyard, new potatoes, peas and pears picked in his garden that morning. He may tell you that the supermarket sells nothing that tastes so good. He may well be right and it would be ungracious to argue. You have enjoyed a luxury. Yet the supermarket foods are also good, can be enjoyed all the year round and are generally cheaper. That canned foods are nutritious is shown by an experiment carried out many years ago by Godden and Thomson (1959). For 18 months they fed one colony of rats entirely on canned foods and another colony on foods brought fresh from shops or grown locally. The growth of the animals, their breeding performance and the chemical composition of their bones, teeth and soft tissues were the same in the two colonies. There was no indication that dependence on canned foods had any adverse effects on health. A similar conclusion can be drawn from the excellent health of several Antarctic expeditions whose members have lived entirely on processed foods for many months.

A food industry is essential to feed the large population of modern towns, whose needs could not be met from markets of the traditional rural type. Further, the food industry continues to grow and is commercially successful because most consumers like its products. In prosperous countries people living in rural areas choose to eat much the same foods as those living in towns. The advantages of modern processed foods are numerous. First, their use greatly reduces the domestic work involved in preparing traditional dishes, and many products are aptly referred to as **convenience foods**; the use of such foods transfers some of a housewife's chores from the home to the factory. Secondly, they provide consumers with a much more varied choice of foods than formerly and choice is no longer restricted by the seasons of the year. Some foods which were once eaten only by the wealthy or on special occasions are now commonplace articles of diet, for example oranges, tomatoes and poultry. Travellers and those who work in foreign countries can in most places obtain foods from their native land and may, if they wish and have the money, feed as they would if they were at home.

FOOD PRESERVATION

Fresh foods may be decomposed by autolysis due to the lytic enzymes which they contain and by the action of putrefactive bacteria and fungi, the spores of which abound in the atmosphere. The ancient methods of food preservation—heating, drying, salting and pickling—are still the basis of modern food technology. Perhaps the most important new factor in determining present diets is the great developments in domestic and commercial refrigeration. In Britain in 1974, 84 per cent of households had a refrigerator and 15 per cent a deep freezer. Canning of food was successfully carried out early in the nineteenth century and has evolved slowly and steadily. The range of foods that are now preserved in cans or in plastic and other synthetic packets is very large, and developments in packaging make many more foods available to consumers.

Chemical preservatives
Sodium chloride, acetic acid, ethyl alcohol and sucrose are preservatives which have been used in the home for generations. Their value is undisputed and they are much used in industry. In the nineteenth century new chemicals were introduced; many of these, such as borate and formaldehyde, have been discarded as they were shown to be potentially toxic in the amounts used. Table 22.1 lists permitted preservatives in the UK. Certain salts and altern-

Table 22.1 Permitted preservatives (UK Preservatives in Food Regulations 1975)

Benzoic acid	Sodium nitrite
Methyl 4-hydroxybenzoate	2-Hydroxybiphenyl
Ethyl 4-hydroxybenzoate	Propionic acid
Propyl 4-hydroxybenzoate	Sorbic acid
Biphenyl	Sulphur dioxide
Nisin	2-(Thiazol-4-yl) benzimidazole
Sodium nitrate	Hexamine

ative forms of these substances are also permitted. Other countries have similar but not necessarily identical lists. As described in Chapter 25, legislation controls the concentrations of permitted preservatives and ensures a wide margin of safety. Permitted concentrations are usually less than one-hundredth of that which might have toxic effects. Sulphur dioxide and the hydroxybenzoates are the most used preservatives and are frequently added to fruit and vegetable products, beer, meat products, sauces and spices. Propionic acid is used mainly for bread and flour confectionery. Sodium nitrate and nitrite are used in cured meats, including bacon and ham, but are not permitted in most other foods.

Although preservation by chemical means is often satisfactory, in general it is better to use physical methods such as heat and refrigeration.

Irradiation of food
Putrefactive bacteria and pathogenic organisms are readily killed by radiation, and hence foods can be preserved and sterilised in this way. As irradiation can be carried out in bulk on packaged foods, this method would have great commercial advantages. However, its use is forbidden in several countries including the UK, although individual foods may be exempted from the ban under very specific conditions. The ban is due to the possibility that irradiation might produce a cytotoxic or mutagenic agent. A Ministry of Health Working Party (1964), whose report led to legislation, commented: 'The treatment of food by irradiation is as new and strange to most people as the cooking of food must have been to our early forefathers. At present the evidence that food treated by irradiation is never harmful is not so complete as might ideally be required, but had we assembled at the Dawn of Time to consider the safety of cooked foods the available evidence would have been much less satisfactory and indeed is still incomplete'. This conservative approach has not changed in Britain despite the fact that an expert international committee (FAO/WHO, 1977) found no evidence that irradiated food was not wholesome.

In at least 18 countries irradiation is now permitted for a restricted list of food items. In the Netherlands these number 14 and in the USSR nine, but in most countries, including the USA, it is restricted to potatoes and one or two other foods (Vas, 1977). The process is not yet applied widely, but, with the lifting of legal restrictions and international assurances of its safety, it may become generally accepted.

COOKING

Most foods of animal origin could probably be digested raw by man but raw meats are unpalatable and seldom consumed; yet in a crisis a hungry man will readily eat the raw flesh of any beast, bird or fish. The cooking of meat makes it easy to chew and so allows the digestive juices a more rapid access to the protein. The heat of cooking coagulates the muscle proteins, which actually thus become less readily digested by proteolytic enzymes *in vitro*. But the tough collagen fibres of connective tissues are converted by heat into gelatin and this increases the tenderness of the meat. The elastic tissue in tendons and sinews is insoluble and virtually indigestible.

Fruits and green vegetables may be eaten raw in limited amounts. Cereals, roots and legumes, however, cannot easily be digested by man unless cooked. Most plant cells are surrounded by a rough cellulose wall which is little disrupted by mastication and through which the digestive enzymes cannot readily pass. The heat in cooking causes the starch within the cells to swell. This bursts the cell walls, and the starch and other nutrients within become accessible to digestive enzymes. Cooking improves the nutritive value of legumes such as soya beans and groundnuts by destroying trypsin inhibitors.

Cooking is, of course, much more than making food more digestible through the action of heat. Ingredients have to be mixed to give the product the correct texture; some foods have to be firm and crisp, others smooth, bland and fluid. Tenderness and succulence are important and above all taste and flavour. A good cook can achieve all these aims using as ingredients only natural foods from the countryside and two artificially purified chemicals, sodium chloride and sucrose. This is seldom practical except in remote rural areas. Elsewhere many ingredients and foods are products of the food industry and contain chemicals added by manufacturers which facilitate a cook's work and improve the quality of the meal when it is served.

Cooks use the same processes whether they are preparing foods at home or in the kitchen of a restaurant or in the plant of large food manufacturer. Methods vary according to the scale of the operation, but fundamental principles are the same.

FOOD ADDITIVES

The food industry could not provide us with satisfactory food products without using a large number of chemical additives. The types of additives needed and the benefits that they provide are set out in a small monograph *Why Additives?* produced by the British Nutrition Foundation (1977). Here we give only a brief outline of the main classes of additive. In Chapter 25 the principles of testing additives are described and the reasons why some additives formerly used are no longer permitted. Chapter 26 gives a brief account of the legal and other measures that protect consumers against possible dangers.

Preservatives
Chemicals which are permitted preservatives have already been listed in Table 22.1.

Colouring agents
The art of cooking includes making food attractive to the eye. Cooks have long been familiar with some natural colouring agents such as cochineal (from crushed insects), caramel (from burnt sugar) and saffron (a plant pigment). Tomatoes, parsley, mustard and cress and cherries are used to give colour to a dish. It would be difficult nowadays to sell a food product unless the colour was pleasing. This applies especially to cakes and sweets. Large numbers of organic dyes have been used to colour foods. Many have been discarded after prolonged tests have shown that they may cause cancers in experimental animals. Thirty-one colours, which have been shown to be harmless in exhaustive animal tests, are permitted colouring matter under the UK Colouring Matter in Food Regulation 1973 (amended 1976) and may be added to foods. Most of these are synthetic organic dyes, but products of natural origin such as chlorophyl, caramel, several carotenoids and beetroot red are included. The Regulations also state permitted concentrations. Other countries have similar but not identical lists.

Flavouring agents
The flavour of most common fruits and many vegetables may be mimicked by synthetic chemicals. Examples are benzaldehyde, *n*-propyl acetate and diethyl sulphite with the flavour of almond, pear and peppermint respectively. Such substances are much used in the food industry, particularly in the manufacture of sweets. Monosodium glutamate, the salt of a natural amino acid, is also much used because it brings out the flavour of the meat in stews, meat pies, etc. Hence it is an ingredient of many sauces.

Flavouring agents make up the largest number of permitted food additives. Over 2000 are on the EEC list. The reasons why there are so many are: (1) these are mostly extracted or synthesised natural flavour components or closely related chemically, (2) natural food flavours consist of many different chemical components, and (3) the amounts concerned are minute and varied.

Sweetening agents
Sucrose from cane or beet is the classical sweetener but, as

it is a rich source of energy, intake has to be restricted especially by persons liable to put on weight. Of artificial sweeteners saccharin is the most used; it is 400 times as sweet as sucrose and provides no extra energy. Diabetic patients and weight-watchers sweeten their drinks with it, but it is not used extensively by the food industry because it is destroyed by heat. Cyclamate, which is 30 times as sweet as sucrose, is heat-resistant and formerly provided an alternative to sugar in pastries, canned foods, jellies, sauces pickles and other foods. Its use was banned in 1969 in the USA, UK and other countries, following a report that some rats receiving very large doses had developed tumours of the urinary bladder. There are those who think that the ban was inadvisable, as the benefit derived from cyclamate far outweighed the possible hazard from the amounts likely to be consumed by any individual. The dipeptide L-aspartyl-L-phenylalanine, aspartame, is 180 times sweeter than sugar; it is broken down in the body to its two constituent amino acids, which are then metabolised in the normal way. In 1974 its use as a food additive was approved in the USA but with certain restrictions.

The search for new sweeteners goes on. The fruit of the climbing vine *Dioscoreophyllum cumminsii*, which grows in tropical forests, contains a substance reported to be 1500 times sweeter than sucrose (Inglett and May, 1969). It is known as the serendipity berry. As yet it has not found a place in western diets.

Emulsifiers and stabilising agents
A number of substances, of which the best known is glyceryl monostearate, are used in the manufacture of cakes, ice-cream and salad creams. They enable fats to be used more economically, and act by allowing fat to be emulsified with more water and by making the emulsions more stable. Glyceryl monostearate is a normal product of digestion in the human small intestine.

Antioxidants
Most natural fats and oils contain substances which prevent the slow oxidative changes leading to rancidity. The best known of these are the tocopherols (vitamin E). Such substances may be removed or destroyed in manufacturing processes. Hence artificial antioxidants are added to the refined products in order to prevent rancidity. Fats used for making biscuits and cakes often contain gallic acid or butylated hydroxyanisole (BHA) or butylated hydroxytoluene (BHT) added for this purpose. Antioxidants are important in the oils used for frying potato crisps.

Flour improvers
These have an effect on the rheological properties of doughs and batters similar to what occurs when flour is stored for some weeks. They are said to 'strengthen' the flour and allow the baking of bread which is well risen and stays fresh longer. For this purpose chlorine dioxide is added to flour used for making bread in the UK and USA. L-Cysteine hydrochloride is an improver added to flour for making cakes. Benzoyl peroxide may be used as a bleaching agent for white flour.

Miscellaneous food additives
Acids give a sour or tart taste and in some foods are needed to achieve the optimal pH for technical purposes. They are compounds which occur in nature, such as citric, tartaric or malic acids or hydrochloric.

Humectants prevent foods from drying out. Sorbitol and glycerine are examples.

Thickeners, including pectins, vegetable gums and gelatins, give foods their uniform texture and desired consistency, as in ice-cream.

Polyphosphates are used to process meats, especially poultry meat and fish, because some taste panels have found that this improves the flavour of the product and makes it more tender and juicy. Many manufacturers do not use phosphates as they are not satisfied that these confer benefits. The treatment carries no toxicological hazard, but inevitably increases the water content of the product.

Micronutrients are sometimes added to restore losses during processing. Some manufacturers add ascorbic acid to dehydrated potato powder or to fruit-based drinks. Enrichment of foods with nutrients is discussed on page 483. A number of food additives used mainly for technical reasons have nutritional value as an incidental bonus, e.g. vitamin E and ascorbic acid as antioxidants, and sugars and organic acids are sources of energy.

23. Losses of Food and Nutrients in Food Processing

WASTAGE

Physiologists who attempt to assess human needs for nutrients naturally use as their data measurements of amounts of food that are actually eaten. On the other hand the data for administrators, whose duty it is to see that a country or district has sufficient food to satisfy requirements, are the statistics of the size of the crops in the fields and of the amounts of food in the holds of ships in the ports and in trucks at the frontiers. These two sets of data cannot be directly compared, for it is inevitable that a proportion of the crop in a field or of a cargo of food in a ship is never eaten but is wasted.

In some countries, two sets of figures should be available for annual food consumption. Food moving into consumption is derived from records of foodstuffs leaving the farms and arriving in the ports, less the food that is exported; this is divided by the population and the number of days in the year. Then there are measurements of actual consumption of samples of families or individuals. For example, in Britain for the five years 1972–76 the food moving into consumption daily per head of population ranged between 12.2–12.8 MJ (2910 and 3060 kcal) with an additional 0.59–0.67 MJ (140–160 kcal) from alcohol. Together they add up to 12.8–13.5 MJ (3070–3200 kcal). However, over the same period the National Food Survey showed that the food brought into the home in a large sample of families averaged 9.6–10.4 MJ (2290–2490 kcal)/head, excluding alcohol and meals consumed outside the home. The weighted physiological requirement for energy calculated from the 1969 recommended daily intakes (p. 152) for the different categories of people in the UK is 9.7 MJ (2325 kcal) per person. This is only 74 per cent of the food moving into consumption. Thus about 25 per cent of food leaving the farms and imported is unaccounted for. There is no reason to suppose that the gap would be smaller in any other industrial country. Some is eaten in catering establishments. Where does the rest of this food go?

It is not possible to give exact figures partly because this is an unglamorous and neglected field of research. Losses of food vary greatly with the food and the circumstances. The Ministry of Agriculture, Fisheries and Food has set up a Food Waste survey unit to try and obtain more figures. In the meantime a small book by Roy (1976) sketches an outline. He suggests that **waste** should be used for a potential source of food that has, knowingly, been discarded or destroyed (kitchen scraps, food not sold in shops or restaurants and food discarded in factories) while **loss** is used for potential food that has inadvertently been destroyed or spoiled, e.g. stored grain eaten by rats, meat spoiled by bacterial growth and nutrients destroyed or going into solution in vegetable canning. These suggested usages seem sensible but are not yet generally adopted; there are overtones of guilt to the word 'waste'. If we start at the farm gate or port, food may be lost during storage. In Britain this is small for milk and cereals but about 10 per cent for potatoes and more for some vegetables. Some potential food is wasted in processing e.g. parts of vegetables and fruit, trimmings of meat and fish, whey in making cheese and blood in abattoirs. Food is also wasted in markets and shops, particularly fruit and vegetables.

Once the food has been brought into the premises where it will be cooked and eaten, waste can occur in the kitchen, from food not used during serving and from food left on the plate. In large-scale catering like school meals overall losses are usually about 10 per cent but caterers are often reluctant or unable to discuss detailed figures. Larger losses are to be expected in expensive restaurants and in hospitals. Platt et al. (1963) in a classic study of hospital catering found 25 to 35 per cent of food sent from the kitchen was leftover in serving dishes, and plate waste averaged an additional 10 per cent.

In the home, plate waste should be less. Dowler (1977) made a small study of 25 households in London over 7 days, measuring the nitrogen, fat and energy in all leftover food. The mean loss of energy was 4 per cent, of protein 4 per cent and of fat 6 per cent with ranges from 0.5 to 14 per cent. Meat fat and children's leavings were the main sources of waste. Wenlock and Buss (1977) report a similar average of 5 per cent of the energy of the food used, or 6 per cent counting food fed to pets or wild birds, in the homes of 52 civil servants who volunteered to collect all waste for analysis over a week. The range of waste was from 2 to 22 per cent. Wasted food contained more fat, 55 per cent as against 44 per cent of fat in the total food used.

When an investigator is scrutinising a family in this way its behaviour is likely to be distorted. Harrison et al. (1975) of the Anthropology Department at the University of Arizona therefore set up a Garbage Project, in which they examined household refuse in Tucson 'as a non reactive measure of behaviour', a sort of instant archaeology. Households in 1974 threw on average $100 worth of food into their garbage bins. More meat, fish and vegetables were discarded than other foods. Average estimates of waste of different types of food ranged from 1 to 12 per cent. Food poured down the drain, put on compost heaps or fed to household pets was not counted.

In communities living at or near the hunger level there is virtually no waste. Anyone who has been a prisoner-of-war can relate elaborate precautions taken to prevent any loss of the meagre rations and may describe how men habitually licked their plates clean. Similarly in many poor homes, especially in Africa and Asia, nothing is wasted. In a survey of 5000 households in Madagascar, waste in the home was estimated to be for rice 3.4 per cent, for maize 5.6 per cent, for manioca 1.6 per cent, for sweet potato 3.2 per cent and for bananas 0.3 per cent.

Food fed to pets
In the USA it has been estimated that 22 million dogs and 30 million cats eat food equivalent to 5 per cent of the total human energy requirement and 14 per cent of the protein requirement. In Britain 4.8 million dogs and nearly 5 million cats may eat 3 per cent of human energy requirement and 2 per cent of protein requirement. In 1970 the pet-food market was estimated to be worth one billion dollars in the USA and £40 million in Britain. It would be improper to suggest that this food was wasted and some of it would legally be 'unfit for human consumption'. Yet these rough estimates do indicate that a significant proportion of the food supplies available for man are diverted to another use in these countries.

LOSSES OF NUTRIENTS DURING FOOD PROCESSING AND COOKING

Wastages of food are obvious to all who witness them, if seldom measured. They are the responsibility of the community, the management or the individual. Invisible chemical losses of nutrients that occur during food processing and cooking are the special responsibility of, and common ground between, nutritionists and food scientists.

PROTEINS, FAT AND CARBOHYDRATES
Many changes in the chemical structure of molecules of proteins, fats and carbohydrates are brought about by heat; some of these may diminish nutritive value, others may lead to the formation of potentially toxic substances. In general there is little difference except in scale between heating processes in industry, in catering and in traditional domestic preservation and preparation of food.

Proteins
The flavour and aroma of roast meat and the golden-brown crust of freshly baked bread are delicious but the complicated chemical reaction underlying these culinary delights reduce the availability of one or more essential amino acids in the food protein. This is the Maillard reaction between reducing sugars and amino acids (Fig. 23.1). In food proteins most amino groups are taken up in peptide bonds, but there are free ϵ amino groups on the dibasic lysine and these may react with sugars and the amino acid is then no longer biologically available. With mild heat treatment causing only a little browning the loss of available lysine is small; but with severe heat, causing pronounced browning, it may be large and accompanied by small reductions of availability of other amino acids (Hurrell and Carpenter, 1977). During the baking of bread, biscuits and breakfast cereals, 10 to 15 per cent of the available lysine is lost; spray-drying of skimmed milk reduces it less than 10 per cent but roller-drying can produce losses up to 40 per cent. The total lysine, measured by amino acid column chromatography, after hydrolysis of the protein may be little changed. Deterioration in nutritive values of the protein

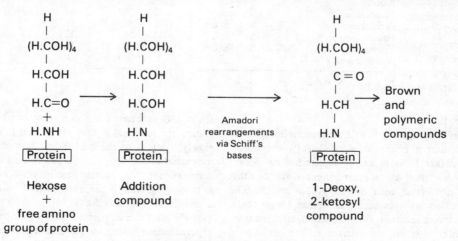

Fig. 23.1 Simplified outline of the Maillard reaction.

can be assessed by biological measurements (p. 41) in animals or man but these are expensive and take time. Available lysine can, however, be measured by microbiological assay with *Tetrahemena* or, more simply, by a chemical method using fluorodinitrobenzene (Hurrell and Carpenter, 1975).

Fats

Changes occur in frying oils and fats when they are used repeatedly or overheated. Part of the fatty acids are oxidised or form cyclic compounds or polymers. Artman and Smith (1972) found 136 monomeric components by multiple chromatography in cottonseed oil that had been heated for 8 hours on 6 days. Most of these are present in tiny amounts and the question arises whether any of them have deleterious biological effects. Overheated or 'abused' frying oils depress the growth of rats. The responsible component is in fatty acids which do not form adduct compounds with urea, the non-urea adduct forming acids (Perkins, 1960). There is also some loss of linoleic acid and of vitamin E when oils are used for frying. All these changes can be minimised by avoiding high temperatures, frying for short times and not repeatedly using an oil. Antioxidants are often incorporated in oils used to manufacture snack foods. Olive oil has a reputation for quality in cooking. Unrefined olive oil does not undergo oxidative deterioration on moderate heating. Morton (1977) find that a minor sterol in the unsaponifiable fraction, Δ^5-avenasterol acts as a natural antioxidant.

VITAMINS AND MINERALS

Losses occur in two ways. First, nutrients may be leached out of the tissues of either plant or animal foods and discarded in the cooking water. Losses of minerals and water-soluble vitamins may result. Secondly, heat may destroy some of the vitamins present.

Table 23.1 summarises the lability or stability of selected vitamins in different conditions. The most sensitive vitamins are ascorbic acid, folate and thiamin but losses of riboflavin, vitamin A, pyridoxine, vitamin B_{12} and vitamin E occur in particular conditions. Nicotinic acid is the most stable of the vitamins and information about vitamin D is incomplete.

Ascorbic acid

Losses in the kitchen may be large and significant. It is readily oxidised and, if this proceeds beyond the stage of dehydro- ascorbic acid, all vitamin activity is permanently lost. Oxidation may be accelerated by enzymic action, by heat, by an alkaline medium, by traces of copper and by free access to atmospheric oxygen. These facts have practical application in preserving and cooking food.

In most plant tissues there is an enzyme, ascorbic acid oxidase, which is separated from ascorbic acid in the intact cells. When leaves or fruits are bruised, pounded or chopped, cell structures are damaged and the enzyme gains access to the vitamin and begins to destroy it. However, the enzyme is rapidly inactivated at temperatures of 60° C and above. The destruction of ascorbic acid is minimal when

Table 23.1 Stability of selected vitamins in different conditions (based on van der Meer, 1972)

	pH <7	pH ±7	O_2	Light	Heat	Metals	Reducing agents
β-Carotene	L	S	L	L	L		
Thiamin	S	L	L	S/L	L	L	L
Riboflavin	S	S	S	L	S/L	L	L
Nicotinic acid	S	S	S	S	S	L	
Pyridoxine	S	S	S/L	L	S	S	L
Folate	L	S	S/L	L	S/L		L
Vitamin B_{12}	S/L	S	S/L	L	S/L		L
Ascorbic acid	S	L	L	L	L	L	S

L, labile;   S, stable.

Carbohydrate

The effects of heating on carbohydrates are predominantly beneficial in that it breaks down cell walls, solubilises starch and makes it more easily digested. Raw potato starch produces lethal caecal enlargement in rats but this effect does not occur with heated potato starch. The Maillard reaction involves sugars as well as amino acids. Another browning reaction, caramelisation, affects sugars alone and fructose is the most sensitive. The loss of food energy from this is negligible with a careful cook.

fruits and vegetables are immediately placed in boiling water, but maximal if they are placed in cold water and slowly brought to the boil. Some loss of the vitamin is inevitable in cooking, but can be reduced if the cooking is carried out for the shortest possible time. Access to oxygen is reduced greatly if the water is first boiled to drive off dissolved oxygen and if a lid is placed on the saucepan to exclude air. Copper pots should not be used for cooking vegetables nor baking soda added to preserve their colouring. Similarly when potatoes are fried, losses of ascorbic acid are less if they are rapidly immersed in hot deep fat than if they are fried slowly in a shallow pan. Losses due to heat continue if vegetables or fruit are kept on a hot-plate after cooking and not served immediately. Ascorbic acid is very soluble in water, and the more cooking water used, the greater the amounts of the vitamin leached out and discarded.

If all these rules are disobeyed, as they frequently are in many homes and even more often in canteens, vegetables and fruits may be served almost devoid of vitamin C. This applies particularly to potatoes, often the most important source of ascorbic acid in the diet. Thompson (1946) showed that less than 30 per cent of the vitamin that survives cooking may be retained after a period on a hot-plate in a canteen. However, if the proper precautions are all taken, it is possible to preserve as much as 70 per cent of the ascorbic acid. In the absence of any accurate knowledge of the cooking methods used, it is advisable to assume a destruction of 50 per cent of the vitamin.

In small domestic pressure-cookers the temperature is raised well above the normal boiling point, but the time of exposure to heat is greatly reduced. These two effects tend to cancel out. Potatoes cooked in a pressure cooker may retain 80 per cent of the ascorbic acid, and such cookers can be used with confidence.

Vitamin C keeps well in frozen vegetables but about 25 per cent is lost in the preliminary blanching and the next step down occurs after the frozen storage period, during the final cooking. In the canning sequence losses may be comparable but are often greater (Benterud, 1977). Dehydration of potatoes in making instant potato granules destroys most of the vitamin C.

Thiamin.

Losses in the preparation of rice are important. In parts of Asia where the diet is predominantly of rice the method of preparation may determine whether the cooked product retains sufficient thiamin to prevent beriberi. Rice, as purchased in any bazaar, has to be washed and this washing water is then discarded. The rice is then cooked in water and this cooking water is usually discarded, though it is sometimes consumed. About 50 per cent of the thiamin (and other B vitamins) that has escaped the miller can be lost. If the rice is clean it does not need to be washed before cooking; the minimum of cooking water should be used and consumed.

In other foods thiamin is sensitive to heat at neutral and alkaline pH though less labile than vitamin C. Losses are usually around 10 to 20 per cent but can be greater. They are hastened by alkaline baking powder and the preservative sulphite (or SO_2).

Other vitamins

Riboflavin is sensitive to light. About 50 per cent of the vitamin in milk can be destroyed in 2 hours by exposure to bright sunlight and 20 per cent on a dull day.

Vitamin B_6 is sensitive to heat and activity is substantially reduced in canning and sterilisation or drying of milk. Loss of pyridoxal and pyridoxamine are greater than those of pyridoxine.

Folate is rapidly destroyed by heat in alkaline or neutral conditions. About 50 per cent is lost in canning and after cooking of vegetables; most of the total folate loss is free folate. Losses in cooking meat and eggs are usually less. More analyses are needed.

Vitamin B_{12} is stable when meat or liver are cooked under ordinary conditions but it can of course dissolve into cooking water or drip. In milk, pasteurisation destroys 7 per cent, boiling for 3 minutes destroys 30 per cent and ultraheat treatment 20 per cent of the vitamin activity.

Vitamin A and carotenes are stable during mild heat treatment but are oxidised at high temperatures in the presence of oxygen. Antioxidants in foods are protective. Only a small proportion of the carotenes pass into cooking water because they are not water-soluble.

Vitamin E is slowly destroyed by heat during frying and is sensitive to light. It is also, unlike other vitamins, unstable in fried foods during frozen storage (Bunnell *et al.*, 1965).

Minerals, including trace elements may be dissolved out in cooking water, but such losses are usually small. Schroeder (1971) reports losses of some trace elements during canning but acquisition of others, presumably from contact with metal surfaces. Losses of iodine in marine fish during freezing have been reported (Gurevic, 1966) but this needs to be confirmed.

COMMENT

Bender (1977) puts the losses of nutrients during food processing into perspective.

1. Some loss is inevitable, but for most nutrients losses are small.
2. Manufacturing losses, when they occur, are often in place of similar cooking losses at home.
3. The importance of the losses in a particular food has to be considered in relation to the whole diet. If a food makes only a small contribution to the intake of nutrients, processing losses are not of practical significance. On the other hand changes in any food which makes a major contribution to nutrient supply, e.g. milk and cereal products for babies, and cereals in many countries need continual vigilance.
4. There are beneficial effects—destruction of trypsin inhibitor in legumes and liberation of bound niacin in cereals.
5. Other advantages of food processing are protection from pathogenic organisms, better flavour and cheaper price. Often the ultimate choice is between dried, canned or frozen peas (say) in mid-winter or no peas at all.

24. Infective Agents in Foods

The dangers from pathogenic organisms in food far exceed those of toxic agents, either natural poisons or manmade chemicals. There are at least 30 species of worms, protozoa, bacteria and viruses which may gain access to food and so enter the body and cause a well-defined disease.

Meats, eggs and milk from infected animals may contain pathogens and, when eaten, can cause disease in man. Helminth infections, e.g. tapeworms, brucellosis (undulant fever), tuberculosis and salmonella infections are familiar examples of diseases of both animals and man.

There are more than 1600 types of Salmonellae which have been identified and distinguished by their serological reaction. These are the commonest cause of **bacterial food poisoning.** They infect most species of vertebrates and are especially widespread in poultry. *Salmonella typhimurium* (mouse typhoid) is the type most frequently responsible for human infections. Salmonella may enter the blood steam and invade the tissues, causing an enteric fever like typhoid, but usually in man they are confined to the intestines where they cause an acute gastroenteritis with diarrhoea and vomiting as the main features. Mice and rats infected with *S. typhimurium* commonly excrete the organism in their faeces and urine and so many infect human food to which they have access.

Many pathogenic bacteria and viruses are excreted in human faeces and some in urine. Infection may spread by transfer of the pathogen by flies or the human hand to foods or food utensils. Infections spread in this way are known as **faecal-oral diseases.** They include the dysenteries and acute gastroenteritis which are often caused by infection with various viruses and serotypes of *Escherichia coli.*

All pathogens are destroyed by heat, and food which has been properly cooked and handled is safe. However, in cooking, the heat may not penetrate the food sufficiently; particularly a large joint of meat, and undercooked foods are dangerous. Furthermore, food may be contaminated after cooking. Meat, milk and eggs are excellent growth media for bacteria; foods which have been cooked, improperly stored and then warmed up are especially dangerous.

Prevention of infections spread by food and the faecal-oral route depends on scrupulous attention to cleanliness along the whole food chain—abattoirs, food manufacturers, warehouses, retail shops, catering establishments, restaurants, and domestic kitchens and larders. In all these places care is required to prevent small rodents and flies from getting access to food. All food handlers should be scrupulously clean in their personal habits and be provided with clean lavatories and opportunities for washing their hands. Some persons harbour a pathogen and excrete it continuously in either faeces or urine without having any symptom of disease. Such **carriers** are particularly dangerous and have been responsible for many outbreaks of disease.

Food-borne infections and faecal-oral diseases are especially prevalent in poor urban communities with poor facilities for storing foods, inadequate water supplies and lavatories. In such circumstances infections are common and contribute to the high death rates, especially in young children. But the wealthy are by no means assured of protection. Anyone who thinks that only the poor are exposed to dirty foods should read George Orwell's *Down and Out in Paris* and find out what may go on in an expensive restaurant out of sight of the patrons.

In the prevention of outbreaks of bacterial food poisoning it is valuable to identify accurately the responsible bacteria and to demonstrate the presence of a specific bacterium both in the patients and in the food responsible for the outbreak. The public health laboratory services have the expertise for precise bacteriological diagnosis.

Public health authorities also have the duty to inspect abattoirs, the premises of food manufacturers, wholesale and retail shops that sell food, and all catering establishments and restaurants. They have the legal right to close any premises that are not up to acceptable standards of hygiene. Unfortunately, few public health departments have sufficient staff to carry out adequate inspections.

BACTERIAL FOOD POISONING

This produces an acute gastroenteritis which is usually short and self-limiting. Between 8000 and 12000 cases are notified each year in England and Wales, but many are unreported. The incidence rises in years when there is prolonged hot weather (Gilbert and Roberts, 1977). There are between 20 and 50 deaths each year, resulting from severe dehydration and loss of electrolytes; these deaths occur mainly in the very young and very old and in those with debilitating diseases.

Salmonella infections. These account for over 70 per cent of reported cases of food poisoning. *Salmonella typhimurium* is the organism most commonly responsible, but over 1600 serotypes of Salmonellae are now known. Many of these are very rare, but two formerly rare, *S. agona* and *S. virchou*, have now become established in the food chain in Britain. An accurate bacteriological diagnosis of the cause of an outbreak is essential to establish its source. This is usually meat or poultry. Imported raw eggs and egg powders have also been responsible. Salmonella may multiply in foods which have been inadequately cooked, but usually infection follows contamination of cooked foods from a raw food via food handlers or kitchen utensils. The incubation period is usually 12 to 36 hours and the disease lasts for 1 to 7 days, being nearly always accompanied by fever.

Clostridial infections. *Clostridium welchii*, known as *Cl. perfringens* in the USA, is responsible for about 20 per cent of infections in Britain. This is an anaerobic organism which forms spores resistant to heat. Spores are widespread in soil and dust. Infection occurs typically after eating meat which has been cooked on the previous day and allowed to cool under conditions which enable surviving spores to form vegetative forms. The victim then ingests what is a broth culture of the bacteria, which then multiply in the gut and produce an enterotoxin. The incubation period of the disease is 8 to 24 hours. Diarrhoea is often accompanied by abdominal pain, but vomiting and fever are uncommon.

Staphylococcal infections. *Staphylococcus aureus* is widespread. Up to 30 per cent of healthy people are carriers and it is frequently recovered from nasal swabs. But it is potentially pathogenic and responsible for many skin infections and may enter the blood stream to form abscesses in deep tissues. Foods are readily contaminated by carriers and may, under suitable conditions, provide a good culture medium for growth of the organism. Some strains produce a powerful enterotoxin which is resistant to heat. Ingestion of a contaminated food may be followed very quickly in 2 to 4 hours by vomiting and diarrhoea, which may be severe and accompanied by collapse due to dehydration.

Other organisms. The three types of infection described above have been well known for 50 years or more. However, in a large majority of outbreaks of gastroenteritis, none of the three can be identified and other organisms have been incriminated in many cases. *Escherichia coli*, one of the predominant members of the normal bacterial flora of the gut, was formerly considered to be non-pathogenic. However, some serotypes have been shown to be responsible for severe watery diarrhoea and these are often responsible for acute gastroenteritis in young children and also for traveller's diarrhoea (p. 403). In these instances the victim may not have built up a specific immunity to a particular serotype not previously encountered.

Bacillus cereus is a saprophytic spore-bearing organism widely found in nature. It can be recovered from many samples of uncooked rice. The spore may survive normal cooking and produce vegetate forms during cooling. These produce an enterotoxin which causes severe vomiting one hour after ingestion or diarrhoea later. Infection occurs usually in those who eat in Chinese restaurants. Incidence is unknown as it is often not reported. Fortunately, recovery is usually rapid.

Vibrio parahaemolyticus is an organism related to the cholera vibrio which grows in sea water. It is responsible for profuse diarrhoea and dehydration which may follow the consumption of raw or undercooked seafoods.

Yersinia enterocolitica under its old name of *Pasteurella pseudotuberculosis* has long been known to cause various disorders in many species of animals. Chinchillas have been much infected and spread from a farm may have been responsible for the first reports of human cases in 1963. Gastroenteritis and mesenteric adenitis due to this organism have now occurred many times (Morris and Feeley, 1976).

Many viruses, especially rotaviruses, echoviruses and reoviruses, can be isolated from the faeces. Viruses, unlike bacteria, cannot multiply in foods, but food handlers and dirty utensils are means whereby small doses may be transferred to foods and subsequently ingested. Then they may multiply in the intestinal tract. To what extent viruses are responsible for attacks of acute gastroenteritis is uncertain. It would seem probably that they are a common cause of attacks in young children when often no bacteria can be held responsible. In early life there is not the immunity to the common viruses which is built up by repeated exposure. For technical reasons the isolation and culture of viruses is a long way behind that of bacteria, but it is catching up fast. The future may show that viruses have an important role in gastrointestinal disease.

OTHER BACTERIAL DISEASES SPREAD BY FOOD

Botulism. This is a severe, often fatal form of food poisoning, fortunately now very rare. First described in Germany in 1817 as 'sausage' poisoning (Latin *botulus*, sausage), it has followed eating canned meats, liver and other pastes and also large hams. These foods under certain circumstances are an ideal medium for the growth of *Clostridium botulinum*. This is a saprophyte which is widespread and found in soils. It forms heat-resistant spores. If these are not destroyed by adequate heat in cooking, vegetative forms may grow anaerobically, and these produce one of the most potent toxins known, the lethal dose for mammals being less than $1\,\mu g/kg$. It blocks transmission at the neuromuscular junctions. Early symptoms of poisoning are weakness of the eye muscles and difficulty in swallowing; paralysis of the muscles of respiration leads to death. The food industry is well aware of the dangers of botulism and uses nitrites as a preservative which prevents anaerobic growth. No case had occurred in Britain for over 20 years until July 1978, when four members of a family in Birmingham became ill after eating tinned salmon. In the USA cases continue to occur occasionally through eating home-canned meat.

Brucellosis. Infection in man gives rise to a continued fever in which remissions and relapses are common (undulant fever). The responsible organisms, *Brucella melitensis* and *B. abortus*, affect goats and cows respectively and are found in their milk. Bruce was an army doctor who first isolated the former species in 1886 from soldiers suffering from 'Malta fever' who had been drinking goat's milk. Eradication of the disease in cattle has proved very difficult. Effective pasteurisation makes milk safe, but cream and cheese made from unpasteurised milk may contain *Brucella*, and those who buy these products from small farmers run a risk of infection. Several hundred cases are notified yearly in Britain; many patients are stockmen or veterinary surgeons for whom the disease is an occupational risk.

Bovine tuberculosis. Cattle are readily infected with tuberculosis and excrete the organism in their milk. *Mycobacterium bovis*, if ingested by man, causes enlargement of the cervical and mesenteric lymph nodes. It may then enter the blood steam and lead to tuberculous lesions in any organ and especially in bones and joints. Fifty years ago, when the drinking of raw milk in Britain was widespread (in part due to opposition to pasteurisation on spurious nutritional grounds), human infection was common in children. Today many elderly people have scars in their necks and some have orthopaedic deformities, as reminders of past illnesses. Tuberculosis has now been almost eradicated from cattle in Britain and all milk is pasteurised. As a result, this dangerous disease is now almost unknown in man. Continual watchfulness is necessary. In south-west England there is a focus of infection in badgers which has been held to be responsible for some occasional cases in cattle. Steps have been taken to control the spread.

HELMINTH INFECTIONS

Many helminths have complicated life cycles in which they live as parasites in more than one host. Man may be infected by eating undercooked pork and beef and raw salads.

Undercooked pork and beef

The pig and beef tapeworms, *Taenia solium* and *T. saginata*, form cysts which are present in muscle. If these are eaten by man, the adult worms develop in the gut. Segments of the worm may be passed in the faeces and cause alarm, but the adult worms are not responsible for any symptoms. If a person harbours *T. solium*, he may infect himself with ova passed in the faeces. These may then develop into larval forms which penetrate into muscles and other tissues where they form cysts. The condition is known as **cysticercosis** and may lead to epilepsy and other neurological disorders if cysts are in the brain. Fortunately this is very rare.

Undercooked pork may also contain larvae of *Trichinella spiralis*, which after ingestion can penetrate the tissues and cause a febrile illness with muscle pain and other symptoms of **trichinosis**, which is usually mild and brief.

Undercooked and raw fish

A fish tapeworm, *Diphyllobothrium latum*, has a worldwide distribution in freshwater fish. Man may be infected by raw fish. The adult worm is very long, up to 15 metres. It competes with the host for limited supplies of ingested vitamin B_{12}, and infection may lead to megaloblastic anaemia. This is not uncommon in Finland and in some other countries.

Raw fish and crabs are sometimes eaten in the Far East and may be considered a delicacy by some Chinese. Visitors are warned not to partake, as they become infected by two flukes. Metarcercaria of *Clonorchis sinesis* enter the biliary tract, where they may survive for many years and lead to a variety of symptoms and liver disorders, **clonorchiasis.** Larvae of *Paragonimus westermanii* burrow through the intestinal wall and in the lungs develop into adult worms which form fibrous cysts; they may communicate with a bronchiole and sputum containing ova may be coughed up. The condition is known as **paragonimiasis.**

Raw salads

The liver fluke *Fasciola hepatica* is common in sheep. Human cases occur occasionally and two small outbreaks of **fascioliasis** have been reported in England after eating watercress. The adult flukes live in the liver and biliary system, where they may be responsible for a variety of disorders. Salads may be responsible for infection with roundworms, *Ascaris lumbricoides*, whipworms, *Trichuris trichura*, and the protozoon *Giardia lamblia*. These parasites spread by the faecal-oral route (see below). In the East the practice of Chinese and other gardeners of using human night soil as fertiliser had led to heavy contamination of lettuce and other salad crops. An article in *The Guardian* (22 April 1978) reports that 9000 tons of human manure leave Shanghai daily for surrounding rural areas. As the population of Shanghai is only 6 million, this is an example of Chinese statistics overestimating the productivity of the people, but it serves as a warning to visitors that they should avoid salads and all uncooked foods.

FAECAL-ORAL INFECTIONS

In these diseases the infective agent is excreted in the faeces and enters the body via the mouth. Mechanisms for transfer of the agent from faeces to mouth vary widely and are often not known. Contamination of drinking water with sewage is a well-known means and food may be contaminated by flies and food handlers. Amoebic and bacillary dysentery are faecal-oral diseases and their incidence is high in many tropical countries where flies abound, and outbreaks often occur in temperate climates when a spell of hot weather allows the fly population to increase. As already mentioned, rota- and other viruses may cause gastroenteritis. Two major diseases, poliomyelitis and infectious hepatitis, are caused by viruses which are excreted in the faeces. In both diseases the virus is excreted by symptom-free carriers, and it has been estimated that a million people in the USA are carriers of hepatitis virus. How these two diseases spread is unknown. Large outbreaks of hepatitis occurred in troops in World Wars I and II and in the Vietnam war. It is not unlikely that these outbreaks were due to poor hygienic conditions in army cookhouses.

CONCLUSION

Brief summaries have been given of common pathogens that may be spread by foods and of the more serious diseases that may arise. A fuller account of the diseases can be found in medical textbooks, e.g. Passmore and Robson (1974), and of how their spread can be prevented by food hygiene in a monograph by Hobbs and Gilbert (1978). Enough should have been said to have impressed on the reader the potential dangers of infection from foods. Prevention depends on 'clean food handled by clean people in clean premises with clean equipment and protection from flies and vermin.' 'Cleanliness is, indeed, next to Godliness,' as John Wesley said in a sermon. It is a virtue which many try to achieve in the domestic life and yet remain all too tolerant of, or unaware of, dirt in public places.

25. Food Toxicity

At a very early age a child learns from his parents that he cannot eat everything and that certain substances are poisonous. An older child hears and reads stories of romance in which kings and courtiers, afraid that their enemies may poison them, employ food tasters at banquets. It is not surprising that many adults have an ingrained fear of poisons in food nor that the widespread dissemination of chemicals in an industrial society and their deliberate addition to food, though proper causes of concern, raise irrational fears and emotions.

A poison is difficult to define and many substances present in food would have adverse or toxic effects if taken in large doses, but the amounts normally present in foods are harmless.

Table 25.1 gives a classification of the ways by which toxic substances may be present in foods.

Toxins naturally present in plant foods, and infection of food by pathogenic bacteria have caused more human disease and mortality than the other categories. Accidental chemical contamination and environmental pollution have been responsible for local disasters from time to time. The intentional additives used in food processing today in well-

Table 25.1 Toxic substances in foods

NATURAL	
Inherent	Usually present in the food and affects everyone if they eat enough, e.g. solanine in potatoes, and lathyrus toxin (p. 221)
Toxin resulting from abnormal conditions of animal or plant used for food	For example, neurotoxic mussel poisoning (p. 221), honey from bees feeding on Rhododendron or Azalea nectar
Consumer abnormally sensitive	Constitutional, e.g. coeliac disease from wheat gluten (p. 405), favism from broad beans (p. 430), allergy to particular food (p. 437), or drug-induced, e.g. cheese reaction (p. 196)
Contamination by pathogenic bacteria	Acute illness, usually gastrointestinal, e.g. toxins produced by *Staphylococcus aureus* or *Clostridium botulinum;* food may not appear spoiled
Mycotoxins	Food mouldy or spoiled, e.g. aflatoxin B₁ from *Aspergillus flavus* is a liver carcinogen
ACCIDENTAL CHEMICAL CONTAMINATION OR POLLUTION	
Unintentional additives—man made Chemicals used in agriculture and animal husbandry	For example, fungicides on grain, insecticides on fruit, antibiotics or hormones given to animals
Environmental pollution	For example, organic mercury (p. 115), cadmium (p. 115), PCB and PBB (p. 225) and radioactive fall-out can affect any stage of food chain
Intentional food additives Preservatives, emulsifiers, flavours, colours, etc.	Some have been in use for centuries; many are naturally based and used in small amounts; the most thoroughly tested and monitored of all chemicals in food

organised countries are those considered safe by authoritative bodies. Standards of safety are strict and may be getting stricter. The public and their food safety administrations tend to set higher standards of safety for pure synthetic chemicals than for the complex of substances present in natural foods.

As Pyke (1971) has put it, the tests for new foods and additives are now so stringent that if Sir Walter Raleigh turned up *now* with the potato, as a new and unknown food, he would never stand a chance of having it accepted because of the solanine which it contains.

Disposal of ingested foreign substances

As foreign substances differ greatly in their chemical nature, their fate in the body varies. In general a substance may follow one of five possible sequences, each of which has variants:

1. It may pass through the gastrointestinal tract and not be absorbed. Pectin and other food thickeners are examples. It may, however, be digested by enzymes in the upper gastrointestinal tract or broken down by bacteria in the colon. Even if a substance is not absorbed it can affect the motility of the gastrointestinal tract and cause vomiting, diarrhoea or constipation. It can also irritate the mucous membrane and produce ulceration. Chronic irritation, if caused by a substance ingested over a long period, could lead to cancer formation. Cancer of the gastrointestinal tract occurs at sites where movement is slowed down and gut contents are in prolonged contact with the mucous membrane, e.g. the lower end of the oesophagus, the pyloric end of the stomach, the ileocaecal valve and the descending colon.
2. A substance may be absorbed and pass in the portal vein to the liver. Here it may be metabolised and then excreted back into the gastrointestinal tract in the bile. This sequence may be repeated, in an enterohepatic cycle. The substance or its metabolites can be recovered in the faeces but it has been inside the body and could damage the liver.
3. Water-soluble substances may be absorbed and pass through the liver into the general circulation. In the blood the substance may be partly bound to one of the plasma proteins, but it is excreted by the kidneys and passes into the urine. An example of a substance which follows this sequence is saccharin, which is excreted unchanged. If such a substance should be oncogenic, the organ most likely to be affected is the urinary bladder.
4. Fat-soluble substances after absorption reach the liver. There they are often metabolised in two stages and usually the metabolites are more water-soluble and so more easily excreted and less toxic. The first stage is oxidation by the non-specific microsomal enzyme oxidising system (MEOS) in the hepatocytes. Cytochrome P-450 is an integral part of this system. The second stage is conjugation of the oxidation product, usually with glucuronic acid or sulphate. Some substances wholly or partly bypass the first stage and are conjugated directly. The metabolites are then excreted in the urine or the bile. An example is the antioxidant BHT (butylated hydroxytoluene); its three butyl groups are partly oxidised and it is excreted mostly in the urine as glucuronic acid conjugates.
5. A substance may be absorbed but neither metabolised nor excreted; it stays in the body and accumulates. Even if harmless in small amounts in acute or subacute tests, it may lead to long-term harmful effects. Toxicologists are naturally concerned about substances that behave in this way. Examples are fat-soluble compounds like DDT (p. 224) and PBB (p. 225). These are not only stored in the adipose tissue but pass into the milk fat in lactating women. Substances handled like calcium can stay in bone for a long time, e.g. fluoride and radioactive strontium.

Toxicity testing

Safety is always relative. Despite numerous statutory safety regulations, travellers on land, sea and air are still killed by accidents, and no food can be guaranteed safe. The most an authority can do is to define an acceptable risk. In general, authorities permit substances to be present in foods when the maximum amount likely to be consumed daily is 100 times less than the minimum amount shown to have an adverse effect on experimental animals with due allowance for the body weight of the animals. Experimental animals are used for toxicity testing of pharmaceuticals, including cosmetics, and foods; such tests form the large majority of over 4 million vivisections carried out annually in the UK. Antivivisectionists protest strongly against this use of animals. The tests are also expensive and add to the price of many products. Hence attempts are being made to find alternative tests which use tissue cultures or isolated cells. These tests may be the main method of testing for toxicity in the future, but cannot wholly replace animal testing until much more is known about their reliability.

Species differ in their tolerance of many poisons, and an equivalent dose of a chemical shown to be harmless in one species of experimental animal may not be safe for man. Most substances are first tested on rats, but none is considered safe for man until the tests have been repeated on a species which is not rodent: rabbits, cats and dogs are most commonly used. Preferably, tests should also be carried out on a primate.

The signs of acute poisoning are usually obvious and it is not difficult to determine the maximum amount of a single dose of a substance that can be taken with safety. Since a potential food toxin is likely to be consumed throughout the life span of consumers, it has to be tested for long periods in animals and over at least two generations. The fetus is especially sensitive to some toxins, as is the ability of mature animals to reproduce. Malignant disease frequently does not arise until an animal has been exposed to an oncogenic agent for a major portion of its life span. A WHO Technical Report (WHO, 1967) outlines procedures for investigating intentional and unintentional food additives.

Examples are now given of poisoning in man due to natural and artificial toxins in foods. The accounts are of necessity anecdotal and many, it is hoped, are only of historical interest. Characteristically the illnesses present with an unusual combination of symptoms and signs in a community over a considerable time, and the possibility of their being due to a food toxin has been overlooked at first. In any outbreak of an unusual disease, it is wise to consider this possibility.

NATURAL FOOD TOXINS

There are people who are so alarmed at the possible chemical hazards from eating foods grown and prepared with the aid of modern chemical industry that they wish to return to a simple life and eat only natural foods. Unfortunately the chemical hazards in the fields and woods are also numerous. Table 25.2 gives a list of foods containing pharmacological agents known to have adverse effects on man. The list is far from complete and monographs are available prepared by the Committee on Food Protection (1973) of the US Food and Nutrition Board and by Liener (1969, 1974) all of which contain much curious information and are very readable. Here it is only possible to give a brief account of a few somewhat arbitrarily selected toxins which appear of special interest in medicine.

Table 25.2 indicates that there are natural poisons which have a great variety of acute and chronic pharmacological effects. Presumably many of these evolved in plants as protective mechanisms against animals feeding on them. Animals in turn have evolved elaborate biochemical reactions and cellular responses for disposing of the toxins or of at least partially neutralising their effects. Man and many other animals have also learnt by experience to avoid eating

Table 25.2 Some possible toxic effects of foods

Source	Active agent	Effects
Bananas and some other fruits	5-Hydroxytryptamine; adrenaline; noradrenaline	Effects on central and peripheral nervous system
Some cheeses	Tyramine	Raises blood pressure; enhanced by monoamine oxidase inhibitors
Almonds, cassava and other plants	Cyanide	Interferes with tissue respiration
Quail	Due to consumption of hemlock	Hemlock poisoning
Mussels	Due to consumption of dino-flagellate, *Gonyaulax*	Tingling, numbness, muscle weakness, respiratory paralysis
Cycad nuts	Methylazoxymethanol (cycasin)	Liver damage; cancer
Some fish, meat or cheese	Nitrosamines	Cancer
Mustard oil	Sanguinarine	Oedema (epidemic dropsy)
Legumes	Haemagglutinins	Red cell and intestinal cell damage
Some beans	Vicine β-Aminopropionitrile β-N-Oxalyl-amino-l-alanine	Haemolytic anaemia (favism) Interferes with collagen formation Toxic effects on nervous system, Lathyrism
Ackee fruit	α-Amino-β-methylene Cyclopropane propionic acid	Hypoglycaemia, vomiting sickness
Brassica seeds and some other Cruciferae	Glucosinolates, thiocyanate	Enlargement of thyroid gland (goitre)
Rhubarb	Oxalate	Oxaluria
Green potatoes	Solanine; possibly other sapotoxins	Gastrointestinal upset
Many fish	Various, often confined to certain organs or seasonal	Mainly toxic effects on nervous system
Many fungi	Various mycotoxins	Mainly toxic effects on nervous system and liver

some of the foods containing potent toxins. Some of the most potent toxins are found in fungi which may contaminate otherwise healthy foods.

LATHYRUS POISONS

Tares is the traditional English name for the vetches and an old word used loosely for various pulses and legumes. In Biblical times they were poorly regarded. 'But while men slept, his enemy came and sowed tares among the wheat' (St Matthew, xiii. 25). Why the sowing of tares was regarded as an unfriendly act is not wholly clear. The tendrils by which these plants climb up the wheat stalks certainly hamper reaping. But they may also have been known to be nutritionally unsatisfactory.

For a long time one species of tare (*Lathyrus sativus: Khesari dhal* in Hindustani) has been deliberately sown with the wheat by farmers in dry districts of many countries in Asia and North Africa where the rainfall is uncertain. If the rains are good, the wheat overgrows the lathyrus, of which little is harvested. If the rains fail and there is a poor crop of wheat, a useful harvest of lathyrus may be reaped. Eaten in small quantities, lathyrus seeds are a valuable food. But if they are the main source of energy (providing more than 50 per cent), a severe disease of the spinal cord (lathyrism, p. 000) may result, causing crippling and permanent paralysis. An excellent account of the disease and the circumstances under which it arises has been given by a soldier, General Sleeman (1844). A neurotoxin has been isolated from seeds of *Lathyrus sativus* and shown to be β-N-oxalyl-amino-l-alanine. This substance, known as BOAA, has been found in samples of seeds in amounts up to 2 g/100 g (Nutritional Research Laboratories, Hyderabad, 1968). Other neurotoxins have been isolated from seeds of the common vetch (*Vicia sativa*), which frequently grows as a weed in lathyrus crops. The relation between intakes of BOAA and the clinical features of lathyrism has not been worked out.

Allied vetches, notably the sweet pea, *Lathyrus odoratus,* when fed to rats, readily give rise to a severe disturbance of collagenous structures throughout the body, notably in skin and bones, known as osteolathyrism (Weaver, 1964; Liener, 1966). Osteolathyrism, or odoratism, has not been described as a natural disease of either man or animals and appears to have been produced only in the laboratory.

SEAWATER FISH

Ciguatera is an old Portuguese word introduced in 1787 to describe poisoning that arose after eating fish from the Pacific Ocean and the Caribbean Sea. The clinical features are those of an acute neuromuscular disorder with weakness and sensory changes. Most attacks are of moderate severity and the symptoms clear up in a few days, but itching may persist for several weeks and occasionally widespread paralysis is followed by coma and death. Captain Cook (1777) describes a typical attack.

5 September, 1774, Cape Colnet, New Caledonia. This afternoon a fish being struck by one of the natives near the watering-place, my clerk purchased it, and sent it to me after my return on board. It was of a new species, something like a sunfish with a large, long, ugly head. Having no suspicion of its being of a poisonous nature, we ordered it to be dressed for supper: but, very luckily, the operation of drawing and describing took up so much time that it was too late, so that only the liver and roe were dressed, of which the two Mister Forsters and myself did but taste. About three o'clock in the morning we found ourselves seized with an extraordinary weakness and numbness all over our limbs. I had almost lost the sense of feeling; nor could I distinguish between light and heavy bodies, of such as I had strength to move; a quart pot full of water and a feather being the same in my hand. We each of us took an emetic, and after that a sweat, which gave us much relief. In the morning, one of the pigs which had eaten the entrails was found dead. When the natives came on board and saw the fish hang up, they immediately gave us to understand it was not wholesome food.

A large number of species of fish may be poisonous. Some of these are always poisonous and others may usually be eaten with safety, but are poisonous at certain times of the year. Poisonous fish have usually been feeding on a coral reef; deep-sea fish are generally safe. The toxin or toxins responsible have not been identified. Fish becomes poisonous because of factors in their environment which get into their food supply. Jardin (1972) has suggested that the toxins may be organo- minerals. It is possible that natural disturbances in ocean beds may affect the amounts of trace elements in rocks and sediment, which become incorporated into organic material and so into the algae and other basic components of the food of fishes.

Scombrotoxism results from bacterial spoilage of tunny and related fish. Disrupted muscle liberates histidine from which histamine is formed, and this together with other toxins produce headache, palpitation, flushing and diarrhoea a short time after ingestion. An outbreak, affecting over 200 people, from canned tuna in the USA is reported by Merson *et al.* (1974).

Other toxins which may be present in seawater fish are described by Bagnis *et al.* (1970).

Mussel poisoning

A toxin, saxitoxin, may be present in plankton, particularly the dinoflagellate *Gonyaulax tamarensis* which is ingested by bivalves such as mussels. The toxin is stable and remains in the tissues of the shellfish which appear to be resistant. It is not destroyed by cooking. Dinoflagellates at times multiply to such an extent that they may colour the sea and such 'red tides' cause a heavy mortality among seabirds, especially shags (Clark, 1968). Mussels, a delicacy usually safe to eat, may then become toxic. These conditions occur occasionally off the eastern seaboard of the USA and Canada (Meyer, 1953), and more rarely during summer off the coast of Britain between Aberdeen and Yorkshire (Gemmil and Manderson, 1960; McCollum et al., 1968). People who are unfortunate enough to eat mussels at such a time develop, within 30 minutes paraesthesiae, weakness of limbs, ataxia and vomiting. Death can occur from respiratory paralysis.

FRESHWATER FISH

Fishermen and their families around the Koenigsberg Haff in East Germany during the period between World Wars I and II suffered outbreaks of acute paroxysmal myoglobinuria, preceded by severe pain in all muscles. Always on the day before an attack fish, usually eel or burbot, had been eaten. The condition became known as Haff disease, and German investigators concluded that the fish eaten contained a toxin which had entered the Haff with the effluent from nearby industrial works. However, a small outbreak in Sweden affected persons who had eaten burbot from a lake uncontaminated by industrial waste (Berlin, 1948). Berlin suggested that thiaminase present in the fish might be the cause, but this seems unlikely. Haff disease is rarely reported nowadays and the toxin responsible remains unidentified.

MISCELLANEOUS TOXINS IN FOODS

Argemone contamination of edible oils

In Bengal and Bihar mustard oil is the chief cooking fat. In the same part of the world epidemic dropsy has been endemic for a long time. In a series of investigations in which the clues were analysed in the best detective manner, Lal and his colleagues (1937, 1940) showed that mustard oil was responsible for this disease. The toxin was not present in the oil from the mustard seeds themselves, but in oil from the seeds of a poppy weed (Argemone mexicana). This weed commonly grows in the mustard crops. Its seeds contain an alkaloid, sanguinarine, which is toxic (Sarkar, 1948). Sanguinarine inhibits the oxidation of pyruvic acid and, as in wet beriberi, cardiomyopathy may follow (p. 284). Other edible oils, such as groundnut oil, can be contaminated with argemone oil.

Ackee fruit (Blighia sapida)

The fruit grows profusely in Jamaica and is eaten by large numbers of people, especially children. Yet it is widely credited with being responsible for a form of food poisoning, 'vomiting sickness' (Hill, 1952; Jelliffe and Stuart, 1954). Dr Cicely Williams (1954) undertook an investigation of the disease for the Jamaican Government. She was able to study numerous patients and a few outbreaks in detail. In some, the symptoms could be attributed to other diseases. Yet there were several patients in whom no definite cause could be found, despite thorough investigation. A specific poison from the ackee fruit could not be

excluded. She concluded that if such poison were indeed responsible, large amounts would have to be consumed, and the patients must be peculiarly susceptible to the poison, probably because of their undernourished state. Ackee fruit contains a water-soluble substance, α-amino-β-methylene cyclopropyl-propionic acid, that causes accumulation of branched short-chain fatty acids and acute hypoglycaemia and is known as hypoglycin (Holt et al., 1964). This substance is now believed to be responsible for the clinical features of vomiting sickness.

Brassica species

Brassica is a large genus which includes cabbages, mustards and rapes. Rabbits and other laboratory animals fed large amounts of raw leaves develop goitre, which may also occur after feeding the seeds. This is due to the presence of glucosinolates and thiocyanates. Glucosinolates act on the thyroid gland like thiouracil by preventing the synthesis of thyroxine. Thiocynates reduce the concentration of iodine in the thyroid gland. Some of the brassicas, notably cabbage, are common human foods, but there is no evidence that when eaten in normal amounts, as part of a balanced diet, they are anything but beneficial. Goitrogens in foods are further considered in Chapter 30.

Cycads

There has been a high incidence of a form of motor neurone disease and of a disease known as Parkinsonism dementia among the Chamorro people on the island of Guam and the neighbouring Mariana islands. It has been suspected that the traditional high consumption of the seeds of the cycad, Cycas circinalis, might be responsible. Certainly cycad seeds contain a toxin, cycasin, which in experimental animals is a potent hepatotoxin and also carcinogenic (p. 510). Yet hepatic disease, including carcinoma, is only slightly more common in Guam than in the USA; feeding adult animals with cycasin has not produced neurological damage, and it has not been shown that the victims of the motor neurone disease have eaten more cycad seeds or prepared them in a different way from unaffected islanders (Kurland, 1972).

Spices

Spices and flavouring agents contain volatile and essential oils and hydrocarbons which stimulate glandular secretion and may have a weak action on the nervous sytem. Many of them if taken in large doses have toxic actions. For instance nutmeg, mace and dill contain myristicin. In 1832, the Czech physiologist Purkinje ate three nutmeg seeds and became delirious and went into a deep stupor. Smaller amounts of nutmeg may cause vomiting and colic.

Wormwood oil obtained from an African tree, Artemisia absinthium with a sweet-smelling wood is used as a flavouring agent in the liqueur absinthe and in vermouth and other wines. Its active principle, thujone, stimulates the nervous system and may cause convulsions.

Worcester sauce contains acetic acid, black pepper, garlic and other spices. Several patients who had acquired the habit of consuming up to one bottle a day have developed renal failure, and in some cases renal calculi (Murphy, 1971). Complete recovery may occur when the habit is given up. The toxin has not been identified.

Oestrogens

Some plant foods, including soya bean, contain traces of oestrogens, but the amounts are so small that no adverse effects follow the consumption of such foods. Larger amounts may be present in meat from animals previously dosed with oestrogens to promote growth. This practice is now not permitted in most countries.

Carcinogens

Many natural foods have been shown to contain substances which produce tumours in experimental animals. The extent to which they may be responsible for malignant disease in man is discussed in Chapter 60.

Antivitamins

Attention was first drawn to the antivitamins in veterinary practice. Cattle fed on spoiled sweet clover develop a haemorrhagic disease. This is due to the presence in the clover of dicoumarol, a substance chemically related to vitamin K (Link, 1944). It produces haemorrhages by causing vitamin K deficiency in the tissues. Synthetic analogues of dicoumarol are used in clinical practice to reduce the liability to coagulation.

Natural substances can act an antivitamins by preventing their absorption or by destroying them in the gut. For example in 1936 an outbreak of paralysis, 'Chastek paralysis', developed in silver foxes on a farm in the USA belonging to Mr Chastek. The foxes had been fed on carp. The presence of a thiaminase was demonstrated in the flesh and viscera of these fish (Green et al., 1942). Additional thiamin both prevented and cured the disease. Thiaminase has been found in several species of fish. A different substance (3, 4-dihydroxy cinnamic acid) with thiaminase activity occurs in bracken and other plants. Thiamin deficiency due to consumption of thiaminase has not been reported in man. Fish is used as a food in zoos and nature reserves, as well as in commercial animal production, and those who use it should be aware of the hazard from thiaminase.

Hallucinogenic substances

In 1676 British soldiers engaged in putting down a rebellion in Virginia ate a salad containing the Jimson weed Datura stramonium. Some of them were reported to have been turned into natural fools performing many simple tricks, but they remembered nothing of this when they recovered. The weed contains alkaloids, such as scopolamine, which produce hallucinations. Cases of poisoning have been reported in 'beatniks' who have eaten the weed for its psychic effects (Blood and Rudolph, 1966). Children who taste the fruit of the weed may also be poisoned.

In Britain an occasional error is the eating of the fly toadstool, Amanita muscaria. This contains muscarine, but only in small amounts. The characteristic symptom of poisoning is cerebral excitement, which is due to mycetoatropine (Ramsbottom, 1953). Horne and McCluskie (1963) describe a young man who was admitted to a Glasgow hospital in a confused and drowsy state. By occupation he was a salmon poacher, and he and his brother used to eat deliberately A. muscaria, because they enjoyed the feeling of unreality and detachment which it gave. Others have become addicted, including apparently the Russian Empress Catherine the Great. Far more dangerous is the Death Cap toadstool, Amanita phalloides. This can be confused with the edible field mushroom Agaricus campestris. Elliot et al. (1961) describe a severe attack of poisoning and also give notes on the identification of poisonous fungi. Their patient, a farmer who had eaten Amanita phalloides in error, was acutely ill when admitted to Cumberland Infirmary. He became unconscious, had watery diarrhoea and was jaundiced. After 48 hours his urine was suppressed, but with the aid of the artificial kidney he recovered. Penicillin to hasten excretion of the toxin and cytochrome c are also helpful (Lancet, 1972).

The Mexican plant peyote, which contains mescaline, and the hemp plant, Cannabis indica, widespread in Asia and Africa, are two examples of plants which have been consumed deliberately for their psychic effects.

TOXINS OF FUNGAL ORIGIN

Ergot

When rye was widely cultivated in Europe, outbreaks of a disease known as 'St Anthony's Fire', or ergotism, were not uncommon. In the Middle Ages sufferers made pilgrimages to St Anthony's shrine. It is now known that rye is liable to infection with ergot, a rust or fungus which contains a number of toxic alkaloids. Barger (1931), who with Sir Henry Dale elucidated their chemical nature and pharmacological action, describes in his book both the properties of the alkaloids and the history of the epidemics. Sir Edward Mellanby (1934) pointed out that outbreaks of ergotism have usually been associated with times of food scarcity. Outbreaks of ergotism are still occasionally reported, most recently from a part of India; millet (bajra) was infected (Indian National Institute of Nutrition, 1976). Again it must be emphasised that rye is a wholesome food. Poisoning results from its consumption only when the grain is infected by rust.

Aflatoxins

In 1960 a widespread outbreak of a fatal disease characterised by acute enteritis and hepatitis occurred in England among young turkeys which had been fed a ration containing imported groundnut meal (Sargeant et al., 1961). The groundnuts concerned had been harvested, stored and processed under conditions of high humidity. The toxic factors were produced by Aspergillus flavus, a mould contaminating the nuts. They are brightly fluorescing furanocoumarin compounds known as 'aflatoxins'. Aflatoxins are now known to contaminate human foods. Nuts and grains produced and stored in warm moist climates are most likely to be affected. Aflatoxins damage the liver and lead to carcinoma in many animals. Aflatoxin B_1 is the most potent known natural hepatocarcinogen, at least in susceptible species such as the rat and duckling. The toxic dose in primates is about 0.05 mg/kg daily (Campbell and Stoloff, 1974). There has been much conjecture about the possible role of aflatoxins in primary carcinoma of the liver in man in Africa and Asia (p. 512).

Maize contaminated with aflatoxin appeared to be responsible for an epidemic of an acute illness which occurred in 1974 and affected 200 villages in Gajarat and Rajasthan, India. The clinical features were jaundice, ascites, portal hypertension and a high mortality. It was estimated that patients had consumed from 2 to 6 mg of aflatoxin daily for one month (Krishnamachari et al., 1975). Aflatoxins have also been detected in autopsy liver samples from some cases of the Reye-Johnson syndrome, acute encephalopathy with fatty liver (Chaves-Carballo et al., 1976). Aflatoxins are of great importance in animal husbandry, and a monograph is available (Goldblatt, 1969).

Other mycotoxins

The discovery of aflatoxins means that mouldy food and fodder is not merely unattractive; it may be dangerous. There has followed a period of search for other potentially dangerous mycotoxins which may be produced by moulds that can grow on foods. Sterigmatocystin from Aspergillus versicolor on maize is carcinogenic in animals but much less potent than the aflatoxins. Patulin from Penicillium expansum, which is found in rotten apples and may occur in apple juice and cider, is also carcinogenic, and so are two toxins which Japanese workers have found on rice infected with P. islandicum—luteoskyrin and cyclochlorotine.

The trichothecenes, produced by species of Fusarium on mouldy cereals, appear to be responsible for a human disease, alimentary toxic aleukia, in Russia. Ochrotoxin from Aspergillus ochraceus on mouldy barley has been responsible for kidney disease in swine in Denmark, and zearalenone from Fusarium graminearum causes genital hypertrophy and reproductive difficulties in swine. Evidence is accumulating that Balkan nephropathy, a slowly progressive nephropathy without hypertension which is endemic in parts of the Danube valley, may be due to toxins from Penicillium cyclopium on stored maize (Barnes et al., 1977). Mouldy sweet potatoes cause lung or liver disease in animals; four different toxins have been isolated.

The list of mycotoxins is long and still being added to. It will take a long time to work out which are of importance in human disease. Meanwhile all mouldy food should be regarded with caution. It would be salutary for the enthusiasts for natural foods to ponder that mycotoxins are more likely to contaminate foods grown and processed without fungicides, preservatives and chemical additives.

AGRICULTURAL CHEMICALS

A farmer has to worry about his crops. Weeds, insects, fungi, bacteria and viruses can all seriously reduce the yield in the fields. After harvest, rodents, moulds and putrefying bacteria may cause further loss. His animals may suffer from external parasites, ticks, lice and maggots in the skin and many species of worms and other organisms in the alimentary canal and internal organs. These dangers can be prevented or at least reduced by chemical agents which, if improperly used, can reach a final food product in amounts which may be toxic to consumers. Modern farming is a highly technical business which depends on the chemical industry. The very high yields now obtainable (Table 50.1) would be impossible without the use of chemicals.

PRESTICIDES AND WEED KILLERS

The danger from these is mainly to manufacturers, distributors and farm workers; acute poisoning is well known to occur amongst them and has been responsible for several deaths. Only very rarely has the residue left on a crop been responsible for acute poisoning. One such outbreak is now described.

One evening in 1959, 13 children and one adult were admitted to a hospital in Singapore. They had been taken ill suddenly and most of them had collapsed. Examination showed signs of overactivity of the parasympathetic system—sweating, dilated pupils, excessive salivation and increased secretions in the lungs. Many had fits and those severely affected became unconscious; four children died. Acting with commendable speed, the medical staff of the hospital suspected organophosphate poisoning and warned the public health authority. Early on the next morning, after it had been discovered that all the patients had eaten barley recently imported from Europe, instructions were issued making 'barley poisoning' notifiable. Subsequently the barley was found to be contaminated with the insecticide Parathion, which is a powerful anticholinesterage agent. Prompt action contained the outbreak to 38 cases with nine deaths. Kanagaratnam et al. (1960) tell this story dramatically.

There are over 100 pesticides in use in the UK. chief interest lies in the organochlorine insecticides, DDT (dichlorodiphenyl trichlorethane) and dieldrin. These substances or their degradation products persist on agricultural products and so find their way into our food. As they are very slowly eliminated from the body and are fat-soluble, they accumulate in adipose tissue. In 1972 in the UK, samples of human fat contained about 2.5 mg/kg of DDT and its derivatives and about 0.2 mg/kg of dieldrin. Substantially higher figures have been found in the USA and other countries. Thus modern man carries around in his adipose tissue a few milligrams of pesticide. We know of no evidence that this does us any harm. The government chemist reviewing the situation in Britain (Egan, 1966) wrote, 'The facts do not give cause for complacency; neither do they merit alarm.' In the 10 years since then, the, dietary intakes of pesticides have fallen substantially (Egan and Weston, 1977).

In 1970 the US Department of Agriculture restricted the use of DDT for livestock, food crops and ornamental plants and gardens. This decision was reached when it was judged that the benefits derived from its use in the USA did not justify a risk to health. In countries where DDT is part of a malaria control programme, the benefits from DDT might be judged to far outweigh the risk.

The widespread use of DDT has had adverse effects on hawks, eagles and other birds that live on the flesh of small animals. In some areas many of their eggs have not hatched and this has lead to a reduction in numbers. The eggs may be defective due to a deficiency of oestrogens which may be metabolised at an increased rate by microsomal enzymes of the liver induced by DDT.

ANTIBIOTICS

Antibiotics are used to treat infectious diseases in farm animals. They have also been incorporated into animal foodstuffs because in some way, not yet fully explained, they promote growth; thus they are of economic value in the rearing of pigs and poultry. They have also been used in food preservation. In these ways foods may become contaminated, but there is no evidence that this has had any direct adverse effect on man.

A serious indirect effect of the indiscriminate use of antibiotics in animal husbandry is the development of bacterial resistance to their action. Strains of *Salmonella typhimurium* and *Escherichia coli* which may infect both man and livestock are liable to acquire such resistance. This is carried in the genetic material of the bacteria and may be transferred to different bacteria, which then become resistant, although not previously exposed to the antibiotic.

Acquired bacterial resistance is a complex phenomenon of the utmost importance to animal husbandry and human medicine. It was considered in detail by a committee under the chairmanship of Swann (1969) and the report is fascinating reading. While appreciating the great value of antibiotics in veterinary practice and in some circumstances in animal husbandry, the committee makes detailed recommendations for preventing their abuse.

HORMONES

Steroid sex hormones act as anabolic agents in beef cattle. **Diethylstilboestrol** (DES) was used in the USA between 1954 and 1972. It hastened growth, reducing feed requirements and producing animals with more protein and less fat in the carcass. Anxiety grew about its use because by 1971 radioactive techniques became sensitive enough to detect DES at 2 μg/kg in livers from a small minority of animals. At the same time in cases of the rare adenocarcinoma of the vagina occurring in young women, it was found that their mothers had been treated with DES in large dosage during pregnancy. It was used then to reduce the risk of miscarriage. The ban on oestrogens in beef production is not really logical. Comparable amounts of oestrogens are naturally present in soya beans and in eggs; endogenous production in women and the amounts used in oral contraceptives are much larger. The ban is being challenged but meanwhile hormonal feed additives are not permitted in the EEC except for a combined DES/androgen preparation still used in pig feeds in Britain.

FUNGICIDES ON SEED GRAIN

Several tragic accidents have affected peasant farmers who were supplied with new types of seed grain that had been treated with chemicals to prevent fungus disease of the young wheat plant. If the previous harvest was small and instructions poor, people have eaten some of the seed grain. Alkyl mercury poisoning in Iraq (in 1972) is described on page 115. In Turkey hexachlorobenzene was used as the fungicide. Ingestion of treated grain led to 3000 cases of a new type of porphyria in the late 1950s (Peters, 1976).

INDUSTRIAL WASTE AND ACCIDENTAL CONTAMINATION

Foods may become contaminated in various ways by industrial waste. Examples of outbreaks of poisoning by lead, mercury and cadmium due to failure to dispose of industrial waste in a safe manner are given in Chapter 12. Accidents may also occur and it is a consequence of industralisation that the bigger the process the wider the effect if something goes wrong. In 1973 an illiterate truck driver in Michigan delivered 2000 lb of Firemaster, a fire retardant made of **polybrominated biphenyls** (PBB), instead of Neutromaster, a magnesium oxide supplement, from a chemical firm to an animal feed depot. Here the employees assumed it was an improved version of the feed supplement. In consequence, poisoned grain was delivered to hundreds of farms and fed to many thousands of animals. Animals became ill but it took a year before the poison was identified. By that time much farm and dairy produce had become contaminated with PBB, which is metabolised extremely slowly and tends to accumulate in the body. Some people in the area lost weight and became disorientated. Three years later PBB could be detected in most samples of mother's milk in Michigan State. The full account of the accident has not yet been compiled.

RADIOACTIVE FALL-OUT

For 18 years from 1945 when an atomic bomb was dropped on Hiroshima until 1963 when the Nuclear Test Ban was signed by the governments of the United States, the Soviet Union and the United Kingdom, atomic explosions periodically liberated radioactive dust into the atmosphere. This dust rose into the stratosphere, where it might drift for many hundreds of miles before sinking into the lower atmosphere and finally to the earth's surface. After each nuclear explosion, fall-out contaminated a large area determined mainly by local meteorological conditions. In an affected area, cereal crops, vegetables and fruits which may be eaten by man were contaminated, and also grasses and herbage eaten by cattle. Their milk and meat then contains radioactive material. In general, foods of animal origin become more dangerous to man than those of plant origin because the radioactive material is concentrated in milk and meat.

The main potentially dangerous radioisotopes in fall-out are iodine-131 (^{131}I), strontium-90 (^{90}Sr) and caesium-137 (^{137}Cs). ^{131}I has a half life of only 8 days and so most of that liberated by an explosion becomes inactive in the upper atmosphere. Nevertheless, unacceptable amounts were found in some samples of milk. ^{90}Sr and ^{137}Cs have half lives of 28 and 30 years respectively and so are potentially greater dangers. The absorption, storage and excretion of strontium is similar to that of calcium and so ^{90}Sr is concentrated in milk. The body deals with caesium as it deals with potassium and so caesium is concentrated in muscle and all meats may be contaminated. ^{90}Sr is especially dangerous because it is stored in bone, and the adjacent bone marrow is very susceptible to damage by radiation. The concentration of ^{90}Sr in milk makes it especially dangerous to infants and children.

Before 1963 radioactive fall-out caused significant contamination of foods in many countries and was a real cause of concern. Accounts of the situation in the United Kingdom at that time are given by Hawthorn (1959) and the Medical Research Council (1960). The Nuclear Test Ban Treaty was an event of major importance to the world. Since 1963 over 100 countries have joined the original signatories, but these do not include China and France. The protection provided by the ban is as secure, and no more, as any other international treaty. The radioactive fall-out in the UK and the amounts of ^{90}Sr and ^{137}Cs in our milk are now slowly diminishing.

An accident in a nuclear power station can also be followed by contamination of foods produced in its vicinity. Such accidents have happened, e.g. at Windscale in the North of England in 1957, but are fortunately rare.

In 1969 WHO and the International Atomic Energy Agency (IAEA) established an International Reference Centre for Environmental Radioactivity at Le Vesignet, France. This assists national governments in collecting information about all forms of radiation in the environment which are a potential danger to health and gives advice on control measures. It publishes periodically reports on the concentrations of ^{90}Sr and ^{137}Cs in samples of milk from various countries.

In an emergency, it is safe to eat foods which have been stored or packed in airtight tins or jars or otherwise protected from atmospheric dust. Tinned foods which have been exposed to intense radiation do not become radioactive. Other remedial measures are uncertain. Since calcium and strontium use the same transport mechanism, increasing the dietary calcium might be expected to reduce intestinal absorption of ^{90}Sr.

FOOD ADDITIVES

No chemical can be deliberately added to foods until it has been through extensive tests for toxicity. Yet, experience may lead to reassessment. Three examples are given.

Agene

For many years nitrogen trichloride, known as agene, was added as an improver to most of the flour used to make bread in the United Kingdom. There was no suspicion that it was in any way toxic. Mellanby (1934) investigated a neurological disorder than prevalent in fox hounds and known as canine hysteria. He was able to show that the disorder affected only dogs whose diet consisted mainly of bread; he then showed that it was agene in the bread which damaged the nervous system. As a result, the use of agene as a flour improver was no longer allowed and it was replaced by chlorine dioxide. Nitrogen trichloride is an example of a substance which is much more toxic for one species, the dog, than for most other species including man. Nevertheless, the decision to ban its use in human foods seems wise.

Cyclamate

The Soft Drinks Regulations (1964) permitted the use of cyclamate as an artificial sweetener. The maximum amount that could be added to soft drinks was 1.35 g/litre. The Regulation was based on the advice of the Food Additives and Contaminants Committee, who were aware that cyclamates were already permitted in the USA and in a report published in 1966 they give extensive evidence based on tests on rats, mice, cats, dogs, rabbits and man that cyclamate is not toxic. In 1969 it was reported that in tests in the USA eight out of 240 rats who were given cyclamate in daily doses of over 2 g/kg body weight developed tumours of the urinary bladder. As a result, cyclamate was banned immediately in the USA and soon after in the UK. The dose shown to be carcinogenic in the rats was very high. To achieve it, a 12 year old boy weighing 40 kg would have to drink daily about 60 litres of a soft drink containing the maximum permitted amount of cyclamate. The ban was the result of a hasty decision and further more careful appraisal seems to be needed. Diabetics, who were taking more cyclamate than the general population, have not shown any excess of cancer of the urinary bladder (Armstrong et al., 1976).

Monosodium glutamate

The 'Chinese restaurant syndrome', first reported by Kwok (1968) and now well known, consists of the following symptoms: pains in the neck and chest, palpitations and headache, all occurring after eating in a Chinese restaurant. It has been deduced that these are due to monosodium L-glutamate (MSG). The Chinese have used seaweeds and soya beans, both of which contain sodium glutamate, as natural condiments for generations. MSG is a permitted flavouring enhancer widely used for savoury foods in the food industry. There is no certainty that it is responsible for the symptoms, but the evidence against it is strong. As the symptoms are transient, only affect a minority of consumers, lead to no permanent damage, are early associated by the sufferer with excess consumption of highly flavoured foods and so can be avoided, there seems no case for banning the use of glutamate as a flavouring agent—at least for adults. Glutamate has been added to many infants' foods, but most manufacturers of these foods have now ceased to use it. This seems a wise decision until more is known about its possible actions.

The stories of agene, of cyclamate and of monosodium glutamate are worth pondering on for they have several messages for nutritionists. First, they show the uncertainty of contemporary knowledge; reports of new observations may at any time challenge accepted opinions of the day. They illustrate the value of a careful study of unusual and unexplained symptoms when these appear either in man or in any other animal species. The difficulty in making a decision as to what is an acceptable risk, and the need to proceed slowly before making a judgment on any chemical, is well demonstrated. Consumers may take comfort from the fact that we are unable to provide evidence that any human being has suffered in health in any serious way as a consequence of taking a permitted food additive. This, of course, must not be used as an excuse for relaxing present standards of toxicity testing. The need to make present tests more precise and to devise better tests continues.

26. Consumer Protection

The records of history show that there have always been men who are ready to make a fast buck by trick or fraud. Short weight and the dilution of milk with water are ancient practices and almost everywhere there have been laws against them; these practices still continue in countries which lack adequate means of enforcement. In Europe in the Middle Ages pepper and other costly spices imported from the East were frequently adulterated by mixing with local seeds, leaves or flour or even with sand. Sugar, coffee and tea were similarly diluted. There were also old laws against the sale of unsound meat and other foods.

In the period 1750–1850 the Industrial Revolution caused large numbers of people to leave the countryside and work in the new towns. Separated from the fields where their food was grown and from the local markets and shops where they could purchase it, industrial workers became increasingly dependent on food manufacturers, some of whom were fraudulent. Foods were often adulterated and some of the adulterants were new chemicals which were poisonous. The medical profession then knew little about toxicology, and analytical methods for detecting and identifying adulterants did not exist. In Britain the problem came to a head in 1851 when Dr Wakley, the owner and first editor of the *Lancet*, published the names of over 3000 tradesmen whose wares had been found by private investigators to be adulterated. Many people thought that libel actions would kill the *Lancet*, but it was never sued, probably because it had the support of the medical profession. Instead, his crusade led to the passage by Parliament of the 1860 Adulteration of Food and Drink Act and, when this proved ineffective, of the 1875 Sale of Food and Drugs Act, the basis from which our modern laws have developed. By 1875 new chemical knowledge had enabled the science of food analysis to develop, and the appointment of public analysts to local government authorities enabled the law to be enforced. Similar laws were passed in other countries and fraudulent adulteration of food on a large scale ceased. The same situation has, however, arisen again since 1950 with the rapid growth of towns in Africa and Asia where many countries lack suitably trained inspectors and analysts who are needed to ensure that laws and regulations are enforced.

In 1875 knowledge of bacteriology was rudimentary, but the next 25 years was a golden age and by 1900 most of the bacteria commonly causing food poisoning had been identified, together with useful knowledge of how they may spread and the nature of the diseases which they cause. Food hygiene then became a science and this made possible the control of the spread of food poisoning by inspection of slaughterhouses, food warehouses, retail shops and kitchens in restaurants, hotels and other public institutions. Today this control is only partially effective and, as shown in Chapter 24, many infective agents continue to contaminate food. Together they constitute far and away the greatest danger to health from food, against which consumers need protection.

The twentieth century has seen the rise of new chemical hazards from food. As already described, food manufacturers deliberately add chemicals to foods to assist manufacture and storage, and farmers use pesticides, weedkillers and antibiotic agents on their crops and animals, some of which may carry over into the final food product. From these practices consumers derive much benefit; without them, food supplies would be less secure, more monotonous and of poorer quality. However, they are and will always remain a potential hazard. The chemical contamination of foods by industrial wastes which pollute our atmosphere and water supplies is probably increasing, and some examples have already been given in Chapters 12 and 25. As will be described later in the present chapter there are government agencies in the larger countries which ensure that there is toxicological testing and assessment of the risks involve in these hazards. It is our opinion that the risks run at present are slight and acceptable.

In an agricultural community food is bought and sold in local markets and small shops. The customer can see what he or she is purchasing and judge its quality. Formerly retail shops bought most of their food in bulk from wholesalers and a purchase was weighed and wrapped before the customer's eyes. Now the housewife shopping in a supermarket sees nothing of what she buys, and can only get information by reading the label on the pack. It is therefore essential that this information be accurate and not misleading. This is particularly important when a pack contains a food preparation with many ingredients or consists of a whole meal. Customers are also greatly influenced in their choice by advertisements and especially those on television. A main concern of contemporary food legislation to protect consumers is with the control of labelling and advertisement.

Although fraudulent tradesmen and manufacturers were responsible for the introduction and growth of food legislation, their modern counterparts must not be cast in this role. Big manufacturers and retail stores are concerned with the quality of their goods, and in a competitive market any disclosure of an unsatisfactory product would have disastrous consequences for the firm. Modern legislation arises out of continuing dialogues between trade associations, consumer associations and enforcement authorities. These dialogues are in general harmonious because each party is concerned that foods should be safe and of good quality.

In a country the size of Britain there are tens of thousands of people whose work in one way or another ensures the quality of our food. Most of these have specialist knowledge and some have experience in judging complex issues. The rest of this chapter is a brief résumé of how their work is organised. There are many large books which deal with technical aspects. One small book which can be recommended to the general reader and to all students of nutrition is *Food Quality and Safety: a Century of Progress* (Ministry of Agriculture, Fisheries and Food, 1977). It records a symposium to celebrate the centenary of the Sale of Food and Drugs Act 1875. Papers were prepared by workers with experience in several countries, and the discussions in which many joined were lively and informative.

LEGISLATION

The Sale of Food and Drugs Act 1875 was replaced in turn by the Food and Drugs (Adulteration) Act 1928 and later by the Food and Drugs Acts of 1938 and 1955, which latter is still in force. The drugs aspects of the 1955 Act were superseded by the passing of the Medicines Act in 1968. Discussions are now taking place which will lead to a new Act concerned only with food. The 1955 Act is amplified by regulations and orders which cover most of the common foods or groups of food, e.g. the Bread and Flour Regulations, the Condensed and Dried Milk Regulations, the Soft Drinks Regulations. There are also separate Food Hygiene Regulations. All of these have been reviewed and amended at intervals. Proposals for new legislation are put before Parliament by the Minister of Agriculture, Fisheries and Food. Before legislation is drawn up, the Minister takes advice from interested parties, and since 1948 this has been channelled through a Foods Standards Committee, in respect of composition labelling, advertising, additives and contaminants. Since 1964 a separate committee, the Food Additives and Contaminants Committee, has taken over reviewing additive and contaminant measures.

Foods Standards Committee
The members of this committee are appointed by the Minister of Agriculture, Fisheries and Food on behalf of all ministeries concerned with foods, but they are not civil servants. There are ten members and at present three come from the food industry, three are drawn from consumer and enforcement interests, and four, including the Chairman, are from the scientific field. The composition of the Committee changes slowly and many members have served for over 10 years and so have acquired much general experience. Officials of the Ministry adminster the Committee and provide expert advice on legislative matters. The Committee receives advice on health and nutritional matters from the Department of Health and Social Security and its advisory committees. Assessors may be appointed from the food industry and scientific institutes to give technical advice on particular subjects. The Committee is asked periodically by ministers to review existing legislation or to consider new areas and make recommendations for changes on specific subjects. Recent reports have been on Bread and Flour (1974), Novel Protein foods (1974), Yogurt (1975), Soft Drinks (1976), Beer (1976) and Water in Food (1978). Reports on Labelling, Meat and Meat Products, Infant Foods and Table Spreads and Margarine are being prepared.

Before starting a report the Committee invites interested organisations and individuals to submit written evidence and some of these later give oral evidence. Committee reports are published and interested parties may send comments to the Minister. After receiving these, the Minister draws up new legislation which does not always follow the recommendations of the Committee. Reports now provide a general account of manufacturing processes and of the nutritive value of the various products and aim to be of general educational value. They are recommended reading for students of nutrition.

Food Additives and Contaminants Committee
This was set up as a body independent of the Foods Standards Committee in 1964 and has since operated in a similar way to carry out duties previously under the single committee. Recent reports have been on Emulsifiers and Stabilisers (1970), Packaging (1970), Preservatives (1972), Solvents (1974), Antioxidants (1975), Lead (1975), Flavourings (1976) and Additives and Processing Aids in Beer (1978). As regards food additives the Committee operates by recommending permitted lists of those that may be used for specific purposes, and these lists are reviewed at intervals.

Two criteria are considered before a substance is put on the permitted list. The first is its safety and the second the technical need in the manufacturing process. The first criterion is overriding, and no substance is considered safe until the Committee is satisfied that it has been tested for toxicity in an elaborate series of trials using several species of animals and that it has no adverse effects on growth and reproduction.

As regards contaminants the Committee aims to encourage good agricultural, manufacturing and handling techniques, so as to reduce possible contamination at all stages of food production to a minimum. For example, there are legal limits to the amounts of arsenic and lead that may be present in a food.

Enforcement

Enforcement of food legislation is in the hands of local government authorities. They inspect, analyse and take legal action. Inspection is by environmental health officers, who are derived from the old sanitary inspectors under the Medical Officer of Health, and by consumer protection officers, formerly known as inspectors of weights and measures. It is the duty of these officers of district councils to inspect regularly all premises handling food in their district, to obtain samples of foodstuffs offered for sale and have them analysed, and to investigate complaints made by individual members of the public. Complaints about composition, labelling and advertising are made to local authorities, who either have their own analytical laboratories run by public analysts or use consultant public analysts. Cases are brought before a magistrate's court.

Local government organisation evolves slowly and usually haphazardly. With the reorganisation of local government in the UK following the 1972 Act, it is too early to say how effective enforcement is at the moment. The general impression is that in many areas it works but that regionalisation might be more sensible. One criticism is that magistrates who for a long time have dealt competently with cases of short weight and other simple frauds have not sufficient knowledge and experience to deal with the complex law on labelling and advertising (see below). It has been suggested that special new courts be set up by central government to deal with such cases.

EUROPEAN COMMON MARKET

The Treaty of Rome established the European Economic Community (EEC) whose members are bound by Article 2 of the Treaty to establish a common market. A common market implies that goods can move freely in it and that their sale throughout the market is not restricted by regional regulations governing their nature and composition or the methods of manufacture, packaging and labelling. Although all the member countries have such regulations with the same aim of protecting consumers, it is surprising how much they differ in detail. Many of these differences arise from long-established preferences by consumers in different countries for particular products. There are, for instance, well-known differences in the bread, beer, chocolate and jam commonly consumed in the various countries. It is not the intention to prohibit the sale of any local product in its country of origin, but to ensure that products can be sold freely within the market. This in practice means that all products are adequately defined and sold with the appropriate label. This process of removing trade barriers is known as **harmonisation.**

The decision-making body in the EEC is the Council of Ministers. Suggestions for legislation are originally put up by the Commission. There are 13 commissioners appointed by national governments and Britain appoints two. They are assisted by some 5000 administrative staff who work in Brussels and are divided into 19 directorate-generals. The European Assembly is an advisory body whose members are at present nominated by national parliaments, but the intention is that in 1979 they should be elected by universal suffrage. It considers and comments on suggestions put up by the Commission to Council. Its headquarters are in Strasbourg, but it sometimes meets in Luxembourg.

The Commission has produced over 20 draft directives affecting specific classes of foods. When these have been approved by the Council, which only follows detailed argument in committee by government representatives, each member government has to amend its national laws if they are at variance with the directive. These new rules are then part of each national law and affect all member countries. In contrast the Council may make 'regulations' which have immediately the force of law throughout the EEC. These are often introduced for new foods. There are already regulations relating to the grading of eggs and of fruit and vegetables, water in frozen chicken and to the categories and labelling on wine. There are directives on chocolate, honey and sugar which have or should soon become national regulations. Most of the draft directives are still under discussion and some have been withdrawn. There are also directives on food additives, most of which are now national regulations.

The process of harmonisation is slow and involves endless committees who receive evidence and information from manufacturers, trade associations and consumers. Imagination, patience and a pragmatic outlook are needed. However, there can be little doubt that as a result of this great expenditure of time and money individual customers in Common Market countries will have better information of the nature of the foods which they purchase and more assurance that whatever their origin they are of good quality.

UNITED STATES

The first settlers soon had to take action against fraud, and in 1630 the Massachusetts Bay Colony prosecuted Nicholas Knopp from Holland 'for taking upon him to cure the scurvy by a water of noe worth nor value which he sold att a very deare note.' He was fined £5 and declared liable to prosecution by his defrauded customers. Various laws were passed modelled on those in the home countries and these include many ordinances to ensure that flour and other foods for export were not adulterated.

Insistence on States' rights delayed the first federal Food and Drugs Act until 1906. This followed a crusade by the chief food chemist to the Department of Agriculture, Dr Harvey W. Wiley. He had a 'poison squad' of volunteers, who were fed for five days large doses of borax, formaldehyde, salicylic acid, copper sulphate and sulphurous acid with the aim of finding the dose sufficient to produce symptoms. The great depression of the 1930s showed up the weaknesses of the Act and led to the Federal Food, Drug and Cosmetic Act (1938). The deaths of at least 73 persons in 1937 from a drug sold as Elixir Sulfanilamide was the final factor in the passage of the Act. The Act set up the Food and Drug Administration (FDA), which is still responsible to the Secretary of the Department of Health, Education and Welfare for protecting public health. The FDA is divided into six sections, one of which is the Bureau of Health.

In the 1938 Act the FDA had to prove that a drug or additive was harmful before it could be removed from the market. But the 1958 Food Additives Amendment changed the responsibility. The onus now lies with the manufacturer to prove the safety of a new additive before it receives clearance for marketing. Additives that may be used are on a list of 'generally recognised as safe' (GRAS) substances. This numbers several hundred and includes natural and traditional additives that have been used for many years, but never subjected to intensive toxicological scrutiny, like sugar, pepper, mustard, cinnamon as well as more modern compounds like MSG, BHA and sulphur dioxide which appear to be safe after multiple animal tests and short-term human studies. The largest number of substances are flavour ingredients, which are mostly natural derivatives and used in very tiny amounts. If new evidence suggests a compound is not safe, it may be removed from the GRAS list. This happened with cyclamate, amaranth and saccharin.

For many fresh foods e.g. meat, poultry, dairy products, fruit and vegetables, the US Department of Agriculture is the regulatory authority.

A feature of modern US food laws, known as the Delaney Clause, is a proviso in the 1958 Food Additive Amendment which states: 'No [food] additive shall be deemed safe if it is found to induce cancer when ingested by man or animal.' This clause is a veto which prevents the FDA from exercising its judgment and was directly responsible for the ban on cyclamates when a few of the rats receiving huge doses developed cancer of the bladder. Americans will probably have to live with the Delaney Clause for some time as any Congressman who tried to repeal it would be interpreted as asking for a vote for cancer and this would not help his political career.

The main risk against which the American public have to be protected is that of food-borne infections. As in Britain, the true incidence is not known because many instances are not reported. In America a higher proportion of meals are eaten outside the home than in Britain; these have been prepared and cooked in restaurants, and although the proportion of these that are unhygienic may be small, the total number is large. Further, botulism, unknown in Britain for decades, continues to occur and causes deaths in the USA although this usually arises from errors in home canning.

The second major concern of FDA is with food labelling owing to the great increase in sales of packaged precooked meals. Enthusiasm for nutritional labelling (p. 152) is much greater in America than in Britain.

DEVELOPING COUNTRIES

The great increase in the growth of cities in Africa, Asia and Latin America in the last three decades has led to problems in food hygiene and adulteration similar to those in Europe and North America in the nineteenth century. It is much easier to pass legislation than to train and support the large staff of skilled people needed to enforce it.

Another factor is that a large part of the exports of many of these countries consists of food products. Importing countries properly require that these conform with their own standards. To facilitate international trade and to assist the advance of food technology in developing countries, FAO and WHO started jointly in 1963 preparing a *Codex Alimentarius*. This is concerned with standards for the composition of all major foods and also with provisions concerning food hygiene, food additives, pesticides and residues, methods of sampling and analysis and labelling. The Codex aims to set standards for some 200 foods. In this immense task most progress has been made with milk and milk products. A Code of Principles dealing with the use of proper designations and ethical practices in the international trade of milk products has been accepted by more than 70 countries. Codex standards have to be considered and adopted by each country. Agreement on a Codex Standard does not compel any country to adopt it.

LABELLING

A housewife often cannot see the goods, which she wishes to purchase, because they are ready packed in the shop. She has to select her goods by using the information on the labels. Consumers in Britain are protected against false information by the Trades Description Act which applies to all goods and, more specifically in the case of foods, by the Labelling of Food Regulations (1970). The latter is based on the Foods Standards Committee report on Labelling (1964) and on Claims and Misleading Descriptions (1966). This whole area is now being reviewed afresh.

With a few exceptions all foods have to be labelled with an 'appropriate designation' defined in the regulations as a 'name and description sufficiently specific, in each case, to indicate to an intending purchaser the true nature of the food to which it is applied and, as respect of any ingredient or any constituent, a specific (and not generic) name or description.' When a food contains more than one ingredient the appropriate designation of each ingredient must be given in a list, setting out the ingredients in the order of the amounts present in the food. It is not necessary to specify the added chemicals and a permitted additive may be described as an antioxidant, colouring matter, preservative, etc.

It is not necessary for a manufacturer to give the amounts of nutrients present in a product, but some like to do so, notably for breakfast cereals. This information is useful and educative for consumers with some knowledge of nutrition but may easily mislead the ignorant, by implying falsely that there is a specific benefit from the amount of a particular nutrient in the product. The advantages and dangers of 'nutritional labelling' are now the subject of much discussion in many countries and the regulations are likely to change.

In Britain there are lists of scheduled vitamins and minerals for which claims can be made. At present these are vitamin A, thiamin, riboflavin, nicotinic acid, vitamin C and vitamin D and the minerals calcium, iodine and iron. Statements of content would be of use to many more people if expressed not as mg nutrient/100 g food but as a proportion of the recommended daily intake present in a usual serving of the product. However, usual servings are not yet defined in Britain.

The labelling of foods designed for those who wish to reduce weight presents problems. In the UK it is illegal to refer to them solely as slimming foods but they may be described as foods useful as part of a slimming diet. A food may only be described as 'starch-reduced' when its starch content is substantially less than that of a similar natural food and its total carbohydrate content is less than 50 per cent of the dry matter. A claim that a food is a source of protein may not be made unless 12 per cent of the energy from such food comes from protein.

Pictures on labels and advertisements may be misleading. They may show fresh fruit when the product contains only fruit flavouring or depict other foods commonly consumed with the product without explicitly stating that these are not present in the container. Adjectives such as 'natural', 'fresh', 'pure' and 'homemade' may be misused. Language is continuously changing and such words as butter, cream, cutlet, steak and chop are now used to describe products different from the original. Some of these extended uses seem legitimate and others appear deliberately misleading. Legislation in these fields is difficult and control is effected mainly by manufacturers and advertisers using codes of practice. Fortunately the big manufacturers are concerned with the good name of the food industry as a whole and through their associations can apply pressure on any manufacturer whose labels and advertisements might bring the industry into disrepute.

Labelling in the USA

In the labelling system introduced between 1973 and 1975 the rules about what is fair description of the product and its ingredients are complex but similar to those in Britain already described. For most foods nutrition labelling is optional but it is mandatory whenever nutritional claims are made or a nutrient is added to a food. When it is used, the manufacturer must put on the label the measurement that he is taking as a serving, how many servings there are in the container and the calories, protein, carbohydrate and fat (all in grams) per serving. This is followed by eight nutrients that all have to be listed, expressed as a percentage of the recommended daily allowance in a serving— protein, vitamin A, thiamin, riboflavin, niacin, vitamin C, iron and calcium. When a serving contains less than 2 per cent, no figure is given for this nutrient. There are three recommended daily allowances that may be used as denominators, one for infants and another for children under 4 years, but the one commonly used is for adults, the US RDA of the Food and Drug Administration. It uses the highest figures for any adult group in the 1968 Recommended Dietary Allowances of the Food and Nutrition Board of the National Academy of Sciences.

In addition to these nutrients that must be listed, there are another 15 optional pieces of nutritional information, any number of which can be shown if the manufacturer wishes. These are the content of saturated and polyunsaturated fat, dietary cholesterol, sodium, vitamins D, E, B_6, B_{12}, folacin, biotin and pantothenic acid, and the minerals phosphorus, iodine, magnesium, zinc and copper. All values have to be expressed as the percentage of the US RDA per serving. When the type of fat or cholesterol is put on the label there must be a footnote saying that, 'This information is provided for individuals who, on the advice of a physician, are modifying their total dietary intake of fat (or cholesterol).'

The American system can only be used by an informed public. A book to educate laymen, *Nutrition Labeling: How It Can Work For You*, has been written by the National Nutrition Consortium of six scientific societies concerned about nutrition. Its address is 9650 Rockville Pike, Bethesda, Maryland 20014. Even for those people who can understand it the present system is cumbersome, it gives unnecessary information, e.g. riboflavin deficiency is rare in the USA, and labels fail to list dietary components that could be important, e.g. dietary fibre.

ADVERTISING

All advertising in Britain including that of food is supervised by the Code of Advertising Practice (CAP) Committee, which is made up of representatives of advertisers, advertising agencies and the media. The Committee, whose address is 15–17 Ridgmount Street, London WC1E

7AW, has a code of practice, regularly updated. It advises advertisers, checks copy and deals with complaints from consumers. The Advertising Standards Authority is a higher authority and about 50 per cent of its members are independent. The Authority deals with the government departments and other outside organisations and with complaints from firms and trading authorities and those from consumers which the CAP Committee may pass on. Advertising on television and radio is the responsibility of the Independent Broadcasting Authority, 70 Brompton Road, London SW3.

SUMMARY

Consumers in the industrialised countries are protected by complicated systems involving government, manufacturers, advertisers and the media, and operating through statutory regulations and voluntary codes of practice. It involves a series of compromises, in many of which the balance may change over the years. The government and manufacturers in general work well together and are rarely at loggerheads on major issues. Manufacturers like to have some guidelines laid down by statute, but prefer details to be left in voluntary hands. They continuously and rightly oppose any proposed change in the law which might restrict technical developments. Consumers may be assured that the system protects them adequately against hazards to health which might arise from chemicals added to foods and from loss of nutrients in foods as a result of processing. Labels and advertisements may not always be as informative as they might be, and on occasions are still positively misleading. However, in this respect they are better than formerly; the system of control is not fixed, but subject to continuing review and we may hope for improvements. It still remains true that the most frequent hazards to health arise not from additives or from processing but from poor hygiene and its associated microbiological risks, which can arise in shops, in restaurants, cafés and canteens in institutions and, all too frequently, in the home.

PART III

Primary Nutritional Diseases

27. Starvation and Anorexia Nervosa

Starvation arises (1) when there is not enough food to eat, for instance in times of famine, (2) when there is severe disease of the digestive tract, preventing the absorption of nutrients, as in the malabsorption syndrome and cancer of the oesophagus, or (3) when there is a disturbance which either reduces appetite or interferes with the normal metabolism of the nutrients by the tissues; such a disturbance might be metabolic in origin (e.g. in renal or hepatic failure) or due to severe and long-continued infection. In all these circumstances there is wasting of the body with much loss of both muscle and fat. This gives rise to a clinical picture with an underlying morbid anatomy and chemical pathology which is essentially similar whatever the primary cause. Substantially the same processes occur in two other conditions, both of which have special features. (4) Starvation, or near-starvation, is sometimes used as treatment for gross and intractable obesity, and this is considered on page 252. (5) People may greatly reduce their food intake and become very wasted for psychological reasons. The condition known as **anorexia nervosa** is described at the end of this chapter.

This chapter is concerned primarily with the clinical features, pathology and treatment of starvation in adults. Its effects in children are described in Chapter 29, and the metabolic changes are discussed from a different viewpoint in Chapter 8. Other relevant material is the effects of diseases of the digestive tract (Chap. 46), special feeding methods (Chap. 52), the numerous causes of a failure in food supply (Chap. 54) and some administrative measures in famine relief (Chap. 58).

HISTORY

There have been three distinct phases in the scientific investigation of undernutrition and starvation during this century. In the period before World War I there were several professional fasting men. These strange creatures were prepared to go for periods up to 30 days without food. They were much studied by physiologists and from their experiments valuable information was obtained, especially in regard to the importance of the obligatory protein losses; this was ably summarised by Lusk (1928) in successive editions of his classic book. Between the two wars the subject attracted little attention; in this period vitamins dominated nutritional research. World War II brought about widespread undernutrition and starvation in many parts of the world. They

became matters of practical importance to many doctors and much valuable new information was obtained. Five excellent monographs are available. Smith and Woodruff (1951) and Helweg-Larsen et al. (1952) describe their own experiences in Japanese and Nazi prison camps; Burger et al. (1948) report on starvation in Holland during the winter of 1944–45, and the workers in the Department of Experimental Medicine, Cambridge (1951), give an account of the undernutrition in Germany in the immediate post-war years. Keys et al. (1950) describe a laboratory experiment in which 32 young men volunteered to live for six months on a diet providing only 7.7 MJ (1600 kcal)/ day. As a result they became severely undernourished, losing about 25 per cent of their body weight.

Since 1945 the concept of the division of the body into compartments (Chap. 2) has been increasingly useful. Measurements of their size in relation to the state of nutrition have led to a clearer understanding of the chemical pathology of undernutrition. As a result more precise methods of treatment are available for patients who are undernourished following serious medical and surgical disorders. It is significant that an important book dealing with undernutrition comes from the department of surgery at Harvard (Moore, 1959).

MORBID ANATOMY

Wasting of the tissues is the most characteristic feature of starvation. At autopsy a patient who has died of starvation may have little or no remaining adipose tissue. As a result the skin is loose. There is also marked atrophy of the skeletal muscles. Superficial oedema is usually present; its distribution is largely determined by gravity. Fluid may also be found in the peritoneal and pleural cavities.

There is also atrophy of all the viscera except the brain, which is spared. Atrophy of the heart is marked. In an adult man in health the heart weighs about 350 g. Porter (1889) who performed 459 autopsies on victims of an Indian famine found that in 45 per cent of the men the heart weighed less than 170 g and in some cases no more than 100 g. This atrophy, if severe, is often irreversible and the subsequent failure of the circulation is a frequent cause of death. Atrophy of the small intestine, which affects both the mucous membrane and the muscular walls, is always present and may be very severe. Donovan (1848), writing of his experiences in the great Irish famine, states that he observed: 'Total disappearance of the omentum, and a peculiarly thin condition of the small intestines which (in such cases) were so transparent that if the deceased had taken any food immediately before death, the contents could be seen through the coats of the bowel.' In 1945 one of us (S.D.) saw a similar picture in persons dying of starvation in Belsen concentration camps. The virtual loss of the power to absorb nutrients by the atrophied intestinal mucous membrane greatly prejudices the chances of recovery. Ramalingaswami (1971) gives an account of autopsies on victims of the 1966–67 Bihar famine which emphasises the extent of the cardiac atrophy.

A monograph by Jackson (1925) reviews past literature on the effect of starvation on the organs of man and experimental animals, and one by Follis (1958) the pathological changes.

ADAPTIVE CHANGES

The wasting and loss of weight are at first rapid if food supplies are suddenly reduced, but gradually slow down even though there is no change in the amount of food eaten. There are three reasons for this slowing down:

1. With the wasting of the body, the cell mass of actively metabolising tissue is reduced and therefore requires less energy to maintain its activities.
2. The body, being lighter, requires less mechanical work to move it about.
3. All unnecessary voluntary movements are curtailed.

In these ways the body is able to achieve an important degree of biological adaptation to a restricted food supply. Indeed were it not for this adaptability, the human species might well have become extinct long since.

Twenty-five per cent of the weight of a healthy, non-obese body can usually be lost without immediate danger to life. With greater losses the hold on life is slender, but some have survived losses up to 50 per cent of their initial weight.

An excellent review of the adaptive changes in response to starvation is by Grande (1964).

CHANGES IN BODY COMPOSITION IN STARVATION

The wasting of tissues during starvation greatly affects the chemical composition of the body. Table 2.1 (p.6) sets out the chemical composition of the body of a normal man. In Table 27.1 the alterations which may occur after he has lost 25 per cent of his original weight are given. The most obvious change is the disappearance of over 70 per cent of the body fat.

Stores of energy and survival

Table 27.1 indicates that a normal man may lose about 3 kg of protein, 6.5 kg of fat and 200 g of carbohydrate. These amounts of protein, fat and carbohydrate represent a reserve or store of about 310 MJ (75 000 kcal). It must be emphasised that these figures apply to a normal man. In an obese subject the reserve is much greater and in a small thin person much less. If the normal healthy man is

Table 27.1 The changes in body composition of a man who in health weighed 65 kg and then lost 25 per cent of this weight as a result of partial starvation

	In health (kg)	After starvation (kg)
Protein	11.5	8.5
Fat	9	2.5
Carbohydrate	0.5	0.3
Water:		
Extracellular	15	15
Intracellular	25	19
Minerals	4	3.5
	65.0	48.8

These figures describe what might occur to the hypothetical man described in Chapter 2. For reported changes see Keys et al. (1950) and Moore (1959)

deprived of all food, but not required to take any exercise, energy expenditure is at about 6.7 MJ/day and at this rate the reserve lasts for 45 to 50 days.

A man does not die quickly of starvation. Many healthy people have taken no food for 14 days. The experience is unpleasant, but involves no serious impairment of physiological function and leaves no permanent effect on health.

Table 27.1 shows that the reserves of carbohydrate are insufficient to meet energy needs even for a day. Wherever possible it is desirable to provide a starving man with at least 100 g of carbohydrate daily. This will prevent the onset of ketosis and also reduce the breakdown of endogenous protein. Measurements of the differences between the O_2, CO_2 and glucose content of the arterial and venous blood of the brain indicate that normally it only utilises carbohydrate and not protein and fat. The oxygen consumption of the human brain is about 45 ml/min. This involves the combustion of 80 to 90 g/day of glucose. During complete starvation part of this comes from the conversion of protein to carbohydrate, i.e. gluconeogenesis in the liver.

Of the 310 MJ reserve in the example quoted above, about 17 per cent is provided by endogenous protein. This corresponds to the breakdown of 66 g/day of protein, and amounts of protein of this order are catabolised during brief fasting (Table 27.2). But in prolonged fasting or starvation adaptive mechanisms come into play which slow down the breakdown of protein to only about 20 g/day after 5 or 6 weeks (Cahill, 1970). Adaptation occurs in the brain so that it can utilise keto acids, particularly β-hydroxybutyric acid (Owen et al., 1967). This spares the need for glucose and consequently gluconeogenesis. Secondly, gluconeogenesis in the liver falls off greatly, probably because the amount of alanine coming from muscle is less; alanine is much reduced and this is the principal substrate that the liver uses for gluconeogenesis. Most of the glucose synthesised in the liver now comes from lactate, pyruvate and glycerol. Meanwhile the kidney has to continue to form ammonia from amino acids to maintain acid–base homeostasis. In the process glucose is produced. Thus the major share of the reduced gluconeogenesis takes place in the kidney.

Changes in body water

Table 27.1 shows estimates of the substances lost from the bodies of young men submitted to partial dietary restriction for two to three weeks, while a regime of physical activity involving an expenditure of about 10.9 MJ (2600 kcal)/day was maintained.

There is a large loss of body water, about 1.5 kg, in the first three days. This is a characteristic immediate response to dietary carbohydrate restriction and is responsible for the greater part of the weight loss that occurs in the first week, when dietary intake is restricted, either by illness or voluntarily at the start of a reducing regime. The mechanism is discussed on p. 251.

Famine oedema. Table 27.2 also shows that in the second week of restriction losses of body water were small and had stopped altogether by the end of the third week. Table 27.1 showed that after six months of partial starvation, the water content of the body had fallen much less than the body weight; the loss was of intracellular water and the amount of extracellular water remained virtually unchanged. Thus as the tissues waste, the size of the extracellular compartment becomes relatively greater, and this gives rise to oedema. Famine oedema is a characteristic feature not only in victims of famine, but also in patients severely undernourished as a result of disease. It has been known and studied since the time of Hippocrates, and McCance's review (1951) has over 500 references; its cause is still not properly understood.

Protein deficiency, always associated with starvation, may cause the concentration of plasma albumin to fall and this contributes to the oedema in some cases. However, there is no correlation between the severity of the oedema and the plasma albumin concentration (Beattie et al. 1948) and this cannot be the main cause. There is surprisingly little disturbance of renal function, although the excretion of a large water load may be delayed. This is probably the

consequence of a slight reduction in glomerular filtration rate resulting from a reduced cardiac output. Again this might be a contributory factor in some cases of famine oedema, but is not the main cause.

A possible explanation, first suggested by Youmans (1936), is a fall in tissue tension. When fat is lost and the tissues shrink, the skin is not sufficiently elastic to contract to the new body size. This may lead to a fall in tissue tension with seepage of water from the blood into the interstitial spaces. The body may be said to get too small for its skin. This explanation could account for the fact that famine oedema is most common and severe in old people, whose skin is less elastic than the young. Pressure in the interstitial tissue is normally subatmospheric and about minus 6 mmHg. A vacuum of over 15 mmHg has to be applied to the arm before oedema occurs (Guyton et al., 1971).

Associated with the constancy of the extracellular fluid volume, there is little change in the amount of sodium in the body. The total exchangeable sodium may be over 2000 mmol and within the normal range. Thus there is an excess of sodium relative to the reduced size of the body.

With the shrinkage of the cells and loss of intracellular water, there is loss of total body potassium. The potassium deficiency may amount to more than one-third of the 3500 mmol normally present in the body.

Unless the period of starvation has been very long, many months or even years, there is only a small loss of minerals from the skeleton.

Hormone production

Secretion of pituitary gonadotrophins is impaired and plasma concentrations of testosterone and urinary 17-oxosteroids fall. Plasma insulin is low during fasting because glucose and amino acids, which stimulate its secretion, are not being absorbed; in addition, the concentration after an overnight fast is below the normal value (Marliss et al., 1970). Secretion of pituitary growth hormone tends to be increased and this favours fat mobilisation. Plasma concentrations of pancreatic glucagon increase early in starvation and remain at a high level (Marliss et al., 1970). Plasma cortisol is elevated because of

Table 27.2 Losses of body weight and fat, protein and water on low energy diets, (a) 4.3 MJ (1020 kcal)/day (13 men) and (b) 2.4 MJ (580 kcal)/day (6 men) (data from Brozek et al., 1957)

Days	Mean daily loss in grams							
	Weight		Fat		Protein		Water	
	a	b	a	b	a	b	a	b
1–3	800	733	200	198	40	66	560	469
4–6	—	500	—	200	—	50	—	250
7–13	233	367	161	194	28	48	44	125
22–24	167	—	142	—	25	—	0	—

a slowed rate of turnover (Alleyne and Young, 1967). Starvation leads to changes in triiodothyronine (T$_3$). Concentration of the active form goes down while there is a reciprocal rise of inactive 'reverse T$_3$' (Vagenakis et al., 1975). Thyroxine secretion is reduced in marasmic children (Graham et al., 1973).

CLINICAL FEATURES

The patients are thin and the lax skinfolds give evidence of recent loss of weight. The hair is dry and lustreless. The eyes are dull and sunken, yet wasting of the orbital tissues may make them appear unduly prominent, particularly since the sclerae are unusually avascular. The skin is thin, dry, inelastic; often there is peripheral cyanosis, even in warm weather. Dirty brown splotches of pigmentation may appear over the face and trunk; these were recognised during the last century as one of the stigmata of famine.

Polyuria at night is a frequent and troublesome symptom of impending famine oedema. When oedema begins to appear it is usually first noticed in the face if the patient is lying down, giving the patient a puffy appearance which may falsely suggest adequate nutrition. When the patient gets up and walks about, the fluid gravitates to the legs, causing ankle oedema.

The blood pressure is low; the diastolic pressure may be impossible to estimate, while the systolic pressure may be as low as 70 mmHg. The pulse rate usually falls progressively during prolonged partial starvation. In severe cases it is often below 40/min. When wasting becomes marked, the heart appears small on a radiograph.

Although hydraemia and a mild anaemia (Hb 9 to 12 g/dl) are common, severe anaemia is not a feature of starvation. If found, it is an indication of other co-existent disease. Associated vitamin deficiencies seldom give rise to clinical signs in starving people; the need for vitamins is probably reduced when the metabolism of the body is lowered by starvation.

Clinical evidence of hormonal disturbance is not lacking in starvation. Amenorrhoea and delayed puberty are common features but lactation is sometimes maintained. Men lose their libido and may become impotent; they may develop enlargement of the breasts (gynaecomastia). In children there is often a growth of lanugo hair, especially over the forearms and back, as may be seen in other gross endocrine disorders.

Symptoms related to the psychological state of starving people are of practical importance. Although the intellect is usually clear, the personality may be seriously deranged. The mind is never fixed for long on a single subject, except the desire for food. Mental restlessness is combined with physical apathy. The patient becomes self-centred and indifferent to the troubles of others, even those of his dearest friends and relatives. He worries and becomes hypochondriacal, even hysterical, about his own disability. He is sensitive to noise and other petty irritations which

may make him quarrelsome. These symptoms may intensify rather than diminish in the early stages of treatment; consequently the starving patient is difficult to manage. This feature of the disorder should be remembered and treated objectively by people engaged in famine relief, otherwise they may lose sympathy with those whom they are trying to help. They must never expect thanks for their kindness.

In the last stages of starvation, the personality may disintegrate completely. A mother may steal from her child. Donovan (1848) described in elegant language the horrible results of breakdowns in family ties which occurred in a small town during the great Irish famine. Cannibalism has been reported in many countries of the world (including Scotland) in times of famine.

Starving patients often suffer from infections—malaria, cholera, typhus, relapsing fever, pneumonia, gastroenteritis—to name only a few. Tuberculosis may add to the clinical signs present, often in unusual ways, for infection in starvation may give rise to little or no fever. These infections further aggravate the plight of a starving person. Their relationship to famine is discussed in Chapter 58.

Cancrum oris, an infective gangrene of the mouth eroding the lip and cheeks, is a dreadful catastrophe which occasionally occurs in famines both among children and adults. The sufferers are usually not only malnourished but also severely dehydrated by diarrhoea or lack of nursing care. Large areas of the mouth and face may be destroyed before the patient succumbs. The only possible treatment is surgical excision of the dead tissues after a period of re-feeding and medical care.

The terminal event in starvation is usually intractable diarrhoea. The atrophied intestinal glands and the paperthin walls of the digestive tract are unable to digest and absorb properly even a bland diet, much less the kind of food on which people during famine may hope to survive, such as roots, leaves, and bread made from coarse grain. In almost all famines, outbreaks of diarrhoea have been reported, but bacteriologists have seldom found organisms that could be held responsible. Once diarrhoea has begun, it is a serious sign.

DIAGNOSIS

In times of famine the signs of starvation may be all too obvious, so much so that other causes of emaciation can be overlooked. However, a similar clinical picture may be produced by tuberculosis, dysentery or other severe chronic diseases. In the early stage of anorexia nervosa the psychogenic origin of the weight loss is easily overlooked.

Famine oedema has to be distinguished from other primary causes of oedema—cardiac, renal or hepatic.

TREATMENT

In simple undernutrition, all that is needed is suitable food. Its management is more an administrative than a medical problem. When the patient suffering from starvation is seriously ill the nature of the treatment depends essentially on the facilities available. Here only measures possible under famine conditions, when the nursing staff is inevitably limited, are described. Under these circumstances methods such as intravenous feeding are often impractical. This and other special feeding methods which may be used when the number of patients is limited, the nursing staff sufficient and well trained and when expert laboratory help is available are described in Chapter 53.

Most famine victims, because of alimentary dysfunction, cannot deal with large quantities of food. The patient's desire for food is often immense and no guide to his digestive capacities. Limitation of the food intake may be necessary. This is essential if there is diarrhoea or severe cachexia.

The choice of food is difficult. Many starving people in the prison camps of World War II died from diarrhoea and collapse after the well-meaning attentions of those who rescued them. They were given any food that happended to be available—bully-beef, baked beans—which they could not readily digest. Only bland foods can be tolerated by the thin-walled intestines lacking essential digestive enzymes.

Frequent small feeds of skimmed milk, 100 ml or so at a time—as often as the patient is willing and able to take them—is a good way to avert death from starvation. This requires constant personal attention and nursing care. It is entirely impractical to prescribe for the needs of the patient in terms of calculated energy needs. Skimmed milk powders are normally reconstituted to give a mixture of 10 to 15 per cent strength. However, if the patient is very weak, a more dilute mixture may be preferable. A variety of mild flavouring essences may be useful to stimulate the appetite. Slightly sour foods are usually acceptable; yogurt or other kinds of curdled milk may be tried. There is a possibility of lactose intolerance if large amounts of skimmed milk are given and starving patients may tolerate moderate amounts of fat or edible oils, which provide a larger energy intake. Mason *et al.* (1974) report good results in children in the Ethiopian famine with a mixture of 42 per cent dried skimmed milk, 32 per cent edible oil, 25 per cent sugar, plus potassium, magnesium and vitamins. As the patient begins to recover he should be encouraged gradually to take semisolid foods, along the lines followed in weaning a baby. With refeeding there may be a temporary increase in oedema, and so the intake of salt should be restricted.

There may come a time in severe starvation when the patient, although still fully rational, refuses all food. The outlook is then very grave. Nasogastric feeding (p.445) provides the only hope. Spectacular improvement may follow, but some patients are beyond recovery.

PROGNOSIS

Most people with primary undernutrition recover rapidly,

once they have a free access to food. Appetites may be enormous. Over 21 MJ (5000 kcal)/day may be consumed and be associated with a weekly gain in weight of 1.5 to 2 kg. In some patients, despite careful nursing and a good diet, low blood pressure and diarrhoea may persist. If, after one or two weeks, they show little improvement, this suggests strongly that irreversible changes in the myocardium or small intestine have developed and that the prognosis is poor. After any severe famine there are some who may linger on in this condition for many months if supported by good medical and nursing skill. But death rather than recovery is the usual end.

ANOREXIA NERVOSA

This is a psychiatric disease arising from a refusal to eat which often leads to severe emaciation. It was first described in 1874 by Sir William Gull of Guy's Hospital, London, who attributed it to a 'morbid mental state'. The disease characteristically occurred in young women aged 15 to 25 years and was uncommon. Since about 1970 it appears to have become much more prevalent and the publication of two important books reflects present interest. The proceedings of a conference at the National Institute of Health, Bethesda (Vigersky, 1977) contains 37 contributions including two from London, where Crisp and Russell have both much experience of the disease. Hilde Bruch of Texas has written a book (1978) which describes the circumstances under which the disease arises and the underlying psychiatric disorder. Entitled *The Golden Cage, The Enigma of Anorexia Nervosa*, it can help the families and friends of patients to get the understanding of the nature of the disease which they need to support the patient.

Patients are usually middle class and often above average intelligence. They come from homes where plenty of food is available and taken for granted, and often some of the family are obese. The disease affects mainly adolescent girls and young women, but cases are seen in older women and also in men.

PSYCHOPATHOLOGY

The central abnormality is a desire to obtain and then maintain a low body weight. The patient may have been through a phase of obesity early in adolescence. Often she has been an obedient and compliant child, but is intelligent, highly strung and insecure. A history of psychological disturbance and conflict with one or both parents during puberty is common, but there is no specific setting which precipitates the onset of the disease (Crisp, 1977a). Both the patient's and the family history may be difficult to obtain, as there may be denial that there is anything wrong or abnormal.

Whether the patients are truly anorexic, i.e. without

desire for food, is uncertain. It is more probable that they repress the sensation of hunger or fail to act on it. Some are tormented by their physiological need and haunted by the thought of food. Insatiable appetite (bulimia) may lead to occasional orgies of eating when large quantities of any food that is available are consumed. Some patients deliberately induce vomiting and others purge themselves repeatedly. Information about these habits may be deliberately withheld from the family and the physician.

A pathognomic feature is 'the vigour and stubbornness with which the often gruesome emaciation is defended as normal and right and the only possible protection against the dreaded fate of being too fat' (Bruch, 1974). There is a distortion of the body image. This can be measured using an apparatus in which two lights on a screen are moved various distances apart. The patient is asked to state the distance which she thinks corresponds to the width of her body at various sites. Hips, waist and bust are often overestimated by 50 per cent. The extent of the overestimation may be so great that it constitutes a delusion.

An important question is whether the compulsive starvation which reduces the body to its size before puberty is due to fear of fatness or fear of feminity. When Freud's influence was dominant, the retreat from sexual maturity was attributed to early sexual trauma or even a confusion between oral sexuality and eating. Today a well-rounded shape is unfashionable among young girls and large numbers of them attempt to slim by controlling their carbohydrate intake. Patients have usually subsisted on a diet based on fruit, vegetables, cheese or yogurt and black coffee. One group of patients admitted to a metabolic ward and allowed a free selection of foods consumed on average 4.3 MJ (1030 kcal) of energy, of which 49 per cent came from fat, 18 per cent from protein and only 33 per cent from carbohydrate (Russell, 1967). Thus they had put themselves on a diet commonly chosen by girls who wish to slim. In anorexia nervosa has the fashionable wish to slim turned into a pathological obsession?

CLINICAL FEATURES

The weight may be reduced to 35 kg or less and the loss of subcutaneous fat sharply delineates underlying muscles. These may be maintained by restless activity. This may be promoted by a high intelligence and take various forms, including sports at which some patients have excelled. Gull remarked of one patient, 'It seemed hardly possible that a body so wasted could undergo the exercise which seemed so agreeable.' Patients often deny all normal sense of fatigue.

Nutritional state

All the usual features of starvation may be present. The pulse is slow, the blood pressure, peripheral blood flow and skin temperatures are all low. These changes have been accurately measured in 33 subjects under controlled conditions by Fohlin (1977). There is usually no anaemia and no hypoalbuminaemia. There may be fine downy hair, lanugo, over the body. Amenorrhea is a characteristic feature but secondary sexual characteristics are present. Urinary excretion of gonadotrophins and oestrogens (testosterone in males) is diminished. Plasma oestradiol is low; plasma luteinising hormone (LH) is low in the day and high at night, the opposite of the normal. The response to LH-releasing hormone depends on the patient's weight and the critical figure is about 47 kg, depending on height. Menstruation starts at puberty when it rises above this, and stops in anorexia nervosa when it falls below (Frisch and McArthur, 1974).

Biochemical tests show a normal fasting plasma amino acids pattern (Russell, 1970). There may be hypercarotenaemia (Robboy *et al.*, 1974) and a high plasma cholesterol with the increase confined to the low-density lipoprotein fraction (Mordasini *et al.*, 1978). The plasma potassium may be abnormally low and this is an indication that the patient may have been taking purgatives or may have been inducing vomiting.

DIAGNOSIS

Anorexia is common in patients with an anxiety state, a depressive illness and some forms of schizophrenia. It may arise from a focal lesion of the pituitary-hypothalmic axis caused by trauma, haemorrhage or a neoplasm, but such lesions are very rare. Occasionally it is the presenting feature of tuberculosis or other general infections. In all of these conditions the obsessional concern with food and the physical and mental overactivity, characteristic of anorexia nervosa, are normally absent. However, the differential diagnosis may be difficult and the pitfalls are more fully described by Crisp (1977b).

TREATMENT

The primary aim is to get the patient to eat. Severe cases should be treated by a psychiatrist and under close supervision in hospital until a satisfactory weight has been achieved. The nursing staff and dietitian have to be skilled and forbearing, for these patients are notoriously slow eaters and many cunningly get rid of food by forced vomiting or concealment. It is unrealistic to expect a patient to eat a large diet at once. Diet No. 2 (p. 550), appropriately modified to the patient's tastes, may be tried at the start. Many patients have eaten no bread, potatoes or cereal products for a long time and it may be difficult to persuade them to try these foods again. This and other practical problems in dietetic management are discussed by Day (1974).

Chlorpromazine in doses up to 150 to 200 mg three times daily makes the patient more amenable, counteracts vomiting and is claimed to increase appetite. The doctor's efforts should be directed to exploring the life situation, and in particular the events immediately antedating the onset, and to supplying explanations and reassurance. In no condition is it more important to have only one therapist in direct charge who must be prepared to follow up the patient over a long period of time.

Disturbed relationships within the family need attention. It is often easy but unhelpful to blame a parent for expressing exasperation or a patient for misinterpreting the concern of others. Regular interviews with relatives conducted by a social worker over many months should aim to reduce guilt, misunderstanding and intolerance. The interviews should promote reassurance and prevent rejection of affection.

PROGNOSIS

Recovery, which implies restoration of weight and menstruation, occurs within several months in favourable cases.

Those who had been previously obese reach their target weight sooner than other patients (Stordy *et al.*, 1977). A disquietingly high proportion, estimated at 50 per cent, make only a partial recovery, continuing to restrict their diet and remaining abnormally thin. There is a mortality of about 5 per cent from suicide or inanition in the five years from first diagnosis.

28. Obesity

Obesity is the most common nutritional disorder in present-day Britain and gives rise to more ill-health than all the vitamin deficiencies put together. The skill of a trained dietitian is invaluable in its treatment. Even if there were no other practical problems in human nutrition, the dietitian would more than justify her training and knowledge by the help she can give to fat people. A nationwide attack on obesity would employ more dietitians than are at present in Britain. The same general statement is true for most other countries in Europe and North America.

DEFINITION AND ASSESSMENT

Obesity is a state in which an excess of fat accumulates. In most cases it can be detected by visual inspection, which usually suffices for diagnosis. It is important to be able to assess the degree of obesity for purposes of regulating treatment. This is customarily done by relating the patient's weight to tables of standard weights for height, e.g. those on page 472, and then referring to patients as 10, 20 or 30 per cent overweight.

However, normal weight depends on body build; some people inherit a large frame and bulky muscles and may be 20 per cent over the standard without being obese. Present weight may be compared with the patient's weight at the age of 20 years; but this may not be remembered and also the patient may have been obese from an early age.

A scientific assessment of obesity is given by the proportion of fat in the total body weight. Mean values of body fat for normal young men are about 12 per cent and for young women about 26 per cent (p. 9). A man whose body fat amounts to more than 20 per cent of his total weight may be considered obese and for a woman a figure of more than 30 per cent represents obesity.

SKIN CALIPERS

Unfortunately determinations of body fat based on measurements of body water, body potassium or body density (Chap. 2) are not possible in clinical practice. However, an assessment can be made from measurements of skinfold thicknesses. For this purpose various calipers are available. The Harpenden calipers (British Indicators Ltd, St Albans, Herts) or the Holtain calipers (Holtain Ltd, Crymmych, Dyfed, Wales) are recommended. Measurements should be made at four sites:

1. Triceps, at a point equidistant from the tip of the acromion and the olecranon.

2. Subscapular, just below the tip of the inferior angle of the scapula.
3. Biceps, at the mid-point of the muscle with the arm hanging vertically.
4. Suprailiac, over the iliac crest in the mid-axillary line.

Durnin and Womersley (1974) made measurements of skinfold thickness at these four sites and of body density by underwater weighing on 209 men and 272 women aged from 16 to 72 years. The relations between the sum of the four skinfolds and the percentage of body fat, derived from density were calculated from regression equations. Table 28.1 gives the results. The higher body fat corresponding to a given skinfold in women than in men is attributable to a higher proportion of the total fat being over the thighs and hips. Durnin and Womersley conclude that the use of their table 'for assessing total body fat with relative ease and reasonable accuracy on men and women of widely differing age should make it of common use in many fields of medicine, physiology, nutrition and anthropology.' Our experience in practical classes with students confirms this view. Skinfold calipers quantitate pinching the skin, as a sphygmomanometer quantitates feeling the pulse. Both instruments should be in common use.

To make the measurements at four sites, the patients have to be undressed; for survey work in which large numbers of people are being studied, this may be impractical. Then a single measurement over the triceps is useful and Table 28.2 relates triceps skinfold thickness to obesity.

EPIDEMIOLOGY

Age

Obesity is often looked upon as a disease of middle age, but it can occur at any time of life. In a poor community it is indeed uncommon in the young and characteristically occurs in successful business men or civil servants who have prospered, and in their wives. In wealthier communities it is becoming an increasingly important problem in the young. Adolescent obesity is common in many countries and is discussed on page 529 It is often attributable to lack of physical activity. Obesity is now common in infants and young children as a result of changes in methods of feeding. Juvenile obesity is sometimes followed by obesity in adult life (p. 528).

Table 28.1 The equivalent fat content, as a percentage of body weight, for a range of values for the sum of four skinfolds (biceps, triceps, subscapular and suprailiac) of males and females of different ages (Durnin and Womersley, 1974)

Skinfolds (mm)	Males (age in years)				Females (age in years)			
	17–29	30–39	40–49	50+	16–29	30–39	40–49	50+
20	8.1	12.2	12.2	12.6	14.1	17.0	19.8	21.4
30	12.9	16.2	17.7	18.6	19.5	21.8	24.5	26.6
40	16.4	19.2	21.4	22.9	23.4	25.5	28.2	30.3
50	19.0	21.5	24.6	26.5	26.5	28.2	31.0	33.4
60	21.2	23.5	27.1	29.2	29.1	30.6	33.2	35.7
70	23.1	25.1	29.3	31.6	31.2	32.5	35.0	37.7
80	24.8	26.6	31.2	33.8	33.1	34.3	36.7	39.6
90	26.2	27.8	33.0	35.8	34.8	35.8	38.3	41.2
100	27.6	29.0	34.4	37.4	36.4	37.2	39.7	42.6
110	28.8	30.1	35.8	39.0	37.8	38.6	41.0	43.9
120	30.0	31.1	37.0	40.4	39.0	39.6	42.0	45.1
130	31.0	31.9	38.2	41.8	40.2	40.6	43.0	46.2
140	32.0	32.7	39.2	43.0	41.3	41.6	44.0	47.2
150	32.9	33.5	40.2	44.1	42.3	42.6	45.0	48.2
160	33.7	34.3	41.2	45.1	43.3	43.6	45.8	49.2
170	34.5	34.8	42.0	46.1	44.1	44.4	46.6	50.0
180	35.3	—	—	—	—	45.2	47.4	50.8
190	35.9	—	—	—	—	45.9	48.2	51.6
200	—	—	—	—	—	46.5	48.8	52.4
210	—	—	—	—	—	—	49.4	53.0

In two-thirds of the instances the error was within ± 3.5 per cent of the body-weight as fat for the women and ± 5 per cent for the men.

Sex

Obesity may occur in either sex, but is usually more common in women, in whom it is liable to occur after pregnancy and at the menopause. A woman may be expected to gain about 12.5 kg (27.5 lb) during pregnancy (p. 518). Part of this is an increase in adipose tissue which serves as a store against the demands of lactation. Many women gain more and retain part of this weight, becoming progressively obese with each succeeding child.

Social class

Obesity is not a disease of very poor communities, but in Western cities it is commoner in those in the lower socioeconomic classes. Thus in a survey in Manhattan, 30 per cent of those graded of low social class were obese, 17 per cent of the medium social class and only 5 per cent of the high social class (Penick and Stunkard, 1970). A similar but less marked gradient was found in London (Silverstone et al., 1969). Obesity is also seen in top class executive men and here the business lunch and the accompanying alcohol may be the main cause.

Countries

There are no comparative international statistics but the observant traveller can notice more obese people in the streets of some countries than others. Two studies, not primarily on obesity, have compared samples of people in two or more countries, using standard procedures for weight, height and skinfold thickness. The Seven Country

Table 28.2 Obesity standards in Caucasian Americans (Selzer and Mayer, 1965)

Age (years)	Minimum triceps skinfold thickness indicating obesity (mm)	
	Males	Females
5	12	14
6	12	15
7	13	16
8	14	17
9	15	18
10	16	20
11	17	21
12	18	22
13	18	23
14	17	23
15	16	24
16	15	25
17	14	26
18	15	27
19	15	27
20	16	28
21	17	28
22	18	28
23	18	28
24	19	28
25	20	29
26	20	29
27	21	29
28	22	29
29	22	29
30–50	23	30

Study (Keys *et al.*, 1972) showed there were more obese adult men in the USA sample than in the samples from European countries. A sample of Edinburgh men had more adiposity than a sample of Stockholm men (Logan *et al.*, 1978). The scanty data on the prevalence of obesity in Britain are summarised by James (1976), who notes that no nationwide representative survey has ever been made. Obesity is widespread in Eastern Europe (Hejda, 1978).

AETIOLOGY

Obesity arises only when the intake of food is in excess of physiological needs. Patients have to be made to realise that adipose tissue comes only from excess food; it is not made out of air. Yet the amount of additional food which produces obesity is small. If a healthy man or woman eats only an extra slice of bread (20 g) at breakfast, this provides a surplus of 200 kJ or 48 kcal of energy, which is stored as triglyceride. If he continues with this as a daily habit, after 10 years the store has grown by 20 kg and he has become very obese. Alternatively, if he takes his car to work instead of walking for 10 minutes each way and does not reduce his food intake, the same surplus of energy has to be stored.

In relation to a person's daily habits of eating and physical activity, 200 kJ is a small amount of energy and this makes the study of the energy balance in relation to obesity very difficult. Experimental studies on man are summarised and reviewed critically in a monograph by Garrow (1978).

Because the daily offset of the energy balance needed to produce obesity is so small, the study of its aetiology is beset with difficulties. Very rarely obesity arises directly due to damage to the controlling centres in the hypothalamus, e.g. following a severe head injury or by pressure from the growth of an intracranial tumour. No other primary cause is known, but there are many predisposing factors which may be genetic, endocrine or behavioural in origin.

Genetic factors

Obesity often runs in families. It is, however, difficult to sort out the genetic from the environmental factors. No one single gene is responsible for human obesity, which is an example of a multifactorial disease. Some groups of people that have had to struggle to obtain enough food in harsh environments and had repeated famines in their history appear to be unusually liable to become obese when they move to a sedentary surburban way of life. Australian Aborigines, the islanders of Nauru and Indians now in Natal in South Africa are examples. Natural selection may have favoured metabolically 'thrifty genotypes' in these groups (James and Trayhurn, 1976). Those of us who can only avoid obesity by eating less than other people may console themselves that, if food were ever very scarce, they would stand a better chance of surviving.

Obesity is determined by a defect in a single gene in some animals, e.g. the ob/ob strain of mice and the Zucker strain of rats, but no such genetic defect is known to occur in man. The literature on genetic obesity in animals is reviewed by Hunt *et al.* (1976).

Endocrine factors

Obesity frequently accompanies hypothyroidism, hypogonadism, hypopituitarism and Cushing's syndrome, but it is not an essential feature of these conditions. The fact that in women obesity commonly begins at puberty, during pregnancy or at the menopause suggests an endocrine factor. Yet the overwhelming majority of obese patients show no clinical evidence of an endocrine disorder and the function of their endocrine glands is normal on routine tests.

There are certain well-defined changes in metabolism associated with obesity which are described below. It is probable that these changes are a result of obesity and not its cause. Yet tests of endocrine function have been crude until recently. It is possible that new methods may lead to the discovery of small, but important deviations of endocrine or metabolic functions that contribute to obesity.

Behavioural factors

Obesity may be the result of either gluttony or sloth, two of the seven deadly sins. Those who do not believe in sin would say that in such cases the obesity is due to emotional disturbances caused by stresses from the psychological and social environment operating on an individual with some defect of personality. However, the great majority of obese people are neither gluttons nor sluggards; they do not appear to suffer more emotional disturbances than persons whose weight remains unchanged. Such field studies as are available indicate that the obese eat on average rather less than those of normal weight, but that they are less physically active. If inactivity is a more important predisposing factor than big eating, this has implications for both prevention and treatment.

Physical activity. Obesity is unusual in those who follow occupations or recreations demanding hard physical exercise. It is common in those whose lives are largely sedentary. Dorris and Stunkard (1957) got obese patients and normal subjects to wear a pedometer for a week. The mean reading for the normals was 34.3 miles/week and for the obese 14.4 miles/week. With the mechanisation of industry and improved transport facilities, in particular the development and widespread use of motor vehicles, the proportion of people who take adequate exercise has declined and the number of sedentary workers, including office workers and business executives, has increased. The farmer who walked behind his plough using up 1670 kJ (400 kcal) an hour now rides a tractor, using only 540 kJ (130 kcal) an hour. The housewife who used to wash clothes by hand, using 1050 kJ (250 kcal) an hour now uses the washing machine at a fraction of that amount. Television, in so far as it may divert people from active recreation, contributes to obesity. Hence inactivity may be an important factor in explaining the frequency of what has been described as 'creeping' overweight in modern Western societies. Although it was once fashionable to decry exercise as a means of reducing weight, a combination of exercise and diet is to be strongly recommended.

Eating habits and cultural factors. In several surveys (Swanson *et al.*, 1955; Johnson *et al.*, 1956; Stefanik *et al.*, 1959; Maxfield and Konishi, 1966), obese people were found to eat on average no more than thin people. Many eat less. When the food intake is high this may be due to nibbling between meals. This contributes to the obesity of many housewives who are fond of cooking and of others who work in kitchens. On the other hand, in Prague, Fabry (1967) found that those who ate only three times a day were more likely to be overweight than those who ate five or six times. Laboratory rats who like to nibble all through the night also become obese, if their access to food is limited to a short period in the 24 hours.

An ingenious set of experiments has been carried out by Schachter (1968) in which the food consumed by subjects who were overweight and by those of normal weight were measured in various artificial situations. Compared with the controls, the amounts eaten by obese subjects were little affected by previous food intake, i.e. by hunger and satiety, and depended more on the taste and appearance of the food and on psychological and physical factors in the environment in which the food was served. Schachter postulates that feeding is determined by internal or physiological cues, to which the obese are relatively insensitive, and by external cues, to which they are more sensitive than normal persons. He supports his theory with observations in real-life circumstances, e.g. the factors which affect how well obese subjects keep a religious fast.

This theory appears convincing, except for reservations about its general applicability. Schachter's subjects were New Yorkers, most of them university students or graduates and many of them Jews. Thus, like the Viennese subjects on whose experiences Freud built his theories of psychoanalysis, they were not typical representatives of mankind. It would be interesting to see if similar results were obtained with middle-aged working-class women in Glasgow or with the shopkeepers of East Africa. Cultural factors may contribute to obesity in various ways. Thus in parts of Africa and the West Indies moderate obesity in women is desired by their menfolk and admired by their sisters. The Sumo wrestlers of Japan weigh 120 kg or more, not all of this muscle.

Another behavioural difference that has been reported between obese and normal people is that the obese eat faster and spend less time chewing each mouthful of food (Wagner and Hewitt, 1975). This, too, needs confirmation.

Although it is difficult to describe the causes of obesity with scientific precision, it is usually possible to give a patient practical advice about predisposing factors arising from his way of life. It is also important to clear his mind of false ideas about the causes of obesity which are prevalent in many communities.

METABOLISM IN OBESITY

Basal metabolism.
Many years ago Strang and Evans (1929) reported that the basal metabolism of obese people was within normal limits. All subsequent work has confirmed this. The difficulty of relating the measured rate of resting oxygen consumption to body size is discussed on page 19; in obese people it was higher than in non-obese controls of the same height (James *et al.*, 1978).

Luxus consumption
It has frequently been suggested that the normal individual can dispose of a dietary excess by increasing the metabolic rate and so burning it off (Grafe and Graham, 1911; Grafe, 1933). Obese individuals are said to lack this physiological control system for regulating body weight. The experimental evidence purporting to support this luxus consumption control is unconvincing. After reviewing it, Garrow (1978) states: 'It is impossible to conclude either that thermogenesis, or luxus consumption, does occur in man or that it does not.' With this we agree, but our studies on 16 subjects, some fat and some thin, under carefully controlled conditions in a metabolic ward (Strong *et al.*, 1967) failed to show any consistent or significant rise in metabolic rates following overfeeding. It is possible that one or other of the potential futile cycles (Chap. 8) may operate to dispose of excess substrate by oxidation rather than storage in some individuals. If so, the effect must be small, as it cannot be demonstrated easily.

Fat metabolism
Many physicians have recorded that obese patients do not readily develop ketosis on reducing regimes. Kekwick *et al.* (1959) measured the level of ketoacids in the blood after a period on a ketogenic diet; they found little or no change in obese subjects even after 10 days, whereas in normal controls, the level rose markedly in two to four days. Thomson *et al.* (1966) starved obese patients for many weeks, and although they found some degree of ketonuria, none of them had any symptoms which could be attributed to ketoacidosis.

Free fatty acid (FFA) concentration in blood after an overnight fast is on average higher in obese than in normal subjects (Opie and Walfish, 1963). This may reflect a priority for fat rather than carbohydrate metabolism.

Plasma triglycerides are often moderately raised in obesity but high-density lipoproteins may be reduced (Truswell, 1978).

Carbohydrate metabolism

Obese subjects appear to handle a glucose load in a way quantitatively different from that of normal subjects. Glucose tolerance is often lower and plasma insulin higher than normal. These may be an early manifestation of the diabetes that frequently develops; yet when fasting the plasma insulin concentration is higher in obese patients than in persons of normal weight. Gordon and Goldberg (1964) and Shreeve (1965) have shown that after giving ^{14}C-glucose, more $^{14}CO_2$ appears in the expired air in normal than in obese subjects. After giving ^{3}H-glucose, more ^{3}HOH was found in the body water of the normal subjects. These findings indicate a diminished rate of carbohydrate utilisation in the obese. There is also evidence (Gordon et al., 1962) that if two isotopes of glucose labelled in the C-1 and C-2 positions are given to normal and obese subjects, the obese expire a greater proportion of CO_2 bearing the C-1 label. This is the carbon atom of glucose which is involved in oxidation in the hexose monophosphate pathway. The use of this pathway leads to the formation of $NADPH_2$ which is needed for the synthesis of fat. In this way lipogenesis may be favoured in the obese.

Adipose tissue metabolism

The chemical composition of adipose tissue has already been discussed (p. 54) where it was stated that even in obesity its fat content is not more than 90 per cent. The remaining 10 per cent or more of fat-free adipose tissue consists of cell material which is metabolically active. An obese person with 50 kg of adipose tissue has thus at least 5 kg of fat-free adipose tissue, equivalent in weight to three livers.

This extra mass of adipose tissue has potential enzymic activity similar to that of normal adipose tissue, as shown by in vitro studies on biopsy samples (Salans et al., 1968; Galton and Wilson, 1970), though there were quantitative differences in the samples studied.

CLINICAL FEATURES

The diagnosis should be made on the observation that there is too much adipose tissue in some part of the body. The distribution of this tissue is variable and attempts have been made to distinguish different types of obesity on the basis of it, but it is doubtful if they serve any useful purpose. It may be confined to the trunk, leaving the extremities slim, or, in the extreme case of the rare disease, progressive lipodystrophy, it centres round the hips and thighs, leaving the rest of the body thin or even emaciated.

The extent to which obesity may progress is amazing. Mr William J. Cobb, who featured in Time (30 July 1965) weighed 802 lb (365 kg) and used to eat 15 chickens at a sitting. After persevering with a 1000 kcal diet for 83 weeks, he lost 570 lb (260 kg): this shows what can be done.

The explorer Speke (1863) in his journey to the source of the Nile stayed with an African tribe whose men greatly appreciated the charms of fat women. His diary records:

After a long and amusing conversation with Rumarika in the morning, I called on one of his sisters-in-law. She was another of those wonders of obesity, unable to stand excepting on all fours. I was desirous to obtain a good view of her and actually to measure her.... After getting her to sidle and wiggle into the middle of the hut, I took her dimensions: round arm 1 ft 11 in; chest 4 ft 4 in; thigh 2 ft 7 in; calf 1 ft 8 in; height 5 ft 8 in. All of these were exact except the height, and I believe I could have obtained this more accurately if I could have laid her on the floor. Not knowing what difficulties I should have to contend with in such a piece of engineering, I tried to get her height by raising her up. This after infinite exertions on the part of both of us, was accomplished, when she sank down again fainting. Meanwhile the daughter, a lass of 16, sat stark naked before us, sucking at a milk pot, on which the father kept her at work with a rod in his hand, for as fattening is the first duty of a fashionable female life, it must be duly enforced by the rod, if necessary. I got up a bit of a flirtation with missy and induced her to rise and shake hands with me. Her features were lovely, but her body as round as a ball.

Complications

Apart from aesthetic considerations, obesity leads to mechanical disabilities, predisposes to metabolic and cardiovascular disorders, and so reduces the expectancy of life.

Psychological. Aesthetic considerations are sufficient to make many people aware of the threat of obesity and anxious to avoid it; those who do not succeed may become unhappy and a problem for their doctor. Thus obesity creates emotional problems in addition to any that may nave been partly responsible for it. Rarely a patient develops a well-defined neurosis, known as disturbance of body image (Stunkard, 1976). Such patients whose obesity usually starts in adolescence have a distorted view of their own body and are revolted by the sight of it in a mirror.

Mechanical disability. The structure of the human skeleton is not well adapted to carry an extra load, consequently flat feet and osteoarthrosis of the knees, hips and lumbar spine are common in obese people. The abdominal muscles that support the viscera, and those in the legs, which help by their contractions the venous return of blood to the heart, are infiltrated with fat. Hence their mechanical action is impaired, with consequent abdominal hernias and varicose veins. Adipose tissue around the chest and under the diaphragm interferes with respiration and predisposes to bronchitis.

Metabolic. Diabetes mellitus arising for the first time in middle life occurs commonly in the obese although many obese people escape it. Obesity tends to be associated with a high plasma urate and also with cholesterol stones in the gall-bladder.

Cardiovascular. Obese people suffer from high blood pressure more commonly than those of normal weight. With increased arm girth, the use of the standard sphygmomanometer cuff may lead to falsely high figures for blood pressure. Pickering *et al.* (1954) calculated correction factors that could be used to allow for this and Trout *et al.* (1956) advised taking blood pressures with the cuff around the forearm in obese people. However, subsequent studies have shown that blood pressure correlated better with relative weight than arm girth, and blood pressure measured at the forearm is still significantly related to relative weight (Kannel *et al.*, 1967). Furthermore, in a prospective study obese people who started normotensive developed hypertension more often than people of normal weight (Kannel *et al.*, 1967) and when obese people succeed in losing weight their blood pressure usually falls (Fletcher, 1959).

The work of the heart is increased by the extra mechanical work needed in moving the overweight body and by the increased peripheral vascular resistance in patients with hypertension. This extra load on the heart, coupled with the tendency to atherosclerosis in the coronary arteries, no doubt contributes to angina pectoris and cardiac failure among obese people in middle life. The increased incidence of varicose veins has been mentioned already.

Respiratory. Increased difficulty in breathing may lead to CO_2 retention and subsequent somnolence. This is known as the Pickwickian syndrome, after the fat boy Joe in *Pickwick Papers*.

Skin. The excessive deposits of subcutaneous fat predispose to skin infections, particularly at the flexures, e.g. intertrigo below the breasts.

Accidents. Obese people are often slow and ungainly; they are therefore liable to accidents of all kinds. At home they may trip over the carpet and spill kettles of boiling water over themselves; at their work they have difficulty in avoiding the moving parts of machinery and in the street cannot quickly escape the traffic.

Life expectancy. In view of these manifold complications it is not surprising that obese people are poor risks from the standpoint of life insurance. The statistics of the Metropolitan Life Insurance Co. (USA) have shown that for a man of 45, an increase of 25 lb above standard weight reduces his life expectancy by 25 per cent. The risks of obesity in women are somewhat less.

DIAGNOSIS

This apparently obvious disorder is frequently overlooked because the doctor is often preoccupied with one of its many complications. A regular practice of weighing patients and examining them for evidence of excessive fat would prevent this. A definition of obesity in quantitative terms is given on page 244.

Excess weight is not necessarily adipose tissue. It may be due to pregnancy, to muscular hypertrophy in athletes, to oedema in patients with diseases of the heart, kidneys or liver and to myxoedema. All of these should become apparent at a careful clinical examination, but mistakes have been made.

TREATMENT

General

There are three essential points in treatment.

First the patient should be made to understand the reasons why she should reduce her weight. No patient follows a weight-reducing regime unless she is motivated to persevere and can see rewards ahead, such as better health and a more attractive appearance.

Secondly the patient should be instructed in some elementary physiological principles in regard to appetite, exercise and the expenditure of energy. False knowledge, often acquired from popular papers and books, must be eradicated. The patient should be taught that there are no 'slimming foods' and no successful 'slimming diets' which do not depend on a reduced intake of energy. The essence of treatment is to reduce the energy content of the day's diet.

Thirdly, to stick to a weight-reducing diet is a battle of the will—the patient's own will! Though some deny it, most people experience periods of hunger, suffer from temptations and are deprived of their accustomed amount of oral gratification. Psychological understanding and behavioural advice are essential weapons, more important than dietary details. Any dietitian or doctor who wants to take on the challenge of helping obese people needs to have some training in the techniques of behavioural modification. These were pioneered by Stuart (1967), and there are manuals available (Stuart and Davis, 1972; Ferguson, 1975). Some of their techniques have been adopted by lay groups like Weight Watchers.

A dietary history shows the pattern of meals normally eaten and the kinds of foods that are taken in excess. These are often sugar, bread, cakes, pastry, chocolates, ice creams, thick soups and fried food. She should also learn that snacks or aperitifs taken between meals cannot be permitted. Chocolate, sweets, cocktail 'pieces', beer, stout and other alcoholic drinks all add to the energy intake and hence cannot be permitted unless the patient is prepared to make a corresponding reduction in her diet.

The successful treatment of obesity requires a strict regime. This is often difficult for people with irregular habits with regard to both food and exercise, such as many doctors, commercial travellers and company directors. An evening with friends, a business lunch, a banquet or a holiday, if care is not taken, may undo the good habits established by weeks of conscientious dieting.

The essential regime for the treatment of obesity is to regulate the daily intake of energy. It is therefore wise that patients who are seriously overweight should at first make a practice of weighing what they are about to eat. This should be continued until they become accustomed to judging correctly quantities of food. A suitable balance for this purpose, on the sideboard or kitchen table, is needed. Adherence to an exact diet necessitates good discipline.

Diets should not depart too much from established food habits. An obvious absurdity is to advise an obese rice-eating Indian to take for breakfast one thin slice of wheaten bread. He may not take any breakfast, and wheaten bread may be unavailable. The art of the dietitian is to provide a diet suitable to the needs and habits of the particular patient. A printed diet sheet, handed out to a patient at a single interview without adequate discussion and explanation, seldom achieves results.

Weighed diet

Energy output has been determined for people undertaking various activities. Sedentary clerical work requires about 8.3 to 10.5 MJ (2000 to 2500) kcal/day, light work 10.5 to 12.5 MJ (2500 to 3000 kcal), while heavy work, such as felling trees, may need 16.7 MJ (4000 kcal) or even more. It is obvious therefore that dietary requirements vary greatly according to occupation and that a business executive might require only about half the energy of a man doing heavy work.

An obese middle-aged housewife usually loses weight satisfactorily on a diet providing about 4.2 MJ (1000 kcal)/day, such as Diet No. 3. This is based on sound physiological principles. If her daily energy expenditure is 9.2 MJ (2200 kcal)/day the negative balance will be 5.0 MJ (1200 kcal). The energy value of obese tissue is about 31 kJ (7.5 kcal)/g. The weekly negative energy balance is therefore equivalent to

$$\frac{5000 \times 7}{31} \text{ g or } 1.1 \text{ kg (2.4 lb)}$$

A weekly weight loss of 2 to 3 lb should be the general aim.

An obese man engaged in active physical work cannot tolerate a diet providing only 4.2 MJ (1000 kcal)/day. Satisfactory weight loss should occur if 6.3 MJ (1500 kcal) is taken daily. Diet No. 3 can be used with the addition of three carbohydrate exchanges, two protein exchanges and half a fat exchange (p. 560) and by increasing the milk allowance to 500 ml/day. With these additions the diet provides approximately 160 g of carbohydrate, 85 g of protein and 65 g of fat.

Protein. The protein content of the diet should be sufficient to maintain the body in nitrogen equilibrium. Usually 50 g/day is sufficient for this purpose. Some weight-reducing regimes have been based on the principle of eating mostly meat and other foods rich in protein. The specific dynamic action of the proteins raises the metabolism by less than 830 kJ (200 kcal)/day and this is of little help in the prevention or treatment of obesity. High protein diets are expensive and so often impractical. However, many people find that the onset of hunger is delayed for a longer time when a meal containing ample protein is taken as compared to one rich in carbohydrate.

Carbohydrate. The intake of foods rich in carbohydrates should be reduced since overindulgence in such foods is a common cause of obesity. Diet No. 3 contains 100 g of carbohydrate, providing 40 per cent of the 4.2 MJ (1000 kcal). Nearly all is complex carbohydrate and, as in all weight-reducing diets, there is little or no sugar. This is because sugar provides 'empty calories' or energy and, when energy intake is reduced foods that are good sources of protein, vitamins and minerals are needed. Furthermore, cutting sugar out of a diet calls for less culinary reorganisation than eliminating the other main sources of energy; it is also common experience that when sugar is given up, people often lose their 'sweet tooth'. Diets in which the carbohydrate is drastically reduced to less than 40 per cent of the total energy are not recommended. One such, *Dr Atkins' Diet Revolution* has provoked a critical review of the dangers of carbohydrate restriction by the American Medical Association (1973). These diets are inevitably high in fat and protein. A high protein content makes such diets expensive. A high fat diet raises the plasma cholesterol (Kouwenhoven and Drijver, 1973), a risk factor for coronary heart disease; it may also produce mild ketosis which can cause complaints of headache and nausea, and in the long term may result in demineralisation of bone (Cahill, 1975). Severe ketoacidosis does not develop as a result of any reducing diet, unless the patient is diabetic. Up to 100 g of carbohydrate-rich foods such as bread and potatoes may be taken and these are cheap and useful sources of many essential nutrients. It is a major popular misconception that carbohydrates are specially fattening.

Fibre. Dietary fibre (usually associated in foods with complex carbohydrates) appears to be helpful in the prevention and management of obesity. Haber *et al.* (1977) compared the same amount of carbohydrate (60 g) in whole apples, apple purée and apple juice, each consumed in turn as a test meal by 10 normal adults. The juice was less satisfying than purée, and purée than whole apples. Plasma insulin rose higher after juice and purée than after the whole fruit. This experiment showed neatly that the removal of fibre from food, and also its disruption, can result in faster, easier digestion and decreased satiety.

Fat. A diet providing 4.2 MJ and containing 100 g of carbohydrate and 60 g of protein, cannot include more than 40 g of fat. This allowance of fat, though small, is sufficient to make the diet palatable and acceptable to the patient. It includes half a pint of milk from which the cream has been poured off first thing in the morning. If whole milk is used the energy value of the diet is about 4.6 MJ.

Alcohol. Whether or not to allow a single drink as a

consolation or reward in a weight-reducing regime is a difficult decision. Weight Watchers (1975) state: 'Any food that supplies only empty calories, such as alcohol or sugar, can have no place in a weight-loss programme.' Furthermore, alcoholic drinks often function as behavioural reinforcers to eating. Nevertheless, some doctors make a concession for individual patients.

Popular books and newspaper articles have stated that there is no need to restrict the intake of fat in obese patients. 'Eat fat and get slim' is advice which has an obvious appeal. It arose from the observation of Kekwick and Pawan (1956) that when patients are treated in hospital on 4.2 MJ diets, the initial weight loss is greatest if almost all the energy (up to 90 per cent) is supplied in the form of fat. This observation is of scientific interest, but has no therapeutic value since this regime ultimately causes no greater loss of weight than the balanced diet described above. The rapid loss of weight which was as much as 2 to 4 kg in a few days was probably due to loss of water. Similar rapid losses of weight occur in the first three days of complete starvation and whenever the carbohydrate intake is drastically cut, even if the energy requirement is met by extra fat or protein (Passmore, 1961). The explanation is that 1 g of glycogen binds 3 to 4 g of water and this water is freed and excreted in the urine as the glycogen store is reduced (Garrow, 1978).

All popular 'slimming regimes' involve a restriction in dietary carbohydrate and in this way it is possible to explain their immediate, but only temporary, success.

Unweighed diets
For patients who are only moderately overweight and for those who have already reduced themselves substantially, careful weighing of the food is unnecessary. It is also impractical for persons with severe visual defects and sometimes because of mental or physical incapacity. Others may be unable or unwilling to co-operate in the accurate regulation of the energy intake by means of a weighed diet. Such persons should be instructed in those foods which all obese persons should avoid (p. 551). They should be told to take no sugar in tea and coffee or on sweets and desserts, and to cut down on their special favourite foods and tempting dishes. It is important that they reduce their customary size of helpings of all foods, perhaps by as much as half. If they are social drinkers, they should be warned of the energy content of alcoholic drinks.

Vitamins
Properly constructed reducing diets should contain plenty of green vegetables and fruits, since they provide little energy while their bulk helps to fill the stomach and relieve hunger; they also help to relieve constipation, common on a low food intake, and to produce satiety. Hence the vitamin A and vitamin C should be sufficient to meet needs. With meat, fish and eggs in the diet and little or no refined cereals and sugar, it is improbable that deficiency of any component of the vitamin B complex will arise. A good reducing diet meets the patient's needs for vitamins. Multivitamin tablets should be unnecessary.

Minerals
The only minerals that need serious consideration are calcium and iron. Provided that the diet includes half a pint of milk, there is little likelihood of a negative calcium balance in an adult. The supply of iron is best ensured by including a portion of lean meat in the diet each day.

Water and salt
At one time patients were often advised to restrict their intake of water, but there is no sensible reason for keeping fat patients thirsty. Plain water or unsweetened tea can be taken but not sweetened 'juices'.

In obese patients with oedema from congestive heart failure or other causes, there is both water and sodium retention. For all such patients, salt restriction is necessary and suitable diuretics should be given.

Diet No. 3 is in general suitable for the treatment of an overweight middle-aged housewife in Great Britain. But it may be unsuitable in other circumstances and cultures. Dietitians with knowledge of food values and local eating habits can achieve a great deal of good by devising diets, suitable to the established customs of their own community, which also provide about 4.2 MJ (1000 kcal) made up from about 60 g protein, 100 g carbohydrate and 40 g fat, or somewhat more for active men.

Proprietary powdered food products
Various firms make such products and promote them by vigorous advertising campaigns. They consist of a balanced mixture of protein, carbohydrate and fat for the treatment of obesity with the addition of essential vitamins and minerals. Half a pound (230 g) of one proprietary preparation is stated to provide 3.8 MJ (900 kcal) daily. It is mixed with water and taken in divided quantities in four, five or six feeds in the day. On such a diet the loss of weight is similar to that achieved by a patient taking a diet of natural foods, as in Diet No. 3. Since these proprietary food products are more expensive, less palatable and more monotonous than this diet, they are not recommended for the routine treatment of obesity. They can only be justified as a novel alternative to a conventional system for those who are either unwilling or unable to adhere to a weighed diet.

Exercise
The value of physical exercise has been underestimated. It is sometimes stated (but without evidence) that exercise promotes appetite in excess of energy needs and so may aggravate obesity. But there is evidence from experiments

on animals that the reverse is true (Mayer et al., 1954). A certain minimum amount of exercise may be necessary for the accurate regulation of food intake.

Most obese patients lead sedentary lives and the full extent to which urban and industrial life restricts activity is only now being realised. In many obese patients it is impossible to prescribe anything but the mildest of physical exercise. Walking, however, is good exercise and an hour's walk at 3 miles an hour will expend about 1.3 MJ (300 kcal) (or more for a heavy person) which represents approximately the energy value of 30 g of fat. This may seem a small amount but, if the daily walk becomes a habit, it adds up to a weight loss of over 9 kg (20 lb) in a year. Obese women who did not restrict their diet lost weight when they took up walking, provided this was at least 30 minutes each day (Gwinup, 1975). There is little doubt that most obese people could benefit from exercise, e.g. walking, swimming, gardening, provided it does not exceed their cardiovascular capacity. Regular daily exercise is much more valuable than spurts of activity at the week-end.

Juvenile obesity

Treatment, as in adults, consists in restricting the diet and altering the child's way of life so that the dietary energy is less than the energy needs for physical activity and the metabolic processes. This is often difficult especially as there are often underlying psychological difficulties in the family. A psychiatric social worker as well as a dietitian is often needed to cope with problems in the home.

Intensive treatment

The regime of dietary restriction and increased regular exercise already described aims at a rate of weight loss of just over 1 kg (2 lb) a week. Very fat patients would have to persist with such a regime for many months before achieving a satisfactory weight loss. Such slow progress may be disheartening and lead to the abandonment of treatment. Provided there are no orthopaedic or cardiovascular complications, it is possible to increase the physcial activities and cut down the diet still further. Patients have been kept for up to six weeks on diets providing only 1.8 MJ (400 kcal)/day, whilst they walked 10 miles daily (Strong et al., 1958). This regime involved negative balances of the order of 12.5 MJ (3000 kcal)/day. The patients lost weight at rates of up to 3 kg (7 lb) a week, yet they remained fit and well able to carry out the exercise. Ashley and Whyte (1961) have also kept obese patients for long periods on diets providing 2.1 MJ (500 kcal)/day or less with no adverse effects and good immediate results.

A period of several weeks of starvation in hospital, has been recommended for very obese patients who have failed to respond to orthodox antiobesity treatment (Bloom, 1959; Thomson et al., 1966). This, although generally safe, is not without its dangers. A cardiovascular complication has caused one death (Spencer, 1968). Disturbances in electrolyte homeostasis also occur (Runcie and Thomson, 1970).

If for any reason a very low energy diet is prescribed, the patient should be carefully supervised and preferably in hospital. The daily requirement of protein should be given, as casein, and also supplements of vitamins and potassium. The regime should not be continued for more than 8 weeks.

The majority of obese patients do well if they persist in a regime of one hour's walk and a diet of 4.2 MJ (1000 kcal)/day, and this is the regime which we recommend.

Other physical measures

Turkish baths have been a popular means of reducing weight. Though they achieve a temporary success in bringing the weight down by a few pounds, this is due solely to loss of body water which is very soon replaced. They provide no escape from the inevitable necessity of dietary restriction. Numerous massage machines are advertised as a means for removing unsightly local deposits of fat. Unfortunately purchasers lose nothing but their money.

Drugs

Anorectic drugs

Amphetamine and its derivatives have been much used as 'slimming agents'. They are psychomotor stimulants and also have an anorectic action. By stimulating higher cortical centres they may overcome feelings of fatigue and depression and create a sense of well-being. They may also cause insomnia, irritability, increased heart rate, raised blood pressure and severe psychotic reactions. Patients rapidly become habituated to them and sometimes develop dependence. Serious withdrawal symptoms may occur on discontinuing the drug. For these reasons amphetamine should not be prescribed.

Diethylpropion, phenmetrazine and fenfluramine are three drugs which have some chemical resemblance to amphetamine. They are also psychomotor drugs, but safer than amphetamine. They have some anorectic action but physicians' assessments of their value in a reducing regime vary greatly. They may be prescribed for cases of refractory obesity for periods of up to six weeks. After this period their appetite-suppressing effect usually wears off. Patients with a history of depression or other psychological disturbance should not be treated thus unless they can be supervised carefully.

Anorectic drugs are no substitute for a dietary regime and radical alteration of food habits. At best they are an aid which may help some patients to adhere more strictly to their diets. It is never justified to use these drugs at the beginning of treatment. If an obese person has failed to adhere to a diet then an anorectic may be tried.

Other drugs

Thyroxine stimulates metabolism and for this reason it has had an extensive trial in the treatment of obesity. However it is contraindicated except in those rare cases in which obesity is associated with evidence of hypothyroidism. In euthyroid people thyroxine produces no increase in metabolism unless given in doses which cause tremor, diarrhoea, palpitation and tachycardia. The latter is particularly undesirable in elderly patients with myocardial weakness. Hence the administration of thyroxine to obese euthyroid patients is not only useless but potentially dangerous.

Methyl cellulose is indigestible and adds bulk to the diet. In clinical trials it has had little if any effect in promoting weight loss, and it is very doubtful if this product is of any value as an adjunct to dietary therapy. However, it is quite harmless.

Sedatives and tranquillisers can play no part in the treatment of obesity *per se* but they may be useful for some obese patients who suffer from an anxiety state.

Diuretics have been extensively tried in the treatment of obesity. They are potentially dangerous and are of no value in promoting weight loss unless the patient has oedema due to cardiac failure or other organic disease.

SURGICAL TREATMENT

Some patients whose life has been made miserable by severe obesity benefit from a jejunoileostomy which, by creating a bypass of the small intestine, leads to malabsorption. After the operation they reduce their food intake to prevent the diarrhoea, flatulence and abdominal discomfort that follows if they persist with previous dietary habits. The operation is unphysiological and there is an operative mortality which has been on average 4 per cent. Any of the features of the malabsorption syndrome (p. 403) may follow and in addition liver failure and oxalate stones in the urinary tract have been reported. The operation should only be considered when a surgical and medical team with special experience is available. All aspects of the operation were discussed at a symposium on Jejunoileostomy for Obesity (1977).

A surgical procedure which reduces the food intake, does no permanent harm and is readily reversible is to wire the jaws together with a special dental splint. The patient can then speak and drink but not eat; he is then limited to a liquid diet based on milk with a low-energy density. The method was introduced by Garrow (1978), who reported some successes, but the Adelaide Obesity Study Group (1978) found that most patients put on weight again when their jaws were unwired.

Plastic surgery to reduce and resuspend enlarged and pendulous breasts may be of great psychological benefit to some patients, and the fat in a pendulous abdominal wall can be removed, although the skin remains undesirably lax. Attempts to reshape unsightly arms and legs are contraindicated, as any operation is likely to be followed by the appearance of irregular ugly lumps of fat.

Neurosurgeons have been able to modify human behaviour making discrete lesions in the brain using stereotatic methods. Aphagia may readily be induced in rats by making such lesions in the hypothalamus (p. 77). Knowledge of the neuronal pathways responsible for feeding behaviour are not sufficiently well known in the rat brain, let alone in the human brain, to justify such operations in man except under exceptional circumstances, but a few have been done in Denmark (Quaade, 1974). With more precise knowledge of human neuroanatomy, it is possible that neurosurgery may come to have a place in the treatment of intractable obesity.

PROGNOSIS

If the patient is well motivated and is persistent in following medical advice, she should be able to lose up to about 15 kg (33 lb) in two or three months without undue difficulty. Almost certainly she will feel better as the loss of weight progresses and this should encourage her to persevere. A reduction in weight reduces the risk of the development of diabetes, coronary heart disease and hypertension. The prognosis for a person only moderately obese and well motivated is therefore good, provided she follows advice.

The prognosis in severe obesity was bad until recently. Stunkard and McLaren Hume (1959) reviewed the published results of seven obesity clinics in the USA, each under the direction of physicians who were experienced and interested in the treatment of obesity. Taking as an index of success the loss of 25 lb or more, satisfactory results in these clinics ranged from 12 to 28 per cent. With a stricter standard (the loss of over 40 lb) the successes amounted to only 2 to 8 per cent. In Edinburgh, Rose (1959) reported a large number of failures. In a series of 407 patients, 148 (36 per cent) did not report again after the first interview and only 15 per cent were discharged after having achieved the desired loss of weight.

Results of treatment have been poor because the majority of patients have a constitutional predisposition to obesity that remains throughout their life. They have a tendency to relapse that can only be overcome by strong motivation and willpower. Prognosis has been improved by psychotherapy, often of groups of patients, that is directed at modifying behaviour and encouraging self-help (Levitz and Stunkard, 1974). A family doctor has reported that his successes were basically happy people, often with a medical condition which could be improved by weight loss; those who did badly often lived in unsatisfactory situations and had a neurotic personality as judged by their responses to a questionnaire (Craddock, 1975).

MANAGEMENT

The obese patient is treated usually by a dietitian on reference from and in consultation with her doctor. The doctor should assure himself that there is no physical disease causing or complicating the obesity. He should make clear that the common type of obesity is a constitutional trait, the nature and origin of which is complex, but the treatment of which is simple—to make energy intake less than energy expenditure until desirable weight is reached and then be kept equal for the rest of the patient's life. The motivational difficulty must be emphasised.

The details of dietary treatment are well left to a dietitian or to an organisation which is in regular consultation with the medical profession and orthodox nutritionists. Much quackery is practised in the popular handling of obesity, often at great cost to the health of the patient and to her pocket.

The patient should weigh herself at the same time of day and unclothed at weekly intervals or more frequently; day-to-day variations in weight are not important and may be due to retention of urine or faeces, or to increase in body water that sometimes precedes menstruation. The weight on each occasion should be recorded in a notebook.

On a low energy diet weight is at first lost rapidly, often partly due to a loss of body water. After a week or so, the rate usually declines even if the patient keeps strictly to her diet. This is partly due to a fall in a previously high resting metabolic rate. The patient should be warned of this, so that she is not disappointed when her initial rapid progress slows down.

The doctor should discuss with the patient a target weight as an objective. The prescribed diet should be carefully explained. The patient has to do her homework to learn the varieties and quantities of food allowed, including alcoholic and sweetened drinks, and the legitimate substitutions. Inexpensive booklets giving the energy values of common foods are available in most bookshops. Weighing servings of food regularly for a short period helps some patients, but is not essential. There must be opportunity for frequent consultation about unusual foods and their energy and nutrient values.

The patient should be seen at first not less than once a week by a dietitian or suitably trained person, to check progress and to give encouragement. If she complains of any symptoms, she should be sent to her doctor at once.

A useful summary of methods available for the treatment of obesity, with emphasis of the underlying psychological considerations, has been made by Guggenheim (1977).

LAY ORGANISATIONS

The formation of Alcoholics Anonymous, which consists of groups of cured alcoholics dedicated to the cause of helping new members to abandon the use of alcohol, and helping old members should they relapse, has been a major advance in the treatment of alcoholism. Similar groups for obese patients have been formed. Weight Watchers and other groups have achieved many successes (Stunkard et al., 1970; Ashwell and Garrow, 1975). When well organised, such groups are capable of greatly improving the depressing results which were achieved with obese people in the past. They are valuable in their emphasis on companionship in stress and group appreciation and reward of success.

29. Protein-Energy Malnutrition

Protein-energy malnutrition (PEM) describes a range of clinical disorders. At one end, marasmus is due to a continued restriction of both dietary energy and protein, as well as other nutrients. At the other end is kwashiorkor, due to a quantitative and qualitative deficiency of protein, but in which energy intake may be adequate. These two syndromes are the extremes. Between them are forms in which the clinical features are due to varying combinations of deficiency of protein and energy together with deficiencies of minerals and vitamins and with associated infections. These less well-defined forms provide the majority of cases. PEM is the most important public health problem in underdeveloped countries in the world today. It is largely responsible for the fact that in many areas up to half the children born do not survive to the age of 5 years. Death rates in these children may be 20 to 50 times the rate in rich and prosperous communities in Europe and North America.

This chapter describes PEM as it occurs in children. It is much less common and usually less severe in adults. This is because adults do not need protein for growth and in most adult diets proteins provide 10 per cent of the energy. Typical kwashiorkor may occur in an adult secondary to malabsorption and following surgical resections of the gut (Krikler and Schrire, 1958; Neale *et al.*, 1967). Evidence of PEM can be found in patients in both the medical and surgical wards of hospitals in North America, if it is looked for carefully (p. 475). It is important for physicians and surgeons to recognise the condition as it occurs in adults.

Cicely Williams introduced the word kwashiorkor into modern medicine. It is the name used by the Ga tribe, who live around Accra in Ghana, for a disease which is the 'sickness the older child gets when the next baby is born'; this indicates the circumstances in which the disease most commonly develops, namely an ignorance of the best foods to give children during the weaning period, or an inability to provide them for one reason or another.

Her first report on kwashiorkor was in the 1931 Annual Medical Report of the Gold Coast colony, which has now been reprinted (Williams, 1973). This was only read locally, but a paper soon followed in an international journal (Williams, 1933).

There was a long incubation period before the disease became generally recognised. This was partly because international communication was disrupted during World War II, but Dr Williams had been transferred to Malaya in 1936, and in Africa the disease was confused with pellagra. Trowell (1975) tells the story of this phase. He writes, 'Experts should never be consulted about the status of a new idea in medicine. They are almost always wrong.' At the first session of the FAO/WHO Expert Committee on Nutrition in 1949 there was no place for protein malnutrition on the agenda. The subject was raised indirectly under the heading of pellagra; the committee asked WHO to conduct an enquiry into the various features of kwashiorkor. To this end Brock and Autret (1952) toured Africa and wrote a report which drew together the common features in different countries and set out questions that required research. In Uganda Trowell *et al.* (1954) wrote the classic textbook on kwashiorkor. Only after this did kwashiorkor start to appear in the textbooks, and in a few years protein malnutrition was being considered the most important nutritional disease in the world. Jelliffe (1959) introduced the term 'protein–calorie malnutrition' because of the close association between kwashiorkor and marasmus. Marasmic children have also received low protein intakes; in kwashiorkor anorexia leads to inadequate energy intake.

AETIOLOGY AND EPIDEMIOLOGY

PEM occurs characteristically in children under 5 years, wherever the diet is poor in protein and energy. No age is immune, but in older persons the disease is much less frequent and the clinical manifestations not so obvious and usually less severe, because both protein and energy requirements are reduced relative to body weight as age advances.

Typically the marasmic form of the syndrome occurs mostly in infants under 1 year and is more frequently found in towns; kwashiorkor is mainly a disease of rural areas occurring in the second year of life. Figure 29.1 emphasises these distinctions, which are often far from clear cut.

Marasmus

During the nineteenth century in the industrial towns in Europe and North America marasmus, resulting from the poor diets and numerous infections, took a toll of infant lives probably as large as it is taking in many Asian, African and South American towns today. The urban influences which predispose to marasmus are a rapid succession of pregnancies and early and abrupt weaning, followed by dirty and unsound artificial feeding of the infants with very

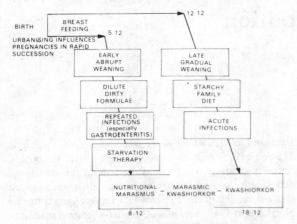

Fig. 29.1 Paths leading from early weaning to nutritional marasmus and from protracted breast feeding to kwashiorkor (McLaren, 1966).

dilute milk or milk products, given in inadequate amounts to avoid expense. Thus the diet is low in both energy and proteins. In addition poor houses and lack of equipment make the preparing of clean food almost impossible. Repeated infections develop, especially of the gastrointestinal tract; these the mother often treats by starvation for long periods, the infant receiving water, rice water or other non-nutritious fluid.

In marasmus, weaning has often been early. The mother may be induced to stop breast feeding for various reasons, including the presence of infections in herself or in the infant. Unfortunately she may have been influenced unwisely by advertisements in the press or on the radio which advocate, for commercial reasons, the advantages of artificial food products. A frequent reason for stopping breast feeding is the beginning of another pregnancy. There appears to be a widespread belief among poor, uneducated women that the milk of a pregnant woman is bad for her child. A common reason in towns is the necessity or desire to return to paid work.

Kwashiorkor

Kwashiorkor arises when, after a prolonged period on the breast, the child is weaned onto the traditional family diet; this may be low in protein because of poverty, insufficient land and poor agricultural practice. There is no supplement of milk or a totally inadequate one. Custom, sometimes reinforced by taboos, determines that the limited supply of foods of animal origin is given mainly to the men of the family. In many rural areas, where kwashiorkor is endemic, the food supply becomes scarce each year before the harvest; at this 'hungry season' the incidence of kwashiorkor and other nutritional diseases increases.

If the customary diet of a population is limited in protein and in energy to around the minimum requirements, a child may be in moderate health until his protein and energy needs are raised by an infection. Kwashiorkor is frequently precipitated in epidemic proportions by outbreaks of febrile illnesses such as malaria, measles or gastroenteritis. A heavy load of intestinal helminths also contributes to the disease.

Both marasmus and kwashiorkor arise as a result of poverty and ignorance. Even if food is available and there is the money to buy it, many mothers have received no satisfactory instruction in infant feeding. Eggs, fish, meat and sometimes milk may not be given to children because custom or taboos do not allow them. Unsuitable commercial food preparations may be purchased or good preparations misused.

Reports on the prevalence of PEM have been collected and summarised by Bengoa and Donoso (1974). In parts of many underdeveloped countries surveys have shown that between 0 and 5 per cent of children or more have severe PEM and up to 50 per cent have moderate forms, which usually means underweight children. Average (median) figures for the Third World countries are 2 per cent with severe and 19 per cent with moderate PEM. The type of severe PEM differs greatly. In large cities, in South America and in Asia, marasmus is generally commoner than kwashiorkor, but in Africa south of the Sahara kwashiorkor is often commoner (FAO/WHO, 1971). There traditional children's diets are often based on cassava and have a low protein/energy ratio (Alleyne et al., 1977). Accurate figures for the incidence of severe PEM can be obtained only by special arrangements, as neither kwashiorkor nor marasmus are notifiable. Surveys show predominantly the marasmic forms because wasting lasts longer than oedema; hospital admissions and death certificates may not record that a child with diarrhoea or other infection was underweight.

The principal features of kwashiorkor are due to protein deficiency. This was shown by Hansen et al. (1956), who treated cases with a mixture of 18 amino acids and glucose, but gave no vitamins, and observed full initiation of cure in a few days.

Associated nutrients deficiencies. Deficiencies of retinol, folate, iron, magnesium and potassium are commonly found in PEM and may be the presenting clinical feature. Deficiencies important in some areas are thiamin (E Asia), riboflavin (SE Asia), nicotinic acid (Africa), iodine (goitrous regions) and vitamin D (when exposure to sunlight is insufficient). Research reports suggest that lack of zinc, copper, chromium, selenium, pyridoxine, vitamins E and K and essential fatty acids may each be important in some circumstances. Thus in individual cases the cause of the child's disease and the clinical features may vary greatly.

CLINICAL FEATURES
The clinical presentation depends on the type, severity and duration of the dietary deficiencies. The five forms, sum-

Table 29.1 Classification of PEM

	Body weight as percentage of standard	Oedema	Deficit in weight for height
Kwashiorkor	80–60	+	+
Marasmic kwashiorkor	<60	+	++
Marasmus	<60	0	++
Nutritional dwarfing	<60	0	minimal
Underweight child	80–60	0	+

Based on Joint FAO/WHO Expert Committee on Nutrition. 8th Report, 1971.

marised in Table 29.1, are described separately, but each is part of the whole PEM spectrum. When describing the metabolic disorders and morbid anatomy, and the treatment, and prevention of the disease, the different forms are considered together.

Nutritional marasmus

There is a failure to thrive, irritability, fretfulness or, alternatively, apathy. Diarrhoea is frequent. Many infants are hungry, but some are anorexic. The child is wizened

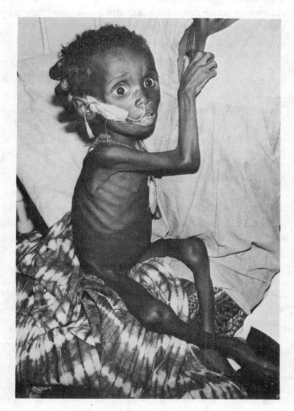

Fig. 29.2 A marasmic child. Some skin lesions can be seen on the shoulders, and the hair is thinned over the temples. Tube used for nasogastric feeding is strapped to the cheek. (Photo by Dr R.G. Whitehead.)

and shrunken and there is little or no subcutaneous fat (Fig. 29.2). He is often dehydrated. The weight is much below the standard for his age. The temperature may be subnormal. If the disease is of long duration, the length of the child is also below the standard, but less so than the weight. There is usually watery diarrhoea with acid stools. If infective gastroenteritis is added, the diarrhoea is severe. The abdomen may be shrunken or distended with gas. Because of the thinness of the abdominal wall, peristalsis may be easily visible. The muscles are weak and atrophic and this, together with the lack of subcutaneous fat, makes the limbs appear as skin and bone.

The skin and mucous membranes may be dry and atrophic, but the characteristic changes found in kwashiorkor are not usually present. Evidence of vitamin deficiencies may or may not be found.

Nutritional marasmus presents a clinical picture similar to marasmus produced by infections or other wasting diseases. Indeed in any infant with PEM there is usually more than one cause and each must be diagnosed if treatment is to be successful.

Psychological disturbances, resulting from a lack of a mother's love and care, can depress the appetite, and hence may be a factor in the causation of marasmus.

Kwashiorkor

There is oedema together with failure to thrive, anorexia, diarrhoea and a generalised unhappiness or apathy. An infection often precipitates the onset and may be the reason for bringing the child to the doctor.

Failure of growth is an early sign, though oedema and the presence of some subcutaneous fat make the weight loss less striking than in marasmus.

Oedema may be slight or gross depending partly on the amount of salt and water in the diet. It may be distributed over the whole body, including the face, but is usually more marked on the lower limbs (Fig. 29.3). Ascites and pleural effusions are usually slight and, if detected clinically, suggest the presence of an infection.

The characteristic **dermatosis** consists of areas of pigmentation and desquamation. In the first stage the skin becomes pigmented and thickened as if varnished. This then peels and appears like 'flaky paint', leaving cracks or

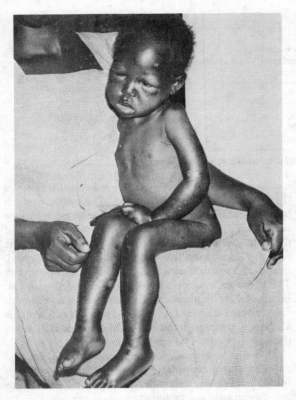

Fig. 29.3 A child with kwashiorkor in Uganda, showing oedema of face, feet and hands, and skin lesions. (Photo by Dr R.G. Whitehead.)

usual. The liver can generally be palpated and is firm and not tender. The hepatomegaly is sometimes marked.

The muscles are always wasted and as a result many children regress in their physical development and may no longer be able to walk or crawl.

Some degree of anaemia is always present and may be severe, though this is unusual. Every variety of haematological picture may be found. As discussed on page 44, protein deficiency itself may give rise to anaemia, but the diets of the children have often been lacking in iron and folic acid and in addition there may be impaired absorption of these nutrients from the gut.

Apathy is a characteristic feature and the child appears constantly unhappy. Neurological features are unusual, but some children during recovery have unexplained tremors resembling Parkinsonism.

Kwashiorkor has to be distinguished from marasmus and from oedema arising from renal or hepatic disease, heart failure or severe anaemia. A careful history and clinical examination including examination of the urine for protein should suffice to exclude these.

Marasmic kwashiorkor

In areas where PEM is endemic, many patients coming to a

denuded areas of shallow ulceration. In moderate cases the dermatosis resembles crazy paving; when severe, the desquamated part of the child's body looks as if there has been a burn. The lower limbs, buttocks and perineum are usually most affected but ulcers can occur over pressure points and deep cracks in skinfolds. The lesions are determined in part by associated skin infections and trauma. In maize-eating areas pellagrous features may also be present in parts of the skin that are exposed to light. The skin lesions heal with areas of depigmentation. Figure 29.4 shows moderately severe skin lesions on the buttocks which are starting to heal.

The **hair** is sparse, soft and thin. Negro children lose their characteristic curl. There may be changes in pigmentation with diffuse patches or streaks which may be red, blond or grey in colour. This is seen more often in Negro than in Asian children. Because hair takes time to grow it reflects the child's nutrition one to three months earlier. The reliability of the hair signs are summarised by Bradfield and Jelliffe (1974).

Angular stomatitis, cheilosis and a smooth atrophic tongue are commonly seen, as is ulceration around the anus.

Watery diarrhoea or large semisolid, acid stools are

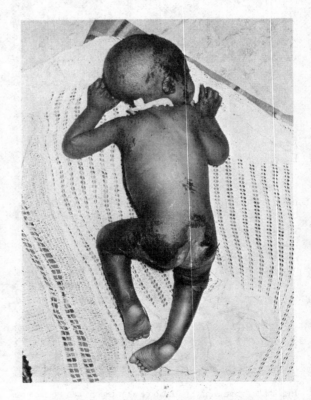

Fig. 29.4 A child with kwashiorkor, showing pigmented skin lesions especially over the buttocks, thighs, side of head and backs of hands. (By courtesy of Professor Walter Gordon.)

hospital or clinic show a mixture of some of the features of both marasmus and kwashiorkor. These children are sometimes said to have marasmic kwashiorkor, but their condition is often referred to simply as protein-energy malnutrition. As already explained, this is due to the varying nature of the dietary deficiency and the social factors responsible for the disease and the presence or absence of infections.

Nutritional dwarfing

Some children adapt to prolonged insufficiency of food—energy and protein—by a marked retardation of growth. They are light in weight for age but their stature is reduced proportionally so that they appear superficially normal. When their weight or height is checked against standards for normal children (p. 471) it is seen that they resemble children a year or more younger.

The underweight child

For every florid case of kwashiorkor or marasmus there are usually several children with mild to moderate PEM. Like an iceberg, there is more malnutrition below the surface than is visible above. Children with subclinical PEM can, however, be detected by their weight for age, which is less than 80 per cent of the standard. In areas where kwashiorkor is the predominant form of PEM, they may have reduced plasma albumin and sometimes other biochemical signs of protein deficiency (Alleyne et al., 1977). These children are growing up smaller than their genetic potential, but of greater importance they are very susceptible to gastroenteritis, respiratory and other infections, which in turn can precipitate frank malnutrition. Mild to moderate PEM is probably the major reason why the mortality in children from 1 to 4 years of age in some parts of Africa, Asia and Latin America is 30 to 40 times higher than in Europe or North America.

For the above reasons doctors, medical assistants and nurses should recognise growth retardation in its early phase. Failure to appreciate its presence and significance, when a child is brought to a clinic for what may be at first a minor ailment, leads to ineffective therapy. This may be followed by repeated outpatient visits, subsequent hospitalisation and all too often a fatal outcome.

Growth retardation can be recognised by weighing and measuring the child and referring to standard charts or tables (p. 471). Nutritional dwarfing must be distinguished from other causes of dwarfing such as renal disease, endocrine disorders, various forms of the malabsorption syndrome and congenital metabolic disorders. In the majority of cases, the dietary and clinical history and a physical examination suffice to make the diagnosis clear.

BIOCHEMICAL AND METABOLIC DISORDERS

The clinical features of PEM are a consequence, direct or indirect, of an insufficient supply of energy and of amino acids to the tissues, which need them for protein synthesis. As a result there is a failure of function of the different organs. Effective treatment of the disorder depends on some understanding of the biochemical lesions and of the effects of associated vitamin and mineral deficiencies. A preliminary account of how the body reacts to protein deficiency has been given on page 44. Laboratory tests are reviewed in the Lancet (1973).

Body composition

A high body water content, loss of the fat stores and loss of protein from the wasted muscles and other tissues greatly alter the chemical composition of the child. Table 29.2 illustrates the differences which may be found. Children with PEM are not only underweight, but their tissues are abnormal in composition. With treatment dramatic gain of weight is associated with a return to normal body composition.

A further point has been brought out by careful chemical analysis of the bodies of children who had died of PEM (Picou et al., 1966). The total protein in the body amounted to 62 per cent of the expected value in a normal child. Of this protein 42 per cent was collagen. In a normal child collagen amounts to 27 per cent of the total protein. Hence the collagen protein, which turns over very slowly, is mostly retained, but a large part of the cellular protein is lost. A study of the chemical composition of organs of children who have died of malnutrition has been made by Alleyne et al. (1970).

General metabolism

The metabolic rate is reduced (Ablett and McCance, 1971), but probably no more than cell mass; there is no evidence of any economy in the utilisation of energy by the cells. Adaptive changes in the utilisation of protein are described on page 44. The tissues have a full capacity to utilise both energy and protein, once these become available. This is well shown by the high intake of both energy and protein when a child with PEM has free access to food and is encouraged to eat (Table 29.3). The figures after recovery are representative of a normal child, but during the period of rapid recovery energy utilisation was nearly

Table 29.2 The chemical composition which might be found in a normal child and in one severely ill with PEM, each aged 1 year

	Normal		PEM	
	(kg)	(%)	(kg)	(%)
Body weight	10.0	100	5.0	100
Water	6.2	62	4.0	80
Protein	1.7	17	0.6	12
Fat	1.5	15	0.1	2
Minerals	0.6	6	0.3	6

Table 29.3 Mean daily intakes of energy and protein and percentage of feed refused by 8 children aged 10 to 36 months during recovery from PEM (Ashworth, 1969)

	Energy kJ/kg	Energy kcal/kg	Protein (g/kg)	Feed refused (%)
Period of rapid recovery	670	160	3.7	0.5
Intermediary period	636	152	3.5	3
Full recovery	485	116	2.7	27

40 per cent above normal. Those children did not begin to refuse feeds until body weight approached the normal for their age, a good example of the regulatory mechanism for control of body weight.

Another study in Jamaica (Ashworth *et al.*, 1968) showed that for every gram of weight gain a dietary intake of 57.8 kJ (13.8 kcal) was required. Assuming a value of 11.3 kJ (2.7 kcal)/g for the tissue laid down, the recovery process has a thermodynamic efficiency of 20 per cent.

In an acute case in an infant or young child, provided electrolyte disturbances are corrected and infections are treated, the cells are well able to utilise nutrients to restore the lost tissues. The above figures provide background information for drawing up dietary schedules for use in treatment (p. 263).

Protein metabolism
The disorder in the supply of amino acids is illustrated by characteristic changes in the pattern of plasma amino acids (Holt *et al.*, 1963; Saunders *et al.*, 1967). Plasma concentrations of branched chain amino acids and tyrosine are low, presumably as a result of adaptive metabolic changes (Lunn *et al.*, 1973). However, concentrations of some non-essential amino acids are higher than normal. As soon as treatment with protein starts, the concentration of amino acids in the plasma rises and there may be an overflow aminoaciduria (Saunders *et al.*, 1967).

The plasma albumin concentration is low, owing to a failure of synthesis in the liver. In patients with severe kwashiorkor it is usually below 20 and sometimes below 10 g/1. In marasmus the concentration is also lowered, but not to the same extent, and values around 25 g/1 are common. A rise in plasma albumin is a useful sign of recovery. A low concentration certainly is in part responsible for the oedema which is often present.

The concentration of γ-globulin is often raised if infections are present, but β-globulins are lowered. Plasma transferrin is lowered, especially in severe cases, and may be a better guide to prognosis than plasma albumin. Plasma retinol-binding protein is also lowered and this may be a contributory cause of keratomalacia.

Concentrations of some plasma enzymes are reduced, reflecting depletion of these enzymes in the tissues and organs. Low values for cholinesterase, alkaline phosphatase, amylase and lipase have been reported.

The blood urea is usually low and may fall to 1 mmol/1 (6 mg/100 ml). This reflects a reduced protein intake rather than a lowered rate of protein catabolism. Urinary creatinine is also reduced, reflecting decreased muscle mass.

Lipid metabolism
A fatty liver is characteristic of kwashiorkor. In a study of biopsy material Chatterjee and Mukherjee (1968) found an average lipid content in cases of kwashiorkor of 390 g/kg, but of only 35 g/kg in marasmus. The phospholipid content was the same in the two syndromes and usually below 20 g/kg. The excess fat in the liver is triglyceride. In kwashiorkor, but not in marasmus, plasma triglyceride and plasma cholesterol are low. There is a decreased ability of the liver cells to mobilise lipid in the form of lipoproteins (Truswell, 1975).

In all forms of PEM, concentrations of FFA in the plasma tend to be high. This probably is a result of the state of partial starvation.

Carbohydrate metabolism
In kwashiorkor hypoglycaemia is an early complication, seen in some countries but not in others (Truswell, 1975). In severe PEM an intravenous glucose tolerance test, which eliminates the intestinal factors, raises plasma insulin less than normally and glucose leaves the blood more slowly. In marasmus results are usually normal. The impaired early response of insulin in kwashiorkor has been corrected by potassium treatment (Mann *et al.*, 1975). In Jordan, Nigeria and Turkey (but not in Egypt) glucose tolerance has improved after giving 0.25 mg of chromic chloride (Gurson and Saner, 1971).

Electrolyte and water metabolism
A deficiency of potassium arises as a result of the diarrhoea and losses in the stools can amount to 20 to 30 mmol/day (Hansen, 1956). The plasma potassium is often below normal, and very low values, less than 2.5 mmol/1 may be found. Measurements of the natural isotope ^{40}K with a total body counter in Jamaican children have indicated a total body potassium concentration of 35 mmol/kg body weight rising to 45 in three to four weeks on treatment with a daily potassium supplement of 6 to 8 mmol/kg (Alleyne, 1970). This made good the depleted potassium levels in the

tissues and thereafter the concentration in the tissues remained constant, but the total body content rose further in the next 8 to 10 weeks as the wasted muscle and other tissue were replaced. Similar results have been obtained in Cape Town (Mann *et al.*, 1975).

A deficiency of magnesium also arises from increased losses in the stools, and plasma magnesium concentrations are generally low.

Plasma sodium concentrations are usually normal. Low values are found if there have been large losses in the sweat, or in association with diarrhoea or a diminished intake of salt with a large intake of water. In this last circumstance the kidneys' ability to conserve sodium may be insufficient to prevent depletion. Thus sodium deficiency is a possible complication of PEM, but is not a usual feature. If the water intake has been restricted and dehydration is marked, plasma sodium may be above normal.

Plasma hydrogen ion concentration may be either raised or lowered. Acidosis is probably due to poor circulation and consequent tissue hypoxia. Alkalosis is known to be associated with potassium depletion and a failure of the kidneys to excrete bicarbonate.

The total body water increases (Garrow *et al.*, 1965; Hansen *et al.*, 1965). Values from 65 to 80 per cent of body weight are found, whereas the value in normal children is 60 per cent. The very high values around 80 per cent occur in marasmic children, whose body fat had been greatly reduced. The increase is mainly in extracellular water; the cells are also overhydrated. The direct effects of PEM on body water and electrolytes are complicated by acute or chronic diarrhoea, leading to dehydration. This may be hypotonic, isotonic or hypertonic depending on the balance of losses of water, electrolytes and nitrogen (Prinsloo and Kruger, 1970).

The severity of the clinical oedema is not closely associated with the size of the increase in total body water or with the level of plasma albumin. The cause and nature of the oedema still remains in part a mystery. Increases of urinary aldosterone, of antidiuretic hormone and of plasma renin have been provisionally reported by different investigators. The oedema may shift from one part of the body to another. Indeed, clinical dehydration and shock may be found in a child, associated with gross oedema in parts of the body. It is of interest that on therapy there may be an increase in oedema coincident with marked improvement in the general clinical condition. It is often several days before diuresis sets in and the oedema disappears.

Drug metabolism

Malnourished children are likely to have infections and may have other complications requiring drug treatment. With each drug that is given, no matter how well known it is, the question should be asked: 'How is this drug metabolised and in what way may it be altered in a malnourished child?' Some antibiotics and antimalarials act by interfering with nutrition more in the microorganism than in the human host, and they need to be used with care in PEM. Chloramphenicol interferes with mitochondrial protein synthesis and tetracyclines cause negative nitrogen balance even in well-nourished adults. The antimalarial trimethoprim can antagonise folate metabolism and there is evidence that this occurs in PEM (Poskitt and Parkin, 1972). Some antibiotics are given as esters in syrups but, despite low pancreatic lipase, plasma concentrations of chloramphenicol after oral administration of the palmitate are as high as in well-nourished children and decline more slowly (Mehta *et al.*, 1975)

Drugs carried in the circulation bound to plasma proteins may be more active in patients with hypoalbuminuria because more is in the free form. Kwashiorkor plasma has a reduced binding capacity for digoxin (Buchanan *et al.*, 1976), salicylates (Eyberg *et al.*, 1974) and thiopentone (Buchanan and van der Walt, 1977). The implication is that a standard dosage per kilogram body weight may be too high in kwashiorkor. Most drugs are detoxicated in the liver microsomal enzyme-oxidising system. Its function can be tested by measuring the half-life of intravenous antipyrine, which is broken down by this system, and has been shown to be impaired in PEM (Narang *et al.*, 1977). More research is needed on the clinical pharmacology of PEM.

CHANGES IN THE ORGANS AND SYSTEMS OF THE BODY

Digestive organs

The cells of the pancreas and of the intestinal mucosa atrophy and cannot produce digestive enzymes in normal amounts. Barbezat and Hansen (1968) aspirated duodenal contents and measured the concentrations of pancreatic enzymes present. They found very low values for amylase, trypsin and lipase in samples from children with kwashiorkor and marasmus. Biopsy specimens of jejunal mucosa show that the activity of many enzymes, especially the disaccharidases, lactase, sucrase and maltase, are greatly reduced in the atrophic mucosa commonly found in PEM (Cook and Lee, 1966; James, 1968). The mucosal atrophy is associated with impaired absorption of nutrients (James, 1971). Although activities of most enzymes rise with treatment, it may take many months before that of lactase returns to normal.

Liver

The clinical and biochemical features of the fatty liver found in kwashiorkor have already been described. The fat first accumulates in small droplets within liver cells, situated at the periphery of the lobules. The droplets increase in size and extend from the periphery to the centre of the lobules. In severe cases all the liver cells may be filled, each with a big fat droplet, pushing aside the cell nucleus and reducing the cytoplasm to a narrow rim.

Despite the marked structural change liver function is well maintained and severe liver failure is unusual. Plasma bilirubin is usually normal; prothrombin concentrations are often reduced, but return to normal on treatment with vitamin K. Plasma concentrations of alanine aminotransferase and isocitric dehydrogenase are usually normal and, if found raised, suggest the presence of damage from a bacterial or viral infection.

With proper treatment the lipid accumulated in the liver cells is all cleared with return to a normal structure. This is the usual course of events. The possible development of cirrhosis is discussed on page 265.

Endocrine organs

There is no evidence of primary hypofunction of the endocrine glands in PEM. Indeed the reverse may be the case. Plasma concentrations of growth hormone may be raised in kwashiorkor (Pimstone et al., 1966), as the pituitary responds effectively to the stimulus of protein depletion. Many studies have shown that plasma concentrations of cortisol and other adrenocorticosteroids are normal or raised. Alleyne and Young (1967) showed that children with PEM responded to stimulation with corticotrophin with higher concentrations of plasma cortisol than normal; there was a prolongation of the half-life of radioactive cortisol in the plasma, which indicates some impairment of cortisol metabolism in the tissues. They suggest that several of the metabolic disturbances found in PEM may be related to the high concentration of circulating cortisol. There is no specific disturbance of thyroid function. Owing to reduced plasma concentrations of thyroxine-binding protein and prealbumin in kwashiorkor total plasma thyroxine is often low, but free T_4 is usually normal or raised. In marasmus it is normal or low. Impaired insulin secretion after glucose tolerance tests has already been described.

Endocrine function in PEM is reviewed by Pimstone (1976), who has himself made important contributions.

Cardiovascular system

Atrophy of the heart, as found in starvation (p. 240), may be seen at autopsy or on radiographs of children with severe chronic PEM. This leads to a reduced cardiac output and a poor circulation. In many severe cases the extremities are cold and cyanosed and the pulse small or impalpable. The signs are associated with a high mortality but recovery may occur and, when it does, no cardiac disabilities remain.

The electrocardiogram shows low-voltage changes in the QRS complex and the T-wave may be depressed or inverted. Some of these changes are rapidly reversed by potassium therapy. The myocardial changes are described by Wharton et al., (1969).

Kidneys

Mild albuminuria may be found but there is no specific structural or functional abnormality of the kidneys. The glomerular filtration rate may be low, but this is probably due to dehydration or reduced cardiac output. The concentrating power of the kidneys is often poor, but this may be the result of depression of tubular function by electrolyte deficiencies. Aminoaciduria occurs when protein is fed. These signs of renal dysfunction are not severe enough to complicate the clinical picture and are not responsible for the oedema. They are all reversible by treatment.

Immunological system

The expected increase of body temperature with infection is often absent in severe PEM and there may be no leucocytosis. The function of leucocytes is defective, as shown by reduced activities of several of their enzymes. Plasma concentrations of immunoglobulins IgA, IgG and IgM are normal or raised and the response to antigenic challenge is usually adequate. Synthesis of plasma γ-globulin, unlike that of albumin, is maintained in kwashiorkor. While humoral antibodies are not depressed, concentrations of several components of complement are subnormal and rise with refeeding (Sirisinha, 1975). The thymus is markedly atrophic and the tonsils and spleen less so (Smythe et al., 1971). Thymus-dependent lymphocytes appear to be reduced, as is lymphocyte transformation in response to phytohaemagglutinin (Sellmeyer et al., 1972) and also delayed cutaneous hypersensitivity responses, e.g. to tuberculin or BCG. Cell-mediated immunity thus appears to be depressed more severely than humoral immunity. These abnormalities may result from other nutritional deficiences as well as protein. Zinc may play a part in the thymus atrophy (Golden et al., 1977) while iron or folate deficiency may contribute to the poor polymorph leucocyte response to infection. These changes lead to decreased resistance to infections, especially those like measles in which cell-mediated immunity is most important in the body's defence. There is also difficulty in diagnosing infections because pyrexia, leucocytosis and the tuberculin skin response may not appear when infection occurs.

TREATMENT

Treatment is required for four different circumstances. First, there are those children who are dangerously ill and need resuscitation; good results depend on high standards of clinical skill and nursing care and adequate laboratory support. Secondly, when a child has been resuscitated or if he has been admitted to hospital not dangerously ill, cure can be initiated by a special diet and the treatment of any infectious or other illness; the care of such children is relatively less exacting. Thirdly, there are children who are convalescent but still undernourished who may need a long period of rehabilitation; these do not need to be in hospital and may be cared for in a home. Fourthly, there are the many underweight children who need nutritional support and often simple medical treatment which can be provided at a clinic without admission to hospital.

Resuscitation

The immediate tasks are to correct the water and electrolyte disturbance and to provide glucose as an easily assimilable form of energy. For this purpose half isotonic Darrow's solution with added glucose is recommended:

Na	60 mmol/l
K	15 mmol/l
Glucose	140 mmol/l
Cl	50 mmol/l
Lactate	25 mmol/l

This may be given by mouth in small frequent doses up to a total of 100 to 200 ml/kg daily. The smaller amount is given if there is oedema. If there is vomiting or signs of severe dehydration, such as a dry tongue or weak pulse, the larger dose may be needed and should be given intravenously. Plasma in the same dosage is also useful if there is severe peripheral circulatory failure. If acidosis is marked, isotonic sodium bicarbonate solution should be given in addition and if the haemoglobin is less than 6 g/dl, a small blood transfusion.

In seriously ill patients there is always a deficiency of both potassium and magnesium. Supplements of 4–8 mmol/kg of K and 1–2 mmol/kg of Mg should be given daily and by the intravenous route if there is diarrhoea and vomiting. Such high doses may be needed for many days to replete the tissues and, owing to the danger of overdosage, plasma concentrations should be measured regularly. There is often a relative excess of sodium in the body and plasma Na should also be measured. Although hypernatraemic dehydration is uncommon, it is dangerous and needs energetic treatment with hypotonic solutions when it occurs.

Hypothermia and hypoglycaemia are often present and always need to be treated urgently.

Antibiotic therapy. PEM is so frequently associated with infection that most cases require treatment with antibiotics or chemotherapeutic agents. Where infections are widespread all cases admitted to hospital should be given a regime such as procaine penicillin 300 000 units i.m./day in a single dose and a sulpha drug such as sulphadiazine 180 mg/kg daily in divided doses as a routine even if infection is not clinically apparent.

Details of the resuscitation of dangerously ill patients are given by Waterlow *et al.* (1978).

Initiation of cure

Once the patient is out of danger, which should be within 24 to 48 hours, intravenous therapy can be stopped or curtailed and attention directed to restoring the tissues by dietary means. Most hospitals with experience of PEM have evolved their own routine of dietary and other treatment. Methods differ depending partly on local patterns of nutritional and infective disease. Specific therapy consists in providing the child with sufficient of a good dietary source of protein and energy and in controlling infection. Milk is excellent for this purpose. Some children who are seriously ill cannot tolerate whole milk and require treatment with skimmed milk or a preparation of casein. Where PEM is endemic supplies of liquid milk are never available in amounts sufficient to treat the large numbers of less serious cases or to prevent the disease.

Dried skimmed milk. When pancreatic functions are impaired, fat is poorly digested and whole milk may aggravate the diarrhoea. Fortunately dried skimmed milk, a byproduct of the butter industry, has been made available in large quantities by international and other agencies. Most skimmed milk powders contain about 50 per cent carbohydrate and 35 per cent protein. If 60 g (2 oz) are reconstituted with water to make 600 ml (20 oz), this provides 21 g of protein which is sufficient to meet the daily protein needs of an infant. This amount supplies only about 1.0 MJ (240 kcal) and extra energy must be given in the form of carbohydrate or fat, if tolerated.

Unless the powder is reconstituted with boiled water, and the feeding bottle likewise sterilised, it is liable to become contaminated with pathogenic organisms. Milk is then an excellent culture medium for bacteria. For this reason it is potentially dangerous; it is safer to advise the mother of a child old enough to take solid foods not to reconstitute the powder, but to sprinkle it on the cereal or any other part of the child's meal.

Casein preparations. The carbohydrate present in milk is the disaccharide, lactose. When the gastrointestinal tract has been seriously damaged and is unable to produce adequate amounts of the enzyme lactase, the infant or child cannot digest the lactose, which is fermented by bacteria in the large bowel. In this way milk aggravates the diarrhoea. In these circumstances a casein preparation must be used and Casilan (Glaxo) has proved effective. It is possible to dissolve 40 g in 800 ml of water, which more than meets the protein needs of an infant. Energy must be provided in the form of glucose and 35 g may be added to the solution; fat in the form of cream can also be added if tolerated. A little salt, about 1 to 2 g of NaCl, should be added. Fortunately the digestive powers improve rapidly with a high protein intake; hence it is usually unnecessary to rely on casein for more than a few days.

In the majority of cases there is no deficiency of lactase or the enzyme is not completely absent and cure can be initiated and completed with skimmed milk and later whole milk.

Milk substitutes of vegetable origin. Vegetable proteins if carefully selected and combined give a mixture of amino acids with a satisfactory pattern. As the available sources of vegetable protein differ greatly throughout the areas where PEM is prevalent, many different protein food mixtures have been made and successfully used in the treatment and prevention of PEM in various parts of the world. A list of some 40 protein-rich foods was given in our last edition. These were commercial products manufactured from locally available material in various countries where PEM was prevalent. It is now clear that most of these have not been a commercial success and the impact of most of them has been small. However, there have been good sales of *Incaparina*, a maize–cottonseed flour product made in Guatemala, and of *Pronutro*, a soya–maize-groundnut product in South Africa. The future of such products and their potential cost-effectiveness in the treatment and prevention of PEM is discussed by Orr (1977). Preparations should be fully tested and approved before being released for general use. It is essential to show that the mixture has an effective NPU value of at least 70, that it is easily digestible, non-toxic and acceptable to children and that it is not adversely affected by storage under normal conditions.

When commercial preparations conforming to these standards are not available in sufficient quantities or are too expensive to buy with a limited income, preparations based on the staple cereal or other food supplemented by locally available high-protein vegetables can be used. An example is 2:1 mixture of maize with bean or pea flour. Such a mixture can be easily adapted to local cultural patterns of eating. Utilisation of the protein depends on an adequate dietary supply of energy.

Dose of protein. This is best related to the observed weight of the child. Recovery and weight gain are not accelerated by daily intakes over 3.5 g/kg. Many infants recover well on the recommended daily intake for the normal infant of 0 to 3 months of age, namely 2.3 g/kg. Infants who are seriously ill with impaired digestive functions may improve with a daily intake of 1 g/kg and this is often sufficient to initiate cure though larger amounts are necessary for full recovery.

It is useful to remember that 30 ml (1 oz) of liquid cow's milk, either skimmed or full cream, contains about 1 g protein. An intake of milk of 100 ml/kg daily thus provides 3.3 g protein/kg. It is unnecessary to give more protein than this.

Diet

After resuscitation, or immediately if this is not necessary, the child is given a milk diet or more rarely a casein preparation. Skimmed milk powder alone cannot meet a child's energy needs for growth and moreover is liable in excessive amounts to cause diarrhoea. It must therefore only be used as one component of the diet. The following recipe is from Jamaica.

Ingredients. Sixty g (2 oz) skimmed milk powder; 15 g (1½ teaspoons) butter; 20 g (2 teaspoons) flour; 250 ml water. About 250 ml of this mixture contains 22 g protein and 1.05 MJ (250 kcal).

Method. Add skimmed milk powder to cold water gradually while stirring. Pour mixture through a strainer. Melt butter in saucepan and add flour to form a smooth paste. Add 2 to 3 tablespoons of liquid skimmed milk. Stir and cook for 2 minutes. Add remaining milk and continue to cook and stir until the flour and butter mixture is well distributed throughout the milk, and the flour is cooked.

The mixture should be given in divided doses four to six times a day so as to provide the patient with about 3.5 g of protein/kg of the ideal weight of a child of the same age. On the second or third day it should be possible to start on a banana/milk or cereal/milk diet. In countries such as Uganda and Jamaica where bananas are a staple article of diet, they should be used because they mix better with skimmed milk powder than do flours made from cereals or roots (cassava) and the mixture is very palatable.

When bananas are not available, semolina, rice, cassava or cereal flours have to be used. Then some fat (butter or margarine) or an edible oil should be added as it makes the mixing of the flour and milk powder easier. Some patients are able to digest fats better than carbohydrates and the mixture is more palatable and of higher energy value.

Anorexia may be serious, but often can be overcome by feeding the child slowly in the mother's lap and not in bed. Food may be taken better cold than hot.

As the clinical condition improves the food intake should be increased gradually. Whole milk powder can be substituted for skimmed milk powder; eggs, fish, flour and bean flour can be added to the diet until the child is eating a satisfactory diet of local pattern, including adequate amounts of easily digested protein-rich foods.

Mineral supplements. Supplements of K and Mg in the doses recommended on page 263 should be given for about two weeks. Iron in medicinal doses is needed for all anaemic patients.

Vitamin concentrates. The diet of a child admitted to hospital is likely to have been poor in vitamins. For the first 10 days in hospital all children should receive a multivitamin preparation. Large doses are not required unless there is clinical evidence of a specific vitamin deficiency. Extra retinol should be given in areas where xerophthalmia is common.

After 10 days the child's appetite should have returned and vitamin requirements are then best met from natural foods in a good mixed diet. A supplement of vitamins and minerals may be needed throughout convalescence in some circumstances.

General measures

As the child's temperature may be subnormal, a heated room, electric blanket or hot cradle may be necessary even in the tropics, especially where there is a large fall of atmospheric temperature at night.

Appetite should return soon and the child be feeding well in a few days. The stay in hospital for a moderately severe case is usually two to three weeks, by which time the plasma albumin should be 35 g/l and a significant gain in weight achieved. Cure may be said to be initiated and the child can be discharged. Very severe cases may need to be hospitalised for two or three months.

Rehabilitation

When a child is fit for discharge from hospital, a period for consolidation of the cure is needed. It may be three months or more before normal weight is reached. This period can be spent at home, after teaching the mother how to feed her child properly. When, as is often the case, home conditions are unsatisfactory, admission to a **rehabilitation centre** is indicated. These have been set up in a number of countries where PEM is common. The buildings are inexpensive; they have usually been sited near to the people's villages. They use less specialised staff than hospitals and the mothers live in and each helps to look after her child. These centres are ideal for new cases of only moderate severity and for rehabilitation of severe cases, transferred after two to three weeks in hospital. They combine the advantages of saving resources and of bringing treatment nearer to the mother and her family. She feels at ease, able to understand what is being done to her child and so is much more likely to acquire lasting and sound habits of feeding this and her other childreh. Sister Joan Koppert, after setting up a rehabilitation centre in Zambia, visited 23 different centres in five African countries and has written a manual based on her experiences (Koppert, 1977).

As already stated, in endemic areas many children who are brought to the doctor with a variety of illnesses and injuries are seriously underweight for age, but have no other clinical features of PEM. A careful dietary history as well as a full clinical examination is needed. If mild or moderate PEM is present, it must be treated since such children are at great risk of developing severe forms of the disease. In outpatients, all the specific therapy needed is the simple dietary advice that more food, especially milk, should be given to the children. This is usually well understood by the parent, but difficulties arise in putting it into practice. The supply of liquid cow's milk is almost certainly limited and the mother may need to be warned that it cannot be made good by further dilution. Skimmed milk powder may be used and a suitable dose is 30 g/day, providing about 11 g protein. This is best given mixed with or sprinkled over solid food. When the patient is an infant requiring liquid milk, the mother must be given detailed instructions on how to reconstitute the powder using boiled water.

If a protein food mixture is used as a milk substitute, the instructions must be explained to the mother. Additional protein can also be provided by eggs, fish and meat if these are available. Eggs may be boiled or scrambled. For very young children the fish or meat may need to be sieved. In the absence of these foods of animal origin, beans and pulses must be used to supplement the cereal protein in the diet.

As many of these children are likely to be on diets lacking in vitamin A, the mother should be advised to add vegetables, especially green leafy vegetables, and fresh fruit as frequently as possible.

PROGNOSIS

A child may suffer for a short period of its life from one of the forms of PEM and make a complete recovery. If growth has been retarded for a short period or only slightly, the child may reach the normal size for its age quickly, provided the dietary supply is satisfactory. If growth is retarded for a long period, the child may develop into a small, but healthy adult. Kruger (1969) measured 154 children treated in Kampala six to 11 years earlier and found them small compared with a control group of Baganda children. Bone age, assessed by X-ray of the wrist, was one or two years less than chronological age.

If the disease is so severe as to demand treatment in hospital, the prognosis is uncertain and often bad. Thus out of 343 children admitted to hospital in Jamaica, 15 per cent died, 12 per cent recovered slowly, 30 per cent at an intermediate rate and 43 per cent rapidly (Garrow and Pike, 1967). Children are often only brought to hospital by their parents as a last resort, and then even with good treatment the mortality rate may be high.

Garrow and Pike (1967) were able to follow up some of their patients, admitted to hospital below 2 years of age. When these children returned home and ate the usual diet for poor Jamaican families, they gained height and weight between the ages of 2 and 10 years comparable to controls in the same families and not greatly below Boston standards for height but less for weight.

Two aspect of prognosis merit further discussion.

The liver disorder

The fatty degeneration of the liver may heal completely without fibrosis and in the vast majority of treated cases this occurs. However, cirrhosis and other disorders of the liver (p. 415) in adolescents and adults are relatively common in many parts of the tropics where PEM is endemic. It is probable that an infection, e.g. virus hepatitis, schistosomiasis or a chemical toxin, e.g. alcohol or iron, or a plant poison is more likely to lead to progressive liver disease if it is acting on a liver damaged by chronic malnutrition.

Mental retardation

The possibility that severe early malnutrition may permanently impair mental development is of great importance. In pigs and rats severe underfeeding early in postnatal life leads to a permanent decrease in myelination of nerve cells, and reduced DNA content and other biochemical changes in the brain (Dobbing, 1968, 1969). This may be associated with impaired learning ability and poor performance in tests of behavioural activity.

There are dangers in extrapolating from these results, well established in animals, to man. The time relationship between brain development, birth and weaning differs in babies, piglets and young rats. In studying the processes of learning in man it is inevitably difficult to separate the effects of malnutrition from those of deprivation of parental and other social care.

Growth of the brain
Growth of the human brain has been measured by Dobbing and Sands (1973) by comparison of a large number of normal brains obtained at postmortem from fetuses and young children. Rapid increase of total cell number starts at midgestation and continues past one year of postnatal life; neurones appear during intrauterine life and neuroglial cells multiply later. Myelination is reflected by the cholesterol content of the brain. It starts to increase before birth and continues past the second year of postnatal life. Compared with the rest of the brain the cerebellum has a more rapid growth spurt, which all takes place in the first year after birth.

In 1963 Stoch and Smythe in Cape Town reported that children who had been severely malnourished in the first year of life had at the age of 7 years a smaller head circumference, reflecting reduced brain growth, and a lower IQ than a control group. Rosso *et al.* (1970) found that the brains of children who died in the first year of life weighed less than normal and had proportional reductions of DNA and cholesterol. However, a small brain in a wasted child may be capable of catch-up growth.

Intellectual development
Many observers have reported that children who had survived severe PEM in early childhood performed less well in intelligence tests than controls. However, a poor performance could be due to their growing up in an unfavourable psychological environment rather than to a short period of malnutrition in early life.

The severe famine in Dutch cities from December 1944 to April 1945 (p. 473) affected the nutrition of large numbers of infants during their last months *in utero* and early months after birth. Stein *et al.* (1972) examined cohorts of Dutch males born between March 1943 and February 1946 at the age of 19 years, when they had to register for military service. They found no effect of the famine on either the incidence of mental retardation or the distribution of measurements of the IQ in any cohort.

In a sibling study of Jamaican children Hertzig *et al.* (1972) found that IQs at ages 6 to 10 were lower in children

who had been admitted for malnutrition in their first two years, and these children tended to be withdrawn in their behaviour. There was no difference in the performances of children who had PEM in the first and the second year of life, but those who grew up in the towns did better than children who returned to homes in the country (Waterlow, 1973). In Uganda a follow-up of children admitted to hospital with acute kwashiorkor showed no correlation between the severity of the disease and subsequent intelligence tests, but those admitted with chronic malnutrition scored less well than controls (Hoorweg and Stanfield, 1976). A symposium of the Swedish Nutrition Foundation (Cravioto *et al.*, 1974) and monographs by Winick (1976) and Lloyd-Still (1976) review the whole subject of early malnutrition and mental development.

In the present state of knowledge it is proper to warn governments that failure to provide adequate nutritional services for mothers and young children may well lead to a school population with a diminished capacity for learning. On the other hand, a mother whose child has for any reason suffered a period of severe malnutrition and made a good recovery may be reassured that subsequent mental development is not likely to be impaired seriously, if at all.

PREVENTION
Ignorance and poverty are the two main causes. Education in nutrition is necessary not only for mothers and potential mothers, but for the whole community including doctors and nurses. An excellent manual by Cameron and Hofvander (1976) gives 75 recommended weaning recipes from many developing countries and much practical information. It is obtainable free of charge from the Protein Advisory Group of the UN or from FAO.

PEM affects from under 5 to over 70 per cent of the pre school children in different areas of underdeveloped countries (Bengoa and Donoso, 1974). It has been estimated that 500 million children now alive will suffer from the disease in one form or another during the course of their development. This estimate is without doubt of the right order.

Family planning should be integrated with child health both in the clinic and in the minds of mothers (Morley and Cutting, 1974).

To overcome poverty in rural areas new methods of animal husbandry, the increased use of irrigation and fertilisers and the introduction of improved varieties of seeds for the main crops are needed. Only a social, educational and economic system that provides employment and a fair wage for all sections of the working population can prevent large numbers of children dying from malnutrition. All these factors are discussed in Chapter 56.

30. Endemic Goitre

Julius Caesar was impressed by the enlarged necks of people living in some Alpine regions. In Renaissance paintings the Madonna and court ladies were often painted with necks which suggest moderate enlargement of the thyroid glands. The British anatomist Thomas Wharton, who gave the thyroid gland its name, thought that it served to beautify the neck particularly in women, to whom for this reason a larger gland had been assigned. But Paracelsus in the fifteenth century pointed out that in areas where goitres were large and frequent some of the children were cretins.

The term 'goitre' is used to denote enlargement of the thyroid gland of whatever kind. Simple goitre is said to be present when the gland is visible and palpable, but the subject has no symptoms either of hypothyroidism or hyperthyroidism. It is endemic in many parts of the world and in these areas it is estimated that 200 million people are affected. Such goitres do not usually affect health, but they sometimes result in complications which may have serious consequences (p. 269). There can be no doubt that environmental rather than hereditary factors determine the prevalence of most simple goitres—especially dietary factors, of which iodine deficiency is the major one. A history of iodine and its relation to the thyroid gland is given on page 107.

Two monographs on endemic goitre by the World Health Organisation (1960) and by Stanbury (1969) are recommended.

GEOGRAPHICAL DISTRIBUTION
Endemic goitre occurs chiefly in three types of terrain:
1. In mountainous areas of Europe, Asia, the Americas and Africa, such as the Alps, Himalayas, Andes, Rockies and Cameroon mountains and the Highlands of New Guinea.
2. On alluvial plains that were recently covered by glaciers, such as the area round the Great Lakes of North America and in some areas of New Zealand.
3. In isolated localities where the water in common use is obtained from wells or springs originating in limestone, as in Derbyshire and the Cotswolds in England.

The condition has always been most prevalent in remote rural areas where there is much poverty and sanitation and water supplies are primitive. In many endemic areas in underdeveloped countries goitres and their associated complications are still a major public health problem, but in prosperous communities, although small goitres may still be found in moderate numbers, the severity of the condition is much less than formerly.

It used to be thought that goitre occurred only in areas remote from the sea. It was even suggested that iodine vapour was carried inland by sea breezes to fertilise the neighbouring land. This idea is now discredited. First, the sea itself contains a very low concentration of iodine; secondly, edible plants grown near the sea have been found to contain no more iodine than those grown elsewhere; thirdly, goitre is quite common in some seaboard regions. It is true, however, that seafoods, fish and shellfish, are the richest food sources of iodine; so also is seaweed, from which iodine was first isolated. Carrigeen 'moss' a seaweed still used as food on the west coast of Scotland, may have unsuspected nutritive value in this regard; also in some parts of the Orient seaweed is used as food.

Derbyshire neck found a place in textbooks of medicine in the nineteenth century because goitre was so prevalent in the rural population of the Peak district, who at that time were greatly impoverished. The West Derbyshire Medical Society (1966) found that in a total population of 30 000, simple goitres with symptoms were present in 6.6 per cent of the females and that 2.5 per cent had been treated for thyroid abnormalities, mostly on account of evidence of hyperthyroidism. Endemic goitre is thus still a problem in Derbyshire, though much less than formerly. The decline probably began with the arrival of railways in the valleys, which made the people less dependent on locally grown foods.

The sporadic form of simple goitre may occur in persons born and raised far from areas where goitre is endemic. This can be caused by inherited dyshormonogenesis (Stanbury, 1966), by autoimmune or infective thyroiditis or by goitrogenic substances, or drugs, as well as by a low intake of iodine in a susceptible individual.

AETIOLOGY
The importance of iodine in relation to the thyroid gland is discussed on page 107. The normal thyroid gland contains about 8 mg of iodine. In simple goitre this amount may be reduced to about 1 mg, even though the gland is larger. There can be little doubt that the essential cause of simple goitre is an inability of the thyroid gland to make sufficient thyroxine, which contains 64 per cent of iodine. Simple goitre arises most commonly at those periods in life when

there is a general alteration in hormonal activity in the body, notably during adolescence and pregnancy. In endemic areas if the prevalence is low, only the women have goitres; but if the prevalence is high, the men may be almost equally affected.

Iodine deficiency. Marine in the USA carried out experiments on trout in which the addition of iodine to the water prevented enlargment of the thyroid gland. He was the first to use iodised salt to prevent the appearance of goitre in schoolgirls living in an endemic area. The evidence that he collected (Marine, 1924) focused attention on the iodine intake and proved that endemic goitre is essentially a deficiency disease. In general, the distribution of endemic goitre in the world goes hand in hand with signs of low iodine intake; these are a low iodine in water, low urinary excretion or low plasma concentrations of inorganic iodine. But the correlation is incomplete. Some individuals and some areas have less or more goitre than would be expected from indices of iodine intake. Evidently dietary and other factors can interfere with the availability of iodine for the thyroid gland.

Dirty water. An early advocate of the belief that simple goitre results from multiple causes, including iodine deficiency, was Sir Robert McCarrison. In Gilgit, in the foothills of the Himalayas, there were eight villages in series, each deriving its water supply from the same stream—progressively contaminated with sewage from the village above. The incidence of goitre was highest in the lowest village. But a neighbouring village was entirely free from goitre; this village had an independent water supply from a spring. McCarrison (1908a, b) himself and some army volunteers drank the filtered silt in the polluted water from the goitrous villages. A third of them developed goitre in one to two months, whereas others who drank the silt after it had been boiled failed to do so. McCarrison's investigations suggest that faecal bacteria can produce a goitrogenic substance. The occurrence of goitre in the same valley was reinvestigated over 60 years later by an Anglo-Pakistan team (Chapman et al., 1972). They did not confirm a correlation between goitre and bacterial counts in the water. They suggest that the silt McCarrison drank adsorbed the small amount of iodine in the water. It is still hard to see how the goitres could have appeared in such a short time. McCarrison's publications on goitre have been collected and edited by Sinclair (1953)

Goitrogenic substances in food. In 1928 Chesney and his colleagues (1928) at Johns Hopkins Hospital made the chance observation that rabbits raised in the laboratory for the study of syphilis and fed largely on cabbage developed goitres. This observation was followed up by Sir Charles Hercus and his colleagues in New Zealand. They established the goitrogenic properties of cabbages, turnips and particularly the seeds of cabbage, mustard and rape (Hercus and Purves, 1936).

The identification of natural inhibitors of the thyroid gland opened up a whole new concept of toxic dietary agents in the causation of disease, by contrast with the idea of deficiencies. The best known of several goitrogenic substances in brassica seeds, and in small amounts their leaves and roots, is the glucosinolate progoitrin. This is itself inactive but can be converted to the active goitrin (5-vinyloxazolidine-2-thione) by an enzyme thioglucosidase. This enzyme is destroyed by cooking. It was therefore assumed that brassicas could not be goitrogenic in man unless eaten in large quantities. However, when Greer and Deeney (1959) fed pure progoitrin, goitrin appeared in the plasma and radioiodine uptake by the thyroid gland was depressed. Intestinal bacteria can produce the thioglucosidase. However, it has not been proved that goitres arise in humans from eating brassica plants (van Etten, 1969) though they certainly can in farm and experimental animals. Since the goitrogens occur principally in the seeds and are associated with their characteristic pungent volatile flavours, it is unlikely that mixed human diets would contain sufficient to produce goitres.

Cattle consume much larger amounts of brassica, depending on the forage, and some of the goitrogen passes into the milk. In Tasmania the incidence of goitre among children increased despite the distribution of potassium iodide tablets. At the same time the consumption of milk increased, and 'many-headed kale' was introduced to feed the dairy herds. It was thought that milk from these cows carried with it goitrogens derived from the kale (Clements and Wishart, 1956). However, Vikki et al. (1962) in Finland found that milk from cows fed on large amounts of brassica forage did not affect uptake of radioiodine by the thyroid gland in human subjects; they considered that the dose of goitrogen that could pass into milk was too small to affect man. Clements et al. (1970) reported that attempts to isolate a substance with sufficiently strong goitrogenic properties were unsuccessful.

Several other foods besides *Brassicae*, such as groundnuts, cassava and soya beans, have goitrogenic properties. The active substances in these plants are not glucosinolates.

Goitre continues to be endemic in areas of Sri Lanka (Mahadeva et al., 1968). This may be in part due to a dietary goitrogen, but there is evidence of iodine deficiency in the water in these areas (Deo and Subramanian, 1971).

Simple goitre in non-endemic areas

In all parts of the world, patients can be found with simple goitres. Glasgow for instance is not an endemic area, but many patients are seen with non-toxic goitres, for which there is no obvious cause. Wayne et al. (1964) gave convincing evidence that iodine deficiency was at least a contributory cause of the goitre in these patients. Their estimated dietary intake of iodine was only 60 per cent of the intake of controls and their urinary iodine excretion was only 50 per cent of the control level. Some of the other aetiological factors discussed above may also be operative in individual cases, but there is little doubt that the customary diet of most communities contains iodine in amounts which provide only a small margin of safety and that iodine deficiency, particularly in adolescents and young women, can occur in any locality.

CHEMICAL PATHOLOGY

Iodine is well absorbed from food (Harrison *et al.*, 1965). After absorption about half of it is normally taken up by the thyroid gland and the rest is excreted in the urine. Whereas the kidneys reduce clearance of chlorides when plasma concentration tends to fall, they cannot do this with iodide (Wayne *et al.*, 1964). Adaptation has to take place in the thyroid. If dietary iodine is insufficient, plasma inorganic iodide falls; urinary excretion falls too and may be used to indicate iodine intake. The pituitary responds by increasing the secretion of thyrotrophin (TSH) and plasma TSH concentration is abnormally high in endemic goitre (Delange *et al.*, 1971). This stimulates increased uptake of iodine by the gland and usually leads to enlargement of the gland. In mild cases normal plasma concentrations of thyroid hormones (T_3 and T_4, p.270) are maintained, but the proportion of T_3 to T_4 may be increased. This may be due to an adaptive change with increased synthesis of T_3 (Karmarkar *et al.*, 1974).

PATHOLOGY

The normal thyroid gland is composed of a multitude of follicles filled with eosin-staining colloid. This material consists of thyroglobulin, an iodine-containing protein, from which the normal hormonal secretions of the gland are derived. Each follicle is surrounded by a layer of cells which synthesise the hormones.

Simple goitre. The enlargement of the gland is due to both overgrowth (hyperplasia) of the cells lining the follicles and to an excess of colloid. The hyperplasia and accumulation of colloid in the iodine-deficient gland can perhaps be compared with the overgrowth of osteoblasts and accumulation of osteoid tissue that take place as a result of lack of calcium at the growing points of the bones in rickets.

Colloid goitre. Simple goitres that have been present for years may become very large, due to a massive accumulation of colloid in thin-walled follicles, and interfere with breathing. However, goitres which appear superficially to be small may cause serious respiratory embarrassment and other pressure effects by retrosternal growth. To most people a prominent goitre is unsightly, but in certain areas of Africa where the condition is endemic such tumours are considered a sign of beauty.

Nodular goitre. In long-standing cases of simple goitre another change sometimes takes place: the development of nodules which are localised areas of cellular proliferation within the gland. Similar nodules sometimes occur—perhaps for other reasons—in people who have never lived in a goitre area. Hyperthyroidism and malignant changes occur in rare instances in patients with nodular goitre.

CLINICAL SIGNS

The thyroid is the only endocrine organ apart from the testes that is readily accessible to clinical examination. The normal gland in an adult weighs 20 to 25 g. A very large goitre is obvious to everyone; recognition of small goitres is also simple and reproducible between observers. Difficulty arises in grading the size of goitres that lie between the just detectable and the very large. In field studies goitres may be graded on the classification of Stanbury *et al.* (1974).

Grade O a	Thyroid not palpable or if palpable not larger than normal.
Grade O b	Thyroid distinctly palpable but usually not visible with the head in a normal or raised position; considered to be definitely larger than normal, i.e. at least as large as the distal phalanx of the subject's thumb.
Grade I	Thyroid easily palpable and visible with the head in either a normal or a raised position. The presence of a discrete nodule qualifies for inclusion in this grade.
Grade II	Thyroid easily visible with the head in a normal position.
Grade III	Goitre visible at a distance.
Grade IV	Monstrous goitres.

Observer variation is considerable and can make comparisons of grades meaningless, e.g. in a group of people before and after prophylactic iodine. In Derbyshire one family doctor recorded three small goitres and 78 of medium size and his neighbour 14 small ones and 12 of medium size (West Derbyshire Medical Society, 1966). Anyone planning a goitre survey needs to take steps to minimise the observer error. It is preferable to have two examiners. Some workers mark the outline of the thyroid on the skin (Fig. 30.1). Others have practised with plasticine models of the gland in a range of sizes (MacLennan *et al.*, 1969). Before going into the field it is recommended that examiners have some training sessions with a specialist in thyroid diseases.

CLINICAL EFFECTS AND COMPLICATIONS

In the great majority of cases of simple goitre there are no clinical manifestations due to hypofunction or hyperfunction of the thyroid gland. Simple colloid goitre may require surgical treatment either for aesthetic reasons or because of pressure effects on the adjacent structures. The following complications occur rarely: (1) hypothyroidism, (2) hyperthyroidism, (3) cretinism, and (4) deaf-mutism. Such complications are more likely to be encountered in regions where endemic goitre is prevalent. These undesirable

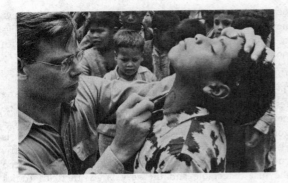

Fig. 30.1 A goitre survey in Guatemala.

clinical effects and complications can be greatly reduced by the appropriate prophylactic measures described below. Figure 30.2 shows grades I and II goitres in Egyptian children.

TREATMENT

A simple goitre in a non-endemic area rarely requires treatment. The patient may be assured that no harm is likely to arise and that in time it will probably get smaller. If this does not occur and the goitre becomes disfiguring, iodine therapy is seldom effective, but thyroxine 0.2 to 0.3 mg/day may be given. This inhibits production of TSH by the pituitary gland and so reduces the size of the thyroid gland. If there is no response to thyroxine and the goitre continues to be disfiguring, thyroidectomy should be considered, and this is indicated if the size of the goitre leads to obstruction of the trachea or if there is retrosternal extension.

Endemic cretinism

In places where endemic goitre is severe, cretinism may

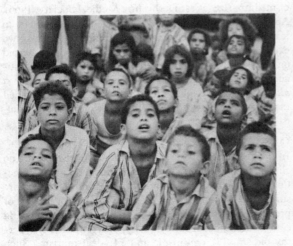

Fig. 30.2 Endemic goitre in children at an oasis in Egypt. (By courtesy of Dr I. Abdou.)

affect as many as 1 to 5 per cent of the population (Bengoa, 1973). This occurs in a few isolated areas in Nepal, the Andes, Zaire and New Guinea. Endemic cretinism presents in two types. In **nervous cretinism** there is mental deficiency, deaf mutism, spasticity and ataxia but features of hypothyroidism are hard to find. In **myxoedematous cretinism** there are dwarfism, signs of myxoedema and no goitre. The nervous type predominates in New Guinea (Pharoah et al., 1971) and some parts of the Andes (Fierro-Benitez et al., 1974), while the myxoedematous type is seen in Zaire. Pharoah et al. (1971) were able to prevent nervous cretinism by giving a single injection of iodised poppy-seed oil to the women of childbearing age but it must be given before pregnancy starts. It thus appears that iodine is required for the early development of the nervous system before the fetal thyroid appears in the third month of gestation. In myxoedematous cretins the nervous system develops normally in the critical early months but the thyroid gland fails to adapt adequately by hypertrophy to severe iodine deficiency. The thyroid glands are small and uptake of radioiodine very low. Consequently such cretins have low plasma T_3 and T_4 with clinical signs of hypothyroidism, including dwarfism (Dumont et al., 1969). Both types of cretinism are seen in endemic areas but the proportion of the two varies from region to region.

PREVENTION

There is no new evidence to alter the view expressed by the Study Group on Endemic Goitre of WHO (1953) that 'when iodine prophylaxis has been introduced and efficiently carried out, endemic goitre is practically abolished'. Iodisation of table salt greatly reduced the prevalence of goitre in many countries, including the USA, Switzerland, Yugoslavia, New Zealand and countries in South America. In the USA iodised salt must contain 76 µg of iodine/g salt and daily consumption of salt by most people is between 2 and 6 g. Lower levels of iodisation are used in most other countries but have been effective. Salt is not iodised in the UK. On account of its stability potassium iodate is preferable to potassium iodide for the iodisation of the crude moist salt consumed in many countries.

In Tasmania potassium iodate was added at 2 parts per million (dry weight) to all the bread made in the island from 1966. The prevalence of goitre declined in schoolchildren and urinary iodide increased. Clements et al. (1970) estimated that an average daily consumption of 180 g bread provided 195 µg of iodine, or rather more than the recommended daily allowance. However, the number of patients with hyperthyroidism seen at Launceston Hospital increased and reached a peak in 1967 (Stewart et al., 1971). There was an unusually high proportion of cases in elderly men. The Tasmanian experience is the first clear demonstration of a temporary wave of hyperthyroidism following iodine prophylaxis, though it has been suspected previously in a few other places. Stewart et al. (1971)

regard it as an acceptable price to pay for eradication of endemic goitre

Unfortunately, the above measures are seldom feasible in those parts of the world where endemic goitre is most severe and accompanied by cretinism. These are isolated communities with few if any roads and no large markets. The mountainous regions of Bolivia and Ecuador, many parts of Nepal and the highlands of New Guinea are examples. There a vicious circle exists. Goitres are not merely a cosmetic problem, but impair the vitality of many of the people by causing hypothyroidism, and cretinism retards the intellectual development of children. The people are unable to do much to help themselves to break out of their bondage to iodine deficiency and the poverty that goes with it. It is for such communities that iodised oil injections offer promise as a medical measure to be applied to vulnerable groups, e.g. young adult women. In the mountainous regions of New Guinea, a single injection of iodised poppy-seed oil has been shown by Buttfield *et al.* (1965) to correct the deficiency for a period of two to three years. It also produced significant regression of goitre in a high proportion of cases within three months of the injection. A similar conclusion has been drawn by Stanbury (1970).

31. Xerophthalmia

Xerophthalmia (Greek *xeros*, dry; *ophthalmos*, eye) is a condition caused by vitamin A deficiency. In its mild form it is confined to the conjunctiva and this is very common in many countries. As long as the condition is confined to the conjunctiva there is no disability, but it is a clear warning of the probability of vitamin A deficiency. When it spreads to the cornea there is danger of corneal ulceration and a permanent defect in vision. In severe cases there is softening of the cornea, keratomalacia, which, if not immediately treated, soon leads to permanent blindness. Keratomalacia is frequently associated in young children with protein-energy malnutrition. When this occurs, the mortality is high even with the best treatment.

For fuller accounts of all aspects of xerophthalmia a report by WHO (1976) and a monograph by McLaren (1963, 1980) are recommended.

HISTORY

Night blindness and its cure by liver, rich in vitamin A, was mentioned in Egyptian and Chinese writings going back to 1500 BC. It was well known to Greek and Roman physicians. European mediaeval literature has many accounts of the condition.

Keratomalacia was described many times in the nineteenth century by physicians and ophthalmologists, as occurring in children in the industrial slums of Europe. The first account of the condition in the tropics is a description in 1866 of an outbreak in the children of Negro slaves on a coffee plantation in Brazil.

The outbreak of xerophthalmia in Denmark from 1916 to 1920 is instructive. Some 700 children were affected and over 400 had keratomalacia despite the fact that Denmark had many large dairy herds, and ample supplies of vitamin A should have been available. However, in the early years of World War I most of the butter was exported to Germany where it fetched a high price. Consequently the price of butter and whole milk rose in Denmark. The poor could only obtain separated milk and vegetable margarine (at that time not enriched with vitamins). Oatmeal gruel and vegetable broth from barley were the main items of the diet of many poor children. In 1918 rationing of butter was introduced and a weekly allowance of 0.25 kg of butter/head abolished the disease. When rationing was lifted prematurely, prices again rose and the disease returned (Bloch, 1921, 1924a, b). Xerophthalmia was prevalent in Singapore after World War II, associated with the widespread use of dried and condensed milk containing little or no vitamin A (Williamson and Leong, 1949).

The World Health Organisation now gives priority in its action programmes to the treatment and prevention of xerophthalmia, along with protein-energy malnutrition, nutritional anaemias and endemic goitre.

EPIDEMIOLOGY

A global survey, sponsored by WHO, was carried out by Oomen *et al.* (1964) and information is given in a further report (WHO, 1976). In Asia xerophthalmia is a major problem in Indonesia, Bangladesh, southern India, parts of the Philippines and Thailand, and in Sri Lanka, Afghanistan and Nepal. It has disappeared from Hong Kong, Singapore, Japan and apparently from the People's Republic of China. Occasional cases are seen in poor communities throughout the Middle East. In Latin America xerophthalmia occurs in north-east Brazil and in Haiti. Low plasma vitamin A concentrations are common in Central America, but a survey in the small country of El Salvador showed very few cases of xerophthalmia.

In Africa seasonal night blindness and some xerophthalmia is reported from Upper Volta and other parts of the Sahel. Xerophthalmia was thought to be uncommon in Africa, but it has been reported from East and Southern Africa and Nigeria.

Keratomalacia is closely associated with PEM. The peak age, when blindness is most likely to occur, is between 2 and 5 years, when kwashiorkor is so common. but cases can occur in the first year of life in association with marasmus.

Blindness is not a notifiable condition and it is difficult to know the incidence of keratomalacia but it is estimated that up to 250000 young children become permanently blind every year from this cause. Figure 31.1 shows one of these tragedies.

The disease is almost unknown in Europe today. Occasional cases have arisen in the United States in unfortunate children reputedly allergic to cow's milk, who were fed on various artificial milk substitutes from which vitamin A had been omitted by oversight.

AETIOLOGY

Xerophthalmia arises when the diet contains practically no whole milk and butter and very limited amounts of fresh vegetables and fruit and so lacks both retinol and carotenes. Xerophthalmia and keratomalacia both occur in the first year of life amongst artificially fed infants but are rare

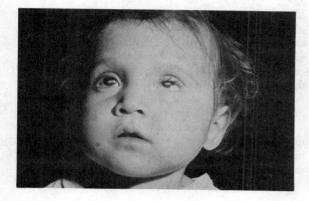

Fig. 31.1 Child blinded in infancy by keratomalacia. (By courtesy of Dr D.S. McLaren.)

amongst the breast fed. Children in poorly nourished communities are born to mothers who have had small intakes of vitamin A and consequently their liver stores are small at birth. Protein-energy malnutrition further aggravates the partial deficiency because absorption and plasma transport of vitamin A are impaired.

PATHOLOGY

When vitamin A deficiency is produced in experimental animals the epithelial cells of the cornea undergo the squamous metaplasia characteristic of vitamin A deficiency (p. 119). There have been no reports of the histopathology of the condition in man for many years. This is probably due to the difficulty in getting permission for autopsies in those countries where xerophthalmia is common.

CLINICAL FORMS

Five clinical manifestations of vitamin A deficiency and three associated conditions are described by WHO (1976) and these have been given code numbers to assist reporting (Table 31.1).

Conjunctival xerosis

The bulbar conjunctiva is dry, thickened, wrinkled and pigmented (Fig. 31.2). The first three signs are due to a failure to shed the epithelial cells, and consequent keratini-

Table 31.1 Forms of xerophthalmia and associated conditions

Code	
X1A	Conjunctival xerosis
X1B	Conjunctival xerosis with Bitôt's spots
X2	Corneal xerosis
X3A	Corneal xerosis with ulceration
X3B	Keratomalacia
XN	Night blindness
Xf	Xerophthalmia fundus
XS	Corneal scars

sation. The pigmentation gives the conjunctiva a peculiar 'smoky' appearance. The pigment is diffuse and especially marked in the interpalpebral fissure. Dryness, thickening and pigmentation, characteristic of the condition, are also caused by long periods of exposure to glare, dust and infections. It is extremely common in older children and adults in the tropics, in whom it often has no nutritional significance, or only reflects a past deficiency of vitamin A. In children under 5 years it is more likely to be due to a dietary deficiency.

Bitôt's spots are commonly associated with conjunctival xerosis, but are also found in children and adults in whom there is no evidence of vitamin A deficiency. They are described on page 305.

Corneal xerosis

When dryness spreads to the cornea, this takes on a dull, hazy, lacklustre appearance. This is due to the keratinisation which is the result of vitamin A deficiency on all epithelial surfaces. The cornea often becomes insensitive to touch with a wisp of cotton wool. Slit-lamp examination may show cellular infiltration of the cornea, which intensifies the haziness and may have a bluish, milky appearance; it is usually most marked in the lower central portion.

Corneal ulceration may occur from many causes and be unrelated to vitamin A deficiency. The characteristic feature is a loss of substance (erosion) of a part or the whole of the corneal thickness. Unless there is secondary infection, there are no signs of inflammation. The lesion only heals by scarring.

Corneal xerosis may progress suddenly and rapidly to keratomalacia.

Keratomalacia

Softening and dissolution of the cornea follow and are known to ophthalmologists as colliquative necrosis. This presents a grave emergency. When the process involves only part of the cornea, there is ulceration but the inflam-

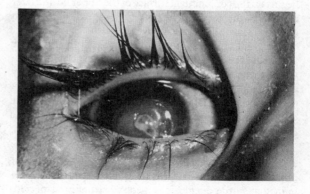

Fig. 31.2 Keratomalacia in a child from Jordan. (By courtesy of Dr D.S. McLaren.)

matory reaction is mild. Effective treatment at this stage is followed by corneal scarring and opacity. If the process is not stopped by treatment, perforation of the cornea leads to prolapse of the iris, extrusion of the lens and infection of the whole eyeball which almost invariably occurs (Fig. 31.2). The chances of saving any useful vision are slight. Healing results in scarring of the whole eye and frequently in total blindness.

The retinol content of the plasma is below 100 μg/l, the lower limit of the range (p. 120). Reserves of retinol are exhausted and none may be detectable in the liver at autopsy.

Night blindness
The role of retinol in night vision has been described on page 119. Night blindness is an early symptom of vitamin A deficiency and is often present without any signs of xerophthalmia. The symptom is also caused by several other conditions and is discussed on page 305.

Xerophthalmia fundus
In schoolchildren or young adults with prolonged vitamin A deficiency ophthalmoscopic examination may show lesions appearing as spots, either white or yellow, scattered along the sides of the blood vessels. The spots may fuse and the lesions are most numerous on the periphery of the fundus and never appear on the macula.

Corneal scars
These are white, opaque patches on the cornea and the result of healing of an older ulcer. Vision may be seriously affected, depending on the size of the scars. There are other possible causes of corneal scars but, in an area where vitamin A deficiency is known to have existed, their prevalence is an indication of its severity.

DIAGNOSIS
Keratomalacia must be distinguished from other diseases causing corneal lesions such as exposure, trauma, bacterial infections, measles and trachoma. Trachoma usually begins on the conjunctival surface of the upper lid and later extends to the cornea. The opacity (pannus) comes down like a window blind from above.

The child often has some other illness at the time, like gastroenteritis, kwashiorkor, measles or respiratory infection, which can distract attention from the eyes unless they are examined. Measles may precipitate or aggravate xerophthalmia in a malnourished child. If in doubt about the eyes of a malnourished child, it can do no harm to give a course of treatment with vitamin A.

TREATMENT
The administration of vitamin A in a dose of 30 mg of retinol (100 000 i.u.) daily for three days should be started immediately the diagnosis is made or strongly suspected. It is recommended that half the dose should be given orally in the form of halibut oil or other oil solution and half

intramuscularly as water-miscible retinol palmitate. An oil solution should not be injected as the retinol is then absorbed very slowly from the injection site. The practice of instilling cod-liver oil directly into the eye is not recommended. During convalescence 9 mg of retinol in the form of a fish liver oil orally is adequate. It is also essential to ensure that the diet is satisfactory in regard to other nutrients.

For the prevention and treatment of secondary bacterial infection, antibiotics are of great value. Local treatment of the eye will only be required if disorganisation is already present, in which case the services of an ophthalmic surgeon should be obtained.

PREVENTION
Medical students in Britain cannot learn to recognise xerophthalmia with confidence by the traditional clinical method of being shown a patient, because the last case reported was in 1938. However, doctors planning to work in underdeveloped areas and medical students in countries where xerophthalmia occurs must be trained to recognise it. The Nutrition Section of the Royal Tropical Institute, Amsterdam in the Netherlands, has made two sets of colour slides of xerophthalmia for this purpose, which they have offered to supply at moderate cost. Colour photographs, 'Know the signs and symptoms of xerophthalmia', are obtainable free by health workers who write to American Foundation for Overseas Blind, 22 West 17th Street, New York, N.Y. 10011, USA.

Training the doctors is only the start of prevention because most cases occur in the urban poor and rural peasants in under-doctored areas, and keratomalacia develops without the children being seen by a doctor. Therefore to extend prevention, nurses, midwives, and other paramedical staff associated with maternal and child health clinics, must be actively involved.

First, pregnant women should be advised to eat dark green leafy vegetables and if possible given nutritional supplements rich in vitamin A in prophylactic doses. This helps to build up stores of retinol in the fetal liver and should be continued during lactations. Secondly, mothers should be advised to include in the weaning foods dark green leafy vegetables or yellow and orange fruits, which are locally available, cheap and known to be good sources of β-carotene. Bangladesh issued two postages stamps in 1976 which show an eye and foods to prevent xerophthalmia, with the caption: 'Foresight prevents blindness.'

Where blindness from keratomalacia is a major public health problem single large prophylactic doses of 60 mg (200 000 i.u.) of retinol in oily solution are recommended for all children. This has to be repeated every six months. Large-scale trials of this procedure started in 1970 and are now going on in India, Bangladesh, Indonesia, the Philippines and El Salvador with varying degrees of success. The dose is safe and adverse effects are rare. The main difficulty and expense is in obtaining and training personnel, and operational costs may be high. Where possible, existing health staff should be used. Any prophylactic programme should be evaluated by periodic field surveys of the prevalence of xerophthalmia.

In Guatemala a different approach is being tried: fortification of table sugar with water-miscible vitamin A. Preliminary studies by INCAP have shown that this is technically feasible. In the Philippines fortification of monosodium glutamate with vitamin A is being tested because MSG is consumed by the whole population, including children.

A newsletter, the Xerophthalmia Club Bulletin, has been started, to keep those working to prevent xerophthalmia in touch with what is being done in other countries. The bulletin's secretary is Mrs A. Pirie, Nuffield Laboratory of Ophthalmology, Oxford, England.

Blindness

Nutritional disorders of the eye are only one of several causes of blindness. There are probably more than 10 million blind people in the world. That most of these became blind before the age of 5 and that probably in two-thirds of the cases the blindness is preventable makes the situation the more tragic. We feel that a far more energetic attack on the problem should be made, especially in the underdeveloped countries. In India there are over two million blind people: in Bangladesh, Vietnam and Indonesia there are very large numbers; in parts of East Africa 90 per cent of the population have eye disease. Throughout much of Latin America eye diseases and blindness are widespread.

Causes of blindness common in some parts of the world are as follows. Trachoma, a virus infection, is still the most important eye disease in the world. The countries around the Mediterranean Sea are severely affected. It is common in children and, if untreated, often causes progressive loss of vision and blindness. Smallpox often affected the eyes and was reputed to be responsible for one-fifth of the blindness in India. Onchocercosis is caused by a small nematode which is transferred from man to man by flies. It causes nodules in the skin and in the conjunctiva which leads to blindness. The disease commonly affects people in Central America and in Central Africa who live beside rivers. In some villages, all the adult population are blind. Venereal diseases, congenital syphilis and gonococcal ophthalmia neonatorum are important causes of blindness in parts of the world where the maternity services are inadequate or totally lacking. Accidents in the home and at work are common causes of blindness. Many young children lose their sight in this way. Diabetes, cataract and glaucoma are important causes of blindness in elderly people.

Vitamin A deficiency is thus one of seven important causes of blindness and the most easily preventable. A former Director-General of WHO has stated: 'If one-tenth of the money we now spend to support unnecessary blindness was spent to prevent it, society would gain in terms of cold economy, not to mention considerations of the happiness of humanity.'

32. Rickets and Osteomalacia

Rickets, a word derived from the Anglo-Saxon *wrikken* to twist, is a disease of children in which the bones are softened and deformed. It arises as a result of deficiency of vitamin D and a failure to absorb calcium from the small intestine.

Osteomalacia, which means softening of bone, arises when there is vitamin D deficiency in adults. The resultant calcium deficiency leads to demineralisation of the bones.

RICKETS

HISTORY

Although rickets was described in ancient times, it was not well known until the seventeenth century. The first clinical description in Britain was that of Daniel Whistler, an Oxford man who wrote his D.M. thesis on rickets in 1645. This was followed in 1650 by the better known description of Glisson, a Cambridge graduate and physician in London. Contemporary writers described the thick pall of smoke that began to overcast London in the seventeenth century. Industrial smoke and high tenement buildings together shut out the sunlight and, as industrial cities grew, so rickets spread. Sunlight provides the ultraviolet rays which facilitate the synthesis of vitamin D in the skin. Although rickets may occur in children living in the country, it is never widespread unless local custom confines them indoors. Prior to 1900, in many of the great industrial cities of the world, up to 75 per cent of the children of the poorer classes were affected. Rickets came to be known as 'a disease of poverty and darkness'. Glasgow, Vienna and Lahore each acquired an unenviable reputation as homes of the disease. In Lahore, as in many other eastern cities, the purdah system confined women and children in narrow courtyards where the sun seldom penetrated. Milk (providing calcium) and cream, butter and eggs, the only common foods providing vitamin D were too expensive for poor urban families. Wealthier families, on the other hand, could enjoy these foods and usually also had access to gardens in which the children benefited from sunlight. The diet of poor families consisted predominantly of cereals and the inhibitory effect of phytic acid in the cereals on the absorption of calcium was possibly rachitogenic (p. 94).

The discovery of vitamin D in 1918 did not immediately resolve the confusion that existed about the aetiology of rickets. Lack of sunshine and lack of vitamin D each had their supporters. Chick and her colleagues (1923) in Vienna after World War I established the importance of both of these factors and explained for the first time the pathogenesis of the disease. Dame Harriette Chick (1976) after her hundreth birthday recalled this work for the British Nutrition Foundation. Her paper presents the chemical, clinical and sociological aspects of her story. It is a masterpiece which all nutritionists will enjoy reading.

Between the two world wars the incidence of rickets declined. This was due to the increasing use of cod-liver oil as a supplement for children and also increased exposure to sunshine due to slum clearances and the reduction in industrial and domestic smoke. Also, sunbathing became fashionable at this time.

EPIDEMIOLOGY

It has been known for over 50 years that rickets can be prevented either by administering cod-liver oil, and now medicinal preparations of vitamin D, or by adequate exposure to sunlight. As one or other of these is readily available in most countries, it might be thought that rickets would have been eradicated as effectively as we have diphtheria, poliomyelitis and smallpox. Yet the disease continues to occur in significant numbers in a number of countries, rich and poor alike. Whereas a child may be protected against many infectious diseases by immunisation procedures, carried out by the medical services on a few isolated occasions, his protection against rickets depends on continuing care and attention from his mother. The epidemiology of rickets is mainly, but not entirely, the epidemiology of maternal ignorance and so a measure of the failure of health education.

In Britain

Severe cases with gross bony deformities are occasionally seen in large children's hospitals but are uncommon. Mild cases in young children are probably numerous in large industrial cities, but not in the country and the outer suburbs of towns. Many cases probably go unrecognised because their doctors are not familiar with the early forms of the disease. Furthermore, both biochemical and radiological evidence of the disease is often equivocal and it may be difficult to decide whether a child has rickets or hypovitaminosis D (see below). The prevalence of rickets has been most studied in Glasgow (Arneil, 1975; Goel *et al.*, 1976), where it is probably highest. From five to ten cases of florid rickets are seen at the main children's hospital each year, but survey indicates that up to 7 per cent of children aged 1 to 3 years have 'minimal' rickets. To what extent this affects their health is uncertain. The great majority reach school age without any deformity of bone. The prevalence of rickets in Birmingham, Manchester and other big industrial cities is probably only a little less than in Glasgow.

Children whose parents come from India and Pakistan are the most liable to develop rickets in Britain. This cannot be entirely due to their skin pigment since West Indian children, usually of Negro origin and more heavily pigmented, are much less frequently affected and perhaps no more often than white children. In one survey the mean daily dietary intake of vitamin D by Asian, West Indian and European children was estimated to be 1.5, 1.8 and 1.6 µg respectively (Ruck, 1973). In London Asian women at the time of delivery had a mean plasma concentration of 25-hydroxycholecholesterol of 7.6 µg/l whereas the corresponding figure for European women was 18.3 (Dent and Gupta, 1975). Hindus have lower vitamin D status than other subgroups of British Asians (Hunt *et al.*, 1976)

Subclinical vitamin D deficiency. There are in Britain a number of children, possibly as many as 25 per cent, whose dietary intake of vitamin D is less than 2.5 µg (100 i.u.) daily which is far below the recommended intake of 10 µg. About 10 per cent of these have a plasma alkaline phosphatase of 250 King-Armstrong units/litre or higher, and these usually fall when vitamin D is given. Plasma 25-hydroxycholecalciferol is usually below 5 µg/l (12 nmol/l). These children do not have clinical rickets and on radiographs their bones usually appear normal, though in some the radiological findings are equivocal. Such children may be said to have hypovitaminosis D and hence are in danger of developing clinical rickets if their supplies of the vitamin remain inadequate while growth continues.

In other countries

Our information is that although sporadic cases of rickets occur, it is no longer an important public health problem in Europe, North, South and Central America, Australia and New Zealand, Hong Kong, the Philippines and Malaysia. However, even in a wealthy country such as Canada Dr Scriver writes that rickets occurs not infrequently in poor families, especially French-Canadians in Montreal and those of Italian origin in Toronto. The children of such families are not provided customarily with a supplement of vitamin D in any form.

Rickets has for long been prevalent in Muslim countries where women and young children have been confined in dark rooms and in high-walled courtyards and are not exposed to the sun. The disease is not uncommon in Pakistan, Egypt and northern Nigeria. We have no information about its incidence in Indian cities. Severe classical rickets is seen commonly in the children's hospital in Addis Ababa (Marian and Sterky, 1973).

With its abundant sunshine South Africa should be free from rickets yet many cases can be seen in infants below the age of 1 year. The dietary intake of bottle-fed infants is inadequate because of the low content of vitamin D in cow's milk and because of failure of parents to provide a supplement, either in the form of cod-liver oil or as calciferol-fortified dried milk powder. In addition, mothers, in order to prevent their children acquiring a dark complexion, wrap them in swaddling clothes and keep them out of the sunlight. Increasing numbers of mothers go out to work and leave their infants indoors at home.

In Kenya, Uganda and Tanzania there is abundant sunshine to which the children are exposed at an early age, and rickets is stated to be very rare. We have also been informed that rickets is a rare disease in Rhodesia and Malawi and this is probably true if one is looking for the clinical features as encountered in Britain in children between the ages of 1 and 3 years. However, Professor Hansen of Johannesburg, who has visited these countries, informs us that he has seen cases of rickets in infants under 10 months of age.

ANTICONVULSANT DRUGS

There have been numerous reports of rickets and osteomalacia arising in children and adults who are under long-term treatment for epilepsy with phenobarbitone, phenytoin, and other drugs. These drugs induce changes in liver microsomal enzymes which lead to conversion of cholecalciferol to inactive metabolites (Stamp *et al.*, 1972). Requirements of such patients for the vitamin are raised. It is important to ensure that preventive measures (p. 280) against deficiency are adequate.

MORBID ANATOMY

The morbid histological changes in the bones in active human rickets are essentially the same as those in experimental animals as described on page 123.

CHEMICAL PATHOLOGY

Failure to absorb calcium causes the plasma calcium to fall from its normal value of about 2.5 mmol/l. It may fall as low as 1.3 mmol/l or even less, which usually causes tetany (see below). More commonly the plasma inorganic phosphorus falls from the normal value of over 1.3 mmol/l in childhood to 1.0 mmol/l. This may be due to the activity of the parathyroid glands which respond to a slight reduction in plasma calcium by increasing the excretion of phosphorus in the urine, with consequent fall in inorganic phosphorus in the blood. In mild cases calcium and phosphorus concentrations in the plasma are usually within normal limits. A more constant change is an increase in plasma alkaline phosphatase. This enzyme is formed by the large number of osteoblasts which accumulate in the osteoid tissue at the growing points of the bones. These cells, unable to make bone without a sufficient supply of calcium, probably liberate into the circulation the excess of enzyme which they cannot use. Alkaline phosphatase in plasma is measured in King-Armstrong units; the normal value in the first three years of life is from 120 to 250 units/l. However, higher values are occasionally found in children receiving supplements of vitamin D and with no radiographic or clinical evidence of rickets (Stephen and Stephenson, 1971). In early mild cases of rickets 300 to 400 units/l are frequently found, but there is not necessarily an increase as the disease progresses.

CLINICAL FEATURES
The infant with rickets has often received sufficient dietary energy and may appear well nourished. Indeed it used to be a commonplace that the fat, flabby child, 'crammed with distressful bread', which won the prize at the local baby show by virtue of being so much heavier than its competitors, was usually rachitic. But the child is restless, fretful and pale, with flabby and toneless muscles which allow the limbs to assume unnatural postures ('acrobatic rickets'). Excessive sweating of the head is common. The abdomen is distended as a result of the weak abdominal muscles, the atony of the intestinal musculature and the intestinal fermentation that may arise from excessive carbohydrates in the diet. Gastrointestinal upsets with diarrhoea are common. The infant or child is prone to respiratory infections. Development is delayed so that the teeth often erupt late and there is failure to sit up, stand, crawl and walk at the normal ages.

The bony changes are the most characteristic and easily identifiable signs of rickets. There is extension and widening of the epiphyses at the growing points, where cartilage meets bone. The earliest bony lesion is often craniotabes—small round unossified areas in the membranous bones of the skull, yielding to the pressure of the finger, with a crackling feeling, like parchment. Another early sign is enlargement of the epiphyses at the lower end of the radius and at the costochondral junctions of the ribs, the latter producing the clinical sign known as 'beading' of the ribs or 'rickety rosary'. Craniotabes is now rarely seen in British children as rickets usually develops when the child is between 1½ and 3 years of age. In contrast, in countries, where the disease occurs within six months of birth, both craniotabes and the rickety rosary are early and important diagnostic features. Later features seen in British children with rickets are 'bossing' of the frontal and parietal bones and delayed closure of the anterior fontanelle. Later too, there may be deformities of the chest such as undue prominence of the sternum ('pigeon chest') and a transverse depression, passing outwards from the costal cartilages towards the axillae which deepens with inspiration. This was very familiar to us in our student days as Harrison's sulcus. It was apparently caused by the sucking in of the softened ribs on inspiration during whooping cough, or other respiratory infections to which rachitic children are prone. Even today in unusually severe cases, respiratory function can be seriously impaired by the combination of respiratory infection and a rachitic chest. Twenty such cases with acute heart failure, aged 1 to 2 years, are described from Ethiopia by Marian and Sterky (1973).

If rickets continues into the second and third year of life, these signs may persist or be magnified. Deformities such as kyphosis of the spine develop as a result of the new gravitational and muscular strains, caused by sitting up and crawling. At the same time there may be enlargement of the lower ends of the femur, tibia and fibula. When the rachitic child begins to walk, deformities of the shafts of the leg bones develop, so that 'knock knees' or 'bow legs' are added to the clinical picture. Anterolateral bowing of the tibiae at the junction of the middle and lower thirds is frequently noted in young children with rickets (Fig. 32.1). The spinal kyphosis is often replaced by lordosis. Pelvic deformities may follow and lead years later to serious difficulties at childbirth.

When ionised calcium in the plasma is reduced, infantile tetany may result, with spasm of the hands and feet and of the vocal cords. The latter causes a high-pitched, distressing cry and great difficulty in breathing. In bygone days—when florid rickets was common—tetany was sometimes associated with alarming general convulsions.

DIAGNOSIS
In a fully developed case this is easy. But in countries where the disease is now rare and medical students and family doctors are no longer familiar with it, there is an increasing likelihood that mild cases will be missed. A flabby baby towards the end of its first year, unable to pull itself up, fretful and easily irritated, with too few teeth showing and liable to profuse sweats, should always be suspected of rickets. The diagnosis may be supported by the dietary history. Early evidence of rickets may be overlooked in a child ill with bronchopneumonia or diarrhoea and this is particularly true in a country where the disease usually develops during the first year of life. If there is any doubt or suspicion, a radiograph of the wrist may show characteristic changes at the epiphyses; the outline of the joint is blurred and hazy, and the epiphyseal line becomes broadened. Later, in older children, as a result of decalcification of the metaphysis and the effects of movements and stresses the classical concave 'saucer' deformity is clearly shown radiographically. The opinion of an experienced radiologist may be needed to distinguish the picture from that of infantile scurvy. The diagnosis is supported by a raised plasma alkaline phosphatase, and confirmed if no 25-hydroxycholecalciferol can be detected in the plasma.

It is sometimes necessary to distinguish rickets from other rare disorders involving the bones, such as congenital syphilis, achondroplasia and osteogenesis imperfecta.

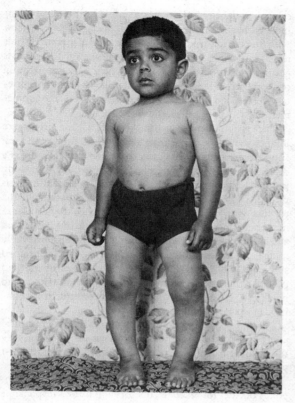

Fig. 32.1 Rickets in a child from the Asian community in Glasgow. Note the marked bowing of the tibiae. (By courtesy of Dr M.G. Dunnigan.)

Radiographs of the bones are helpful in differentiating these disorders.

TREATMENT

The two essentials are adequate doses of vitamin D and an ample intake of calcium. The therapeutic dose of vitamin D varies from 25 to 125 μg (1000 to 5000 i.u.)/day, depending on the severity of the disease. For comparison the prophylactic dose is 10 μg/day or less. Children can be given halibut-liver oil in a very small dose (1 ml) since it contains 30 to 40 times the concentration of vitamin D of cod-liver oil. Many proprietary preparations are available which contain standard amounts of vitamins A and D dispensed as capsules or palatable syrups. For severe cases needing 125 μg/day, synthetic calciferol is useful. One millilitre of the B.P. solution contains about 75 μg of vitamin D.

In times of social upheaval, such as may be occasioned by war, floods or pestilence, when an infant or young child may be seen once by an emergency medical service and perhaps not again for months, a single massive dose of vitamin D, e.g. 3.75 mg (150 000 i.u.) (three strong calciferol tablets, B.P.), can be given by mouth with reasonable safety and curative effects. The single dose can be given by intramuscular injection, but this has no proved advantage over the oral route. A daily small dose is recommended for normal practice because of the danger of overdosage.

The best source of calcium is milk and a young child with rickets should drink at least 500 ml/day. For a severe case a supplement of calcium lactate should also be given orally. The diet after weaning can include with advantage an egg daily and butter or margarine fortified with vitamin D.

Vitamin D and diet are not the whole solution to the treatment of rickets. An attempt should be made to improve the hygienic environment of the child. This often requires the tactful education of the mother in feeding practices and general care. Unnecessary clothing should be removed and the child allowed out as much as possible to enjoy the sunshine. This is particularly important in countries where supplements of vitamin D are not provided.

The earliest evidence of healing in rickets comes from radiographs of the growing ends of the bones. Concentrations of calcium and phosphorus in the plasma provide an inconstant and unreliable guide. A decrease in the plasma alkaline phosphatase does not usually occur for several weeks after adequate treatment is initiated; the therapeutic dose of vitamin D should be continued so long as the phosphatase level remains elevated; thereafter it may gradually be reduced to the prophylactic dose of 10 μg daily.

Occasionally cases of rickets are encountered that are resistant to ordinary therapeutic doses of vitamin D. The disease persists into late childhood ('late rickets') or even adult life, producing the clinical appearance of osteomalacia, unless adequately treated. The cause of this resistance is not always understood, although in many cases it is due to a defect in the reabsorption of phosphate by the renal tubules, e.g. the Fanconi syndrome. Classification of the different types is discussed by Dent (1969). A similar state may sometimes arise as a conditioned deficiency resulting from malabsorption or renal failure. Whatever the cause, treatment consists in giving large doses of vitamin D by mouth in the form of calciferol, together with calcium salts, e.g. calcium lactate in pill or powder form, 5 g three times daily, or 2 tablets of calcium gluconate effervescent B.P.C. three times daily. The initial dose of calciferol may be 3.75 mg (3 B.P. tablets) daily or even more, but it should be reduced at the first suspicion of toxic symptoms (p. 124).

PROGNOSIS

Rickets is not a fatal disease *per se,* but the untreated rachitic child is a weakling with an increased risk of infections, notably bronchopneumonia. The skeletal changes usually tend to heal spontaneously as the child gets older. The bony deformities, if mild, usually right themselves as growth proceeds, but in severe cases pigeon chest, contracted pelvis, knock knees or bow legs may persist. With early and sufficient treatment these changes are entirely avoided.

PREVENTION

As most children probably obtain the greater part of their supply of vitamin D by synthesis in the skin, adequate exposure to sunlight is important. Slum clearances, the provision of open-air playgrounds and smoke abatement schemes are taking place in most big cities and their value in the prevention of rickets must not be underestimated. In addition mothers should be educated in the need to keep their infants out in the sunshine as much as possible. Nevertheless, for reasons already discussed and particularly in northern countries, the supply of the vitamin from this source is uncertain and attention must be paid to the dietary supply.

It cannot be too strongly emphasised that none of the common foods, including milk, in a child's diet is a good source of the vitamin. In Britain, despite fortification of infant milks and other foods with vitamin D, as already described, many infants and young children consume amounts of the vitamin far below the recommended intake of 10 μg (400 i.u.) daily. We would not recommend fortification at a higher level of the foods already fortified because of the risk of hypercalcaemia which is a much more serious disorder than rickets. Of unfortified foods, liquid milk is a main article of the diet of children and both human and cows' milk contain only a small amount of the vitamin. This could be raised by (1) feeding dairy cows concentrates of the vitamin, (2) irradiating the milk with ultraviolet light and (3) the addition of this vitamin to milk, as is often done in North America, or to chapattis for Asian families in Britain. Each of these possibilities merits consideration in the future, but each presents technical and administrative difficulties, not least expense.

Many children whose dietary intake of the vitamin is inadequate require a supplement. Cod-liver oil is of proven value. The prophylactic dose is one teaspoonful (about 4 ml) which contains not less than 9 μg (360 i.u.) of vitamin D. Infants and young children take it readily, though older children may find it distasteful. Many mothers object to the smell and it is difficult to prevent some of it being spilt on the child's clothing. For this reason some mothers refuse to give it to their children. Preparations of vitamin D also containing vitamin A and C are available.

Cod-liver oil and other fish liver oils contain vitamin A as well as vitamin D and medicinal preparations of vitamin D should also contain vitamin A. This is especially important in countries where protein-energy malnutrition is prevalent, because this is not infrequently accompanied by xerophthalmia and keratomalacia.

Rickets can be prevented by giving a child a single massive dose of vitamin D. The vitamin is stored in the liver and liberated for use as required. As this procedure carries a slight risk of hypervitaminosis, it is not recommended for use under normal conditions.

Before deciding on a prophylactic dose of vitamin D, it is necessary to consider how much of the vitamin the infant is getting from other sources. Thus if he is being brought up on a preparation of fortified dried milk (or given a proprietary cereal food fortified by the manufacturers) the supplement of cod-liver oil should be reduced.

The prophylactic dose of vitamin D for premature infants should be twice that for full-term infants and the supplement should be started soon after birth. There is a divergence of view among paediatricians about how long prophylactic administration of vitamin D should be continued. Obviously the social and economic status of the parents and the climate in which the family lives are matters of importance. It seems reasonable to suggest that at least in temperate climates with limited sunshine a daily intake of about 10 μg (400 i.u.) should be continued summer and winter for the first five years of life and possibly beyond this during the winter in groups known to be at risk. It is probably advisable to continue it indefinitely in epileptic children on anticonvulsant drugs.

A supplement of vitamin D is also essential in tropical and semitropical countries, if mothers insist on keeping their children wrapped up and out of the sun in the first year of life.

All forms of prevention depend on education of mothers. A booklet for teachers, doctors and nurses responsible for health education has been prepared (Darke and Stephen, 1976).

OSTEOMALACIA

AETIOLOGY

Osteomalacia is the adult counterpart of rickets. In its fully developed form, which affects especially women of childbearing age who become depleted of calcium by repeated pregnancies, it may cause great deformity and suffering. Formerly this was seen commonly in China, northern India and Pakistan and in Middle East countries. The main factors responsible include the purdah system and a cold winter, keeping women indoors and out of the sun, and a very poor diet with little or no milk, providing no vitamin D and often low in calcium. Wilson (1929) has given a good account of the disease in Kashmiri women, in whom all these factors were operative.

In Europe in the nineteenth century and early years of this century, many women who developed rickets in infancy continued to be deficient in vitamin D throughout childhood, adolescence and adult life. In consequence progressive deformities of the pelvis developed and these led to great obstetric difficulties. There was a severe outbreak in Vienna, when in the winter of 1918–19 after the war, food supplies were greatly restricted. Both old and young were affected and their condition is described by Dalyell and Chick (1921).

Table 32.1 The differential diagnosis of osteomalacia and osteoporosis

	Osteomalacia	Osteoporosis
Clinical features		
Skeletal pain	A major complaint usually persistent	Episodic and usually associated with a fracture
Muscle weakness	Usually present and producing disability and, when severe, a characteristic gait	Absent
Fractures	Relatively uncommon; healing delayed	The usual presenting feature; heals normally
Skeletal deformity	Common, especially kyphosis	Only occurs where there is a fracture
Radiographic features		
Loss of density of bone	Widespread	Irregular and often most marked in the spine
Loss of bone detail	Characteristic	Not a feature
Looser's zones	Diagnostic	Absent
Biopsy		
Histological changes	Excess osteoid tissue with bone present in normal quantity	Bone reduced in quantity but fully mineralised
Biochemical changes		
Plasma Ca and P	Often low	Normal
Plasma alkaline phosphatase	Often high	Normal
Urinary calcium	Often low	Normal or high
Response to treatment		
Vitamin D	Dramatic	None

PRESENT POSITION

Osteomalacia is still an important disease in north India (Mathew *et al.*, 1975) and the biochemical abnormalities are common in Pakistan (Rab and Baseer, 1976), although the clinical disease is not often seen. The disease is not uncommon in old women in Scotland (Anderson *et al.*, 1966; Chalmers *et al.*, 1967) and probably in many northern countries where the winter sunlight is insufficient to allow sufficient synthesis of vitamin D to make good dietary deficiency. This particularly applies to old people who cannot go out easily owing to physical incapacity. It is probable that in some patients with severe senile osteoporosis the symptoms and disabilities are in part due to co-existent osteomalacia. In England, Aaron *et al.* (1974) examined iliac-crest biopsy specimens in 102 women and 35 men over 50 years of age with fractures of the femur: 34 per cent of the women showed histological features of oesteomalacia and 34 per cent showed severe osteoporosis including 10 per cent with osteomalacia as well. This has important consequences since osteomalacia, unlike senile osteoporosis, is readily treated and prevented. The present position is uncertain because, although severe osteomalacia is not likely to be overlooked, mild forms associated with osteoporosis are not easy to diagnose and may be overlooked, especially by doctors working in areas where the disease is considered rare.

Occasional cases of osteomalacia in younger women have been reported from several of the large industrial cities in Britain. Most of them have been in Indian and Pakistani women (Ford *et al.*, 1972; Holmes *et al.*, 1972). The condition may present during pregnancy.

Osteomalacia is a common consequence of chronic diseases of the digestive system which cause steatorrhoea, and so prevent absorption of the fat-soluble vitamin D. It also occurs in rare forms of chronic renal disease in which urinary losses of calcium are excessive.

PATHOLOGY

The changes in the blood are essentially the same as those in rickets. The progressive decalcification of the bones leads to the replacement of bony substance with soft osteoid tissue. This process goes on all over the skeleton, but the effects are greatest in the spine, ribs, shoulder girdle, pelvis and lower limbs. As already discussed, a combination of osteomalacia and osteoporosis is not uncommon.

CLINICAL FEATURES

Pain is usually present and ranges from a dull ache to severe pain. Sites frequently affected are the ribs, sacrum, lower lumbar vertebrae, pelvis and legs. Bone tenderness on pressure is common. Muscular weakness is often present and the patient may find difficulty in climbing stairs or getting out of a chair. A waddling gait is not unusual. Tetany may be manifested by carpopedal spasm and facial twitching. Spontaneous fractures may occur, independent of the pseudofractures described below.

RADIOGRAPHIC FEATURES

There is rarefaction of bone and commonly translucent bands (pseudofractures, Looser's zones), often symmetrical, at points submitted to compression stress. Common sites are the ribs, the axillary borders of the scapula, the pubic rami and the medial cortex of the upper femur. Looser's zones are diagnostic of osteomalacia.

DIAGNOSIS

The early symptoms may resemble those present in osteoporosis and rheumatic disorders. Table 32.1 lists the distinctions from osteoporosis. In mild cases these may not be clear. Then the presence or absence of response to treatment with vitamin D should clinch the diagnosis.

TREATMENT

This is essentially the same as for rickets when osteomalacia is primarily due to a defective intake of vitamin D, namely 25 to 125 μg (1000 to 5000 i.u.) daily. If there is evidence of malabsorption the dose should be up to 1.25 mg (50 000 i.u.) daily and it may have to be given intramuscularly at weekly or monthly intervals. If the disease is secondary to renal disorders double this dose may be required or more.

Maintenance treatment with vitamin D is required for all cases of osteomalacia in which the cause cannot be removed. In addition a good diet should be given which includes milk, eggs, fortified margarine or butter. This may be difficult or impossible under the conditions in which the disease arises in the East. In all cases of osteomalacia a supplement of calcium should be given orally, e.g. calcium lactate 1 to 2 g/day. Within four to eight weeks of starting treatment the pain and weakness have usually disappeared. The decision to reduce or discontinue the dose of vitamin D and calcium is based on the improvement in the clinical features and the disappearance of biochemical and radiological abnormalities. The dangers of vitamin D intoxication should be kept in mind.

PREVENTION

Once major deformities are established they cannot be corrected by diet or drugs but only by an orthopaedic surgeon. Hence the great importance of early and correct diagnosis and proper treatment. Free access to sunshine and an adequate intake of dairy produce, with a vitamin D supplement when necessary prevents nutritional osteomalacia. It is important for old people to get out of doors and exposed to sunlight. When for any reason they cannot do this regularly, they should take a vitamin D supplement daily.

33. Beriberi and the Wernicke-Korsakoff Syndrome

Beriberi is a nutritional disorder formerly widespread in the rice-eating people of the East. The etymology of the word 'beriberi' is obscure; it probably comes from a word in a Malay dialect, *beri,* meaning weak. The epidemiology, chemical pathology and response to therapy all suggest that its main features are due to deficiency of thiamin, although other factors in a poor diet contribute. Three forms of the disease occur: (1) wet beriberi, characterised by oedema often associated with high-output cardiac failure, (2) dry beriberi, a polyneuropathy, and (3) the infantile form. Characteristically beriberi has occurred in outbreaks or epidemics in a community, whose members are all eating similar diets based on the same type of rice.

Thiamin deficiency is also an aetiological factor in three conditions which are not uncommon in chronic alcoholics and occurs in all parts of the world. These are (i) alcoholic polyneuropathy clinically indistinguishable from dry beriberi, (ii) a thiamin-responsive cardiomyopathy, and (iii) an encephalopathy, the Wernicke–Korsakoff syndrome.

Classical oriental beriberi is first described and then thiamin deficiency as it presents in non-rice eaters.

ORIENTAL BERIBERI

HISTORY AND AETIOLOGY

A Japanese naval surgeon, Takaki (1885, 1906), was the first to demonstrate that beriberi is essentially a nutritional disease arising when the proportion of polished rice in the diet is excessive. After studying the disease for a number of years he persuaded the Japanese authorities in 1883 and 1884 to replace a part of the rice in the ration by wheaten bread and to increase the allowance of vegetables and milk.

Table 33.1 Beriberi in the Japanese Navy

Year	Force	Cases of beriberi	Deaths from beriberi
1878	4528	1485	32
1879	5081	1978	57
1880	4956	1725	27
1881	4641	1163	30
1882	4769	1929	51
1883	5346	1236	40
1884	5638	718	8
1885	6918	41	0
1886	8475	3	0
1887	9106	0	0

Table 33.2 Observations on patients in Kuala Lumpur asylum (Fletcher, 1907)

Diet	Number of patients	Cases of beriberi	Deaths
East ward: mainly raw polished rice	124	34	18
West ward: mainly par-boiled rice	123	2	0

There was a striking reduction in the incidence and mortality of the disease as shown in Table 33.1. Takaki himself attributed this improvement to an increase in protein intake.

Further observations in the Far East also showed that beriberi was associated with the consumption of rice that had been highly polished in the raw state and that it could be prevented either by adding other foods, as Takaki had done, or by substituting parboiled rice for raw-milled rice. The observations made by Fletcher (1907) in the asylum at Kuala Lumpur (Malaya) shown in Table 33.2 illustrate this.

Beriberi was also endemic in the Philippine Scouts: in 1909 there were 618 cases. Then 20 oz of polished rice in their rations was changed to 16 oz of unpolished rice and 1.6 oz of dried beans (Vedder, 1913). In 1911 there were only three cases of beriberi and in 1913 none. Numerous other reports have described the spectacular reduction of beriberi in China, Japan, the Philippines, Thailand, Malaysia, Singapore, Indonesia and Burma amongst people living on diets composed chiefly of highly milled rice. In India, beriberi was an important endemic disease only in the coastal region between Madras City and Vishakhapatnam where rice is usually raw-milled. In all other parts of India, Pakistan and Sri Lanka rice is usually parboiled before milling and this conserves the vitamin B complex (p. 173) and so prevents beriberi.

Although beriberi is usually associated with a rice diet, this is not invariably the case. The disease may occur in groups consuming excessive amounts of highly milled wheat. A striking example of this was found in the fishermen of Newfoundland and Labrador (Aykroyd, 1930). These men and their families were often cut off through the long winter from all sources of fresh provisions. When their winter stores consisted mainly of large quantities of refined wheat flour, beriberi used to be common. Another example of the disease afflicting wheat-eaters occurred in 1916 when the Third Indian Division was besieged by the Turks at Kut-el-Amara (Hehir, 1922). During the siege the Indian sepoys ate whole-wheat chapattis and did not develop beriberi. The British troops ate white bread made from refined wheat flour and beriberi broke out among them.

The present position

Beriberi is much less common in South-East Asia than formerly. The disease has virtually disappeared from prosperous Asian countries such as Japan, Taiwan and Malaysia, as well as in the big cities such as Hong Kong, Singapore, Manila, Bangkok, Rangoon and Jakarta and their surrounding countryside.

The position is not so clear in the remote country areas. Here accurate information is difficult to obtain. Infants and young children who are ailing from any cause but without fever, are sometimes reported to have beriberi but the diagnosis has seldom been made by a doctor. It is common in some remote villages in Thailand but is seldom seen in hospitals. Eating raw fermented fish, which contains thiaminase, and chewing fermented tea leaves both reduce the availability of the small amount of thiamin in the diet (Tanphaichitr et al., 1970; Tanpaichitr, 1976). There may well be areas where it is still endemic.

There are several factors which may be responsible for the virtual disappearance of beriberi from many places and its marked decline in others. These are discussed on page 286.

CHEMICAL PATHOLOGY

In wet beriberi a specific biochemical lesion arises as a result of the dietary deficiency of thiamin. Carbohydrates are incompletely metabolised because thiamin pyrophosphate (TPP) is an essential coenzyme for the decarboxylation of pyruvate to acetyl CoA, which is the bridge between anaerobic glycolysis and the citric acid cycle. TPP is also the coenzyme for transketolase in the hexose monophosphate pathway and for decarboxylation of 2-oxoglutarate to succinate in the citric acid cycle. Consequently pyruvic acid and lactic acid accumulate in the tissues and body fluids. Platt and Lu (1936) found elevated concentrations of blood pyruvate in patients with wet beriberi. The local accumulation of these metabolites dilates peripheral blood vessels especially in the muscles, as in normal subjects during exercises. In beriberi this vasodilation may be extreme and so lead to capillary leakage. To maintain the circulation the cardiac output is increased. This adds a burden on the heart muscle which is already impaired through lack of thiamin. As the disease progresses the heart dilates and congestive heart failure accentuates the oedema. This is an example of 'high output' failure. Sudden death may result from myocardial failure.

The best method of detecting thiamin deficiency in the tissues is by measurement of transketolase activity in the erythrocytes (Tanphaichitr et al., 1976) (p. 137).

In chronic dry beriberi the blood pyruvate is usually within normal limits.

MORBID ANATOMY

In wet beriberi the heart at autopsy is greatly dilated; there is general oedema of the tissues and serous effusions into the body cavities, often most marked in the pericardium. Microscopic examination usually shows loss of striation of myocardial fibres, which are also finely vacuolated and often fragmented.

In dry beriberi there is severe wasting of muscle. In long-standing cases there is degeneration of peripheral nerves, both sensory and motor, with extensive demyelination and destruction of the axons. The vagus and other autonomic nerves may be affected. Degenerative changes both in the tracts and in grey matter of the cord may be found.

CLINICAL FEATURES

The early symptoms and signs are common to wet and dry beriberi. The onset is usually insidious, though sometimes precipitated by unwonted exertion or a minor febrile illness. At first there is anorexia and ill-defined malaise, associated with heaviness and weakness of the legs. This may cause some difficulty in walking. There may be a little oedema of the legs or face and the patient may complain of precordial pain and palpitations. The pulse is usually full and moderately increased in rate. There may be tenderness of the calf muscles on pressure and complaints of 'pins and needles' and numbness in the legs. The tendon jerks are usually sluggish, but occasionally slightly exaggerated. Anaesthesia of the skin, especially over the tibiae, is common. Such a condition may persist for months or even years with only minor alterations in the symptoms. In areas where beriberi is endemic it is often extremely common. Patients are only mildly incapacitated and may continue to earn their living even as manual labourers, but at a low level of efficiency. At any time this chronic malady may develop into either of the severe forms.

Wet beriberi

Oedema is the most notable feature and may develop rapidly to involve not only the legs but also the face, trunk and serous cavities. Palpitations are marked and there may be breathlessness. Anorexia and dyspepsia are commonly present. There may be pain in the legs after walking, similar to the pain that results from ischaemia in muscle. The calf muscles are frequently tense, slightly swollen and tender on pressure.

The neck veins become distended and show visible pulsations. The apex beat of the heart is displaced outwards. In the arteries there is often a lowered diastolic pressure and a proportionally higher systolic pressure. In consequence, on auscultation over the femoral and other large arteries, a curious 'pistol shot' sound may be heard. The pulse is generally fast and bounding as in aortic regurgitation. Walters (1953) described an outbreak of beriberi amongst pearl divers in Kuwait in which the most striking clinical feature was high blood pressure. Systolic pressures up to 200 mmHg were recorded. If the circulation is well maintained, the skin is warm to the touch owing to the associated vasodilation. When the heart begins to fail the skin becomes cold and cyanotic, particularly on the face. Electrocardiograms often show no changes but in some cases there are low voltages of the QRS complex, inverted T waves or evidence of disturbed conduction. The volume of the urine is diminished, but there is no albuminuria. The mind is usually clear. The patient is in danger of sudden increase in the oedema, acute circulatory failure, extreme dyspnoea and death.

Dry beriberi

The essential feature is a polyneuropathy. The early symptoms and signs are described above. The muscles become progressively more wasted and weak, and walking becomes increasingly difficult. The thin, even emaciated patient needs at first one stick, then two, and may finally become bedridden. The disease is essentially a chronic malady, which may be arrested at any stage by improving the diet. Bedridden patients and those with severe cachexia are very susceptible to infections. When bacillary dysentery or tuberculosis accompanies dry beriberi, a fatal result may rapidly occur unless prompt and efficient treatment is given.

The older accounts of beriberi record that cerebral manifestations are uncommon. However, amongst the British prisoners of war in Japanese camps, where beriberi was endemic, there were many cases of Wernicke's encephalopathy (p. 288).

Infantile beriberi

This occurs in breast-fed infants, usually between the second and fifth months. The mothers may have no clinical signs of beriberi although they must have been eating a diet and secreting milk with a low thiamin content. However, frank beriberi can develop in late pregnancy and the puerperium. The clinical features in infants differ somewhat from the adult disease. It exists in an acute and chronic form. In the former cardiac failure may develop abruptly; the mother may have noticed that the infant is restless, cries a lot, is passing less urine than normal and shows signs of puffiness. The infant then may suddenly become cyanosed with dyspnoea and tachycardia and die within 24 to 48 hours. Other serious signs are convulsions and coma. One characteristic sign, usually encountered only in severe cases, is partial or complete aphonia; the infant's cry becomes thin with a plaintive whine. In the few cases in which it has been measured, the TPP effect in the transketolase test has been high (Pongpanich *et al.*, 1974).

In the chronic form, which is much less common, the main symptoms are due to gastrointestinal disturbances. There is obstinate constipation and vomiting, repeated irregularly throughout the day and unrelated to meals. The child is fretful and sleeps poorly. The muscles are soft and toneless, but not markedly wasted. There is often intense pallor of the skin with cyanosis round the mouth. Cardiac failure and sudden death are common.

Infantile beriberi has been the chief cause of death between the ages of 2 and 5 months in rice-eating rural areas, and may still be an important cause in some. The diagnosis of the disease in public health practice and the difficulties in prevention are discussed by Aykroyd (1957). Postmus (1958) has described the problem in Burma. Thanangkul and Whitaker (1966) report 45 cases seen in a hospital in northern Thailand.

DIFFERENTIAL DIAGNOSIS

A large number of diseases may closely resemble the various forms of beriberi. In endemic areas the diagnosis is usually not difficult. Outside these areas it is unwise to make the diagnosis unless there is a history of a poor diet based on polished rice or other refined cereal or of alcoholism and poor food intake (see below).

In mild and chronic cases there may be few or no physical signs and the diagnosis may have to depend on the interpretation of symptoms and the dietary history, often inaccurately described. In prisons and labour forces, such patients may be accused of malingering. The symptoms also closely resemble the manifestations of anxiety states common amongst Europeans.

The oedema of wet beriberi has to be distinguished from that associated with hepatic and renal disease and heart failure. The warm extremities in cardiac beriberi and the absence of protein in the urine are useful diagnostic points. Famine oedema should seldom be a diagnostic difficulty if a proper dietary history is taken. In the past there has been much confusion with epidemic dropsy (p. 222).

Cardiovascular beriberi has to be distinguished from other causes of high output cardiac failure, notably hyperthyroidism and severe anaemia.

In all doubtful cases of wet beriberi the therapeutic response to thiamin usually settles the diagnosis.

The features of dry beriberi are sometimes indistinguishable on clinical examination from other forms of polyneuropathy (p. 287). The diagnosis is based mainly on the dietary history, and the absence of other aetiological factors. In endemic areas the disease may be confused with neuritic leprosy, but this is characterised by palpable, cord-like superficial nerves and areas of skin anaesthesia. These two diseases not infrequently occur together and when they do, dry beriberi, if mild, may be overlooked.

The diagnosis of infantile beriberi may be difficult. Neither oedema nor paralysis is an early sign and sudden death may occur before either is present. In cases of doubt the presence of minimal signs or symptoms of beriberi in the mother may decide the issue. A history of the sudden death of a previous child between the ages of 2 and 5 months is suggestive. In public health practice among a rice-eating community a rise in death-rate of infants of this age group should suggest the possibility that infantile beriberi has become endemic. Infantile beriberi may be confused with PEM and the two may occur together.

Laboratory confirmation of the diagnosis of beriberi is by RBC transketolase and TPP effect (p. 137). The test requires a sample of fresh heparinised whole blood, which must be taken before thiamin treatment is started.

TREATMENT

Wet beriberi. Treatment must be started as soon as the diagnosis is made, because fatal heart failure may be sudden. Complete rest is essential and thiamin should be given at once, intramuscularly, 25 mg twice daily for three days. Thereafter an oral dose of 10 mg two or three times a day should be continued until convalescence is established. Smaller amounts would probably be adequate. Many prisoners of war in Malaya during World War II responded excellently to a daily dose of 5 mg allotted from the short supply.

The prompt response of a patient with cardiovascular beriberi to thiamin is one of the most dramatic events of medicine. Within a few hours the breathing is easier, the pulse-rate slower, the extremities cooler and a rapid diuresis begins to dispose of the oedema. Within a few days the size of the heart is restored to normal. Muscular pain and tenderness are also dramatically improved. The ECG may show characteristic paradoxical changes while the patient improves. In a typical case the tracing is normal while heart failure is severe, then as recovery starts T-wave inversions appear in some precordial leads for a few days.

During convalescence and rehabilitation a good mixed diet with less emphasis on rice is needed. Another cereal should, if possible, be substituted for part of the rice in the diet. Pulses have a well-deserved reputation for curing and preventing beriberi, e.g. 120 g (4 oz) of beans or lentils.

Dry beriberi. Thiamin should be given in the same doses as for wet beriberi in order to refill the depleted tissue stores of the vitamin. However, no spectacular improvement is likely to follow as with other nutritional neuropathies. Patients are generally undernourished and, if they take sufficient of a good mixed diet to enable them to gain weight, slow improvement may be expected. Provided the dietary intake is adequate, there is no need to continue with supplementary thiamin. Infections and intercurrent disease should be treated and appropriate physiotherapy given.

Infantile beriberi. The simplest way to treat infantile beriberi is via the mother's milk. The mother should receive 10 mg thiamin twice daily—in severe cases this should be by injection. In addition the infant should be given thiamin in doses of up to 10 to 20 mg intramuscularly once a day for three days. This should be followed by 5 to 10 mg orally twice a day. With severe heart failure or convulsions and coma the initial dose may be increased to 25 to 50 mg given intravenously very slowly.

PREVENTION

Beriberi can be prevented by the use of undermilled, home pounded or parboiled rice, by the fortification of rice with thiamin or by increased use of pulses and other foods containing thiamin. Medicinal preparations of thiamin are also available and cheap.

It is difficult to say which of these factors has been responsible for the widespread decline in the disease. Changed milling practices are probably the most important and in many areas rice is not so highly polished as to remove all the bran. There are government regulations controlling milling in several countries, but these are largely ineffective owing to the difficulty of enforcing them. There is a move to replace the steel rollers in mills with ones made of rubber or other soft material, which prevents a high degree of polishing, but this is likely to be resisted by the millers.

There is no evidence of an increased use of home pounded or parboiled rice. Indeed the increasing number of small village mills has reduced home pounding. Such mills are potentially dangerous as they can produce a highly polished product and since the millers usually retain the bran as commission and sell it for cattle food, they have an incentive to produce an overmilled polished rice.

Fortified rice is available in Japan; it is supplied to the armed forces in Taiwan, but not to the civilian population. In the Philippines the only manufacturer of fortified rice has gone out of business. In Papua/New Guinea, there is a law that only fortified white rice may be imported, but this may not be enforced. In northern Thailand a trial programme of rice enrichment is in progress. In other countries there is no programme of fortification.

Improvement in social and economic conditions and the consequent consumption of a better diet with more thiamin-containing foods has certainly occurred in Japan, Taiwan and Malaysia, and in the larger cities, where beriberi was formerly common.

Medicinal thiamin is more widely used owing to the extension of medical services. The establishment of Maternal and Child Health Centres has led to many pregnant and lactating women getting good advice on diet as well as vitamin supplements; infants may also receive them or extracts of rice bran (in the Philippines).

The reasons for the decline of beriberi remain obscure. Clearly no single preventive measure has been applied effectively over a wide area. In most rice-eating countries, levels of thiamin intake appear to provide little margin of safety. There is no cause for complacency among public health authorities and efforts to increase thiamin intake by the measures described above should be pursued energetically.

THIAMIN DEFICIENCY IN THOSE WHOSE STAPLE DIET IS NOT RICE

Although outbreaks of beriberi have occurred in groups with highly milled wheat flour as their staple food (p. 286), this is most unusual. Thiamin deficiency in countries where rice is not the staple food arises in the great majority of cases in persons whose diet has been greatly restricted usually as a result of chronic alcoholism. It also arises, but rarely, secondary to carcinoma of the stomach, severe and recurrent vomiting in pregnancy and treatment of obesity by prolonged starvation. Hence there is always a lack of other essential nutrients and this together with the effects of the primary disease affects the clinical picture, which is seldom as clear-cut as in oriental beriberi.

It is important to realise, both in the pathogenesis and the management of these syndromes of thiamin deficiency, that intravenous infusions of dextrose can precipitate or aggravate the condition unless thiamin is given as well.

Alcoholic neuropathy
Alcoholics who have restricted their food intake for many weeks often develop a disorder of peripheral nerves sometimes indistinguishable from dry beriberi. In the days when the US Navy was supplied with liberal amounts of spirits, alcoholic neuritis was often diagnosed in ratings, but not in officers, who suffered from beriberi. This social distinction was not supported by any differences in the clinical and laboratory findings. Strauss (1935) showed conclusively that alcohol was not the direct cause of the nerve lesions. These may improve on dietary therapy without altering the intake of ethanol. Biochemical tests on the blood when the patient is seen do not necessarily reflect the nutritional state of the peripheral nerves when the condition was developing.

Treatment is as for dry beriberi. The administration of thiamin leads to no dramatic improvement, but if the patient takes a good diet and gives up alcohol completely a slow diminution of the symptoms may be expected.

Polyneuropathy
Dry beriberi and alcoholic neuropathy are often clinically indistinguishable from other types of neuropathy, in which more than one nerve is involved. The lesions are symmetrical and the nerves of the lower limbs are affected more severely than those in the upper limbs. Usually there is dysfunction of both sensory and motor fibres. The effects on sensory nerves may be paraesthesiae (pins and needles) or sometimes severe nerve pains, as in the burning feet syndrome; there may be loss of sensation, either numbness of the extremities or loss of position sense. Signs of motor nerve involvement are foot drop, muscle wasting and impaired knee and ankle jerks.

The causes of polyneuropathy are as follows.

1. Deficiency diseases—beriberi (p. 286), pellagra (p. 291), subacute combined degeneration (p. 300), burning feet syndrome (p. 299), alcoholic neuropathy and pyridoxine deficiency (p. 148).
2. Metabolic diseases—diabetes mellitus (p. 360), uraemia, porphyria, etc.
3. Chemical poisoning—many heavy metals (lead, arsenic and mercury), tri-o-cresylphosphate, which has caused outbreaks from contamination of edible oil, and some drugs, e.g. large doses of isoniazid (over 300 mg/day) for the treatment of tuberculosis, may cause neuropathy, probably because of excessive urinary losses of pyridoxine.
4. Infective—Guillain–Barré syndrome, diphtheria, leprosy, etc.
5. In association with carcinoma.
6. Rare genetic types include Refsum's disease (p. 326).

Occidental beriberi heart disease
Cardiac failure may set in rapidly over a few days, usually in a patient who has been taking large amounts of alcohol but very little food for several weeks. Cardiac symptoms predominate, with peripheral oedema in some patients. Others present with dyspnoea and pulmonary congestion. On examination the heart is enlarged and there are usually signs of a high cardiac output, with warm skin and a bounding pulse. Haemodynamic studies with cardiac catheterisation, arm plethysmography and kidney function tests are reported by Blacket and Palmer (1960). The electrocardiogram is usually normal before treatment, thus differing from other forms of cardiomyopathy, and T-wave inversions appear as the patient is improving clinically (Schrire, 1966). Patients respond rapidly to 50 to 100 mg thiamin intramuscularly but sometimes diuretics or digoxin are required as well at first. Provided the right diagnosis is made and the patient does not succumb in the acute illness there is usually no residual cardiac disease.

Less commonly the cardiac failure is sudden and the patient is very distressed, with signs of a low cardiac output and cold extremities. The fulminating form is called **shoshin beriberi**, following the original Japanese descriptions. In Japanese *sho* means acute damage and *shin* means heart. Majoor (1978) reports cases from Holland and shows how lactic acid acidosis contributes to the severity of shoshin. Cases of the usual form and of shoshin beriberi have been reported from England (McIntyre and Stanley, 1971) and the USA (Jeffrey and Abelmann, 1971).

WERNICKE-KORSAKOFF SYNDROME

Wernicke in 1881 described a neurological disorder occurring in three patients, two of them alcoholics and the third a seamstress who had persistent vomiting after ingestion of sulphuric acid. It is characterised by weakness of eye muscles (ophthalmoplegia), so that the patient cannot look upwards or sideways, and a state of disorientation and apathy. Sometimes there are jerky, rhythmical movements of the eyes (nystagmus) and if the patient can stand he is unsteady (ataxia). The mortality was very high until thiamin became available, when it was found that many of the cases recovered dramatically after large doses.

Korsakoff in 1887 described a psychosis, also occurring in alcoholics, characterised by a severe defect in memory and learning, but with other thought processes relatively little affected. Confabulation is a characteristic feature, though not always present. The patient can remember past events with verifiable accuracy. He cannot remember what he did earlier in the same day but tends to provide a superficially convincing tale rather than say he has forgotten.

As a result of studying 245 patients in Boston, Victor et al., (1971) concluded that Wernicke's disease and Korsakoff's psychosis are manifestations of the same pathological process and attributable to thiamin deficiency. They were able to carry out postmortems on 82 cases. There were symmetrical lesions in various parts of the brain stem, diencephalon and cerebellum, the areas commonly affected being the mamillary bodies, the nuclei of the thalamus and the periaqueductal grey matter. In the most advanced lesions there was virtually complete tissue necrosis; the less severe lesions were characterised by destruction of myelin with less damage to neurones. Small haemorrhages are characteristic but not always present.

The same histological features were seen in cases of Wernicke's disease and of Korsakoff's psychosis. Most of the patients who recovered from the acute confusional state subsequently developed some memory defect; patients with Korsakoff's psychosis had nearly always had some ocular and ataxic signs. It is postulated that Korsakoff's psychosis develops later in a patient who has recovered from Wernicke's encephalopathy. As Victor et al. put it, 'The response of the Korsakoff's psychosis to thiamin is slow and in almost 80 per cent of cases is incomplete. This does not necessarily mean that the pathogenesis of the memory defect is different from that of the ophthalmoplegia and ataxia but may simply reflect the fact that the structural changes in the diencephalon which are responsible for the memory defect are more severe (and less reversible) than those in the ocular and vestibular nuclei and the cerebellum.'

To be effective thiamin therapy has to be given early in the disease and in the same large doses as for wet beriberi. Early diagnosis is therefore essential. The clinical features usually suggest the syndrome but, because of its rarity in many communities, it may easily be overlooked. Confirmation may be obtained by showing a quick response of the ophthalmoplegia and disorientation to thiamin therapy or demonstrating thiamin deficiency by the RBC transketolase test (p. 137). The TPP effect is very high in Wernicke's encephalopathy (Truswell et al., 1972) but in suspected cases thiamin should be given as soon as blood has been taken, without waiting for the result.

Although the syndrome usually occurs in alcoholics, it may arise, as already mentioned, secondary to any disorder which seriously impairs nutrition. It is perhaps the human counterpart of the severe brain disturbances that occur in pigeons fed on polished rice. It is strange that the syndrome is not described by early writers in the Orient; there is no mention of it in the classical monograph on beriberi by Vedder (1913). However, De Wardener and Lennox (1947) describe 52 cases in Europeans on rice diets in prison camps in Singapore, where outbreaks of beriberi were occurring.

COMMENT

Thiamin deficiency can thus lead to Wernicke's encephalopathy or to beriberi cardiomyopathy or to peripheral neuropathy. Two, or rarely all three, diseases can occur together in a patient but it is surprising how often they do not. We cannot yet explain why the brain is affected in one person, the heart in another and the peripheral nerves in a third. Possibly the cardiomyopathy occurs in people who use their muscles for heavy work and so accumulate large amounts of pyruvate, producing intense vasodilation in the muscles and increasing cardiac work, while encephalopathy is the first manifestation in less active people. Because alcoholism is widespread and body stores of thiamin in alcoholics are likely to be small, all doctors should be aware of thiamin deficiency. It is treatable if not left too late.

34. Pellagra

Pellagra is a nutritional disease endemic among poor peasants who subsist chiefly on maize, among whom it is chronic and relapsing, with a seasonal incidence. The typical clinical features are loss of weight, increasing debility, an erythematous dermatitis characteristically affecting parts of the skin exposed to sunlight, gastrointestinal disturbances especially diarrhoea and glossitis, and mental changes. Pellagra has been called the disease of the three Ds: 'dermatitis, diarrhoea and dementia'. This is a useful mnemonic for medical students but diarrhoea and mental changes are not always present in mild and early cases and the mental symptom is usually depression and not dementia.

Features of protein-energy malnutrition and sometimes other nutritional deficiencies are often present.

HISTORY

Pellagra was unknown to classical and mediaeval physicians. After the introduction of maize into Europe from the Americas, it was first described by Casal as occurring in Spain in 1735. An Italian physician Frapolli named it in 1771 (*pelle* = skin; *agra* = rough). The disease spread with the cultivation of maize. In the nineteenth century it was common in Spain, Italy, France, Serbia (Yugoslavia), Romania, Bulgaria and the Ukraine. Great epidemics occurred in North Africa, especially in Egypt. Later it spread to other parts of Africa. Thus in 1897 there was a large epidemic of rinderpest in South Africa which decimated the cattle. Before this disaster milk, and especially 'amasi', a sour milk preparation, were important items of the Bantu diet. With the loss of this milk the children had to be weaned on to maize paps; the reduced supply of meat led to a much bigger proportion of maize in the diet. Large numbers of children and adults began to suffer from pellagra.

The disease first became prominent in the USA after the Civil War. The consequent social disruption and poverty led to many Negro and poor white families in the Southern States becoming increasingly dependent on maize. Pellagra was so widespread that it was held to be an infectious disease. The Federal Government sent a physician, Goldberger, to investigate the outbreaks and much of the credit for demonstrating that pellagra is a deficiency disease belongs to him. A selection of his papers written between 1913 and 1928 has been edited by Terris (1963). This book provides a classical example of how the nature of a disease may be elucidated by a combination of epidemiological and experimental studies. Pellagra remained an important disease in many Southern States until the USA entered World War II; then consequent upon full employment and the rise in wages, poverty and the dietary dependence on maize were reduced. Maize meal has subsequently been enriched with nicotinamide in the USA. A good account of the factors that led to the disappearance of endemic pellagra from the USA is given by Davies (1964). Roe (1973) has written an interesting book on the social history of pellagra in different parts of the world.

EPIDEMIOLOGY

Africa appears to be the only continent where there are areas in which it remains an important public health problem. In parts of southern Africa, it remains endemic and there are large outbreaks in the spring and summer months. More than half the patients who attend clinics in some Bantu homelands have pellagrous skin lesions, and pellagra accounts for a proportion of the admissions to the Bantu Mental Hospital in Pretoria. The prevalence of pellagra in South Africa is probably due to the maize being machine-milled in factories and not pounded by the women in their villages. Refined machine-milled maize flour contains less tryptophan and much less nicotinic acid than wholemeal maize flour. Pellagra is endemic in Lesotho. The people have their own name for it, 'Lefu-la-pone', which means the disease of the mealies (maize). In Egypt pellagra is much less common than formerly, but still occurs in some areas. Farmers are encouraged by government subsidies to grow wheat and its production now exceeds that of maize. In many villages in which the disease was prevalent no cases are found today. In the Sudan, Kenya and Tanzania the disease sometimes occurs but is not widespread.

Pellagra has disappeared from many countries where it was once endemic, and in areas where it remains the incidence is much less than formerly. In Europe and North America the disease is rarely seen, and usually a complication of chronic alcoholism or the malabsorption syndrome.

It occurs sporadically in those parts of India where maize is the staple cereal; 128 cases, all maize-eaters, were admitted to the Udaipur Hospital in one year (Shah and Singh, 1967). Pellagra also occurs in jowar (sorghum) eaters in Hyderabad, where it is responsible for up to 10 per cent of admissions to mental hospitals in certain seasons. Jowar, like maize, contains a high proportion of leucine in its proteins and Gopalan (1969) considers that this plays a role in the development of pellagra. Against this hypothesis are the low plasma leucine concentrations in Hyderabad pellagrins (Ghafoorunissa and Rao, 1975) and excess leucine neither precipitates nicotinic acid deficiency in beagles on low intakes of the vitamin (Manson and Carpenter, 1974), nor affects urinary excretion of niacin metabolities in normal human subjects (Nakagawa et al., 1975). Aggravation of mental symptoms and deterioration of the ECG in pellagrins when they were given leucine (Srikantia et al., 1968) could, we suggest, result from competitive interference with transport of tryptophan into the brain, where it forms the neurotransmitter 5-hydroxytryptamine (see Chap. 47). Krishnaswamy et al. (1976) now suggest that low intakes of pyridoxine on jowar diets may complicate the picture.

AETIOLOGY

The history of the search for the cause of pellagra well illustrates how the growth of knowledge can bring together apparently opposing theories and shows in the end that each has a substance of truth.

The maize theory

Casal himself believed that the disease was connected with eating maize. With the discovery of bacteria in the nineteenth century it became a common idea that any disease in which no causative infective organism could be found was probably due to 'toxins' made by bacteria, either inside or outside the body. Pellagra was attributed to some hypothetical toxin in the maize, perhaps produced by bacterial fermentation during storage.

The protein deficiency theory

It was soon clear that the diet of impoverished pellagrins was poor in protein and this deficiency was first suggested as the cause of the disease nearly a century ago. This theory gained support when Wilson (1921) in Egypt showed how closely pellagra was linked to an insufficient intake of good quality protein.

The vitamin deficiency theory

The above concept of the cause of the disease was altered by the discovery that extracts of yeast and liver contained a heat-stable, non-protein factor that would cure both human pellagra and black-tongue in dogs. The investigation of black-tongue in dogs ultimately led to the identification of nicotinic acid as the pellagra-preventing (P-P) factor (p. 138).

Reconciliation of the three theories.

The dramatic therapeutic effects of nicotinic acid in pellagra at first seemed the final proof of the last of these theories, with the result that the two alternatives were temporarily forgotten, until revived by the results of subsequent research.

It still remained to be explained why the disease is so closely associated with maize. Maize actually contains more nicotinic acid than oats, rye and white wheaten bread though less than whole wheat. Aykroyd and Swaminathan (1940) pointed out that maize diets in a part of India where pellagra is endemic contain more nicotinic acid than poor rice diets in other regions where it is rare. The explanation is that most of the nicotinic acid in maize is present in a bound form, unavailable to the consumer (Kodicek, 1962); also the major protein of maize, zein, is deficient in tryptophan, from which the body is able to make nicotinic acid (p. 139).

Goldberger recognised the therapeutic value of milk in pellagra and milk, as we now know, contains little nicotinic acid, but is rich in tryptophan.

A review of the history of the development of ideas about the aetiology has been written by Dame Harriette Chick (1951).

Other aetiological factors

Although the most outstanding feature—the dermatitis and diarrhoea—respond rapidly to nicotinic acid, as do acute and recent mental changes such as confusion, depression and even mania, there are others sometimes present that respond less readily, or not at all. The improvement in dementia and psychotic disorders under nicotinic acid therapy is often disappointing, probably because of the prolonged preceding state of severe malnutrition which may include thiamin deficiency. The orogenital and spinal cord changes, the anaemia and hypoproteinaemia, which are all recognised features of the syndrome, may be due to deficiencies other than that of nicotinic acid. In the words of McLester and Darby (1952): 'While lack of nicotinic acid dominates the picture, pellagra is in truth a disease of multiple deficiencies—nicotinic acid, protein, riboflavin and perhaps haemopoietic factors'.

CLINICAL FEATURES

The patient is often underweight, and presents the general features of undernutrition.

Skin

The diagnosis is generally first suggested by the appearance of the skin. Characteristically, there is an erythema resembling severe sunburn, appearing symmetrically over the parts of the body exposed to sunlight, especially the backs of the hands, the wrists and forearms, face and neck. Exposure to trauma or mechanical irritation of the skin, especially over bony prominences, may also determine the site of the lesion. The skin in the affected areas is at first red and slightly swollen; it itches and burns. In acute cases the skin lesions may progress to vesiculation, cracking, exudation and crusting with ulceration and sometimes secondary infection; but in chronic cases the dermatitis occurs as a

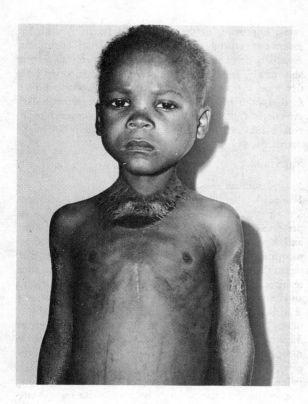

Fig. 34.1 Pellagra in a child, showing Casal's collar and also skin lesions on the arms. (Patient of J.D.L. Hansen and A.S. Truswell.)

roughening and thickening of the skin with dryness, scaling and a brown pigmentation (Fig. 34.1). This is the only symptom or sign in many people in endemic areas in Africa.

Digestive system

Complaints of digestive upset are usual, and diarrhoea is common but not always present. There may be nausea, a burning sensation in the epigastrium, and sometimes constipation in chronic cases. The digestive symptoms may be aggravated by the presence of intestinal parasites. The mouth is sore and often shows angular stomatitis and cheilosis. The tongue characteristically has a 'raw beef' appearance—red, swollen and painful, though usually without loss of papillae. Secondary infection of the mouth with Vincent's organisms is common. A non-infective inflammation followed by mucosal atrophy may involve the gastrointestinal tract and account for the diarrhoea which is characteristically profuse and watery, sometimes with blood and mucus in the stools, and accompanied by tenesmus. The rectum and anus are frequently affected and chronic gastritis with reduction or absence of acid secretion is a common finding. Vaginitis and amenorrhoea may occur.

Nervous system

In mild cases the symptoms consist of weakness, tremor, anxiety, depression and irritability; in severe acute cases delirium is common and dementia occurs in the chronic form. Because of these changes, chronic pellagrins may be admitted to mental hospitals. In chronic cases there may be decreased sensation in the feet to touch and loss of vibration and position sense, often accompanied by hyperaesthesia and paraesthesia. The loss of position sense may give rise to ataxia. Spasticity and exaggerated tendon reflexes give evidence of involvement of the pyramidal tracts. These features are those of subacute combined degeneration of the cord and may be due to associated vitamin B_{12} deficiency. Alternatively there may be footdrop and impairment of tendon reflexes, indicating a peripheral nerve lesion.

Secondary pellagra

A conditioned pellagra can be precipitated when the drug isoniazid is given to patients who have been on poor diets (Roe, 1971). This occurs because isoniazid acts as an antagonist to pyridoxine, which is a necessary coenzyme for the conversion of tryptophan to nicotinamide.

In industrial countries pellagra is occasionally seen in alcoholics and in the malabsorption syndrome. It can also occur as a complication of low and very low protein diets, used in patients with chronic renal failure if prophylactic B vitamins are forgotten, especially when the patient is on intermittent dialysis.

One other cause of pellagrous skin lesions in wellnourished communities is **Hartnup disease,** which was first described from the Middlesex Hospital, London, as 'hereditary pellagra-like skin rash with temporary cerebellar ataxia, and other bizarre biochemical features' (Baron *et al.*, 1956). A prominent biochemical feature is an aminoaciduria including tryptophan, and there is a defect of tryptophan transport not only in the renal tubules but also in intestinal absorption (Milne *et al.*, 1960). The pellagrous skin rash responds promptly to nicotinamide.

DIAGNOSIS

The classical case is easily diagnosed if a careful dietary and social history is taken and the typical clinical signs are present. The skin lesions are of diagnostic importance since they are only found in pellagra, whereas the gastrointestinal and mental features may be present in many other diseases. It is the occasional case in a non-maize eater that may present difficulties. A variety of erythemas and exfoliative skin lesions may mimic pellagra. The two characteristic features of cutaneous pellagra are its symmetrical distribution, determined by the clothes of the patient and exposure to sunlight, and the therapeutic response to nicotinic acid. A nutritional glossitis identical with the tongue changes seen in pellagra may occur without the other signs of the disease in people who have been all the time indoors, out of sunlight. In any unexplained delirium or dementia in a person who has been taking a poor diet for a prolonged period, the possibility of pellagra should be remembered.

PATHOLOGY

The mucous membranes of the mouth, tongue, oesophagus, stomach, colon and vagina shows changes somewhat similar to those on the skin. There is atrophy and inflammation and small ulcers may be found. The most characteristic changes are to be seen in the colon where there may be numerous small ulcers, covered by fibrin, small submucous abscesses and prominent cystic dilations of the mucous glands. The liver may show periportal fatty changes, and patchy non-specific degenerative changes have been reported in the central nervous system.

The content of NAD and NADP is reduced in some tissues, such as muscle and affected parts of the skin. The achlorhydria might be explained by the fact that the oxyntic cells of the stomach normally contain large amounts of pyridine nucleotides.

The mental changes, in which depressive features are prominent, can be explained by reduced synthesis of 5-hydroxytryptamine (5-HT) in the brain. Though this has not been demonstrated directly we know that 5-HT can only be synthesised from tryptophan. Reduced 5-HT concentrations in platelets (Krishnaswamy and Murthy, 1970) and low urinary 5-hydroxyindoleacetic acid (Belavady et al., 1963) are found in pellagrins.

LABORATORY FINDINGS

N-Methylnicotinamide, a normal excretory product of nicotinic acid, appears in reduced amounts in the urine. A level of urinary excretion below 0.2 mg/6 hr or 0.5 mg/g of creatinine indicates a deficiency of the vitamin, but not necessarily a diagnosis of pellagra (Jelliffe, 1966). Reproducibility of the method is not very satisfactory, as other substances sometimes interfere with the fluorimetric procedure. A second excretory product, the 2-pyridone of N'-methylnicotinamide is more difficult to measure but is used in research (de Lange and Joubert, 1964). The ratio of 2-pyridone to N'-methylnicotinamide excretion is normally greater than 1.0.

The fasting plasma tryptophan ranges from 1.0 to 4.8 mg/l in pellagrins and from 6.5 to 8.8 mg/l in healthy adults (Truswell et al., 1968). Plasma tryptophan may prove to be a convenient test for confirming a diagnosis of pellagra.

Examination of the blood may show anaemia and hypoalbuminaemia (Prinsloo et al., 1968) due to the associated dietary deficiencies. The anaemia may be macrocytic or microcytic, depending on the predominant associated deficiency.

PROGNOSIS

In endemic areas the majority of patients are mild cases, improving in the winter and relapsing with the increased sunshine in the spring. Mental symptoms, especially dementia, are perhaps the most serious feature and may be permanent. Occasionally a fulminating form develops, with fever and severe prostration which is often fatal. In the past many deaths were due to secondary infections (notably tuberculosis and dysentery) or to emaciation due to general dietary failure, intensified by the diarrhoea.

TREATMENT

Specific vitamin therapy

For quick relief of symptoms nicotinic acid or nicotinamide are the standard treatment. Nicotinamide is to be preferred because it does not cause the unpleasant flushing and burning sensations that often result from taking nicotinic acid. These are transitory and harmless, but may alarm the patient. A suitable dose for either nicotinamide or nicotinic acid is 100 mg 4-hourly by mouth, although a smaller dose is likely to be effective. The vitamin is rapidly absorbed from the stomach, despite severe digestive disorders. There is therefore no need to give intravenous or intramuscular injections. The immediate response to nicotinamide is usually dramatic; within 24 hours the erythema diminishes, the tongue becomes paler and less painful and the diarrhoea ceases. Often there is striking improvement in the patient's behaviour and mental attitude. But nicotinamide alone is usually insufficient to restore health, because of other associated deficiencies, notably of protein and other components of the vitamin B complex. Preparations of vitamin B complex should be given as a routine and if there are signs of peripheral neuropathy or subacute combined degeneration of the cord larger doses of thiamin or vitamin B_{12} are indicated.

Diet

The first aim should be to compensate for the qualitative and quantitative deficiencies of the previous diet. To restore the patient to normal weight, the diet should provide ample energy and good quality protein, as is present in milk, eggs, meat or fish. In severely ill patients it is necessary to climb the dietetic ladder cautiously. The food should be low in bulk at first in order to avoid further diarrhoea. The diet may be poorly tolerated because of the mental state of the patient and the sore mouth which may make eating difficult. Alcohol should be forbidden.

General measures

Rest in bed and sedation are necessary for severely ill pellagrins, especially those with marked mental symptoms; they are often troublesome patients who need understanding. If the dermatitis is associated with much crusting or secondary infection, gentle washing with a bland solution is indicated.

PREVENTION

The remarkable fact that pellagra has vanished from the southern states of America, whereas formerly it afflicted tens of thousands of poor country folk, demonstrates in a dramatic way that the disease is preventable. Its disappearance has sometimes been attributed to the fortification of bread and maize with nicotinic acid in the USA, but this is only one of several factors which have produced this satisfactory result. The most likely reason is the general improvement in the economic state, the education and the nutrition of the population.

Enrichment of maize meal with a suitable vitamin supplement is technically simple and inexpensive but is difficult to implement for subsistence farmers who grow their own maize.

From the standpoint of agricultural policy, it is clearly wise to avoid dependence on a single cereal crop, such as maize, or to devote too great an acreage of fertile land for the cultivation of cash-crops, such as cotton or tobacco. Animal husbandry should be encouraged in all areas where pellagra is endemic so that the production of milk and milk products and meat is increased. In the shorter term, encouraging the planting of opaque-2 maize (p. 174) may help. It contains about three times as much tryptophan and twice as much lysine as conventional maize.

35. Scurvy

Scurvy is a nutritional disease which results from prolonged subsistence on diets practically devoid of fresh fruit and vegetables. Lack of ascorbic acid causes a disturbance in the structure of connective tissue, leading to swollen, bleeding gums and haemorrhages into the skin and elsewhere.

HISTORY

Scurvy was not clearly recognised by Greek, Roman or mediaeval physicians. In 1453 Constantinople was sacked by the Turks, so that Venice lost naval control of the Eastern Mediterranean, and the overland trade route between Europe and Asia was blocked. This disaster for Christian merchant adventurers stimulated the Portuguese to find a sea route to India. In 1497 Vasco de Gama sailed round the Cape of Good Hope and established a trading centre on the Malabar coast. Scurvy broke out among his crew on the voyage and 100 out of his 160 men died. For the next 300 years scurvy was a major factor determining the success or failure of all sea ventures, whether undertaken for purposes of war, trade or exploration. As early as 1535 the French explorer Jacques Cartier, whose crew was severely affected in Newfoundland, discovered that the juice of the leaves of a certain tree had remarkable antiscorbutic properties. An account of this discovery, as recorded in Hakluyt's *The Principall Navigations* (1600), was reproduced in earlier editions of our book.

Later Canadian explorers, suffering from scurvy, attempted to identify the curative Ameda tree without success, probably because the Indians by then were less communicative. The tragedy was that as they died of the disease the tree was probably standing right beside them; for as Lind suggested, it was probably the spruce fir. The value of a decoction of spruce or pine needles as an antiscorbutic remedy was well known to the Swedes at least as early as the sixteenth century, and subsequently used by the Russians in their repeated attempts to find an Arctic sea-route to the Pacific. Curiously the antiscorbutic value of pine needles was rediscovered in the USSR in 1943.

The subsequent history of scurvy is of great interest. Many writers showed that the disease could be cured by a variety of fresh fruits and vegetables, but medical learning was so constricted by Galen's classical pathology of 'humours' that the conception of a deficiency disease was not realised till long after. In 1753 Lind, a Scots naval surgeon, published *A Treatise of the Scurvy,* in which he showed not only that the disease could be cured by fresh oranges and lemons, but also that it could be prevented by adequate dietary and other hygienic measures. His own account of the first controlled therapeutic trial ever undertaken is as follows:

On the 20th of May 1747, I took twelve patients in the scurvy, on board the *Salisbury* at sea. Their cases were as similar as I could have them. They all in general had putrid gums, the spots and lassitude, with weakness of their knees. They lay together in one place, being a proper apartment for sick in the fore-hold; and had one diet common to all.... Two of these were ordered each a quart of cyder a-day. Two others took twenty-five gutta of *elisir vitriol* three times a-day, upon an empty stomach; using a gargle strongly acidulated with it for their mouths. Two others took two spoonfuls of vinegar three times a-day, upon an empty stomach; having their gruels and their other food well acidulated with it, as also the gargle for their mouth. Two of the worst patients, with the tendons in the ham rigid...were put under a course of sea-water. Of this they drank half a pint every day, and sometimes more or less as it operated, by way of gentle physic. Two others had each two oranges and one lemon given them every day. These they eat with greediness, at different times, upon an empty stomach. They continued but six days under this course, having consumed the quantity that could be spared. The two remaining patients, took the bigness of a nutmeg three times a-day, of an electuary recommended by an hospital-surgeon, made of garlic, mustard-seed, *rad. raphan.*, balsam of Peru, and gum myrrh; using for common drink, barley-water well acidulated with tamarinds....

The consequence was, that the most sudden and visible good effects were perceived from the use of the oranges and lemons; one of those who had taken them, being at the end of six days fit for duty.... The other was the best recovered of any in his condition; and being now deemed pretty well, was appointed nurse to the rest of the sick. (Lind, 1753.)

Lind was aware that an adequate supply of fresh vegetables or a suitable fruit juice could prevent the occurrence of scurvy. He states that abstinence from them is 'the occasional (i.e. apparent) cause of the evil' but other factors such as exposure to cold and wet, drunkenness, putrid air and overcrowding below decks were 'predisposing causes'. Such factors, often today loosely called 'stress', are now known to have important effects on ascorbic acid metabolism (p. 133).

Captain James Cook was the first person to demonstrate that a long voyage could be undertaken without the crew developing scurvy. In his voyage round the world from 1772 to 1775 in which he explored Australia and New Zealand, none of his men developed the disease, thanks to the care with which he seized every opportunity to provide them with fresh vegetables and fruit (including oranges and lemons) whenever they touched land. But it was not until 1795, 42 years after the publication of Lind's treatise, that his pupil Sir Gilbert Blane persuaded the Lords of the Admiralty to put his precepts into practice and thus immediately abolished scurvy from the Royal Navy. This was at the beginning of the Napoleonic wars when Great Britain's command of the sea was of paramount importance to her. The application of Lind's teaching doubled the fighting force of the Navy at sea without adding a penny to the naval estimates. For a further 50 years however, the disease lingered on in the merchant navies of the world. The long interval between the discovery of the new knowledge and its application to the benefit of humanity makes a sad story in history.

When scurvy ceased to be an important disease of sailors, it developed in another section of the community; the knowledge of the chemistry of foods obtained in the nineteenth century enabled a variety of preserved and artificial milks to be manufactured. These provided an adequate substitute for the protein, fat and carbohydrate in human milk and so removed the wet nurses from our society. But these substitutes for human milk contained little or no ascorbic acid, so scurvy in infants became an important disease. The heyday of infantile scurvy was in the last 20 years of the nineteenth century.

EPIDEMIOLOGY

In Britain. Scurvy is an uncommon disease which is most likely to be seen in old people. Usually the patient is a bachelor or widower who is living alone. Very occasionally scurvy is seen in a chronic alcoholic, a migrant labourer, or a food crank.

Infantile scurvy is also rare, but sometimes occurs in a family where the mother is feckless and the social and economic background poor. During 1960–62, consultant paediatricians reported 78 cases (British Paediatric Association, 1964). The incidence today is not known, but is probably less.

Although frank scurvy is rare, there are many persons, especially old people, living alone and on poor diets with no fresh fruit and little vegetables, who have low levels of ascorbic acid in their blood and tissues. This condition is often referred to as subclinical scurvy. Some geriatricians

consider that it is in part responsible for the anaemia not uncommonly found in old people and for other clinical features of vague ill health. The importance of subclinical scurvy is disputed and there are some who think that it is a misleading term.

In other countries. The reports that we have received from many countries in America and Europe, from North, South and East Africa, Australia, New Zealand, India, Malaysia, Hong Kong and the Philippines, all indicate that scurvy is a rare disease and is not an important public health problem. This satisfactory position is partly due to the more widespread knowledge of its aetiology and also to the increased production of citrus and other fruits and green vegetables, and to their distribution in the canned or frozen state; this makes them available at all seasons of the year.

In all countries, sporadic cases are seen, under circumstances similar to those in Britain. In South Africa, it is found in migrant labourers. This arises from the fact that at home the Bantu women collect wild plants for the main meal, a task which young men would not undertake. In Johannesburg it is often associated with alcoholism (Seftel et al., 1966).

In countries where the Maternal and Child Health Services are inadequate, infantile scurvy may be more common than reports indicate, especially in infants who for one reason or another are weaned from the breast prematurely.

AETIOLOGY

Scurvy results from the prolonged consumption of a diet devoid of fresh fruit and vegetables. Lack of ascorbic acid is responsible for the characteristic features of the disease, but such diets are likely to lack other nutrients such as iron, folic acid, vitamin A and sometimes protein. Thus although ascorbic acid relieves the predominant signs of the disease it does not always completely cure the patient. Further, although a diet may seem from the history to contain adequate amounts of ascorbic acid, it may in fact be scorbutic if practically all the vitamin has been destroyed in its cooking. Another factor may be the influence of 'stress' which increases the utilisation of ascorbic acid.

PATHOLOGY

Haemorrhages either large or microscopic may be found anywhere in the body. They are most common in the gums if the teeth are still present, in subcutaneous tissues, and beneath the periosteum of bones and the synovia of joints. These are sites of minor trauma. Haemorrhages into the brain or heart muscle may cause sudden death. Haemorrhages are due to defective collagen formation in the basement membranes of capillaries arising from lack of ascorbic acid needed to convert proline to hydroxyproline. There is also a failure of wound healing and old wounds which have healed may break down (p. 133).

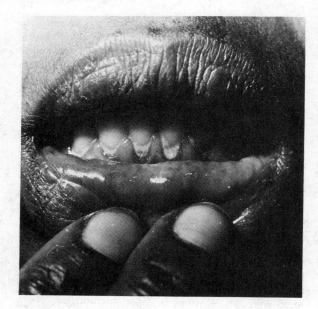

Fig. 35.1 The gums in scurvy.

As deaths from scurvy are now rare, there is seldom an opportunity for a postmortem and the classical account of autopsy findings is by Aschoff and Koch (1919).

CLINICAL FEATURES

The best clinical account of scurvy is that given by Lind, who had greater experience of the disease than any modern physician and described his observations with the clarity and elegance characteristic of his time.

Lind said that the pathognomonic sign of the disease was the appearance of the gums and certainly the characteristic gingivitis often first suggests the diagnosis. The gums are swollen, particularly in the region of the papillae between the teeth, sometimes producing the appearance of 'scurvy buds' (Fig. 35.1). These may be so extensive that they project beyond the biting surface of the teeth and almost completely conceal them. The spongy gums are livid in colour and bleed on the slightest touch. There is always some infection; indeed this seems necessary for the production of the scorbutic gingival appearances since human volunteers suffering from ascorbic acid deficiency did not develop it if their gums were previously healthy. Associated with the infection there is an offensive foetor. In patients without teeth the gums appear normal.

The first sign of cutaneous bleeding is often to be found on the lower thighs, just above the knees. These haemorrhages are perifollicular—tiny points of bleeding around the orifice of a hair follicle. For some time beforehand the follicle can be seen to be raised above the general surface of the skin, giving the appearance of folliculosis, which is quite commonly seen in varying degrees in people apparently well supplied with ascorbic acid. The condition in scurvy can be distinguished by its appearance from the follicular keratosis sometimes associated with vitamin A deficiency. In the latter condition there is usually a horny plug of keratin projecting from the orifice of the hair follicle. In scurvy there is a heaping up of keratin-like material on the surface around the mouth of the follicle, through which a deformed 'corkscrew' hair characteristically projects. Perifollicular haemorrhages may subsequently appear on the buttocks, abdomen, legs and arms; they are often followed by petechial haemorrhages, developing independently of the hair follicles, due to rupture of capillary vessels. Such purpuric spots are usually first seen on the feet and ankles. Thereafter large spontaneous bruises (ecchymoses) may arise almost anywhere in the body, but usually first in the legs. In dark skins these changes are not always easily seen and may be overlooked. African patients often present with pain in a leg due to haemorrhage into intermuscular septa in the thigh or calf. In volunteers with experimental scurvy Hodges et al. (1971) and Hodges (1971) describe several additional clinical features. These include (1) ocular haemorrhages, especially in the bulbar conjunctiva; (2) Sjögren's syndrome, i.e. loss of secretion of salivary and lacrimal glands and swelling of the parotid glands; (3) femoral neuropathy; (4) oedema of the lower limbs with oliguria; and (5) psychological disturbances, hypochondria and depression.

Before the changes in the gums and skin appear, the patient has usually felt feeble and listless for some weeks. By the time the disease is fully developed the patient is often anaemic. As anaemia has not occurred in experimental scurvy in man, this is not directly attributable to lack of ascorbic acid. Deficiencies of other nutrients, blood loss and perhaps unidentified factors may be responsible (Goldberg, 1963). Usually there is normoblastic hyperplasia of the bone marrow with reticulocytosis (Bronte-Stewart, 1953; Goldberg, 1963). Loss and destruction of red cells in muscle haematomata may lead to mild jaundice and increased urobilinogen (Bronte-Stewart, 1953; Bothwell et al., 1964). Sometimes the marrow is megaloblastic and this is not corrected by ascorbic acid but requires folic acid (Zalusky and Herbert, 1961). Iron is also needed in some cases (Goldberg, 1963).

Ascorbic acid is necessary for the synthesis of collagen in all parts of the body, including the bones. Scurvy in adults may be associated with the radiological changes in bone characteristic of osteoporosis (Joffe, 1961). The combination of osteoporosis, scurvy, siderosis and alcoholism in middle-aged Bantu men is well known in Johannesburg (Seftel et al., 1966). In these cases, ascorbic acid deficiency may have been a factor causing the osteoporosis. It is possible that in old people in Britain hypovitaminosis C may contribute to the demineralisation of the skeleton.

Examination of a patient with scurvy usually reveals no abnormal physical signs of disease except gingivitis and cutaneous haemorrhages and hence the gravity of his

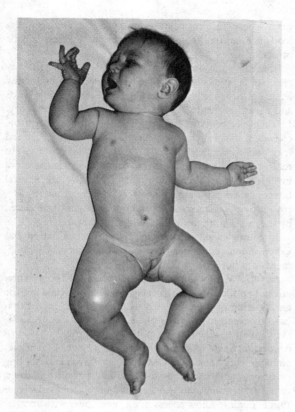

Fig. 35.2 Infantile scurvy. The frog-like position is due to large painful subperiosteal haemorrhages in both femurs. There are haematomata in the scalp and also beading of the costochondral junctions. (Patient of J.D.L. Hansen.)

condition may not be appreciated. Yet in fact he may die suddenly and without warning, apparently from cardiac failure. Lind himself described how a sailor afflicted with scurvy fell dead while working at a windlass.

Scurvy in infants

Until the teeth have erupted, scorbutic infants do not develop gingivitis. When this occurs the gums have the classical appearance of 'scurvy buds' described above, a diagnostic feature. The first sign of bleeding is usually a large subperiosteal haemorrhage immediately overlying one of the long bones—frequently the femur—producing the characteristic 'frog-legs' position (Fig. 35.2). This gives rise to intense pain, especially on movement. The infant may cry continuously and agonisingly, and scream even louder when lifted.

DIAGNOSIS

The distinctive appearance of the gums must be distinguished from other causes of gingivitis, the commonest of which is periodontal disease (p. 392). In the latter condition there are usually accumulations of tartar on the teeth,

with retraction of the gum margin. The inflamed rim of the gums is bright red in colour, in contrast to the cyanotic appearance in scurvy, and there is usually much less swelling. In Vincent's angina the gums are acutely inflamed, ulcerated and painful, but here again the bright red appearance of the lesions is distinctive. Poisoning with heavy metals, particularly lead and mercury, produces a gingivitis in which the gum margin is stained blue; but there is usually little swelling and the appearance is easily distinguished from scurvy. Phenytoin, a drug used in epilepsy, may cause marked swelling of the gums, but they preserve their normal colour and do not bleed.

The perifollicular haemorrhages of scurvy are distinctive in appearance. But if only petechiae are visible, other causes of purpura must be excluded, e.g. blood dyscrasias, drug poisoning or prothrombin deficiency. If ecchymoses are the chief manifestation, the patient may be seen first by a surgeon, on the suspicion of some undisclosed trauma.

Scurvy in infants and children may sometimes be mistaken for rheumatic fever or osteomyelitis, because of the pain caused by a subperiosteal haemorrhage. The refusal of the child to use one leg may cause the disease to be mistaken for poliomyelitis.

The dietary and social history establishes the diagnosis in doubtful cases. Old solitary people may insist that they fend very well for themselves, but careful questioning shows that they do not bother to buy fresh fruit or vegetables. In other instances the proper foods may be purchased but they are so badly cooked that the diet is made scorbutic.

Special investigations. Capillary fragility may be increased. This can be shown by the application of a sphygmomanometer cuff to the arm and leaving it inflated for five minutes, half-way between the systolic and diastolic blood pressure. A shower of petechiae then appears over the area of skin below the cuff (Hess test). But this is not a specific test for scurvy.

Ascorbic acid can be estimated with relative ease either in blood plasma or whole blood. This is useful only in excluding the diagnosis, since if any measurable amount of ascorbic acid can be detected in the blood, the case is not one of scurvy. The absence of detectable ascorbic acid, however, does not necessarily indicate that the patient has scurvy, since the blood level of the vitamin falls to unmeasurable levels long before the disease develops.

A better index of the body reserves of the vitamin is its concentration in the white blood corpuscles. The method of Denson and Bowers (1961) is suitable. If none can be measured, the diagnosis of scurvy is practically certain.

The estimation of ascorbic acid in the urine provides no reliable aid to diagnosis, because small amounts of the vitamin, or some other substance reducing 2,6-dichlorophenolindophenol, continue to be excreted in the urine, even in manifest scurvy. In 'loading' tests one or more doses of ascorbic acid are given by mouth and the amount excreted in the urine subsequently measured. But results of such tests are subject to so many variable factors that they are seldom used.

TREATMENT

Because of the danger of sudden death, synthetic ascorbic acid should be given at once and in adequate amounts. The vitamin is very soluble and rapidly absorbed from the digestive tract. It can be given intravenously, but a large part of the dose is immediately lost in the urine. The aim should be to saturate the body with ascorbic acid with as little delay as possible. The fully saturated body contains about 5 g of the vitamin, so that a dose of 250 mg by mouth four times daily should achieve this within a week, despite some loss in the urine.

It sometimes happens that scurvy arises among people far removed from supplies of synthetic ascorbic acid (e.g. among prisoners of war); in such situations valuable therapeutic effects are obtained by the use of natural sources of the vitamin such as fresh fruit and vegetables, sprouting peas or extract of pine needles.

Once the danger of sudden death is averted by giving ascorbic acid, attention should be paid to correcting the general deficiencies of the patient's former diet. A liberal diet, including fresh fruit and as much properly cooked vegetables as are available and the patient will accept, should be given. If the patient is anaemic, ferrous sulphate and folic acid tablets by mouth are indicated.

With adequate treatment no patient dies of scurvy; but if treatment is delayed he may die. If the measures recommended above are applied, recovery is usually rapid and complete.

PREVENTION

Scurvy tends to occur at the two extremes of age. The prevention of scurvy in infants has been accomplished by the better education of mothers and helped by the distribution of cheap, concentrated orange juice of standard ascorbic acid content.

For old people living alone, the provision of proper meals is the best means of preventing scurvy. This should be the responsibility of their family. If there are no relations or these are unable or unwilling to care for the old person, responsibility falls on the social services. So far, however, the Welfare State has failed to find any simple administrative means of preventing scurvy among the old and solitary, who are largely unresponsive to education. In cases where an old person is unwilling or unable to eat foods containing the vitamin, ascorbic acid tablets may be prescribed.

Special provision against scurvy is desirable for any group of people living on packed, preserved rations for any length of time such as the explorers of inaccessible lands and oceans, or armed forces defending a barren territory. In such circumstances the bulk of the rations is a prime consideration, especially if airlifts are involved. Tinned fruit and vegetables provide little energy in proportion to their weight. Synthetic ascorbic acid tablets are therefore invaluable under such conditions, although some natural but concentrated source of ascorbic acid, e.g. orange juice, rose-hip or blackcurrant syrup may be better appreciated by the men and therefore more likely to be taken regularly.

In countries where there is rapid industrialisation and urbanisation, education and sometimes dietary supplements are needed for migrant labourers.

In times of drought and famine, when fresh vegetables are not available, ascorbic acid can be obtained by the germination of pulses or cereals. A well-tried recipe that has prevented many cases of scurvy in India is: 'A sufficient quantity of whole (unsplit) dhal or gram (say 1½ to 2ᵉ oz per man) is soaked in water for 12 to 24 hours. A container big enough to allow for expansion and holding sufficient water should be used. Then pour off the water, remove the grains and spread on a damp blanket in a layer thin enough to allow access of air, and cover with another damp blanket. Keep the blankets damp by sprinkling with water. In a few hours small shoots will appear, and when these are ½ to 1 inch long the process is complete. Vitamin C content is maximal after about 30 hours of germination.' Pulses normally contain no ascorbic acid but 30 g of dried pulse on germination yield 9 to 15 mg, sufficient to prevent scurvy.

On his solo sailing voyage around the world (1966–67) Sir Francis Chichester grew mustard and cress in trays and avoided scurvy by eating this. Visitors to his 54-foot yacht, *Gipsy Moth IV*, can still see mustard and cress growing in the galley.

The distribution of synthetic ascorbic acid tablets on a large scale to civilian populations is seldom warranted. Ascorbic acid is rarely the sole nutrient lacking in a defective diet; so to give this vitamin alone is an inadequate preventive measure and distracts attention from the essential need of improving the diet.

36. Other Nutritional Disorders of the Nervous System

In addition to conditions due mainly to thiamin deficiency, there are other primarily neurological disorders directly attributable to dietary factors. With the exception of vitamin B_{12} neuropathy, the precise cause is unknown. Most patients have been on poor diets deficient in many nutrients and sometimes in addition there may be evidence of a toxic factor in the food. These disorders are described in this chapter. The relation of diet to neurological and psychiatric disorders in general is discussed in Chapter 49.

Burning feet syndrome

Outbreaks of this distinct clinical syndrome have occurred at various times in Europe, Central America, Africa and India among people living on very poor diets. It was common during the Spanish Civil War and among European prisoners in the Far East during World War II. Excellent descriptions of the condition have been provided by Peraita (1942), Smith and Woodruff (1951) and Cruickshank (1952). It is sometimes seen in elderly people in Britain.

The earliest symptom is aching, burning or throbbing in the feet. This becomes more intense and is followed by sharp, stabbing, shooting pains, which may spread up as far as the knee like an electric shock, causing excruciating agony. They come on in paroxysms and are usually worse at night. Most patients get some relief by walking about, and sufferers may spend the night limping up and down outside their quarters. Some manage to get relief by wrapping their feet in cold wet cloths or sitting with their feet in a pail of cold water. Continuous pain and loss of sleep produce a thin, exhausted, irritable patient.

In contrast to the striking symptoms, objective signs of neuropathy are seldom marked unless the polyneuropathy of beriberi co-exists. The tendon jerks are usually normal but may be exaggerated. In the great majority of cases there is no demonstrable sensory change; indeed there is some doubt whether the syndrome should properly be classified as a neuropathy. It may be due chiefly to peripheral vascular changes (Cruickshank, 1952). On the other hand there seems to be no constant change in skin temperature. Some patients develop a transient hypertension during the course of an attack. Smith and Woodruff (1951) hold the view that the probable sites of the lesion are the dorsal root and sympathetic ganglia.

The syndrome has been associated with the prolonged consumption of a diet deficient in protein and the B group of vitamins. Patients who suffer from it may also develop the orogenital syndrome (p. 304) or nutritional amblyopia see below, but rarely beriberi. World War II prisoners improved when given yeast, Marmite, rice polishings and other foods rich in the vitamin B complex and a well-balanced high protein diet. The nutrient responsible was not identified. Subsequently Gopalan (1946) reported improvement of the same symptoms in Indians when pantothenate was given but Bibile *et al.* (1957) in Sri Lanka could not confirm this. Lai and Ransome (1970) report a case with malabsorption who responded to riboflavin.

The syndrome can be seen sometimes in chronic alcoholics and patients with other neuropathies, e.g. diabetic and in chronic renal failure on dialysis. It has also been reported in a case of nerve entrapment, the 'tarsal tunnel syndrome' (*Lancet,* 1972) and in circulatory disorders such as polycythaemia vera (Fitzgerald *et al.,* 1976) and ergotism.

Nutritional amblyopia (Nutritional retrobulbar neuropathy)

A progressive failure of vision attributable to a retrobulbar neuropathy occurred among prisoners of war in World War II. Denny-Brown (1947) reported a number of cases in British and Indian soldiers admitted to military hospitals in India after release from Japanese camps. In Egypt also, about a hundred cases occurred among German prisoners of war who had suffered for some time previously from chronic dysentery. Fitzgerald Moore (1937) reported many cases in Nigeria between 1930 and 1940. Disturbances of vision, however, are seldom mentioned in accounts of pellagra and beriberi. The incidence of the condition in prisoners of war aroused renewed interest and discussion, though little new was learned about its aetiology.

All the patients appear to have had one feature in common—a period of many months on diets grossly deficient in respect of many essential nutrients. There are thus good reasons for thinking that the disorder is nutritional in origin. The nature of the diets held to be responsible has been very variable. It would appear unlikely that a deficiency of any single nutrient is responsible.

A typical history is that over a period of three weeks or so there is a growing inability to see the colours of small objects. A mist obscures the central field of vision and gradually becomes so intense that it is impossible to recognise acquaintances. There may be retrobulbar pain, but this is often absent. Sometimes the eyes smart. Tinnitus, deafness and dizziness—apparently due to associated involvement of the eighth nerve—may occur. In Japanese camps none became completely blind, but several were severely incapacitated.

A central or paracentral scotoma is always present but there is little or no peripheral contraction of the visual fields. The visual acuity varies greatly; in some there is little impairment; in others it may be as low as 6/60. In mild cases the retinae appear normal on examination with an ophthalmoscope. When the loss of vision is severe, temporal pallor of the optic discs is usually present.

When the symptoms are not severe they are relieved rapidly by a good diet supplemented by yeast or Marmite, but when vision is markedly affected little or no improvement results from any form of treatment (Clarke and Sircus, 1952; Rodger, 1952).

Optic atrophy also occurs in heavy smokers and then is often effectively treated with hydroxocobalamin. It probably arises from the neurotoxic effect of cyanide present in tobacco.

Retrobulbar neuropathy and spinal ataxia occur together in Western Nigeria among people who subsist largely on cassava. The syndrome, called tropical ataxic neuropathy, appears to be caused primarily by chronic ingestion of small amounts of cyanide from the cassava. It is dealt with more fully in the following section.

Spinal ataxia

Patients who have been living for long periods on unbalanced diets occasionally develop neurological signs which indicate that the principal lesion is in the dorsal columns of the spinal cord, involving particularly proprioceptive sensation. The gait is unsteady and the patient is unable to stand upright without swaying when the eyes are closed (Romberg's test). Vibration sense in the legs is often lost. The condition has been described in association with nutritional amblyopia by Landor and Pallister (1935) in Malaya and by Spillane and Scott (1945) in prisoners of war. We ourselves have seen two cases in strict vegetarians who ate no foods of animal origin and in such cases the essential dietary abnormality is lack of vitamin B_{12}, which occurs only in foods of animal origin or in foods fermented by microorganisms. In other words, the disease may be a form of subacute combined degeneration of the cord, but due to a direct dietary deficiency of vitamin B_{12}, in contrast to the conditioned deficiency that occurs in pernicious anaemia.

In tropical ataxic neuropathy, seen in Western Nigeria (Osuntokun, 1968) and Tanzania (Makene and Wilson, 1972), vitamin B_{12} plays only a secondary role. In the fully developed syndrome there is sensory spinal ataxia, retrobulbar neuropathy or optic atrophy and sometimes bilateral nerve deafness. Signs indicating mild involvement of

the lateral or pyramidal tracts may be found. Epidemiologically the condition is found in people who regularly consume large amounts of cassava (Osuntokun et al., 1969). Cassava contains a cyanogenic glycoside, linamarin, which can be broken down to yield free hydrogen cyanide by enzymes in the plant tissue if it is crushed or left standing in water. Ingested cyanide is detoxified by sulphur-containing amino acids, which convert it to thiocyanate, and by hydroxocobalamin which forms cyanocobalamin. Patients with tropical ataxic neuropathy have increased plasma concentrations and urinary excretion of thiocyanate (Osuntokun, 1968) with increased vitamin B_{12} and reduced cystine in the plasma (Osuntokun et al., 1968). These findings strongly suggest that this nutritional neuropathy results from chronic ingestion of small amounts of cyanide from cassava in people whose diet does not contain sufficient sulphur-containing amino acids and vitamin B_{12} to detoxify it. The condition can be prevented in part by cooking methods which wash out the glycoside or boil off the HCN.

Cerebellar cortical degeneration

This condition in which the characteristic clinical feature is ataxia of the legs arises from degenerative changes limited to the anterior superior part of the vermis of the cerebellum. It is associated with alcoholism and poor nutrition but the response to vitamin therapy and nutritional rehabilitation is less consistent than in Wernicke-Korsakoff syndrome.

Vitamin B_{12} neuropathy

This was commonly associated with pernicious anaemia before the introduction of treatment with vitamin B_{12}. Known as subacute combined degeneration of the cord it affected mainly the dorsal and lateral columns and was often severe and incapacitating. The full clinical picture of the disease is now rarely seen but some evidence of involvement of the spinal cord is not uncommon when a patient first presents with pernicious anemia and is occasionally found before anaemia develops. Vitamin B_{12} neuropathy also arises from lack of vitamin B_{12} in the diet, e.g. in some castes of strict Hindus and in vegans. In such people anaemia is characteristically not seen, presumably because a vegetable diet supplies sufficient folic acid.

Clinical features. Early symptoms are tingling, coldness and numbness in the extremities due to peripheral neuropathy. Motor weakness and ataxia appear later and become increasingly severe as the cord is involved. The physical signs depend on the relative involvement of the peripheral nerves and the dorsal and lateral columns of the cord. In severe cases ataxia is the outstanding feature with loss of reflexes especially in the lower limbs. Sometimes the pyramidal tracts are involved and spasticity, increased reflexes and an extensor plantar response are present. If the brain is affected there may be an organic psychosis and this may be the first evidence of vitamin B_{12} deficiency.

Treatment and prevention This is the same as for pernicious anaemia and is described on page 427. If treatment is begun early, recovery is complete, but in severe cases the damage is irreparable.

Spastic paraplegia

Lathyrism. *Lathyrus sativus*, or Kesari dhal, is a drought-resistant pulse, widely grown in parts of the Indian subcontinent (p. 221). If eaten in excessive amounts and for a long period, it gives rise to lathyrism.

The onset of lathyrism is usually sudden and is often preceded by exertion or exposure to cold. A patient may go to bed well and wake up paralysed; or he may fall down at the plough. Sometimes backache and stiffness of the legs precede the onset of the paralysis by a few days. The condition is a spastic paralysis of the lower limbs, due presumably to a precisely localised lesion of the lower parts of the pyramidal tracts. The motor nerves to the muscles of the trunk, upper limbs and sphincters are spared. The sensory nervous system is not involved. In mild cases there is only stiffness and weakness of the legs and exaggerated knee and ankle jerks. In more severe cases the patient walks with bent knees on tiptoe. The legs are often crossed; a 'scissors gait' develops and walking is only possible with the aid of sticks. In severe cases paraplegia in flexion follows, and walking becomes impossible. The patient can only move about by pushing himself along, supporting his body on his hands, buttocks and heels. The paraplegia is typically spastic with greatly increased ankle and knee jerks, and with clonus. The final stage of the disease is completely incapacitating and the sufferers may move to the cities where they are easily recognised amongst the beggars.

The toxic factors responsible for lathyrism are discussed on page 221.

Epidemic lathyrism is essentially a disease of famine since the pulse is only eaten in large quantities when the main crops have failed. It would appear then that long periods on an inadequate diet, deficient in energy, proteins and vitamins, predispose to the disease. The clinical and epidemiological findings of an outbreak in West Bengal are reported by Chaudhuri *et al.* (1963).

There is no specific treatment. All patients need a good diet. Minor cases may make a complete recovery following satisfactory dietary and physical rehabilitation. In most cases the pathological changes are irreversible and, as already stated, the patients drift into beggary.

As a preventive measure, it has been found that most of the toxin can be extracted if Kesari dhal is heated in four volumes of water for an hour and the water discarded (Nagarajan, 1971). Thiamin and some other water-soluble vitamins are lost in the process. A programme of selective breeding to develop strains of *L. sativus* low in toxin is needed.

Other forms of spastic paraplegia

Spastic paraplegia in adults has often been reported in Asia and Africa. Thus out of 2530 consecutive neurological patients admitted to hospital in Baghdad, 84 had spastic paraplegia of uncertain origin (Al-Witry *et al.*, 1950). Many Indian hospitals could probably provide the same experience. In the former Belgian Congo, Lucasse (1952) found 34 cases in 117 villages. Spastic paraplegias, very similar to lathyrism, were reported amongst prisoners of war both in the Far East and in Egypt. The great majority of these patients had never at any time in their life eaten lathyrus, but had subsisted for many months on an inadequate diet. Cruickshank (1962) and Montgomery *et al.* (1964) report on 200 patients in Jamaica, of both sexes, between the ages of 10 and 70 with pyramidal tract damage. A quarter of the patients showed evidence of retrobulbar neuropathy and a few suffered from nerve deafness. The diet of Cruickshank's patients varied from good to very poor; they showed no overt signs of vitamin deficiency or malnutrition.

Toxic dietary factors may have a precipitating role in these cord syndromes but they have not yet been identified. Since 1965 there appears to have been little interest in this disease and it may now be much less common.

37. Lesser Nutritional Disorders

In this chapter an account is given of a variety of clinical conditions which are commonly found in malnourished people. For the most part they do not result in severe disability and are rarely a primary cause of complaint. They are usually found on the routine examination of school children, the medical inspection of a labour force, or at maternity and child welfare clinics.

Much has been written about the aetiology of each of these conditions. In general it may be said that the majority can arise from a variety of causes, both dietary and otherwise. The practical importance of these stigmata is that their presence should draw attention to the diet. A single case found in a prosperous community is likely to be due to a cause other than a dietary deficiency. When many cases are found in a poor community the diet is probably responsible, but accurate diagnosis can only be made by biochemical studies and the results of appropriate therapeutic trials.

DISORDERS OF THE SKIN

Follicular hyperkeratosis

The normal human skin contains pores, which are the openings of microscopic follicles. The secretions of the sebaceous and sweat-producing glands enter the follicles and reach the surface through these pores. Hairs emerge from their roots through the same follicles. In follicular hyperkeratosis the follicles become blocked with plugs of keratin derived from their epithelial lining which has undergone squamous metaplasia (Fig. 37.1). This pathological change has been attributed to vitamin A deficiency. Therapeutic trials in the East and in Africa have repeatedly shown that halibut-liver oil, red-palm oil or other oils rich in vitamin A or carotene may produce a striking clinical improvement in follicular hyperkeratosis; yet other factors may contribute to its development, such as exposure to sunlight, lack of cleanliness and deficiency of essential fatty acids and pyridoxine (Chowdury et al., 1954). Certainly follicular keratosis was not a regular feature in experimentally induced vitamin A deficiency in British adults (Hume and Krebs, 1949). It is rarely seen in very young children, the vulnerable age for xerophthalmia. A further difficulty is that slight follicular keratosis is not uncommon in British and other people who are adequately nourished in respect of vitamin A. Thus the condition is not a specific or constant feature of vitamin A deficiency.

The WHO (1976) report on vitamin A deficiency advises caution in assessing the significance of the occurrence of follicular keratosis.

The typical distribution is over the backs of the upper arms and the fronts of the thighs, but it may extend over the buttocks and indeed over the whole trunk. Only the feet, hands and face may be spared. Some degree of xeroderma (see below) is commonly associated. The horny plugs that project from the follicular orifices can often be pulled out with a fine pair of forceps; they give the skin a characteristic feeling of roughness, like that of a nutmeg grater. Because of its appearance, the condition has been called 'toad-skin' or phrynoderma. The appearance is distinct from the condition sometimes seen in scurvy, in which the hyperkeratosis is superficial and perifollicular—often with a small underlying haemorrhage—but without any projecting horny plug (Chap. 35).

Folliculosis This is sometimes mistaken for follicular hyperkeratosis. The follicles are raised above the surface, but no horny plug projects from the follicular orifices. It is

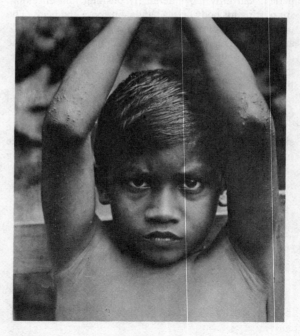

Fig. 37.1 Follicular hyperkeratosis. (By courtesy of Dr K. Mahadeva.)

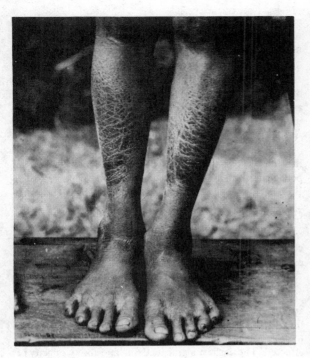

Fig. 37.2 Crazy-paving skin.

common on the backs of the arms of well-nourished British school children, and although its cause is unknown, there is no evidence that it has any nutritional significance.

Xeroderma
This means dryness of the skin. Instead of the normal smooth, moist, velvet texture, the skin feels dry and often rough. On uncovering the legs, a cloud of fine, branny dandruff is often seen. Xeroderma is commonly but not constantly associated with follicular keratosis and 'crackled skin'.

Crazy-paving skin
In this condition the appearance suggests a layer of lacquer painted on the surface, which on drying has broken up into individual islands of varying size (Fig. 37.2). There is often some desquamation from the borders of each island, while the intervening gaps may become fissured. The commonest site for this lesion is the shins, and it seems probable that exposure to dirt and alternate heat and moisture is often responsible.

Flaky paint dermatosis
This is characteristic of PEM. The skin becomes hyperpigmented and keratin separates in flakes which are larger than those in crazy-paving skin. It is common in the napkin area and often secondarily infected. Cure has been effected by an amino acid mixture devoid of vitamins.

Pachyderma (elephant skin)
This word was introduced by Nelson (1952) to describe a condition common in malnourished people. The areas of skin affected are thick, rough and thrown into folds like the skin of an elephant. It starts as a roughness of the skin on the back of the hands and feet, and the skin of the whole body may be affected. The changes are most marked at the back of the elbows and front of the knees. Fissures may occur round the heels. The condition is seen most often in boys and in the dry season.

It is obviously unwise to suggest that 'elephant skin', 'crazy-paving' and xeroderma are due solely to poor nutrition. On the other hand Nicol (1949) has demonstrated their probable nutritional significance by showing that these conditions are less common among Nigerians who eat red-palm oil (rich in vitamin A activity) than among those who do not.

Dyssebacea (nasolabial seborrhoea)
This term has been given to the appearance of enlarged follicles around the sides of the nose and sometimes extending over the cheeks and forehead. The follicles are plugged with dry sebaceous material which often has a yellow colour, for which reason Stannus originally coined the name 'sulphur flake' in describing the condition in malnourished Sudanese. It is commonly found in Africans with pellagra and may be related to riboflavin deficiency.

Atrophy of skin
In starving people and those suffering from serious undernutrition as a result of debilitating disease, the skin may be thin and inelastic. Over the front of the legs it appears shiny and tightly stretched. This is due to a general failure in the nutrition of the cells that are normally concerned with maintaining the skin in health and replacing losses of epithelium from the surface. It cannot be ascribed to dietary deficiency of any single nutrient.

Pigmentary changes and colour
Nutritional failure can affect the colour of the skin in many different ways. The dirty brown pigmentation of the skin in chronic undernutrition has already been described, as well as the patchy hyperpigmentation and depigmentation often associated with kwashiorkor. In pellagra there is typically an erythema with subsequent desquamation and pigmentation. The areas of skin especially involved are those exposed to sunlight or affected by friction. In anaemia the skin may be unduly pale. The hands of underfed children are often cyanosed, even in warm weather; while in cold, damp climates they may be affected by chilblains.

Chilblains, once common in Great Britain in wintertime, are seldom seen in North America where the houses are centrally heated. Nutritional deficiencies have often been blamed for chilblains, on no good grounds. Calcium, nicotinic acid, vitamin K and others have all been recommended for their treatment. Nicotinic acid may help by its vasodilator properties.

Tropical ulcer

Tropical ulcers were once of considerable interest to nutritionists but are now rarely discussed, probably because their prevalence is much reduced. They are chronic ulcers, affecting chiefly the lower limbs, occurring in hot, damp climates among people whose tissues are vitiated by malnutrition. They are often caused by minor injuries in people living in poor hygienic surroundings, debilitated by diseases such as dysentery and malaria. They used to be common in coolies employed on plantations; European prisoners of war working on the Burma-Siam railway were severely affected. *Fusobacterium fusiformis* and *Borrelia vincenti* are commonly present in the lesions. Tropical ulcers are not attributable to lack of a single nutrient, but their presence in any community or labour force is an indication that the diet and hygienic conditions are unsatisfactory.

Angular stomatitis

This is an affection of the skin at the angles of the mouth, characterised by heaping-up of greyish-white sodden epithelium into ridges, giving the appearance of fissures radiating outwards from the mouth (Fig. 37.3). Secondary infection and staining by food may give the lesion a yellowish colour. It may extend across the mucocutaneous boundary and produce whitish patches on the mucous

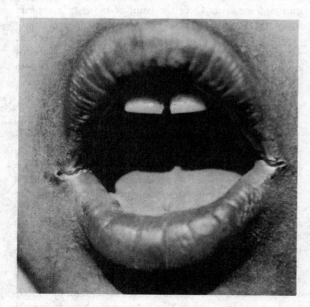

Fig. 37.3 Angular stomatitis. (By courtesy of Dr K. Mahadeva.)

membrane lining the cheeks. In differential diagnosis it must be distinguished from other lesions in the same site, notably herpes labialis, syphilitic rhagades and lichen planus.

Angular stomatitis often responds rapidly to large doses of riboflavin and sometimes to pyridoxine. It occurs in association with iron deficiency anaemia and other debilitating diseases. The most common cause in Britain is ill-fitting dentures.

Cheilosis. This is a zone of red, denuded epithelium at the line of closure of the lips. It is frequently seen in pellagrins and is often associated with angular stomatitis. Both lesions may have a seasonal incidence and only appear during periods of drought and lack of fresh foods; but it is unlikely that lack of any one specific vitamin or nutrient is the sole cause. The condition overlaps with chapped lips, seen in healthy people who have been exposed to cold winds or excessive sunlight.

Orogenital syndrome

In this condition there is angular stomatitis, but in addition there are changes in the epithelium of the mouth, tongue and lips, and other mucocutaneous junctions are affected. The earliest sign is oedema and milky opacity of the buccal mucosa which goes on to patchy or diffuse desquamation of the lips, tongue and sometimes soft palate. These areas are red and sensitive. Capillary oozing, with crusted blood on the lips and secondary infection with superficial ulceration may occur. Soggy, whitish patches at the outer angles of the eyes, within the ears, at the vulva or prepuce of the penis, and around the anus are often present. Associated with these changes there is often corneal vascularisation and a scaly, greasy eczema at the angles of the nose, on the lips, chin and behind the ears. A dry, intensely itching, erythematous dermatitis, with a well-defined edge, may appear on the genitalia—the scrotum or mons pubis, over the perineum and down the inner sides of the thighs. There is often secondary infection. The syndrome caused much distress among British prisoners of war in Japanese hands. It responds well to natural preparations of the vitamin B complex such as yeast extract (e.g. Marmite), though not to any single synthetic vitamin.

DISORDERS OF THE HAIR AND NAILS

In health the hair is sleek and glossy, often with a natural wave or curl. In malnourished or undernourished people the hair frequently becomes dull and lustreless; it is not easily brushed and tends to stand up straight ('staring hair'). At the same time the colour of the hair may change. In fair people it may turn to a dirty brown, while in black-haired people there may be loss of pigment, with a change of colour ranging from brown, rusty red to almost white.

This occurs in kwashiorkor (p. 258). The depigmentation is sometimes seen in bands across the length of each individual hair, corresponding to previous alternating periods of poor and relatively satisfactory nutrition—the flag sign.

Dietary factors such as deficiency of pantothenic acid (p. 150) or biotin can change the colour of the hair of black rats to grey, but the white or grey hair of human middle age has no nutritional significance. Nor is baldness a manifestation of nutritional failure.

In chronic iron deficiency anaemia the fingernails may be spoon-shaped (koilonychia). In other forms of malnutrition the nails may be brittle or thickened or lined on the surface, either transversely or longitudinally; but these changes may also be seen in well-nourished people. Severe protein deficiency may result in transverse white bands in the nails, occurring symmetrically on both hands (Muehrcke, 1956).

COMMENT

Until more is known about the chemical pathology of the skin, hair and nails it will continue to be difficult to assess the significance of certain clinical changes in these structures which are sometimes seen on examination of underfed or malnourished people. There have been many varying descriptions given of these signs, and equally many interpretations offered for them. A classic review of the large literature on the subject is by McCance and Barrett (1951).

DISORDERS OF THE EYE

Night blindness

It has already been explained in Chapter 13 that retinol plays an essential part in the mechanism of vision in dim light. Night blindness is a frequent complaint in underdeveloped communities who have no night lights and where the diet is grossly lacking in retinol and β-carotene. Children who stray from home after dark may get lost, or fall down a well or injure themselves in other ways. However, many factors besides retinol deficiency may contribute to complaints of night blindness. These include fatigue, emotional disturbances associated with acute danger and also chronic anxiety states. Moreover, there are organic causes such as retinitis pigmentosa. Night blindness arising from vitamin A deficiency always responds to suitable vitamin therapy and it is unwise to make the diagnosis before adequate therapeutic trials have been carried out.

In the past, night blindness has been a common complaint of the malingerer and is quickly learnt by others unless promptly dealt with. Unless the diet is known to be grossly deficient, or therapeutic trials have been carried out, it is best to assume that the cause is not nutritional.

Conjunctival xerosis

This has already been discussed as a manifestation of vitamin A deficiency (p. 273).

Bitôt's spots

Charles Bitôt was a French physician who first described, over 100 years ago, greyish or glistening white plaques formed of desquamated thickened conjunctival epithelium, usually triangular in shape and firmly adherent to the underlying conjunctiva. Sometimes the spots are covered with material resembling dried foam which can be scraped away but forms again. It consists of epithelial debris, fatty globules and often masses of xerosis bacilli. The spots are generally bilateral, on the temporal sides of the corneae, and in coloured races are often surrounded by dense brown pigmentation. In the past Bitôt's spots have often been associated with vitamin A deficiency and they are frequently present in children whose diet has been grossly lacking in this vitamin. However there is good evidence (Darby et al., 1960; Rodger et al., 1963; and others) that the condition can be present when there are no other signs of lack of vitamin A, including no impairment of dark adaptation, and the diet provides ample quantities of the vitamin or its precursor, β-carotene.

Pigmentation of the conjunctiva is frequently associated with xerophthalmia. Pigment may be deposited (1) round the cornea (pigmented ring), (2) in the lower eyelid (pigmented gutter), and (3) over the sclera equatorially in the area commonly occupied by Bitôt's spots. The nutritional significance of this pigment formation is uncertain. Various forms of irritation appear to play a major role in its causation.

Corneal vascularisation

The essential lesion in this condition is an invasion of the normally avascular cornea by capillary blood vessels. These vessels cannot be seen with the naked eye, nor with an ordinary hand lens. A slit-lamp microscope in the hands of an experienced observer is needed for positive identification. Small greyish-white opacities may also be seen on the surface of the cornea. The patient usually complains of a burning sensation in the eyes, misty vision, lachrymation and photophobia—the latter symptom may make slit-lamp examination difficult. Associated with the condition there is often injection of the conjunctiva with dilated blood vessels which are easily visible on simple inspection, without the use of a slit-lamp. However, the presence of an injected conjunctiva should not allow the assumption that a vascular cornea is also present. Corneal vascularisation may be associated with the orogenital syndrome, with keratomalacia and with ariboflavinosis.

Nutritional amblyopia (p. 299) is a major nutritional disorder of the eyes.

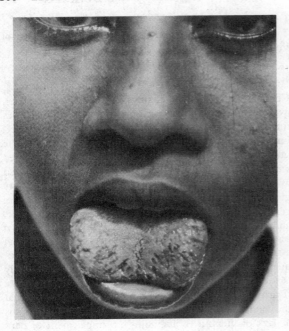

Fig. 37.4 Nutritional glossitis.

DISORDERS OF THE MOUTH

Angular stomatitis and cheilosis are described earlier in this chapter.

Nutritional glossitis

Deficiencies of nicotinic acid, riboflavin, vitamin B_{12}, folic acid and iron may all give rise to glossitis. It is a feature of pellagra, sprue and the various types of nutritional anaemias. The tongue seems to be particularly susceptible to metabolic disorders of all kinds. When a sudden and severe restriction in the supply of one or other of the above nutrients occurs, acute glossitis develops. If the deficiency is partial and extends over months or years, chronic atrophic glossitis is more often seen. In acute glossitis the tongue is swollen, sometimes to such an extent that it is continually pressed against the lower jaw and well-marked dental impressions are visible. The papillae are usually very prominent. The colour of the tongue is characteristically red, but in some cases it may have a purplish hue. The mucous membrane sometimes desquamates in patches leaving areas of red raw surface. Deep irregular fissuring is common and shallow ulcers may occur, especially on the sides or tip (Fig. 37.4). The tongue may be extremely painful, so much so that fear of pain may prevent the patient from eating.

There are those who claim to be able to distinguish the appearance of the tongue in nicotinic acid deficiency from that of vitamin B_{12}, folic acid or riboflavin deficiency; the last is said to be magenta in colour. But the distinction is not important as in nearly all cases there has been a multiple dietary deficiency of vitamins.

In chronic atrophic glossitis the tongue is small, with an atrophic mucous membrane and small or absent papillae so that its surface appears smooth, moist and abnormally clean. Fine fissuring may be present. It is usually not painful.

In pellagra the tongue responds dramatically to nicotinic acid, as is the case with the acute glossitis of pernicious anaemia treated with vitamin B_{12} or the glossitis of the sprue syndrome treated with folic acid.

The tongue of different individuals varies considerably. Some healthy people have patches on the tongue where the filiform papillae are absent. This geographical tongue is not related to disease. Others have a fissured or pigmented tongue. These normal variations can be confused with nutritional glossitis by inexperienced observers. The tongue is affected too by prolonged or severe dehydration.

Parotid gland enlargement

Swelling of the parotid glands is found among children in some parts of Africa and Asia. Raoul *et al.* (1957) made an extensive study of the condition in French West Africa and produce convincing evidence that the swellings are nutritional in origin, and lack of adequate protein a probable cause. The swellings may increase slowly and persist for years; on the other hand, with an improvement in the diet they may disappear quickly. The condition may readily be confused with mumps. Histological examination of the swollen gland shows hypertrophy of the acini. In the final state, fibrosis develops with cystic dilation of the ducts—a parotid cirrhosis.

The parotid glands are sometimes enlarged temporarily during the refeeding of people who have been severely undernourished.

COMMENT

The observing and recording of the signs described in this chapter is a useful aid to nutritional assessment, as discussed on page 464.

Diet and Other Diseases

38. Nutritional Aspects and Dietetic Treatment of General Diseases

Part III deals with nutritional diseases which are called primary because the principal or most obvious causation is the consumption of a diet with insufficient or excess sources of energy or lacking a proper balance of protein or other nutrients. In Part IV a number of diseases, many of which are common and well-known, are considered for one or both of two reasons: (1) the nature of the previous diet may play some part in aetiology which is multiple and complex, and (2) modification of the usual diet or the provision of a special diet reduces the metabolic burden on disordered organs or relieves symptoms and other manifestations of disease.

DIET AND DISEASES OF MULTIPLE AETIOLOGY

Most of the diseases described in Part IV cannot be attributed to a single major cause. Figure 38.1 may help understanding of the complexities of their aetiology. Its essence is a triad, inheritance (the genotype), favourable environmental influences (nurture) and unfavourable environmental influences (stress). The genotype represents inheritance which is complete at the moment of conception. From then onwards, including the intrauterine period, the constitution evolves under the continuing interaction of favourable and unfavourable factors in the environment. The nutritionist and dietitian should notice that the first item in the left-hand column of favourable environmental influences (nurture) is food. While it is true that 'we are what we eat' it is also true that 'we are what we are born' or in the language of biology 'we are what our environment allows our genotype to become'. Here the role of nutrition in the promotion of health and the role of malnutrition in the causation of a number of diseases are stressed, because these are the themes of the book. The perspective shown in Figure 38.1 is discussed more fully by Brock (1972) in a Croonian lecture.

Another feature shown in the figure is that the actions of nurture, including good diet, and of stress, including bad diet, often have to operate over very long periods of time before their effects become evident in an unhealthy constitution or a recognisable disease. Constitution is never fixed; in the same individual it may be healthy in one decade and unhealthy in another. Over short periods of time, the patient may fluctuate between health and disease,

even if he has a healthy constitution but, of course much more readily if he has an unhealthy constitution.

In the diseases known as **inborn errors of metabolism** (Chap. 39), a term introduced by Garrod in 1908, the major cause is a deficiency or error in a single gene. This is usually the result of spontaneous or induced mutation in one or both of the parents and becomes part of the genotype of the fetus. These diseases are therefore at least potentially present at the moment of conception. A concept 'one gene, one enzyme' evolved from Garrod's ideas

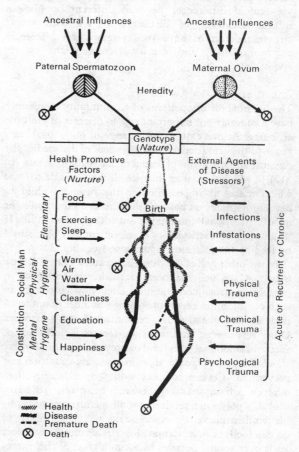

Fig. 38.1 Diagram illustrating relationships between genotype and environment, both favourable and unfavourable, in determining the development of constitution and life expectation, and of experience of health and disease.

and was first expressed by Beadle (1948). Several hundred such inborn errors of metabolism have since been described and probably many hundreds more remain to be discovered. Some of these undoubtedly account for idiosyncrasies of food preference, digestion and assimilation which come within the notice of dietitians. Although theoretically one enzyme is deficient because of one gene error, in many of the inborn errors there is evidence of aberration of several enzymes and presumably more than one gene is involved. These inborn errors of metabolism have to be sharply distinguished from **acquired congenital diseases** which though present at the time of birth are not due to genetic errors but to defects of the intrauterine environment exerted through the maternal tissues. Examples are the defects which have arisen when during pregnancy a mother has contracted rubella or received thalidomide.

Congenital defects can be produced in animals by feeding grossly defective diets during pregnancy. There are tenfold differences between different populations in the incidence of births of babies with severe structural defects of the nervous system. These differences are unexplained and dietary factors might be responsible.

HABITUAL DIETARY PATTERNS
The habitual dietary patterns of a community or a family have a complex but important role in diseases of multiple aetiology. At one extreme of a range of nutritional relevance to the causation and management of disease lies the classical inborn error of metabolism, galactosaemia (p. 317), in which there is an inherited lack of a single enzyme which makes it impossible for the newborn child to develop normally on nature's diet, human breast milk, or on the traditional community substitute, cow's milk. If diagnosed early, satisfactory development may be ensured by feeding the infant on a galactose-free diet.

In the other half of the range lies coronary heart disease (Chap. 41) which has been increasing in incidence in prosperous urban communities. Diets now customary in such communities constitute one of a number of unfavourable environmental causes responsible for this increase. Other responsible environmental factors include lack of exercise, emotional stress and cigarette smoking. All these should be given consideration in assessing causation and prevention. Certain families suffer more heavily than others which suggests that there may be an inherited basis, probably polygenic, rendering some members of susceptible families unable to metabolise normally high intakes of certain foods such as saturated fats. This metabolic defect leads over several decades to accumulation of cholesterol and the development of atherosclerosis in the coronary arteries. In the fourth and fifth decades of life other adverse environmental factors, which may include short periods of relative overindulgence in rich foods, may precipitate a thrombus in the atherosclerotic coronary arteries (coronary thrombosis).

Between the two extremes of this spectrum there lies a great range of diseases of multiple and uncertain origin in which conditioning may occur over decades in subjects who are rendered vulnerable by their basic inherited gene pattern (genotype); susceptible, that is, to the effects of unfavourable factors in their environment which would be better resisted by another genotype. The resultant phenotype or constitution is a diathesis or state of undue susceptibility to later events which precipitate a disease. The constitutional diathesis leads to few if any symptoms until the disease is precipitated, which may be in early childhood, in middle life, or only late in life.

The aetiology of gout (Chap. 43) might be represented somewhere in the middle of the range of nutritional relevance. Gout is clearly based on an inherited metabolic aberration which permits excessive endogenous purine synthesis. This aberration often does not become manifest until the fifth decade of life or later. It may be suggested by a family history of gout and diagnosed while still asymptomatic by a high concentration of plasma uric acid. It may remain undetected throughout life if the environment is favourable. If, on the other hand, this gouty constitution or diathesis is taxed by high intakes of exogenous purines, as in repeated overindulgent eating of rich protein meals and by much consumption of alcohol, an attack of acute gout is precipitated. If the dietary overindulgence is continued or periodically repeated, chronic gout may follow.

It is difficult to place diabetes mellitus (Chap. 42) at an appropriate point in the spectrum of relevance of diet to causation, although diet is of outstanding importance in management. It would appear that diabetes mellitus in its common juvenile and adult forms is a constitutional disease of multiple aetiology. There is evidence that, in the common clinical type associated with obesity in middle age, an important provoking cause is long-continued overconsumption of energy-yielding foods in relation to energy expenditure. This hypothesis underlies orthodox advice to people to avoid obesity particularly if they have a family history of diabetes. In juvenile diabetes it is likely that constitutional susceptibility (diathesis) is more important than habitual diet.

The common deficiency dyshaemopoietic anaemias (Chap. 48) fit well into the principles represented by Fig. 38.1. Dietary deficiency of the more important haemopoietic nutrients, iron, folate and vitamin B_{12} may be absolute or may be conditioned by other environmental factors. Chronic blood-loss and repeated pregnancies drain the iron stores of the body and increase the need for dietary iron. In idiopathic chronic iron-deficiency anaemia there is evidence of constitutionally impaired ability to absorb iron from the intestine. In classical pernicious anaemia there is a failure of intestinal absorption of vitamin B_{12}. This is classically constitutional; it has inher-

Table 38.1 Constitutional aberrations of which the effect may be neutralised or prevented by a diet, dietary modification or nutrient therapy

Aberration	Recommendation
Phenylketonuria	Low phenylalanine intake
Galactosaemia	No milk
Lactose intolerance	Limited milk
Sickle cell trait	Iron and folic acid supplements
Glucose-6-phosphate deficiency (favism)	No broad beans
High blood uric acid	Moderation at all times and especially at feasts
High plasma cholesterol	Low saturated fat
High blood pressure	Salt restriction
Gluten sensitivity	No wheat or wheat products
Various hypersensitivity states	No shellfish, eggs, milk or wheat etc.
Obesity	Low energy

ited roots and develops over decades in the form of gastric mucosal atrophy, probably the result of autoimmune mechanisms. Folate deficiency may be dietary or follow imparied digestion and absorption, and lead to megaloblastic anaemia. Increased demands arising from a constitutional disorder (sickle-cell trait) or in pregnancy may contribute in varying proportions to folic acid deficiency.

The figures given for recommended intakes of nutrients (Chap. 15) should not be taken to imply that the dietary needs of all men are alike if physiological and other stresses allowed for in the tables are the same. Such an assumption is of course demonstrably wrong in the case of some inborn errors of metabolism where 'one man's meat may be another man's poison'. Moreover there are among apparently healthy people many variations in response to daily diets which fulfil 'recommended intakes' of nutrients. Some grow fat and some stay thin (Chap. 25). Some are flatulent and some comfortable after meals. With further knowledge it may well appear that constitutional idiosyncrasies of digestion, assimilation and metabolism are responsible for a great variety of unidentified symptoms and minor ill-health and eventually contribute to certain chronic and degenerative diseases of middle age.

PROPHYLACTIC DIETARY REGIMES

Table 38.1 lists some constitutional aberrations, in which the expression of the genotype may be prevented or mitigated and the individual enjoy good health if he lives within certain dietary restrictions.

Emphasis is laid, because this is a book on nutrition and diet, on those dietary measures which can prevent or delay the onset of the symptoms of the disease. However in dealing with any of these constitutional abnormalities the physician should correct any apparent overemphasis on food and diet against the general perspective of other environmental or inherited factors which determine the development of healthy and unhealthy constitutions. In other words habitual dietary patterns, although important, constitute only a part of the total environment which shapes the constitution towards susceptibility to manifestations of disease. Prophylactic diets nevertheless constitute an important responsibility of physicians, paediatricians, nutritionists and health administrators. In the section on coronary heart disease (p. 337) it is shown that the nature of the diet probably contributes to the length of the life span in millions of people; this is one example of the potential value of the diet in prophylaxis.

THERAPEUTIC DIETARY REGIMES

Table 38.2 lists some disturbances of physiological function imposed upon the organs and tissues of the body by organic diseases. In each of these conditions the functional state of the organs and the patient's health can be made better or worse by the nature of the diet. Table 38.3 lists some symptoms which may be relieved by appropriate changes in diet. The elaboration and application of the above dietary regimes is particularly the sphere of dietitians. These diets and regimes have wide application but opinions have changed greatly about the value of some of them in the last two decades. For example, in many disorders of the gastrointestinal tract, such as peptic ulcer, therapeutic diets are now thought to have value in the relief of symptoms rather than in the cure of the disease. On the other hand, interest in therapeutic diets in chronic renal disease has grown following the success of haemodialysis and transplantation in prolonging the lives of many patients.

Whereas medical and nutritional science has provided a firm basis for some aspects of dietetic therapy, there remains much that is empirical. It is tempting to reject certain diets as having no scientific validity but the art of medicine is wider than the science. A patient is sometimes benefited by a remedy which has little or no scientific basis. The diets listed in Tables 38.1 and 38.2 all rest on some scientific basis. Some of those in Table 38.3 are used empirically.

GENERAL DIETETIC CONSIDERATIONS

When prescribing a diet it is essential to bear in mind the following points.

1. Be sure that the diet is well balanced and satisfactory in relation to energy, carbohydrates, protein and fat, with adequate minerals and vitamins. The recommended daily intakes of nutrients vary with age, sex, physiological state and activity. The energy intake has to be adjusted to the individual if the patient is not to gain or lose weight. Remember that if attention is directed solely to the dietetic treatment of a particular symptom, e.g. diarrhoea or gastric pain, the general nutrition of the patient may suffer.

2. Consider the patient's economic status and occupation and see that the dietary regime is suitable for each

Table 38.2 Disturbances of physiological function that may be mitigated by a dietary regime

Disturbance of physiological function	Disease	Therapeutic diet
Uraemia	Renal failure	Low protein
Excess protein loss in urine	Nephrotic syndrome	High protein
Oedema, generalised	Heart failure, renal disease, liver disease	Salt restriction
Failure to digest and absorb fat	Pancreatic disease, biliary obstruction, malabsorption syndromes	Low fat
Diminished glucose tolerance	Diabetes mellitus	Low sugar, often low energy
Excess acid and pepsin secretion by stomach	Peptic ulcer	Bland regime
Gluten enteropathy	Coeliac disease	No wheat or wheat products

case. Obviously different schemes will be required for an office worker, a miner and a night watchman.

3. The diet may need to be adjusted for the patient's religious practice. It is no use prescribing a midday meal for a Muslim during Ramadan, or pork for an orthodox Jew or a chicken curry for a strict Hindu.

4. Give due consideration to the individual's likes and dislikes for different articles of food. Never prohibit an article from a diet unless there is a clear history of a personal idiosyncrasy to it, or unless there is adequate clinical or experimental evidence for its exclusion.

5. The dietetic requirements of acute and chronic disease may be very different. Thus, in intense diarrhoea, excessive vomiting or infections which are severe in degree but short in duration (e.g. acute food poisoning and lobar pneumonia) the essential need is for fluids, glucose and salt to prevent or correct dehydration, ketosis and loss of electrolytes. In long-continued diseases, such as ulcerative colitis, the diet should be adequate both in quantity and quality, and if possible in variety.

6. Foods consumed away from home must be taken into account. This includes alcoholic drinks, sweets and confectionery and advice about eating in a restaurant.

Food idiosyncrasy

In medicine idiosyncrasy is a term used to describe an unusual effect not met with in a normal person. Idiosyncrasies to individual drugs and foods are common. Established causes of food idiosyncrasy are immunological disorders or allergies described in Chapter 50 and genetic abnormalities of specific enzyme systems described in Chapter 39. Some of these are serious disorders and major modifications of a patient's diet is necessary to prevent them.

Patients often say that a particular food does not agree with them. In most cases a dietitian drawing up a therapeutic diet should respect this view and may be able to plan a diet that excludes the food, and elaborate investigations of the cause of its adverse effect are not needed. While in some cases there may be an underlying organic disorder, often the patient simply dislikes the food and any symptoms which may arise from taking it are psychological in origin.

DIET SHEETS

The details of prophylactic and therapeutic dietary regimes are given in an appendix (p. 548); in various parts of the text the reader is referred to a numbered diet as one example of a type diet. Such type diets require to be modified by dietitians to suit the needs of individual patients in different parts of the world. The diets are based on British or North American foodstuffs which may be too

Table 38.3 Symptoms that may be relieved by dietary modifications

Symptom	Diseases present in	Recommendations
Dysphagia	Various diseases of the pharynx and oesophagus	Semifluid diet
Dyspepsia	Many causes, including peptic ulcer	Bland regime
Nausea	Liver disease, gallbladder disease etc.	Low fat
Chronic constipation	Dyschezia	High fibre
Chronic diarrhoea	Many causes	Bland regime
Loss of weight	Wasting diseases, burns, trauma	High energy

expensive, unavailable or not appreciated in other countries; then it is the task of dietitians to adapt the specimen diets to comparable local foodstuffs. A glossary on page 543 is designed to help dietitians and doctors to talk to patients who come from other areas or parts of the world and to understand diet sheets from the other side of the Atlantic.

In general, strict and rigid adherence to a dietary regime with accurate weighing of all foods is seldom needed except for short periods. As it requires close supervision by a dietitian, it is usually best done in hospital. A short period in hospital on a strict diet is often beneficial in that it teaches a patient what foods to avoid and how to judge the weight of a helping of food by eye. Thereafter he may be able to follow easily at home a less severe regime. This gradation is exemplified in diets for diabetes. Many patients who require dietary treatment have chronic diseases and the treatment may have to continue for a long time and often for life. Dietary restrictions are always irksome, but to a varying degree depending on the personality of the patient. When patients are seriously ill and cannot be expected to survive for a long period, it is seldom justifiable to add to their trouble by imposing a rigid adherence to a strict diet.

Therapeutic diets have an important role in modern medicine. Many patients do not get adequate advice and instruction, and as a result they may fail to derive full benefit from other forms of treatment. On the other hand therapeutic diets should always be used with common sense. The benefit to the patient likely to arise from improvement in his physical condition should outweigh the tedium of the restrictions on his enjoyment of food.

'There's many a slip twixt cup and lip.' Merely to hand a printed diet sheet to a patient across a desk is no guarantee that there will be any change in what the patient eats. Communication, though sometimes difficult, is the easiest first step in the complex and difficult task of persuading the patient to change his dietary habits. Diet sheets are only one tool in this task and should be supported by talks, demonstrations, sometimes group sessions and home visits, and then reinforced by arrangements for follow-up at suitable intervals.

39. Inborn Errors of Metabolism

Sir Archibald Garrod (1908) in his Croonian lectures to the Royal College of Physicians described four conditions: albinism, alkaptonuria, cystinuria and pentosuria. He produced evidence that these conditions were characterised by being genetically determined, present at birth and not constituting a disease, although persons with cystinuria might develop renal stones. He called these conditions inborn errors of metabolism and distinguished them from metabolic diseases, determined in part by genetic constitution, of which he gave gout, diabetes and obesity as examples.

This distinction has now been blurred. More than two hundred conditions have been described in which there is a metabolic defect, genetically determined and usually demonstrable at birth. In a few, as in Garrod's original cases, the defect does not lead to disease, but in many it is so severe that symptoms are manifest soon after birth. Such defects are often incompatible with normal development, especially of the nervous system; in such cases an infant may survive for only a few weeks or months, and, if adult life is reached, there is severe handicap. In other conditions the defect becomes manifest much later in life, perhaps as a result of metabolic strains imposed by environmental factors which may include diet.

Metabolic diseases form an important part of medicine and there are two large and deservedly famous textbooks devoted to them (Stanbury, Wyngaarden and Fredrickson, 1972; Bondy and Rosenberg, 1974) and there is a monograph on disorders of amino acid metabolism by Scriver and Rosenberg (1973). Our book deals with only part of the field. Diabetes, gout, the hyperlipidaemias and obesity are considered in separate chapters. Here we deal only with those other inherited metabolic diseases in which dietary treatment is or may be of value. First diseases of amino acid metabolism which may be treated by formula diets are considered. Then a brief summary is given of disorders which respond to vitamin therapy, usually in doses far above normal requirement. Lastly a brief account is given of certain disorders of carbohydrate metabolism in which diet therapy may be useful. As these diseases are rare, few doctors or dieticians have much experience of any one of them. A book by Francis (1975) describes the diets used at The Hospital for Sick Children, Great Ormond Street, London.

DISORDERS OF AMINO ACID METABOLISM

Over 50 conditions are known in which there is a defect in an enzyme system responsible for the intermediary metabolism of one of the amino acids. Table 39.1 lists those in which treatment by a diet with a reduced content of the amino acid concerned may be recommended. This may be either a low protein diet or a formula diet based on a suitable mixture of amino acids. The list may well be extended in the future. Phenylketonuria is the only one of these disorders in which a large number of patients have been successfully treated for over 20 years. This is described together with the lesser disorders of phenylalanine and tyrosine metabolism. The other disorders in Table 39.1 are all rare and there is only limited experience of their treatment.

Phenylketonuria

Phenylketonuria (PKU) is due to a genetic deficiency of phenylalanine hydroxylase, an enzyme essential for the conversion of phenylalanine to tyrosine. In consequence the blood and cerebrospinal fluid contain phenylalanine and its pyruvate, lactate and acetate derivatives greatly in excess of normal. As a result, damage to the brain occurs which may be severe and irreversible unless treatment is started at an early stage.

Clinical features. Mental deficiency, usually severe, is the most important clinical feature, but convulsions, tremor, rhythmic rocking of the body and posturing of the hands in front of the eyes also occur. Skin lesions such as dryness, roughness and eczema are common. However, the infant may progress normally at first and none of these changes may be observed before the age of 5 or 6 months. In addition to these mental, neural and dermal changes, the hair and skin of PKU children are often fairer and their eyes bluer than their unaffected siblings.

If effective treatment is begun in time, i.e. within the first few weeks or months of life, the clinical features can be prevented or, if already present, can be ameliorated. Unfortunately the results are far less satisfactory, especially in regard to the mental state, if treatment has been delayed beyond the first few months. Mental development may be restored but the early retardation can never be compensated for. In consequence early diagnosis is essential.

Table 39.1 Examples of inborn errors of amino acid metabolism which may be treated by formula diets

	Amino acids or organic acids increased in plasma	Biochemical lesion	Clinical features and treatment
PHENYLALANINE AND TYROSINE			
Phenylketonuria	Phenylalanine	Phenylalanine hydroxylase deficiency	Usually severe mental retardation, tremors, reduced skin and hair pigmentation. Treat with low-phenylalanine diet
Hyperphenylalaninaemia	Phenylalanine	Not known precisely; phenylalanine aminotransferase deficiency in some cases	May be normal depending on type. Treat if plasma phenylalanine above 200 mg/l
Hypertyrosinaemia	Tyrosine, phenylalanine	Transient p-hydroxyphenylpyruvic acid oxidase deficiency	Several clinical varieties and some forms asymptomatic; failure to thrive, cirrhosis and jaundice, renal tubular defects. Treat with low-phenylalanine, low-tyrosine diet
DEFECTS IN THE ORNITHINE CYCLE			
Argininosuccinic aciduria	Argininosuccinic acid citrulline	Argininosuccinate lyase deficiency	
Ornithine transcarbamylase deficiency		Ornithine carbamyl transferase deficiency	
Citrullinuria	Citrulline, methionine	Argininosuccinate-synthetase deficiency	Episodes of vomiting, restlessness, ataxia, convulsions, coma
Argininuria	Arginine	Liver arginase deficiency	
Carbamyl phosphate synthetase deficiency	Glutamine; also ammonia	Carbamyl phosphate synthetase deficiency	
Hyperornithinaemia	Ornithine, lysine, ammonia	Unknown	
BRANCHED-CHAIN AMINO ACIDS			
Maple-syrup urine disease	Leucine, isoleucine, valine and corresponding ketoacids	Branched-chain ketoacid decarboxylase deficiency	Neonatal difficulty in feeding, anorexia, convulsions, and other CNS signs
Hypervalinaemia	Valine	Not identified	Failure to thrive, vomiting, nystagmus
Propionic acidaemia			
Type A	Propionic acid	Propionyl CoA carboxylase deficiency	Neonatal severe acidosis
Type B	Glycine + +; also serine, alanine, glutamic acid	Propionyl CoA carboxylase deficiency	Neonatal vomiting, ketosis, neutropenia, thrombocytopenia, osteoporosis
HISTIDINE			
Histidinaemia	Histidine	Histidine ammonia lyase	Mental retardation; slurred, inarticulate speech. Low-histidine dietary treatment has been advised; results questionable
DIBASIC AMINO ACIDS			
Hyperlysinaemia	Lysine, ammonia	Lysine acyclase, lysine dehydrogenase, or lysine ketoglutarate reductase	Convulsions and coma related to protein feeding
SULPHUR-CONTAINING AMINO ACIDS			
Homocystinuria	Methionine	Cystathione synthetase deficiency	Mental retardation, ectopia lentis, skeletal features resembling Marfan's syndrome thromboembolic disease

Screening. As clinical diagnosis is impossible in the first weeks of life, mass screening of all infants is advised. This is done by determining blood phenylalanine at the end of the first week of life when feeding is well established. Testing, if carried out earlier, may yield false results or, if later, some brain damage may have already occurred. The Guthrie microbiological test is used in hospitals all over the world. It has displaced urine tests for phenylketones because these do not become positive until later and may even be negative when the blood phenylalanine level is dangerously high. In Scotland 105 cases of PKU were detected in 863 330 tests in 1965–77 and prevalence is just over 1 in 8000. Each year between 1 and 2 per cent of babies are not screened, and it is the important and difficult task of the health services to see that all babies are tested.

Treatment. This consists in giving the infant or child a diet containing a very small amount of phenylalanine. Since phenylalanine is one of the essential amino acids, normal growth does not occur if it is entirely excluded from the diet. However, if the daily intake of an infant is reduced from the normal of about 100 mg/kg body weight to between 20 and 60 mg/kg body weight, the child grows satisfactorily and the plasma phenylalanine concentration falls to between 30 and 100 mg/l. If it falls below 20 growth is likely to be impaired, and if it rises above 100 mental development may be retarded. The intake of phenylalanine should be adjusted to keep the concentration within this range. Since phenylalanine is present in all dietary proteins (2 g of milk protein contains about 100 mg) a baby has to be bottle-fed. Special infant foods with a low phenylalanine content are Minafen (Trufood Ltd) and Lofenalac (Mead Johnson Ltd). For older children complete synthetic diets are available commercially. A diet can also be made up using a phenylalanine-free preparation of beef serum albumin (Albumaid XP) or an amino acid mix (Aminogran) together with cream, butter, margarine, sugar and golden syrup as sources of energy. Phenylalanine-free rusks, bread and biscuits are also available commercially.

Children with PKU vary in their tolerance of phenylalanine. The tolerance of a child may also change from time to time, especially when he is suffering from an infection or any other disease in which there is a breakdown of tissue protein with release of phenylalanine. The plasma concentration of phenylalanine should be determined at frequent intervals and the diet adjusted, if necessary, to keep it within the range quoted above.

Tolerance rises with age and it is probably safe to stop dietary treatment at the age of 8 years (Smith and Wolff, 1974). This relieves the child of the severe emotional strains, inevitable with an artificial diet. The risk of subsequent mental deterioration is certainly slight, but has not yet been fully assessed. If in adult life a girl who has PKU decides to have children, the risk of her child having PKU should be pointed out. If she becomes pregnant, she should return to a low phenylalanine diet to avoid the risk of damage to the fetus.

Bringing up a child with PKU is a long arduous task beset with technical difficulties. A mother requires continuing advice and support from a paediatrician and a dietitian who both have specialised knowledge of this rare disease. With their help her child should grow up to be a physically and intellectually normal adult.

Variant forms. Screening has brought to light some cases of hyperphenylalaninaemia in which the biochemical defect differs from that in PKU. Such cases may be benign and not need treatment. However, it is recommended that all infants with a plasma phenylalanine above 200 mg/l should have their dietary intake restricted.

Hypertyrosinaemia

Screening has shown that a disorder of tyrosine metabolism is the commonest abnormality of amino acid metabolism in infants. Tyrosine is transaminated to *p*-hydroxyphenyl pyruvic acid (*p*-HPPA) which is then oxidised to fumarate and acetoacetate.

Activity of the enzyme responsible (*p*-HPPA oxidase) is often subnormal at birth and may be detected by finding a plasma tyrosine concentration above 50 mg/l. This occurs in about 0.5 per cent of breast-fed babies, in 5 per cent of those artificially fed and in 50 per cent of infants born preterm. Normal activity of the enzyme is in the vast majority of cases reached before the age of 4 months. This **transient hypertyrosinaemia** is accentuated by deficiency of vitamin C and by a high protein intake. In the majority of these children there are no clinical effects and the prognosis is good. However, it is possible that there may be some impairment of development of the brain. For this reason it is important to ensure that all preterm and artificially fed infants have a supplement of vitamin C.

Partial *p*-HPPA deficiency is a rare but serious condition which leads to failure to thrive and disorders of the liver and kidneys. Such children should be given a formula diet low in tyrosine and phenylalanine.

DIETARY TREATMENT OF OTHER DISORDERS

The disorders listed in Table 39.1 may all in theory be treated by restricting the intake of a specific amino acid or the total protein intake. However, they are all rare and, except for PKU and hypertyrosinaemia, knowledge about their natural history and response to treatment is limited.

Propionic acidaemia

This leads to severe and often fatal attacks of ketoacidosis in the neonatal period. These may be prevented by a formula diet in amounts providing only 0.5 g of protein/kg body weight and biotin (5 mg twice daily) may be effective. It is difficult to raise a child on such restricted intakes of protein and the long-term effects of treatment have not yet been evaluated.

Defects in the ornithine cycle

As the amino acids involved in this group of disease are non-essential and produced endogenously, restriction of specific amino acids is useless. Treatment by lowering the protein intake to 0.5 to 1.0 g/kg body weight has been effective in some cases.

Maple-syrup urine disease

Beneficial results follow the use of a formula diet low in leucine, isoleucine and valine. As the intake of each of these branched-chain amino acids has to be adjusted in relation to plasma concentration, control of the abnormality is much more difficult than in PKU. Nevertheless some infants have been successfully reared, and older children's diets can be devised based on gelatin, gluten-free flour, butter, margarine, sugar and fruits with a low protein content. In hypervalinaemia, in which only one amino acid is affected, a formula diet low in valine has been used.

Hyperhistidinaemia and hyperlysinaemia

These may also be treated with formula diets, but the results of restricting histidine intake in this way have not always been satisfactory. On the other hand, it has been found that approximately half of the late diagnosed and untreated cases are not mentally retarded. The decision whether to treat a child found to have hyperhistidinaemia in the neonatal period is a difficult one and it has been suggested that an international collaborative study is needed (Popkin et al., 1974).

Homocystinuria

A low protein, low methionine diet can reduce the raised plasma methionine, and infants in which the diagnosis has been made at birth are being successfully raised on such diets. Some but not all infants with cystathione synthetase deficiency respond to large doses (200 to 500 mg/day) of pyridoxine. Homocystinuria may also arise from other genetic or acquired defects, and the condition is not a clinical entity. For the precise diagnosis and a decision as to what form of treatment to give, an affected child should be referred to a special centre.

DISORDERS RESPONDING TO VITAMIN THERAPY

Table 39.2 lists conditions which usually respond to treatment with a vitamin, often in doses far above the physiological requirement. Some present in infancy, others later in life. In most of them a specific defect in an enzyme system has been identified. Almost certainly all are genetic in origin, but this has not been established in some instances where only two or three cases have been observed.

The evidence suggests strongly that each case has a specific defect and is not the extreme end of a normal distribution curve. If the latter was correct, then it would be expected that a much larger number of cases with less severe symptoms would have been identified.

DISORDERS OF CARBOHYDRATE METABOLISM

Pentosuria, one of the four inborn errors described by Garrod, is benign and requires no treatment. The various abnormalities that may lead to glucose appearing in the urine and to lactose intolerance are discussed in the chapters on diabetes and gastrointestinal diseases. Here an account is given of disorders affecting the metabolism of galactose and fructose, and of those varieties of glycogen storage disease in which dietary treatment may be given.

Galactosaemia

Galactosaemia is due to a specific deficiency of galactose-1-phosphate uridyl transferase, the enzyme required for the conversion of galactose to glucose. The metabolic block occurs between galactose-1-phosphate and glucose-1-phosphate.

It is probable that the clinical and pathological features of galactosaemia are not due to the excess galactose in the body fluids, but to toxic effects resulting from intracellular accumulations of galactose-1-phosphate or one of its derivatives.

Clinical features. The clinical picture varies in severity from case to case. In its severe form the disorder may be manifest in infants within two or three weeks after birth, as indicated by vomiting, difficulty in feeding, loss of weight and the onset of jaundice. In such patients the spleen may be palpable and the liver greatly enlarged and very firm, and ascites may be present. Examination of the urine shows the presence of sugar (galactose) and also protein. Without immediate dietetic treatment of such severe cases death rapidly occurs. In mild to moderate cases the diagnosis may be missed because of the failure of the doctor to examine the urine of an infant who has infrequent vomiting and who is not thriving. If the disorder is allowed to continue for months, cataracts are likely to develop and these may lead in time to blindness. Mental and physical retardation are also likely to occur.

Screening. This can be carried out on the sample of blood used for PKU testing. In Scotland six cases were detected in 1969–79 and prevalence is about 1 in 80 000.

Treatment. Succesful treatment requires early diagnosis and involves the complete exclusion of lactose and galactose from the diet. If this is accomplished successfully and in time, the hepatic, mental, physical and ocular changes may be prevented. Even when pathological alterations have occurred in the liver, kidney and eye, these may be reversed or improved. In addition the proteinuria and

Table 39.2 Examples of inherited metabolic diseases which involve or respond to vitamins

Name of condition	Description	Numbers and genetics
Thiamin		
Thiamin-responsive maple-syrup urine disease (Scriver et al., 1971)	Delayed neurological development; increased branched-chain As in plasma; response to thiamin, 10 mg/day; TPP is coenzyme for oxidative decarboxylation of branched-chain oxo-acids. (Most cases of MSU disease do not respond to thiamin)	One female infant
Thiamin-responsive lactic acidosis (Brunette et al., 1972)	Hypoglycaemia on and off from birth, acidosis with accumulation of lactate; dramatic response to thiamin; deficient pyruvate carboxylase activity in liver biopsy	One female infant
Nicotinamide/tryptophan		
Hartnup disease (Jepson, 1966)	Intermittent pellagra-like skin rash with temporary cerebellar ataxia; renal aminoaciduria of characteristic pattern (the monoamino, monocarboxylic As, including tryptophan); indicanuria; impaired intestinal absorption of tryptophan and other As; skin and neurological features appear to respond to nicotinamide	23 cases reported, first from England; recessive inheritance
Hydroxykynureninuria (Komrower et al., 1964)	Mild mental deficiency, short stature, rash on buttocks and stomatitis; hydroxykynureninuria on ordinary diet; response to nicotinamide	One female child; mother showed biochemical abnormality
Pyridoxine		
Pyridoxine-dependent infantile convulsions (Coursin, 1964)	Convulsions, hyperirritability and hyperacousis immediately after birth; normal tryptophan load test, no biochemical abnormalities found; responds to 10 mg pyridoxine daily by mouth which must be continued for years	Cases reported from several countries; some familial; recessive, commoner in girls
Cystathioninuria (Frimpter, 1966)	Large amounts of cystathionine in urine and plasma reduced by pyridoxine; mental retardation and congenital defects, pituitary abnormalities and bleeding tendency; pyridoxal phosphate is coenzyme for cystathioninase	11 cases, each a single case in a family; heterozygotes have mild cystathioninuria
Pyridoxine-responsive hypochromic anaemia (Harris et al., 1964)	Hypochromic anaemia, with high serum iron and increased iron stores; no response to iron treatment; may show increased xanthurenic acid after tryptophan; bone marrow hyperplastic; respond, but not always, to large doses of pyridoxine (20 to 100 mg/day); affected enzyme is presumably δ-aminolaevulinic acid synthetase	Usually presents in young adults; 22 out of 72 cases were familial; onset can be in early childhood or even infancy; males preponderate
Homocystinuria (Brenton and Cushworth, 1971)	Some cases respond to very large doses of oral pyridoxine, 200 to 500 mg/day	Autosomal recessive
Xanthurenic aciduria (Tada et al., 1968)	Exaggerated urinary excretion of xanthurenic acid after oral tryptophan; some response to large doses of pyridoxine; a few cases mentally defective	Familial, and 15 of the 18 reported cases have been female
Biotin		
Propionic acidaemia (some cases) (Barnes et al., 1970)	Severe neonatal ketoacidosis; accumulation of propionic acid; defect in propionyl-CoA carboxylase; responded to biotin, 10 mg/day	One case reported
Folic acid		
Congenital isolated defect in folate absorption (Lanzkowsky, 1970)	Megaloblastic anaemia in first year of life, low plasma and RBC folate; mental retardation, seizures, and extrapyramidal symptoms; defect in folate absorption and transport into CSF; haemoglobin and blood folate normal on 40 mg/day folic acid by mouth but fits more frequent	One case, and two others in the literature which differed in some details

Table 39.2—*continued*

Name of condition	Description	Numbers and genetics
Folic acid (contd.)		
Congenital formimino; transferase deficiency (Arakawa, 1970)	Retarded mental and physical development; increased plasma folate (over 50 μg/l), normal vitamin B_{12}; megaloblastic anaemia in only 1 case; increased urinary FIGLU after oral histidine; formiminotransferase activity in liver decreased but other THFA enzymes normal	Four cases, two of whom were siblings whose parents appeared healthy but showed increased FIGLU after histidine (Japan)
Vitamin B_{12}		
Familial selective vitamin B_{12} malabsorption with proteinuria (Mackenzie *et al.*, 1972)	Megaloblastic anaemia in late childhood, responsive to parenteral vitamin B_{12}; normal transcobalamin II; malabsorption of vitamin B_{12} but other intestinal functions normal, with intrinsic factor and acid in gastric juice; normal ileal mucosa. Renal function normal	Thirty four cases in literature many of them familial
Congenital lack of intrinsic factor (McIntyre *et al.*, 1965)	Vitamin B_{12}-responsive megaloblastic anaemia; gastric mucosa and acid normal but no intrinsic factor; no antibodies to intrinsic factor; onset in early life	Several case reports; familial tendency
Neonatal megaloblastic anaemia due to inherited transcobalamin II deficiency (Hakami *et al.*, 1971)	Onset within a few weeks of birth; failure to thrive, megaloblastic anaemia with normal serum vitamin B_{12}; response to injections of 1 mg vitamin B_{12}; low plasma unsaturated B_{12} binding capacity and virtually absent transcobalamin II	Two siblings affected; several other members of family had reduced transcobalamin II only (USA)
Deficiency of vitamin B_{12} binding alpha globulin (transcobalamin I) (Carmel and Herbert, 1969)	Persistent lack of transcobalamin I, manifested only by low plasma vitamin B_{12} with few or no other signs of deficiency	Two affected brothers
Vitamin B_{12} responsive (dependent) methyl malonicaciduria (Mahoney and Rosenberg, 1970)	Ketoacidosis in neonatal period; large amounts of methylmalonic acid in urine; normal plasma vitamin B_{12} and no anaemia; responds well to pharmacological doses of B_{12} (e.g. 1 mg I.M. bi-weekly); biochemical defect in forming 5'-deoxyadenosyl coenzyme of B_{12}	Six cases, all unrelated; autosomal recessive inheritance suggested
Vitamin A		
Failure of enzymic cleavage of β-carotene (McLaren and Zekian, 1971)	Night blindness, Bitôt's spots; very low plasma retinol with high β-carotene, no retinyl ester in plasma after β-carotene by mouth	One case, a girl with consanguineous parents (Lebanon); onset at age 7 years
Vitamin D		
Hereditary vitamin D-resistant rickets with hypophosphataemia (Williams *et al.*, 1966; Glorieux *et al.*, 1972)	Hypophosphataemia always present; plasma calcium not reduced and no aminoaciduria; primary abnormality of phosphate re-absorption in renal tubule; rickets in early childhood can lead to deformities and dwarfism or osteomalacia; responds to large doses of vitamin D (e.g. 2.5 mg/day), but vitamin D intoxication can occur; best treatment probably with oral phosphate	Transmitted as an X-linked dominant; many reported cases
Fanconi group of conditions with rickets/osteomalacia and renal tubular defects (Dent, 1969)	Rickets or osteomalacia with hypophosphataemia, resistant to vitamin D in usual doses; renal glycosuria and a generalised aminoaciduria; usually a defect of renal acidification and hypokalaemia; cystinosis in affected children	May be inherited as a recessive, or acquired (e.g. heavy metal poisoning)
Primary renal tubular acidosis (Seldin and Wilson, 1966)	Persistent form usually affects females in late childhood; chronic acidosis; osteomalacia, nephrocalcinosis, and nephrolithiasis; increased urinary phosphate and calcium, serum calcium and phosphorus normal or reduced; treatment of acidosis with citrate; vitamin D not usually required	Sporadic or familial; inheritance dominant in some of latter

galactosuria disappear. Until recently the preparation of a galactose-free diet for infants presented great difficulty as this entails the rigid exclusion of milk, which is the main dietary source of galactose. Many technical difficulties are encountered when an attempt is made to remove all the lactose from casein. Fortunately, there are now available commercial synthetic milk powders in which lactose has been replaced by dextrin, dextrose and maltose (Galactomin—Trufood Ltd; Low Lactose Milk Food—Cow and Gate). For those infants with a hypersensitivity to even very small amounts of lactose in the diet, a malt and soya flour food (Wanderlac) manufactured by A. Wander Ltd has been recommended. When suitably diluted with water this forms a vegetable milk equal in value to cow's milk. Mixed feeding should be started early and, as a child gets older, it becomes much easier to provide a lactose-free diet. Older children may acquire some tolerance, perhaps by the development of an alternative pathway for galactose metabolism in the liver. Details of treatment are given by Donnell and Lieberman (1970).

Galactokinase deficiency

Lack of the enzyme galactokinase also causes galactosaemia and galactosuria, but mental development is normal and enlargement and damage to the liver does not occur. Galactokinase catalyses the conversion of galactose to galactose-1-phosphate. However, cataracts leading to blindness develop in childhood. They can be prevented by strict exclusion of lactose from the diet.

Fructose intolerance

This condition is due to lack of the aldolase which converts fructose-1-phosphate to dihydroxyacetone phosphate and glyceraldehyde. When fructose is ingested, fructose-1-phosphate accumulates in the liver; this interferes with release of glucose from the liver and leads to severe hypoglycaemia. Infants are free of symptoms unless given sugar (sucrose). Then there may be vomiting and hypoglycaemic fits, and a series of episodes may lead to jaundice and enlargement of the liver. Treatment consists of excluding sucrose and fruit from the diet. This is easy in an infant, but is a formidable problem for a mother as her child grows up. Fortunately the condition is very rare. It has been noticed that the teeth of patients with fructose intolerance do not show caries.

Glycogen storage diseases

Ten types of this group of rare disorders are now recognised. Precise diagnosis depends on finding in a biopsy of liver or muscle a defect in one of the several enzyme systems concerned with glycogen storage.

Type I is due to a low activity of glucose-6-phosphatase in liver. Under its old name of von Gierke's disease, it is the best known of the group because, although very rare, many patients survive into adult life. Growth is retarded and there is marked enlargement of the liver, so that the abdomen is protruded. There is a history of episodes of ketosis and hypoglycaemia. Mental development is retarded only if episodes of hypoglycaemia have been frequent and severe. Dietary management consists in preventing such attacks, which arise as a result of inability to maintain the concentration of blood sugar by mobilising glycogen. A diet high in protein promotes gluconeogenesis from amino acids and so helps to maintain blood sugar. In severe cases frequent feeds, every 3 to 4 hours may be required. A moderate amount of carbohydrate is permissible, but this should be in the form of glucose or its polymer, starch. Both sucrose and lactose should be avoided, because fructose and galactose are readily converted to glycogen in the liver. As the child grows up attacks of hypoglycaemia become less severe.

Similar dietary measures may be tried in types III, VI and X in which hypoglycaemia may also occur due to diminished activity of other enzyme systems. In these conditions, all very rare, experience of the value of dietary treatment is limited.

MANAGEMENT IN GENERAL

Screening may detect a plasma concentration of an amino acid or other compound slightly above normal; then it may be uncertain whether this will lead to any impairment of development; if so, lowering the concentration by dietary restriction serves no purpose. On the other hand, the defect may be so severe that without treatment the infant would not be expected to live more than a few months or years. Treatment may prolong life, but not lead to a normal life. It is not right to ask a mother to undergo the great strain of raising an infant on a formula diet, if the end result is likely to be little better than a deformed cabbage. Only time and experience will enable appropriate advice to be given to mothers. There is also the question of cost-effectiveness to the community. To raise a PKU child on a formula diet costs many thousands of pounds, but this a much smaller sum than that required to keep an untreated child in an institution for many years. As most of the diseases listed in Tables 39.1 and 39.2 are very rare, it will inevitably be many years before the long-term effects of treatment are fully known, and can be properly appraised.

Most of the disorders briefly mentioned in this chapter are so rare that a doctor might spend a lifetime in practice without having to be responsible for the care of a single case. Whenever it appears possible that a patient is suffering from one of them, the advice of a special centre should be sought both for diagnosis and treatment. As a result of knowledge slowly accumulated, worthwhile therapy is becoming available for a small but increasing proportion of these diseases.

40. Hyperlipidaemias. Diet and Plasma Lipids

Three metabolic disorders are common in prosperous communities; they are elevation of blood glucose, i.e. diabetes mellitus (Chap. 42), elevation of plasma urate, which is associated with gout (Chap. 43) and elevation of one or more plasma lipids, hyperlipidaemia. All affect especially middle-aged, sedentary people and tend to occur in combinations of two or three in the same individual. Thus some types of hyperlipidaemia are common in diabetics, and hyperuricaemia is associated with diabetes and some types of hyperlipidaemia. All three disorders are associated with obesity.

The triad have other features in common. Their appearance is partly determined by inheritance, partly by a rich diet. Though often asymptomatic and detected only by a blood test, each has acute complications, which respond promptly to treatment; in some types of hyperlipidaemia eruptive xanthomatosis and severe abdominal pain occur and these clinical features are analogous to the coma and acute arthritis which may complicate diabetes and hyperuricaemia respectively. All three disorders also have long-term complications. These affect mostly the cardiovascular and renal systems; coronary atherosclerosis is the most important and is common to diabetes, hyperuricaemia and most of the hyperlipidaemias. Late complications cannot be easily treated and the need to develop scientifically based methods of prevention is the main reason for detection, understanding and judicious management of the hyperlipidaemias. Most people with hyperlipidaemia have no symptoms and often the only sign is that one of the plasma lipids is above the normal range. The questions a doctor has to answer are what type of biochemical abnormality is present, what are the probable chances of late complications such as atherosclerosis and what treatment should be advised and persevered with in the absence of present symptoms. As with diabetes and hyperuricaemia, an appropriate diet is a major and sometimes the only necessary treatment for hyperlipidaemia.

Unlike hyperglycaemia and hyperuricaemia there are several distinct types of hyperlipidaemia. There are two major neutral lipids that may be present in increased concentrations in the plasma, cholesterol and triglycerides. They are often accompanied by an increased concentration of phospholipids but phospholipids are not elevated on their own. In the early 1960s the hyperlipidaemias were classified into hypercholesterolaemia, in which the plasma is clear; lipaemia or hypertriglyceridaemia in which the plasma is milky or creamy in appearance, and a combination of hypercholesterolaemia and hypertriglyceridaemia. Ahrens *et al.* (1961) pointed out that lipaemia may be exogenous and induced by dietary fat or endogenous and induced by carbohydrate via the liver. We now know that endogenous hypertriglyceridaemia is much the commoner and that it is induced not only by carbohydrate. In 1967 Fredrickson *et al.* published a classic series of papers in which they classified the hyperlipidaemias into five types (Table 40.1) depending on which lipoprotein was increased in concentration in the plasma. They recommend the name hyperlipoproteinaemia for these conditions because lipids only occur in plasma carried on lipoprotein molecules, and the ratio of cholesterol, triglycerides and phospholipid in the different hyperlipoproteinaemias can be predicted from the lipid composition of the major lipoprotein classes (Table 6.2, p. 51). Although hyperlipoproteinaemia is the more correct term, these disorders are nearly always detected by measuring plasma lipids as such and we generally use the shorter term hyperlipidaemia.

This systematic description of the hyperlipidaemias showed that hypercholesterolaemia and hypertriglyceridaemia were not complete biochemical diagnoses, and stimulated the setting up of lipid or hyperlipidaemia clinics in many medical centres. With experience it became clear that it was not possible to fit every case into one of the five types. There are intermediate and mixed types, the most common of which is the combination of raised low density lipoproteins (LDL) with some elevation of very low density lipoproteins (VLDL). This was designated type IIB in an extension of the classification to six types (Table 40.1) published in 1970 by WHO in collaboration with Fredrickson (Beaumont *et al.*, 1970).

As a rule a patient's lipoprotein type can be worked out from serum or (EDTA) plasma cholesterol and triglyceride, and paper electrophoresis of lipoproteins, together with the clinical findings. The blood should be taken before breakfast and 12 hours after a meal, which allows complete clearing of normal alimentary lipaemia. The patient should be on his usual diet. It is no use determining the lipoprotein type during an acute illness. For example, plasma cholesterol falls after a myocardial infarct (Watson *et al.*, 1963) so accurate typing can only be done one to two months after the infarct; triglycerides are increased by inactivity and both lipids can rise following mental stress.

Table 40.1 Hyperlipoproteinaemias

Type	Names	Lipoproteins increased in plasma	Lipids increased in plasma	Main features
I	Hyperchylomicronaemia. Fat-induced or exogenous hypertriglyceridaemia or lipaemia	Chylomicrons	Triglycerides	Rare, usually recessive disorder, presenting in childhood; eruptive xanthomata, abdominal pain, enlarged liver and spleen; responds to very low fat diet
IIA	Pure hypercholesterolaemia. Familial hypercholesterolaemia	LDL (β)	Cholesterol	Usually a genetic dominant disorder; heterozygous form common in young adults; tendon xanthomata, corneal arcus, accelerated coronary atherosclerosis
IIB	Mixed hyperlipidaemia (one form)	LDL (β) +VLDL (pre-β)	Cholesterol Triglycerides	More often acquired than genetic; may be due to rich diet; common in affluent countries; xanthomata and tendency to CHD similar to type IIA
III	'Floating β' or 'broad β' disorder	Floating β lipoprotein	Cholesterol Triglycerides	Uncommon, genetic recessive disorder seen in adults; tuberose and palmar xanthomata as well as tendon; associated with atherosclerosis
IV	Endogenous or carbohydrate-induced hypertriglyceridaemia or lipaemia	VLDL (pre-β)	Triglycerides	Common, especially in middle-aged men in affluent countries; often associated with obesity and glucose intolerance; usually no clinical manifestations, appears to predispose to atherosclerosis
V	Mixed lipaemia	VLDL (pre-β) + chylomicrons	Triglycerides (cholesterol)	Uncommon, usually secondary to metabolic disease, e.g. uncontrolled diabetes; eruptive xanthomata, sometimes abdominal pain; often an acute disorder which changes to type IV as plasma lipids fall with treatment

In any patient who is reported to have an increased plasma cholesterol or triglycerides, the first action should be to arrange for the measurements to be repeated after an overnight fast.

Estimations of cholesterol by methods used in routine clinical biochemistry laboratories have a fairly high variance (Whitehead *et al.*, 1973). For reference and research purposes the method of Abell *et al.* (1952) is commonly used; in this the lipids are extracted and saponified and the colour produced by the Lieberman-Burchard reaction is a measure of the cholesterol. Moderate and severe degrees of hypertriglyceridaemia can be detected by the milky appearance of the serum or plasma. When this is seen, triglycerides should be measured by a method such as that of Van Handel and Zilversmit (1957). If the lipaemia results from chylomicrons the plasma develops a layer of cream after standing for some hours in a refrigerator; in type IV this does not happen, the plasma remaining turbid throughout. Plasma for lipoprotein electrophoresis should not be kept in the deep freeze because freezing breaks up chylomicrons and some other lipoproteins. The simplest way of demonstrating the lipoprotein pattern is by electro-

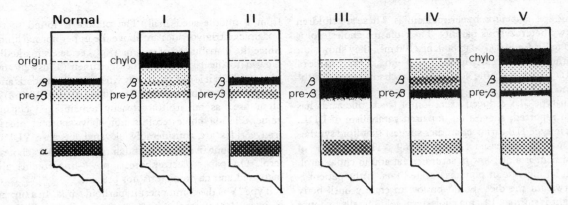

Fig. 40.1. Paper electrophoresis in five types of hyperlipoproteinaemia (Roberts *et al.*, 1970).

phoresis, e.g. on paper in buffer containing plasma albumin. Other support media, such as cellulose acetate or agarose, can be used. The stained bands give a semiquantitative idea of which lipoproteins are increased; with experience they can usually be interpreted provided the quantitative cholesterol and triglyceride values are known. Only in a minority of cases is it necessary to use more elaborate techniques such as ultracentrifugation or immunochemical precipitation of specific lipoproteins. The pattern of lipoproteins shown by paper electrophoresis in the different types of hyperlipidaemia is illustrated in Fig. 40.1.

THE HYPERLIPIDAEMIAS

Type I hyperlipidaemia

The alimentary lipaemia, seen after a meal containing fat, is not cleared at the normal rate and chylomicrons persist in the blood on an ordinary diet. This rare type usually presents in childhood; it is often familial and appears to be the homozygous form of a rare autosomal mutant. The child may present with abdominal pain, and pancreatitis can occur. The liver and spleen are enlarged. There are eruptive xanthomata, small yellow skin nodules on a faintly erythematous base, which appear when the plasma triglycerides are very high. Lipaemia may be visible in the retinal veins (lipaemia retinalis). Plasma triglycerides are very high and though cholesterol may be moderately elevated the TG:cholesterol ratio is about 10:1. There is a massive band of chylomicrons at the origin on paper electrophoresis. Post-heparin lipolytic activity of the plasma (p. 52) is grossly defective. Treatment is with a very reduced fat intake, usually 25 to 30 g/day or sufficiently low to keep the patient asymptomatic (e.g. Diet 10). Medium-chain triglycerides can help make the diet more palatable because they do not form chylomicrons. However, they are expensive and there is little knowledge of their long-term effect. No drugs are effective. Type I

hyperlipidaemia is not associated with diabetes and does not predispose to atherosclerosis. Affected children appear to grow out of the disturbance to some extent as they get older.

Type II hyperlipidaemia

Type IIA is usually a dominant genetic disorder which can be detected if the blood is examined early in childhood and sometimes in cord blood (Kwiterovich *et al.*, 1973). It persists throughout life. Affected members in a family with this disorder can be recognised by comparing their plasma cholesterol with the normal for age, which is lower in children than adults, and cases can be recognised with greater precision by measuring plasma LDL. Type IIB may be either genetic (Nikkilä and Aro, 1973) or acquired. It has been suggested that mild degrees of this type commonly result from a rich diet. Both types may be secondary to other diseases, including diabetes, the nephrotic syndrome and hypothyroidism. In heterozygous adults the plasma cholesterol is usually 7.8 to 9.0 mmol/l (300 to 350 mg/100 ml). With increasing age, clinical signs of hypercholesterolaemia may be detected. These are tendon xanthomata, corneal arcus and xanthelasma of the eyelids. Tendon xanthomata most commonly affect the Achilles tendons, which show a uniform thickening; xanthomata may also cause nodules in the extensor tendons of the fingers. Corneal arcus suggests hypercholesterolaemia if seen in a young adult; over the age of 40 it is more likely to be a non-specific degenerative change. The presence of xanthelasma is an indication for measuring the plasma cholesterol but this lesion sometimes occurs in people with normal plasma lipids. The most important characteristic of types IIA and B is their association with accelerated atherosclerosis, particularly of the coronary arteries. Slack (1969) estimates that men with type II have a 5 per cent chance of a first attack of CHD by the age of 30, 51 per cent by the age of 50 and 85 per cent by age 60.

Because familial hypercholesterolaemia is fairly common, homozygotes are encountered occasionally in any clinic specialising in hyperlipidaemias. These are children of two heterozygous parents. Their plasma cholesterol is 18.5 to 21 mmol/l (700 to 800 mg/100 ml), they show skin xanthomata from early in childhood and are likely to die of CHD before reaching adult life (Khachadurian and Uthman, 1973).

In type IIA reduced excretion of faecal bile acids has been reported, suggesting impaired catabolism of LDL. But in type IIB turnover studies suggest that lipid synthesis may be increased (Kottke, 1969). The first line of treatment is a diet low in saturated fat and in cholesterol, with an increase of polyunsaturated fats. If the patient is overweight the diet should be low in energy until body weight is normal. Plasma cholesterol seldom falls by more than 25 per cent and diet is often ineffective in patients with type IIA so that it needs to be supplemented with drugs. An oral resin such as cholestyramine, which binds bile acids and removes them from the bowel, is usually effective. If this is taken for a long time it is advisable to give a supplement of fat-soluble vitamins. For type IIB clofibrate or a related drug is usually effective. Homozygous patients are very difficult to treat even with diet and a combination of two drugs. Operative procedures such as ileal by-pass and even portocaval shunt have been tried (Starzl et al., 1973).

Type III hyperlipidaemia

This is a less common type but not rare. It is usually familial and transmitted as a recessive trait. In adult life tendon xanthomata may occur, as in type II, but the characteristic xanthomata are palmar and tuberoeruptive. In the former the palmar creases show as yellow lines from infiltration of lipid, while tuberose xanthomata appear as masses round the elbows or knees. CHD or arterial disease in the legs is common, particularly in men. Patients are often overweight. Both cholesterol and triglycerides are moderately elevated in the plasma, appearing in approximately equal concentrations. Lipoprotein electrophoresis shows a broad band extending forward from the normal position of ß-lipoprotein. This lipoprotein has the immunological features of ß-lipoprotein but the ultracentrifugal flotation of VLDL. The abnormal lipoprotein in type III appears to be an intermediate in the transformation of VLDL to LDL (Levy et al., 1971a).

The response to treatment either with diet or drugs is very gratifying. The diet used is a combination of that for type II with that for type IV, i.e. it is low in energy and cholesterol; carbohydrate and fat each provide about 40 per cent of the energy and saturated fat is replaced by polyunsaturated oils. This is often so effective (Levy et al., 1971b) that it is sufficient therapy, but if a drug is needed clofibrate is usually given.

Type IV hyperlipidaemia

This is often an incidental finding when blood is taken from a middle-aged man. The plasma is found to be lipaemic or triglycerides are above the upper normal limit. Since the distribution of plasma triglycerides is markedly skewed to the right in middle-aged men (Truswell and Mann, 1972), it is difficult to say where normality ends and type IV begins. In practice 2.3 mmol/l (200 mg/100 ml) is often used as an arbitrary, easily remembered cut-off value. Plasma cholesterol is not above normal unless triglycerides are considerably elevated, because VLDL contains about five times as much triglycerides as cholesterol. On paper electrophoresis pre-ß-lipoproteins are increased and chylomicrons not present.

Type IV is the commonest hyperlipidaemia. In a survey of over 1000 normal people in California, Wood et al. (1972) found the prevalence in adults 25 to 80 years of age was 13 per cent in men and 4.8 per cent in women. It is uncommon in children. Type IV is often associated with overweight and glucose intolerance. Families have been reported in which it is transmitted as a dominant trait (Glueck et al., 1973). Secondary type IV can be associated with diabetes, alcoholism, the nephrotic syndrome, pregnancy, the use of oral contraceptives, a change to a high carbohydrate diet and with several other diseases and metabolic states. In some patients synthesis and release of VLDL from the liver is increased, but in others peripheral removal of VLDL appears to be inadequate. The two mechanisms often operate together. Triglyceride turnover studies in diabetes are discussed by Nikkilä (1974).

Type IV is about three times as common in survivors of myocardial infarction as in comparable controls. This retrospective association was supported by the first prospective study in Stockholm (Carlson and Böttinger, 1972) but in eight subsequent studies, in which other risk factors were included, plasma triglycerides were found not to be independently related with the development of coronary heart disease.

The first line of treatment is a diet low in energy and in carbohydrate (about 45 per cent). It is also helpful to replace saturated fat by polyunsaturated oils. Careful enquiries should be made about the patient's alcohol consumption. If his social drinking appears excessive, he should be advised to reduce it to one or two drinks daily. Another valuable measure is to encourage the patient to take more exercise if he is physically able to do so. Type IV is much less common in middle-aged office workers who take regular strenuous exercise in their leisure time (Truswell and Mann, 1972). Where these simple measures are insufficient, drugs such as clofibrate or nicotinic acid (in pharmacological dosage) can be used.

Type V hyperlipidaemia

This is uncommon though not rare. Like its number the disorder is the sum of types IV and I. There is an increase of VLDL and an accumulation of chylomicrons in the plasma. It occurs in patients with diabetic lipaemia, with pancreatitis, in some alcoholics, in the nephrotic syndrome and in some other diseases. Occasionally it is familial and type IV hyperlipidaemia may be present in other members of the family. Unlike type I it does not occur in childhood. The plasma is lipaemic and the triglyceride concentration higher than in type IV, over 11 mmol/l (1000 mg/100 ml). With treatment the abnormality usually reverts to type IV, indicating that this is the principal abnormality. A very high VLDL concentration evidently interferes with clearing of chylomicron triglycerides as well.

Patients often have eruptive xanthomatosis and may have abdominal pain, a large liver and spleen and bouts of pancreatitis. They are often obese, and glucose tolerance is usually abnormal. In secondary forms of this type the most important part of the management is to treat the underlying disorder, e.g. diabetes or alcoholism. Drugs such as clofibrate, nicotinic acid or norethindrone are often effective symptomatic therapy. The therapeutic diet should be low in energy if the patient is overweight. Fat should be restricted to about 30 per cent of energy because it is fat that causes the abdominal pain, and carbohydrate should be controlled, at approximately 50 per cent of energy (Levy et al., 1971b).

The principles of dietary therapy for the six types of hyperlipidaemia are shown in Table 40.2, which is from the frontispiece of a handbook (Fredrickson et al., 1973b) recommended to those seeking more dietetic details than those given in Diet 14. A monograph on the hyperlipidaemias by Lewis (1976) is also recommended.

OTHER LIPID DISORDERS

Abetalipoproteinaemia

In this rare, recessive disorder there is absence of low density ß-lipoprotein. It presents in early childhood with steatorrhoea, spiky red blood cells, a progressive neuromuscular ataxia and retinitis pigmentosa. Plasma total cholesterol averages only 0.9 mmol/l (35 mg/100 ml) and chylomicrons do not appear after a meal of fat. There is malabsorption of fat-soluble vitamins, particularly A and E, which may be partly responsible for some of the clinical features. This is one human situation in which severe deficiency of vitamin E occurs (Lloyd and Muller, 1971; Molenaar et al., 1973).

Tangier disease

In this rare, recessive disorder there is absence of high

Table 40.2 Summary of diets for types I-V hyperlipoproteinaemia (from Frederickson et al., 1973)

	Type I	Type IIA	Type IIB and Type III	Type IV	Type V
Diet Prescription	Low fat 25–35 g	Low cholesterol Polyunsaturated fat increased	Low cholesterol Energy about 20% from pro. 40% from fat 40% from CHO	Controlled CHO, about 45% of energy Moderately restricted cholesterol	Restricted fat 30% of energy Controlled CHO 50% of energy Moderately restricted cholesterol
Energy	Not restricted	Not restricted	Achieve and maintain 'ideal' weight, i.e. reducing diet if necessary	Achieve and maintain 'ideal' weight, i.e. reducing diet if necessary	Achieve and maintain 'ideal' weight, i.e. reducing diet if necessary
Protein	Not limited	Not limited	High protein	Not limited	High protein
Fat	Restricted to 25–35 g Kind of fat not important	Saturated fat intake limited Polyunsaturated fat intake increased	Controlled to 40% energy; polyunsaturated fats recommended in preference to saturated fats	Not limited other than control of patient's weight; polyunsaturated fats recommended in preference to saturated fats	Restricted to 30% energy; polyunsaturated fats recommended in preference to saturated fats
Cholesterol	Not restricted	As low as possible; the only source of cholesterol is the meat in the diet	Less than 300 mg —the only source of cholesterol is the meat in the diet	Moderately restricted to 300–500 mg	Moderately restricted to 300–500 mg
Carbohydrate	Not limited	Not limited	Controlled—concentrated sweets are restricted	Controlled—concentrated sweets are restricted	Controlled—concentrated sweets are restricted
Alcohol	Not recommended	May be used with discretion	Limited to two serings (substituted for carbohydrate)	Limited to two servings (substituted for carbohydrate)	Not recommended

density or *a*-lipoprotein (HDL). The name comes from Tangier Island in Chesapeake Bay, USA, where it was first discovered in an inbred community. The plasma total cholesterol is around 2.3 mmol/l (90 mg/100 ml). Deposits of cholesterol occur in many organs, notably the tonsils which are enlarged and yellow. This suggests that HDL normally play a role in maintaining an equilibrium between tissue and plasma cholesterol. There is no treatment except tonsillectomy.

Familial lecithin-cholesterol acyltransferase (LCAT) deficiency

Some seven cases have been described from Norway in which the plasma enzyme that catalyses the formation of cholesterol esters is absent (Norum *et al.*, 1970). The clinical features, which are proteinuria, anaemia and corneal opacity, occur only in adult life and are benign. In the plasma, cholesterol esters are greatly reduced as are *ß*-lipoproteins while concentrations of triglycerides, lecithin and unesterified cholesterol are increased. Paper electrophoresis shows a band in the *ß*-position with tailing. A low fat diet is under trial (Glomset *et al.*, 1974). The condition illuminates the role of the plasma LCAT enzyme.

Refsum's disease

In this recessive disorder there are hypertrophic peripheral neuropathy, cerebellar ataxia, nerve deafness, retinitis pigmentosa, ichthyosis and a raised protein in the CSF. Patients have been found to accumulate a branched chain fatty acid, phytanic acid (3,7,11,15-tetramethyl-hexadecanoic acid) in plasma and tissues. Phytanic acid is derived from phytol, a terpene obtained on hydrolysis of chlorophyll. Patients have therefore been treated with a diet from which vegetables, fruits, butter and ruminant fat were excluded. The plasma phytanic acid fell to a quarter of the original value after a year and conduction velocities in nerves increased (Eldjarn *et al.*, 1966).

Other lipoidoses

There is a group of disorders in which sphingomyelins and other lipids accumulate in the tissues especially in the central nervous system. At least 10 are now well defined chemically and some, e.g. Tay-Sach's disease, Gaucher's disease and Niemann-Pick disease, have been known for many years. They cause a variety of disabilities, which usually shorten life. No dietary treatment is of value.

EFFECT OF DIET ON PLASMA LIPIDS

Possibly no other blood constituent varies as much between normal people as the plasma cholesterol. In different parts of the world the mean value in healthy adults ranges from 100 mg in New Guinea (De Wolfe and Whyte, 1958) to 268 mg/100 ml in East Finland (Keys *et*

al., 1958b) (i.e. 2.6 to 6.9 mmol/l). These differences between populations are almost entirely environmental in origin. When people migrate from one country to another they soon assume the plasma cholesterol of the new country. This is well illustrated by the plasma cholesterols of Japanese who are living in the USA (Keys *et al.*, 1958c). The customary diet is the most important of the environmental influences on the plasma cholesterol.

Diet is also the principal method of treating all the hyperlipidaemias, as outlined above. The plasma lipid concentration at which treatment is started depends on judgment, which takes into account among other factors the level of plasma lipids in the population and the patient's age. In practice the concentration at which a plasma cholesterol is called type II or a plasma triglyceride called type IV is likely to be the concentration at which a doctor starts a mild form of lipid-lowering therapy. Some dietary modification is then probably needed. Drugs should be reserved for cases with higher lipid concentrations that have proved resistant to a thorough trial of diet.

Dietary manipulation is not only used for cases of hyperlipidaemia. As discussed in Chapter 41 the chance of a healthy individual developing CHD correlates with his concentration of plasma cholesterol and possibly triglycerides as well. There are therefore activists who recommend that all or most of the adult population in prosperous countries should modify their diet so as to produce some lowering of plasma lipids. According to this school of thought the mean plasma cholesterol of normal people in, say, East Finland is not normal and the population needs treatment. Wynder and Hill (1972) wrote to investigators engaged in research on atherosclerosis in several countries, asking them what they considered to be normal levels for plasma lipids. The mean value in the replies for normal cholesterol for men aged 30 years was 4.5 mmol/l (174 mg/100 mg); all thought a normal cholesterol in this age and sex should not be over 5.7 mmol/l (220 mg/100 ml). This controversial subject is discussed on page 328. A review (Truswell, 1978a) gives an account of recent observations on the relation between diet and plasma lipids in man.

While the indications for a lipid-lowering diet are a matter of opinion, the effects of dietary components on plasma lipids are largely matters of scientific fact from which appropriate diets can be constructed and prescribed whenever the decision is made to do so. We concentrate on these facts in the following section and discuss in the next chapter whether or when they should be used.

EFFECT OF DIET ON PLASMA CHOLESTEROL

Dietary components that lower chiefly cholesterol do so by lowering LDL. There is no qualitative difference in this effect whether the individual has type II hyperlipidaemia or a 'normal' plasma cholesterol for his community. Dietary fat has very little effect on HDL, which contributes some 1.0 to 1.3 mmol/l (40 to 50 mg/100 ml) to plasma cholesterol, and there is much less cholesterol than triglycerides in VLDL and chylomicrons.

Dietary fats (glycerides and their fatty acid pattern)

It has been known since before World War I that the addition of cholesterol to rabbits' feed produces a large increase in their plasma cholesterol. But in man early attempts to change plasma cholesterol by varying dietary cholesterol were disappointing and inconclusive. Keys (1952) found that human plasma cholesterol can be reduced by eating a diet low in total fat, but this is unpalatable. Kinsell *et al.* (1952) discovered that much the same result could be achieved by avoiding animal fats, yet continuing to eat vegetable oils. Bronte-Stewart *et al.* (1956) showed that marine oils lower and coconut oil raises cholesterol; what affects plasma cholesterol is not whether a fat is of animal or plant origin, but the degree of saturation of the fatty acids in the dietary triglycerides.

The next step was to work out from multiple feeding trials that saturated fatty acids raise the plasma cholesterol about twice as much as polyunsaturated fatty acids lower it, while monounsaturated fatty acids have no effect (Keys *et al.*, 1958a). Keys expressed this mathematically in an equation.

$$\Delta \text{Cholesterol} = 2.76\ \Delta \text{sat} + 0.05\ \Delta \text{mono} - 1.35\ \Delta \text{P} - 1.68$$

(where Δ means change of and sat, mono and P are saturated, mono and polyunsaturated fatty acids respectively). Subsequently, workers at Harvard (McGandy *et al.*, 1970) and at Unilever Research in Holland (Vergroesen and de Boer, 1971) showed that chain length influences the cholesterol-elevating effect of saturated fatty acids. Palmitic ($C_{16:0}$) and myristic ($C_{14:0}$) have the major effect while acids with chain lengths shorter than 12, i.e. medium-chain triglycerides; and stearic acid ($C_{18:0}$) have little effect. This is shown schematically in Table 40.3.

Sinclair (1956) suggested that the cholesterol-lowering effect of polyunsaturated fatty acids is an essential fatty acid (EFA) effect. But the vast majority of people whose cholesterol falls on polyunsaturated fat diets show no signs of EFA deficiency (p. 55) and Ahrens *et al.* (1959) found that a fish oil rich in marine polyunsaturated fatty acids ($C_{20:5}$ and $C_{22:6}$) but containing hardly any EFA ($C_{18:2}$ or $C_{20:4}$) reduced plasma cholesterol about as effectively as maize oil which is rich in linoleic acid ($C_{18:2}$).

Much work has been done on the mechanism by which polyunsaturated fats lower plasma cholesterol. This requires cholesterol balance experiments which are extremely difficult to carry out and interpret in man because of the different metabolic pools of cholesterol, including enterohepatic cycles and the large variety of neutral steroid and bile acid excretory products in the faeces. On the whole the evidence shows that polyunsaturated fats increase faecal excretion of bile acids, indicating accelerated catabolism of cholesterol. However, this does not occur in patients with type IIA hyperlipidaemia (Connor, 1970); in this disorder there is probably an abnormality in the degradation of cholesterol to bile acids.

The long-term effect of a diet low in saturated fats and high in polyunsaturated fats on plasma cholesterol is shown in Fig. 40.2. Provided that patients persist with the diet the plasma cholesterol remains at a lower level for years. The question naturally arises whether there are any side effects, other than culinary inconvenience, from taking large amounts of polyunsaturated fat over a period of years. A suggestion from one trial (Pearce and Dayton, 1971) of some increase in cancer was unconvincing because most of the cancer cases had not adhered to the diet; it was not confirmed in other dietary trials (Ederer *et al.*, 1971; Heady, 1974).

Dietary sterols

Cholesterol. The effects of fatty acid patterns of dietary glycerides on plasma cholesterol overshadowed any effect of dietary sterols for several years. Keys maintained that dietary cholesterol had no apparent effect (Keys *et al.*, 1956). However, it has become clear that dietary cholesterol does have some plasma cholesterol-elevating effect and in 1965 Keys added to his equation for predicting plasma cholesterol a term which uses the square root of the cholesterol intake (Keys *et al.*, 1965). In other words the first 200 to 300 mg of cholesterol in a diet has

Table 40.3 Effects of different dietary fatty acids on plasma cholesterol and triglycerides, as demonstrated in acute experiments on man

Dietary fatty acid		Plasma Cholesterol	Triglycerides
MCT	$C_{8:0}$ to $C_{10:0}$	0	↑
Lauric	$C_{12:0}$	↑	0
Myristic	$C_{14:0}$	↑↑	0
Palmitic	$C_{16:0}$	↑↑	0
Stearic	$C_{18:0}$	?↑	↑
Oleic	$C_{18:1}$	0	0
Linoleic	$C_{18:2}$	↓	↓
Other polyunsaturated		↓	

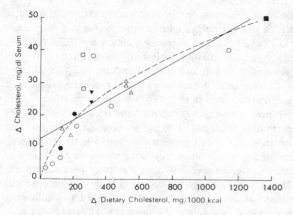

Fig. 40.2 Plasma cholesterol concentrations in 200 survivors of a myocardial infarct while taking a diet low in saturated fat and rich in soya bean oil (ratio of polyunsaturated to saturated fatty acids approx. 2.0). The three lines show the group divided roughly into thirds, depending on whether the starting level of cholesterol was high, medium or low (modified from Leren, 1966).

much more effect in raising plasma cholesterol than further increments (Fig. 40.3). The cholesterol content of Western diets is of the order of 500 mg/day. Patients with type II hyperlipidaemia are often advised to keep cholesterol intake below 300 mg/day (Levy *et al.*, 1971b). In general, dietary cholesterol is reduced when less saturated fats are eaten but vegetable sources of saturated fats, e.g. coconut oil and plain chocolate, contain no cholesterol. Among food of animal origin, eggs, brain and, to a lesser degree, glandular organs are rich in cholesterol but not in saturated fat, while adipose tissue is the opposite and contains only traces of cholesterol. Most food tables do not give the cholesterol content of foods. Bernice Watt and colleagues who are responsible for the US Handbook on the composition of foods give a useful provisional table of values (Feeley *et al.*, 1972).

Phytosterols. The occurrence and chemistry of the plant sterols is discussed in Chapter 6. The best known is ß-sitosterol, which differs in structure from cholesterol only in having an extra ethyl group on the side chain. In large doses, e.g. 3 to 6 g thrice daily, it lowers plasma cholesterol in man (Farquhar and Sokolow, 1958) and has been used as a cholesterol-lowering agent under the trade name Cytellin. It probably acts by competitive inhibition of cholesterol absorption and reabsorption (Salen *et al.*, 1970) but may have systemic actions as well (Ravi Subbiah, 1971). Diets rich in polyunsaturated fats usually contain some phytosterol in the vegetable oils, but the amounts in refined oils are small compared to the doses needed for clear-cut effects on plasma cholesterol.

Other dietary components

Energy balance. This affects plasma VLDL and triglycerides more than cholesterol, as does an increase in

dietary carbohydrates. Plasma cholesterol is usually reduced after some months of semi-starvation (Keys *et al.*, 1950) but tends to be high in patients with anorexia nervosa (Crisp *et al.*, 1968). For a review of plasma lipids in different states of energy balance see Truswell (1978b).

Dietary protein. Reduction below minimum requirements usually lowers the plasma lipids, as is seen in kwashiorkor, but populations who habitually live on low protein intakes usually eat very little saturated fat. In controlled human experiments the effect of short-term changes of dietary protein on plasma cholesterol appear to be negligible, provided that the intake exceeds the minimum protein requirements (Anderson *et al.*, 1971). Individual amino acids which impinge on pathways of cholesterol metabolism or which alter plasma cholesterol in animal species have not had an effect in human experiments provided, again, that the minimum requirements are supplied.

Meal frequency. In Prague an examination of 440 middle-aged men showed that those who ate one to three meals daily were heavier and had higher plasma cholesterol and more impaired glucose tolerance compared with those who ate five or six meals daily (Fabry *et al.*, 1964). Several investigators have given subjects a constant daily amount of food while varying the number of meals. Plasma cholesterol tends to be a little higher when all the food is eaten at one meal, compared with eating it divided between more

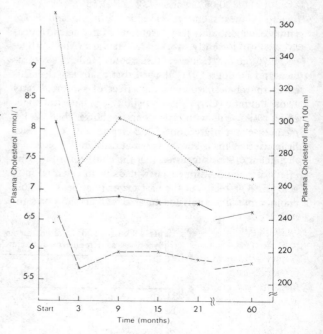

Fig. 40.3. Change in plasma cholesterol in response to change in dietary cholesterol in man. Data from six different experiments. The interrupted, curved line, calculated from the square root of change in dietary cholesterol, fits the points better than the linear regression line (Keys *et al.*, 1974).

than three meals a day (Gwinup et al., 1963; Young et al., 1972). However, in about half the published experiments the changes in plasma cholesterol have been insignificant.

Dietary fibre. Communities that eat high fibre diets usually have low plasma cholesterols and vice versa. There are, of course, many other environmental differences between peasant communities who live on unrefined staples and industrial societies who eat refined foods. Under controlled conditions plasma cholesterol falls with diets high in legumes (Grande et al., 1965; Mathur, 1968). Legumes have a substantial content of fibre but they also contain pharmacologically active substances, one or more of which might affect plasma cholesterol. Wheat fibre does not lower plasma cholesterol (Truswell and Kay, 1976) but pectin does if taken in large doses (Kay and Truswell, 1977).

Vitamins. Nicotinic acid (not nicotinamide) is a cholesterol-lowering agent but only in pharmacological dosage, e.g. 1 to 2 g thrice daily. Hypercholesterolaemia is a feature of human biotin deficiency but only three spontaneous cases have ever been reported (Scott, 1958). Low plasma cholesterol has been reported in scurvy (Chap. 35); moderate or large doses of vitamin D are associated with some increase of plasma cholesterol (Linden, 1974).

Minerals. Plasma cholesterol is often low in patients with iron-deficiency and other forms of anaemia (Rifkind and Gale, 1967; Elwood et al., 1970). Large oral intakes of calcium, e.g. 2 g/day, lower plasma cholesterol (Carlson et al., 1971; Bierenbaum et al., 1972). The effects of trace elements have been little studied in man, but vanadium and zinc can lower plasma cholesterol in animals.

The pattern of fatty acids in the dietary fat is the major dietary influence on plasma cholesterol but by no means the only one. The foregoing account summarises an extensive literature and although the outlines are now apparent we expect more details to emerge from research in progress or to come, particularly on the influence of non-nutrient material in foods, of fermentation of foods, and of the physical and stereoisomeric forms of fats.

EFFECT OF DIET ON PLASMA TRIGLYCERIDES

Because plasma triglycerides, unlike cholesterol, are affected by meals containing fat it is necessary to measure them under standard conditions, before breakfast, after no food overnight. In the following account we consider dietary influences on these fasting triglycerides, which are predominantly VLDL. Before doing so we should not forget the exogenous triglycerides or chylomicrons which appear in plasma after a meal containing fat. The degree of alimentary lipaemia is enhanced when sucrose (Mann et al., 1971) or alcohol (Barboriak and Meade, 1971) is taken with the fat.

Carbohydrates

The fasting concentration of triglycerides increases when either starch or sugar is added to an experimental diet and also when carbohydrate replaces fat isocalorically. Carbohydrate induction of plasma triglycerides was first described by Ahrens et al. (1961) and has been confirmed repeatedly. The rise of triglycerides on changing from a 40 to an 80 per cent carbohydrate diet averaged 1.1 mmol/l (100 mg/100 ml) in normal people but was two to three times as great in patients with types III and IV hyperlipidaemia (Glueck et al., 1969). The lipoprotein which increases is VLDL with more triglyceride per unit of protein and a larger particle size (Mancini et al., 1973). Hepatic synthesis of triglyceride is probably increased.

There is evidence that the effect does not last for more than a few months. People who subsist on diets high in starchy foods, like rice or maize, do not appear to have high plasma triglycerides unless they are obese (Florey et al., 1973). Most human metabolic experiments last only a few weeks but Antonis and Bersohn (1961) made long-term observations on prisoners in South Africa. When white prisoners changed from a European diet to an African one based on maize, which contained more carbohydrate and less fat than they were used to, their plasma triglycerides rose and cholesterol fell; however, after 8 months they had returned to their original level.

Plasma cholesterol usually falls during carbohydrate induction. The plasma triglycerides are actually lower during the day, because there is less alimentary lipaemia on a low fat intake, and climb during the night (Schlierf et al., 1971).

Sucrose

Whether sucrose has more than the general effect of carbohydrates can only be tested by measuring triglycerides when starch (or other carbohydrate) is replaced isocalorically by sucrose or vice versa. Macdonald and Braithwaite (1964) demonstrated that plasma triglycerides rose when sucrose was substituted for starch in a diet in which 70 per cent of the energy came from carbohydrate. This effect was found in male medical students, but not in women. Fructose had a similar effect but other sugars did not. When ^{14}C-labelled sugars were given, radioactivity in plasma triglycerides was much greater after fructose than after glucose (Macdonald, 1967), indicating that fructose in the sucrose was being preferentially metabolised towards lipid synthesis. When the amount of sucrose exchanged for starch is 20 to 25 per cent of the dietary energy, the amount present in many British diets, the plasma triglycerides of men did not change (Dunnigan et al., 1970; Mann and Truswell, 1972). Thus sucrose at the usual level of intake does not appear to have a specific triglyceride-inducing effect in normal people but may have in a minority of patients with type IV hyperlipidaemia (Mann and Truswell, 1974).

In practice, patients with type IV (and type III) are treated with a low carbohydrate diet and sugar is more restricted than starch largely for culinary convenience.

Energy balance

In the general population fasting plasma triglycerides correlate with indices of obesity such as weight-height index (Carlson and Lindstedt, 1968) and skinfold thicknesses over the trunk (Allbrink and Meigs, 1964). The dietary treatment for most patients with type IV hyperlipidaemia includes weight reduction.

Fatty acid pattern of dietary fat

Fasting plasma triglycerides are somewhat lower if dietary fat is polyunsaturated rather than saturated. Table 40.3 summarises the effect of different fatty acids. The saturated fatty acids that tend to increase plasma triglycerides are those in medium-chain triglycerides together with stearic acid (Grande *et al.*, 1972), i.e. not the saturated fats which raise plasma cholesterol. Replacement of saturated by polyunsaturated fats is a subsidiary part of therapeutic diets for type IV hyperlipidaemia (Table 40.2). It is not yet settled whether synthesis of VLDL is increased or its catabolism decreased on polyunsaturated fat diets.

Alcohol

Generous intakes of ethanol may lead to hypertriglyceridaemia, of type IV, or sometimes IIB or even type V in predisposed individuals, Chait *et al.* (1972) found that alcoholism was the third commonest cause of hypertriglyceridaemia in Hammersmith Hospital. Alcohol favours hepatic lipogenesis, and this stimulates the synthesis of VLDL as well as leading to a fatty liver (Chap. 7). There are individual differences in sensitivity of plasma triglycerides to alcohol. In some persons even small amounts increase triglycerides (Ginsberg *et al.*, 1974) while on the other hand some alcoholics do not have hyperlipidaemia (Mendelson and Mello, 1973). In any patient with types IV, V or IIB hyperlipidaemia it is advisable to make a therapeutic trial of giving up social drinking.

EFFECT OF DIET ON PLASMA HDL

For a long time no dietary effects on plasma high-density lipoproteins were known. Amount and type of dietary fats do not affect HDL, only LDL and total cholesterol. Mean values for plasma HDL (or α-lipoprotein cholesterol) do not parallel epidemiological differences in mean values of total cholesterol in different countries. However, two dietary influences on HDL are now known. Obesity is associated with reduced concentrations that rise after weight reduction (Wilson and Leeds, 1972). A low concentration of HDL is undesirable, judged by epidemiological associations with coronary heart disease. The second dietary component now known to raise HDL is alcohol. There is a consistent correlation of HDL with individual alcohol consumption in several communities (Castelli *et al.*, 1977) and in controlled human experiments 60 g ethanol/day as beer raised the HDL of healthy students over five weeks (Berg and Johansson, 1973).

ENVIRONMENTAL AND OTHER FACTORS

The season of the year affects plasma cholesterol and values tend to be lower in the summer. Mental stress may increase plasma cholesterol or triglycerides. Strenuous muscular exercise may have a pronounced effect on plasma triglycerides. Holloszy *et al.* (1964) reported that a three-mile run lowered the concentration markedly and the effect lasted at least two days. Exercise has less effect on plasma cholesterol. Drugs which are used as lipid-lowering agents have already been mentioned. Others, such as aspirin, used for quite different purposes, also affect plasma lipids in addition to their main action and these have been reviewed by Truswell (1974).

In the first part of this chapter genetic factors and certain diseases which lead to hyperlipidaemia were considered. In the second part we have described the effects of dietary factors on plasma total cholesterol, triglycerides and high-density lipoproteins. The chapter has been concerned mainly with facts. The reader should now be equipped to move on to the more difficult subject of the causes of coronary heart diseases and the role of dietary and other measures in its prevention.

41. Diseases of the Cardiovascular System

Coronary heart disease and hypertension are the two most common disorders of the cardiovascular system in Britain. The role of dietary factors in their aetiology and treatment has been the subject of much study and still remains contentious.

CORONARY HEART DISEASE (CHD)

Coronary heart disease or ischaemic heart disease (IHD) are synonymous terms for a group of syndromes arising from failure of the coronary arteries to supply sufficient blood to the myocardium. These syndromes are in most cases associated with atherosclerosis of the coronary arteries. They include myocardial infarction, angina pectoris and sudden death without infarction.

Myocardial infarction. This is necrosis or destruction of part of the heart muscle due to failure of the blood supply (ischaemia). It may lead to sudden death or heal, leaving a scar. Patients with healed lesions may be severely disabled or may be able to return to their normal life with little or no restriction of their physical activities, but they carry an increased risk of a second infarct. The infarction is usually due to a thrombus forming in an atherosclerotic coronary artery and blocking the lumen. Sometimes there is no thrombus and the infarct arises because the lumen of a coronary artery has been so narrowed by atherosclerosis that the blood flow is insufficient to supply the oxygen needed to maintain the cardiac muscle. However, occasional cases of myocardial infarction are seen in which neither thrombosis nor significant narrowing of the lumen can be recognised.

Angina pectoris (Latin, pain in the chest). In this condition exercise or excitement provokes severe chest pain and so limits the patient's physical activities. Patients may live for many years and remain free of further disability, so long as they keep within the limits of their exercise tolerance. However they carry an increased risk of sudden death or infarction, especially if they undertake any unusual exertion. Emotional stress may also bring on angina.

Sudden death. A high proportion of cases of sudden death occur in people who have had angina pectoris or myocardial infarction. Their death is presumed to be due to CHD. In others death is unexpected but autopsy shows evidence of old myocardial infarction or extensive atheroma of the coronary arteries; they are also presumed to have died of CHD. In a third group the cause remains unexplained after autopsy. Some of these may be due to cardiac arrest or ventricular fibrillation resulting from minor or painless ischaemia sufficient to interrupt the electrical conduction system of the heart.

CLINICAL FEATURES

The dominant symptom is a severe, pressing or constricting pain, poorly localised deep in the centre of the chest and characteristically radiating down the left or both arms. In angina pectoris this pain comes on with exertion or excitement; it forces the patient to stop and when he does so the pain passes off in a few minutes. It is relieved by sublingual glyceryl trinitrate. Patients with angina can suffer several attacks of pain in a day and they can go on like this for long periods of time.

In myocardial infarction the pain often comes on at rest; it is very severe, lasts for hours and is only relieved by strong opiates like morphine. It is accompanied by general symptoms such as weakness, collapse, cardiac arrhythmias and circulatory shock.

The pain is not always typical in CHD. Some unusual patients have a mild myocardial infarction without noticing pain ('silent coronary'). On the other hand there are several other causes of pain in and around the chest which can mimic CHD.

While the electrocardiogram often changes temporarily during an attack of angina, it can be unremarkable between attacks. But soon after the onset of myocardial infarction the ECG usually undergoes a permanent change and shows the infarct pattern. In the first few days after an infarct raised plasma concentrations of aspartate aminotranferase and other myocardial enzymes are of diagnostic value.

Patients with angina or who have had a myocardial infarct are liable to develop cardiac failure or arrhythmias.

PATHOLOGY (ATHEROSCLEROSIS)

The pathological basis of CHD is atherosclerosis in one or both coronary arteries. This is usually associated with atherosclerosis in the aorta and often in other major arteries. Atherosclerosis, the most important of the degenerative diseases of arteries, consists of focal accumulation in the intimal lining of arteries of a variable combination of lipids, complex carbohydrates, blood and blood products, fibrous tissue and calcium deposits; there are associated changes in the media of the arteries. Arterioles are relatively unaffected.

Atherosclerotic narrowing of the carotid or basilar arterial system leads to strokes and other forms of cerebral vascular disease. In a femoral artery it can result in intermittent claudication. The three major forms of atherosclerotic disease arise from involvement of the coronary arteries, the cerebral arteries and the femoral artery and its branches, but other arteries can be affected, such as the renal or mesenteric, with the possible consequences of disease in the organ supplied by the artery.

Coronary atherosclerosis is almost invariably associated with aortic atherosclerosis. Although it tends to be associated with disease in other arteries most of the epidemiological and experimental work has been concerned with atherosclerosis in the coronary rather than other arteries. Less is known about atherosclerosis of the cerebral arteries but its natural history and epidemiology differs in some respects from that of CHD (p. 432).

Stages of development
It is customary to separate the lesions of atherosclerosis into fatty streaks, plaques and complicated lesions.

Fatty streaks are short, thin, slightly raised yellow lines running longitudinally along the internal surface of arteries and consist of an intracellular accumulation of lipids within the intima. Electron microscopy has shown that the affected cells are probably smooth muscle cells. Fatty streaks differ somewhat in their anatomical and epidemiological distribution from plaques and it would seem that, while they may progress to plaques in some situations, they may be reversible in others.

Plaques are the established lesions of atherosclerosis. They are raised, focal, circumscribed lesions up to 1 cm in diameter, consisting of various amounts of fibrous tissue and lipid. The lipid accumulates mostly in extracellular amorphous masses; plaques in which this process is prominent are called **soft** or **atheromatous plaques.** In others fibrous tissue is prominent and lipid is widely scattered or localised to the deeper portions of the lesion; these are called **hard** or **fibrous plaques.** The plaques increase the thickness of the intima and thus encroach on the lumen of the artery. As individual plaques become larger they tend to coalesce. Large lesions destroy the internal elastic lamina and involve the inner layer of the media.

Four other processes may now occur to complicate the lesions. First, the endothelium may be lost so that the surface ulcerates and the fatty contents may be exposed to the blood stream. Secondly, fibrin is commonly deposited and thrombosis occurs on the plaque surface, probably because of the roughening produced by ulceration. Organisation of the thrombus is followed by its incorporation into the plaque and it may become eventually covered by endothelium. Thirdly, free blood can be found in a plaque. It is often difficult for the pathologist to decide whether

this has come from rupture of small vessels deep in the lesion or from the lumen of the artery through a surface fissure. Finally calcification may occur.

Distribution of lesions
Some atherosclerotic lesions can be found at almost all postmortems. A few small lesions are seen in most adolescents and they increase in number and size throughout life. In some communities there are fewer lesions than in others and within a community some individuals have accelerated atherosclerosis while the arteries of others are relatively spared. Atherosclerosis does not usually lead to clinical disease, such as myocardial infarction, until middle age. Figure 41.1 shows the extent of atherosclerotic lesions of the different grades in the aorta in two communities from the same genetic stock. In young men most of the aorta is unaffected and the few lesions are chiefly fatty streaks. With advancing age an increased area of the aorta is covered by plaques but the process is more extensive in the USA than in rural Ireland. There is a corresponding difference in mortality from CHD.

Although our understanding of the natural history of atherosclerosis comes from postmortem material, it is possible to demonstrate narrowing of susceptible arteries in living patients by arteriography. However, since this carries some risk it is only performed when disease is suspected on clinical grounds and in patients for whom arterial surgery is contemplated.

Chemical pathology
That atherosclerotic lesions contain large amounts of fatty material, a big proportion of which is cholesterol, has been known since the time of Virchow in the middle of the nineteenth century. Detailed chemical characterisation of the lipids was first carried out by Böttcher *et al.* (1960). It requires delicate microdissection of the lesions, followed by extraction and thin-layer or gas chromatography. The tiny amount of lipid in fatty streaks or plaques is easily

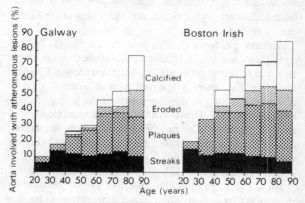

Fig. 41.1 The extent of involvement of aortas with four types of atherosclerotic lesions in Galway (Eire) and Boston subjects. (Brown *et al.*, 1970.)

diluted by the structural lipid of the unaffected intima and media and by the adipose tissue in the adventitial coat of the artery. It has been found that the lipid in fatty streaks is quite different from that in plaques.

The largest class of lipid in atherosclerotic plaques is cholesterol ester, in which the fatty acid pattern resembles that of plasma cholesterol ester, with linoleate the most abundant followed by oleate (Lawrie et al., 1964; Smith et al., 1968). Phospholipids are reduced in plaques, compared with plasma lipoproteins, and the predominant type is sphingomyelin. This is presumably synthesised in the arterial wall (Abdulla and Adams, 1965). The plaques are usually coloured yellow or orange by carotenoids (Blankenhorn et al., 1956) which cannot be synthesised by the tissues; these pigments must have come from the plasma and originally from the diet.

The fatty streaks in intracellular lipids are mostly cholesterol esters, with a bizarre fatty acid pattern. They contain a high proportion of oleic acid, low linoleic acid and raised $C_{20:3}$ (Smith et al., 1968; Lang and Insull, 1970). Fatty streaks contain less low density lipoprotein than the normal intima (Smith and Slater, 1972) and it would appear that their lipids have mostly been esterified in situ.

Mode of formation

There are two main hypotheses for the pathogenesis of atherosclerosis, which are not mutually exclusive.

Filtration theory. This postulates that the principal lipids of the plaque reach the intima by passing through defects in the endothelium carried on low density lipoproteins (LDL). Immunoassays show that plaques contain more LDL than the surrounding normal intima (Smith and Slater, 1970). In normal intima the concentration of LDL is seven times that of albumin, yet albumin with its smaller molecular weight is known to diffuse through endothelial membranes more rapidly than LDL (Smith and Slater, 1972). Some structural or chemical property presumably retards the passage of LDL out of the intima. This could be the glycosaminoglycans (mucopolysaccharides) of the ground substance, some of which can precipitate LDL in vitro.

Thrombogenic theory. This originated in 1842 when Rokitansky, the famous Viennese pathologist, put forward the view that atherosclerosis was derived from material deposited on the intimal wall from the blood. Duguid (1954) placed the theory on a more secure basis. In its simplest form it postulates that a minute lesion of the intimal surface occurs, perhaps as a result of mechanical trauma. At this point a platelet aggregation forms a small thrombosis which sticks to the vessel wall. The fibrin in this thrombus becomes organised; fibrous tissue is formed, it eventually becomes covered with endothelium and the lipid in the thrombus becomes the lipid of the atherosclerotic lesion. An extension of the theory is that minute lesions of the intima, followed by local mural thrombosis, are common but are normally cleared by fibrinolysis. Hence the primary fault responsible for atherosclerosis might lie in an increased tendency to thrombosis or in an inefficient fibrinolytic mechanism.

All would agree that thrombosis may occur as a complication, on top of an atherosclerotic plaque, and that this can become organised. On histological examination some fibrous plaques show a layered appearance, which suggests they were formed from repeated thrombosis and organisation. But other lesions can be found, sometimes in the same patient, in which the dominating feature is an amorphous extracellular collection of cholesterol-rich lipid. When platelet thrombi are produced in experimental animals and become organised, the fat which they accumulate differs from that of spontaneous atherosclerosis. It contains very small amounts of cholesterol esters and their fatty acids are saturated (Craig et al., 1973).

Dietary factors may be responsible for the development of filtration atherogenesis. Lesions resembling human atherosclerosis can be produced in many species of experimental animals by dietary manipulations which raise the plasma cholesterol concentration. This was first shown in Russia as long ago as 1913 by Anitschkow, who fed cholesterol to rabbits (Anitschkow, 1933). The effective diet varies greatly with the cholesterol feedback mechanisms of the different species. In rats it is necessary to feed not only cholesterol and saturated fats but also to give cholic acid and thiouracil.

There are also indications from both animal and human experiments that the tendency to thrombosis (Renaud et al., 1970; Hornstra et al., 1973) and fibrinolysis (Dalderup and van Haard, 1971) can be influenced by the long-term diet or even by single meals rich in particular foods. Again there are important differences between species, for example in platelet function (Mills, 1970). Techniques are difficult, partly because they are all artificial to a greater or lesser extent and because the measurements are affected by much variability (Merskey and Nossel, 1957).

While there is a close association between myocardial infarction and the degree of coronary atherosclerosis there must be other factors, chiefly superimposed thrombosis and the state of the myocardium, which determine whether there is sudden death, an infarct or no permanent damage when the blood flow in a coronary artery is reduced below a critical level. These other factors may sometimes be more important than the degree of atherosclerosis in determining differences in the frequency of clinical CHD between different communities or with time in the same community. Morris (1951) reported that coronary atheroma had not changed in severity in the postmortem material of a London hospital during the first half of the twentieth century but that obstruction of the lumen had increased. Likewise coronary atherosclerosis does not appear to be more extensive in Finland than in Norway, although the mortality from CHD is twice as high in Finland (Rissanen and Pyörälä, 1974).

EPIDEMIOLOGY

Any doctor who has been in practice for more than 30 years will have seen a remarkable increase in coronary heart disease. Forty years ago it was essentially a disease of men belonging to the well-to-do classes, successful businessmen and members of the professions. It was uncommon to find a woman affected. Between 1950 and 1965 an increase in mortality in Britain and in many other countries occurred, sufficiently great to be called the 'modern epidemic' (Morris, 1975). The increase affected men of all social classes and was most marked in those aged 35 to 44 years; little or no increase occurred in women. Between 1966 and 1975 mortality rates in the different age groups of men in Britain have remained high; there have been slight tendencies for those in the young age group to fall and in the older age groups to continue to rise slowly; there have also been small rises in rates for women. The epidemic had reached a plateau and may be beginning to fall. A fall began earlier in the USA (Gordon and Thom, 1975).

Interest in the epidemiology and possible prevention of myocardial infarction started with the observation by Strøm and Jensen (1951) that mortality from arteriosclerotic heart disease in Norway during World War II declined after the German invasion but returned gradually to its former level with returning prosperity after the war was over. The same phenomenon occurred in several other European countries including England and Wales and suggests that austere rations more than counterbalance the effects of the stresses of war on the coronary arteries.

Table 41.1 shows the mortality rates for coronary heart disease in middle-aged men and women in selected countries when the world epidemic may have reached its height. Finland, the United States, Scotland, Australia and Canada head the list. These are prosperous countries. There is no doubt that atherosclerosis and its sequelae are associated with prosperity. However, there are many anomalies. Swedes and Englishmen do not appear to live less well than Finns and Scots.

For countries in Asia and Africa, where there is still much poverty the incidence is low, even less than that recorded for Japan in Table 41.1. Postmortem examination of the hearts of American and Korean soldiers of the same age group showed a much higher prevalence of atherosclerosis in the American hearts. Korean soldiers also had a low concentration of plasma cholesterol and a low intake of dietary fat in comparison with American soldiers.

There is no evidence that Asians and Africans possess any racial immunity to the disease. Prosperous Asians and Africans who adopt American or European ways of life are frequently affected. The incidence of ischaemic heart disease in Japanese who live in California is 10 times that of those who live in Japan (Keys et al., 1957).

There are many differences in the mode of life between those who live in prosperous countries and those who live in underdeveloped areas of the world. Some of these differences were analysed in parallel studies of three population groups resident in the environment of Cape Town (Bronte-Stewart, 1958; Brock, 1972).

RISK FACTORS

The large differences in CHD between people living in different environments (Table 41.1) have stimulated many people in different parts of the world to search for risk factors or characteristics associated with an increased frequency of CHD by epidemiological techniques. The quickest and the cheapest method is a **retrospective study.** A doctor may notice, for example, that several of his patients with myocardial infarction have an impaired glucose tolerance. To investigate this further he could measure glucose tolerance on 100 consecutive patients and compare the results with an equal number of controls of the same sex and similar age. He may find that impairment of glucose tolerance is more frequent in the myocardial infarction patients. But there are three big weaknesses of such a retrospective study. First, patients with myocardial infarction in hospital are only a minority of all the cases in a community who develop CHD. Some die suddenly or within a few days of the attack. Others have angina pectoris or a silent infarct and are not admitted to hospital. Secondly, myocardial infarction and the physiological and psychological disturbances that attend it could themselves impair glucose tolerance. Thirdly, the choice of controls for a doctor able to collect a selection of patients with a particular disease in hospital is very critical. If patients with other diseases are chosen these may themselves influence glucose tolerance; while if healthy persons outside hospital are chosen, it is difficult to get a truly random sample.

For these reasons a retrospective study can only be regarded as a screening procedure for risk factors. Characteristics which appear to be associated with CHD need to be further tested in the more stringent conditions of a **prospective study.** The most famous prospective study has been conducted in the small town of Framingham, Massachusetts, in the USA. Over 5000 healthy men and women over 30 years of age were taken into the study in 1949. They were questioned about their way of life and examined clinically and a number of biochemical and other investigations were carried out. Thereafter they were re-examined every two years, and the staff of the study, who maintained a permanent office in the town, made careful records of all illnesses. As the years passed some developed one of the forms of CHD, others had other illnesses and some died. The accumulated records of these have been related to the habits and findings noted in the earlier

Table 41.1 Deaths per 100000 of the population from ischaemic heart disease in people aged 45–54 years in 1970 (from *WHO Statistics Annual* for 1970)

Country	Men	Women
Finland	403	55
USA	346	83
Scotland	343	81
Australia	297	77
New Zealand	273	18
Canada	270	48
England and Wales	259	42
Norway	213	23
Netherlands	201	25
Czechoslovakia	194	38
Israel	194	59
Federal German Republic	148	26
Hungary	146	38
Sweden	137	25
Italy	106	21
Bulgaria	72	26
France	66	12
Romania	61	20
Spain	50	10
Hong Kong	34	12
Japan	34	14

examinations. Some 20 other prospective studies have been carried out around the world but none has run for as long as the Framingham study. From these studies we now have quantitative information about several risk factors for CHD—and for some other diseases of later life as well—which provide a basis for preventive measures.

A number of risk factors are well established (Table 41.2), some are obviously interrelated and others apparently independent; clearly many factors contribute to the aetiology of CHD.

Maleness
CHD is about 10 times as common in men as in women up to the age of 45. After the menopause there is a greatly increased incidence in women, and by the age of 70 there is no difference between the sexes. The relative immunity of women during their reproductive life is almost certainly due to the secretion of the ovarian hormones. The concentration of plasma total cholesterol is lower in women aged 20 to 45 years years than men of the same age group but HDL cholesterol is higher. If both ovaries are removed before the age of 35, this is often followed by a rise in plasma total cholesterol and the incidence of CHD is greatly increased.

Age
In both sexes death rates from CHD rise with age.

Family history
In homogeneous communities there are families which are relatively more or less susceptible to CHD. Family clustering of any disease may be due either to inherited suscepti-

bility or family sharing of environmental experience, e.g. an atherogenic diet. In families susceptible to CHD there is often a high incidence of other diseases which have multiple aetiology, e.g. hypertension, diabetes mellitus, gout and hyperlipidaemia.

Knowledge of the genetic basis of CHD and its relationships to the associated diseases is still fragmentary. An excess of blood group AB over O in CHD patients has been reported (Bronte-Stewart *et al.*, 1962) and an excess A/O ratio in patients with aorto-iliac and femoro-popliteal atherosclerosis (Kingsbury, 1971). National death rates from CHD are correlated with the frequency of the HLA-8 antigen in the population (Matthews, 1975).

Somatotypes or body build
Endomorphs are most susceptible, followed by mesomorphs and ectomorphs in that order.

Behaviour patterns and personality traits
Friedman and Rosenman (1969) have claimed that people with what they call Behaviour Pattern A have an increased incidence and prevalence of CHD. Such people show an excessive sense of time urgency, a preoccupation with vocational deadlines and enhanced aggressiveness and competitive drive. This behaviour pattern is probably constitutional, i.e. it results from the interaction of inheritance and environment.

Hyperlipidaemias
These disturbances are discussed in Chapter 40. Some are

Table 41.2 Risk factors in coronary heart disease (modified from Brusis and McGandy, 1971)

Factors known to increase the risk of coronary heart disease but not necessarily 'abnormalities' *per se* and not amenable to preventive intervention.
1. Maleness
2. Increasing age
3. A family history of premature vascular disease
4. Endomorphic body build
5. Certain behaviour patterns and personality traits.

Factors known to increase the risk of coronary heart disease which are, or merge into, disease entities *per se*.
1. Hyperlipidaemias
2. Hypertension
3. Diabetes mellitus
4. Obesity
5. Hyperuricaemia and gout
6. Certain electrocardiographic abnormalities.

Factors known to increase the risk of coronary heart disease which are primarily due to culture and environment.
1. Cigarette smoking
2. Dietary habits (high intakes of saturated fats, etc.)
3. Lack of physical exercise
4. Occupational hazards.

Less well demonstrated
5. Emotional stress and tension
6. Large coffee intake
7. Soft drinking water.

almost purely genetic and others almost purely environmental in origin. With the exception of Fredrickson's type I the hyperlipoproteinaemias represent risk factors and justify attempts at correction by diet and drugs. The risk of developing CHD rises stepwise with the plasma total cholesterol (Fig. 41.2). More specifically this relates to an elevation of low density or β lipoproteins (LDL).

An association between elevated plasma triglycerides has also been reported (Carlson and Böttiger, 1972). These are carried mainly on very low density or pre-β lipoproteins (VLDL). There is less data about the relationship of plasma triglycerides to CHD as they were not measured in the earlier prospective studies. However, in the last eight prospective studies, although plasma triglycerides were sometimes higher in patients with CHD, computer analysis shows this is not an independent association but due to mutually associated risk factors such as lack of exercise, diabetes, hypercholesterolaemia and obesity (Truswell, 1978). High density lipoprotein (α-lipoprotein cholesterol) has a negative association with the development of CHD of about the same magnitude as the positive association with total cholesterol and appears to be independent (Truswell, 1978).

Only a small percentage of all patients with CHD have a true inborn error of lipid metabolism, in which plasma total cholesterol is often grossly elevated, between 350 and 1000 mg/dl (9 to 26 mmol/l) at an early age. In the great majority of CHD cases, the lipid abnormality is probably mainly acquired, with the possibility of some genetic or constitutional tendency, plasma cholesterol is seldom much above 300 mg/dl (7.8 mmol/l) and often between 250 and 300 mg/dl.

Hypertension
In the Framingham study, the incidence of CHD in men aged 45 to 65 years with blood pressures exceeding 160/95

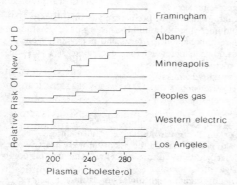

Fig. 41.2. Relative incidence of CHD at different levels of initial plasma cholesterol concentration in US males, as observed in six prospective epidemiological studies. Incidence among men with plasma cholesterol <200 mg/dl was given the same arbitrary value in each study, and rates among men with higher levels were plotted in relation to that group (Dayton, 1971).

was more than five times that in normotensive men (blood pressure 140/90 or less). Elevations in both diastolic and systolic pressures correlate positively with CHD, the diastolic pressure perhaps being more important in younger people.

Diabetes mellitus
This disorder is an important risk factor both in its clinically recognised and latent forms. This association is not due solely, or evenly mainly, to blood lipid disturbances. Diabetics are particularly prone to hypertension and proliferative lesions of the small blood vessels.

Obesity
All official and expert bodies that have made recommendations for prevention of CHD advise that obesity should be prevented or treated, often as one of the first measures. Yet epidemiological data indicate that obesity is a relatively weak risk factor especially if it is separated from diabetes, hypertension and hyperlipidaemia. In Framingham, for example, obesity was only associated with an increased risk of angina pectoris and of sudden death in middle-aged men; it was not a risk factor in women or for myocardial infarction (Kannel et al., 1967). In the Seven Countries prospective study (Keys et al., 1972) obesity was associated with CHD in the USA and southern Europe but not in northern Europe. Though obesity is a weak and inconstant predictor of CHD as an independent variable, it predisposes to the development of hypertension and diabetes, which are themselves important risk factors, and to a lesser extent it is associated with hyperlipidaemia. In addition, obesity directly increases the work load of the heart and, by interfering with chest movement, may restrict pulmonary ventilation.

Hyperuricaemia and gout
There is a positive association between these abnormalities and CHD (Chap. 43), although not all hyperuricaemia represents pre-gout. The mechanisms are unknown.

Electrocardiographic abnormalities
Persons with ECG changes of left ventricular hypertrophy and with certain arrhythmias have an increased risk of developing CHD. If the changes are present when the patient is at rest, they may represent early CHD rather than predisposing factors. But abnormalities that appear on exercise can sometimes be corrected by careful training.

Cigarette smoking
Statistical data (Dawber et al., 1957; Doll and Hill, 1964) show that peripheral vascular disease and CHD, particularly myocardial infarction, occur much more frequently in heavy cigarette smokers than in those who do not smoke. There is a clear relationship between CHD and the amount of smoking; in men aged 45–54 years mortality increases

tenfold as the number of cigarettes smoked daily rises from 0 to 40 (Ball and Turner, 1974). The mechanism(s) by which nicotine or some other constituent of tobacco causes this adverse effect is not clear. It may be due to the vasoconstrictor action of nicotine, to inhalation of carbon monoxide, or to some undesirable effect on the coagulability of the blood. Alternatively, heavy smoking may be a manifestation of a susceptible personality and a reaction to stress and strain. What is clear, however, is that patients with CHD should give up smoking.

DIETARY HABITS

Fats. In prosperous countries the intake of fat is high and a major proportion is of animal origin, containing large amounts of saturated fatty acids. Keys (1953) first suggested that differences in incidence of CHD between different countries can be largely explained by the fat intakes of their populations and, as described in Chapter 40, it is well established that the plasma cholesterol can be reduced in normal people by switching from a Western diet to one low in saturated fats with or without polyunsaturated fat. In the Seven Countries prospective study (Keys et al., 1970) the incidence of CHD in 13 communities was strongly correlated ($r=0.84$) with intake of saturated fats. There were also strong correlations between dietary saturated fat and plasma cholesterol and between plasma cholesterol and CHD. Masironi (1970) compared death rates from atherosclerotic heart disease in 37 countries with their estimated average dietary consumption; the best correlation was with saturated fat. The dietary fat hypothesis states:

High intake of saturated fats
↓A
Raised plasma cholesterol (LDL)
↓B
Atherosclerosis
↓C
Coronary heart disease

The hypothesis arose from considerations of measurements of plasma total cholesterol. It is not changed essentially by later knowledge that it is mainly the cholesterol carried in low density lipoproteins which is increased and that cholesterol carried in high density lipoproteins is reduced.

Significant statistical correlation does not necessarily mean cause and effect. Other factors operate at each step so that while the sequence may be a sensible explanation of the average differences between communities with different ways of life, it is less reliable in predicting which individual in a community will develop CHD and who will not. At stage A, in addition to saturated fat, other dietary components affect plasma cholesterol as can several non-dietary factors (some diseases, season, exercise, drugs, etc)

and the genotype is also important. At stage B plasma cholesterol is only one factor determining atherosclerosis; hypertension is another that is well established. At stage C, as we have said earlier, the appearance of clinical CHD does not only depend on the degree of atherosclerosis but on thrombotic mechanisms and the state of the myocardium as well.

In a homogeneous group of men it has not usually been possible to demonstrate that dietary habits correlate with plasma cholesterol (Morris et al., 1963) unless repeated measurements are made (Easty, 1970) or a large group examined. In 1500 Finnish children saturated fat intake was found to increase stepwise from the lower third to the upper third of the distribution of plasma cholesterol (Räsänen et al., 1978). In Framingham (Kannel and Gordon, 1970) and in other prospective studies the development of CHD could not be related to any dietary factor. But in Framingham the usual dietary intake was estimated from a single interview, and assessment of fat, fatty acid pattern and cholesterol in diets are subject to more variation than are most other constituents (Balogh et al., 1971).

Carbohydrates. Increased consumption of sucrose may have contributed to the increase of CHD. Yudkin (1967) pointed out three types of evidence which he believes incriminate sucrose. First, our primitive ancestors evolved eating the meat and fat of animals but were not accustomed to eating sucrose except for a little in fruits and occasional wild honey. Secondly, the largest change in the diet of prosperous countries in the last 100 years has been a striking rise in sugar consumption (p. 179). Thirdly, Yudkin and Roddy (1964) reported that in a retrospective study patients who had had a myocardial infarction took larger quantities of sugar than control patients. However, the opposite case can be argued. The wild meat that our hunter-gatherer ancestors ate was probably very lean and its small amount of fat relatively unsaturated, as it still is today in wild African bovids (Crawford, 1968). The greatest increase of sugar consumption in Britain and the USA occurred in the second half of the nineteenth century, long before the modern epidemic of CHD started, around 1925. Subsequent measurements of sugar intake in CHD patients have mostly not shown a significant increase over matched controls (Medical Research Council, 1970). In the Seven Countries prospective study sucrose intake was correlated with the incidence of CHD but it was also correlated with the saturated fat intake. A multivariate analysis (Keys, 1973) showed that the partial correlation coefficient of sucrose with CHD was not significant when saturated fat was held constant, but saturated fat was still significantly correlated with CHD with sucrose held constant. There are some countries, such as Mauritius and Venezuela, where sugar intakes are as high as in Britain but CHD mortality is low, as is the intake of saturated fat (Masironi, 1970).

A review of the literature (Truswell, 1977) shows that most writers consider that no direct link between sucrose and CHD has been established.

By contrast, the epidemiological data suggest that if starchy foods have any effect it is a beneficial one. Countries where the intake of starches is high tend to have low rates of CHD. These are technologically underdeveloped countries and their consumption of saturated fat is low. The fibre associated with some starchy foods, if unrefined, may have a lipid-lowering effect (p. 329).

Proteins. There are no grounds for believing that a high intake of animal protein increases the risk of CHD (Brock, 1964). However, there are suggestions that milk consumption could be a risk factor. Davies et al. (1974) reported that 74 per cent of patients with severe myocardial infarction had antibodies to milk in the serum, compared with 36 per cent of hospital control patients of the same age. In rabbits substituting casein and other animal protein for vegetable proteins in the diet raises plasma cholesterol (Carroll and Hamilton, 1975). In human experiments replacing animal protein with vegetable protein has been followed by a fall in plasma cholesterol, but this was probably due to an increased intake of dietary fibre from the vegetable foods (Truswell, 1978).

Drinking water
In at least nine countries a significant negative association between the hardness of the drinking water and mortality from all cardiovascular diseases has been reported. The harder the drinking water the lower the death rate from cardiovascular disease (Crawford et al., 1968). No explanation of this extraordinary finding is as yet established. Calcium or magnesium in hard waters could have a protective action and there are several trace elements in hard waters that might be beneficial. On the other hand, soft waters, being more acidic, are more likely to dissolve potentially toxic trace elements like lead and cadmium from pipes or rocks. The possibilities are reviewed by Masironi et al. (1973). For various reasons the water supply in 11 towns in England and Wales has been changed, making the water harder in five cases and softer in six cases. Coincident with these changes the mortality from CHD amongst men has increased much more in those towns with the softer water than in those with the harder water (Crawford et al., 1971). However, no association between the quality of the water supply and the incidence of CHD has now been reported in many countries. Heyden (1976) lists these reports and after reviewing the evidence in favour of the 'water story' concludes that, because of the inconsistencies and controversies, it would be premature to advise modification of water supplies in the hope of preventing cardiovascular diseases.

Large coffee intakes
In the Boston Collaborative Drug Surveillance Program (1972), a multicentre retrospective study, it was found that patients with myocardial infarction consumed significantly more coffee than matched controls. A similar result had been reported earlier from a prospective study in Chicago (Paul et al., 1963). The Boston group extended their survey to over 1200 patients in 24 hospitals (Jick et al., 1973). The same result was found and could not be explained by other factors such as sugar intake, smoking or occupation. Tea showed a slight but not significant negative association with myocardial infarction. However, this effect of coffee was not confirmed in reported prospective studies (Yana et al., 1977; Truswell, 1978).

LACK OF EXERCISE
Prosperity certainly leads to a reduction in the amount of manual work done by members of a community. As the wealth of a country increases, the 'pick and shovel' men decline and are replaced by those who flick switches and occupy office chairs. An increase in private cars and public transport reduces the number who rely on walking and the push bicycle to get them from place to place. There is some evidence that physical activity protects against CHD. There are occupations in which the risk of developing CHD is less than in others. Thus Morris and his colleagues (1953, 1966) showed that London bus conductors (on double-decker vehicles) have a lower incidence than bus drivers, and postmen who deliver letters have a lower incidence than telephonists and post-office clerks. Further, when the disease was present in conductors and postmen, it was less severe. Morris and Crawford (1958) in a national survey in Britain correlated the extent of the atherosclerosis found in coronary arteries at postmortem with previous occupation. They concluded that physical activity at work was a protection against CHD. 'Men in physically active jobs have less coronary heart disease during middle age, what disease they have is less severe, and they develop it later than men in physically inactive jobs'.

OCCUPATIONAL HAZARDS
In three rayon factories Tiller et al. (1968) showed that the mortality from coronary heart disease was 42 per cent among the process workers as compared to 24 per cent in the non-process workers in the same factories and 17 per cent among other men living in the locality. During the manufacture of viscose rayon, cellulose produced from wood pulp is mixed with carbon disulphide (CS_2). Further, the death rate from coronary heart disease was significantly higher than expected only in those men with more than 10 years employment in the spinning department and it was in this department that the concentration of carbon disulphide in the atmosphere was greatest.

EMOTIONAL STRESS AND TENSION
It is often suggested that the stress and strain of modern life predispose to atherosclerosis. The stress and strain to

which the prosperous business executive or professional man is exposed are well known. A cartoon in the *New Yorker* showed two middle-aged men in shorts on the verandah of a luxurious holiday hotel. One says to the other 'If I were the type to relax could I afford to be here?' The stress and strain of poverty receive much less publicity, but perhaps only a minor proportion of the poor rest content with their lot. It is difficult to be certain that the modern prosperous communities suffer from more stress and strain than their less wealthy predecessors. The behaviour pattern described by Friedman and Rosenman (1969) as type A is associated with increased risk of myocardial infarction and the association could be due to acute or chronic adrenergic overdrive. Possible mediating factors include plasma noradrenaline and FFA. Taggart and Carruthers (1971) reported that the stress of racing driving raised plasma triglycerides and FFA but not plasma cholesterol. The same reaction probably occurs in some urban drivers.

However, there is no doubt that once atherosclerosis is established, emotion, especially anger, can be the immediate cause of clinical symptoms. Long ago the great anatomist, John Hunter, who suffered from angina pectoris, said that he was at the mercy of any knave who chose to enrage him. President Eisenhower described how his symptoms of coronary thrombosis developed on the golf course when for the third time in one morning he was recalled to the clubhouse to answer an unnecessary telephone call from the State Department.

EFFECTS OF DIETARY CHANGES

Trials have been made of the effect of reducing the amounts of dietary saturated fats and increasing the amounts of polyunsaturated fats on the morbidity and mortality from CHD of men who have already had a myocardial infarct or other evidence of the disease (secondary prevention trials) and of apparently healthy men (primary prevention trials). The more important primary trials are those by Rinzler (1968), Dayton *et al.* (1969) and Miettinen *et al.* (1972a), and the main secondary trials are those by Lyon *et al.* (1956), Morrison (1960), Rose *et al.* (1965), Leren (1966), and the Medical Research Council (1965, 1968).

These trials leave no doubt that the dietary changes reduce concentrations of plasma cholesterol, but the effects on morbidity and mortality have been equivocal. In three of the secondary trials (Rose *et al.*, 1965; Medical Research Council, 1965, 1968), there were no differences in the mortality of the experimental and the control group. In others the dietary changes appeared to give some advantages, but each has been criticised because the conditions in the experimental and control groups might not have been precisely comparable. By the time clinical features of CHD first appear, there may be irreversible changes in the myocardium. A dietary change that slows the rate of atherogenesis should be more effective in apparently healthy people.

The best primary prevention trials are by Dayton *et al.* (1969) and Miettinen *et al.* (1972a). The former studied 424 men on an experimental diet and 422 controls in a Los Angeles domicile for veterans. The total deaths from atherosclerosis over a five-year period were 63 in the experimental group and 82 in the control. Miettinen *et al.* (1972a) conducted a 12-year primary prevention trial in two mental hospitals in Helsinki. In one hospital the inmates were given a diet with a P/S ratio over 1.4. Plasma cholesterol values fell and over six years there were fewer coronary events in this hospital than in the control hospital which provided the usual diet, high in saturated fat. The diets were then switched over and in the next six years coronary events were less in the other hospital. Although this experiment is a remarkable achievement, details of the design have been criticised (Rivers and Yudkin, 1972; Malperin *et al.*, 1973) and defended Miettinen *et al.*, 1972b, 1973).

The difficulties in carrying out these long-term trials are enormous. The American Heart Association (1969) has made a study of the feasibility of mass field trials. The plans for seven studies which might give a definite answer are set out. The cheapest, which is not recommended, involves the study of 11 000 men for five years and would cost 19 million dollars. The best, involving 319 000 men, would cost 379 million dollars (both estimates at 1969 prices).

PROPHYLAXIS AND MANAGEMENT

Thus physicians have inadequate information about the probable benefits which their patients are likely to receive from dietary modifications. Depending on their interpretation of the above reports some may conclude that there is little justification for troubling their patients with dietary changes and restrictions and others that diet is a very important factor in determining the risk of development of CHD. Both these views can be sustained by selected reading. In the present state of uncertainty, which is likely to continue, a *via media* seems necessary.

When a man's life is threatened or he has disabling consequences of CHD, it is enough that preventive measures recommended to him should have a reasonable basis of probability. On the other hand, when recommendations are made for the primary prevention of atherosclerosis, a process which is known to start in the second or third decades of life, and these recommendations are intended for whole populations threatened by a serious epidemic of CHD, some certain bases are expected.

Advice on prophylaxis differs under three circumstances. First, there is general advice applicable to all adults who live in prosperous communities; this is discussed on page 531. Secondly, there is advice to persons who are apparently healthy but in whom one or more of the risk factors described above is found. Thirdly, there is advice to persons who already have signs or symptoms of CHD and face the possibility of severe disablement or death in the near future; such persons are said to be coronary prone.

Apparently healthy persons at special risk

Such persons may first need to be convinced that they are at special risk. A physician has the task of explaining to him or her the reasons for this and urging the advantages of a programme of prophylaxis. Such a programme need not be onerous.

All modern studies lend support to the old advice given by many physicians of moderation in all things. 'Take regular daily exercise out of doors, stop smoking or smoke only a few cigars or a pipe; plan a daily routine that causes no undue stresses; and avoid dietary excesses, especially of animal fat and energy.' This advice does not involve great changes in traditional food habits or bizarre diets. In simple language such persons should be advised to limit their intake of dairy fats. Polyunsaturated fats should be used for frying. Bacon and eggs for breakfast should be taken exceptionally and not regularly. They should choose chicken, fish or lean portions of meat and remove all excess fat. They should be advised to take regular physical exercise. Walking is specially to be recommended, as are recreations such as golf, gardening and cycling, provided they are carried out sensibly and in moderation. However, strenuous exercise is usually contraindicated in middle-aged or elderly persons, since this may lead to rupture of diseased vessels or to subintimal haemorrhage in the coronary arteries with a subsequent myocardial infarct.

A doctor is in a good position to advise patients on their general habits as outlined above. In addition he has an important role both in the prevention of atherosclerosis by treating hypertension, diabetes, obesity and thyroid deficiency, diseases known to be associated with CHD. All these persons should have their plasma cholesterol measured and in appropriate cases plasma triglycerides should be measured and lipoprotein electrophoresis done. Doctors have the responsibility of presenting the facts and theories with sufficient force to persuade those who are at risk to modify their way of life but without creating coronary phobia.

Coronary-prone persons

For patients with signs and symptoms of CHD and a markedly raised plasma cholesterol much stricter control of the quantity and nature of the fat in the diet should be considered. Diet No. 14 (p. 568) shows how intake of saturated fat can be reduced with partial substitution by oils rich in polyunsaturated fatty acids. In the majority of cases this produces a significant fall in plasma cholesterol. For patients who do not respond to this strict diet treat-

ment with cholestyramine or other drugs which lower plasma cholesterol may be indicated.

Far fewer physicians than formerly keep patients who have had a myocardial infarction on anticoagulant drugs. The possible prevention of recurrence of thrombosis has to be offset against the risk of inducing a haemorrhage. Clinical trials have been equivocal. Their use necessitates repeated laboratory tests of the blood prothrombin and this may induce or aggravate an anxiety state.

Finally the patient requires reassurance and psychological support. The risks of serious consequences and a fatal recurrence after a myocardial infarct may be far less than the patient has been led to think. Many patients continue to live useful and active lives for many years, as do many patients after the onset of symptoms of angina pectoris.

The controversial and rapidly evolving views on surgery both in prophylaxis and management have been left out of this book. They have in common an attempt to revascularise (or even replace) hearts which have various degrees of coronary atherosclerosis.

SUMMARY

We believe that the following characteristics of prosperous urban living all contribute to the rising incidence and prevalence of CHD: a sedentary life, reduced physical activity, a high consumption of saturated fats, cigarette smoking and emotional disturbances. The effects of individual factors are independent and additive. Fortunately these factors offer scope for preventive measures. The fact that the epidemic appears to have reached a plateau and may be declining (p. 334) suggests that many individuals may already have benefited from the wide publicity given to these measures.

HYPERTENSION

Some degree of hypertension in the systemic arteries is a common finding in middle age when the pressure in the brachial artery is measured with the sphygmomanometer. Because hypertension can be asymptomatic for many years, because it it is an important predisposing cause of several major diseases and because it is amenable to treatment, measurement of the blood pressure is a part of all routine clinical examinations of adults.

The pathological changes which accompany established hypertension are a thickening of the arterioles with hyaline material and, later, hypertrophy of the myocardium of the left ventricle. If untreated, moderate hypertension eventually leads to cardiac failure, with dilation of the left ventricle and congestion of the pulmonary or systemic veins. It also causes ischaemic changes in the kidney, nephrosclerosis. However, before these direct consequences of prolonged hypertension develop the patient may suffer from vascular accidents to which hypertension is an important predisposing factor. It is one factor increasing the risk of coronary atherosclerosis (as discussed above) and is a strong risk factor for cerebral vascular disease (Chap. 49).

In a minority of patients blood pressure is very high. This is called malignant hypertension. The heart, kidneys, retinal and other arteries are quickly affected; there is an immediate risk of a dangerous vascular accident, thus vigorous treatment is required.

In about 80 per cent of cases clinical examination and special investigation do not demonstrate a cause for the condition. This is essential hypertension. Treatment has to be symptomatic. In the remaining cases the hypertension is secondary to renal disease, e.g. glomerulonephritis or pyelonephritis (Chap. 44), or, less commonly, to an endocrine disorder, e.g. Cushing's syndrome, phaeochromocytoma, primary aldosteronism or acromegaly, or to the rare congenital malformation, coarctation of the aorta. Pregnancy also predisposes to hypertension. Ideally it should be possible to treat these secondary types of hypertension radically by eradicating the underlying disease, but this is not always possible.

Essential (idiopathic) hypertension
In most cases of hypertension the cause is obscure, and for these the term 'essential' hypertension is used.

In healthy young adults the systolic blood pressure is about 120 mmHg and the diastolic pressure about 80. There is usually a gradual rise of blood pressure as age advances and at 65 years the mean figure is about 160/90. The rise with age is very variable. In some people it is more rapid and reaches a higher level than the above figure. It is difficult to state at what point the level ceases to be normal and hypertension begins. The diastolic pressure is a more reliable guide to the presence or absence of hypertension than the systolic pressure. Without qualifications, e.g. age, obesity and the circumstances in which the blood pressure is recorded, blood pressure figures *per se* are often of little value. Nevertheless the following figures may be used as a rough guide to severity, if present persistently. Mild hypertension may be said to be present when the diastolic pressure is 90 to 105, moderate hypertension when the diastolic pressure is 105 to 120 and severe hypertension when the diastolic pressure exceeds 120. The association of severe hypertension with renal failure or papilloedema is characteristic of malignant hypertension.

In some individuals there is no rise of blood pressure as age advances. This is also the case amongst some isolated groups of primitive people, e.g. in New Guinea (Whyte, 1958), in some Pacific Islands (Maddocks, 1964) and in Kalahari bushmen (Truswell *et al.*, 1972). On the other hand, Japan has the highest incidence of hypertension in the world.

The causes of the gradual rise in blood pressure which usually occurs with advancing age and the excessive rise which develops in some patients are not fully known. Of various possibilities, genetic factors are certainly important. The blood pressure appears to be inherited in much the same way as height (Pickering, 1968). However, genetic factors cannot account for all the variations.

Environmental factors are also responsible. Two which may operate in some patients are dietary in origin. Excess energy intake leading to obesity is associated with hypertension. This old clinical observation was confirmed at Framingham (Kannel *et al.*, 1967). However, thin people may develop hypertension.

It is well known that a low salt diet reduces the blood pressure of normal people and of patients with hypertension. Whether a high salt intake predisposes to hypertension is less certain. It is difficult to get reliable estimations of salt intakes by a population group, but the literature contains records, not all reliable, of mean salt intake and mean blood pressure of 27 populations scattered throughout the world (Gleibermann, 1973). The data indicate that there is a direct positive correlation between the two variables, and in some culturally homogeneous groups in Japan and Taiwan salt intake appears as the major environmental factor affecting blood pressure. In Europe and North America much salt is added to foods in manufacturing processes and salt intakes are generally high. There is a case, well set out by Dahl (1972), that this is an important factor in the prevalence of hypertension in industrialised countries (see also p. 88).

Psychological factors often cause an immediate and temporary rise in blood pressure, but whether the stress and strain of life can be held responsible for permanent rises is uncertain. Many patients with anxiety states have normal or even low blood pressures and many well-balanced individuals become hypertensive.

TREATMENT
There is no specific remedy, and hence, at present, no permanent cure. Yet hypotensive drugs are effective in controlling most progressive cases and so reduce morbidity and mortality.

Mild hypertension (diastolic pressure 90 to 105). The condition may be found accidentally in the course of a life insurance or routine medical examination and the patient may complain of no symptoms. Then usually no mention of the finding need be made but it is good practice to check the blood pressure again at future opportunities in case it shows a tendency to rise.

Moderate hypertension (diastolic pressure 105 to 120). The common symptoms are headache, cardiac discomfort and breathlessness. These are often improved by simple dietary treatment and advice. If the patient is overweight, treatment of the obesity so as to cause loss of .1 to 1.5 kg a week often relieves the symptoms and brings about a significant fall in blood pressure. This is very important since the chance of developing CHD is greatly increased if hypertension and obesity co-exist.

Many patients need to be told how to organise their lives so as to avoid emotional stress and excessive physical activity. Moderation in all things is the guiding principle to be adopted.

If these simple measures are not sufficient, hypotensive drugs or a diuretic should be given alone or in combination. Morgan *et al.* (1978) have shown that in some cases reduction of sodium intake may be as effective in reducing diastolic blood pressure as the use of drugs.

Severe hypertension (diastolic pressure over 120) and malignant hypertension. For patients with moderate hypertension who have failed to respond to the measures discussed above, and for patients with objective evidence of severe hypertension, namely disease of the heart, retina, kidneys or peripheral arteries, two lines of treatment are available:

Hypotensive drugs. These lower the blood pressure by producing vasodilation through a central or peripheral action and block selectively the peripheral sympathetic nervous system. There is no hypotensive drug that is entirely satisfactory, as all may have unpleasant or serious side-effects. Nevertheless such drugs offer the best hope of controlling severe hypertension.

Decreased intake and increased excretion of sodium. If the sodium content of the body is significantly reduced there is usually a fall in blood pressure and relief of the symptoms. This can often be achieved by the use of the restricted salt regime (p. 85) combined with the administration of a diuretic. As the use of a diuretic often leads to hypokalaemia, it is usual to give a potassium salt as well. As sodium restriction depresses renal function there is a danger that it may precipitate uraemia in patients whose kidneys are already damaged.

OTHER VARIETIES OF HEART DISEASE

In many forms of heart disease, e.g. congenital, valvular, pulmonary, endocrinal and infective, dietary factors appear to play no part in the aetiology and they are not considered here except under heart failure.

The variety most clearly associated with malnutrition and most amenable to nutrient therapy is described under beriberi (p. 287). Rheumatic fever is a common cause in childhood, adolescence and early adult life but its incidence is falling. In some industrial areas, notably in Britain, chronic bronchitis is common and frequently leads to pulmonary heart disease. In some communities in tropical and temperate climates, especially in Africa, cardiomyopathy of complex and unknown aetiology is common.

The heart is affected both in hypothyroidism and in hyperthyroidism and both conditions are more prevalent in endemic goitre regions than elsewhere (Chap. 30). However iodine when used in hyperthyroid heart disorders is used pharmacologically rather than as a nutrient.

Myocarditis (inflammation of the heart muscle) is part of the clinical and pathological picture of a variety of infective, parasitic and hypersensitivity diseases which include rheumatic fever, diphtheria, pneumonia, typhoid fever, typhus, malaria, Chagas' disease (South American trypanosomiasis) and infections with viruses.

Cardiomyopathies

This hodge-podge has been classified by Schrire (1972) and defined as 'a primary involvement of the myocardium, non-inflammatory in nature'. Certain varieties are common in tropical and developing areas, especially in the African continent. Because of their geographical distribution and the absence of a clear cut aetiology they are sometimes referred to as 'nutritional cardiomyopathies' although the role of nutrition in their causation is uncertain and they do not show any dramatic or specific response to diet therapy or vitamins. Schrire (1966) described four varieties of 'nutritional cardiomyopathies'.

Endomyocardial fibrosis In some African regions this is the most common form of heart disease. Various hypotheses of causation have been postulated, e.g. that it is a viral disease, that it is due to filariasis, that it is due to the 5-hydroxytryptamine found in the banana diet of East and West Africa or that it is due to a hypersensitivity response to infection. Apart from its geographical distribution, there is no direct evidence of nutritional causation.

The clinical presentation is with congestive cardiac failure, cardiomegaly, triple rhythm and very rarely with systemic emboli. The onset is usually insidious. Involvement of the atrioventricular valves produces murmurs which are easily confused with those of rheumatic heart disease.

Myocardopathy of unknown origin (MUO) Attention was directed to this group of cases by Gillanders (1951) among Bantu patients in Johannesburg, which is not even subtropical. He described a very large heart, massive oedema and associated hepatic damage. The disease in his experience did not respond to thiamin, but only to a good general diet. However the favourable response probably was due as much to a prolonged period of bed-rest as to the diet, since cardiac failure returns in most cases on resumption of work, and becomes chronic and irreversible.

The cause of this condition must be regarded as unknown. There has been reasonable speculation that chronic malnutrition, alcoholism, particularly with doctored liquors, or long-continued consumption of small quantities of food contaminants, e.g. mycotoxins, may be responsible. Similar cases have been described in many parts of Africa and in other parts of the world. The geographical incidence overlaps that of endomyocardial fibrosis but only to a slight degree, and the two conditions are probably distinct.

Alcoholic cardiomyopathy Alcohol can affect the heart, either by producing a vitamin deficiency heart failure, beriberi, or by directly poisoning the heart as in alcoholic cardiomyopathy. In high dosage alcohol has widespread toxic effects on myocardial cells which have been well investigated. Mitochondrial function and lipid metabolism are impaired (Bing and Tillmans, 1976). Beriberi heart disease occurs when alcoholism has led to anorexia, usually in people living on poor diets. Alcoholic cardiomyopathy occurs after prolonged high intakes of spirits or beer. The disease is insidious in onset, taking months or years to develop, but ending in heart failure that is usually irreversible although a few patients who can be persuaded to abstain from alcohol may improve. Palpitations are common, usually due to atrial fibrillation or ectopic beats; dyspnoea occurs early and this is followed later by congestive failure with cardiomegaly, triple rhythm, functional systolic mitral or tricuspid murmurs, pulmonary and systemic congestion (Demakis et al., 1974).

Postpartum heart disease Obscure cardiac failure during and after pregnancy has long been known in most parts of the world. The usual background for this disorder is a history of multiple pregnancies occurring in rapid succession. Some of these may be due to chronic after-effects of viral myocarditis. Usually the symptoms of cardiac insufficiency develop in the puerperium although they may be present during pregnancy and recur in the puerperium (Stuart, 1968). Apart from the association with pregnancy there is nothing to distinguish these cases from MUO. A large series has been described from New Orleans, where it has been claimed that bed rest lasting for as much as a year may allow ultimate recovery. In regions where MUO is endemic, usually among males, this variety may present during the puerperium.

Occasional cases of cardiomyopathy occur from accidental contamination of foods with toxic plants. *Argemone mexicana* has caused epidemic dropsy in India (p. 222) from contamination of mustard-seed oil; it has also caused some cases of cardiomyopathy in South Africa from contamination of wheat (Brink et al., 1965).

HEART FAILURE

Whatever the cause of heart disease, it will, unless very mild, lead to some impairment of the efficiency of the heart as a pump. In severe CHD and in cardiomyopathies the heart fails because its muscle is weakened; in hypertension and valvular disease it fails because the muscle is working against an increased load. In mild degrees of heart failure the only manifestation is an inability to increase the cardiac output in response to strenuous exertion and the patient has dyspnoea on exertion. In moderate grades there is venous congestion, either in the pulmonary circulation causing dyspnoea or in the systemic veins causing oedema and hepatic enlargement. Acute and severe cardiac failure causes pulmonary oedema and cardiogenic shock.

TREATMENT

As already indicated heart failure may occur in hypertensive, coronary, valvular, pulmonary or other cardiac disease. Irrespective of the cause, the aim of treatment is to secure the maximum of rest for the heart and to remove the oedema. The basis of treatment is (a) complete rest, (b) the administration of diuretics and a digitalis preparation, and (c) a diet low in sodium, and also in energy if the patient is obese.

It is important to realise that when heart failure first presents this is often not a terminal event. It has usually been precipitated by a respiratory infection, arrhythmia or some other complication. If these are diagnosed and effectively treated at the same time as symptomatic treatment is given for the heart failure, the patient may well get over the episode and be able to lead a relatively normal life, sometimes for years before heart failure becomes incapacitating.

DIETARY MANAGEMENT

The diet should be constructed on the following principles.

1. As the oedema fluid has the same sodium concentration as plasma, oedema is always associated with retention of sodium. In severe oedema the excess fluid retained may amount to 10 litres or more, containing 1400 mmol of sodium, equivalent to over 80 g of sodium chloride. The removal of this is greatly facilitated if the sodium intake is reduced. Details of how to reduce the sodium intake are given on page 85.

2. Rigid restriction of the fluid intake, as was formerly recommended, is not necessary if the intake of sodium is adequately reduced and its excretion increased. Sufficient fluid to quench thirst and make the patient comfortable, i.e. 1.5 to 2 litres daily, may be allowed.

3. Owing to the congestion of the digestive organs, each feed must be small in quantity and easily digestible. In the initial treatment, fluid or semifluid food is advisable for patients who are seriously ill.

For most patients with mild or moderate degrees of cardiac failure the restricted salt regimen described on page 85 is suitable.

For the severe grades of failure, the Karell fluid diet has been recommended. This is simple and effective. It consists of 800 ml of milk, given in four feeds each of 200 ml (one small glass). No other food or fluid is given. It provides about 2.2 MJ (550 kcal), 28 g protein and about 0.45 g (20 mmol) of sodium. This diet should only be employed for two or three days as the patient will complain of monotony and thirst.

Alternatively the patient can start with a light diet (Diet No. 13) which provides about 3.8 MJ, 40 g protein and 1 g

(45 mmol) of sodium. No table salt should be added. Care should be taken not to prescribe medicines containing sodium, e.g. stomach powders, and to avoid baking powder in cooking.

With improvement in the clinical condition a light ward diet can be given and the protein intake increased, but the salt intake must still be restricted. The restricted salt regimen keeps the sodium intake to about one-third of normal. If a diuretic is prescribed for a long period, a potassium supplement is needed.

Compensated heart disease. When recovery has taken place or in less severe cases, the patient may be up and about and able to continue his normal occupation. Heart disease, however, always involves some curtailment of physical activities, and the more arduous recreations must be given up. This reduction in energy expenditure should always be balanced by a corresponding reduction in food intake. If the diet is not reduced appropriately, obesity will inevitably follow. Obesity is common in patients with heart disease and requires to be treated in the usual way.

Chronic congestive failure. Some patients, especially those with hypoxia from respiratory disease, become pathetically thin and undernourished. This cardiac cachexia is largely the result of poor appetite, resulting from hypoxaemia, compression of the stomach by the congested liver and the tendency of high doses of digitalis to produce nausea. In addition specific deficiencies of nutrients may arise in patients with chronic congestive cardiac failure. Hypoalbuminaemia may occur due to leakage of plasma albumin into the congested gastrointestinal tract (Davidson *et al.*, 1961). Malabsorption of fat can sometimes be demonstrated (Vaughan Jones, 1961) and biochemical tests may show evidence of subclinical folate deficiency (*British Medical Journal*, 1970). Thus, even if the prognosis is hopeless, at least protein, potassium and vitamin deficiencies should be looked for and corrected.

42. Diabetes Mellitus

Diabetes mellitus is a syndrome characterised by a raised glucose concentration in the blood, due to deficiency or diminished effectiveness of insulin. The disease is chronic and also affects the metabolism of fat and protein. Glucose usually spills over into the urine and this is associated with polyuria and loss of weight. There is always the hazard of the acute complication of ketoacidosis, which is a dangerous, but treatable, medical emergency. Diabetics have an increased risk of atherosclerotic diseases and of certain obstetrical difficulties. In longstanding cases specific changes can occur in the eyes, feet, nerves and kidneys. Fuller accounts of the disease are given by Irvine *et al.* (1974) and Oakley *et al.* (1974).

EPIDEMIOLOGY

Diabetes mellitus is the commonest endocrine disorder. Of the two types described on page 349 the 'juvenile-onset type' is less common; its incidence reaches a peak between 10 and 12 years of age (Bloom *et al.*, 1975). The maturity-onset type contains the great majority of diabetics who first become ill in middle age or later (Fig. 42.1). For this reason the frequency of diabetes in different communities can only be compared when rates are standardised for age. Because the onset is often insidious, in any large group of people there are some who know they have diabetes and others with mild or early diabetes who are as yet unaware that they have it; these can be detected by finding glucose in the urine and a high blood glucose. In Britain about 1 per cent of the population have 'known' diabetes and a similar proportion may be 'discovered' by biochemical screening. Criteria for diagnosis are becoming standardised (p. 356) and there are now sufficient comparable surveys to show that the prevalence of the maturity-onset form of diabetes varies greatly between different populations.

Probably the highest rate in the world is in the Pima tribe of American Indians among whom half of all people over 35 years of age have known plus discovered diabetes (Bennett *et al.*, 1971). Prevalence is nearly as high in some other tribes of American Indians but not in all (West, 1974). Polynesians and Micronesians have a genetic predisposition and where they have become prosperous, inactive and overweight prevalence may be high, as on the island of Nauru where one-third of all people over 15 years of age have diabetes (Zimmet *et al.*, 1977). Other groups with a high prevalence are Asian Indians in South Africa (Jackson, 1970), Maoris in New Zealand and some Aborigines in Australia. These races have been through famines or periods of prolonged food shortage in their history; natural selection may have led to survival of a 'thrifty genotype' which may predispose to obesity and to diabetes in conditions of affluence (Neel, 1962).

AETIOLOGY

Two types of diabetes are recognised, primary and secondary.

Primary diabetes
Most cases belong to this group. Although several contributing factors are known, the precise aetiology is still uncertain.

Heredity. A familial tendency to diabetes undoubtedly exists but neither the specific biochemical defect nor its mode of inheritance has yet been identified. This is shown by the association of insulin-dependent diabetes with tissue antigens HLA-B8 and DRW3. Genetic factors are probably more important in those who develop diabetes before the age of 40, but in both young and old, environmental and other factors also operate and may determine which of those with a genetic predisposition develop the clinical syndrome, and when this occurs.

Sex. There are rather more young male diabetics than female; in middle age women are more often affected. Pregnancy and increasing parity add to the likelihood of developing diabetes.

Obesity. The association of obesity and diabetes has long been recognised, but it is still uncertain whether obesity is the result or the cause of diabetes. The majority of middle-aged diabetic patients are obese (Fig. 42.1) but only a minority of obese people develop diabetes. There is a clinical impression that the incidence of clinical diabetes is rising and this may be related to increasing prevalence of obesity. West and Kalbfleisch (1971) examined the prevalence of diabetes in relation to income, diet, obesity and race in ten different countries, using standardised diagnostic criteria. The correlation coefficient, between average percentage of standard weight and prevalence of diabetes, was 0.89.

The view that obesity is diabetogenic in those genetically predisposed to the disease is based on the fact that in simple obesity there is insulin resistance (Rabinowitz and Zierler, 1961), particularly in muscle (Butterfield and Whichelow, 1968) and hyperinsulinaemia (Karam et al., 1963). The mechanisms which induce this increased secretion of insulin and resistance to its action are being investigated, but it is clear that obesity acts as a stress on the endocrine pancreas. It is postulated that genetically poorly endowed ß cells may be unable to meet this stress, and that when someone with this inherited liability becomes obese, clinical diabetes results.

Estimates of plasma immunoreactive insulin (IRI) in patients with symptoms of diabetes immediately after diagnosis support this concept. Although some of those who are obese have an abnormally high plasma IRI, most show some degree of insulin deficiency (Perley and Kipnis, 1966; Seltzer et al., 1967; Baird, 1973). In general, the more carbohydrate tolerance is impaired in obese diabetics, the more deficient the insulin response to various stimuli.

Studies of diabetic sibships (Baird, 1973) also suggest that although an inherited liability to diabetes is the most important single factor leading to the development of clinical diabetes, obesity, acting as a diabetogenic agent, is also a critical factor in many instances. In all social classes and in both sexes, the percentage of obese subjects was found to be significantly higher among diabetic propositi compared with their non-diabetic siblings and with non-diabetic controls (Fig. 42.2).

Diet

Himsworth (1949) recorded the fall which occurred in

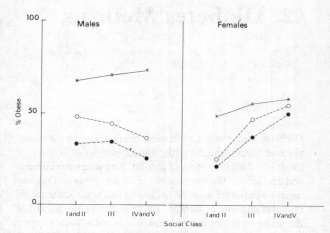

Fig. 42.2 Comparison of percentage obese (see legend to Fig. 42.1 for definition of obesity) among diabetic patients (×), their non-diabetic brothers and sisters (O), and the non-diabetic brothers and sisters of controls (●) engaged in the same type of employment. From data of Baird et al. (1973).

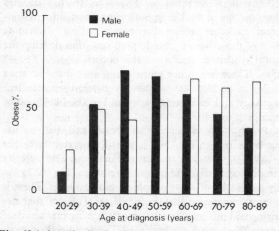

Fig. 42.1 Age distribution of all new cases of diabetes mellitus occurring within a defined geographical area over 2 years by age and obesity. A diabetic patient was classified as obese if he weighed 10 per cent or more above the mean weight of all persons in the population of the same sex, height and age, or had been more than 10 per cent overweight for more than half his adult life. From data of Baird et al. (1973).

mortality from diabetes in Britain in the two world wars and related this to the fall in the national consumption of certain foodstuffs. There was a closer association with fat than with total carbohydrate, protein or energy. Trowell suggests that the fall of diabetes mortality in Britain during World War II fits well with increased intake of dietary fibre from use of flour with a higher extraction rate (Chap. 17). The reliability of such studies depends on the accuracy of the information on death certificates, which is usually seriously deficient as far as diabetes is concerned (Cameron, 1966). There is often a striking increase in the incidence of diabetes in hitherto isolated populations used to hard physical work and limited food when they are exposed to affluence and civilisation, and this may be due to a change in diet, particularly to an increased consumption of refined carbohydrate (Cohen et al., 1961; Politzer and Schneider, 1962; Campbell, 1963; Wicks et al., 1973). However, under these circumstances many things change and other factors may be more important than diet in the development of diabetes (Gelfand, 1967). Dietary factors may act indirectly, e.g. through an increased incidence of obesity.

Direct observations in both man and animals are scarce. In man the various components of the diet have been altered under controlled conditions, and the changes in metabolism monitored (Brunzell et al., 1971; Grey and Kipnis, 1971; Mahler, 1972) but since these are short-term studies their relevance to the aetiology of diabetes mellitus is questionable. In longer studies using animal models (Stauffacher et al., 1972), there is the problem that at least two dietary components have to be altered at any one time, if diet is to remain isoenergetic.

There are no primary prevention studies in man in which the composition of the diet has been altered over a prolonged period and the effect on the incidence of diabetes followed up. It would be extraordinarily difficult and expensive to set up such a study.

Forty years ago Himsworth (1935) attempted to make a direct approach to the problem in another way by experiments with diabetic patients involving a 'preferment-choice' technique. This depends on the doubtful assumption that the choice of food of an individual, who knows that he suffers from 'sugar diabetes', is an accurate index of his dietary habits prior to the diagnosis. Such a technique is particularly unreliable for the quantitative aspects of dietary habits.

Another attempt has been made to assess the relative importance of heredity and environmental factors such as diet by comparing newly diagnosed, middle-aged diabetics with their non-diabetic siblings and with non-diabetic control subjects (Baird, 1972, 1973). In all social classes and in both sexes, diabetic patients were found to eat significantly more than non-diabetics (Fig. 42.3). The food consumed by diabetics did not appear to differ in any way from that consumed by non-diabetics, except in quantity, and no relationship was found between glucose tolerance and any dietary constituent. This does not lend support to the idea that any specific dietary factor is diabetogenic; nor does it fit with the suggestion that hyperphagia results from impaired carbohydrate tolerance. The interpretation which seems to fit the data best is that patients developing maturity-onset diabetes are selected from a larger group with an inherited abnormality of the endocrine pancreas by their high intake of energy. Lack of exercise adds to the difficulty of disposing of excess energy consumed.

Infections. These may unmask latent diabetes. Staphylococcal infections in particular are frequently associated with the development of clinical diabetes.

Stress. Physical injury, severe infection or an emotional disturbance sometimes precedes the onset, as in many other diseases that arise mysteriously and unexpectedly. Stress may act via an adrenocortical response since corticosteroids or ACTH can precipitate diabetes. However, stress probably does not cause diabetes in people who would otherwise never have had it; it unmasks a latent form.

Secondary diabetes

A minority of cases of diabetes occur as a result of diseases which destroy the pancreas and lead to impaired secretion of insulin, e.g. pancreatitis, haemochromatosis, carcinoma of the pancreas and pancreatectomy.

Diabetes may also accompany endocrine disorders which increase concentrations of hormones that are insulin antagonists.

Growth hormone. This, if administered to dogs, produces permanent diabetes and about 30 per cent of patients with acromegaly are diabetic.

Adrenocortical hormones. Cortisol and other corticosteroids raise the blood glucose by increasing protein breakdown and by inhibiting utilisation of glucose by peripheral tissues. Thus, many patients with Cushing's syndrome show impaired carbohydrate tolerance; conversely increased sensitivity to insulin is an important feature of Addison's disease and hypopituitarism, and this can be corrected by corticosteroids.

Adrenaline. This raises blood glucose by increasing breakdown of liver glycogen and by suppressing secretion of insulin. Patients with a phaeochromocytoma frequently show a diabetic glucose tolerance test and the incidence of these rare tumours is relatively high among diabetic patients.

Thyroid hormones. Thyroxine if given in excess aggravates the diabetic state and some patients with hyperthyroidism show impaired glucose tolerance.

Gestational diabetes. This refers to the hyperglycaemia which may occur temporarily during pregnancy in women with an inherited predisposition. During normal pregnancy there is an increased production of hormonal antagonists to insulin which leads to increased rates of secretion and release of insulin. A failing pancreas may be unable to meet this demand.

Drugs, for example adrenocortical steroids and thiazide diuretics, may precipitate diabetes, especially in those genetically susceptible.

Liver disease, particularly cirrhosis and hepatitis, may be associated with impaired glucose tolerance.

CHEMICAL PATHOLOGY

The hyperglycaemia results from the insulin secreted by the pancreas being either insufficient in amount or ineffective in action for one or more reasons. Hence there is an

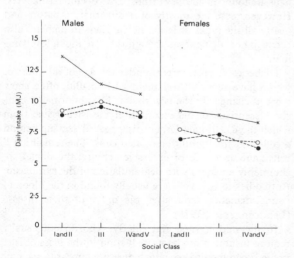

Fig. 42.3 Comparison of the amount of energy consumed daily by untreated diabetic patients (×), their non-diabetic brothers and sisters (○), and non-diabetic controls (●) for all social classes and engaged in the same type of employment. From data of Baird *et al.* (1973).

underlying intracellular lack of glucose, leading to increased gluconeogenesis and lipolysis as compensatory reactions under the influence of such hormones as growth hormone and cortisol. Thus the hyperglycaemia arises from two main sources, a reduced rate of removal of glucose from the blood by the peripheral tissues and an increased release of glucose from the liver into the circulation. Although significant amounts of insulin can often be detected in the plasma of cases of primary diabetes, its concentration is lower than in normal subjects whose blood glucose is raised to comparable heights. It seems likely that the abnormalities in carbohydrate tolerance and lipid metabolism result directly from the lack of insulin. However, the sequence of events which culminate in the development of this insulin-deficient state is still uncertain. It may arise from a primary disorder of insulin secretion. Alternatively the primary defect may not be in the pancreas but in either a circulating antagonist to insulin or a cell-based resistance with secondary deficiency of insulin.

Consequences of hyperglycaemia and glycosuria. When the glucose concentration in the blood exceeds the capacity of the renal tubules to reabsorb it from the glomerular filtrate, glycosuria occurs. In the majority of people the level of blood glucose at which this happens is approximately 10 mmol/l (180 mg/100 ml). Glucose increases the osmolality of the glomerular filtrate and thus prevents the reabsorption of water as the filtrate passes down the renal tubules. In this way the volume of urine is markedly increased in diabetes and polyuria and nocturia occur. This in turn leads to loss of water and electrolytes which results in thirst and polydipsia. In acute cases, or in more slowly progressive cases if the fluid intake has been low, e.g. because of mental confusion or for other reasons, severe depletion of water and electrolytes may occur. As the blood glucose rises the extracellular fluid becomes hypertonic, and water leaves the cells. In the early stages, before the volume of the extracellular fluid is grossly reduced the patient shows few clinical signs, but if the loss of water and electrolytes continues, depletion of extracellular fluid leads to the clinical features of severe dehydration.

Consequences of poor glucose utilisation. Impaired utilisation of carbohydrate results in a sense of fatigue, and two compensatory mechanisms operate to provide alternative metabolic substrate. Both lead to loss of body tissue and wasting may occur in spite of a normal or even an increased intake of food. This is added to any loss of weight resulting from loss of fluid.

Increased glycogenolysis and gluconeogenesis. Glycogen and protein are present in cells associated with water and intracellular electrolytes. As glycogen and protein are catabolised, glucose, water and electrolytes, particularly potassium, are released into the extracellular space. An increased urinary excretion of potassium, magnesium and phosphorus therefore occurs in uncontrolled diabetes.

Increased lipolysis. This is seen as a raised fasting plasma concentration of free fatty acid (FFA), and a diminished fall in plasma FFA in response to a carbohydrate load. The extent to which lipolysis occurs is proportional to the degree of insulin deficiency. If the latter is marked, the normal response to feeding may be completely lost and the plasma concentration of FFA may remain three or four times the normal level.

Fatty acids are taken up by the liver and degraded through stages to acetyl CoA. Normally most of these molecules enter the citric acid cycle, but in severe diabetes more is formed than the cycle can handle. Instead acetyl coenzyme A is converted to acetoacetic acid. Most of this is then reduced to β-hydroxybutyric acid, while some is decarboxylated to acetone. These **ketone bodies** are oxidised and utilised as metabolic fuel, but their rate of utilisation is limited. When the rate of production by the liver exceeds that of removal by the peripheral tissues, then the blood concentration rises. Ketone bodies are strong acids which dissociate readily and release hydrogen ions into the body fluids. The fall in pH causes a decrease in plasma bicarbonate and an increase in $P\text{co}_2$ in the arterial blood. This state is called **ketoacidosis.**

The extent to which the clinical features of dehydration and ketoacidosis are seen in individual cases depends on the speed at which the condition develops and the extent to which the patient himself increases his intake of fluid, as well as on the degree of insulin deficiency present.

MORBID ANATOMY

The pancreas. Abnormalities in the islets of Langerhans are found at autopsy in most cases of clinical diabetes. However these are mostly of a quantitative nature and nearly all the types of lesion in the islets in diabetes also occur in non-diabetics, although they are much less common.

Diabetics at postmortem under the age of 40, most of whom have required treatment with insulin, often show marked changes in the islet tissue. The abnormality consists essentially of degeneration of the islet tissue, from which the β cells have largely disappeared, leaving behind α cells and small undifferentiated cells. The remaining β cells show evidence of excessive activity; the nuclei are commonly enlarged with degranulation of the cytoplasm. Antibodies to islet cells are usually found in the blood of young diabetics soon after the onset of their disease (Lendrum et al., 1976).

In the middle-aged and elderly, who do not usually require insulin, a moderate reduction in the mass of islet tissue is commonly seen which does not appear to account for the degree of impaired carbohydrate tolerance. On the other hand, in many cases the β cells, despite prolonged hyperglycaemia and their reduced number, fail to develop cytological signs of hyperactivity, which suggests that in these diabetics the *ß* cells may be insensitive to the stimulus of a rise in blood glucose. This could result from vascular lesions.

Extrapancreatic tissues. Long-standing diabetes is commonly associated with a disorder of small blood vessels which is seen as an abnormal thickening of the basement membrane of the capillaries throughout the body. It is uncertain whether this occurs in the prediabetic period, but its development thereafter seems to be mainly related to the duration of clinical diabetes. The widespread involvement of small blood vessels appears to be the common denominator of a large group of complications associated with long-term diabetes. The main impact of this microangiopathy is on the retina, the kidneys and the nervous system.

CLINICAL FEATURES

Clinical types

Juvenile-onset types. The diabetes usually appears before the age of 40 years in patients of normal or less than normal weight. Symptoms are usually severe and develop rapidly. Without insulin treatment severe ketoacidosis occurs and is often fatal. Since insulin is required for their survival, an alternative and preferable name for this group of patients is **insulin-dependent.**

Adult (or maturity-onset) type. The diabetes usually appears in middle age or later in patients who are often obese and in whom hyperglycaemia can usually be controlled by dietary means alone or, if not, by an oral hypoglycaemic drug. Some insulin is detectable in the plasma of nearly all patients in this category, and they are therefore less prone to develop ketosis. In this sense the disease is less severe than in the juvenile-onset type; however, the long-term complications occur in both types. Many patients with maturity-onset diabetes have a long history of mild symptoms which may be ignored or misdiagnosed for years.

Potential diabetics. These are persons with a normal glucose tolerance test who nevertheless for genetic reasons have an increased liability to develop diabetes, e.g. the children of two diabetic parents; the children of parents where one is diabetic and the other has a diabetic first-degree relative; the non-diabetic members of pairs of identical twins where one is known to be diabetic.

Latent diabetics. These are persons in whom the glucose tolerance test is normal, but who are known to have given an abnormal result under certain conditions, e.g. during pregnancy, infection or other severe stress, mental or physical, during treatment with cortisone or other diabetogenic drugs, or when overweight.

SYMPTOMS AND PRESENTATION
Diabetes may be discovered in several ways.

1. Many patients are first found to have glycosuria in the course of some routine examination, for insurance, for employment purposes, or pre-operatively. They may have had few or no symptoms.

2. Some patients present complaining of some or all of the classical symptoms which are thirst, polydipsia, polyuria, nocturia, tiredness, loss of weight, reduced visual activity, white marks on clothing, pruritus vulvae or balanitis.

3. Diabetes may first present as a fulminating ketoacidosis. This may have been precipitated by an acute infection but there may be no obvious cause. Epigastric pain and vomiting may be the presenting complaints. These cases are acute medical emergencies and are usually of the juvenile-onset type.

4. Patients may present with symptoms due to one of the complications of diabetes, e.g. failing vision; paraesthesiae in the limbs or pain in the legs due to diabetic neuropathy or to peripheral vascular disease, or to a combination of the two; impotence; infection of the skin, lungs, or urinary tract. Many of these patients also admit to symptoms attributable to glycosuria.

The severity of many of the classical symptoms, particularly thirst, polyuria, pruritus vulvae and balanitis, is related to the severity of glycosuria. If relatively mild hyperglycaemia has developed slowly over many years, glycosuria may be slight, and the symptoms of diabetes correspondingly trivial.

Physical signs
Cases without complications usually show no signs attributable to diabetes. Vulvitis or balanitis may be found, since the external genitalia are prone to infection by fungi (candida) which flourish on skin and mucous membranes contaminated by glucose.

In a fulminating case there is dehydration, with loose dry skin, and a dry furred tongue with cracked lips, and the intraocular pressure may be obviously reduced. Usually the pulse is rapid and blood pressure low. Breathing may be deep and sighing; the sickly sweet smell of acetone may be noticeable in the breath. Apathy and confusion may be present or there may be stupor or even coma.

Evidence of complications of diabetes may be noted. Ophthalmoscopy may show diabetic retinopathy. Early signs of diabetic neuropathy are depression of the ankle jerks, and impaired vibration sense in the legs. The presence of nephropathy may be indicated by proteinuria.

DIAGNOSIS
When the classical symptoms are present, the diagnosis is often beyond doubt by the time the history taking and physical examination are complete, and it may then be confirmed by the finding of marked glycosuria, with or without ketonuria, and a random blood glucose greater than 14 mmol/l (250 mg/100 ml). However, in many

cases, particularly those with diabetes of later onset who have few if any symptoms, and where glycosuria is frequently discovered by chance, the diagnosis is less obvious and a glucose tolerance test is required.

Urine testing

Glycosuria. Glucose-specific dipstick methods are best. Clinistix (Ames and Co.), consists of a paper stick impregnated with an enzyme preparation which turns purple when dipped in urine containing glucose. No other urinary constituent gives this reaction: it therefore provides a rapid and specific test for glucose. A positive response indicates that the urinary glucose concentration exceeds 1 mmol/l, but does not measure the amount accurately. Quantitative measurement of urinary reducing activity can be obtained using copper reduction methods, most conveniently with Clinitest tablets (Ames and Co.).

When Clinitest tablets only are used to detect reducing substances in the urine, it may be necessary to establish the identity of the urinary reducing agent. Glucose can easily be identified with Clinistix paper. Other reducing substances, occasionally present in urine, are lactose, which may be found in the later stages of pregnancy or during lactation, fructose, galactose and pentoses. The three last are manifestations of rare genetic disorders and special methods are required for the identification of these reducing substances in urine.

It is common practice to examine overnight specimens of urine for glucose. Mild cases of diabetes may be missed in this way but are detected if a sample collected during the two hours following a meal is examined.

Some undoubtedly diabetic people have a negative test due to a raised renal threshold, and non-diabetics with a low renal threshold may give a false positive test. In order to distinguish cases of this type from patients with mild diabetes, glucose tolerance tests are required.

Ketonuria. The amounts of ketone bodies normally excreted by healthy persons are not detected by routine side-room methods, but clinically important amounts are detected by the nitroprusside reaction which is conveniently carried out using Acetest tablets or Ketostix test papers (Ames and Co.). Ketonuria may be found in normal people who have been fasting for long periods, who have been vomiting repeatedly or who have been eating a diet high in fats and low in carbohydrate. Ketonuria is therefore not pathognomonic of diabetes, but if both ketonuria and glycosuria are found, the diagnosis of diabetes is practically certain.

Random blood sugar
In many cases diabetes can be diagnosed by a single blood glucose estimation, which may be used as a confirmatory test when the classical symptoms suggest the diagnosis. A random blood glucose exceeding 14 mmol/l (250 mg/100 ml) is almost certain to indicate diabetes. However, a lower random blood glucose does not exclude it, and some degree of standardisation of the conditions under which the blood glucose is measured is necessary. In practice, the oral glucose tolerance test is the cornerstone of the diagnosis.

The oral glucose tolerance test (Fig. 42.4)
The patient, who should have been on an unrestricted carbohydrate intake of at least 150 g for three days or more, fasts overnight. Out-patients should rest for at least half an hour before the test, and should remain seated and not smoke during the test. A sample of blood is taken to measure the fasting blood glucose level and 50 g glucose dissolved in about 200 ml of water is then given by mouth. Thereafter samples of blood are collected at half-hourly intervals for two hours, and their glucose content estimated.

Criteria for diagnosis
The WHO Committee on Diabetes (1965) recommended that the following levels of glucose, either fasting or two hours after the glucose load, should be accepted as normal or diabetic respectively.

	Glucose concentration			
	mmol/l		mg/100 ml	
Sample	Normal	Diabetic	Normal	Diabetic
Venous blood	<6.1	>7.2	<110	>130
Capillary blood	<6.6	>7.8	<120	>140
Plasma	<7.5	>8.6	<135	>155

The particular method of estimating the blood glucose and the precise technique used for carrying out the glucose tolerance test should be taken into account. In elderly persons and in patients after myocardial infarction or with malignant disease, blood glucose concentrations may be somewhat higher than those quoted above, without the patient necessarily having diabetes.

There is still a need for standardisation of the tests used and the criteria for diagnosis in screening apparently healthy populations (West, 1975).

Differential diagnosis of glycosuria.

Renal glycosuria. If glucose appears in the urine when the blood glucose level is less than 10 mmol/l (180 mg/100 ml), the individual has a low renal threshold for glucose or renal glycosuria. This is a benign condition which may run in families and which commonly occurs temporarily in pregnancy.

Renal glycosuria is a much more frequent cause of glycosuria than diabetes in young persons, particularly in the age group 20 to 30 years, when they are commonly examined prior to entering the armed services, professions and industry. In the older age groups the reverse holds, and hyperglycaemia in excess of 10 mmol/l can occur without any glycosuria. Hence if urine tests for glucose are used as a method of screening for diabetes, some cases will be missed.

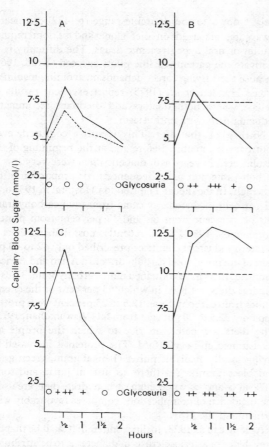

Fig. 42.4 The glucose tolerance test: blood glucose curves after 50 g glucose by mouth, showing (A) normal curve, (B) renal glycosuria, (C) alimentary (lag storage) glycosuria and (D) diabetes mellitus of moderate severity. The dotted line is the renal threshold.

Alimentary (lag storage) glycosuria. In some individuals an unusually rapid but transitory rise of blood glucose follows a meal and the concentration exceeds the normal renal threshold and during this time glucose is present in the urine. Although the peak blood glucose is abnormally elevated, the value two hours after oral glucose is within normal limits (Fig. 42.4). This response to a meal or to a dose of glucose is traditionally known as 'lag storage', although alimentary glycosuria is a better term. It is not uncommon as a cause of symptomless glycosuria and may occur in otherwise normal people or after a partial gastrectomy, when it is due to rapid absorption, or in patients with hyperthyroidism or liver disease. This type of blood glucose curve is usually regarded as benign and unrelated to diabetes.

Starvation. Carbohydrate deprivation can lead to the development of a diabetic type of blood glucose curve with associated glycosuria in normal people. However, the carbohydrate intake has to be less than about 50 g/day

before it has a notable effect and there is no glycosuria. This may be important in interpreting a glucose tolerance test in a person on a reducing diet or with a low intake of food during an acute illness.

MANAGEMENT

Diabetic patients no longer die in ketoacidosis in any number as they once did, but treated diabetic patients still have an overall mortality two and a half times that of the non-diabetic population, largely due to an increased death rate from coronary heart disease (Pell and D'Alonzo, 1970). Moreover, many of those whose duration of life has been extended are chronic invalids. They may live for many years with cerebral, coronary or peripheral vascular disease or with renal disease or serious visual impairment.

LONG-TERM AIMS
The ideal treatment for diabetes would allow the patient to remain not only symptom-free but in good health with a normal metabolic state and to escape the long-term complications.

Although the relation between the degree of control and the development of serious complications is not simple, it would appear that the vascular abnormalities are secondary to the metabolic abnormalities, since they are found in both primary and secondary diabetes and in experimental diabetes in animals. The increased death rate from coronary heart disease is only partly accounted for by increased prevalence of obesity, hyperlipidaemia and hypertension amongst diabetics.

The incidence of diabetic microangiopathy is related to age at diagnosis and duration of diabetes and almost certainly results from metabolic abnormalities present in the majority of patients undergoing treatment (Caird, 1971). It is therefore important to strive to achieve and maintain a normal metabolic state. Unfortunately the degree of metabolic control achieved in most patients by conventional treatment is poor when monitored on a 24-hour basis and compared with normal subjects (Hansen and Johansen, 1970; Baird *et al.*, 1973; Alberti, 1973).

The immediate aims of treatment are therefore:
1. The abolition of symptoms while avoiding hypoglycaemia.
2. The correction of hyperglycaemia and glycosuria and other metabolic abnormalities.
3. The attainment and maintenance of a desirable body weight.

The patient should realise as early as possible that it is upon him that success or failure will depend. The doctor can only advise. As adherence to a diabetic regime demands self-discipline and a sense of purpose, time should be spent on the education of each patient, so that he understands the object of each aspect of his treatment and has sufficient knowledge to undertake the day-to-day management of his diabetes.

As soon as the diagnosis is certain, the patient should be told that he has diabetes, he should be reassured, and instruction and treatment begun forthwith. Many patients have an anxiety reaction on being told that they have diabetes. If he understands what is wrong with him, why he has certain symptoms, and what he should do to correct the abnormalities present, then he is likely to be less afraid and much more co-operative in carrying out the regimen prescribed.

Types of treatment
There are three methods of treatment and each involves an obligation for the patient to adhere to a dietary regimen for the remainder of his life.
1. Diet alone.
2. Diet and oral hypoglycaemic drugs.
3. Diet and insulin.

Approximately 40 per cent of new cases of diabetes can be controlled adequately by diet alone, about 30 per cent require insulin and another 30 per cent will need an oral hypoglycaemic drug. Insulin is needed for juvenile-onset cases; older patients often do not require insulin except when control of their dieabetes is disturbed by an illness, infection or operation.

DIET
In all diabetics the amount and time of food intake, particularly the carbohydrate, should be controlled so as to prevent, as far as is possible, fluctuations of blood sugar beyond the normal range. Intake of refined sugars should be low because their consumption is followed by rapid absorption and a high peak of the blood glucose (Swan et al., 1966). Patients should avoid feasting or fasting; their intake from day to day should be maintained with adjustments for exercise and appetite; they should not miss a meal or overindulge.

Juvenile-onset patients require insulin and their food, especially carbohydrate, should be adjusted to match the time of action of their insulin. This depends on the type of insulin being used and whether the patient is having a single injection or more than one each day. The balance between insulin and meals has to be adjusted from time to time. These patients may still be growing and often start treatment below normal weight. They usually want to take moderate and sometimes strenuous exercise. They therefore require a generous amount of dietary energy.

Maturity-onset patients are usually obese. Being middle aged or elderly they do not usually take much exercise. For both of these reasons the daily energy intake should be restricted to about 4.2 MJ (1000 kcal). For them, Dr Arnold Bloom's dictum is sound advice: 'If you are overweight it doesn't matter what you eat as long as you don't eat it!' Such patients, if only they can bring their weight down to the desirable range (p. 472) can nearly always be managed on diet alone and seldom require insulin or oral hypoglycaemic drugs. The difficulty is to motivate the patient. Airline pilots succeed (Krall, 1969) because their flying career depends on avoiding insulin or drugs. Hadden et al. (1975) report excellent results in Belfast where both doctors and dietitians recommend reducing diets with enthusiasm.

Nature of the diet. This is still a confused, even controversial, matter. Before and at the beginning of the insulin era, 50 years ago, diabetic diets were very low in carbohydrate and in consequence their proportion of fat was high. In the diet at The London Hospital in 1931 only 15 per cent of the energy came from total carbohydrate, but 68 per cent from fat and 17 per cent from protein (Simmonds, 1931). Until recently most diabetic diets in Western industrial countries prescribed only 42 to 40 per cent of energy as total carbohydrate. In Asian and African countries diets have contained more carbohydrate. Thus in Madras diets are used in which 55 per cent of the energy comes from carbohydrate, 12.5 to 25 per cent from protein and only 32.5 to 20 per cent from fat (Viswanathan, 1973). The diets are based on rice to which the people are accustomed and can afford. The protein is increased by giving locally available pulses (Bengal gram, green gram and black gram). Yet there, as also in Japan and some African countries where high carbohydrate diets are used, the incidence of complications compares favourably with Britain and the USA.

As long ago as 1928, Joslin wondered: 'Can it be that the prevalence of arteriosclerosis in diabetes is to be attributed to the high fat diets we have prescribed and more especially if these diets have been rich in cholesterol? I suspect this may be the case. At any rate it is reasonable to maintain the cholesterol in the blood of our patients at a normal level and that I shall strive to do. This may result in the limitation of eggs...this therapeutic procedure is adaptable for experimental investigation and should not require long for solution.' Fifty years later, results from a large multicentre trial are still not available; indeed we are not aware that such a trial has been started. Several individual diabetic clinics have shown, however, that control of glucose metabolism is not more difficult and that plasma cholesterol is lower when diabetic patients are given diets lower in fat and higher in starchy carbohydrate foods than has been traditional. This was first reported by Rabinowich (1935) in Canada and later by Weinzier et al. (1974) in the USA, Ernest et al. (1965) in Sweden and Hockaday et al. (1978) in England.

The Committee on Food and Nutrition of the American Diabetes Association considered that 'there no longer appears to be any need to restrict disproportionately the intake of carbohydrates in the diet of most diabetic patients.... The average proportion of calories consumed as carbohydrate in the US population as a whole approximates to 45 per cent; this proportion or even higher appears to be acceptable for the usual diabetic patient as well' (Bierman *et al.*, 1971).

Since the above statement appeared, evidence is accumulating that one class of total carbohydrate, viz. dietary fibre, has positive benefits in diabetes. The hypothesis was well stated by Trowell (1975). Improved control and less need for insulin has been reported when patients were transferred to a 75 per cent carbohydrate high fibre diet (Kiehm *et al.*, 1976). Urinary glucose excretion fell to half when a small group of patients took 25 guar gum/day with their food (Jenkins *et al.*, 1977). This is a large amount of guar to take; smaller amounts of foods containing viscous and gummy polysaccharides require to be tested in diabetic diets.

At present therefore it is not possible to lay down a detailed dietary programme as the only true way to treat diabetes. Physicians and dietitians need to understand the principles and be prepared to adapt the details in their diabetic regimens as new experimental results emerge.

Exchange systems

Most British diabetic clinics divide foods into three categories—forbidden, freely allowed and foods that may be exchanged on the basis of carbohydrate content. The British Diabetic Association has a List of Carbohydrate Exchanges (p. 558); each item contains 10 g of carbohydrate. Thus 7 oz (200 ml) milk can be exchanged with one orange or half a thick slice of bread (20 g). A difficulty is that these foods are not equivalent in their pattern of other nutrients, and even their carbohydrates are not qualitatively the same. The larger hospitals have their own set of diabetic diet sheets and the foods on the free, forbidden and exchange lists vary. The frequency with which some foods occur in forbidden lists of different clinics is unrelated to the carbohydrate contained in an average portion (Thomas *et al.*, 1974).

In the USA the exchange unit for bread contains 15 g carbohydrate. This is the amount in a full slice of bread. The exchange system is extended to all types of food and, in the 1976 revision, six exchanges are used—for milk, vegetables (non-starchy), fruit, bread (including pasta, other cereals and starchy vegetables), meat (with fish and other protein-rich foods) and fats. For each group the carbohydrate, fat and protein of the exchange unit are different. The exchange unit for each food group is based on the composition of average servings of foods in the group. From these seven food exchanges the American Diabetic and Dietetic Associations have nine standard diet plans. The diets for growing children provide more milk. Where the physician wants to take steps to reduce plasma cholesterol, milk is replaced by skimmed milk and dairy fats replaced by polyunsaturated oils and margarines. The exchanges are shown on page 563.

Method of constructing a daily diet

As the daily intake of nutrients should be fixed, some kind of exchange system is necessary to avoid the monotony of a static diet sheet; this is the basis for the construction of nearly all diets.

The first step in preparing any dietary regimen is to map out a timetable of the patient's day including a description of his usual meals. The daily requirement of energy is next decided. This must be adequate for the patient's needs, and it should be determined for each patient after considering such factors as age, sex, actual weight in relation to desirable weight (Table 55.5, p. 000), occupation and other physical activities. An approximate range for various groups might be (1) an obese, middle-aged or elderly patient with mild diabetes, 4.2 to 6.7 MJ (1000 to 1600 kcal) daily, (2) an elderly diabetic but not overweight, 5.8 to 7.5 MJ (1400 to 1800 kcal) daily, (3) a young, active diabetic, 7.5 to 12.5 MJ (1800 to 3000 kcal) daily. The importance of maintaining the body weight at or slightly below the ideal for the patient's height cannot be overemphasised. The energy range of group 2 may have to be extended if the diet is not sufficient to maintain weight, and young patients in group 3 who are overweight may have to reduce temporarily their daily intake to below 7.5 MJ (1800 kcal).

Next the proportion of energy derived from carbohydrate, protein and fat must be allocated. The average in British household diets is about was carbohydrate 46 per cent, protein 12 per cent and fat 42 per cent. In most diabetic diets the proportion of energy from carbohydrate is between 45 and 48 per cent, from protein between 15 and 18 per cent and from fat less than 40 per cent. As stated above, most clinics in Third World countries and some in affluent countries manage their patients with a higher proportion of carbohydrate, as starch and associated fibre but not as sugar.

Carbohydrate. Most British clinics prescribe from 100 to 180 g of carbohydrate daily (Truswell *et al.*, 1975). A minimum of 100 g is needed to prevent ketonuria. With higher intakes it may be difficult to achieve satisfactory blood glucose concentrations throughout 24 hours. If the daily intake of carbohydrate has to be as high as 240 g to meet energy needs, about 50 g is usually provided in the three main meals, 20 g in three snacks and 30 g in 500 ml of milk. Experience shows that it is difficult to prevent an excessive rise in blood glucose after each meal with amounts larger than this. Foods rich in sucrose and other sugars should be kept to a minimum.

The British Diabetic Association allows diabetics to take up to 2 oz (60 g) of fructose a day. Sorbitol, used for making diabetic jams, is not restricted on the ground that large intakes cause diarrhoea and so are self-limiting. As fructose and sorbitol have the same energy value as other sugars, obese diabetics should not use them. These allowances enable British diabetics to include fruit in their diets but fruit containing (say) 30 g fructose is likely to have a more favourable effect on glucose and insulin metabolism than pure fructose. Though fructose may not raise blood glucose as much as sucrose or glucose, it may raise plasma triglycerides more.

Protein. The consumption of protein is largely determined by social and economic considerations and is frequently lower than desirable. If this is the case, every effort should be made to ensure that some protein is eaten at each meal. As amino acids stimulate insulin secretion, in both normal subjects and in those with maturity-onset diabetes, a smaller rise in blood glucose occurs when carbohydrate is consumed along with protein (Estrich *et al.*, 1967). In both types of diabetes consumption of protein promotes satiety and so helps patients to keep to their carbohydrate allowance. A minimum amount of protein should therefore be specified in all diabetic diets but, unless the patient is obese, more may be taken if desired. Consumption of protein usually lies in the range of 60 to 110 g/day.

Fat. Because diabetic patients have an increased risk of death from coronary heart disease, and because this may be related to the amount of saturated fat in the diet, the total amount of fat should be restricted even in those who are not obese. Plasma lipids should be checked regularly and if high the diet may be modified on the lines indicated on page 568.

When the patient's requirements have been assessed the figures must be translated into practical and comprehensible instructions, using one of the types of diet prescription sheets described below.

Each patient should be given a list of exchanges (p.558) with instructions regarding the meals at which they may be taken. The diet sheet and exchanges should be discussed with the patient repeatedly and with a relative if necessary.

Types of diet

There are two types of diet: (1) measured, in which the amount of food to be eaten at each time of the day is specified, and (2) unmeasured, in which the patient is supplied with a list of foods grouped in three categories: foods with a high carbohydrate content which are to be avoided altogether; foods with a relatively low carbohydrate content which are to be eaten in moderation only; and non-carbohydrate foods which may be eaten as desired. An example is shown on page 562.

Measured diets. In these diets the portions of food may be measured either by weighing with scales or more simply by using household measures. Measured diets are required for patients who are being treated with insulin or an oral hypoglycaemic agent, and also for those who are overweight and on a reducing regimen.

The former should, if at all possible, weigh out the portions of food initially and should be provided with a simple balance (available on NHS prescription). After a

few weeks most patients are capable of assessing the weight of portions with sufficient accuracy by eye, and regular weighing becomes less necessary. However it is often valuable to check visual assessments by weighing from time to time. As a well-tried example of a traditional British diabetic diet the scheme used in the Western General Hospital, Edinburgh, is given on pages 560-561. Many British hospitals do not use the protein and fat exchanges given there.

Diabetics who are obese should be urged to accept a reducing regimen. The method of achieving reduction in weight is the same for obese diabetic patients as for those with simple obesity. Diet No. 3 (p. 551) meets the needs of many. The portions in this diet can be weighed out with scales but usually household measures suffice. It should be explained that such a strict diet has to be followed only until the standard weight is reached; thereafter the diet may be increased, and advice can then be given on how to avoid monotony by using the list of exchanges for diabetic diets.

Unmeasured diets. If insulin or oral hypoglycaemic agents are not required and obesity is not marked, it may not be necessary for the patient to follow such an accurate diet. Sometimes it may be impracticable to do so because of the patient's mental, visual or other physical incapacity or unwillingness to cooperate. Many patients develop the disease when they are already middle-aged or elderly and have a mild type of diabetes often associated with moderate obesity. For such patients an unmeasured diet of the type described on page 562 is used.

Alcohol. Patients need advice regarding the consumption of alcohol. There is no medical objection to taking alcoholic drinks in moderation provided the patient realises that he must take account of their energy value and sometimes of their carbohydrate content. Beer for example may contain 10 to 30 g of carbohydrate per half litre (1 pint approx.) and with the alcohol this provides 630 to 1700 kJ (150 to 400 kcal), depending on the strength of the beer. Sweet wines and cider all have a high sugar content, and spirits such as whisky and gin, while free of carbohydrates, provide about 300 kJ (70 kcal)/30 ml.

Sweetening agents. Advice may also be asked about sweetening agents and diabetic foods and drinks. Saccharin has been employed as a sweetening agent for many years. It has no energy value.

DRUGS

Oral hypoglycaemic drugs

A number of compounds reduce hyperglycaemia in patients who would otherwise require insulin. The sulphonylurea compounds, tolbutamide and chlorpropamide, and to a lesser extent the biguanides, metformin and phenformin, have a place in the management of about 30 per cent of diabetic patients. Although their mechanism of action is different, the action of both groups depends upon a supply of endogenous insulin, and it is therefore futile and dangerous to attempt to control juvenile-onset diabetes with these compounds.

Sulphonylureas. Tolbutamide is the mildest, and probably also the safest, of the sulphonylureas. Since its effective action does not exceed six to eight hours it should be taken two or three times a day. The dose varies between 1 and 2 g/day. It is well tolerated and toxic reactions such as skin rashes rarely occur. Unfortunately, the relapse rate is relatively high.

Chlorpropamide has a biological half-life of about 36 hours, and an effective concentration can be maintained in the blood by a single dose at breakfast. The usual maintenance dose is between 100 and 375 mg/day; larger doses should not be used on a long-term basis, since there is an increased risk of toxic effects, such as jaundice, drug rashes, and blood dyscrasia. Two other effects should be noted. If alcohol is taken following chlorpropamide an unpleasant flushing of the face occurs in some patients. Chlorpropamide may lead to severe hypoglycaemia, which can be refractory to treatment. Care should be taken to avoid this in elderly patients, and once glycosuria has been abolished and symptoms relieved, the dose should be reduced to the minimum. Many patients who require 375 to 500 mg/day initially can later be maintained on 100 mg or less/day.

Sulphonylureas are valuable in the treatment of patients with maturity-onset diabetes who fail to respond to simple dietary restriction and who are not overweight. They should not be given to obese patients since they act by stimulating the production of endogenous insulin and this leads in turn to an increase in weight with a consequent reduction in life expectancy.

Biguanides. These have a higher incidence of adverse effects than the sulphonylureas, particularly gastrointestinal symptoms, but are valuable in two situations. First, they do not lead to an increase in weight, so they are to be preferred for a patient with maturity-onset diabetes who is overweight but in whom hyperglycaemia persists despite efforts to adhere to a diet and reduce weight. Secondly, as their hypoglycaemic effect appears to be synergistic with that of the sulphonylureas, there is a place for combining the two when the sulphonylureas alone have proved inadequate (primary failure), and when, as happens with 5 to 10 per cent of patients, initial success is followed after several months or even one to two years by loss of control (secondary failure).

Metformin is less likely to cause gastrointestinal side-effects than phenformin, and is given with food in two or three daily doses of 0.5 to 1.0 g each. The usual dose of phenformin is 50 to 150 mg/day.

Clinical uses

Patients of normal weight may be started on an oral hypoglycaemic drug as soon as it is clear that dietary measures alone are inadequate. It is usually possible to reach a decision on the success or failure of these drugs within a week, though occasionally a full response may not be apparent for much longer. Diabetics treated successfully in this way for prolonged periods may later need an alteration of dose or a change of regimen temporarily or permanently; in particular they may require insulin to meet the needs created by a severe infection, an operation or other stress.

Risk of coronary heart disease. A report from America (UGDP Report, 1970) suggests that those taking tolbutamide and phenformin are at increased risk of dying from cardiovascular disease. This may be due to a high incidence of ventricular fibrillation in such patients (Soler et al., 1974). This has not yet been confirmed and indeed at least two studies in Europe suggest a significant advantage to patients receiving tolbutamide. In view of this the British Diabetic Association has concluded that the case against tolbutamide is 'not proven' and that there is no reason at present to recommend a change in treatment policy for diabetic patients. However, patients on oral hypoglycaemic drugs who develop a myocardial infarct should have these replaced by insulin during their acute illness and have a longer period of close supervision than non-diabetic patients, preferably in a coronary care unit.

Insulin

Unfortunately no method of giving insulin has yet been found that will maintain the blood glucose within the physiological range throughout the 24 hours without some risk of hypoglycaemia. However, with one or more of the preparations of insulin available it is usually possible to keep the blood glucose within reasonable limits throughout the 24 hours without undue risk of hypoglycaemia.

Two main forms of insulin are available, namely soluble and depot, and there are several varieties of depot preparations. These vary in the rate of onset and duration of their effect.

Soluble insulin. This is a clear solution in contrast to the depot insulins which are cloudy. When injected subcutaneously, soluble insulin begins to lower the blood glucose in 30 min; the effect is maximal in 4 to 6 h and ends after 6 to 10 h. A patient stabilised on soluble insulin alone would therefore need at least two injections in the day.

Soluble insulin is essential in the following circumstances:

1. For new cases with severe dehydration or ketoacidosis.
2. For emergencies associated with ketosis, such as acute infection, gastroenteritis or some surgical operations.
3. For the treatment of nearly all young patients.

Depot insulins. The action of a single injection of insulin can be prolonged by delaying its release from the site of injection into the circulation. For this purpose there are insulin zinc preparations suspended in acetate buffer.

Release of insulin in the tissues depends on the size of the insulin particles. Insulin in the presence of zinc can be absorbed onto a foreign protein (protamine or globin). A protein-zinc and insulin complex forms which breaks up slowly in the subcutaneous tissues. Slow onset/long duration depot insulins do not lower blood sugar before 4 to 6 hours; the effect is maximal at 8 to 14 h and only ends after 20 to 30 h. With intermediary depot preparations, the corresponding times are 2 to 3 h, 6 to 10 h and 10 to 14 h, but with one preparation, isophane, the effect continues for 12 to 22 h. Some, but not all, soluble and depot preparations are miscible and then a single injection of the mixture can be given and provide better control. A small number of cases can be adequately controlled by a single morning injection of depot insulin. These are usually elderly with mild diabetes. Most insulin-requiring diabetics however do best on a depot insulin with one or two supporting doses of soluble insulin. The choice of depot insulin is determined by consideration of the patient's way of life, e.g. his meal pattern, occupation, hours of work and recreation, in relation to the time of action of the various depot insulins. More insulin is required to cover main meals and periods of inactivity, and vice versa.

Highly purified insulins. Most insulin preparations are made from beef pancreas and contain polypeptides other than insulin which are antigenic (Bloom *et al.*, 1976). Antigenicity depends on the animal source, physical properties and above all the purity of a preparation. Monocomponent (MC) insulin preparations are made from pig pancreas and purified in various ways, e.g. anion exchange chromatography. With these preparations there is usually a fall in insulin requirements and cases of severe insulin resistance are rare; further local and general allergic reactions are less frequent. It is possible that they may give better control and so reduce the incidence of the complications of diabetes. The processes for manufacturing MC insulins are more complex than those for conventional insulin and so it would be difficult to meet the insulin needs of diabetics throughout the world with these preparations and it would be much more expensive.

In practice, combinations of the various insulin preparations should be tried, and the time of their administration varied in the light of urine tests and blood glucose estimations at different times of the day until control is smooth over the 24-hour period. It is impossible to forecast the response of a patient to insulin, and the daily dose required varies from 10 to 100 units or more.

A practical point worth mentioning since it may give rise to distress if not anticipated, is that blurring of vision (which may occur in a severe diabetic before treatment) may become noticeably worse after starting treatment with insulin. It is due to transitory osmotic abnormalities in the eye, especially the lens, and may persist for several weeks.

CHOICE OF THERAPEUTIC REGIMEN

The regimen eventually adopted in each case is chosen by a process of trial and error, and changes may be needed as more is learnt about the patient and the kind of diabetes which he has.

The indications for the types of regimen are as follows.

1. Practically all young patients who develop diabetes before the age of 40 require treatment with insulin. The majority are best controlled by soluble insulin in the morning along with one of the depot insulins, usually protamine zinc or isophane insulin. In addition a dose of soluble insulin may be needed before the evening meal.

2. Most patients developing the disease over the age of 40 can and should be controlled by diet alone. This applies particularly to obese patients, but others may do well on dietary therapy alone.

Obese patients should be treated by dietary restriction and weight reduction rather than by insulin or other hypoglycaemic agent. The advent of insulin obscured the remarkable improvement in glucose tolerance which usually results from reduction in weight. Insulin and the sulphonylureas increase the appetite, and thus may increase weight and intensify disability.

3. Those over the age of 40 who are not controlled by dietary measures alone usually respond well to sulphonylurea if they are not obese, or to a biguanide if they are obese. If adequate control is not achieved by one drug, a combination of sulphonylurea and biguanide may be tried. If this fails insulin is needed.

4. Elderly patients who require insulin often do well with a small dose (20 units) of a depot insulin alone. A few, particularly those who would otherwise require more than 40 units a day, should be given soluble insulin in addition.

INITIATION OF TREATMENT

It is seldom necessary to admit diabetic patients to hospital for initial stabilisation. It is desirable that the patient learns to manage all aspects of his disorder as quickly as possible, while leading a normal existence at home and at work and this can best be done as an outpatient. However, patients being stabilised on insulin have to be seen daily at first and if this is not otherwise possible, admission to hospital is necessary. Hospital admission is also needed if there is severe ketoacidosis.

As soon as the diagnosis is made, a careful search is needed for early evidence of complications such as coronary heart disease and hypertension, obliterative arterial disease, peripheral neuropathy, cataract, retinopathy, nephropathy, pulmonary tuberculosis and other infections, particularly of the skin and urinary tract.

Patient's education. 1. All patients capable of learning should be taught how to test urine with a Clinitest set (and sometimes with Acetest tablets also), to keep a record of the results in a notebook and to understand their significance.

2. All patients requiring insulin should learn to measure the dose accurately with an insulin syringe (BS 1619), to give their own injections and to adjust their dose on the basis of urine tests and factors such as illness, unusual exercise and insulin reactions. They should be made to experience an insulin reaction at an early stage, so that they can recognise the early signs and take appropriate action.

3. All patients should have a working knowledge of diabetes, i.e. be able to recognise the symptoms associated with marked glycosuria and to understand their significance. They should be told that many drugs have undesirable effects on the diabetic state, as may also an illness of any kind or an emotional upset. They should be advised to come to the doctor or the clinic at once, without prior appointment, as soon as they are aware of any deterioration in health or urine tests not responding rapidly to simple measures.

4. All patients should know how to take care of their feet, and to respect any infected lesion.

Education of the patient is time-consuming and repeated practical demonstrations may be required, supplemented by appropriate booklets. If the patient is a child, or is blind, mentally defective or otherwise incapable, instructions in these matters should be given to a parent or guardian.

Diabetics who are taking insulin or oral hypoglycaemic drugs should carry a card at all times stating their name and address, the fact that they are diabetic, the nature and dose of insulin or other drugs they may be taking, and giving the name, address and telephone number of their family doctor and their diabetic clinic. Suitable cards are provided by the British Diabetic Association.

SUPERVISION AND ASSESSMENT OF CONTROL

Diabetics should be seen at regular intervals for the remainder of their lives. The object of these visits is to check the degree of control and to watch for complications. The frequency of visits is determined by the biochemical control achieved and the reliability of the patient. At the patient's regular visit to the diabetic clinic or to his general practitioner, the degree of control should be assessed by considering his weight, the results of urine tests, a blood glucose estimation and the presence or absence of symptoms of hyper- or hypoglycaemia. Fasting plasma lipids should also be checked from time to time.

Urine testing

Proper assessment of control is impossible unless in the course of his normal activity the patient tests samples of urine regularly. By selecting suitable times for the tests and tabulating the results, it is easy for the doctor or the experienced patient to decide whether the dose of insulin or hypoglycaemic drug should be adjusted, or whether the carbohydrate content of the diet or the time when it is taken should be altered.

Diabetics taking insulin should test samples of urine obtained before breakfast, before the mid-day and evening meals, and at bedtime. He should empty his bladder and discard this urine about 30 minutes before passing the specimen for the test. Otherwise the pre-meal specimen includes urine passed into the bladder after the previous meal and gives the impression that the blood glucose before meals is higher than it really is.

Patients treated by diet alone or with oral hypoglycaemic agents should test the first morning specimen and samples passed two to four hours after the main meals of the day; the majority of specimens should be either free of or contain only a trace of glucose.

While the patient is being stabilised, tests have to be carried out three or four times daily; when control is established the frequency is greatly reduced. Three to four tests on a single day once or twice weekly are much more informative about the state of control than a daily single test.

Insulin reactions and hypoglycaemia

If soluble insulin is injected into a normal person the blood glucose falls, producing symptoms that may begin to appear when the concentration is about 2.8 mmol/l (50 mg/100 ml) and are fully developed at about 2.2 mmol/l. In diabetics who are constantly hyperglycaemic, the same symptoms may develop at much higher concentrations, e.g. 7 mmol/l.

The symptoms of hypoglycaemia are a feeling of being weak and empty, hunger, sweating, palpitation, tremor, faintness, dizziness, headache, diplopia and mental confusion. Abnormal behaviour, leading occasionally to arrest by the police on a charge of being drunk and disorderly, may also occur. Alternatively, and particularly in children, there may be lassitude and somnolence, muscular twitching, convulsions and deepening coma.

Hypoglycaemia causes secretion of adrenaline which leads to tachycardia and tremor and, by mobilising liver glycogen, combats the hypoglycaemia. This homoeostatic reaction partly explains why patients rarely die of hypoglycaemic coma from too much soluble insulin. By contrast, coma is dangerous when it arises from a large dose of depot insulin or from an overdose of a sulphonylurea, particularly chlorpropamide. Repeated profound hypoglycaemia may lead to permanent mental changes because the brain is dependent on the blood glucose for its energy. For this reason, recurrence of hypoglycaemia should be prevented by prompt reduction of the dose of insulin or of sulphonylurea.

Hypoglycaemia due to overdosage with soluble insulin comes on rapidly, at the time when the insulin is having its maximum effect, and usually passes off soon. Reactions from excessive IZS (lente) given before breakfast usually occur in the late afternoon and those from PZI at night or early next morning. These reactions begin gradually with little adrenaline response and can become persistent and profound unless treated vigorously.

Treatment of hypoglycaemic reactions

Since hypoglycaemia can easily be corrected if recognised early, it is useful for diabetic patients to experience the condition under supervision. In this way they learn to recognise the early symptoms. They should be advised that the most frequent causes of the condition are unpunctual meals and unaccustomed exercise, and try to avoid both or make adjustments to meet these circumstances. They should always carry some tablets of glucose or a few lumps of sugar for use in an emergency. Unless an attack of hypoglycaemia is accounted for adequately, the patient should reduce the next and subsequent dose of insulin by 20 per cent, and seek medical advice.

If the patient is so stuporous that he cannot swallow, he should be given an intravenous injection of 25 g of glucose (50 ml of a 50 per cent solution) which may have to be repeated. Alternatively, the insulin-dependent patient may be given a subcutaneous or intramuscular injection of 1 mg of glucagon, repeated if necessary after 10 minutes.

As soon as the patient is able to swallow, he should be given 30 g of sugar by mouth. Full recovery may not occur immediately, especially if the patient has been in coma for some time.

COMPLICATIONS

Ketoacidosis

Before the discovery of insulin more than 50 per cent of diabetic patients ultimately died of ketoacidosis. Today this complication is preventable and accounts for less than 2 per cent of diabetic deaths. However, both the incidence and the mortality rate are still regrettably high. Failure of the patient to understand his disease, and failure to appreciate the significance of symptoms of poor control are the common causes. A clear understanding of the biochemical disorders involved is essential for its efficient treatment which should aim at having the patient out of danger within 24 hours.

Water and electrolyte depletion The deficit of total body water in a severe case may be about 6 litres. About half of this is derived from the intracellular compartment and occurs early in the development of acidosis when there are few clinical features; the remainder represents loss of extracellular fluid sustained largely in the later stages. Marked contraction of the size of the extracellular space occurs, with haemoconcentration, a decrease in plasma volume, and finally a fall in blood pressure with oliguria.

The concentrations of sodium and potassium in plasma give little indication of total body losses, and may even be raised due to disproportionate losses of water. Sodium loss, mainly from the extracellular space, may amount to as much as 500 mmol. Potassium loss from the cell may be 400 mmol or more. The plasma potassium concentration is dependent on the balance between catabolism of protein and glycogen and haemoconcentration on the one hand, and urinary excretion on the other. Since the former generally exceeds the latter, plasma potassium is likely to be high initially, in spite of a total body deficit. However, within a few hours of beginning treatment with insulin, there is likely to be a precipitous fall in the plasma potassium. This is due to (1) dilution of extracellular potassium by the administration of potassium-free fluids, (2) the movement of potassium into the cells as the result of insulin therapy and (3) the continued renal loss of potassium.

Acidosis is assessed by measuring the plasma bicarbonate and is severe if the concentration is less than 12 mmol/l. The blood pH is a more valuable guide but its measurement may not be so readily available. There are no rapid quantitative methods for the determination of plasma ketones but a Ketostix strip dipped in plasma indicates whether significant ketonaemia is present or not.

Clinical features

Any form of stress, particularly an acute infection, can precipitate severe ketoacidosis in even the mildest diabetic. The most common cause is neglect of treatment due to carelessness, misunderstanding or illness, and failure to adjust the therapeutic regimen in the event of an acute infection.

There is intense thirst and polyuria. Constipation, muscle cramps and altered vision are common, Sometimes, there is abdominal pain, with or without vomiting. Hence diabetic ketoacidosis is important in the differential diagnosis of the acute abdomen. Weakness and drowsiness are commonly present, but the state of consciousness is variable and a patient with dangerous ketosis requiring urgent treatment may walk into hospital. For this reason the term diabetic ketoacidosis is to be preferred to the traditional 'diabetic coma', which suggests that there is no urgency until unconsciousness occurs. In fact it is imperative that energetic treatment is started at the earliest possible stage.

The signs include a dry tongue and soft eyeballs due to dehydration, hyperventilation indicated by long, deep, sighing respirations and a rapid, weak pulse, with low blood pressure and acetone may be smelt in the breath. Sometimes there is abdominal rigidity and tenderness. Ultimately coma supervenes.

Laboratory tests show heavy glycosuria and ketonuria, blood glucose usually between 20 and 40 mmol/l (360 and 720 mg/100 ml), and low plasma bicarbonate and blood pH.

The degree of hyperglycaemia and ketoacidosis do not

always correlate well. Even at a level of blood glucose as low as 20 mmol/l (350 mg/100 ml), life-threatening acidosis may be present; on the other hand coma can occur, usually in elderly patients, with extreme hyperglycaemia and dehydration but no ketoacidosis, **hyperosmolar diabetic coma.**

Treatment

This condition should be treated with the utmost urgency in hospital. Intravenous therapy is required since, even when the patient is able to swallow, fluids given by mouth may be poorly absorbed. Extracellular fluid is repleted first with sodium chloride infusions; large doses of soluble insulin are required, starting with 100 units and as the blood sugar starts to come down potassium is added to the infusion fluid. Intracellular fluid is replaced once the blood sugar has fallen to below 14 mmol/l (250 mg/100 ml) by infusing glucose solution, covered by appropriate doses of insulin. Intensive medical care is needed and the blood sugar, pH, electrolytes and ketones have to be monitored, hourly at first. Details of management are given in textbooks of medicine.

Differential diagnosis of coma in a diabetic. Confusion between coma due to hypoglycaemia and that associated with ketosis should seldom arise; the distinction is usually clear, but diabetic coma may occasionally pass undetected into hypoglycaemic coma through too enthu-

	Hypoglycaemic coma	*Coma with ketosis*
History	no food too much insulin unaccustomed exercise	too little or no insulin an infection digestive disturbance
Onset	in good health immediately before related to time of last injection of insulin	ill-health for several days before
Symptoms	of hypoglycaemia; occasional vomiting from depot insulins	of glycosuria and dehydration; abdominal pain and vomiting
Signs	moist skin and tongue sweating normal or raised blood pressure shallow or normal breathing brisk reflexes plantar responses usually extensor	dry skin and tongue low blood pressure reduced intra-ocular tension hyperventilation ('air hunger') diminished reflexes plantar responses usually flexor
Urine	no ketonuria no glycosuria, provided that the bladder has been recently emptied	ketonuria glycosuria
Blood	hypoglycaemia normal plasma bicarbonate	hyperglycaemia reduced plasma bicarbonate

siastic treatment; likewise, vomiting induced by hypoglycaemia from a depot insulin may continue until diabetic coma develops.

Vascular disorders

Vascular disease, arterial, arteriolar and capillary, is the largest and most intractable problem in clinical diabetes. Arterial disease is much the commonest cause of death in diabetics over the age of 50, and the mortality rate is far higher than expected, while nephropathy accounts for more than half the deaths under 50. Moreover, diabetes is the most important systemic disease causing blindness. Strict control probably offers the best chance of delaying the onset and progress of the vascular complications of diabetes. Unfortunately, however, they may develop despite every effort by both patient and doctor to maintain precise control of the diabetes.

Atherosclerosis occurs commonly and extensively in diabetics. The pathological changes in diabetics are not specific in a qualitative sense but they occur earlier and are more widespread than in non-diabetics. Thus diabetics are more prone at an earlier age than other people to intermittent claudication, gangrene of the toes and feet and myocardial infarction.

The peripheral pulses in the legs are often diminished or impalpable, and particularly in elderly patients, ischaemic changes in the feet are frequently apparent. Defective circulation in the legs resulting in poorly nourished tissues predisposes to the dangerous complication of gangrene. If a painless peripheral neuropathy is present, this may also be of aetiological importance, since the patient tends to ignore or neglect injuries and other damage to the tissue. Diabetic gangrene usually starts in one foot, following a trivial injury—the cutting of a corn, or a burn from a hot water bottle. Toxic absorption from necrotic tissue and secondary infection may kill the patient unless the limb is amputated. Amputation of a toe, a foot, or even a whole leg is sometimes necessary to save life.

Much can be done to prevent this serious complication by instructing diabetics with a poor circulation to wear properly fitting shoes, to use bed-socks rather than hot water bottles, never to cut their own corns and to 'keep their feet as clean as their face'. The services of a skilled chiropodist are invaluable.

Diabetic nephropathy. A specific type of renal lesion may occur as a result of the changes in the basement membrane of the glomerular capillaries. This is known as **diabetic glomerulosclerosis,** and there are two types, diffuse and nodular: the former is the more common and consists of a generalised thickening of glomerular capillary walls. The nodular type is a development of this, and in these cases rounded masses of acellular, hyaline material are super-imposed upon the diffuse lesion in the glomeruli. These nodules are sometimes called Kimmelstiel-Wilson bodies. Diabetic glomerulosclerosis can be seen by light microscopy in about 70 per cent of diabetic patients at autopsy. In the early stages of diabetes there may be little or no clinical evidence of renal involvement, and even with well-established diabetic glomerulosclerosis there may be only slight to moderate proteinuria. In some cases, however, there is marked proteinuria and the nephrotic syndrome with increasing renal failure and uraemia.

There is no way of preventing or modifying the progress of nephropathy once it is apparent as proteinuria. Management is similar to that for other forms of chronic renal disease.

Diabetic retinopathy. This has a specific appearance when seen with the ophthalmoscope and seven elements make up the clinical picture. These are micro-aneurysms of the capillaries; abnormalities of the retinal veins, particularly dilatation and tortuosity; haemorrhages; waxy exudes; new vessel formation; fibrous proliferation, occurring mainly in association with new vessels; and vitreous detachment. They are seen in varying combinations in different patients.

Micro-aneurysms, abnormalities of the veins, and new vessels do not of themselves interfere seriously with vision, but the other elements of retinopathy may do so. Retinal or pre-retinal haemorrhages seriously affect vision if they involve the macula, or if they break through into the vitreous, when sudden severe visual loss is usual. Exudates are also associated with symptoms if the macula is involved. Unfortunately all these lesions occur most frequently in the vicinity of the disc. New vessels appear most commonly at the disc, but can originate anywhere except at the macula. The new vessels in themselves do little harm, but they leak irritative serous products which cause vitreal-retinal adhesions and vitreous contraction. The latter puts traction on the friable new vessels so that vitreous haemorrhage and retinal detachment may occur and cause blindness.

Patients with only micro-aneurysms, retinal haemorrhages and exudates are classified as having simple diabetic retinopathy; those with pre-retinal haemorrhages, new vessel formation or fibrous proliferation are classified as having proliferative diabetic retinopathy.

As with nephropathy, duration of diabetes is the important factor influencing the occurrence of retinopathy, the course of which is very variable. However in general, prognosis for vision is good for patients with simple retinopathy, especially if they are young, and bad for those with proliferative retinopathy, of whom half are blind within five years. This fact has led to numerous proposals for treatment, including pituitary ablation and photocoagulation of new retinal vessels. The variable nature of the natural course makes assessment of the effectiveness of any treatment extremely difficult.

Cataract
The incidence of cataract in old people is considerably higher in those who have diabetes. Very rarely a specific type of opacity of the lens occurs in diabetic children whose disease has not been adequately controlled.

Infections
Lowered resistance to infection is associated with poor control of diabetes. The following forms are especially important.

Carbuncle. The development of a carbuncle may unmask latent diabetes and may even precipitate ketosis and coma. The diabetic state brought on by a carbuncle is not invariably permanent; glucose tolerance may return to normal (at least temporarily) when the infection subsides. Cleanliness is a special virtue in the prevention of skin infection in diabetes. Once infection has occurred a suitable antibiotic is needed.

Pulmonary tuberculosis. If a diabetic under treatment shows unexplained loss of weight, or increase in insulin requirements, a chest radiograph should be taken.

Urinary tract infections. The presence of glucose in the urine provides a favourable medium for the growth of bacteria. Intractable infections of the urinary tract frequently occur, and for this reason catheterisation should be avoided. Once infection has occurred treatment consists in controlling the glycosuria and the administration of suitable antibiotics.

Vulvitis. Pruritus vulvae is very commonly associated with moniliasis in the diabetic woman. *Candida albicans* is nearly always present. In the majority, the treatment is abolition of glycosuria which brings rapid relief. In a few cases local treatment with vaginal pessaries and nystatin cream may be required.

Diabetic neuropathies
Peripheral neuropathy is a frequent complication of diabetes at any stage, which in the majority of cases may be unnoticed by the patient, but in some gives rise to troublesome symptoms. Motor, sensory or autonomic nerves may be involved, usually in a symmetrical manner. The most common types are:

1. Acute peripheral neuropathy occurs usually in poorly controlled severe diabetes and involves one or many nerves. The clinical features are described on page 287. Pain is prominent, especially in the legs at night. This type of neuropathy appears to be metabolic in origin since it often improves rapidly when the diabetes is controlled.

2. Chronic peripheral neuropathy is probably due to ischaemic damage to the sensory fibres of peripheral nerves consequent upon diabetic microangiopathy. It is therefore usually seen in older diabetics with long-standing disease. The clinical features are those of a painless neuropathy affecting the legs, with diminished tendon jerks and vibration sense. In severe cases there may be trophic changes in the feet; ulceration may follow trivial trauma and disorganisation of joints can occur.

3. Involvement of autonomic nerves may cause nocturnal diarrhoea, overflow incontinence of urine, impotence or postural hypotension. This complication occurs in long-standing cases and is unresponsive to treatment.

4. Diabetic amyotrophy is a predominantly motor form and consists of bilateral weakness and wasting of muscles of the pelvic girdle. With good control of the diabetes slow recovery usually takes place.

PROBLEMS IN MANAGEMENT

Children

Fortunately diabetes is not common in childhood, but when it occurs it is relatively severe and always requires treatment with insulin. The therapeutic problem of matching the dose of insulin to the food intake raises practical difficulties.

Food. Since children should be growing, their energy requirements are large in proportion to their size and difficulties may be experienced in meeting them. In children, likes and dislikes for particular foods are often fickle and unpredictable. It is important to make sure that the child does not become too fat; hypoglycaemia due to too much insulin can lead to excessive appetite and hence to obesity. A diabetic child must not have sugar or sweets, but otherwise the composition of his diet need differ little from that of his friends. Everything possible should be done to avoid making him appear different from his contemporaries. As early as possible he should be encouraged to take responsibility for his own care and, once properly trained, can take part in all normal activites. However, he should swim only in supervised pools, and avoid lonely cross-country walks. The British Diabetic Association runs special summer camps for diabetic children.

Insulin. Day-to-day requirements for insulin are often very variable. Children cannot be expected to lead the steady life of a business man or housewife; their emotions and activities fluctuate unexpectedly—sometimes wildly active and sometimes sulking. This affects their daily needs for insulin; excessive activity may result in hypoglycaemia, and lethargy in hyperglycaemia. The latter may also be caused by any one of the numerous infectious diseases to which all children are prone. A combination of one of the depot insulins and soluble insulin before breakfast and usually a second dose of soluble insulin before supper is usually a suitable arrangement.

Pregnancy

If a diabetic woman wishes to have a child there is no reason why she should avoid pregnancy, provided that she suffers from none of the more serious complications and is under close medical care.

Nevertheless pregnancy in a diabetic woman carries certain definite risks; in the later stages she may develop an excessive accumulation of amniotic fluid (hydramnios); in addition the fetus is sometimes unusually large, leading to difficulty in labour. Moreover the chances that she may lose her baby either from a stillbirth or in the neonatal period are greater than those of a non-diabetic mother, even with the most careful supervision.

A pregnant diabetic patient requires close supervision by a team consisting of physician, obstetrician, anaesthetist, nurse and dietitian. The sooner the pregnancy is diagnosed the better. An expectant mother should spend a week as an ambulant in-patient in hospital towards the end of the third month of pregnancy. This enables her and the team to get to know each other and her diabetes can be brought under the best possible control; she may need further education in the management of her diet and insulin while at home. If her diabetes was previously well controlled, at first her diet need not differ from that to which she is accustomed, but later she may need more milk. Practical problems may be created by bouts of vomiting and food fads that commonly occur in the early stages of any pregnancy.

After the diagnosis of pregnancy, the patient should be seen at first at fortnightly and later at weekly intervals. Continued control of the diabetes may be complicated by other factors. First, the renal threshold for glucose often falls as pregnancy advances. This leads to no ill effect but it means that tests for glycosuria at home may cease to be a reliable index of diabetic control. Further, in the later stages of pregnancy, lactosuria occasionally occurs and may lead to confusion. If excessive amounts of glucose are lost in the urine because of the lowered renal threshold, additional carbohydrate feeds may be given between meals and sometimes at night, covered by suitable amounts of soluble insulin. Requirements for insulin often increase as pregnancy advances. Frequent measurements of blood glucose are needed to ensure that extra insulin is not producing hypoglycaemia; or alternatively, that hyperglycaemia is not insidiously building up.

Pregnancy should seldom, if ever, be allowed to proceed to term. The infant has a much better chance of survival if it is delivered between the thirty-sixth and thirty-eighth weeks by induction of labour or by Caesarean section. Following delivery the insulin requirements of the mother fall. Frequent blood glucose estimations and co-operation between the physician and dietitian are needed to ensure an uneventful return to the former regimen.

Diabetes and surgery

Any surgical operation, however minor, and the accompanying anaesthetic, cause a metabolic stress which the diabetic is less well able to meet than the normal person. The stress is temporary and is not aggravated by a mild hyperglycaemia, but an accompanying acidosis prejudices normal recovery. The position is worse if there is tissue wasting with much breakdown of fat and protein. Two points should be kept in mind: first is the need to provide an adequate supply of energy for the tissues, and secondly, the need to be on the alert for acidosis.

In practice there are two separate problems. The first is the management of a stabilised diabetic who has to undergo an operation at a time which can be chosen by the surgeon and physician. The second is that of a diabetic whose disease may not be well controlled and who has to undergo an emergency operation; diabetes is sometimes first diagnosed when the urine is tested before an operation.

Elective surgery in a stabilised diabetic

All diabetics should be admitted to hospital about three days before an operation, even a minor one. During this period the control of the diabetes can be checked thoroughly. Provided he goes to the theatre in good condition, there is unlikely to be any significant change in the blood glucose, plasma bicarbonate or ketone levels during the operation. In fact, hypoglycaemia is more likely to occur than acidosis so it is generally advisable to give no insulin immediately before operation. During the day before the operation the usual diet and morning dose of soluble insulin should be given but doses of depot insulin of more than 20 units should be reduced by half and a supplementary dose of soluble insulin given later that day instead. It is usually possible to arrange for the operation to take place in the morning. The patient should receive no breakfast and nothing by mouth before operation. Before being transferred to the theatre the fasting blood glucose level should be determined. If this lies between 7 and 11 mmol/l (120 to 200 mg/100 ml) then no glucose or insulin need be given. If the level is below 7 then about 25 to 40 g of glucose should be given intravenously, preferably in hypertonic solution, in order to prevent possible hypoglycaemia during the operation. No insulin is necessary. If the fasting blood glucose is over 11 mmol/l which is infrequent, then some soluble insulin is required. About one-third of his usual total daily dose is indicated, but its administration can usually be postponed until after operation.

Recovery from the anaesthetic should be carefully supervised. The sooner the patient returns to his usual diet the better. This interval may be a few hours or several days, depending on the nature and severity of the operation. Within a few hours of recovery from the anaesthetic many patients are able to take a fluid or semi-fluid feed containing 25 g of carbohydrate at three- to four-hourly intervals, covered by suitable doses of soluble insulin. Examples of feeds which may be given are: (1) 100 ml fruit juice plus 15 g sucrose, (2) 200 ml milk plus 10 g cereal plus 7 g sugar, and (3) 200 ml milk plus 20 g Ovaltine, Horlicks or similar preparation.

Some insulin-dependent diabetics after a major operation may need to have most of their energy requirements supplied as glucose, either intravenously or by mouth. If all has gone well, a single determination of the fasting blood glucose each morning suffices. If recovery is stormy, measurements may be necessary at four-hourly intervals or even more frequently.

Each specimen of urine should be tested for sugar and ketone bodies. Determination of the plasma bicarbonate and electrolytes in the blood are also helpful. The insulin dosage depends on these findings, and until stability has been regained only soluble insulin should be used.

Surgical emergencies. Circumstances vary so much that it is impossible to consider them except in the most general way. The essentials are to maintain the oxidation of glucose by the tissues at a sufficient rate and to combat acidosis and electrolyte disturbances when they occur. This can only be done effectively if the state of the diabetic control is assessed continuously and accurately. A laboratory service that can provide rapid results is thus essential. As long as the surgical condition remains untreated and the metabolic stress continues, the diabetic condition is likely to get worse. Once the patient's surgical condition is under control he may be expected to respond promptly to the appropriate therapy for his diabetes.

PROGNOSIS

The prognosis in diabetes has improved steadily since the introduction of insulin, but even with its use the expectation of life is still less than that of a non-diabetic. It is difficult to estimate the prognosis of an individual patient because so many variable factors have to be considered. Thus the child of parents poor in means and education, who is first seen in coma, obviously has a very different future compared with the middle-aged lady in easy circumstances who complains of nothing but a little thirst and pruritus, and can afford the time and the means to follow precisely the diet prescribed. The incidence of the complications of diabetes is mainly related to the duration of the disease but probably also to the precision with which it has been controlled.

PREVENTION

Diabetes is a disease of the prosperous, and in wealthy countries it is one of the major health problems. The hardships of World War II were associated with a marked decline in the incidence of diabetes in European countries; rationing of both food and petrol was probably responsible. The importance for health of sufficient exercise and of avoiding dietary excess has been stated repeatedly. Diabetes, like obesity and atherosclerosis, is likely to arise in predisposed persons who eat too much and exercise too little.

Screening

It is much easier to control the disease and to maintain the health of the patient if the diagnosis is made early. In many patients, the biochemical changes can be detected before symptoms make them seek medical advice. Any screening technique is expensive and should only be used if it is likely that a significant number of new diabetics will be recognised. Groups at high risk are first degree relatives of known diabetics, the obese and mothers of babies weighing more than 4.5 kg at birth. The overall prevalence of diabetes in different communities varies from 0.5 to 5 per cent and sometimes more. About half of the cases may be unaware that they have the disease. These figures vary widely according to the social and economic state of the people and the educational and medical services available.

Urine testing has been used as a screening procedure but is wasteful since up to 3 per cent of people may have renal glycosuria and so have to be recalled for blood tests. Estimation of the blood glucose two hours after 50 g glucose orally is recommended and auto-analysers enable large numbers of samples to be tested daily.

Genetic counselling

Diabetic patients often consult their doctor about the advisability of having children and sometimes it is his duty to warn them of the dangers. They can be told that the risks of pregnancy and delivery are little greater for a diabetic mother than for a normal woman, provided she submits to the strict discipline required. The chances that she will produce a healthy baby are also good, but not quite so good as for a normal mother. The chances that her child will eventually develop diabetes are higher than normal. If both parents have diabetes, the probability is that about 25 per cent of their children will develop the disease at some stage in life. The risk is about half this if only one parent is affected. Many diabetics have healthy children, and how strongly a doctor should word these necessary warnings is a matter for judgment in each case.

CONCLUSION

The management of a patient with diabetes mellitus offers an opportunity for good medical practice, there being few other chronic diseases in which efficient management makes so much difference to a patient's life. The problems presented by the aetiology of diabetes and its long-term complications continue to offer some of the most demanding and fascinating challenges in medical research today.

43. Gout and Hyperuricaemia

Gout is a characteristic arthritis which affects single joints, often the big toe, in painful episodes that last only a few days but are liable to recur. Middle-aged men are chiefly afflicted. It is caused by deposition in the joint of urate crystals, associated with an increased concentration of urate in the plasma, **hyperuricaemia.**

Gout is thus a clinical entity and hyperuricaemia its biochemical basis. Gout was known to the physicians of ancient Greece and Rome. The classical description was written in 1663 by Sydenham, himself a lifelong sufferer, who clearly differentiated it from other joint disorders. Hyperuricaemia was first demonstrated in gouty patients in 1848 by Sir Alfred Garrod, who should not be confused with Sir Archibald Garrod (p. 314). Subsequent research showed that it results from abnormal purine metabolism which is usually primary and then partly of genetic origin. Less commonly it occurs secondary to renal and certain metabolic diseases.

Hyperuricaemia may be, and often is, asymptomatic. Such individuals, however, carry a greatly increased chance of the clinical complications, gouty arthritis, or uric acid stones in the urinary tract. Those who have recurrent gout and hyperuricaemia over a long time are liable to develop tophi, accumulations of urate in tendons or cartilage. Epidemiological studies also show significant associations between hyperuricaemia and several of the common degenerative diseases of affluent societies, such as hypertension and atherosclerotic diseases.

AETIOLOGY

Table 43.1 shows data for a small North American town and probably reflects the prevalence in most Western countries, 3.0 per cent of all men over 30 years and 0.4 per cent of women. The prevalence of gout was directly related to the plasma urate concentration and most cases occurred in association with concentrations over 420 μmol/1 (7.0 mg/100 ml) in men and 355 μmol/1 (6.0 mg/100 ml) in women.

That primary gout is a disease in which both genetic and environmental factors play a part is illustrated by the Maoris (Table 43.2). There is a high prevalence amongst the Maoris on the remote Pacific island of Puka Puka, who live today under the same conditions as their forefathers have for at least 2000 years. The prevalence is nearly twice as high in the Maoris in New Zealand who originally emigrated from islands like Puka Puka and now lead a Westernised life. The European population of New Zealand has a lower prevalence, similar to that in Framingham, USA.

The Maoris and certain other populations around the Pacific—Filipinos, Marianas Islanders and the Blackfoot and Pima Indians of the United States—have high plasma urates. In other parts of the world such as Africa the frequency of gout and hyperuricaemia appears to be less than in Western communities.

Gout tends to be familial and about 25 per cent of the relatives of patients have hyperuricaemia. In some families transmission patterns suggest an autosomal dominant inheritance with low penetrance, especially in females.

Gout is rare in boys before puberty and in women until after the menopause. Hippocrates noted this and added that eunuchs were not affected. The concentration of plasma urate is low in children. It rises in boys at puberty so that the average value is about 90 μmol/1 (1.5 mg/100 ml) higher in men than women. In women plasma urate falls during pregnancy. It goes up at the menopause and

Table 43.1 Serum uric acid concentrations and the prevalence of gouty arthritis in men and women aged 30 years or over in Framingham, Massachusetts (Hall *et al.*, 1967)

		Men			Women		
Serum uric acid		Number	Gouty arthritis		Number	Gouty arthritis	
μmol/1	mg/100 ml	examined	Number	Per cent	examined	Number	per cent
<355	<6	1281	8	0.6	2665	2	0.1
355–410	6–6.9	790	15	1.9	151	5	3.3
420–475	7–7.9	162	27	16.7	23	4	17.4
480–535	8–8.9	40	10	25.0	4	0	—
535+	9+	10	9	90.0	1	0	—

Table 43.2 Prevalence of gouty arthritis in Maori and Causasian men and women over 30 years of age (Prior, 1972)

Race	Habitat	Prevalence of gouty arthritis (per cent)	
		Men	Women
Maori	Puka Puka	7.0	0
Maori	New Zealand	13.3	1.4
Caucasian	New Zealand	2.4	0

thereafter runs only a little below the male average. Plasma urate is lowered by oestrogens, and gout may occur in women given androgen therapy.

It was recognised in the eighteenth century that large enjoyable meals and the consumption of alcoholic drinks were often the prelude to an attack of gout. Doctors often imposed some sort of dietary discipline on their gouty patients. When Garrod showed that gout was characterised by an increase in blood urate this provided an apparent rational basis for dietetic treatment. For a time it was assumed that this increase in urate was derived directly from the diet and patients were advised to restrict meat and other food rich in purines. We now know that dietary nucleoproteins contribute, at most, only 50 per cent of the urate present in the blood of normal people and cannot account for the high concentrations found in gout. Most of the urate is formed endogenously. When effective uricosuric drugs were introduced, starting with probenecid in the 1950s, dietary treatment for patients with gout came to take very much of a second place, and patients were only advised to avoid excessive intake of food rich in purines.

The fact remains, however, that gout is a disease of the wealthy and disappears in times of need. At the end of the Second World War it was exceedingly rare in Germany. Epidemiological and metabolic information has accumulated which shows several ways in which diet can contribute to underlying hyperuricaemia or precipitate an attack of gout.

Overweight. Many patients who first develop gout in middle life are overweight. Table 43.3 shows how the mean blood urate increases as relative weight creeps up in British business executives. At the other end of the world, obesity is thought to be an important factor accounting for the higher plasma urates and frequency of gout in New Zealand Maoris compared with primitive Polynesian islanders.

Alcohol. In an earlier age doctors observed empirically that an acute attack of gout might be precipitated by overindulgence in alcohol. Port and Madeira wine were thought to be especially dangerous. This was probably because of associated social and dietary habits. It is now known that plasma urate is higher in men who habitually consume too much alcohol in any form and that it is raised by a binge. The mechanism is probably that the associated increase in plasma lactate inhibits renal excretion of urate.

Dietary purines. When gouty subjects change to a low purine diet plasma urate falls by about 70 μmol/1 (1 to 1.3 mg/100 ml) but on very large intakes it may rise by a larger amount. Zöllner et al. (1972) have been making a careful re-examination of the effect of dietary purines. They report that on a purine-free formula diet plasma urate fell by 100 μmol/1 (1.65 mg/100 ml) in normouricaemic subjects. With these subjects on a constant lowpurine diet, addition of DNA to the diet produced increases of 24 μmol/1 (0.4 mg/100 ml) for each 1 g nucleic acid added. RNA (from yeast) increased plasma urate by 55 μmol/1 (0.9 mg/100 ml) in normal subjects and by 85 μmol/1 (1.45 mg/100 ml) in hyperuricaemic subjects for each 1 g of nucleic acid. The few existing tables that give the purine content of foods need to be rewritten because of this qualitative difference between nucleic acids and because the available figures for vegetables and 'low purine' foods are extremely variable. Yet some of these contain more purines per unit of utilisable energy than meat.

Starvation. Plasma urate rises strikingly, starting after only one day (MacLachlan and Rodnan, 1967), and can reach 600 μmol/1 (10 mg/100 ml) or more. The hyperuricaemia coincides with the development of ketosis and comes about because ketoacids reduce the renal excretion of urate. Occasional attacks of gout have been reported in obese patients treated by total starvation. This is important when someone with a tendency to gout stops eating because of an acute illness or an operation.

Fructose. Rapid infusions of intravenous fructose produce a temporary increase in plasma urate, which is a hazard, but it also occurs after an oral dose of 0.5 g/kg (Perheentupa and Paivio, 1967). It is due to rapid phosphorylation of fructose causing instability of AMP in the liver. The unstable AMP breaks down to adenosine and ultimately to uric acid (Woods and Alberti, 1972).

Table 43.3 Mean blood urate and weight, as percentage of expected weight, in British male business executives (Phoon and Pincherle, 1972)

	Relative weight							Total
	80	80-	90-	110-	100-	120-	130+	
Number of men	114	616	1996	2660	1415	463	180	7444
Mean blood urate (mg/100 ml)	5.16	5.39	5.72	6.01	6.27	6.46	6.66	5.96
(μmol/l)	300	325	345	360	375	390	400	355

Fat. On high fat diets plasma urate is increased and urinary uric acid excretion falls (Ogryzlo, 1955). The fat intakes that have this effect have been around 200 g/day. The effect is seen regardless of the degree of saturation of the fat.

Many famous men in history suffered from gout, including Alexander the Great, Luther, Newton, Milton, Harvey, Dr Johnson, Franklin and Louis XIV. To Sydenham it seemed that 'more wise men than fools are victims', though there are many exceptions. In our own times its frequency in university professors and business executives has prompted the hypothesis that a moderately high concentration of urate may be a cerebral stimulant. Caffeine, the stimulant in coffee and tea, only differs chemically from uric acid in having three extra methyl groups on the purine ring.

Normal man and the primates are relatively hyperuricaemic compared to most mammals, whose serum urate is about 12 to 18 μmol/1 (0.2 to 0.3 mg/100 ml). This is because during evolution the primates have lost the liver enzyme uricase, which breaks uric acid down to allantoin.

Secondary gout

In some cases gout occurs secondary to another disease, either one which impairs renal excretion such as chronic renal failure, or a condition which leads to overproduction of urate such as proliferative haemopoietic disorders like leukaemia, polycythaemia or myelofibrosis, and the skin disease, psoriasis. A few drugs have the side-effect of reducing urate excretion, the most important being the thiazide diuretics. The Lesch–Nyhan syndrome is an inborn error of metabolism in which an affected boy has choreoathetosis, mental deficiency, and strikingly aggressive personality associated with gout and urate stones (Lesch and Nyhan, 1964). Though fortunately very rare, this condition has illuminated our understanding of the regulation of purine metabolism. The biochemical abnormalities in this and other forms of gout associated with rare genetic enzyme deficiencies are reviewed by Wyngaarden (1974).

CHEMICAL PATHOLOGY

Uric acid is 2,6,8-trioxypurine (Fig. 43.1). It ionises weakly at N-9. Its pK is 5.8 so that at the pH of plasma, it is almost completely dissociated and circulates as the monovalent urate ion. In urine, which usually has a lower pH, it is excreted for the most part as the free acid.

Uric acid is the ultimate oxidation product of the purine bases, adenine and guanine. The enzyme for the last step, xanthine oxidase, contains molybdenum. Adenine and guanine are synthesised as part of the body's nucleoproteins from the simple precursors indicated in Figure 43.1. This summarises the many chemical steps in building up AMP and GMP. Thus purines are synthesised from three non-essential amino acids, glycine, aspartic acid and glu-

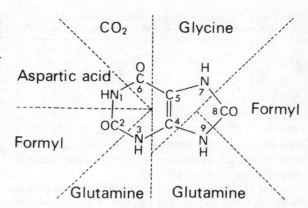

Fig. 43.1 Uric acid and the origins of the atoms of the purine ring.

tamine, and from one-carbon units, which are all freely available in the body's metabolic pools. The formyl units are supplied by THFA (folic acid) derivatives.

Studies with ^{15}N-glutamine indicate that the miscible pool of urate in body fluids is normally about 70 mmol (1.2 g). There are two sources of this pool, exogenous and endogenous. The exogenous source is the diet; a good Western diet contains sufficient purines to provide 30 to 60 mmol (0.5 to 1.0 g) of urate/day. About 20 per cent of the dietary purines are destroyed in the process of digestion; but the greater part goes to form urate in the body's miscible pool. The second, endogenous source is from breakdown of purines made in nucleoprotein synthesis. The extent of endogenous urate production can be judged by the fact that on a purine-free diet the excretion of uric acid is 18 to 60 mmol (0.3 to 0.5 g)/day.

The amount of urate destroyed in the body is small. Studies with ^{15}N-urate show that about 15 per cent of the miscible pool is catabolised daily and this takes place by bacterial action in the gut. Gouty patients may break down rather more than normal people. But the major way in which urate is lost from the body is by excretion in the urine, normally around 45 per cent of the miscible pool daily.

In gout the miscible pool of urate is enlarged and ranges from 120 to 1800 mmol (2 to 30 g). But in tophaceous gout only the peripheral layers of the tophi are readily exchangeable and the body's total urate can therefore be even larger. At least one-third of patients with gout are obvious overproducers of urate with a high urinary excretion on low purine diets. In them there appears to be some acceleration of the first, rate-limiting step in purine synthesis:

5-Phosphoribosyl-1-pyrophosphate+glutamine
→ 5-phosphoribosylamine+glutamic acid
    +pyrophosphate

In other gouty patients evidence of overproduction is more

subtle or absent. Secondly, whether they are over-excretors or excrete normal amounts of uric acid, gouty subjects in general show a somewhat lower rate of uric acid excretion at any given plasma urate concentration than do non-gouty subjects.

CLINICAL FEATURES

The first attack of gout is often a dramatic and alarming experience. The patient has usually enjoyed good health until his early forties, and then suddenly (often in the middle of the night) has an agonising, stabbing pain in one joint, generally the metatarsophalangeal joint of the big toe. The joint selected for attack is thought to be determined by its susceptibility to minor injury; the big toe is easily stubbed or injured by an ill-fitting shoe. The wrists, ankles and knees are much less common sites. As a rule it is peripheral rather than central joints that are affected; the spine is practically immune.

The joint is swollen and exquisitely tender; pain is aggravated by the least movement. The overlying skin is tense, red and shiny with distended veins and may later show oedema. Fever, malaise, loss of appetite, gastrointestinal upset and scanty highly coloured urine are common accompaniments. The patient may with good reason be very irritable. Blood examination often shows a raised erythrocyte sedimentation rate and a polymorph leucocytosis.

Even without treatment the natural tendency is for the attack to pass off after a few days. As the inflammation subsides the skin over the joint becomes scaly and itches. The joint recovers completely. There may be no further episodes for years but if the underlying hyperuricaemia is high and not regulated, attacks tend to occur with increasing frequency and to last longer. Eventually a stage may be reached where there is chronic, persistent, though generally less painful arthritis of several joints. During this phase **tophi** begin to appear; these are crystalline deposits of sodium urate which develop in the lobes of the ear, at the base of the big toe, in other toes or fingers, in the olecranon bursa behind the elbow or in tendon sheaths on the back of the hand. A tophus may vary in size from a pin head to a golf ball. It is usually painless. When tophi develop in joints they erode the neighbouring bone and appear on radiographs as clear, punched-out areas, since sodium urate is not radio-opaque.

Production of arthritis

Acute gouty arthritis is a non-infective inflammation with a polymorphonuclear exudate in the joint and intense congestion around it. Sudden changes in the plasma urate are likely to provoke an attack, whether the concentration is rising or falling from a previously high level. A careful search of fluid from gouty joints usually shows needle-shaped, birefringent crystals of sodium urate. Injection of urate microcrystals into the knees of healthy volunteers brought on in two hours acute arthritis that closely resembled gout in both its local and general effects. Faires and McCarty (1962) who did these courageous experiments on one another were both prostrated with excruciating pain after four hours. When their joints were aspirated many of the urate crystals in the fluid were found to be inside polymorphs. In the pathogenesis of acute gout there appears to be a vicious cycle in which precipitation of sodium urate crystals from supersaturated body fluids evokes a polymorph response. The polymorphs phagocytose the urate crystals and this raises their metabolic activity, increases the local lactate concentration and lowers the pH, which favours further crystal formation in the joint.

Complications

People with hyperuricaemia have a greatly increased liability to form **uric acid stones** in the urinary tract. These can present with renal colic and are one cause of the chronic renal disease that is an important late complication in gout. Uric acid stones are seen in hyperuricaemic patients who excrete normal amounts of uric acid as well as in the overexcretors. The reason appears to be that the urine is unusually acid, thus reducing the solubility of uric acid and this acidity is related to reduced NH_4^+ excretion. The NH_4^+ which is excreted has been formed in the kidneys mostly from glutamine. In gout the kidneys may receive decreased amounts of glutamine because more has been diverted into purine synthesis.

The Framingham prospective study showed an increased incidence of coronary heart disease in persons with asymptomatic hyperuricaemia. Hyperuricaemia is associated with hypertriglyceridaemia, or type IV hyperlipoproteinaemia, which itself may be a risk factor for CHD.

There is also an association between hyperuricaemia and hypertension, which is only partly explicable by the action of some drugs used for hypertension, like thiazide diuretics, that are known to decrease urate excretion. Degenerative renal disease occurs in patients with chronic gout, and hypertension itself appears to reduce uric acid clearance. It is not surprising that raised plasma urates have been reported in patients with cerebral vascular disease.

DIAGNOSIS

When the classic site, the big toe, is affected, clinical diagnosis is usually straightforward and is confirmed by a raised plasma urate. But when other joints are affected it must be borne in mind that asymptomatic hyperuricaemia can coincide with non-gouty arthropathy. The clinical setting for an attack of gout is sometimes confusing. It may come on following some period of stress, such as an injury or a surgical operation or following a myocardial infarction. Response of monoarticular arthritis to a course of colchicine is useful, but not infallible evidence of gout. If tophi are present, urate can be confirmed chemically by the murexide test in a biopsy; tophi and punched out translucent juxta-articular lesions on radiographs are late changes and gout should be diagnosed before this stage.

There is another type of arthritis caused by deposition of crystals of calcium pyrophosphate in joints, sometimes called 'pseudogout'. Large joints are usually involved, especially the knees, which show calcification of articular cartilage. It does not respond to colchicine and the plasma urate is normal.

TREATMENT

Some patients, after a single attack, remain in a state of natural remission for years without further disability. They do not need drugs, but require advice about diet and way of life and arrangements for periodic follow-up of the plasma urate In other patients attacks of gout are frequent and plasma urate is high. Regular and continued medical treatment is needed both to relieve the arthritis and to reduce the risk of late complications.

Drugs

These are used for two purposes. First there are drugs which relieve the acute arthritis, but do not affect plasma urate concentrations. The oldest effective remedy for acute gout is colchicine, the alkaloid from the autumn crocus (*Colchicum autumnale, L.*) This plant has been used as specific treatment for over 200 years and was introduced into America for this purpose by Benjamin Franklin. It appears to act by inhibiting the polymorph response to urate crystals and so breaking the vicious cycle. The dose is 0.5 mg every hour or 1 mg two-hourly until relief is obtained (usually at 4 to 8 mg total dose) or diarrhoea supervenes. If the response to colchicine is too slow or diarrhoea too troublesome, it may be reinforced with or replaced by a short course of phenylbutazone or of corticotrophin or one of the adrenal corticosteroids. During the acute attack the patient gets little rest from pain, which is always worse at night. He should be in bed and the joint made as comfortable as possible by supporting it on pillows and protecting it from pressure and knocks.

The second group of drugs reduce the pool of urate in the body and hence deal with the underlying biochemical abnormality. They have to be given for months or years. Probenecid, introduced in 1952, is a uricosuric agent, i.e. it impairs the reabsorption of uric acid by the renal tubules and so increases uric acid excretion in the urine usually by 30 to 50 per cent. As its administration is continued, plasma urate falls and later the frequency of arthritis decreases and tophi regress. Sulphinpyrazone is another drug of this type. Aspirin should not be given at the same time as uricosuric agents because it interferes with their action on the renal tubules.

The use of uricosuric drugs is difficult if patients already have renal damage or a history of uric acid stones. Ample fluids should be given to reduce the risk of further stone

formation. In such patients and when there is gross overproduction of uric acid the newer drug allopurinol is the preferred treatment. It acts by inhibiting xanthine oxidase so that uric acid production is reduced and the patient excretes instead xanthine and hypoxanthine, which are more soluble.

Neither probenecid nor allopurinol have any direct effect on gouty arthritis; indeed when treatment to reduce the body's pool of urate is started attacks of gout are liable to occur, and prophylactic doses of colchicine, 0.5 mg three times a day, should be given for the first two or three months. Other adverse effects are unusual with these drugs.

Diet

The dietary advice for a patient who has had one or more attacks of primary gout should be based on the following principles, which arise from the epidemiological and metabolic findings discussed earlier.

If the patient is overweight, he should be advised to bring his weight down by a gentle dietary regimen. This has been demonstrated to produce a moderate reduction of plasma urate (Nicholls and Scott, 1972). But fasting, even for short periods, is likely to do more harm than good and may induce an attack of gout.

Feasting should equally be avoided. Heavy, rich meals high in purines or fat are likely to raise the plasma urate and may be followed by an acute attack.

Excessive alcohol is sometimes the underlying stress which precipitates gout. People are prone to understate their alcohol consumption, and the patient should be told that all types of alcoholic drinks need to be restricted. A compromise prescription of 'reasonable amounts' can all too easily be interpreted by the patient with too much latitude. Men who take more than two drinks a day have plasma urate concentrations higher than normal (Phoon and Pincherle, 1972).

For the small minority of patients with severe gout who respond poorly or are intolerant to uricosuric drugs a strict low-purine regimen along the lines recommended by Zöllner may be valuable. But for the majority of patients urate-lowering drugs are so effective and so easy to take that the only modification of dietary purine necessary is to avoid foods rich in purine, e.g. liver, kidneys, sweetbreads, sardines, anchovies, fish roes and meat extracts.

Because of the increased risk of stone in the urinary tract patients should maintain a good intake of non-alcoholic fluids, and take a drink of water before going to bed. Coffee and tea, although they contain methylxanthines such as caffeine, can be drunk because caffeine is not converted into uric acid in the body.

Lastly it is wise to check fasting plasma lipids and treat hyperlipidaemia if present, and to give gouty subjects some advice on dietary and other measures which may reduce the risk of coronary heart disease.

44. Diseases of the Kidneys and Urinary Tract

In the past decade the dietetic treatment of patients with renal disease has undergone many changes as a result of the widespread avilability of artificial kidneys (dialysis) and kidney transplantation. In many centres patients who would have died from terminal renal failure now have a reasonable chance of living for another ten years in good health. With improvements in the use of the artificial kidney, patients on regular dialysis have been liberated from some of the dietary restrictions that were previously thought necessary. The recipient of a successful, well-functioning renal transplant can usually eat normally with few restrictions on food and fluid intake. While these developments have made the task of the dietitian easier in some respects, her role in the treatment of other renal disorders remains unchanged. Dietetics still forms the cornerstone of treatment when renal function is modified or impaired by disease.

PHYSIOLOGY

The management of patients with renal disorders is firmly grounded on an understanding of how the kidneys work in health and how their function is disturbed by disease processes.

The kidneys are each composed of approximately one million similar functional units called nephrons. Each nephron consists of a glomerulus which is a tuft of capillaries invaginated into an epithelial sac (Bowman's capsule), from which arises a tubule. The blood flow through the kidneys is large, amounting to about one-quarter of the cardiac output at rest, i.e. 1300 ml/min. Branches of the renal artery give rise to afferent arterioles which divide to form the glomerular capillaries. These unite to form the efferent arterioles which supply blood to the renal tubules.

The hydrostatic pressure within the glomerular capillaries results in the filtration of fluid into Bowman's capsule. This fluid is similar in composition with plasma, except that it normally contains no fat and very little protein.

The filtrate, formed at the glomerulus at a rate of 100 ml/min, passes first into the proximal convoluted tubule and from there through the loop of Henle and distal convoluted tubule to the collecting ducts. It is modified according to the needs of the body by the selective reabsorption of its constituents and of water, and by tubular secretion. Of the 150 000 ml of water and 225 000 mmol of sodium filtered through the glomerular capillaries during the course of a day, only about 1500 ml of water and 100–200 mmol of sodium remain to be excreted as urine.

The kidneys are essential for maintaining many aspects of the internal chemical environment of the body. Their main functions are indicated in Table 44.1.

As excretory organs they are responsible for the elimination of such waste products of nitrogen metabolism as urea, uric acid and creatinine, as well as hydrogen ions and sulphates which arise from degradation of sulphur-containing amino acids. The kidneys must also excrete surplus quantities of water, sodium, potassium, calcium, phosphate, magnesium and other ions. These substances are taken in by mouth as essential nutrients, often in excess of requirements.

The kidneys regulate the amounts of water, sodium, hydrogen ions and several other electrolytes in the body. By modifying the composition of the urine they maintain not only the volume of the body fluids but also their electrolytic composition within very narrow limits. In the healthy adult, for example, extreme responses to dehydration and overhydration are produced by a change in either direction of only 2 per cent in the water content of the body. The daily urinary volume can be reduced from the usual 1500 ml to only 500 ml, following water deprivation, and increased to approximately 20 litres following the ingestion of a sufficiently large volume of water.

The kidneys also have important metabolic roles. They are the exclusive site for the production of 1,25-dihydroxy vitamin D, the most active metabolite of the vitamin which acts on the intestine to increase calcium absorption, and maintains normal mineralisation of bone. The kidneys also produce erythopoietin and renin. Erythopoietin acts on the bone marrow to increase production of red blood cells. Renin is released from the kidneys in response to a low blood pressure or sodium deficiency; it enhances the production of angiotensin which increases the blood pressure directly and also stimulates production of aldosterone. Several polypeptide hormones, including parathyroid hormone, calcitonin, insulin and gastrin are degraded by the kidneys.

ASSESSMENT OF RENAL FUNCTION

Clinical observation and biochemical analysis of plasma and urine can be used in conjunction to provide a reliable assessment of renal function and the patient's needs. Used in isolation they can be misleading. Many symptoms and signs are not specific, but are often valuable guides to

Table 44.1 Functions of kidneys

	Daily load for an adult	Effects of renal failure
EXCRETION		
Nitrogenous metabolites		
Urea	(dietary protein × ⅓) g	Increased plasma
Uric acid	4 mmol	concentrations,
Creatinine	10 mmol	uraemia
Other metabolites		
Sulphate	25–60 mmol	Acidosis
Hydrogen ions	40–80 mmol	
Surplus nutrients		
Water	1500–5000 ml*	Hypertension,
Sodium	100–200 mmol	oedema,
Potassium	60–80 mmol	Hyperkalaemia
Calcium	2–7 mmol	—
Chloride	100–200 mmol	As for sodium
Phosphate	20–40 mmol	Hyperparathyroidism
REGULATION		
Water — total body content, tonicity		
Sodium — extracellular fluid volume, blood pressure		Loss of
Potassium — plasma concentration, neuro-muscular excitability		homeostasis and flexibility in
Hydrogen — level of acidity in cells and plasma		extreme conditions
Magnesium — plasma concentration		
METABOLIC		
Vitamin D — 1α-hydroxylation		Bone disease
Erythropoietin synthesis		Anaemia
Renin synthesis		?
Hormone degradation		?

* Including 'one over the eight' on Saturday night.

therapy. Thirst, polyuria and polydipsia are features of diabetes mellitus and insipidus as well as of chronic renal failure. In all three conditions they indicate not only that the kidneys are unable to conserve water, but also that the patient has an increased requirement for water which must be satisfied if fluid balance is to be maintained. Peripheral oedema and pulmonary oedema indicate that the extracellular fluid volume is increased by at least 2 litres in adults with a corresponding increase in total body sodium. Both arise from failure of renal regulation of sodium homeostasis, which can result from cardiac failure as easily as from intrinsic renal disease. Whatever the cause, the patient benefits from measures designed to promote net loss of sodium from the body. The absence of oedema, hypertension and polyuria in a patient with biochemical signs of advanced renal failure sometimes indicate the presence of excessive renal sodium loss due to defective tubular reabsorption of sodium. This condition often responds to an increase in sodium intake, with restoration of total body sodium, extracellular fluid and plasma volumes, and with

improvement in renal blood flow, **glomerular filtration rate** (GFR) and overall renal function.

Measurement of plasma concentrations of urea, creatinine, sodium, potassium, bicarbonate, calcium, inorganic phosphate and alkaline phosphatase provides inexpensive and convenient biochemical indices of renal function.

Changes in the excretory function of the kidney are reflected in plasma urea and creatinine concentrations. If their production rates remain unchanged, their concentrations double when GFR is halved. In patients with established renal failure these measurements provide a simple guide to the progress of disease.

A substance that is neither secreted nor reabsorbed in the tubules, e.g. creatinine, can be used to measure GFR. If U and P are the concentrations in the urine and plasma respectively and V is the volume of urine excreted in 1 min, then UV/P is the **clearance** of the substance. GFR is conveniently estimated by measuring creatinine clearance. Its value is about 125 ml/min in healthy young men; it is related to the size of the kidneys, which are related to the size of the body, and so is usually a little less in young women. GFR falls slowly with age and at 70 years is about 75 per cent of the value in youth. There is a large reserve of glomerular function. Kidney failure rarely produces symptoms until the GFR falls below 30 ml/min.

The regulatory function of the kidneys with respect to potassium and phosphate ions is reflected directly in their plasma concentrations, whereas the renal contribution to hydrogen ion homeostasis is reflected in the plasma bicarbonate concentration. The secondary effects of renal dysfunction on vitamin D and bone metabolism are often indicated by changes in plasma calcium and alkaline phosphatase concentrations.

Paradoxically, the plasma sodium concentration reflects a change in body water as often as a change in sodium balance, being increased in dehydration and decreased in overhydration or in water intoxication. Since sodium is an important determinant of extracellular and plasma volumes, changes in body sodium are more reliably assessed clinically in terms of the presence or absence of peripheral oedema and by measurement of arterial blood pressure.

The volume of the urine is variably increased, normal, or decreased at different stages of acute and chronic renal failure. While the urine volume is often the most important factor in determining water balance, other sensible and insensible losses must be taken into account when assessing the fluid requirements of a patient. Since 1 litre of water weighs 1 kilogram, an invaluable guide to changes in body water is to weigh the patient at the same time each day or at each clinic visit under standard conditions.

Abnormal urinary constituents such as blood and protein do not always indicate the presence of kidney disease, but call for further investigation of the kidneys and urinary tract. In glomerulonephritis both the activity of the disease process and the response to treatment can be followed by measuring the quantity of protein excreted in a 24 h collection of urine. The same sample can be used to measure creatinine clearance. The excretion rates of sodium and potassium can be easily measured, and can be used to assess either the response to diuretic therapy or requirements for dietary supplements. In certain primary and secondary disorders of the renal tubules, there may be excessive loss of electrolytes such as sodium, potassium or magnesium which can be diagnosed only by giving the patient a diet low in one of these substances and observing whether the urinary excretion is reduced appropriately.

PRINCIPLES OF DIETETICS IN RENAL DISORDERS

Diseases affecting the kidneys disturb renal function in a limited number of ways. Frequently prescription of appropriate dietetic therapy is a logical way to help a patient compensate for the altered pattern of renal excretion and regulation.

As can be seen in Table 44.1, a major task of the kidneys is the elimination from the body of surplus nutrients taken in by mouth. When renal function is greatly reduced, homeostasis may often be maintained by reducing oral consumption of water, sodium, potassium and magnesium to no more than minimum requirements. In addition, by reducing intake of protein, the production of urea, the principal nitrogenous waste metabolite, is reduced substantially. These dietetic measures form the basis for the conservative management of severe acute and chronic renal failure.

In other renal disorders the capacity of the kidney to excrete sodium is impaired, with little or no loss of other excretory and regulatory functions. This can be treated by reducing the dietary intake of sodium.

Certain diseases, e.g. the nephrotic syndrome, damage the glomerular capillaries and result in massive loss of albumin and other proteins from the plasma into the urine. Increasing dietary intake of protein allows increased hepatic synthesis of albumin which compensates in part for the urinary losses.

Diseases affecting the renal tubules can result in excessive urinary losses of water, sodium, potassium, phosphate and other substances, either alone or in combination. These losses can usually be replaced by an appropriate increase in oral intake.

Dietetic principles are still of major importance in the successful management of the patients with renal disease, despite the introduction of effective diuretic agents which inhibit tubular reabsorption of sodium and water, and the use of the artificial kidney. In sodium-retaining states, for example, the therapeutic effect of diuretics in increasing the urinary excretion of sodium is enhanced if the oral intake of sodium is also limited. In many patients who appear to have refractory oedema, the effectiveness of the diuretic regimen may have been lost by the continued consumption of an unlimited quantity of sodium chloride by mouth. In these circumstances, the only additional measure required for therapy to be successful is to reduce oral sodium intake. Even when renal function is lost completely, dietetic measures alone may hold the patient in reasonable homeostasis for several days before artificial kidney treatment becomes necessary to sustain life and health. Such conservative treatment may be sufficient in a metabolically stable patient with a short self-limiting disturbance in renal function.

Unfortunately, severe constraints upon eating habits are poorly tolerated, not only for social reasons but also because they affect the supply of essential nutrients, and patients often feel hungry. In practice, the need to sustain general nutrition becomes a major consideration. Dietetic measures cannot compensate for other aspects of disordered renal function, and in both acute and chronic renal failure many of the roles played by the dietitian have been taken over by the artificial kidney.

THE ARTIFICIAL KIDNEY

Peritoneal dialysis and haemodialysis refer to the two different ways in which urea, creatinine and other substances of small molecular weight can be removed from the blood by diffusion across a semipermeable membrane into fluid that can be drained away. In peritoneal dialysis fluid is introduced into the peritoneal cavity where it is separated from the blood capillaries by the natural cellular peritoneal membrane. In haemodialysis the blood is taken from the patient and passed through a haemodialyser in which the blood is separated from the dialysis fluid by an artificial cellophane membrane.

Peritoneal dialysis

The first demonstration that peritoneal lavage might benefit both animals and humans with renal failure was in 1923. Peritoneal dialysis is now a standard treatment for both acute and chronic renal failure, but is less efficient and takes longer to perform than haemodialysis. However, it has the valuable advantage for small hospitals of being simpler and the equipment is relatively inexpensive and does not require special installation.

A patient on peritoneal dialysis is shown in Fig. 44.1.

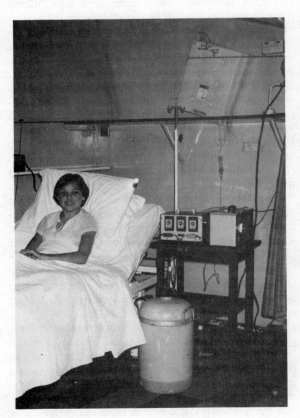

Fig. 44.1 A patient with chronic renal failure on maintenance peritoneal dialysis.

One to 2 litres of sterile dialysis fluid are run into the peritoneal cavity through an indwelling polyethylene cannula from a reservoir above the patient. After an equilibration period of 15–20 minutes, the fluid is drained into a large vat at the bedside, and the cycle repeated. One cycle lasts ½ to 1 hour and is controlled by clamps on the tubing from the reservoir to the patient and from the patient to the drainage vat. Strict asepsis is necessary to avoid peritonitis. For patients with chronic renal failure the treatment typically lasts for 10–15 hours using 20 litres of dialysis fluid, and is repeated three to five times per week.

The dialysis fluid contains sodium, calcium, and magnesium in approximately the same concentrations as in normal plasma. Urea, creatinine, potassium, phosphate and toxic metabolites and certain drugs diffuse from the blood into the fluid in the peritoneal cavity and are 'excreted' into the drainage vat. Acidosis can be corrected by including lactate in the dialysis fluid. Lactate diffuses from the dialysis fluid into the plasma and is metabolised with the consumption of one hydrogen ion for each molecule of lactate. Surplus water is removed osmotically. Glucose is added to the dialysing fluid to increase the osmotic pressure and to draw water across the peritoneal membrane from the plasma. Sodium is removed simultaneously since the water drawn into the peritoneal cavity dilutes the dialysis fluid and causes a fall in the sodium concentration; this generates a concentration gradient for the diffusion of sodium from plasma into dialysis fluid. Sodium can also be removed by using dialysis fluid in which the sodium concentration is somewhat lower than in the plasma.

Haemodialysis

A haemodialysis machine to purify the blood continuously in an extracorporeal circuit was first used successfully by Dr Willem J. Kolff in occupied Holland in 1943. Since then, haemodialysis equipment has been modified extensively with a considerable reduction in size and a corresponding rise in efficiency. The disposable device shown in Fig. 44.2 brings the patient's blood and dialysis fluid together on opposite sides of a cellophane membrane and has an excretory capacity for urea and creatinine of between two and three normal human kidneys. Since blood is pumped through the extracorporeal circuit at a rate of 200 ml/min, the patient has to be protected against the hazards which would arise if a leak developed, a clot formed, or if air was drawn into the system. This is effected by a series of monitors controlled electronically and incorporated into the dialysis machine. This machine also produces dialysis fluid by mixing tap-water in a fixed proportion with a concentrated solution of salts. The fluid is warmed to blood temperature, drawn through the dialyser and pumped off to waste with its additional load of urea and creatinine and other metabolites removed from

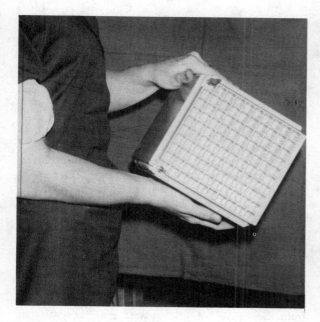

Fig. 44.2 Haemodialyser used in treatment of patients with acute and chronic renal failure.

the blood. Figure 44.3 shows the dialyser and supporting equipment. It can be truly regarded as an artificial kidney, producing a continuous supply of artificial urine!

Haemodialysis works in a comparable fashion to peritoneal dialysis. The dialysis fluid is similar in composition, except that acetate is used instead of lactate for correction of acidosis. Sodium and water are removed by applying a hydrostatic rather than an osmotic pressure differential across the semipermeable membrane.

With improvements in dialyser design, haemodialysis is now much more efficient than peritoneal dialysis. Many patients with chronic renal failure require no more than four hours on dialysis repeated three times a week. The procedure is somewhat more complex for the patient to understand and to learn to use unaided, and the capital costs of the machine and its installation are greater. Access to the blood stream is gained either by the insertion of indwelling cannulae into a peripheral artery and a neighbouring vein or by the surgical creation of a subcutaneous arterio-venous fistula. In a patient with chronic renal failure this can last for many years. The veins are dilated with blood under arterial pressure and are thus more accessible for repeated venepuncture. Patients soon learn to insert their own needles under local anaesthesia and to carry out their own dialysis treatment with little or no assistance.

Peritoneal dialysis and haemodialysis are not without disadvantages. The patient is tied to a kidney machine for hours at a time and treatments must be repeated several times each week under pain of death for non-compliance.

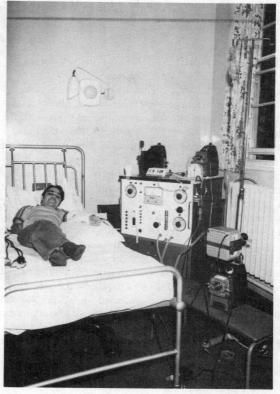

Fig. 44.3 A patient with chronic renal failure on maintenance haemodialysis. The extracorporeal blood circulation through the haemodialyser shown in Fig. 44.2 is controlled by the dialysis machine (centre) with dials and electronic monitors to safeguard the patient. The machine also produces and continuously monitors the dialysis fluid.

Amino acids and water soluble vitamins are removed from the plasma as readily as other small molecules and lost in the dialysis fluid. The peritoneal membrane is not impermeable to plasma proteins, and large quantities of proteins and smaller peptides may be lost from the body. Both forms of treatment replace renal function in terms of the excretion of nitrogenous metabolites and the correction of acidosis to the extent that patients can enjoy a normal intake of protein. Their capacity for the excretion of drugs and surplus quantities of water, sodium, potassium and phosphate is limited, largely because both techniques are used intermittently rather than continuously. Thus some limitation of dietary intake is always necessary and nutrients removed during dialysis must be replaced (p. 375). Neither form of dialysis can replace metabolic functions of the kidney such as the synthesis of erythropoietin and the conversion of 25-hydroxy vitamin D to 1,25-dihydroxy vitamin D. Nevertheless, renal function is sufficiently replaced by these artificial means to enable most patients to stay not only alive but well and able to continue their normal employment and family life for many years.

DIETETICS IN RENAL DISORDERS

In the management of patients with diseases affecting the kidneys, dietetics is of greatest value when renal function is impaired. There is little or no need to interfere with the eating habits and way of life of patients when the kidneys continue to preserve homeostasis, as they usually do in acute and chronic pyelonephritis, asymptomatic glomerulonephritis, mild proteinuria or hypertension. Tubular disorders, such as the Fanconi syndrome, which can result in abnormal losses of phosphate, sodium, potassium or magnesium, may appear to invite dietetic intervention but in most cases can be treated by giving supplements of the appropriate salts on top of a normal food intake.

While the kidneys are affected by many different diseases, the ways in which renal function can be impaired are relatively few and disorders requiring the specialised help of a dietitian are included in four clinical syndromes, (1) acute glomerulonephritis, (2) the nephrotic syndrome, (3) acute renal failure and (4) chronic renal failure.

Acute glomerulonephritis

Acute glomerulonephritis is characterised by acute inflammation of the glomeruli with congestion, cellular proliferation and infiltration of polymorphs. Renal blood flow and glomerular filtration rate are reduced by 50 per cent or more and the damaged glomerular capillaries exude plasma proteins and cellular elements of the blood into Bowman's space. The urine volume falls to between 500 and 1000 ml/day and sodium excretion is greatly reduced. The urine contains moderate amounts of protein, with red and white blood cells in abundance, and casts of the renal tubules formed by precipitation of protein and red cells in the tubular system.

Since the patient continues to ingest normal quantities of sodium and water, oedema develops and the blood pressure rises, leading to complaints of malaise, headaches and swelling of the face and hands in the morning and of the ankles at night. Plasma concentrations of urea and creatinine rise in proportion to the fall in glomerular filtration rate, but acidosis and hypokalaemia are usually mild and only require treatment if renal failure ensues.

In the past, acute glomerulonephritis was common, frequently following infection with β-haemolytic streptococci in children and young adults with tonsillitis or scarlet fever. Today troublesome streptococci are usually rapidly obliterated by penicillin, and acute glomerulonephritis is less common, but it can still follow infection of the upper respiratory tract. In poststreptococcal glomerulonephritis glomerular damage is caused not by direct infection of the kidney but by deposition of soluble immune complexes of streptococcal antigen with antibody formed in response to the foreign organisms. A similar syndrome with a comparable pathogenesis can develop in patients with bacterial endocarditis, and in patients with other manifestations of disordered immunity, e.g. Henoch Schonlein purpura and systemic lupus erythematosis.

In almost all patients the disease is self-limiting. The glomerular inflammation resolves spontaneously and usually full renal function is restored in one to three weeks. In a few patients proteinuria persists and the nephrotic syndrome develops. Infrequently there is a progressive decline in renal function, leading ultimately to chronic renal failure.

Treatment

There are no specific agents known to reverse the glomerular lesion. Dietetics forms the mainstay of treatment, although drugs may be indicated to control hypertension and diuretics are often used to increase urinary excretion.

Fluid intake should be restricted to a volume calculated from the volume of urine passed plus the estimated insensible water loss, usually 500 ml daily. During the first few days of treatment, the fluid given should be less than the requirements to allow for dispersal of oedema fluid. Daily weighing provides a useful monitor of overall fluid balance.

At first it is wise to restrict the sodium intake to 40–60 mmol/day and the protein intake to 40 g/day, although the latter is often unnecessary. Diet No. 6 can be used for this purpose. Restriction of sodium intake can be relaxed when oedema resolves and the blood pressure falls. Restriction of protein is only needed when the blood urea is raised. Diuretics are sometimes used to increase urinary sodium and measurements of the daily output are useful. In the great majority of patients the glomerular lesion resolves completely within three weeks and no further treatment is needed.

A few patients develop severe renal failure and require dialysis. The dietary protein can then be restored to normal or may be increased if there has been heavy proteinuria. If facilities for dialysis are not available, a very low protein diet (Diet No. 4) may be needed. The theoretical and practical difficulties with these measures are discussed in the section on chronic renal failure.

Nephrotic syndrome

The nephrotic syndrome is characterised by heavy proteinuria, hypoalbuminaemia and peripheral oedema. It occurs when damage to glomerular capillaries results in greatly increased losses of plasma proteins from the body into the urine. Normally only small amounts of protein are filtered through the glomerular basement membrane and these are totally reabsorbed by the tubules. Proteinuria develops when the leakage of protein from the glomeruli exceeds the reabsorptive capacity of the renal tubules. The nephrotic syndrome ensues when the loss of protein in the urine exceeds the capacity of the liver to compensate by increasing synthesis of albumin. Daily losses of up to 5 g in the adult and up to 0.1 g/kg in children can usually be tolerated. If the loss of protein is greater or if protein synthesis in the liver is impaired, plasma concentration of albumin falls. The balance of hydrostatic and colloid osmotic pressures across the capillaries throughout the body is altered, favouring the movement of water and solute from the circulating blood plasma to the interstitial fluid. The plasma volume falls and in compensation sodium is reabsorbed avidly from the renal tubules. Sodium is retained in the body and the plasma volume restored at the expense of a greatly increased extracellular volume which is evident clinically as peripheral oedema. Of the plasma proteins albumin with its relatively small molecule escapes most readily through the leak in the glomerular membrane. Plasma globulins with a higher molecular weight appear in the urine in much smaller amounts. In fact, plasma concentrations of lipoproteins are increased and hyperlipaedemia is a feature of the nephrotic syndrome.

The syndrome can arise from diseases affecting the glomeruli alone, and from diseases in which the glomeruli are affected secondarily to changes elsewhere in the body. Indeed, in the world as a whole, the commonest cause of the nephrotic syndrome may be quartan malaria. In temperate climates a frequent cause in children is **minimal lesion glomerulonephritis** in which the glomeruli are primarily involved mysteriously with little or no abnormality to be seen on light microscopy and no sign of damage to the glomerular basement membrane on electron microscopy. In **membranous glomerulonephritis** there is thickening of the basement membrane with deposition of immunoglobulins and complement. In **proliferative glomerulonephritis** there is also deposition of immunoglobulins in the basement membrane and elsewhere in the glomeruli with an increase in the number of cells in a manner similar to that found in acute glomerulonephritis. Minimal lesion glomerulonephritis is distinguished by the consistency with which the proteinuria responds to treatment with corticosteroids and other immunosuppressive drugs. The treatment of membranous and proliferative glomerulonephritis with these agents is much more controversial.

The nephrotic syndrome can arise secondarily from damage to the glomerular capillaries in diabetes mellitus, amyloidosis, multiple myeloma and disseminated lupus erythematosis.

Treatment

Dietetics plays a major part in treatment. The two renal defects are loss of plasma proteins and retention of sodium. All patients benefit from a limitation in sodium intake and an increase in dietary protein, even when the glomerular lesion can be expected to respond to prednisolone. These symptomatic measures are often necessary both before diagnosis can be made by renal biopsy and also while waiting for the kidneys to respond to more specific therapy.

In practical terms the simultaneous manipulation in opposite directions of two prominent constituents of the diet presents a considerable challenge. A daily protein intake of 90–120g for adults and of 2–3g/kg for children is recommended to replenish depleted stores and to enhance hepatic synthesis of albumin. This could be achieved by taking double helpings of meat and fish, at least two and preferably four eggs daily (each contains approximately 7g of protein), an extra half to one pint of milk and cream-cheese in abundance. Unfortunately, as reference to Table 10.3 shows, these foods are classified as moderate sources of sodium even before the addition of salt in cooking or at table.

For many patients, in whom the renal tubules are responsive to diuretic drugs, extreme degrees of salt restriction are not required. Salt should not be added at table and only small quantities added during cooking. Fresh meat and fish can be used to supplement the protein intake, but tinned products and foods preserved with salt, such as ham, sausages and kippers must be avoided. Eggs can be used freely but cheese other than cream-cheese should be reserved for special occasions. There is usually no difficulty in meeting the increased protein requirements of the mild nephrotic by these dietetic means, apart from the ability of the patients to pay for a richer style of living.

Difficulties arise if the patient is refractory to diuretic therapy. Frequently the albuminuria is of greater magnitude, often in excess of 10 g/day and the plasma albumin is reduced to less than 20g/1. Then tubular reabsorption of sodium is so avid, that even by using combinations of diuretics that act at different sites along the nephron the excretion of sodium in the urine may not exceed 50 mmol/day. Under these conditions salt should be avoided in cooking as well as at the table. This can be achieved at home without subjecting the rest of the family to a restricted salt regimen, if the food for the family is cooked together without added salt and the portion for the patient separated before adding salt to the rations for the rest. Food cooked without salt is impalatable. Moreover, at very low salt intakes, even food containing only moderate amounts of salt may need to be restricted. This at once jeopardises attempts to increase protein intake. It may be necessary to use salt-free bread and salt-free butter to allow sodium to be taken in more proteinaceous forms. The good domestic cook can do much to provide a large range of tasty salt-free foods. Herbs, curry powder, paprika and other peppers, onions and garlic can be used to flavour savoury dishes containing meat and fish. Potassium glutamate can be used in cooking and table salt substitutes such as Selora and Theradal which also contain potassium can be used freely unless renal failure supervenes. Salt-free tinned foods such as baked beans and processed peas are available and salt-free tomato ketchup and salad dressing can be obtained from Health Food stores. Salt-free pickles and chutney can be made at home. Salt-free baking powder containing potassium bicarbonate and bitartrate instead of the sodium salts can be used at home to provide salt-free breads, scones and cakes. Recipes and more detailed advice can be found in *Cooking for Special Diets* by Bee Nilson (Penguin).

Frequently the protein intake cannot be sustained by these manipulations and protein concentrates are needed. Salt-free casein, derived from milk, is available in powder form. Casilan, Edosol and Lonolac are preparations which can be added to milk drinks, milk puddings and sauces, or sprinkled on porridge. These must be distinguished from other milk preparations, such as Complan and Carnation Breakfast Food, which provide a palatable protein supplement but contain sodium in abundance. Salt-free mixtures of essential amino acids are now marketed (Aminutrin, Nefranutrin, Geistlich) and are an expensive alternative to supplements of whole protein. The effectiveness of these measures in sustaining the prescribed level of dietary protein can be assessed by measuring the urinary urea excretion rate as well as the total urinary protein. The same 24 h collection of urine can be used to measure sodium and potassium excretion and thus to monitor the effectiveness of the diuretic therapy. Unless the patient is losing abnormally large quantities of nitrogen in the faeces, or is in a strongly anabolic or catabolic state, the urinary urea excretion should reflect changes in the intake of protein by mouth. Thus a daily intake of 90–120 g protein should result in the urinary excretion of approximately 600 mmol (36g) of urea daily.

Dietary salt restriction is aided by the use of diuretics to increase loss of sodium in the urine. There is always an associated increase in potassium excretion and so a supplement of potassium chloride should be given to all patients on diuretic therapy. Excessive use of diuretics may reduce the plasma volume and renal blood flow and so can precipitate acute renal failure.

Patients whose oedema remains refractory to dietary measures and diuretics usually respond to infusions of salt-poor albumin derived from fractionation of human plasma proteins. The albumin infusion is accompanied by an appropriate cocktail of diuretics, and is an important safeguard against the calamity of acute renal failure.

In nephrotic patients with slowly deteriorating renal function a dilemma arises. Should he be given a high protein diet to supplement losses or a low protein diet to mitigate the uraemia? Usually a compromise is reached by moderating the degree of protein restriction. Often the patient solves his own problem when his abnormally permeable glomeruli are obliterated by advancing disease and the urinary loss of protein falls.

A daily intake of 90–120g protein, 80–120 mmol sodium and 10 MJ (2400 kcal) is suitable for most patients with the nephrotic syndrome of mild to moderate severity. Diet No. 7 illustrates how this can be achieved.

Acute renal failure

Acute renal failure is a catastrophic event. When it occurs in a patient whose kidneys were previously healthy, the kidneys can recover functionally provided that the patient can be kept alive during the period when their excretory function is lost and homeostasis is impaired and that the patient does not die from the causative injury or disease. Keeping a patient alive for the two or three weeks needed for recovery is one of the most satisfactory achievements of modern medicine. Unfortunately, acute renal failure has a depressingly high mortality as it is often a complication of an illness which itself presents a grave threat to life.

Acute renal failure was not described in early textbooks of medicine. It was first recognised in 1940 in the London Blitz when it was a common complication of crush injuries and shock caused by falling masonry. Causes found today are:

1. *Loss of blood* from any cause including complications of pregnancy, trauma or gastrointestinal bleeding.
2. *Loss of plasma* as in burns and crush injuries.
3. *Loss of fluid*—(a) *from the gut* in severe vomiting, diarrhoea, acute intestinal obstruction, paralytic ileus and fistulous drainage, (b) *in the urine* in diabetic coma, (c) *from the skin* in excessive sweating (heat stroke).
4. *General anaesthetics and surgical operations* which reduce renal blood flow and may precipitate renal failure in those whose blood volume is precariously balanced.
5. *Serious infections,* especially septicaemia from *Escherichia coli,* may produce shock, and reduce renal blood flow.
6. *Acute haemolytic disorders.*
7. *Nephrotoxins* which may be drugs, industrial chemicals or natural substances. Examples of these are paracetamol, paraquat and mushrooms.

A common factor in many of these conditions is a prolonged episode of hypotension with systolic blood pressure less than 90 mmHg for one hour or more.

The susceptibility of the kidney to ischaemic damage may be related to the high renal blood flow which amounts to one-fifth of the resting cardiac output, and to the critical balance between arterial, venous and capillary pressures which determines the glomerular filtration rate. Blood loss is not the only cause of peripheral circulatory failure. Severe infection and septicaemia can result in shock in various ways. A fall in plasma volume can arise from excessive loss of plasma proteins in inflammatory exudates and from a generalised increase in capillary permeability.

The plasma proteins are consumed at an increased rate in catabolic states, following infection and trauma, especially when the supply of exogenous fuel to provide energy is inadequate for the increased needs.

The serious nature of the underlying condition may explain why the overall mortality in acute renal failure is around 50 per cent, varying from less than 10 per cent in obstetrical cases to over 80 per cent in patients with multiple injuries or abdominal sepsis. Despite these gloomy statistics, there is every reason to expect that the kidneys will recover with little or no residual damage in the great majority of patients, if only the patient can survive and recover from his underlying illness. Rarely infarction of the kidney causes necrosis of the renal cortex and then there is no chance that normal renal function will ever return.

The disturbance in renal function passes through a phase of total renal failure with oliguria, followed by a phase of recovery characterised by diuresis. The oliguric phase immediately follows the precipitating event and can last for a few days or for several weeks. The patient is often very ill with the metabolic distrubances of uraemia superimposed on his underlying condition. Some of the consequences of acute renal failure can be inferred from Table 44.1. The urine volume is low. The excretion of water, sodium, potassium and nitrogenous waste products are all diminished. The patient is at risk from overloading with fluid and electolytes by both oral and intravenous routes. He cannot respond to an increased intake which may be given in the mistaken belief that his kidneys need encouraging. Hyperkalaemia is common and threatens life. Its prominence in acute renal failure may result from the increased breakdown of damaged tissues and extravasated blood with release of intracellular potassium. Acidosis and tissue hypoxia which accompany peripheral circulatory failure may also have a part to play. The blood urea can rise alarmingly, at a daily rate approaching 15 mmol/1. This results both from the breakdown of damaged tissues and also from an exaggeration of the catabolic response to trauma.

The diuretic phase is welcomed like rain after a long drought. After passing little or no urine for two weeks or longer the day arrives that the patient's attendants have been waiting for and a moderate amount of urine is passed. In succeeding days the urine volume reaches supernormal quantities. The patient has now entered the diuretic phase of the illness, which indicates that the tubular epithelium is starting tó regenerate. But the quality of the urine is at first subnormal. It contains too little urea and too much sodium and potassium. When diuresis is established, the urine volume increases progressively to between 3 and 5 litres per day and the excretion of sodium, potassium, urea and other solutes increases in parallel. The blood urea falls to normal over seven to ten days, reflecting the restoration of effective glomerular filtration.

Although the excretory function of the kidney is restored, the regulatory function of the tubules recovers more slowly. The internal environment of the patient is still at risk, but from excessive losses of water, sodium, potassium, bicarbonate and magnesium, rather than from the retention of these substances, as in the oliguric phase. Residual defects of tubular function can sometimes be detected long after the blood urea has returned to normal.

Treatment

During the phase of oliguria or anuria, protein metabolism should be reduced to a minimum, by giving only 20 g/day of protein and appropriate treatment to reduce endogenous protein metabolism to the lowest possible level. A daily intake of 100 g of sugar has a marked protein-sparing effect. If more sugar can be given, e.g. up to 300 g, this helps to reduce the inevitable loss in weight which occurs during the anuric phase. Such large quantities of sucrose and glucose are unpleasantly sweet, but glucose polymers such as Caloreen or Hycal are better tolerated. They are given in about 500 ml of water which is administered daily by mouth. If the patient is vomiting, dextrose in water has to be given intravenously. This amount of water roughly meets the daily obligatory loss of water through the skin and lungs. During the diuretic phase electrolytes are given only to replace losses. The diet should contain potassium chloride by mouth. Usually 2 to 3 g/day are required. With further improvement in renal function a gradual return to a normal diet is made.

The above old orthodox treatment is in some places the only one available. Where there are the facilities, it has been replaced by haemodialysis for the more serious cases, but not all patients with acute renal failure need dialysis. When the precipitating event is short-lived and the disturbance rapidly corrected with incomplete loss of renal function lasting only a few days the above regimen suffices. It is also often advisable in elderly patients who tolerate dialysis poorly. Patients with oliguria lasting from one to three weeks were often treated successfully in the ten to fifteen years before dialysis became readily available and many owed their lives to the above regimen and others derived the same principles.

Haemodialysis. The introduction of haemodialysis has changed the dietetic management of patients in acute renal failure. The dictum 'feed and dialyse' has replaced attempts to reduce protein turnover by restricting dietary protein. There are many reasons for wishing to support protein stores. The most common cause of death in acute renal failure is infection, and protein deficiency is well-known to lower the resistance of the body to invading micro-organisms. Many patients have surgical wounds to heal and damaged tissues to repair. The hypercatabolic patient whose blood urea rises by daily increments of 10–15 mmol/l consumes body protein at rates approaching 100 g/day. There may be additional protein losses into pleural and peritoneal exudates, or from open wounds. Peritoneal dialysis can impose another drain on protein reserves. The failure of earlier approaches to treatment was acknowledged in the traditional expectation that ill patients with acute renal failure would lose lean body weight at rates of 0.5 to 1 kg daily and in the comment that this weight loss should be taken into account when assessing fluid requirements.

The main purposes of dietetic treatment are to maintain stores of protein and to provide an optimal environment for wound healing and the defence against infection. Sufficient energy should be provided to minimise catabolism of body protein and to allow dietary amino acids to be used for protein synthesis. Sufficient protein must be given to balance metabolic and exudative losses. Between 9 and 12 MJ (2000 and 3000 kcal) and 50–100 g protein are usually required. The problems in providing such a regimen vary with the stage of the illness.

During the oliguric phase, the patient is acutely ill and has little appetite for food. Feeding by mouth may not be possible following abdominal surgery, if the bowel has been damaged or if there is peritonitis. Initially intravenous feeding may be the only way to provide nutrients in sufficient quantity. Solutions of amino acids, glucose and other carbohydrates are available in varying concentrations, as well as fat emulsions suitable for intravenous administration. A typical regimen supplying 10 MJ (2400 kcal) and 100 g amino acids is shown in Table 44.2. The potential hazards can be seen immediately in the 2000 ml of water and the 160 mmol of sodium which it provides. The solution to this problem is daily haemodialysis, often necessary in any case to remove nitrogenous waste. For patients maintained by parenteral nutrition for periods longer than a week, attention should be given to the possible need for phosphate, magnesium, zinc and ultimately trace elements. Vitamin supplements are also needed.

As uraemia and infection come under control, feeding by mouth can be resumed. Initially provisions from the hospital kitchen may need to be supplemented at the bedside with imagination and flexibility. A wide variety of different preparations, both new and old, can be tried. Milk forms a useful basis. One or two eggs whipped into half a pint of milk with brandy to taste is surprisingly well accepted. Milk products such as Complan and Carnation Breakfast Food can be made up with a wide range of flavours. Ice-cream is usually well tolerated. Amino acid preparations, e.g. Aminutrin and Nefranutrin (Geistlich) are now available and especially useful for patients intolerant of milk and eggs. The supply of non-protein energy can be increased by adding cream to desserts and breakfast cereals and by the use of starch hydrolysates such as Hycal and Caloreen. Unfortunately, these often give rise to diarrhoea.

In patients with prolonged oliguria the dietetic regimen and dialysis treatment more closely resemble the approach to patients with stable chronic renal failure (see below). The frequency of haemodialysis can often be reduced to three times weekly and normal food can be taken. A normal to high protein intake is encouraged and the diet is limited only with respect to sodium, fluids and foods rich in potassium.

The diuretic phase indicates a return of renal function. Nonetheless, dietetic treatment is still important although the problems are reversed. The patient is at risk from excessive loss of water, sodium, potassium, chloride, bicarbonate, phosphate and magnesium. Normal food and a free fluid intake may need to be supplemented by salts given in tablet or capsule form. As before, the fluid and electrolyte status should be monitored by daily weighing, clinical examination and measurements of plasma electrolytes. Analysis of the urine for sodium and potassium provides a useful guide to replacement therapy.

Chronic renal failure (uraemia)

Chronic renal failure is the final common pathway in many different diseases (Table 44.3). The two commonest causes are glomerulonephritis and pyelonephritis (infection of the urinary tract). Polycystic disease is a congenital disorder, the effects of which are often not manifest until adult life. Analgesic nephropathy follows prolonged use of phenacetin and possibly aspirin and other drugs. **Uraemia** is a term used to describe general renal failure from any cause. As renal function becomes impaired many complex biochemical changes occur some of which are probably more responsible for the clinical features than the elevation of blood urea. These changes include disturbances in hydrogen ion concentration and abnormalities in water

Table 44.2 Parenteral nutrition in acute renal failure

Solution	Volume (ml)	Energy MJ	Energy kcal	Amino acids (g)	Sodium (mmol)
Dextrose 50%	500	4.2	1000	—	—
Aminosol 10%	500	0.8	200	50	80
Intralipid 20%	500	4.2	1000	—	—
Aminosol 10%	500	0.8	200	50	80
Total/24 h	2000	10	2400	100	160

Table 44.3 Causes of chronic renal failure

	Relative* incidence
Pyelonephritis	30
Glomerulonephritis	28
Hypertension	10
Polycystic kidneys	7
Obstruction of the urinary tract	5
Analgesic nephropathy	5
Diabetic nephropathy	3
Miscellaneous disorders	12

* Based on a survey of 500 cases in Scotland (Pendreigh et al., 1972)

and electrolyte balance. In addition, renal failure is accompanied in the majority of cases by arterial hypertension, and this complicates still further the clinical picture.

The kidneys have a large functional reserve, and the body can tolerate a considerable accumulation of waste metabolites. In consequence few patients develop symptoms of renal failure until the glomerular filtration rate has fallen below 10 ml/min and some 90 per cent of the capacity for eliminating urea and creatinine has been lost. Depending on the activity of the original disease process, renal function may be lost slowly or rapidly and the end stage of renal failure may develop over many years or only a few months.

CLINICAL FEATURES

Clinical features depend on the stage of the disease. At first patients may have symptoms and signs of their original disorder. Patients with glomerulonephritis may be hypertensive or nephrotic. In others with analgesic nephropathy the blood pressure may be low from excessive salt loss. An early sign in many patients is loss of renal reserve. As the patient loses the capacity to concentrate urine, the urine volume rises and the requirement for water increases. The normal diurnal variation in urine volume disappears and the patient has to rise at night to pass urine. He has increased thirst and spontaneously increases his fluid intake to compensate for the loss in renal flexibility.

The failing kidney is equally unable to compensate for large fluctuations in salt intake and for other increased metabolic demands. The patient with mild renal failure tolerates poorly intercurrent medical and surgical illnesses which increase urea production and interfere with the normal intake of water and sodium or which cause increased losses of water and sodium from the gastrointestinal tract. Uncompensated losses of water and sodium result in dehydration and salt depletion, with a fall in plasma volume, arterial blood pressure, renal blood flow and glomerular filtration rate. Renal function is lost in proportion and mild renal failure progresses to severe uraemia. It is not uncommon for mild chronic renal failure to present for the first time as acute renal failure following a chest infection or an acute abdominal surgical emergency.

When more than 90 per cent of functioning renal tissue has been destroyed, uraemic symptoms become more prominent (Table 44.1). Tiredness and breathlessness on exertion may arise from anaemia. A tendency to bleed due to abnormal platelet function is common. Anorexia, nausea and vomiting may result from the accumulation of urea, creatinine or an unknown uraemic 'toxin'. When GFR falls below 5 ml/min the kidneys may be unable to excrete even normal quantities of sodium and water. Many patients at this stage develop hypertension, oedema and features of water intoxication. The excretion of hydrogen ions is impaired, the plasma bicarbonate concentration falls and an observer may notice compensatory hyperventilation of which the patient is often unaware (Kussmaul's respiration). Potassium homeostasis is usually maintained until the urine volume falls below 1000 ml/24 h, after which hyperkalaemia can be rapidly fatal. Plasma phosphate rises and plasma calcium falls; the parathyroid glands hypertrophy to compensate for these biochemical changes and the plasma concentration of parathyroid hormone is increased. Metabolic bone disease may lead to bone pain and pathological fractures in patients with renal failure of several years duration.

Hyperlipidaemia is a characteristic feature of chronic renal disease and occurs early in the nephrotic syndrome. The main abnormality is increased plasma concentrations of triglycerides and VLD lipoproteins. This reflects a general metabolic disorder, but the mechanisms responsible for the change in blood lipids are not known (Cramp et al., 1975; Ibels et al., 1975). The abnormality persists on dialysis and after a renal transplant, and is associated with an increased risk of cardiovascular disease.

In the final stages death can result from hypertensive encephalopathy, uraemic coma, pulmonary oedema, gastrointestinal haemorrhage, pericardial effusion, hyperkalaemia or severe infection. Many of these events can be predicted from Table 44.1 and almost all can be prevented by rational therapy based on an understanding of the excretory and homeostatic tasks of the kidney.

TREATMENT

Treatment of chronic renal failure varies according to the stage of the illness. In mild cases, active steps should be taken to control hypertension, to correct salt and water imbalance and to treat active urinary tract infection. During the course of an illness in which oral feeding cannot be maintained, fluids and electrolytes should be given intravenously. Protein restriction may not be necessary in the absence of symptoms. Indeed, a high protein diet may be indicated in nephrotic patients with excessive losses of protein in the urine. Sodium restriction may be necessary in some patients, but others may need extra sodium chloride to compensate for urinary losses of salt. Sodium bicarbonate may be needed for treatment of acidosis. The development of more active analogues of the vitamin D metabolites, such as 1α-hydroxycholecalciferol, indicate that the treatment and prevention of the metabolic bone disease should become more effective (Catto et al., 1975; Tougaard et al., 1976). There is a real risk, however, that an increase in plasma calcium may damage the kidney and accelerate loss of renal function.

As renal failure progresses and the patient develops symptoms of uraemia, more active measures become necessary to compensate for the loss of renal function. Patients may be treated conservatively by dietetic measures alone, by regular haemodialysis or peritoneal dialysis or by renal transplantation.

Conservative treatment
One hundred years ago the patient with renal failure was cupped and bled, and the activity of the bowels and skin promoted by saline purges, hot baths and Dover's powder, which increased the elimination of 'excrementititous substances' by alternative routes. He was advised to travel south in winter and to take the mineral waters at Vichy and other spas in order to flush out the urinary passages. He was instructed always to wear flannel next to the skin and to abstain totally from the use of alcohol. Few of these measures survive today, apart from venesection which is still practised, but for investigative purposes rather than for therapy. By contrast, some aspects of the dietetics practised in Victorian times may still be valid in the treatment of uraemia, although perhaps for different reasons.

Failing kidneys, like tuberculous lungs, were thought to need rest. Thus treatment was directed towards relieving the kidneys as much as possible from 'the labour of elimination'. The volume of the urine and the urea excretion rate were measured and taken as guides to fluid replacemeent and to the quantity of protein given by mouth. Dietary protein was limited and the patient advised to take meat only once daily. Acute illnesses were treated with milk fortified by arrowroot, but the quantity limited to 1–2 pints daily since greater volumes of fluid and the dissolved mineral elements were felt to make dropsical conditions more difficult to treat. The convalescent patient was weaned from beef-tea and mutton broth to fish and fowl and not allowed red meats such as mutton and beef.

Now, as then, in both severe and mild renal failure, regular attention should be given to the state of water and sodium balance, to the correction of acidosis and to control of blood pressure. The principal additional measure as renal failure progresses is to reduce dietary protein, in the first instance to 0.5 g/kg bodyweight, which corresponds to 30–40 g/day in most adults. There is then a parallel fall in urea production and in the blood urea. Gastrointestinal symptoms such as anorexia and vomiting are often relieved. This may result from a reduction in the diffusion of urea from the plasma into the intestinal lumen where it is hydrolysed by bacterial urease to ammonium carbonate. The ammonium ion is a well-known gastrointestinal irritant and could thus mediate the potentially toxic effects of increased blood urea. The ammonia released in the gut is reabsorbed and taken to the liver in the portal circulation where it is either recycled to urea or used for synthesis of non-essential amino acids. This provides an important metabolic pathway which is exploited in patients on very low protein diets and other experimental regimens in the treatment of severe chronic renal failure.

Diet No. 6 (p. 554) provides 40 g of protein and 40 mmol sodium. Protein restriction of this order usually has little effect on the supply of energy or on the provision of essential nutrients. For patients expending more than 8.4 MJ (2000 kcal)/day additional energy can be provided by increasing the consumption of fat and sugar, or by the use of polymeric glucose preparations derived from hydrolysis of starch such as Caloreen and Hycal.

It is customary to restrict protein when the blood urea rises above 30 mmol/1 and the plasma creatinine above 500 mmol/1. Nevertheless, it is debatable whether any benefit is derived from such dietary measures before symptoms develop. The adverse effects of unnecessary protein restriction are illustrated by the experience of Sir Stanley Davidson. He had a kidney removed for hydronephrosis at the age of 12. Despite this handicap he managed to enlist in the infantry in August 1914 and spent the autumn, winter and spring in the trenches in northern France under the dreadful conditions of wet and cold that existed during that period of World War I. In the summer of 1915 he was very severely wounded and developed extensive gas gangrene. His life was endangered from sepsis and cachexia for nearly a year. That his remaining kidney was markedly affected was manifested by the constant passage of albumin, leucocytes and casts in the urine. The diet prescribed and eaten for more than a year after discharge from hospital was low in protein and high in carbohydrate, and alcohol was prohibited. As the albuminuria continued and health was not fully restored, and because the restriction of food and drink proved extremely irksome, he decided to stop all dietary restriction and eat and drink whatever he liked. More than 60 years have elapsed since that decision and the function of the one remaining kidney is satisfactory, as judged by the sense of well-being, a normal blood pressure and pyelogram and the absence of abnormal constitutents in the urine and the blood.

Very low protein diets. On a diet totally devoid of protein but supplying adequate quantities of other essential nutrients and energy, the body continues to produce urea and other nitrogenous metabolites from the breakdown of endogenous protein. In theory, nitrogen balance should be maintained and loss of lean body mass prevented if just sufficient protein is given by mouth to balance these basal endogenous losses, which correspond to approximately 0.25 g of protein/kg body weight, or 15–20 g protein daily in the average adult.

Giovanetti and Maggiore (1964) demonstrated that uraemic patients could be sustained on a basal protein-free diet when this was supplemented with a mixture of essential amino acids or a single protein of high biological value, e.g. egg protein. Another Italian, Giordano, argued that with such a regimen the patient could be induced to utilise his own waste urea nitrogen for synthesis of non-essential amino acids through the enterohepatic cycle of urea. Berlyne and his colleagues (1967) adapted these Italian regimens to British tastes, and showed that patients who would otherwise have required dialysis could be kept well, symptom-free, and even rehabilitated at work for several months. The modified Giovanetti/Giordano diet is illustrated in Diet No. 5. Supplements of methionine, the first limiting amino acid in the diet, and of vitamins are needed and a major problem is the supply of sufficient energy. In practice many patients feel hungry and find it difficult to tolerate large quantities of cream, butter or margarine, cooking oil and sugar. Polymeric glucose preparations, such as Hycal and Caloreen, can be used but, as unabsorbed polysaccharide may cause an osmotic diarrhoea, they are often poorly tolerated.

These dietetic measures can sustain patients in whom the GFR has fallen to 2–4 ml/min long after dialysis would have been necessary if protein intake had not been reduced. Not surprisingly, in patients with less than 5 per cent of their original functioning kidney tissue, other steps have to be taken in addition to protein restriction to preserve fluid and ionic balance. In many ways doctor and dietitian can be regarded as a pair of artificial organs themselves functioning on behalf of the patient to maintain 'renal' homeostasis.

Thus fluid balance needs even more careful attention than before and the patient should be advised to limit fluid intake when the urine volume falls below 1000 ml/day. Varying degrees of sodium restriction become necessary to control hypertension and to prevent peripheral and pulmonary oedema. Hyperkalaemia, often a problem as urine volume falls, can be treated by the oral or rectal administration of cation exchange resins such as Resonium A (Winthrop) (in the sodium and hydrogen phase) or Calcium Resonium (Winthrop) (in the calcium phase). Potassium ions are exchanged for sodium and hydrogen ions with Resonium A, and for calcium ions with Calcium Resonium. In some patients this replaces one problem with another. Acidosis can be corrected by giving sodium bicarbonate by mouth, but dietary sodium may need restricting even further. The rise in plasma phosphate can be limited by using the gastrointestinal tract as a substitute for the artificial kidney. Aluminium hydroxide given by mouth in the form of tablets, capsules, or an antacid gel

(Aludrox) removes phosphate in direct combination as aluminium phosphate. In some patients it may cause flatulence and a sensation of epigastric fullness, as well as producing constipation. Unfortunately, these measures cannot prevent death in terminal uraemia from gastrointestinal haemorrhage, pericarditis and pericardial tamponade or uraemic coma. Despite the best dietetic attention, it is difficult to avoid depletion of protein and other essential nutrients. Patients' resistance to infection is often lowered and wounds heal poorly following surgery and there are a variety of biochemical abnormalities. Previously these features were attributed to the effects of uraemia, but many are found in protein depletion from other causes and it is difficult to exclude the possibility that the dietetic treatment may have a contributory role. This may help to explain why a patient taken on for treatment by dialysis and transplantation after a period of severe protein restriction often has a long uphill struggle to climb out of the grave that almost buried him.

Experimental 'no-protein' diets. Amino acids can be synthesised in the body by transamination of 2-oxo-acid precursors which supply the analogous carbon skeleton of the amino acid.

$$CH_3 \diagdown$$
$$\qquad CHCOCOOH$$
$$CH_3 \diagup$$

2-Oxoisovaleric acid

$$CH_3 \diagdown \quad \downarrow$$
$$\qquad CHCHNH_2COOH$$
$$CH_3 \diagup$$

Valine

The body can synthesise the oxo-acid precursors of the non-essential amino acids but not those of the essential amino acids. In theory, a patient given the oxo-acid analogues of all the essential amino acids in correct proportion should be able to utilise his own waste amino groups to synthesise both essential and non-essential amino acids, and thus could replace endogenous protein losses entirely from waste amino nitrogen. In this way a patient with total renal failure and no loss of urea in the urine could be made self-sustaining with respect to nitrogen and independent of exogenous protein.

There are many practical difficulties facing the patient who attempts to feed on his own flesh and blood in this way. The problems of very low protein diets would be intensified. Moreover, the cost of the synthetic oxo-acid precursors is high. Nonetheless the idea is attractive, and may find a place in future regimens for patients with advanced uraemia.

Dialysis treatment
In the early 1960s when dialysis facilities were scarce and

almost experimental, patients were taken on for treatment only when life was threatened and conservative measures had been unsuccessful. Today it is generally accepted that dialysis treatment is best started when the patient can no longer be maintained on moderate protein restriction, and long before the effects of protein depletion become apparent.

Both peritoneal dialysis and haemodialysis rapidly relieve the patient not only from uraemic symptoms such as tiredness and anorexia but also from many dietary restrictions. The residual limitations depend to some degree on the treatment used and to some extent on the patient.

Treatment with the disposable device shown in Fig. 44.2 for four to eight hours three times weekly removes all the urea generated by a normal dietary intake of protein, and all the creatinine and uric acid produced from the metabolic turnover of a normal lean body mass. Oedema in all patients and hypertension in almost all patients can be corrected by the removal of fluid by ultrafiltration at the time of dialysis. In most patients, however, the urine volume falls below 500 ml daily within the first week of regular treatment, and thereafter the excretion of sodium and potassium in the urine makes little or no contribution towards homeostasis. If dietary intake of sodium and water is not limited in the 2–3 day intervals between treatments, oedema fluid accumulates and the blood pressure rises.

The two criteria of successful management are the control of hypertension and the social rehabilitation of the patient. Unfortunately few patients can walk out of the dialysis unit and return to work unaided after losing more than 2 litres of fluid over a single treatment period. For the majority of patients this means drinking no more than 500 to 1000 ml of fluid and restricting sodium intake to 50 mmol daily. Patients become thirsty if more salt is taken and find it difficult to comply with fluid restrictions.

If blood pressure is normal and oedema absent, the amount of fluid removed in dialysis is determined from the change in body weight between treatments. An increase in weight of 1 kg indicates the consumption of 1 litre of water over requirements. The patient rapidly learns both to adjust the ultrafiltration pressures across the dialyser to remove this fluid and also to regulate his fluid intake to maintain his 'dry' weight stable over weeks and months of regular treatment.

Patients also lose lean body mass and adipose tissue when appetite is impaired during an intercurrent illness and regain their weight during their recovery. These longer term changes have to be distinguished carefully by patient, dietitian and doctor from short-term changes due to indiscretion of salt and water. Patients adapt to severe fluid restriction in various ways. One Scot was happy with his regimen as long as he could take his fluid allowance entirely in the form of neat whisky.

In the past, potassium intake was controlled rigorously and ion exchange resins given to prevent plasma potassium rising to dangerous levels before dialysis. Today the patient should still be cautioned severely against the consumption of large quantities of foods very rich in potassium, e.g. bananas, fresh oranges and dried fruits. However, even these foods may be allowed in small amounts at long intervals and there is no reason to limit dietary intake of potassium below 80–100 mmol/day, which is the average for the general population. This more liberal policy has resulted from a reduction in the potassium concentration of the dialysis fluid, from the use of better dialysers and from more frequent dialysis which gives better control of acidosis. Most of the potassium in the body is located in the cells, and the balance between intracellular and extracellular fluid concentrations of potassium is governed by the prevailing state of acidosis or alkalosis. Between dialysis treatments hydrogen ions accumulate causing a slight shift of potassium from the cells and a substantial rise in plasma potassium. The degree of hyperkalaemia is quite out of proportion to the 10–15 per cent increase in total body potassium represented by the 200–300 mmol ingested over the 3–4 day period between dialysis treatments.

Aluminium hydroxide is required by most patients to maintain plasma phosphate concentrations below 2.0 mmol/l. Above this level calcium and phosphate salts precipitate in extraskeletal tissues, ultimately causing irritation of the conjunctiva and red eyes, vascular calcification, unsightly periarticular swellings and pseudogout. On the other hand, too much aluminium hydroxide and too little dietary phosphorus, which can result from excessive limitation of protein intake, can result in phosphate depletion and skeletal demineralisation resembling osteomalacia. Hyperparathyroidism, which previously was resistent to all medical treatment, can now be controlled in most patients by the administration of minute daily doses of 1–2 μg of 1α-hydroxycholecalciferol. This analogue of vitamin D is ready to be hydroxylated in the liver to form the active metabolite 1,25-dihydroxycholecalciferol.

Iron requirements are increased by blood losses in the dialyser, from cannulation sites and from medical curiosity. It is usually sufficient to give a daily iron supplement by mouth. In most patients haemoglobin concentration is low, between 6 and 10 g/dl, due to deficiency in erythropoetin, but would be lower without iron.

Peritoneal dialysis is less efficient than haemodialysis and may be totally unsuitable for large muscular men. Even in smaller members of the 'weaker' sex, treatments are longer than in haemodialysis and are repeated more frequently. Schedules varying from 10 hours on three nights a week to 15 hours on five nights may be needed to cope with the metabolic load of a normal protein intake. Since amino acids and up to 15 g protein are lost over each 10 h dialysis session, a high protein intake is needed to maintain plasma protein concentrations and lean body mass. Most patients are encouraged to take at least 100 g of protein daily, using eggs, milk and meat to supplement their normal diet. Hypertension is readily controlled by removal of sodium and water on dialysis, and since treatments are repeated frequently most patients can enjoy a free fluid intake with salt in cooking but not at table. In some patients' blood pressure is difficult to control. Fluid intake should then be limited to 500 ml/day and sodium intake to 50 mmol/day. In addition the sodium concentration in the dialysis fluid can be reduced from 140 to 130 mmol/1.

Some limitation in the consumption of foods high in potassium may be needed but, as for patients on haemodialysis, a normal daily intake of potassium can be allowed. Patients require aluminium hydroxide for control of phosphate, and water-soluble vitamins to replace losses on dialysis (see below). Since there are no losses of blood on dialysis, the requirements for iron are less and supplements not essential.

Unwanted losses and gains from dialysis fluids. The natural peritoneal and artificial cellophane membranes used for dialysis are permeable not only to unwanted ions and waste metabolites but also to water-soluble nutrients which could be lost from the plasma. Excessive quantities of mineral salts present in haemodialysis fluid prepared from domestic water may diffuse in the opposite direction. Patients on haemodialysis are exposed each week to 900 litres of dialysis fluid by contrast with more modest requirements of patients on peritoneal dialysis (100 litres) and normal individuals who rarely ingest more than 15 litres weekly.

Loss of glucose is readily prevented by including it in the dialysis fluid. Amino acids and small peptides are lost by diffusion but the combined loss rarely exceeds 30 g weekly on either peritoneal or haemodialysis, and is readily replaced if the patient has a normal protein intake. Patients on peritoneal dialysis lose on average 60 g of plasma proteins each week and require a high protein diet. Even then their albumin is usually slightly reduced.

Vitamins. Plasma concentrations of ascorbic acids, folate and pyridoxine are reduced by dialysis. Losses of 80 to 280 mg of ascorbic acid have been reported in a single haemodialysis treatment. As plasma concentrations fall, so does removal by diffusion across the dialyser membrane. Nevertheless, to maintain normal plasma concentrations daily oral supplements of 100 mg of ascorbic acid, 1 mg of folic acid and 5 mg of pyridoxine are recommended.

Thiamin, riboflavin, pantothenic acid, nicotinic acid and biotin are also lost on dialysis, but in quantities no greater than urinary losses in patients with normal renal function, and plasma concentrations are normal. Supplements are usually given routinely in the form of a multi-vitamin pill.

Although vitamin B_{12} is a large molecule and bound to plasma proteins, significant losses may occur. Plasma concentrations are usually normal, but there may be a slight downward trend in patients maintained on dialysis for several years. As in malabsorption syndromes, plasma concentration may be kept within the normal range at the expense of hepatic stores; the need for supplements may become apparent in the future when more patients have been on dialysis for many years.

Plasma concentrations of vitamins A and D are normal in patients on haemodialysis. Losses across the cellophane membrane would be unlikely in view of their low solubility in water and their binding to plasma proteins. Losses on peritoneal dialysis might be greater in view of the losses of plasma proteins, but there is no evidence to confirm this.

Minerals. Under normal circumstances the dialysis patient neither gains nor loses excessive amounts of copper, molybdenum, lead, cobalt, nickel, zirconium, manganese or bromine. An increased tissue content of fluorine, tin, strontium and cadmium and a loss of rubidium have been reported, but the clinical significance of these changes is not known. In the early days of dialysis copper tubing was used and adverse effects occurred from copper leached into the dialysis fluid. Reports of zinc toxicity and accumulation have been followed by the conflicting suggestion that zinc deficiency may be more prevalent and indeed may be responsible for symptoms of sexual inadequacy. The risks of lead intoxication are greatly reduced by replacing lead in piping by plastic or stainless steel.

A far greater problem is the accumulation of aluminium, now recognised as a major cause of disability and death in patients on haemodialysis. All dialysis patients are given aluminium hydroxide by mouth to bind phosphate in the gastrointestinal tract for treatment of hyperphosphataemia. A far more important source of unwanted aluminium is the water used for making dialysis fluid. Alum is used extensively for the treatment of drinking water, but not all water authorities take steps to ensure the removal of surplus aluminium. Transfer from dialysis fluid to the patient is enhanced by the very low concentrations in plasma water which result from the protein binding of the metal and its rapid dispersal to the tissues, particularly to brain, bone and muscle. The clinical effects are consistent with this distribution. Patients initially develop disturbances of speech and progress to severe dementia and death within months. Skeletal demineralisation, in the form of intractable osteomalacia resistant to treatment even with 1α-hydroxycholecalciferol, may complicate the picture. There is a wide variation in the incidence of these disorders between different centres, which correlates with aluminium concentrations in the water supply. Dialysis dementia disappears when dialysis fluid made from highly purified water is used. In one hospital with a very high incidence of dialysis dementia, the aluminium content of the water delivered to the dialysis unit was 1 part per million, compared with a concentration of less than 0.06

p.p.m. in ordinary tap water. The source of the aluminium was traced to two anodes of aluminium weighing 32.4 kg in the water heating system, which completely disappeared over a two-year period. Most of the aluminium was precipitated at the bottom of the hot-water tank as aluminium hydroxide, but enough was dissolved in the water passing through to intoxicate fatally six patients. No other patients were affected after the unit was transferred to another hospital where the aluminium content of the water was low, despite the continued administration of aluminium hydroxide by mouth (Flendrig et al., 1976).

Transplantation

There are many advantages in having a built-in kidney that works on its own. This is obvious at social gatherings of patients with chronic renal failure. Those with transplanted kidneys look pink, drink beer and have to use the lavatory. By contrast, dialysis patients are pale, drink spirits only and usually have to wait until their next dialysis to achieve salt and water homeostasis.

Unfortunately the body has a built-in reaction to a kidney that once belonged to someone else. Even after great care has been taken to get a compatible donor and with powerful drugs which can suppress the immune response, there is only a 50 per cent chance that a transplanted kidney will be functioning two years after the operation. These depressing statistics are tolerable only because the chances of a kidney, which has survived two years, working for another ten years thereafter are high, and because with careful attention to diet and drugs the mortality and morbidity from the operation is now very low. Many patients come back for a second operation which carries no worse a prognosis than the first.

The most important role for the dietitian is to support the general nutrition of the patient before, during and after the transplant operation in order to counterbalance the side-effects of the drugs, azathioprine and prednisolone, given to prevent rejection. Immunosuppressive drugs as a group impair the resistance of the body to infection. Most of the problems in the transplanted patient arise from the use of prednisolone, which is used in very high dosage during the first few weeks after the operation and also when acute rejection threatens the graft. Corticosteroid drugs even in moderate dosage have pronounced catabolic effects, accelerating protein breakdown and hepatic gluconeogenesis from amino acids. In patients unsupported by an adequate dietary protein, muscle wasting and depletion of tissue proteins results, with delayed healing of wounds and failure to localise infections. While some of these effects on underlying protein metabolism are probably unavoidable, they can be prevented to a large extent by providing sufficient dietary energy and protein to match catabolic losses and maintain tissue protein.

Patients are best prepared for transplantation by regular dialysis for several weeks with restoration of a healthy appetite and a normal way of life. Since the transplanted kidney is placed in the iliac fossa outside the peritoneal cavity, the activity of the gastrointestinal tract is impaired for no more than a few hours after the operation and feeding by mouth should be resumed as soon as possible. Management of the patient thereafter depends on what the kidney does next.

If the kidney functions immediately, the patient can eat normally with free fluids and an unrestricted salt intake. Subsequently the onset of rejection is usually accompanied by a reduction in the urine volume and sodium excretion, then by a deterioration in renal excretory function. The fluid allowance and sodium intake should be reduced to maintain homeostasis. However, it is unwise to restrict protein, since the dosage of prednisolone has to be greatly increased in an attempt to reverse the rejection process; it is better to dialyse the patient if the rejected kidney is unable to meet the metabolic demands of a full diet. Most transplanted kidneys undergo at least one rejection episode of variable severity, but with prompt treatment there is a reasonable chance of full recovery.

If the transplanted kidney does not function immediately, the patient should be fed and dialysed in the manner to which he has been accustomed, until renal function recovers sufficiently to make dialysis unnecessary. Kidneys from cadaver donors have often undergone a period of ischaemic damage between clamping the renal vessels and perfusion with ice-cold preservative. Renal ischaemia following a fall in arterial blood pressure is a common cause of acute tubular necrosis, so it is not surprising that many transplanted kidneys pass little urine in the early days following anastomosis with a different set of blood vessels situated several miles from their original supply. Frequently the onset of recovery is characterised by a diuretic phase, in which supplements of sodium chloride, sodium bicarbonate and potassium may be required.

The functioning transplanted kidney produces erythropoetin and the red cell count and haemoglobin concentration usually rise to normal within 1–3 months. Haematinics such as iron and folic acid should be given to maintain stores and to support the increased activity of the bone marrow. Another metabolic function resumed by the transplanted kidney is the synthesis of 1,25-dihydroxy vitamin D. In most patients bone lesions heal and hyperparathyroidism resolves. In some patients the plasma phosphate concentration falls to abnormally low levels in the first few weeks after kidney function is restored. This may be due to residual hyperparathyroidism or renal tubular damage. Phosphate supplements may be needed if plasma concentrations are very low, so as to ensure normal bone mineralisation. In most patients, however, a full normal diet is sufficient in itself.

After the first month with a new kidney, the most prominent nutritional problem is one of surfeit, resulting from the high doses of prednisolone. As in Cushing's disease, fat stores are increased, partly at the expense of the lean body mass and partly from an increased appetite. Few patients can voluntarily limit their food intake and so do not lose weight until the dosage of prednisolone is reduced even with encouragement from doctor and dietitian. Often control of weight gain is as much as can be expected. The occasional patient is overtly diabetic, requiring insulin in the early stages and subsequently oral hypoglycaemics or carbohydrate restriction alone as the dosage of steroids is reduced.

Treatment of diabetics in chronic renal failure.
Many young diabetics die from chronic renal failure. Recent experience shows that they can benefit from dialysis and transplantation, providing there are no overt signs of ischaemic heart disease. Most of the difficulties in management arise not from the increased complexity of having two metabolic disturbances to treat, but from technical problems relating to vascular access.

In patients on dialysis with little urine and even less glomerular function, the urinary glucose is a poor guide to the state of the diabetes and control depends on measurements of blood glucose. On peritoneal dialysis there is an additional glucose load from the dialysis fluid, but this can be covered with an increased dosage of insulin. Ketoacidosis is rarely a problem, and patients with little or no renal function are largely immune from excessive urinary losses of sodium and water.

After renal transplantation the same principles should be followed as for the surgical diabetic (p. 362). An increased insulin requirement can be expected from the high doses of prednisolone given. Subsequently insulin should be reduced in parallel with the dosage of prednisolone.

RENAL AND VESICAL CALCULI AND NEPHROCALCINOSIS

Urinary stones present problems which have fascinated doctors and chemists for generations and which are still largely unsolved. It has been suggested that dietary factors are responsible, at least in part, for the formation of stones and also that certain dietary restrictions may reduce the likelihood of their formation in susceptible persons.

CHEMISTRY OF CALCULUS FORMATION

Most stones contain calcium, but the nature of the salt varies. Many stones are a mixture of salts, such as calcium phosphate, magnesium ammonium phosphate and calcium carbonate. Such stones form readily in infected urine in which bacteria have converted urea into ammonia, so raising the pH and thereby making the phosphates less soluble. Calcium oxalate is often present in mixed stones and about 25 per cent of stones are pure calcium oxalate. Only about 10 per cent of stones do not contain calcium and nearly all of these are composed of uric acid.

The solubility of a salt in a solvent depends on the product of the concentrations of its cation and anion or more correctly of the ion activities. These are difficult to measure, and are determined in part by the presence of other ions in the solvent. These may allow a salt solution to become supersaturated.

Crystals of calcium oxalate are present in all urines and are probably the result of precipitation from a supersaturated solution of these ions (Robertson *et al.*, 1969). The crystals are small and normally washed out when the urine is voided.

Calcium oxalate crystals grow abnormally fast in the urines of patients with recurrent renal stone formation. This was found to be due to their urine containing reduced amounts of an inhibitor present in all urines (Dent and Sutor, 1971). Citric acid is present in urine in molar concentrations comparable to that of calcium. As it binds calcium ions to form a soluble complex, citrate might allow more free calcium ions to pass into solution. Hodgkinson (1962) has measured citrate excretion in healthy persons and in those with renal calculus. Low rates of excretion were found in 19 per cent of those with calculus, but were always associated with poor renal function. Measures to increase citrate excretion are unlikely to be of use in preventing the recurrence of renal calculi.

Stone formation is rare in the black population of South Africa. They normally have a high intake of salt. Modlin (1967) has produced data to show that stone formation is associated with a low sodium/calcium ratio in the urine.

Clearly the physical chemical factors that determine the initial formation of a crystal and those that subsequently determine its rate of growth each remain a mystery. Perhaps the real question is not 'Why do some people form stones?' but rather 'Why do we not all have stones?'

HISTORICAL AND GEOGRAPHICAL CONSIDERATIONS
Both the history and the geography of kidney and vesical bladder calculi differ markedly; so much so that they may be considered as separate diseases.

Renal calculus
In the medical and surgical wards of hospitals throughout the world patients are to be found suffering from renal colic with stones in the kidney or ureter. Accurate figures for the prevalence of renal calculi in any country are not available. There is a general impression that they are more common in countries with a hot climate than in temperate regions. As far as can be gathered from old textbooks and senior physicians, there is no indication that the incidence has changed either in living memory or in the more remote past.

Vesical calculus
Whereas renal calculus is equally common in men and women, bladder stone usually occurs either in boys, in young men or in old men (in whom it is generally asso-

ciated with prostatic obstruction or other cause of urinary stagnation). Formerly it was common in young boys in Britain, but now it is very rare. A similar decline has taken place in all prosperous countries of Europe and North America.

Excruciating pain often led the sufferers to desperate measures. Relief by operation was sought long before the era of anaesthetics and aseptic surgery. Accredited surgeons fought shy of the risks of the operation. Indeed cutting for the stone was expressly forbidden in the earliest forms of the Hippocratic oath. In consequence many sufferers availed themselves of the services of 'stone-cutters' or lithotomists. These men flourished in Europe between 1500 and 1800. Their craft was often handed down from father to son as a closely guarded secret. Eight generations of the Collot family practised in France, and some by attendance on the King or his family acquired the title 'Royal Lithotomist'. Many lithotomists travelled widely seeking patients or perhaps avoiding the relatives of their less fortunate patients. During the nineteenth century the incidence of stone in the bladder began to decline in Europe. It is now a rare disease (except in elderly men). A fascinating history of bladder stone has been written by Ellis (1969).

In most parts of the tropics stone in the bladder is also uncommon, but there are well-defined 'stone areas' in Southern China, Thailand, Pakistan, Iran and other countries. In such areas the visitor may find a surgeon who has a cupboard full of an assortment of bladder stones of every variety of chemical composition.

One of us had the opportunity to visit such an area in the Ubon province of Thailand (Passmore, 1953). The surgeon-in-charge of the hospital at the capital of the province kindly gave access to his hospital records. During four years he had removed 610 bladder stones. This corresponded to a yearly rate of 1.8 operations per 10 000 inhabitants of the province, but this gives a false impression of the incidence. The disease, in fact, is largely confined to young boys. Between the ages of 4 and 6, the operation rate amongst boys was over 10 per 10 000 boys. The relative immunity of young girls is probably attributable to their anatomy; it is easier for them to pass small stones *per urethram*. The epidemiology of stone in Thailand has now been studied in much more detail by Halstead and Valyasevi (see below).

AETIOLOGY

Climate. A hot climate contributes to the formation of both renal and vesical calculi, for excessive loss of water in sweating diminishes the volume of urine which then becomes more concentrated. Climate can at most be a contributory factor but in the Royal Navy the incidence of stones is about five times higher in sailors serving in tropical stations than in those in Britain, and is higher in engineers and cooks than in other branches.

Dietary factors. The great fall in the incidence of vesical calculus among children and young adults in Britain coincided roughly with improvement in nutrition: the disease affected predominantly the poorer classes. In all the 'stone areas' in Asia the diet is far from ideal and is generally of a poor vegetarian nature. These facts suggest a dietary cause.

Nevertheless there are other facts that are not consistent with this view. In former times prosperous men sometimes suffered from stone. Samuel Pepys was 'cut for the stone' in 1658 when he was 25, and we know from his *Diary* that he lived well. In the 'stone areas' of Thailand the nutritional state of the children is not good, when judged by modern European or American standards. Yet the children compare favourably with those in other parts of Asia, especially in many parts of rural Madras, where deficiency diseases are common, but stone in the bladder is rare.

McCarrison and others produced both renal and vesical calculi in rats by feeding diets low in vitamin A and rich in calcium. These diets had little resemblance to human diets and so his results must be interpreted with caution (Sinclair, 1953).

Unfortunately all these observations leave the problem of the 'stone areas' in the tropics unsolved. However, at least in Thailand there is evidence that the diet may contribute. Halstead and Valyasevi (1967) found marked differences between the diets consumed by 16 farm families resident in a small village in which bladder stone was epidemic, compared to that consumed by 15 families who were predominantly shopkeepers and government workers in Ubol, a town of 27 000 inhabitants in which the incidence of stone was 14-fold lower. The town families consumed ordinary rice predominantly, while the villagers ate glutinous rice. Village diets were monotonous and consisted of rice, vegetables and uncooked 'fermented' fish, with infrequent supplements of fruits and animal protein, while the town families ate rice with cooked fermented fish, a great variety of fruits and other animal protein prepared in a variety of ways. Village children have many more crystals of oxalate in their urine than children in the town. These disappeared when orthophosphate was given. The village diets may contain an excess of oxalate and oxalate precursors and be relatively deficient in phosphate (Valyasevi et al., 1969, 1973).

Infection of the urinary tract. Any chronic infection of the urinary tract is liable to give rise to stones; pus cells, dead bacteria and epithelial cells form a starting point around which a stone may form.

Stagnation of urine. This is a frequent cause of vesical calculi in old men and may be due to prostatic obstruction of the urinary flow or other disease of the urinary passages.

Prolonged confinement to bed. This is a common cause of stone formation. Confinement to bed may lead to rapid decalcification of the bones and increased excretion of calcium in the urine.

Increased urinary excretion of calcium. This undoubtedly predisposes to the formation of calculi. An excretion of above 300 mg/24 hours in men and 250 mg/24 hours in women has been termed 'hypercalciuria'. This is present in about 8 per cent of the healthy population in whom balance studies show low faecal outputs of calcium (Parfitt *et al.*, 1964).

Hypercalciuria also occurs in hyperparathyroidism, after prolonged use of corticosteroids, in renal tubular acidosis, sarcoidosis, malignant disease of bone and in other diseases.

However, in the great majority of cases of renal calculi, no known cause can be found. Of the known causes, hyperparathyroidism is the most common.

Increased absorption of oxalates. The incidence of renal stones has been reported to be increased in patients with Crohn's disease (regional enteritis) and ulcerative colitis (Gelzayd *et al.*, 1968). A possible explanation is increased absorption of oxalates and subsequent oxaluria, which occurs in a variety of gastrointestinal disorders (Andersson and Gillberg, 1977).

Genetic enzymic defects. Cystinuria is due to a failure of the renal tubules to absorb the amino acids, cystine, lysine, arginine and ornithine. Large amounts of these amino acids appear in the urine. Cystine is the least soluble and tends to precipitate out of the urine and form stones.

Primary hyperoxaluria (Archer *et al.*, 1957) is due to an excessive formation of oxalate in the tissues, probably by conversion from glycine. There is no evidence either of excessive absorption of oxalate from the alimentary tract or a failure of absorption by the renal tubules. The increased oxalate precipitates out in the urine and forms stones from early childhood.

Both cystinuria and primary hyperoxaluria are very rare.

Excessive excretion of uric acid. Uric acid and urate stones often arise in patients with gout or hyperuricaemia (Chap. 43). They can also occur when there is no detectable abnormality in uric acid metabolism.

CLINICAL FEATURES

These vary according to the size, shape and position of the stone, and the presence and nature of the underlying condition. Renal calculi may be present for many years and yet give rise to no symptoms. The most common complaint is an intermittent dull pain in the loin or back, increased by movement or a sudden jolt. When a stone is small enough to enter the ureter and large enough to obstruct it, an attack of renal colic develops. The patient is suddenly aware of intense pain in the loin, which soon radiates round the flank to the groin and often into the testis or labia.

TREATMENT AND PREVENTION

The immediate treatment of renal pain and renal colic is rest in bed, the application of warmth to the seat of pain and the giving of analgesic and antispasmodic drugs. Antibiotics may be needed for the prevention and treatment of infections. In many cases the stone passes *per urethram*, while the patient is on this regimen. If the stone is not passed within a few days, an experienced urologist should be called in. He should decide if and when to operate.

The next problem is the prevention of recurrence. Infections, anatomical abnormalities of the urinary tract and underlying causative conditions should be looked for and treated appropriately. Tests for hyperparathyroidism should be carried out. A high level of urinary phosphate and a low level of blood phosphate with or without a high plasma calcium suggest the disease, provided renal function is otherwise normal. Parathyroidectomy is indicated if evidence of hyperparathyroidism is found.

Since the constituents in renal and vesical calculi are all found in (or derived from) articles of food, it is not surprising that physicians have frequently advised dietary restrictions of various kinds depending on the nature of the stone. Their value is now criticised on three grounds. First, the urinary output of oxalates, urates and phosphates, from which stones are usually formed, depends more on endogenous metabolism than on exogenous sources. Secondly, stones seldom consist of a single substance, and the dietary treatment of mixed stones obviously presents practical difficulties. Thirdly, the evidence that dietary restrictions are successful in the prevention of urinary calculi is unsatisfactory. For these reasons some physicians impose no dietary restrictions, but there are circumstances in which they may be advisable.

Idiopathic hypercalciuria. This condition is usually associated with increased alimentary absorption of calcium (Peacock *et al.*, 1968). This may be reduced by limiting the calcium intake by restricting the intake of milk and cheese and by giving 5 g of cellulose phosphate three times daily. This binds calcium in the diet and increases faecal excretion and may thereby reduce urinary calcium. Also, pyrophosphate in urine tends to inhibit crystallisation of calcium salts. Bendrofluazine in a dose of 5 mg/day reduces urinary calcium by about 30 per cent. As calcium salts are more soluble in acid urine, the urine should be kept acid, if necessary by drugs.

Oxalate stones and oxaluria. Usually 80 to 90 per cent of the oxalate in the diet is not absorbed, but passed in the faeces as insoluble calcium salts. Typical British diets contain from 70 to 150 mg of oxalate; over half of this is provided by five cups of tea. Rhubarb and spinach contain large quantities (250 to 800 mg/100 g). Beetroot and parsley contain 100 to 200 mg/100 g and most beans about 25 mg/100 g. Other vegetables and fruits, meats and fish contain less than 5 mg/100 g. Bread and other cereal products have a content of 5 to 20 mg/100 g (Zarembski and Hodgkinson, 1962). Urinary oxalates are mostly endogenous in origin. In patients with hyperoxaluria a third to a half of the oxalate in the urine has been shown to be derived from glycine (Crawhall *et al.*, 1959).

If a patient has passed a stone which is mostly oxalate, and if he continues to pass gravel, or urine with large numbers of oxalate crystals, and if pain and dysuria persist, it is wise to eliminate rhubarb and spinach from the diet and to restrict greatly tea and cocoa drinking. Restriction of other foods containing oxalates is only justified by a process of trial and error. Large (pharmacological) intakes of ascorbic acid are contraindicated (p.134).

Endogenous oxalate is formed from glycine. Glycine may also give rise to serine, a pathway which requires both folic acid and pyridoxine. Patients with oxaluria have been treated with folic acid (5 mg) and pyridoxine (10 mg) in the hope of diverting glycine metabolism towards serine and so away from oxalate. No dietary restrictions are necessary for people who have had an oxalate stone removed and are then free of symptoms, and whose urine contains only a few oxalate crystals. Large quantities of fluids should be drunk.

Uric acid and urate stones. These usually arise as a result of hyperuricaemia and patients are at increased risk of developing gout. They should avoid the foods rich in purines described on p.365.

The maintenance of an alkaline urine by the administration of alkalis is of some value in keeping uric acid in solution. Large quantities of fluid should be drunk to decrease the urinary concentration of uric acid (see below). If these measures are unsuccessful or renal damage has occurred, allopurinol can be used to block the conversion of hypoxathine and xanthine to uric acid. The more soluble xanthines are excreted in the urine and seldom form stones.

Cystine stones and cystinuria. Cystine can be made more soluble by combination with D-penicillamine, an amino acid derived from penicillin which has no antibiotic activity. It acts as a chelating agent and its administration reduces stone formation in cystinuria. Restriction of dietary methionine, alkalisation of the urine and a high fluid intake are probably of value (Stokes *et al.*, 1968).

Phosphates. Phosphatic calculi are formed only in alkaline urine. When there is known to be a tendency for the formation of such stones, the urine should be kept acid with small doses of ammonium chloride. Owing to the wide distribution of phosphorus in foodstuffs, dietary restriction for the treatment of phosphatic calculi is unlikely to be of any value.

The presence of a persistently alkaline urine suggests a focus of infection requiring treatment.

Provision of an adequate fluid intake
This is by far the most important prophylaxis against recurrence of all forms of stone. A daily flow of urine of 3 litres helps to wash out particles of gravel. Urine flow is usually at its lowest during the night. Hence the patient should drink water before going to bed.

If the climate or the patient's occupation leads to much sweating, then the fluid intake should be increased. Europeans who have suffered from renal colic should not be debarred from working in the tropics, but they must see that in all circumstances their fluid intake is sufficient to promote the urinary output recommended. Occasional measurements of urinary output by the patient may be a useful reminder to him of this necessity.

45. Dental Disease

The teeth are a living memorial to the defects of the previous diet. Too often by middle age a few crumbling and unstable tombstones are all that remain to commemorate past errors. This is a misfortune, since there can be no question that good teeth and gums are important for maintaining health. Furthermore the appearance of bad teeth, and the foetor that may come from them, are undesirable for aesthetic reasons.

Two closely associated pathological processes need to be considered: dental caries (decay of the enamel of the teeth) and periodontal disease of the gums (pyorrhoea alveolaris).

HISTORY AND GEOGRAPHICAL DISTRIBUTION
Both caries and periodontal disease occur among people of British ancestry throughout the world and among other people who have adopted their dietary habits. Rickets used to be called 'the English disease', but dental caries has at least as much title to that name. A German visitor to the Court of Elizabeth I left a personal impression of the Queen; he remarked on her hooked nose, narrow hips and bad black teeth; the last he explained as 'a defect the English seem subject to from their too great use of sugar.' George Washington (a man of impeccable British ancestry) was one of the first ever to wear false teeth.

Although the British have always been prone to bad teeth, the evidence of mediaeval graveyards suggests that the standard of dental health was much better a few centuries ago than it was in the nineteenth century (Drummond and Wilbraham, 1939). They concluded that the decline in dental health that took place in the last century was due to the altered eating habits of country people coming into the new industrial towns. The changes which they thought most important were: (1) the decline in the consumption of milk, (2) the general use of refined sugar which had previously been an aristocratic delicacy, and (3) the introduction in the 1880s of roller-milled white wheaten flour which was softer and less nutritious than the traditional wholemeal stone-ground wheat (p. 168). Certainly by 1900 the general state of dentition in Britain was deplorable; bad teeth was one reason that led to such a high rejection of recruits for the army at that time. In 1965, 84 per cent of our 5-year-old children had decayed deciduous teeth and over one-third of the teeth of 13-year-old children had been damaged by caries. Periodontal disease is just as widespread although occurring mainly in adults.

By contrast, good dentition is the rule in certain primitive (though not necessarily uncivilised) people. The Eskimos who live in isolated settlements have excellent teeth with less than 5 per cent affected by caries. Their traditional diet is composed largely of raw walrus meat and fish. In those who live in trading stations where they can buy canned food prevalence of caries is high. The Masai in Kenya, who live almost entirely on milk, meat and raw blood, have little caries, as Orr and Gilks (1931) reported. Their neighbours, the Kikuyu, on the other hand, whose diet is rich in carbohydrates and who readily adapt themselves to European dietary habits, are prone to caries. In many underdeveloped countries such foodstuffs as refined wheat flour and sugar and sweetened soft drinks nowadays form a regular part of the diet of the people, particularly in the towns. The incidence of caries and periodontal disease among the children is often very high (Nicol, 1956). Their parents frequently have lost many teeth, a large number of those remaining being loose and embedded in pools of pus.

In France and Norway (Toverud, 1949) the dental health of children actually improved in World War II during the German Occupation, despite the cruel restriction of food supplies. Sugar and sweets were, of course, almost impossible to obtain; the people reverted to the traditional short commons of the European peasantry— wholemeal bread and such vegetables as they could grow for themselves. Though the supply of milk for children was deficient, they nevertheless developed good teeth.

For many years the people of Tristan da Cunha lived in almost complete isolation in the Atlantic. They were poor, but several investigators who visited the island reported on their excellent dental health. In 1942 a meteorological station was set up on the island. The regular visits of ships and the establishment of a fish canning factory led to a great increase in prosperity, the introduction of imported foods and a rapid decline in dental health. When the islanders were evacuated in 1961, a dental survey showed that both caries and periodontal disease was widespread (Holloway et al., 1963)

DENTAL STRUCTURE
The substance of the teeth is mainly composed of a bone-like material, dentine, which is protected on its outer surface by a thin layer of very hard enamel. Inside is the soft pulp cavity, supplied by a nerve and an arteriole (Fig. 45.1). Enamel is formed by cells known as ameloblasts,

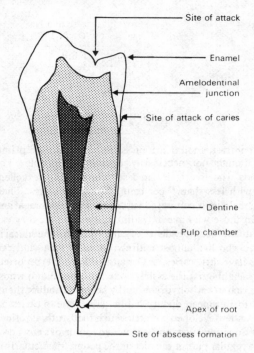

Fig. 45.1 The structure of a tooth showing sites of attack of caries

which are ectodermal in origin; dentine is formed by odontoblasts derived from mesoderm.

Dentine resembles bone in that it is composed of a cellular, protein-containing matrix in which calcium salts are deposited. Whereas bone consists of about 40 per cent of inorganic salts and 60 per cent of matrix, dentine contains about 80 per cent of inorganic salts. Enamel is even more dense, with less than 5 per cent of non-cellular matrix which nevertheless plays an essential part in maintaining its structure. Even the enamel surface of a tooth is a living tissue.

DENTAL HYPOPLASIA

The growth of teeth, like that of any other organ or structure in the body, may be impaired by adverse factors in fetal life, infancy or early childhood. A defective diet or a severe infection which impairs growth may lead to hypoplasia of either enamel or dentine or both. Two types of hypoplasia of the permanent teeth have been described.

G-hypoplasia (gross hypoplasia). In this the enamel surface is seen to be deeply pitted. The pitting is often present in a regular line affecting most of the teeth. This hypoplasia can often be ascribed to an illness in early childhood—such as whooping cough—at the time when the permanent teeth were developing.

M-hypoplasia. This less familiar kind was first described by Lady Mellanby and called after her. There is a general defect in development of the enamel so that the surface of the tooth, instead of being perfectly smooth and hard, has an irregular 'washboard' texture, which is often more easily felt than seen, by running a fine probe over the posterior surface of the tooth. In a long series of investigations, a close association was demonstrated between the incidence of M-hypoplasia and of caries in London schoolchildren (Mellanby and Mellanby, 1954).

Linear hypoplasia of the incisors of the primary dentition has been reported in several underdeveloped parts of the world. It is more common in children with PEM (Sweeney et al., 1971) but development of the enamel is interfered with in the neonatal period, before the teeth erupt. Insufficient vitamin D in the mother is one of several causes (Purvis et al., 1973).

DIETARY FACTORS AND DENTAL DEVELOPMENT

Vitamin D deficiency. Dentine and bone are analogous structures of similar origin and in the absence of vitamin D neither develop normally. The relation between vitamin D deficiency, dental hypoplasia and caries is not clear cut and surveys in the United States and Canada have given conflicting answers (Shaw and Sweeney, 1973). Very few of the children in London studied by the Mellanbys would have had clinical rickets, but for many of them the supply of vitamin D would at best have been only marginally adequate. The much greater prevalence of caries in northern countries than in tropical countries may be in part due to smaller exposure to sunlight and the consequent diminished synthesis of the vitamin in the skin. Eruption of the teeth is delayed in children with clinical rickets.

Protein-energy malnutrition. Widdowson and McCance (1960) and McCance et al. (1961) reported that undernutrition or overnutrition have little effect on the time of eruption of teeth in experimental animals even if growth is stunted. In their book, *Kwashiorkor,* Trowell et al. (1954) remarked on 'the incongruous sight of the tiny child with his mouth crowded with teeth.' It was therefore suggested that the dental age could be used to indicate chronological age in surveys of children living in societies without calendars and birth certificates. The relation between eruption of the deciduous teeth and PEM was examined in a symposium edited by Jelliffe and Jelliffe (1973) which contained reports from fifteen different countries. In general, dental eruption is usually little delayed in mild or moderate PEM but may be in children with severe growth retardation.

DENTAL CARIES

The first lesion is erosion of the enamel. This usually occurs at contact points between teeth, at the gum margins or in pits and fissures of posterior teeth. When the enamel is breached, there is rapid spread along the amelodentinal margin and then penetration of the dentine. This may occur slowly with secondary formation of dentine by the pulp which regresses and may become fibrosed. Alternatively, there may be rapid spread with infection of the pulp (pulpitis) and formation of an apical abcess.

In the early stages there may be no pain or only a vague awareness of the tooth. Later the tooth is sensitive to cold. The classical sharp, stabbing pain is associated with secondary dentine deposition within the pulp. With pulpitis or an apical abscess, the tooth is actually tender to touch. The intensity of the pain varies greatly.

EPIDEMIOLOGY

The standard way of expressing the extent of dental caries is to count the decayed teeth, i.e. those showing caries, together with those that have been filled and those that are missing. This give the **DMF index** (decayed, missing, filled). There should be a total of 20 teeth in the deciduous dentition by the age of 20 to 30 months and eventually 32 teeth in the permanent dentition when the wisdom teeth have appeared. In Massachusetts the DMF index increases from 3.5 at the age of 8 years to 12 teeth at 14 years (Glass et al., 1973). Massachusetts, which has no fluoridation, has more dental disease than most of the USA. The average British experience is 5 to 7 DMF teeth at the age of 12 years. In adults average figures from a national survey in the USA in 1965 are shown in Table 45.1. Caries is the usual cause of loss of teeth up to the age of about 45 and thereafter periodontal disease. The major attack by dental caries takes place before the age of 25 years.

PATHOGENESIS

Production of dental caries depends on bacteria. Streptococci normally reside on and between the teeth and produce lactic acid by fermenting sugars ingested as food and drink. When a sufficient concentration of acid (about pH 5) is in contact with a dental surface for a long enough time, the crystalline material in the enamel starts to dissolve because calcium phosphate is soluble in acid. Unlike bones the enamel of teeth has little or no capacity for regeneration; once a hole is established, it remains and is likely to enlarge because bacteria can lodge in it more securely than on the biting or brushed surfaces of the teeth.

As well as breaking down sugars to lactic and similar organic acids, some bacteria, e.g. Streptococcus mutans, possess enzymes which can build up extracellular accumulations of insoluble polymers of glucose and fructose (dextrans and levans). These adhere to the teeth and form a **plaque** in which the bacteria are protected from the cleansing action of the tongue. After feeds containing sugar, acid is produced in the plaque next to the enamel but inaccessible to neutralisation by saliva.

AETIOLOGY

Four factors determine whether an individual has much or little dental caries.

Table 45.1 Decayed, missing and filled teeth in a National Survey in the USA in 1965 (from Kapur et al., 1972)

Age	Decayed	Missing	Filled	DFM
25–34	1.7	7.3	8.3	17.3
35–44	1.2	10.0	8.1	19.3
45–54	1.0	15.6	5.1	21.6
55–64	0.7	21.4	3.3	25.4
65–74	0.4	24.5	2.1	26.9

1. *The bacterial flora of the mouth.* Caries does not occur in germ-free animals and attempts are being made to develop a vaccine to *S. mutans.*
2. *The substrates for acid production.* These are sugars and are discussed below.
3. *Good oral hygiene.* Brushing the teeth cleans their outer surfaces and can prevent accumulation of bacteria and plaque; the fissures between the teeth are partly cleaned by the flow of saliva, drinking with meals and fibrous foods, but most effectively by using dental floss.
4. *The resistance of the teeth.* Crowded teeth with narrow crevices between them and teeth with poorly developed enamel are more susceptible; fluoride in drinking water or topically applied decreases the acid-solubility of the outer layer of the enamel.

Sugar. Clinical observations, animal experiments and epidemiological studies all show that sucrose is an important but not the only cariogenic food (Shaw and Sweeney, 1973). Confectionary and sweets may lodge in the teeth sufficiently long to allow bacteria to produce acid and, when eaten between meals, increase the time in which teeth are exposed to excess acid. The importance of the physical form of sugary foods and the time at which they are eaten was demonstrated in a long-term experiment carried out between 1945 and 1951 in a mental hospital in Vipeholm, Sweden (Gustafsson et al., 1954). Sucrose in solution with meals had little cariogenic effect, but sticky toffees and caramels between meals produced a sharp increase in dental caries.

The contribution of sucrose to the development of dental caries is strikingly shown by its virtual absence in children who cannot eat sucrose without becoming ill because of a rare inborn error of metabolism (p. 320). Seventh Day Adventists limit their consumption of sugar and avoid sweets between meals. Their children have less dental caries than other American children. The amount of sugar taken with meals may not be important. There was no increase in caries when children in British institutions were given extra sugar at the end of rationing, but only at meal times (King et al., 1955). There is no more caries in children who eat breakfast cereals coated with sugar or with added sugar compared with those who do not (Glass and Fleisch, 1974). Besides sucrose, glucose, fructose, maltose, galactose and lactose are all cariogenic in experimental animals, as is honey, and may be presumed to be so in man. Xylitol (p. 27) is as sweet as sucrose, and is not fermented by oral streptococci. In a controlled trial a group of young adults who used confectionery sweetened with xylitol developed less caries than two groups who used sucrose or fructose as sweeteners (Scheinen *et al.*, 1974).

Even infants and very young children may be exposed to cariogenic foods. Vitamin supplements, dummies and reservoir feeders (small bottles used as comforters) may all be sweetened and their use has been shown to be associated with a high incidence of caries in children aged 3 to 4 years.

Other dietary components. Strongly acid drinks, taken frequently, can gradually dissolve and wear down the enamel. Fibrous foods like apples and carrots have a scouring action which reduces plaque formation when they are eaten after a meal, but they only protect the biting surfaces, not the sides of the teeth or fissures. Several other foods are reported to be protective, including cheese and peanuts which increase the flow of saliva and also have inhibiting effect on dental plaque by raising the pH and increasing its calcium content (Rugg-Gunn *et al.*, 1975). Chewing betel reduces the chance of dental caries.

Fluoride. The salts present in dentine and enamel normally contain, besides calcium phosphate and bicarbonate, traces of other elements including fluoride.

A concentration of fluoride in drinking water between 0.5 and 1 part per million (p.p.m.) protects against caries (p. 108); fluoride ions replace hydroxyls in the hydroxyapatite lattice of the mineral in the enamel. In areas where the fluoride content of the water is low, addition of fluoride may more than halve the incidence of caries (Table 12.1), but if the drinking water in a locality contains more than 2 p.p.m. of fluoride, mottling of the teeth occurs and at higher levels (5 p.p.m.) every tooth may be affected (p. 109 and the enamel surface is often irregular and stained brown at the gum margins. Such teeth are softer than normal and yet unusually resistant to dental decay. The presence of abnormal amounts of fluoride has been demonstrated in these teeth, and it is likely that the bacteriostatic power of this element is the factor that protects them from caries.

Other trace elements. In Heliconia, an isolated village in the Andes in Colombia, the prevalence of dental caries is unusually low. Yet the water is low in fluoride and the population consume plenty of sugar. A team from the Forsyth Dental Center, Boston, with Colombian scientists, examined the trace elements in water, saliva, teeth and dental plaques. Compared with a control village, where the incidence of caries was high, the water of Heliconia contained more calcium, magnesium, molybdenum and vanadium and less copper, iron and manganese (Glass *et al.*, 1973). Hardness of water is often associated with a high fluoride content but here they were separated. There have been reports from other countries which suggest that molybdenum may protect against caries. In 21 villages in Papua-New Guinea analyses of soil and food for minerals and trace elements were compared with the number of carious teeth, which ranged from 0 to 30 per cent. Caries was negatively related with alkali and alkaline earth elements in soils, including magnesium, calcium and lithium, and in staple foods with molybdenum and vanadium. Copper and lead in soils and foods were associated with caries (Barnes *et al.*, 1970).

PERIODONTAL DISEASE

Healthy gums, like the skin of the hands, withstand hard usage. They are covered with a firm epithelium, below which there is dense connective tissue. When periodontal disease is present, the gum margin falls away from its immediate contact with the teeth and may be withdrawn several millimetres from its original point of attachment. The margin is usually intensely red and inflamed, probably because of the bacteria that inevitably accumulate in the pocket that develops between the tooth and the margin of the gum. Their growth is certainly assisted by accumulation of calculus or tartar. This material consists of a deposit of calcium salts, mucin and bacteria. The cause of its formation is obscure. The calculus is first deposited in the pockets between the teeth and the gums. Indeed it has been argued that if the gums are healthy and closely applied to the teeth this would not occur. Lack of saliva is certainly not the usual cause. Whatever may be the aetiological relation between calculus and periodontal disease, the fact remains that they are closely associated. In advanced cases the gingival bone underlying the gum is eroded so that the teeth become loose and ultimately fall out, even though they may be free of caries.

Factors concerned in the causation and prevention of disease of the gums are now considered.

Infection. A soft diet, rich in carbohydrate which sticks around the teeth, forms a good medium for the growth of bacteria. Bacteria can seep down beneath the gum margins and so damage the underlying tissues. This damage is progressive and ultimately affects alveolar bone, which supports the teeth. This process is exaggerated in scurvy, in which there is a distinctive type of inflammation of the gums (p. 296). Scurvy also leads to defective formation of dentine; the teeth may become loose from lack of the cement that normally holds them to the jaw. In severe periodontal disease the teeth also become loose through erosion of the surrounding bone. It is unlikely that lack of ascorbic acid is usually an important factor in the causation of periodontal disease.

Physical effects. It is noteworthy that periodontal disease is rare among primitive people who make full use of their teeth. The massaging effect of rough, tough foodstuffs no doubt quickly removes the earliest deposits of calculus. As an instance, children in Jamaica have excellent gums, perhaps because of their habit of chewing pieces of sugar-cane between meals; the cane, despite its sugar content, seems to keep the teeth and gums healthy by its local abrasive action. Similarly, Eskimo women keep their gums clean and in good health by chewing strands of sealskin which they afterwards use for weaving.

The relation between periodontal disease and caries. Although these two conditions are frequently seen together in the same patient this is not always the case. As a rule, however, the accumulation of calculus in the pockets and crevices of unhealthy gums tends to cause erosion of dental enamel, so that periodontal disease may be a subsidiary cause of caries.

PRESERVATION OF DENTAL HEALTH

Clearly the relationships between dental disease and diet are not simple. Nevertheless there is enough evidence to state several practical principles for the prevention of dental disease.

INFANT NUTRITION

The foundations of the first teeth are laid down before birth. It is therefore important that attention be paid to the nutrition of the pregnant mother (p. 519). For the newborn infant it is necessary to ensure that proper calcification of the teeth and bones continues, as discussed in connection with the prevention of rickets (p. 280). A good maternity and child health service is sound prophylaxis against caries in the next generation.

FLUORIDATION OF WATER SUPPLIES

There can be no question that insufficient fluoride in the drinking water of a community increases the incidence of dental caries among children (p. 109). For reasons already given we have no hesitation in stating that where a public water supply is deficient in fluoride, this deficiency should be made good and that this will reduce the incidence of dental disease in children.

Where the natural water is low in fluoride and a vociferous antiscientific minority makes politicians anxious about introducing fluoride, alternative ways of providing it for children have to be devised by conscientious parents and their health advisers. Fluoride tablets (the dose is one 0.25 mg tablet thrice daily) are available, but have to be paid for and remembered. There have been proposals for fluoridated milk or for small plants which fluoridate a school's water supply. Toothpastes containing fluoride give a little protection; 100 μg F on average gets swallowed with each brushing and traces of the fluoride accumulates on the teeth. Topical applications of more concentrated fluoride solutions have to be administered by dentists or dental nurses because the solution would be toxic if consumed accidentally by a child. The first effective period for fluoride prophylaxis is while the crowns are being calcified within the jaws; for most of the permanent dentition, except the third molars, this is from birth to about 8 years of age. Only ingested fluoride can reach the enamel at this stage. The second effective period is for the first few years after eruption. At this stage the enamel is more susceptible to caries and fluoride, either systemic or topical, hastens maturation. But of all the methods for achieving an enamel with optimal fluoride content and so resistant to caries, fluoridation of public water supply is the most effective and economical, and it benefits all the people.

DENTAL SERVICES.

Every well-organised community should provide services whereby the teeth and gums of pre-school children, schoolchildren and adolescents are inspected at regular intervals and any necessary treatment given. Overcrowded teeth can be drawn apart by orthodontic treatment. This inspection should be carried out not only in schools, but also in training colleges and industrial works that employ young people.

Although our knowledge of how to prevent the onset of caries is far from adequate, there can be no question that proper treatment at an early stage will arrest the progress of the disease and prevent the loss of teeth in later life.

EDUCATION

A good dental service provides opportunities for proper education. In communities where dental disease is common, three points should be stressed. First, that prevention is better than cure; regular attendance at a dental clinic for a prophylactic inspection will save much future trouble. Secondly, the teeth and gums ought to be kept clean at all times. For the modern city dweller the regular use of a toothbrush—properly applied—as soon as possible after meals, should be explained and encouraged. Thirdly, it should be stressed that sticky sweets or soft starch foods between meals are harmful, since they lodge between the teeth and encourage dental decay. A tax on sweets is as logical as taxes on tobacco and alcohol.

There can be no doubt that if dentists, doctors, dietitians and school teachers devoted more time to educating young people in the care of their teeth, much dental disease could be avoided. Children should not be taught about proteins and vitamins until they know how to care for their teeth. At their stage of life how to prevent dental caries is the most important nutritional message that they can be given.

46. Diseases of the Gastrointestinal Tract

Some aspects of the applied physiology of the gastrointestinal tract are discussed before the nutritional and dietetic aspects of clinical syndromes and diseases are described.

1. The lumen of the gut from the mouth to the anus is outside the body. Thus nutrients within it have to be processed and assimilated before they reach the metabolic machine.

2. The intestinal contents are moved along the small intestine by peristaltic waves. The onward movement is delayed by sphincters, the pylorus between the stomach and the duodenum, the ileocaecal valves and the anal sphincters.

3. The absorption of most nutrients depends on active (energy-dependent) transport across the intestinal epithelium. Most nutrients are absorbed from the upper small intestine (jejunum) but vitamin B_{12} and also bile acids are absorbed from the distal ileum and large amounts of water and electrolytes from the colon.

4. Exchange between the body proper and the lumen of the tract through the intestinal mucosa is a two-way process. The tract is not only a mechanism for digestion and assimilation but also for exchange and elimination. Here it has much in common with renal tubular secretion and reabsorption.

5. Metabolic activity of the bacterial flora in the caecum and colon modifies organic compounds which have come through the small intestine, notably those secreted into it by the liver. Some of these are then absorbed and so form an enterohepatic circulation; others pass out in the faeces.

6. The functions of the gastrointestinal tract depend on exocrine glands which discharge into the lumen, e.g. the parotid glands, pancreas and liver. They also depend on hormones secreted into the blood stream by the upper part of the tract which influence other parts of the tract.

7. These hormones are peptides. The main physiological actions of three of them, gastrin, secretin and cholecytokinin are well known. Five other gastrointestinal hormones are now identified (Bloom and Polak, 1978), but their physiological roles are not yet well defined, and it is not known whether over- or underproduction of any of them is responsible for any gastrointestinal disorder.

8. The amount of water and electrolytes secreted into the lumen is large (Table 46.1) so that diarrhoea or vomiting may cause large negative balances requiring oral or parenteral replenishment.

9. Protein enters the gastrointestinal tract not only in the diet but also in the digestive juices and in the shed mucosal epithelium. The daily output of digestive enzyme is equivalent to up to 50 g of protein and the whole mucosa is replaced or turned over every three or four days. Hence usually only about half of the protein entering the lumen is of dietary origin. In digestion the body makes no distinction between native proteins (enzymes secreted by the gut) and exogenous denatured proteins (that is, cooked protein).

10. The intestinal mucosa contains cells which produce antibodies, including the immunoglobulins IgA and IgM. Dysfunction of these cells is a possible basis for gluten enteropathy and may be part of the mechanism leading to pernicious anaemia.

Table 46.1 Estimates of quantities of water and Na , K and Cl⁻ entering the human intestine daily (Parsons, 1967)

	Volume (ml)	Concentration (mmol/l)			Electrolyte load (mmol/24 h)		
		Na	K	Cl⁻	Na	K	Cl⁻
Saliva	1500	30	20	35	45	30	52
Gastric juice	3000	50	10	150	150	30	450
Bile	500	160	5	50	80	3	25
Pancreatic juice	2000	160	5	30	320	10	60
Internal load	7000				595	73	587
Dietary intake	1500				170	65	110
Grand total	8500				765	138	697

11. Some primary nutritional diseases, e.g. protein-energy malnutrition, lead to atrophy of the gastrointestinal tract and impair absorption of nutrients, so setting up a vicious circle.

12. The gastrointestinal tract through its autonomic nerve supply is closely related to centres in the limbic system of the brain concerned with expression of emotion. Worry and anxiety can be expressed as dyspepsia, which is also one feature of depressive illness. Eating is not only a physiological necessity but also a mode of expression of the emotions and social, cultural and religious attitudes. A diet may need to be modified to relieve symptoms in many organic and psychosomatic disorders of the alimentary tract. Every patient with a disorder of the digestive system should be carefully questioned about his dietary and social habits.

DIETARY HISTORY

The dietary history includes information about the number and time of the meals taken daily, whether they are taken regularly, if they are huried and if the food is adequately chewed. A description should be obtained of the various foods eaten and of their effects in alleviating or producing symptoms. Enquiries should be made about the use of alcohol, tobacco and medicines. Some drugs may irritate the gastric mucosa and disturb the neuromuscular function of the gastrointestinal tract. Self-medication with proprietary preparations, especially those containing aspirin, may cause dyspepsia. Questions should be directed to finding out whether the patient is living in a state of anxiety induced by social relations at home or at work. We have repeatedly seen dyspepsia, diarrhoea or other abdominal symptoms developing when a love affair is not proceeding on a satisfactory course, when an employee is being bullied by an employer or when some financial misfortune is causing undue worry. It is also important to question whether the patient has been abroad recently, which may give a clue to the diagnosis of worms or parasites of the gastrointestinal tract.

METHODS OF INVESTIGATION

The oesophagus, stomach, duodenum and small intestine can be visualised by radiography after a barium meal and the colon and rectum after a barium enema. Aspiration of gastric juices allows the secretory activity of the stomach in response to gastrin and other stimuli to be measured. The rectum and descending colon can be examined through a sigmoidscope. These are established techniques in use for more than 50 years.

The upper part of the gastrointestinal tract can now be examined using a flexible fibre optic gastroscope. With this instrument the mucosa of the oesophagus, stomach and duodenum can be observed directly and biopsy samples taken for histological examination. In skilled hands the procedure is now easy and safe. Biopsy material from the small intestine can be obtained using a Crosby capsule.

This is attached to a thin plastic tube and swallowed by the patient. It contains a rotating knife which is triggered by suction applied by a syringe to the end of the tube.

DISEASES OF THE MOUTH

Examination of the mouth may show lesions due to local causes or be indicative of general disease. Lesions primarily nutritional in origin are angular stomatitis, cancrum oris, nutritional parotitis and nutritional glossitis (Chapter 37). Glossitis is often a presenting feature in pellagra, the sprue syndrome, pernicious anaemia and iron-deficiency anaemia of long standing. Primary disease of the oral cavity may cause serious malnutrition and dehydration.

The tongue

Doctors have examined the tongues of their patients since the earliest times. The tongue may be dry in mouth breathers and coated with whitish yellow fur in those persons who smoke excessively. A clean red tongue, which is inflamed and painful (acute glossitis), suggests an acute primary deficiency of some member of the vitamin B complex. A clean pale and smooth tongue (chronic atrophic glossitis) suggests pernicious anaemia in remission or a long-standing iron-deficiency anaemia. Treatment includes a well-balanced diet, supplemented by iron or the appropriate vitamin when indicated. A local ulcer may be due to an ill-fitting denture or malignant disease, but rarely nowadays syphilis or tuberculosis.

The teeth, gums and mouth

Nutrition and dental disease are discussed in Chapter 45. While dental sepsis is no longer considered important as a cause of disease, it stands to reason that infections of the teeth and gums should be treated.

A bad taste in the mouth may be due to pyorrhoea and is rarely due to disease. It often coincides with emotional problems and discussion of these may help.

Inflammatory and haemorrhagic lesions in the mouth and gums can result from many causes, e.g. infections with Vincent's organisms, haemolytic streptococci, Candida albicans (thrush), drug reactions and blood diseases (acute leukaemia, agranulocytosis, aplastic anaemia).

Recurrent aphthous ulcers are the commonest form of mouth ulcers. These are small (2 or 3 mm in diameter), superficial and painful. They may begin as vesicles and crops may come and go for no apparent reason, healing spontaneously. Occasionally this unpleasant condition is the first sign of coeliac disease. Therefore if the ulcers persist or recur repeatedly examination of the jejunal mucosa may be considered (p.405).

Any inflammatory condition of the mouth may contribute to a nutritional disorder, for the pain and difficulty in swallowing may restrict the intake of food.

TREATMENT

The treatment of angular stomatitis, glossitis and other primary nutritional disorders of the mouth has already been described in Chapter 37. There is no satisfactory evidence that any of the other lesions of the mouth mentioned above are improved by dietary therapy, with the exception of aphthous ulcers of the mouth associated with coeliac disease which may resolve with a gluten-free diet. If lesions are causing pain on chewing or swallowing, a fluid or semiliquid diet (Diet No. 16) might be given until the condition is brought under control.

DISEASES OF THE SALIVARY GLANDS

Parotitis

The enlargement of the parotid glands common in Asia and Africa associated with inadequate intakes of protein is described on page 306.

Inflammation of the parotid gland may be due to the virus of mumps (virus parotitis) or to bacterial infection of the glands which tends to develop during severe febrile illnesses and after major surgical operations if adequate attention is not given to oral hygiene.

Acute parotitis from any cause is often so severe as to make chewing and swallowing painful and difficult. A fluid diet, based on Diet No. 16, should be given until the inflammation subsides.

DISEASES OF THE OESOPHAGUS

Diseases of the oesophagus are much less common than diseases of the stomach or intestine. Difficulty in swallowing (dysphagia) is the main feature and may lead to choking and even inhalation of food, causing pneumonia or death. Inhalation may occur, particularly at night. Dysphagia results from a functional defect, with failure of onward movement of the peristaltic waves; alternatively the wave may be adequate but a block caused by spasm, inflammation or malignant disease prevents the food from getting through the affected area.

Swallowing is under voluntary control in the upper third of the oesophagus and is automatic thereafter. The stomach and oesophagus are kept separate by a combination of the muscle fibres of the diaphragm, the oblique entry of the oesophagus into the stomach and contraction of the smooth muscle fibres at the gastro-oesophageal junction, known as the cardia. A peristaltic wave which moves a bolus of food down the oesophagus relaxes the cardia temporarily. Thus appropriate relaxation and contraction of the smooth muscle at the cardia allow food to enter the stomach and prevent regurgitation of stomach contents into the oesophagus. If this neuromuscular mechanism is disturbed, dysphagia or heartburn may ensue.

Dysphagia may be produced by any neurological disorder, which damages the motor pathway between the cerebral cortex and peripheral muscle. Common causes are a stroke and achalasia. Possibly the commonest cause is achalasia.

Achalasia

The difficulty in swallowing is probably due to failure of the muscular relaxation of the lower end of the oesophagus which normally precedes the advancing peristaltic wave. Peristalsis itself is also abnormal as a result of degenerative changes in the neurones Auerbach's plexus in the wall of the oesophagus.

Dysphagia is at first intermittent, but may become more and more persistent. In time the oesophagus becomes dilated and later, as a result of the stagnation of food, an oesophagitis develops and causes substernal pain. Diagnosis depends on characteristic changes in radiology and on manometery, i.e. pressure recordings along the oesophagus.

In early cases relief may be obtained by the use of a bland diet (Diet No.17). If such a simple measure is ineffective either surgical myotomy or mechanical dilation may give permanent relief.

Sideropenic dysphagia (Patterson–Kelly or Plummer–Vinson syndrome)

Most patients are women of middle age who have been living on poor diets. It was common in Britain 50 years ago when malnutrition was much more frequent than it is now. Dysphagia is due to degenerative changes at the junction of the pharynx and the oesophagus which may eventually lead to deformity in the form of a mucosal web in the upper oesophagus. These changes are attributed to iron deficiency because almost all patients have iron-deficiency anaemia. The syndrome may predispose to carcinoma. Treatment consists in improving the diet and giving medicinal iron and thereafter keeping the patient under periodic review.

Stricture

This may be either fibrous or malignant. Difficulty in swallowing, first of solid foods and later of semi-solids and liquids, is the presenting feature. Diagnosis is confirmed by oesophagoscopy using a flexible fibre optic endoscope and taking a biopsy for histological examination. Immediate relief from the danger of inhalation depends on aspirating swallowed fluid remaining in the oesophagus each night and morning. Lasting relief can be obtained only by surgery or radiotherapy or by dilation. Before the operation it is important to restore the patient to a good nutritional state by pre-operative feeding, e.g. by intravenous feeding or by a tube passed through the strictured area with the help of an endoscope. In an inoperable case feeding via a plastic tube introduced through the stricture may prolong life in a merciful way, but a semiliquid diet must be taken as the tube does not drain easily.

A common complication following dilation of a benign stricture of the lower oesophagus is heartburn, a sympton resulting from reflux of gastric contents into the oesophagus.

Hiatus hernia and reflux oesophagitis

These are common causes of dyspepsia and dysphagia and occur more frequently in women than in men. The diaphragm has several openings through which abdominal viscera can enter the thorax. Of these the most important is the oesophageal opening, or hiatus, to which the oesophagus is loosely attached. In middle age this attachment weakens so that thereafter the oesophagus and stomach readily herniates. This occurs more commonly in the obese as the increased bulk of their abdominal contents exerts more pressure on the hiatus. Pregnancy and chronic cough may act in the same way. Many of these hernias are symptomless and discovered accidentally by radiologists. Hiatus hernia usually gives rise to symptoms only in so far as the cardia of the stomach ceases to act as a sphincter and allow acid peptic juice to regurgitate into the oesophagus. This produces **reflux oesophagitis.** The cardinal symptom is heartburn which is felt substernally and may be accompanied by regurgitation of acid fluid into the mouth. Periodicity of the symptoms is an important diagnostic point. Heartburn may occur after meals but typically follows bending, lifting or straining. It may occur when asleep in bed and wake the patient, who may obtain relief by sitting up. Few other pains produced in the alimentary tract are so closely linked to change of posture. The patient may also complain of a more severe pain or the sensation of food sticking. Chronic bleeding is not infrequent and a hiatus hernia should be suspected in any obscure iron-deficiency anaemia. Peptic ulceration of the oesophagus frequently occurs when a hiatus hernia impairs the sphincter and allows acid contents of the stomach to reflux into the oesophagus.

Patients can usually be kept free from symptoms by medical treatment. If there is obesity, weight reduction usually leads to a marked improvement; knowledge of this should motivate the patient to persist with a reducing diet. Corsets and other tight garments should not be worn. Patients distressed with pain at night should sleep with a pillow under the chest and the head of the bed raised on blocks; they should not take solid food before going to bed.

If the pain is severe the regimen should be of the ulcer type with the use of liquid antacids particularly those containing topical anaesthetics in an antacid gel. These should be taken at the onset of pain and one to two hours thereafter.

Anaemia due to bleeding should be treated with oral iron; if severe, blood transfusion may be needed. If pain persists despite medical treatment, there is probably ulceration and some degree of stricture, and surgical treatment is often required. As a result of newly devised operations more patients who fail to respond adequately to medical treatment are being sumitted to surgery than in the past and good results may be expected.

Carcinoma of the oesophagus

The clinical features are those of a stricture. Such carcinomas are either squameous cell carcinomas, which are treated by radiotherapy, or adenocarcinoma arising from the vault of the stomach. Adenocarcinoma may be treated by surgery. The epidemiology is discussed in page 510.

DYSPEPSIA

Dyspepsia is a word of Greek derivation, meaning indigestion or difficulty in digestion. Any gastrointestinal symptom associated with the taking of food is called dyspepsia, e.g. nausea, heartburn, epigastric pain, discomfort or distension. Dyspepsia may be present when there is no structural change in any part of the alimentary canal, in which case it is described as 'functional' and the symptoms may be psychological in origin or due to intolerance of a particular food. On the other hand dyspepsia may be a symptom of any organic disorder of the alimentary canal. It may also be caused reflexly by disease or disorder of structures outside the alimentary tract, e.g. the gall-bladder, pancreas, etc. Dyspepsia may be a symptom of a general disease, e.g. chronic nephritis and cardiac failure.

DYSPEPSIA AND ACID SECRETION

There is a great variation both in the quantity and concentration of acid secreted by the gastric glands. It was once thought that dyspepsia frequently arose as a result of too little or too much acid secretion. However, good digestion may be associated with the whole range of gastric acidity. For instance, patients with pernicious anaemia always have complete absence of acid secretion and yet seldom suffer from dyspepsia when the anaemia has been corrected by treatment with vitamin B_{12}. It is very doubtful if lack of acid alone is ever responsible for digestive disturbances. When dyspepsia occurs with achlorhydria, it is probably due to coincidental conditions such as chronic gastritis, cancer of the stomach or disease of the gall-bladder, or to emotional states.

Likewise, high rates of acid secretion (hyperchlorhydria) may be found in people who have never suffered from dyspepsia. Hyperchlorhydria is frequently found in patients with duodenal ulcer, yet such patients may continue to secrete excessive amounts of acid, not only when they are having symptoms, but during long intervals when they are symptom-free. Hydrochloric acid may be partially responsible for the pain and dyspepsia of the acute stage of peptic ulcer, but this is by no means certain, because these symptoms may be due to hypermotility which so frequently accompanies hypersecretion.

MANAGEMENT OF DYSPEPSIA

A careful enquiry into the dietary history and social habits and a general physical examination are necessary. In young people, unless there is reason to suspect organic disease, it is unnecessary and probably unwise to investigate the stomach by radiography or the response to pentagastrin. Usually the patient has been overworking or overworrying, or is bolting his meals or eating his meals when excessively tired, or has been smoking immoderately or taking too much alcohol. The patient should be assured that if he gives up such habits, his symptoms will probably clear up rapidly. However, dyspepsia occurring for the first time in middle age, especially if accompanied by weight loss, should be carefully investigated without delay.

Patients with functional dyspepsia need dietary advice based mainly on common sense, with no rigid rules. Help is needed to prevent them becoming hypochrondriacs.

Patients may find that certain foods bring on their symptoms whereas others can be taken with impunity. Hence bland diets have been prescribed. However, there is no evidence that any foods are generally irritant and it is important not to restrict a patient's diet unless a particular food has been shown to bring on symptoms in his case. On page 571 a list of ten types of foods that may cause trouble is given, together with a list of foods that can usually be recommended. These lists together with general advice may be helpful in discussing with a patient what he should and should not eat, and so aid him to follow a sensible dietary regimen.

PEPTIC ULCER

Peptic ulcer is one of the most common diseases in civilised countries. Incidence varies widely and population surveys suggest the percentage of adult men likely to be affected is 2.5 in the USA, 6.5 in London, 7.2 in Melbourne, and 15.1 in both Aberdeen and Assam, India (Langman, 1974). The term is used for an ulcer in any part of the digestive tract exposed to acid gastric juice, but the common sites are the stomach (gastric ulcer) and duodenum (duodenal ulcer) above the point of entry of the alkaline pancreatic juice.

The term peptic ulcer is used because it appears to develop from a loss of ability of the mucosa to withstand the digestive action of pepsin and HCl. How the healthy mucous membrane is protected from the action of gastric juices is little understood. Obviously a balance exists between acid pepsin secretion and mucosal resistance. In patients with gastric ulcer the secretion of acid is often within normal limits, but patients with duodenal ulcer nearly always have a high output of acid. This is probably accounted for in most cases by a larger than normal number of acid secreting parietal cells in the gastric mucosa. The great importance of gastric hypersecretion is supported by the intractable pepic ulceration of the Zollinger–Ellison syndrome in which gastrin, produced by a tumour of the non-β islet cells of the pancreas stimulates excessive gastric secretion by day and night.

Less attention has been paid to the response of the gastric mucosa to its own secretion of enzymes and acid. One probable protective agent is the mucoprotein, mucin, which adheres to the stomach wall as a thin but resistant coating. Mucin is secreted in response to local, nervous and hormonal influences. Florey (1955) in a Croonian lecture to the Royal Society reviewed what little was then known about its protective action. Unfortunately not much more is known now, as Schrager and Oates (1978) relate, except for details of the chemical structure of its constituent glycoproteins. Mucin possesses no appreciable buffering power against hydrochloric acid and has no inhibitory effect on pepsin digestion..Hence any protective action which it possesses probably depends on its acting, when gelled by contact with hydrochloric acid, as a physical barrier. Such a barrier would impede the mechanical mixing which brings the gastric juice in contact with surface cells. The lubricant properties of mucin may also help to protect the mucosa from mechanical trauma.

Claims that dietary factors cause peptic ulcer are based mostly on epidemiological evidence. The incidence of gastric ulcer and duodenal ulcers varies so markedly in different populations that they may be taken to be separate diseases. Certainly it is necessary to discuss them separately here. Two excellent reviews are available (Rhodes, 1972; Sircus, 1973).

Gastric ulcer

An argument to support the claim that dietary factors might be responsible for gastric ulcer is the fact that in Great Britain between 1920 and 1940 it was between twice and five times more prevalent in the poorest class than in the upper social class. The poorest social class at this time were consuming diets which were below physiological standards both in quantity and quality. Further, since then there has been a steady fall in the number of deaths attributable to gastric ulcer. How much of this fall in mortality rates is due to better food reducing the incidence of ulcers or to better treatment following new anaesthetics and operative techniques is a matter of speculation. Gastric ulcer is rare in most parts of Asia and Africa, including many districts where the diet is known to be grossly defective.

Duodenal ulcer

In contrast to gastric ulcer duodenal ulcer is uniformly distributed throughout the social classes in Britain. It is about three times as common in men as in women. A great increase occurred after 1940 reaching a peak in the 1950s

(Sussor and Stein, 1962). As during this period, standards of living greatly improved, nutritional deficiency was unlikely to be the cause. Constitutional and other factors such as smoking, feeding habits and the stress and competition of modern living require careful consideration.

On the other hand, duodenal ulcer is very prevalent in some parts of the world where the diet is poor. South India is the most important example; it is also common in some districts in Indonesia and West Africa. Yet in many other parts of the tropics where the diet is equally unsatisfactory, duodenal ulcer is not prevalent.

Hereditary factors

In support of a hereditary factor is the fact that a high proportion of duodenal ulcer patients belong to blood group O, and non-secretors of blood group substances have a higher than expected incidence as well. Possibly the secretion of A and B blood groups substances into the gastric juice have some protective effect. The risk of duodenal ulcer is reported to be 2.9 times greater in men with the HLA 35 antigen than in controls (Rotter *et al.*, 1977). Close relations of ulcer patients are more liable to develop peptic ulcers than are the relatives of normal people.

Occupational factors

Certain occupations appear to predispose to peptic ulcers. It has been suggested that stress and strain and having irregular meals and the consequent bolting of food and inadequate mastication may be important contributive factors. This may be so but Avery Jones (1957) found that bus drivers were not particularly prone to the disease; agricultural workers have a low incidence.

Potential irritants

Caffeine produces an increase in gastric acid secretion and in large doses may cause marked hyperaemia of the gastric mucosa. Alcohol has a similar effect but also stimulates secretion of mucus and, if taken repeatedly in excess may lead to acute damage to the superficial layers of the mucosa. Aspirin and related drugs are potent causes of ulceration and can lead to severe haemorrhages; this effect depends on the amount taken and varying individual responses.

CLINICAL FEATURES AND DIAGNOSIS

The commonest sympton is pain or discomfort in the upper central abdomen. It is usually described as burning or gnawing in character. Characteristically the pain comes and goes and is related to meals. In duodenal ulcer it usually occurs when the stomach is empty and is relieved by meals if they are not too large; the pain of gastric ulcer often comes on shortly after eating. Other symptoms which may occur are loss of weight, heartburn or vomiting. In some patients an ulcer causes no symptoms until a complication such as haemorrhage occurs. Should an ulcer bleed slowly, there is melaena (black stools) and anaemia. With a larger haemorrhage there is usually haematemesis; the blood which is vomited is altered to a dark brown colour.

In addition to the symptoms which are ascribable to acid, spasm of the pyloric canal (pylorospasm) can give rise to a characteristic feeling of sickness and distension; this prevents some patients from taking food which would relieve their symptoms. In addition there may be heartburn, due to reflux of acid into the oesophagus.

The cardinal investigations for peptic ulcer are radiographic examination with a barium meal and endoscopy. Fibre-optic endoscopes have transformed the diagnosis of ulcers, as biopsy of the affected areas is easy and rewarding. These techniques usually demonstrate the ulcer, but even an experienced operator may fail to detect one which is small or in a site where it is difficult to see. Intubation of the stomach and measurement of maximal acid output after stimulation by pentagastrin is a useful further investigation if surgery is contemplated. Acid output is usually above the normal range in patients with duodenal ulcer, and low or absent in patients with carcinoma of the stomach.

MEDICAL TREATMENT

Before discussing the medical and dietetic treatment of peptic ulcer it is necessary to indicate the types of cases for which a surgeon should always be called into consultation.

These are:

1. Perforation of a peptic ulcer.
2. Ulcers which, despite medical treatment, cause recurrent attacks of dyspepsia.
3. Any gastric ulcer in middle-aged patients which does not show satisfactory signs of healing within four weeks while on medical treatment; this is because carcinoma of the stomach can masquerade as a simple ulcer at first. Duodenal ulcers on the other hand are never malignant.
4. Any ulcers suspected of malignancy at gastroscopy.
5. Ulcers which show a persistent tendency to bleed in spite of repeated courses of medical treatment, particularly if the patient is over 60 years of age.
6. Old, indurated duodenal ulcers which are producing pyloric stenosis and marked gastric retention, and gastric ulcers on the lesser curvature producing hourglass contraction of the stomach and obstruction.

Aims of medical treatment

Relief of symptoms. In the absence of complications such as pyloric stenosis or penetration of the ulcer into an adjacent organ, it is usually easy to secure relief of symptoms. In many patients the symptoms disappear spontaneously without any medical treatment; yet medical treatment usually leads to a more rapid and complete relief.

Prevention of recurrence. This is more difficult. Patients have remissions and relapses with or without any treatment. The relapse rate for duodenal ulcer may be as high as 80 per cent in a 5 to 10 year period despite medical treatment, including bed rest. Many of the relapses are mild and can be controlled easily.

Principles of treatment

The traditional principles are: (1) rest, both physical and psychological; (2) a bland diet, given in small amounts at frequent intervals; (3) drugs—antacids and secretory inhibitors; (4) giving up smoking.

Rest. Symptoms are often relieved when a patient curtails his business and social activities. Both physical and mental rest appear to promote healing of an ulcer. The great majority of patients with duodenal ulcer and gastric ulcer do not require admission to hospital but they often have anxiety and emotional difficulties which require simple psychological support.

Diet. As a student in the early 1930s one of us had to learn the pros and cons of difficult strict dietary regimens which were imposed on patients with ulcers at that time. Some 35 years later he was admitted suffering from the effect of a gastric ulcer to a medical ward in a teaching hospital and later to a surgical ward in another teaching hospital. In both he was given a selection from the ordinary ward diet which he enjoyed and did well on. This remarkable change in the therapeutic practice was not entirely due to the whims of fashion.

A generation ago doctors thought, quite reasonably, that strict dietary regimens could produce excess gastric secretion of acid. Only after many years of experience was it realised that any reduction of secretion brought about in this way was insufficient to accelerate the healing of an ulcer or to prevent its recurrence. Further, too rigid an adherence to a strict diet sometimes led to the patients becoming undernourished. To Meulengracht (1939) of Copenhagen belongs the main credit of liberating patients from the old restrictive diets. Nevertheless some lessons have been learned from them.

Although patients may now eat normal foods, they should avoid large meals. By spreading out their food intake, they reduce the risk of exposing the gastric and duodenal mucosa to excessive amounts of acid. Also many patients find that their symptoms are aggravated by certain foods. These they learn by experience to avoid. A regimen for patients with dyspepsia or peptic ulcer is given in Diet No. 17. While a bland diet usually relieves dyspeptic symptoms, controlled trials have not demonstrated acceleration of healing of ulcers, as shown by barium meal (*British Medical Journal*, 1969; *Drug and Therapeutics Bulletin*, 1974). We agree with the advice of Ingelfinger (1966), 'Let the ulcer patient enjoy his food.'

When a patient has severe symptoms with pylorospasm or has had a haemorrhage he should be given several small meals daily. Milk, eggs and fruit juice should be the main ingredients. It is important to ensure a good intake of vitamin C since some patients have low reserves as a result of previous self-imposed dietary restrictions.

Drugs Many drugs have been used to relieve symptoms, promote healing and prevent recurrence, and most have proved disappointing. Two are of proven value. Insoluble antacid powders (aluminium hydroxide, magnesium oxide or trisilicate) are usually effective in relieving pain and are taken by millions of people. The histamine antagonist cimetidine effectively reduces acid secretion and relieves symptoms; it appears to prevent recurrence and to have few adverse effects, but it will be many years before it can be fully evaluated.

Complications of medical treatment

Excessive treatment may cause undesirable results. Scurvy has resulted from too strict adherence for long periods to milk diets prescribed for adults. A rigid dietary regimen may in obsessional persons give rise to emotional disturbances and so aggravate the symptoms. An excess of soluble alkalis can lead to alkalosis with tetany. A condition known as the milk alkali syndrome has occurred in patients with renal or pulmonary disease who take large amounts of milk (more than 1 litre daily) and soluble alkali usually over long periods. Weakness, anorexia and lethargy are the characteristic features and there may be psychological disturbances. Hypercalcaemia is always found and may give rise to calcification in the kidneys and elsewhere. Deaths have been reported. Fortunately all of these undesirable effects are very rare.

SURGICAL TREATMENT

Indications of when surgery may be needed have been given on p.339. The principal operations are shown diagrammatically in Fig. 46.1. The selective vagotomy is now the treatment preferred by many surgeons.

After an operation some surgeons keep the stomach empty by continuous suction until the daily aspirate is less than 250 ml/24 hours, during which time the patient is fed intravenously. Thereafter he is introduced to water, 30 ml hourly, for the second and third day and then given a soup and tea and weaned on to a solid diet over the next 2 to 3 days. Once a patient is free of symptoms and there is no evidence of active ulceration he no longer needs drugs. He should avoid taking alcohol on an empty stomach and tobacco consumption should be reduced.

As soon as convalescence is established, a patient may return to a full normal diet. A follow-up is necessary to see that he does not suffer from any nutritional deficiency. Many patients have lost weight prior to operation and, if this is not made good, it is important to take a careful dietary history and to ascertain the cause if he is not eating properly. This may be mental depression or other co-existing disease.

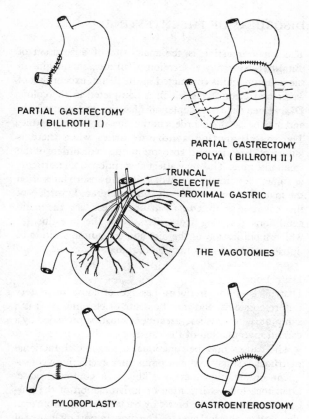

PARTIAL GASTRECTOMY
(BILLROTH I)

PARTIAL GASTRECTOMY
POLYA (BILLROTH II)

TRUNCAL
SELECTIVE
PROXIMAL GASTRIC

THE VAGOTOMIES

PYLOROPLASTY

GASTROENTEROSTOMY

Fig. 46.1 Operations for peptic ulceration. (Macleod, J. (Ed.) (1977) *Davidson's Principles and Practice of Medicine.* 12th edition. Edinburgh: Churchill Livingstone.)

Iron-deficiency anaemia is common after partial gastrectomy, perhaps due to loss of acid which converts the iron to the ferrous state. Megaloblastic anaemia may arise due to loss of intrinsic factor and a failure to absorb vitamin B$_{12}$. Owing to the large reserves in the liver, deficiency of this vitamin may not be apparent for two or three years.

Evidence of deficiency of riboflavin and nicotinic acid (glossitis), of thiamin (peripheral neuropathy) and of vitamin D (osteomalacia) may occur after major gastrectomies and the prolonged use of restricted diets, but are unusual.

Complications of surgical treatment

After any operation on the stomach many patients complain of symptoms after meals. These **post-cibal syndromes** may occur singly or in combination.

Small stomach syndrome. About 50 per cent of patients feel distended and uncomfortable during or after a meal. This occurs not only after partial gastrectomy but also after vagotomy and drainage. The symptoms tend to lessen with time. Management consists of dividing the individual's usual daily intake into a larger number of smaller meals.

Postvagotomy diarrhoea. This occurs in a minority of patients, typically in episodes, and is often severe.

Food intolerance. About 5 per cent of patients find they are unable to eat particular foods such as eggs, milk or tomatoes without discomfort.

Dumping syndrome. This is a feeling of drowsiness, muscular weakness and sometimes palpitations that occurs after a meal. It is probably due to rapid emptying of the stomach and dumping of its contents into the small intestine; there osmosis may move extracellular fluid into the lumen and so reduce plasma volume. The syndrome can be avoided by measures to slow down gastric emptying, e.g. taking small or dry meals and eating them slowly.

Hypoglycaemia. Signs of weakness, tremor and faintness, associated with hunger and an empty sensation in the epigastrium sometimes occurs between 1 and 2 hours after a meal. This is due to reactive hypoglycaemia; it is less common than the dumping syndrome.

Jejunal ulceration may result when the jejunum is anastomosed to the stomach and thus becomes exposed to the effects of acid gastric juice and pepsin. Medical treatment is often unsatisfactory and then further surgical treatment (vagotomy or partial gastrectomy) is necessary.

Gastritis

The introduction of the flexible gastroscope and improvements in radiological technique have shown that gastritis occurs more frequently than was formerly thought. Yet it is a somewhat imprecise diagnosis. The inflammatory lesion may be either an acute erosive gastritis or a chronic atrophic gastritis. It is rarely due to the direct effect of infection by a pathogenic organism. The cause is often unknown but ingestion of alcohol, drugs or other chemical irritants may be responsible. The commonest drug causing gastritis is aspirin, often taken for headaches and menstrual pain. Atrophic gastritis may be due to an autoimmune reaction and this is responsible for the failure to secrete intrinsic factor and HCl in pernicious anaemia. It is also present in half of the patients with severe iron-deficiency anaemia. Gastritis may also be present in metabolic disorders, e.g. uraemia, and an area of gastritis often surrounds peptic ulcer or carcinoma of the stomach.

Clinical features of gastritis vary from mild anorexia, vague discomfort, nausea and heartburn to severe and repeated vomiting accompanied by diarrhoea if there is associated enteritis. Sometimes the clinical picture may stimulate acute peptic ulcer and massive gastric haemorrhage may occur. Nausea, abdominal fullness, heartburn and pain occurring before breakfast and improving as the day goes on are frequently present in chronic alcoholics. Secretory studies indicate an outpouring of mucus and a reduction in the secretion of hydrochloric acid during acute attacks and also in most cases of chronic gastritis.

Acute gastritis

The symptoms are nausea, pain and vomiting and commonly follow an excess of alcohol, aspirin or other drugs, e.g. arsenic formerly used by murderers. They may also follow ingestion of plant or bacterial toxins but are rarely due to infection of the gastric mucosa. The diagnosis is often obvious from the history. Treatment consists of stopping the drug, sometimes washing out the stomach and giving alkalis, Maxolon and a liquid diet for 24 to 48 hours. Since acute gastritis rarely lasts more than two or three days, attention should be focused on the prevention of dehydration and the loss of electrolytes, associated with excessive vomiting. Water or half molar NaCl with or without the addition of glucose and fruit juice should be given frequently. Small amounts, 100–150 ml, may be taken every hour. If fluids given by mouth cannot be retained and signs of dehydration appear, 5 per cent glucose in isotonic NaCl should be given intravenously. With improvement of the condition the patient is given small feeds of milk and gradually returns to a normal diet within 1 to 2 days.

Chronic atrophic gastritis

The aim of treatment is rest to the chronically inflamed mucous membrane. This may be achieved by removal or correction of the underlying cause, e.g. correction of faulty habits of feeding, drinking or smoking; administration of drugs, e.g. antacids, ferrous sulphate for iron-deficiency anaemia or vitamin B_{12} for pernicious anaemia may be needed. Once the cause has been removed and the symptoms have disappeared, a patient can return to an ordinary diet provided he corrects his habits of eating, drinking and smoking.

Carcinoma of the stomach

Epidemiology and aetiology are discussed on page 511.

Permanent cure can only be achieved by radical surgical resection before metastasis has occurred. Unfortunately early diagnosis is often difficult; hence the results are poor when reviewed over a postoperative period of five years. A carcinoma may arise at the orifices or in the body of the stomach. In the former case pain and vomiting with all its evil consequences on nutrition and salt and water metabolism are the principal features. When gastrectomy is contraindicated, a gastroenterostomy may relieve the obstruction. Developments in chemotherapy and radiotherapy, e.g. the cyclotron therapy, may improve the prognosis. In carcinoma of the body of the stomach, weakness, loss of appetite, vague abdominal discomfort and anaemia are the presenting features. Such patients are often diagnosed too late for radical surgery. Then treatment consists of letting them eat such food as they can enjoy and giving iron for the anaemia. If sufficient food cannot be given by mouth, intravenous feeding or gastrostomy or jejunostomy feeding, as described in Chapter 51, should be used.

DISORDERS OF THE INTESTINE

The small intestine is the main site of absorption of nutrients. Normally absorption of all nutrients begins in the jejunum and is completed in the ileum, except that of water and electrolytes which is completed in the colon. **Diarrhoea** leads to depletion of water and electrolytes and may be due to disorders of the small or large intestine. The **malabsorption syndrome** arises when there is failure of digestion and absorption due to disorders of the small intestine. This may affect absorption of all nutrients or sometimes only one or two. Failure to absorb fat is often the main feature and leads to **steatorrhoea.** Disorders of the colon lead to **constipation.** These are the main conditions resulting from diseases of the intestine for which modification of the diet and the administration of nutrients parenterally may be required.

Diarrhoea

Diarrhoea is the frequent passage of loose or watery unformed stools, and may be acute or chronic. As it is a symptom, not a disease, treatment must be preceded by a careful investigation of the cause.

The causes may be functional or organic. Functional diarrhoea results from neuromuscular overactivity consequent on emotional states. This is a common cause. Diarrhoea follows irritation or inflammation of the mucous membrane of the bowel by bacterial, viral, protozoal, chemical or physical agents. The most important causes of inflammation are the microorganisms responsible for food poisoning and faecal–oral infections (Chap. 24), including *Salmonella* and *Shigella*. Acute gastroenteritis is a common cause of diarrhoea in children. In tropical and subtropical countries bacillary and amoebic dysentery are often responsible. Diarrhoea may be a prominent feature of regional ileitis (Crohn's disease) and ulcerative colitis. Diarrhoea may be the presenting symptom of carcinoma of the colon or rectum. It may be a troublesome symptom after operations on the gastrointestinal tract and as a result of various malabsorptive disorders. Diarrhoea may alternate with constipation, and liquid stools can run past impacted hard faeces (spurious diarrhoea). Another important cause of diarrhoea is the excessive use of laxatives which becomes a habit in many people.

Acute gastroenteritis. This is the commonest cause of acute diarrhoea and is usually the result of one of the infections described in Chapter 24. The disease is usually mild and self-limiting but if severe or prolonged, the losses of water may so reduce the blood volume as to cause circulatory collapse with a marked fall in blood pressure (oligaemic shock). Unless this is prevented or treated, death may occur. For this reason acute gastroenteritis is often a serious disease in young children and in old people and others debilitated by chronic diseases. Three types of gastroenteritis require special mention.

Infantile gastroenteritis, as its name implies occurs in the first 12 months of life. In developed countries epidemics sometimes break out in children's wards or institutions; they are usually due to *Escherichia coli* serotypes. In England and Wales gastroenteritis was responsible for 36 000 infants deaths in 1898, compared with 372 deaths in 1966. In many developing countries the incidence is today as high as or higher than it was in nineteenth-century Britain and it is the major reason for the high infant mortality rates. The cause is early weaning and unhygienic bottle feeds.

Weanling diarrhoea is very common in many topical and subtropical rural areas where lactation is prolonged. It occurs characteristically in the second year of life after weaning to a diet of cereal or starchy porridge, often prepared in conditions of poor hygiene. Gordon (1963) reports an epidemiological study.

There is a very close relationship between weanling diarrhoea and infantile gastroenteritis with protein-energy malnutrition. Figure 29.1 shows how repeated attacks of gastroenteritis lead to nutritional marasmus. Gastroenteritis is also one of the acute infections that in series can lead a child on the downward path to kwashiorkor. Secondly diarrhoea is a characteristic symptom of both marasmus and kwashiorkor (Chap. 29). Thirdly, while mild cases are common all over the world there is evidence that in a child with mild to moderate PEM (the underweight child) an attack of gastroenteritis is more likely to be severe and result in dehydration than in a well nourished child (Truswell *et al.*, 1964).

Traveller's diarrhoea. In many parts of the world, particularly in Africa and in Mediterranean, Arabic and Latin American countries, travellers are frequently incapacitated for one to three days by the sudden onset of acute diarrhoea which usually develops soon after the patient's arrival. The clinical features are colic and malaise with the repeated passage of watery stools without blood; usually there is little or no fever. Although traveller's diarrhoea is not a severe illness, it can disrupt a business trip.

In Mexico, Lowenstein *et al.* (1973) asked all the participants at the International Congress of Microbiology to fill in a questionnaire about their experience of 'turista', one of the local names of the disease: 50 per cent of those who came from the USA and Britain suffered an attack, but only about 10 per cent of those from Mediterranean countries in Europe. The preventive measures much used by tourists, such as drinking only bottled water, avoiding salads and taking clioquinol, were of no avail. The disease appears to be due to an immunologically related group of infectious agents, possibly specific serotypes of *E. coli*.

Treatment of acute diarrhoea
The patient's activities are usually sufficiently curtailed by his symptoms. Drugs are unnecessary and antibiotics are probably best avoided unless there is a bacterial diagnosis and the appropriate drug can be given.

In cases of moderate severity, treatment should start with 2 hourly feeds of 5 to 8 oz (150 to 250 ml) of barley water or milk diluted with equal parts of water. Improvement is usually rapid, and then chicken broth, junket and custard, fruit and jellies, proprietary invalid foods, softboiled or scrambled eggs and milk puddings can be taken, and soon the patient should be able to take the bland low roughage Diet No. 17.

In more severe cases it may be advisable, for a period not exceeding 48 hours, to give the patient nothing by mouth except water or, better still, half-normal saline (½ teaspoonful sodium chloride to 1 pint of water) flavoured with fruit juice and glucose. Patients should be allowed to sip small quantities of the fluid as frequently as desired during the waking hours.

Oral rehydration fluid. A prescription for a suitable fluid, which can be given by mouth and is recommended by WHO (Pierce and Hirschorn, 1977) is as follows:

Sodium chloride (table salt)	3.5 g
Sodium bicarbonate (baking soda)	2.5 g
Potassium chloride	1.5 g
Glucose	20 g

Dissolve in one litre of potable water

This has been effective in the tropics for the treatment of children with acute gastroenteritis and also for patients with cholera, and is suitable for patients with severe diarrhoea in any country. It is given in small doses at frequent intervals, assessed by the quantity that can be retained.

Intravenous fluid. If the patient cannot retain oral fluid and is showing signs of shock, no time should be lost before giving intravenous fluid. A solution containing 50 mmol NaCl with 5 per cent glucose may be used. As losses of water are relatively greater than those of sodium, the plasma is likely to be hypertonic and isotonic NaCl should not be used. Intestinal losses of potassium should be replaced and $NaHCO_3$ may be needed to correct a metabolic acidosis due to starvation.

MALABSORPTION SYNDROME

In a number of diseases there is a defect of absorption of one or more essential nutrients. They are associated with some or all of the following features: diarrhoea, steatorrhoea, abdominal distension, loss of weight, anaemia which may be macrocytic or hypochromic, hypoproteinaemia and deficiencies of vitamins and minerals, producing such features as stomatitis, glossitis, dermatitis, paraesthesia, or tetany. Although the difficulty of absorbing fat is usually the most evident feature it is essential to think of defective absorption in more general terms. Hence the title of 'the malabsorption syndrome'. There are several ways in which it may arise.

Reduced absorptive surface
1. Atrophy of the villi, e.g. in coeliac disease and tropical sprue.
2. Intestinal resection
3. Gastrocolic and jejunocolic fistula
4. Damage by radiation and by drugs.

Causes within the lumen
1. Deficiency of pancreatic secretion, e.g. in chronic pancreatitis and fibrocystic disease of the pancreas
2. Deficiency of bile salts, e.g. in obstructive jaundice
3. Too rapid emptying of the stomach and failure of coordination with secretion of bile and pancreatic juice, e.g. after operation for peptic ulcer
4. Inappropriate H^+ concentration in the duodenum, e.g. too low in achlorhydria and too high in the Zollinger-Ellison syndrome
5. Drugs that impair absorption of specific nutrients or interfere with digestion, e.g. neomycin can precipitate bile acids and so prevent their detergent action.

Competition with bacteria for nutrients. In health the duodenum, jejunum and upper ileum are virtually free of bacteria. Acid gastric juice, bile acids and the bactericidal action of intestinal mucus prevents the growth of bacteria swallowed with foods and saliva. The lower ileum is populated by small numbers of bacteria from the caecum and colon. If the protective secretions are deficient or cannot function adequately, due to stasis in the upper gut associated with a jejunal structure or diverticulum or a blind loop following surgery, or if they are overwhelmed as a result of a gastrocolic fistula, colonic bacteria multiply in the upper intestines. There they compete with the host for essential nutrients and may be responsible for signs of deficiency of these. Megaloblastic anaemia due to lack of vitamin B_{12} or folate is the most usual finding.

Defects of the gut mucosa
1. Deficiency of disaccharidases, especially lactase, in the brush border; this may be a primary genetic disorder or secondary to other conditions such as coeliac disease.
2. Deficiency of mechanisms for the transport of amino acids, e.g. cystinuria.

Failure of clearance
1. Lymphatic obstruction, which may be due to lymphagiectasis, tuberculosis or a tumour
2. Venous congestion, e.g. in congestive heart failure.

Steatorrhoea
This is the main clinical and biochemical manifestation of malabsorption and maldigestion of food. Excess of fat is found in the stools. A history of frequent, loose, bulky, offensive stools which float in water and flush with difficulty from the water closet indicates a gross degree of steatorrhoea. When present in a mild degree such obvious abnormalities may be absent, but steatorrhoea is diagnosed when the daily faecal output of fat exceeds 7 g while the patient is on a diet containing 50 to 100 g of fat. For accurate diagnosis faeces should be collected for at least three and preferably five days.

Since steatorrhoea is a feature of many disorders of the gastrointestinal tract, treatment should be preceded by accurate diagnosis. This may be easy or difficult, and may entail radiographic, chemical and haematological tests and a jejunal biopsy.

In forms which do not respond to specific treatment, a low fat diet (Diet No. 11) is necessary. When steatorrhoea is severe it is best to begin with a diet as nearly fat-free as possible, and to add small quantities of fat every few days until the patient's limit of tolerance is reached. Articles of food particularly rich in fat should be rigorously excluded at first. Of all fats, milk fat is often best tolerated; perhaps because it contains a high proportion of fatty acids of medium chain length. Medium chain triglycerides (MCT) (p. 418) are useful in the treatment of intractable steatorrhoea.

Vitamin and mineral deficiencies
Anaemia is almost as common a feature of malabsorption syndrome as is steatorrhoea. It may be due to failure to absorb sufficient amounts of either folic acid or iron and commonly of both. Vitamin B_{12} deficiency is less common. When malabsorption has been present for a long time, signs of osteomalacia are often present, due to failure to absorb vitamin D and calcium. Patients may show signs of deficiency of nicotinic acid and riboflavin and much less frequently of thiamin.

Diagnosis
A test for steatorrhoea should be carried out first because the absorption of fat is so frequently impaired. This is usually followed by a glucose tolerance test since it distinguishes between the steatorrhoea of pancreatic disease and the steatorrhoea of intestinal malabsorption. In the former, there will be either a diabetic or pre-diabetic curve, while in the latter, the curve is flat. Absorption of xylose is a simple and useful test of intestinal absorption since this sugar is normally absorbed actively but once in the blood it is not metabolised. It is excreted in the urine, where it is measured usually in a 5-hour collection.

Chronic pancreatitis as a cause of steatorrhoea can usually be diagnosed by tests of pancreatic function, such as enzyme excretion tests. If, in addition to the features of malabsorption, there is a history of intestinal pain, this suggests organic disease of the small intestine, such as regional enteritis, neoplastic infiltration or the presence of adhesions causing obstruction. The history of a previous operation, with an abdominal scar, may suggest resection or short-circuiting of the small intestine, and also the possibility of a **blind loop** or intestinal fistula. If a gastroenterostomy has been performed, a gastrojejunal

4

ulcer, with a gastrojejuno-colic fistula, is a possibility. In the case of a child, gluten-sensitive enteropathy is the most probable diagnosis, and this is also true of the majority of cases occurring in adults if malabsorption appears spontaneously and insidiously.

Gluten enteropathy (coeliac disease)

Gluten enteropathy arises in individuals who are sensitive to gluten, a main constituent of wheat flour and also present to a small extent in rye, barley and oats but not in rice. Such persons develop lesions of the small intestine which lead to diarrhoea and malabsorption. Symptoms usually arise within the first three years of life, but may first present at any age, even in the elderly. They are relieved if gluten is excluded completely from the diet. This means that many common foods cannot be eaten and, for most patients, life long commitment to a special diet.

Credit for the discovery that an idiosyncrasy or sensitivity to gluten is the cause of coeliac disease goes to the Dutch workers, Dicke (1950) and Weijers (1950). Gluten is a mixture of proteins (p. 33) and gliadin is the component responsible for coeliac disease.

Epidemiology

Prevalence varies in different parts of the world. It appears to be rare in Africa (Trowell, 1960), and unusually frequent in Galway, in the west of Ireland (Mylotte et al., 1973). The Coeliac Society estimate that there are 25 000 patients in the United Kingdom, i.e. prevalence is about 1 in 2000. The disease shows a familial tendency, especially if abnormal intestinal biopsy findings rather than symptoms are used to make the diagnosis (McDonald et al., (1965). Furthermore the HLA-B8 antigen is present in 72 per cent of patients with coeliac disease and only in 23 per cent of the general population.

Pathology

Endoscopy and biopsy of the small intestine show a patchy atrophy of the mucosa. In mild cases the surface appears flat and the villi are blunted. The epithelial cells are flat instead of columnar. The crypts are enlarged and tortuous and the epithelium infiltrated with lymphocytes. In severe cases there are large areas of the jejunum in which there are virtually no villi. Associated with these morphological changes there is a lack of disaccharidases and peptides. The lesions are reversible when gluten is removed from the diet.

The lesions are probably due to a local immunity reaction to a small polypeptide fraction of gliadin. There is evidence that fraction 9 of a peptic-tryptic digest of the gliadin in wheat gluten damages the intestinal mucosa. A defect in the enzyme system which splits this fraction may be the specific cause of the disease (Townley et al., 1973). The difficulties of separating the fractions of gliadin and of defining the methods for testing their toxicity make this a controversial area (Evans and Patey, 1974).

Clinical features

The characteristic feature is a fatty diarrhoea. Children fail to thrive and adults lose weight, mainly due to malabsorption of fat. Malabsorption of iron, folate and vitamin B_{12} may lead to anaemia, of vitamin D to rickets and osetomalacia and of vitamin K to haemorrhages. There is a wide range in the severity of the disease. Characteristically an untreated child presents a pathetic picture of severe undernutrition, but in some cases the disease is mild and anaemia or bone pain from osteomalacia may be the main feature.

Before the work of Dicke and Weijers in 1950 coeliac disease was known only as a disease of children. About one-third of the cases died of malnutrition after a varying period, a third survived into adult life as chronic invalids and about a third appeared to recover. The disease was not known to arise in adults but, with hindsight, we can be sure that many adults diagnosed as 'idiopathic steatorrhoea' were suffering from coeliac disease which had presented for the first time after childhood. Thus the disease, if untreated, varies greatly in intensity and patients are subject to exacerbations and remissions. It may be presumed that patients presenting first in adult life have had the disorder since early childhood but in so mild a form as to escape detection until some factor, nearly always unidentified, provoked symptoms. Although a few patients may revert to a normal diet with apparent impunity, some abnormality of the jejunal mucosa probably always returns and some biochemical evidence of poor absorption of one or more nutrients usually persists. They are also at risk of further exacerbations and complications.

Several diseases may be associated with coeliac disease. In children those include IgA deficiency, diabetes mellitus, allergy to cow's milk, lactase deficiency and dermatitis hepatiformis. Adults are more prone to autoimmune disorders and may be infertile; they are also at increased risk of developing lymphoma and carcinoma of the small intestine.

Diagnosis

The diagnosis should be suspected when any of the above clinical features are present. Confirmation is provided when there is a marked improvement following withdrawal of gluten-containing foods from the diet. It should be firmly established by endoscopy and biopsy, if possible, but this procedure requires experience and in young children is difficult and not without danger.

Treatment

The disease can be completely relieved if gluten derived from wheat or rye is entirely excluded from the diet. This is a formidable task for wheat flour is present in bread, many breakfast cereals, biscuits, cakes, pastries, sausage, macaroni and spaghetti; it is added to many soups, sauces and puddings and to some proprietary milk preparations.

Diet No. 15 sets out a sample menu for a day and on the same page there is a list of foods containing gluten which are forbidden, and a list of foods free of gluten (p. 569) which can be included in the diet. The Coeliac Society supplies a comprehensive list of gluten-free products available commercially.

Children who have suffered from coeliac disease for a short time respond to the gluten-free diet within a few weeks. Patients who have been ill for years, particularly adults, may have a badly damaged mucous membrane. They may require up to three to six months dietetic treatment before full recovery.

Anaemia is usually present. In more than 90 per cent of children it is due to iron deficiency. Folic acid deficiency is also usually present as shown by low plasma levels, but megaloblastic anaemia is uncommon. In adult coeliac disease, a megaloblastic anaemia due to folic acid deficiency is frequently present. Correction of both types of anaemia occurs coincidentally with the improvement in absorption which results from the gluten-free diet. Until this recovery is complete, it is advisable to give iron orally and in some cases parenterally to those patients with hypochromic anaemia, and folic acid by mouth. These preparations will cure not only anaemia but the glossitis and stomatitis which may also be present.

The remarkable success which results from the gluten-free diet in both children and adults suffering from coeliac disease can only be obtained if every trace of gluten is eliminated from the diet.

Once the diagnosis has been firmly established, it is recommended that every patient stays on a gluten-free diet for life, because of the risk of the disease recurring or of malignant disease arising if there is a return to a normal diet (Barry et al., 1974; McCrae et al., 1975). These risks have not yet been and may never be stated in accurate quantitative terms, but tragic cases occur of patients who, after giving up the diet, develop severe osteomalacia or die of one of the complications of the disease. If a patient returns to a normal diet and finds that he remains well, he may decide that the benefit from eating normal foods outweighs the risks of further disease. Such cases should be seen at yearly intervals and examined carefully for clinical and biochemical evidence of the return of the disorder.

Tropical sprue
Sprue is the name which the Dutch in Java gave to a tropical disease in which the presenting features are sore mouth, fatty diarrhoea and associated secondary manifestations of undernutrition and malnutrition. The cause is unknown.

Although delayed and defective absorption of fat is the abnormality most easily recognised, the absorption of water, electrolytes, glucose, vitamins and minerals is also impaired. These defects are associated with atrophy of the jejunal villi, which is a non-specific change similar to that seen in gluten enteropathy.

Sprue is a serious disease, and without proper medical and dietary care may prove fatal. Remissions and relapses are common. With proper treatment the majority of patients make a full recovery and seldom relapse, particularly if they leave the tropics. Nevertheless a few fail to respond to all forms of therapy and become chronic invalids.

Treatment
The principles of treatment are as follows: (1) rest in bed; (2) the administration of vitamins and minerals, if there is evidence of a deficiency, e.g. the vitamin B group (especially folic acid) for glossitis, stomatitis and megaloblastic anaemia, and vitamin K (if a haemorrhagic state is present); calcium and vitamin D for hypocalcaemia and tetany; iron for anaemia; (3) the prescription of diet which is mechanically non-irritating, high in protein and low in fat and carbohydrate, as originally recommended by Hamilton Fairley. Diet No. 11 is suitable for a case of moderate severity. For the few cases which fail to respond to the above measures, improvement usually follows the administration of a wide-spectrum antiobiotic such as tetracycline, 1 g daily by mouth.

Epidemiology and aetiology
Sprue was a common disease amongst Europeans in India and the Far East, but those in Africa were not affected. Many cases occurred during World War II but since then incidence has declined and it is now uncommon. Many studies failed to identify either an infective agent or a dietary toxin (Strong, 1942) and the cause was, and remains, a mystery.

Although the full picture of sprue and, especially the severe steatorrhoea, is seldom seen in natives of the topics, intestinal malabsorption is common and this is now discussed.

Tropical malabsorption
Patients with intermittent chronic diarrhoea who are underweight and anaemic are commonly seen in the tropics. Though the symptoms are usually mild, severe secondary malnutrition may occur which can be fatal. At postmortem marked atrophy of the small intestine is seen. This condition occurring in the indigenous population resembles sprue as seen in Europeans in many ways, but a sore mouth and tongue and steatorrhoea, which are such prominent features in sprue, are much less evident. Biopsy studies on apparently healthy people in several tropical countries have shown villi in the jejunal mucosa to be blunted and shortened with apparent reduction in the absorptive surfaces (Falaiye, 1971). It is suggested that a **tropical enteropathy** is common and may often be subclinical.

The cause is unknown. Many patients have suffered from attacks of dysentery, malaria and other tropical diseases, but the diarrhoea is not usually associated with severe, recent infections. Examinations of the faeces often shows a number of protozoal and helminth parasites. The significance of these is uncertain but opinion is growing that *Strongyloides stercoralis*, a nematode worm, and *Giardia lamblia*, a flagellated protozoa, may be responsible for malabsorption by mechanisms at present unknown. The plasma albumin is often low, perhaps due to increased loss of protein in the faeces. Anaemia may be due to defective absorption of iron and folic acid and not uncommonly of both.

When the symptoms are not severe the diarrhoea may cease and the patient's general condition improve greatly after a few days in hospital on a good diet, with deworming, the treatment of any identified infections and supplements of iron and folate. Some patients do not respond to these simple measures and the diarrhoea persists. The intestinable atrophy is then irreversible and the prognosis poor.

Chronic pancreatitis and failure of bile secretion due to liver disease are also important causes of the malabsorption syndrome in the tropics. Cook (1974 and 1977) reviews the different causes and discusses nomenclature and the problem of whether sprue is a definable pathological entity.

Carbohydrate intolerance

Deficiencies of disaccharidases in the brush border of the intestinal mucosa occur as both genetic and acquired disorders and give rise to failure of absorption and chronic diarrhoea. The clinical features are discussed by McMichael (1975) and the biochemical defects by Dahlquist and Asp (1975). Congenital deficiency of sucrase and maltase is rare but lactase deficiency is not uncommon.

Lactose intolerance

Infants and young children with protein-energy malnutrition often tolerate milk poorly and occasionally this occurs in an otherwise healthy infant. This is due to a failure of the mucosal cells of the small intestine to produce the enzyme lactase; as a result lactose passes unchanged into the large intestine where it is fermented by the bacterial flora with the production of loose stools containing lactic acid. Deficient lactase activity occurs under three circumstances. First, there is the rare congenital lactase deficiency which is inherited and gives symptoms shorly after birth. Secondly, there is the very common racial–ethnic form which affects a majority of the world's population. In Asians and many Africans (Kretchmer, 1972; Cook, 1973) the enzyme disappears at various times between infancy and adult life in most people, as is the case in all other mammals. Symptoms of lactose intolerance are usually mild or absent unless large amounts are taken such as half a litre of milk, which contains 25 g of lactose. In most Caucasians and in some African tribes, mostly Hamitic, who traditionally keep dairy herds and drink milk, the enzyme persists into adult life. Lactase cannot be induced in adults who have lost the enzyme (Gilat *et al.*, 1972) and the world distribution of lactase in adults is thought to be the result of natural selection. The third cause of lactase deficiency, only of importance in populations who retain their lactase and consume milk regularly, is disease of the small intestinal mucosa.

Tolerance is tested by giving 50 g of lactose and measuring the response of the blood glucose, a flat curve indicating intolerance, and by observing if the test dose causes any intestinal disturbance. An alternative method is to measure the breath hydrogen. The usual breath hydrogen is up to 20 p.p.m. Lactose passing into the colon results in the production of increased hydrogen in the breath in subjects who do not have lactase activity. Confirmation of the absence of lactase can be obtained by a jejunal biopsy and measuring the lactase activity directly. The reason why people with lactase deficiency can often tolerate moderate intakes of milk fairly well is that there are three lactase enzymes. It is the brush border lactase which disappears, but two other, less active, enzymes persist in the lysosomes and cytoplasm.

Enthusiasm for milk and milk diets should be tempered by the knowledge that many people cannot tolerate large quantities of lactose, in whom it may cause unpleasant digestive symptoms.

Short bowel syndromes

With improvements in surgical technique and aftercare, there are now many patients who have survived a massive resection of the small bowel for Crohn's disease, intestinal ischaemia or other cause. Nearly all have diarrhoea or a steatorrhoea with other features of the malabsorption syndrome. Because of the limited area for absorption, patients frequently have to be maintained on a restricted diet of easily assimilable foods. Artificial diets providing energy in the form of casein hydrolysate, sucrose and MCT are often of benefit and may promote weight gain. Diarrhoea may be due to irritation by unabsorbed bile salts and is relieved by cholestyramine, an anion exchange resin which binds the excessive bile salts in the intestine.

Radiation injury

Radiotherapy, particularly for carcinoma of the uterus and vagina, may damage the ileum and large intestine. Injury to the mucosa and the formation of sinuses and fistula may lead to malabsorption. The folic acid antagonist methotrexate and other drugs used in tumour chemotherapy may also damage the intestinal mucosa and commonly cause diarrhoea.

Intestinal obstruction

Intestinal obstruction may arise in many different ways. It is essential to decide in every case whether the cause of the obstruction is mechanical or due to paralysis of the intestinal muscle (paralytic ileus), as treatment in each type is entirely different. It is also important to determine whether the obstruction is high, i.e. in the jejunum or upper ileum, or low, i.e. in the lower ileum or colon, and whether strangulation of the bowel has occurred.

The common causes of mechanical obstruction are external hernias, volvulus, tumours of the colon, bands or adhesions due to previous inflammatory disease or operation and, in children, intussusception. Paralytic ileus is usually a consequence of peritonitis, resulting from any cause, e.g. a gastric or intestinal perforation or an abdominal operation.

The chief features of intestinal obstruction are vomiting, complete constipation and colicky pain which may be absent or slight in paralytic ileus. A serious loss of water and electrolytes results from the vomiting and from the stagnation of intestinal secretions in the dilated paralysed loops. The loss of fluid from the circulation from this latter source may be several litres in the 24 hours and this may lead to prerenal uraemia. The loss of potassium contributes to the apathy, mental confusion and muscular weakness, which usually follows intestinal obstruction.

Intestinal obstruction is always serious and so it should be treated only in a hospital where surgical and biochemical help are available. Immediate operation is required for the relief of mechanical obstruction, while it is strongly contraindicated in paralytic ileus. In the latter the distension of the paralysed gut must be treated by continuous suction through a tube passed into the stomach or jejunum, and continued until the bowel recovers from its paralysed state. In both types of obstruction the loss of fluid and electrolytes must be made good by appropriate infusions and intravenous feeding is often needed.

Chronic regional enteritis (Crohn's disease)

This is a chronic inflammatory disease which may arise anywhere along the alimentary tract but classically, the ileocaecal region is most frequently affected, then the colon and, less commonly, the small intestine. The inflammatory process is focal, with normal tissue between affected areas. It usually presents in early adult life with chronic ill-health, diarrhoea, abdominal pain, anaemia and weight loss. There may be chronic intermittent obstruction and even fistula to the skin, bladder or vagina. Systematic manifestations are arthritis, iritis, skin lesions (erythema nodosum) and liver disease.

Crohn first described the disease in 1933. It was apparently unknown before but it is now not uncommon and its prevalence appears to be still increasing. The aetiology is obscure and there is no evidence that any dietary factor is responsible. There is no specific treatment.

Diet is an important part of the management of the patient, who is usually unwell and off his food. He should be given a diet which provides sufficient energy, protein, vitamins and minerals. Good nutrition is essential in a disease which is characterised by malabsorption. A recurrent problem is that of intermittent obstruction. When obstruction occurs, the fruit and vegetables in the diet should be stopped immediately and omitted for up to a week after the attack has ended. It is not necessary to reduce intake of fruit and vegetables in intervals between attacks of obstruction.

When fistulae develop, then there is a case for placing the patient on a formula diet, or intravenous feeding. There are two arguments for this. First, it reduces losses of nutrients through the fistula. Secondly, it reduces potential allergenic materials in the intestinal tract. There is no doubt that those patients who have recurrent obstruction feel better for such a diet in the short term. It is yet to be proven that they benefit in the long term as most of them ultimately require surgical excision of the affected area of the gut. Before operation a few days on a formula diet cleanses the bowel and helps to restore nutrition.

Crohn's disease is a chronic, remitting disease; it is important to follow up all patients and assess regularly their state of nutrition by clincial examination and biochemical tests.

Ulcerative colitis

This is a common cause of chronic diarrhoea in temperate climates. There is blood and mucus in the stool due to an inflammatory reaction and ulcers in the mucosa of the large intestine. The ulcerations are superficial in contrast with Crohn's disease. Colitis is most frequently situated in the rectum and may extend as far as the caecum but this is uncommon. No cause is known, though there are many theories. No microbial pathogen has been identified but there is evidence in many cases of an autoimmune disorder.

The tendency of this disease to remit and relapse has become somewhat less frequent since the introduction of effective treatment with sulphasalazine. In the acute stage treatment is with corticotrophin and corticosteriods, and in the long term, sulphasalazine. The complication of toxic dilation is dangerous since it may be followed by perforation of the gut wall. Then the only treatment is to remove the entire colon and fashion an ileostomy. This operation is also recommended for some patients who have much diarrhoea and in whom conventional therapy has proved ineffective. Occasionally, patients who have had the entire bowel affected by colitis from their youth may develop cancer of the colon, but this is much less frequent since safe and effective drugs became available. Mild cases confined to the rectum may be treated by corticosteroid enemata. The very sick patient requires skilled nursing and medical care with replacement of fluid, electrolytes and blood. In general, a patient who is mobile yet passing several stools a day or who is under control with drugs, does not need dietary constraints or recommendations. He should eat a diet which is adequate in all usual ways. When there is associated diverticulosis or, curiously, constipation, the diet may have to be modified appropriately.

Diet and ileostomies and colostomies
After operation to the whole or part of the colon, the proximal part of the gut is sutured to the skin of the abdominal wall. This artificial stoma serves as a passage for the removal of unabsorbed material which has passed through the ileum.

Patients with an ileostomy can usually eat a normal or nearly normal diet fairly soon after operation, It is important that a patient who has been troubled by diarrhoea for a long period of time or has been ill from toxic dilation should be encouraged to eat exactly what he likes as soon as possible. Where patients find that particular items of food, for example rhubarb, alcohol, onions, lettuce, fried fish or soup cause trouble, that item should be removed from the diet. At some later time—say, after one or two weeks—this item of food can be returned to the diet to see whether this coincides with recurrence of symptoms. One problem is that of flatulence, and eating beans and onions may cause an unpleasant smell. Each patient must, however, judge for himself by trial and error. Because of the risk of water and sodium depletion, plenty of water and an increased salt intake are advisable. Some practical advice for patients is given by Bingham *et al.* (1977).

Colostomies are the result of a portion of the large bowel being brought up onto the surface and the faecal material passing out into a bag at that point. Usually such an operation is for cancer of the colon or for complicated diverticular disease. A low-residue diet is sometimes advised postoperatively but it is again important to achieve a normal diet rapidly. Some patients find loose stools may be caused by certain vegetables but this is variable and each patient must experiment for himself. After either an ileostomy or a colostomy it is important that the patient should never resort to eating or drinking less than he requires in an attempt to alter the functioning of the stoma.

Diverticulosis and diverticulitis
Diverticula are blind pouches which may be present in the oesophagus, stomach and small and large intestines. They may be congenital in origin or be acquired during life. They are found most frequently in the colon, and especially in the sigmoid section. The presence of diverticula is known as diverticulosis; when they are inflamed the condition is called diverticulitis. About up to 30 per cent of all persons over the age of 60 in Britain and America have diverticulosis, but only 5 or 10 per cent of these develop diverticulitis. Diverticulosis is less common in many of the countries of the Third World. Painter and Burkitt (1971) suggest this is because people in affluent societies eat too little fibre in their diets. If stagnation in diverticula is followed by infection, an inflammatory reaction occurs.

Repeated attacks of diverticulitis result in a chronically inflamed bowel, with narrowing of the lumen and pericolic adhesions.

Treatment
If symptomless diverticula are discovered during routine radiological examination, no treatment is required, except to advise the patient to include more dietary fibre in his diet. This should be on the same lines as the diet recommended for patients liable to constipation. The addition of wheat bran to an ordinary Western diet improves bowel habits (Painter *et al.*, 1972) and reduces colonic pressures in patients with diverticulosis (Findlay *et al.*, 1974).

Many cases of diverticulitis have periodic attacks of mild left-sided abdominal pain, fever and irregularity of the bowels. These should be treated medically by giving two tablespoons of bran three times a day to increase the bulk of the stools and eating a high fibre diet (Diet No. 18). When there are signs of active inflammation a broad-spectrum antibiotic, e.g. ampicillin, may be given. Pain may be relieved by giving antispasmodic drugs. Purgative should not be used.

A few cases require surgery because of obstruction, perforation or abscess formation, or for severe and extensive involvement of the intestine.

Irritable bowel syndrome
Mucomembranous colic, spastic constipation, spastic colon, 'mucous colitis' and nervous diarrhoea are probably all manifestations of the syndrome of the 'irritable bowel'. The term 'mucous colitis' is particularly unfortunate, as the condition is emphatically not an inflammation of the colon.

Nervous diarrhoea occurs in highly strung individuals and is characterised by the passage of loose stools after meals or as a result of some situation producing emotional strain. The sufferer may become so conscious of, and so obsessed with his condition that visits to a theatre or travel in a train without access to a toilet become impossible. The patient may appear tense with signs of general reactivity such as tachycardia and brisk reflexes and the descending colon may be tender and palpable. Examination by barium enema and sigmoidoscopy are normal.

All these disturbances of the function of the colon may be regarded as abnormal responses to emotional stimuli and so are psychosomatic disorders. The first essential is to see that the symptoms are not due to simple constipation and then to exclude an inflammatory disorder or cancer. Psychotherapy is needed; often simple reassurance and explanation of the nature of the symptoms is all that is required, but sometimes expert psychiatric treatment is required. The patient should be helped to develop regular bowel habits by following the regimen recommended for patients liable to constipation (see below). The regular use of drugs should be avoided. Circumstances may require the use of tranquillisers, laxatives or drugs to control diarrhoea, but these should be discontinued as soon as possible and the patient should not be allowed to become dependent on any drug.

Carcinoma of the colon and rectum

The causes are discussed in Chapter 60. The only treatment of value is resection of the tumour, preceded if necessary by colostomy for the immediate relief of colonic obstruction.

The diagnosis may be missed when there has been longstanding constipation or other chronic disease of the colon. It should always be considered when there is a change of bowel habits in a middle-aged or elderly person.

Constipation

Constipation is delay in passage of the faeces. Defaecation is a reflex action, stimulated by distension of the rectum with faeces, but it is under voluntary control and normally takes place only when time and circumstances are suitable. The presence of food in the stomach is a stimulus to a gastrocolic reflex which causes movements of the colon, and these may lead to faeces entering the rectum. The reflex usually occurs after the first meal of the day. In some people the presence of liquid in the stomach initiates the reflex and a drink on rising may be sufficient to stimulate defaecation. Some healthy people do not defaecate every day and a few do so only once or twice a week. They should not be considered constipated, and constipation should only be diagnosed when delay in defaecation causes discomfort and indigestion.

The two common causes of constipation are a small faecal bulk and persistent neglect of the call to defaecate. Many diseases are associated with constipation.

The daily faecal output ranges normally from 75 to 200 g of which 50 to 175 g is water. The bulk of the faeces is mainly water, and the amount of water depends on the amount of dietary fibre present and the capacity of the fibre to bind water. Low fibre diets predispose to constipation.

If the call to defaecate is persistently neglected, the reflex mechanism becomes less sensitive and constipation results. This is likely to happen when there are insufficient toilets or the toilet is cold, dirty or inaccessible. Children are readily put off from going to the toilet, and parents should see that they do. Going to the toilet should become a habit early in life.

Gastrointestinal diseases that commonly give rise to constipation are diverticulitis and the irritable bowel syndrome. Carcinoma of the colon and rectum sometimes present as constipation and, when a middle-aged or elderly person develops constipation for the first time, it is essential to make a thorough examination of the large bowel. Constipation is common in psychiatric disorders which cause depression. Any neurological disease causing lesions

in the lumbar cord may affect the reflex centres responsible for defaecation and lead to constipation.

Pregnant women and old people are often constipated. The reasons for this are not known. Perhaps the pressure of the gravid uterus on the colon may delay movements of the contents. In old people the sensitivity of the neuromuscular reflexes in the colon may be impaired or they may become less aware of the presence of faeces in the rectum.

When constipation is due to a low intake of dietary fibre, there is often pain in the left side of the abdomen along the line of the descending colon, and the faeces may be passed as hard pellets. Passage of faeces relieves the pain. When the call to defaecate has been repeatedly ignored, a mass of inspissated faecal matter may accumulate in the descending colon. Then fluid contents of the colon may run down the side of the mass and cause a watery diarrhoea.

Treatment

Diet. The intake of dietary fibre should be increased by eating whole cereals and increasing consumption of fruit and vegetables. The most important factor is the water-holding capacity of the fibre. Coarse bran has a capacity of 6 g water/g of fibre, but fine bran holds only 2–3 g water/g (Kirwan *et al.*, 1974). Patients should be encouraged to take coarse bran as a breakfast cereal. One tablespoonful of bran may be taken in the first week and two thereafter. The bran may be made more palatable by adding cooked fruits Fruits and vegetables whose fibre hold waters effectively are oranges, apples, carrots and the cabbage family. The diet should contain a helping of vegetables and two such fruits each day. These measures were shown to increase faecal weight and reduce transit time in subjects on controlled diets (Cummings *et al.*, 1978). As these fibres also bind metallic cations, faecal loss of these may be increased, but the danger of deficiency arising is slight. Diet No. 18 is suitable for patients with constipation and incorporates the advice above. When obesity is present, Diet No. 3 may be prescribed.

Correction of faulty habits. It is important to see that a young child goes to the toilet at a regular time each day. An adult may lose the habit from laziness, hurry or a lack of suitable accommodation. Once the reflex has been lost, it can only be regained by persistent and unhurried attempts to move the bowels at the same time each day. Worry, anxiety, fatigue and change of occupation may each effect the normal rhythm of evacuation, and a patient may need advice on his whole way of life. Sufferers from constipation have often been exhorted to drink more water and take more outdoor exercise; these are two healthy practices but may not relieve constipation.

Drugs. Many laxatives are available. Their continued use may lead to excessive losses of potassium, sodium and water in the faeces and is not recommended. Two mild laxatives that are recommended for short periods on occasions are lactulose and senna. Lactulose is a sugar which is not absorbed in the small intestine but passes to the colon where it may be partially broken down by bacteria. It reduces absorption of water from the colon by increasing the osmolality of its contents, and so increases the bulk of the faeces. Senna is a glycoside which is broken down in the small intestine to emodin; this is absorbed into the blood stream and stimulates the muscles of the colon for 6 to 12 hours after administration of the senna.

47. Diseases of the Liver, Biliary Tract and Pancreas

The liver is made up of lobules which each contain a small branch of the hepatic vein in the centre. These drain the blood into the systemic circulation via the inferior vena cava. At the periphery of the lobules the branches of the portal vein bring blood to the liver cells from the abdominal viscera. Running with the portal veins are branches of the bile duct and hepatic artery. The liver cells are arranged in columns radiating out from the hepatic vein at the centre of the lobule to the portal system.

The liver is responsible for some 25 per cent of the basal metabolism and is intimately concerned with the metabolism of carbohydrates, protein, fat and vitamins. Over 90 per cent of ingested ethanol is metabolised there. The liver inactivates many hormones and detoxicates exogenous drugs and poisons; it may also convert some non-toxic substances into toxic metabolites.

The production of bile and the excretion of bile acids and cholesterol are other essential functions. The common bile duct discharges its contents into the duodenum where they play an important part in digestion. On its way the duct passes through the head of the pancreas and receives the main pancreatic duct; this close relation is important as pancreatic disease may obstruct the common bile duct.

Three pathological changes may follow damage to the liver. **Fatty infiltration** is the deposition of droplets of fat in the cells. This process is completely reversible, but if the damage is severe or long-lasting it may be accompanied by necrosis followed by fibrosis. **Necrosis** or death of the cells may be slight and only involve part of the lobule, e.g. ischaemia due to heart failure causes central necrosis around the hepatic vein, or it may be massive and cause widespread destruction of the organ. Fibrosis is the end result of any liver damage which leads to necrosis and sometimes occurs in the absence of obvious preceding necrosis. It gives rise to the condition **cirrhosis.** This term was introduced by Laennec in 1826 and refers to the colour (Greek *kirros,* orange yellow) of nodules of regenerating liver cells between the fibrous strands. This capacity to regenerate permits survival even after severe liver damage. However, fibrous tissue contracts with time and then may obstruct either the flow of blood in the portal vein system causing portal hypertension, or the outflow of bile in the bile duct, leading to jaundice.

In experimental animals severe damage to the liver can be caused by deficient diets. In man the main known causes of acute liver damage are viral infections and exogenous poisons, particularly alcohol, but in many cases of liver cirrhosis there is no obvious cause.

Therapeutic diets have an important place in the treatment of symptoms arising from failure of liver function and diminished entry of bile into the duodenum.

EXPERIMENTAL LIVER DISEASE IN ANIMALS

A monograph by Himsworth (1950) described how rats fed on diets low in protein developed fatty infiltration and necrosis of the liver, and how both could go on to fibrosis and cirrhosis. The fatty infiltration was perhaps due to lack of methionine, which is necessary for the synthesis of choline. Choline was shown to be a lipotropic factor by its action in preventing the fatty infiltration of the liver which occurs in depancreatised dogs maintained on insulin (Best *et al.*, 1956). Massive necrosis of the liver only occurs if the diet is deficient in vitamin E as well as protein; protection against this effect of vitamin E deficiency may be provided by an adequate intake of selenium.

Monkeys fed on low protein diets also developed fatty infiltration of the liver (Ramalingaswami, 1972). This has been shown to be associated with a reduced capacity of the liver to synthesise and secrete lipoprotein. However, no fibrosis or cirrhosis developed in these monkeys. Indeed protein deficiency appeared to delay fibrous tissue proliferation not only in the liver, but in other tissues.

AETIOLOGY OF LIVER DISEASES

How far these conditions in experimental animals are analogous to human liver disease is uncertain. The fatty infiltration occurring in rats and monkeys on protein-deficient diets closely resembles that seen in kwashiorkor (p. 256). In each case the periportal areas of the lobules are mainly affected, and on a good diet the histological picture of the liver returns to normal. Truswell and Hansen (1969) provided evidence of reduced synthesis of β-lipoprotein by liver in children with kwashiorkor and this appears to be the major cause of the fatty infiltration. There is, however, no evidence that deficiency of choline causes any liver disease in man. The facts that phosphatidylcholine forms about 60 per cent of the plasma phospholipids in both healthy children and those with severe fatty infiltration of the liver due to kwashiorkor (Truswell *et al.*, 1966) suggests that there is no deficiency of lipotropic factor.

Cirrhosis of the liver. The prevalence of cirrhosis of the liver is not accurately known but Table 47.1 gives death rates in some countries. There is no reliable data from

412

Africa or Asia, but probably more patients with cirrhosis are seen in hospital wards in tropical countries than in Britain. Factors known to be responsible for cirrhosis are alcohol, toxic chemicals and previous infections; however, there is sometimes no obvious cause.

Table 47.1 Death from cirrhosis of the liver per 100 000 of the population in 1965

West Berlin	44.7	Denmark	7.5
France	34.2	Canada	6.4
Austria	26.9	Australia	4.8
Italy	22.9	Scotland	4.2
Spain	18.0	Holland	3.5
USA	12.8	England and Wales	2.9

Alcohol. In those countries where the death rate from cirrhosis is high, most of the cases occur in chronic alcoholics. There is no doubt that regular and continued consumption of alcohol either as wine or spirits may lead to cirrhosis. Since 90 to 95 per cent of ethyl alcohol is oxidised in the liver, it is not surprising that large doses are liable to lead to hepatic damage. Even a single large dose of alcohol given to a healthy volunteer can cause a significant rise in the plasma ornithine carbamoyl transferase which is almost a specific sign of liver damage. Lieber and Rubin (1968) showed that subjects with a history of alcoholism, but whose hepatic morphology had returned to normal, developed a fatty liver with the ingestion of alcohol either in addition to, or as isocaloric substitution for, carbohydrate in an otherwise adequate diet. Rubin and Lieber (1968) gave human volunteers alcohol in large doses (200 g) daily for 18 days; biopsy specimens of the liver showed fatty infiltration and changes in the ultrastructure of liver cells. They also gave 13 baboons large doses of alcohol for periods of nine months to four years, and two of the animals developed cirrhosis (Rubin and Lieber, 1974).

Although alcohol can play an important role in the production of fatty infiltration of the liver, there is less certainty about its relation to cirrhosis of the liver. Only a minority of heavy drinkers develop cirrhosis, while the structure and function of the liver in others may remain normal. The reasons for individual susceptibility are not all known. The daily intake and duration of drinking are important. The incidence rises steeply when the daily dose exceeds 80 g in men and 60 g in women (Péquignot, 1962) and women are more susceptible than men (Morgan and Sherlock, 1977). The probability of cirrhosis rises to 50 per cent after 22 years of heavy drinking (Thaler, 1977). A high prevalence of HLA type B40 antigen in patients with cirrhosis indicates a genetic predisposition (Bell and Nordhagen, 1978).

Toxic chemicals. Many drugs and industrial chemicals are known to cause cirrhosis, but they are responsible for only a small proportion of cases. Numerous substances present in plants can damage the liver. Herbs of the genus *Senecio* (ragwort) contain an alkaloid which damages the liver in experimental animals and in horses and cattle. Such herbs are frequently consumed as bush teas and herbal remedies in Jamaica, where there is strong evidence that they are responsible for a form of cirrhosis known as **veno-occlusive disease of the liver (VOD).** In this condition degenerative processes start around the hepatic veins in the centre of the lobule. Occlusion of the hepatic veins may occur owing to thickening of the intimal lining; venous drainage is thus impaired. Cirrhosis may follow with scarring distributed around the central veins in the lobules and its pathology is quite different from that of portal cirrhosis (Bras and Hill, 1956). Clinically VOD resembles other forms of cirrhosis and patients who are often children, present with hepatomegaly and ascites. It has a high mortality. Cases closely resembling, if not identical with VOD, have been reported in several African and Asian countries. In Afghanistan an outbreak arose after a drought when the wheat was contaminated with seeds of a heliotrope present in the crop as a weed (Mohabbat *et al.*, 1976).

Aflatoxins are known to have caused liver disease in domestic animals and it is probable that they are responsible for some cases of human cirrhosis. Methylazoxymethanol present in cycad nuts and nitrosamines present in fish, meat and cheese are other substances present in natural foods which are known to damage the liver. These substances are further discussed as possible causes of cancer of the liver in Chapters 25 and 60.

Infective agents. Schistosomiasis is the only important infection which commonly gives rise to cirrhosis. This occurs when eggs of *Schistosoma mansoni* are held up in the liver where they cause multiple granulomata and subsequent fibrosis.

Viral hepatitis causes acute degenerative changes in the liver and very occasionally cirrhosis has developed soon after an infection. However, soldiers who contracted the disease in epidemics during World War II and the Korean war have been shown not to have been at increased risk of developing cirrhosis. It is possible that a combination of kwashiorkor and viral hepatitis may be responsible for some cases of cirrhosis. **Indian childhood cirrhosis** is a condition in which there is fibrosis around the central veins of the lobules. Many cases closely resemble VOD and it has often been suggested that it is nutritional in origin. However, Chandra (1970) has found raised levels of immunoglobins in the disease and suggests that it is due to infection with a virus early in the life of a genetically predisposed child.

Malarial parasites may damage the liver, but are not known to be a direct cause of cirrhosis. However, in Gambia, Walters and Waterlow (1954) found that cirrhosis was most common in areas where malaria was hyperendemic.

Most cases of cirrhosis in tropical countries occur in

people who have been living on poor diets, which may have contained unknown plant toxins, and been exposed to a great number of infections. Ramalingaswami and Nayak (1970) have written an admirable account of malnutrition in relation to liver disease in India.

Cirrhosis of the liver arises in several rare inborn errors of metabolism, e.g. haemochromatosis, Wilson's disease, glycogen storage disease and galactosaemia.

JAUNDICE

Jaundice is due to an increase in the bilirubin content of the blood above the normal range of 3.4 to 13.6 μmol/l (0.2 to 0.8 mg/100 ml) of plasma. When the increase is slight (<34 μmol/l) it can often be detected only by plasma analysis, and biochemical jaundice is then said to exist. When the increase is greater, there is visible yellow colouration of the skin and the sclerae of the eyes, and the urine usually becomes dark yellow or brown; this is clinical jaundice.

Haemolytic jaundice
Excessive destruction of red blood cells results in increased bilirubin formation and anaemia. A healthy liver can handle a bilirubin load six times greater than normal before unconjugated bilirubin accumulates in the plasma. This accounts for the fact that except in the newborn, jaundice due to haemolysis is usually mild. Because the bilirubin is unconjugated it does not pass into the urine, but the urine contains urobilinogen. The condition may arise from congenital defects in the red cells which renders them unduly fragile (spherocytosis, sickle-cell anaemia, thalassaemia) or because of the action of extracorpuscular factors on the red cells. These include infections, drugs and red-cell antibodies as in incompatible blood transfusion.

Obstructive jaundice
This occurs when there is a block to the pathway between the site of conjugation of bilirubin in the liver cells and the entry of bile into the duodenum. Stasis occurs within the dilated bile ducts and canaliculi, and conjugated bilirubin is retained and enters the blood stream. The urine is darkly pigmented from conjugated bilirubin. The stools on the other hand are abnormally pale. Pruritis results from retention of bile salts.

Obstructive jaundice may be divided into two categories: (a) extrahepatic where there is obstruction in the main bile ducts, and (b) intrahepatic, where the lesions lie within the liver between the cells and the main bile ducts. The most common extrahepatic causes are impaction of gallstones in the common bile duct and carcinoma of the head of the pancreas or ampulla of Vater.

Hepatocellular jaundice
This is usually associated with damage to the liver cells by toxic or infective agents particularly viral hepatitis. This interferes with the uptake of bilirubin by the cells and also with its conjugation and excretion. In this form of jaundice the patient feels unwell, with anorexia often a prominent symptom. Jaundice is variable, but the stools are usually pale and the urine dark.

HEPATOCELLULAR DISEASE

Disease of the liver may arise as a result of damage to the liver cells (hepatocellular disease) or to the cells lining the biliary passages within the liver. Injury to the liver cells may cause acute, subacute or chronic hepatitis. In some cases chronic hepatitis may be attributable to previous acute disease; in others it arises insidiously and no history of an acute attack can be obtained.

Infections. The liver cells are particularly susceptible to invasion by the viruses responsible for infective hepatitis and yellow fever. The former is the most common cause of acute hepatitis. Bacteria (e.g. pyogenic cocci and in typhoid fever), protozoa (amoebic hepatitis) and spirochaetes (leptospirosis) may parasitise and provoke inflammatory reactions but do not invade the hepatocytes. Although there is no evidence that susceptibility to any of these diseases is increased by malnutrition, their hepatotoxic effects may be augmented by any preceding condition which leads to hepatic damage, e.g. protein deficiency or alcoholism. Viral hepatitis can occur in one of four forms. First, it may be so mild that it is not recognised clinically and can only be diagnosed by laboratory tests. Secondly, and this is the most common, the illness is of moderate severity. Complete recovery is the rule in the vast majority of such patients, but the time taken varies from a few days to many months. Thirdly, and very occasionally, the clinical course from the onset may be that of subacute or acute necrosis of the liver, death usually occurring within a few days or weeks. Fourthly, and again rarely, the final pathological result may be portal cirrhosis (chronic hepatitis).

Toxic agents. The adverse effects of drugs and other foreign compounds on the liver can be classified into several types.

Direct toxicity. This is dose-related. There is fatty change progressing to necrosis of hepatocytes. The causes include carbon tetrachloride, used as a solvent for dry cleaning and in industry, and heavy metals.

Hepatitis-like drug reactions. These are not related to dose or duration of exposure but to individual susceptibility. The picture resembles that of acute viral hepatitis. A number of drugs occasionally have this effect.

Hypersensitivity cholestasis. This only occurs in a small minority of individuals taking certain drugs, e.g. chlorpropamide and chlorpromazine. There is an obstructive type of jaundice with little disturbance of other hepatic functions.

Non-sensitivity cholestasis. This is the most benign of these conditions. There is intrahepatic cholestasis with no disturbance of other hepatic functions. It is caused by C_{17} alkyl derivatives of testosterone and rarely by oral contraceptives.

Liver cells have a remarkable regenerative capacity. Great improvement in liver function may occur spontaneously or consequent on treatment, even when there are widespread structural changes. Patients with severe ascites or hepatic coma have made remarkable recoveries. Hence treatment should be vigorous and persistent even although it is largely symptomatic. The course of parenchymal disease of the liver is so unpredictable that it is extremely difficult to assess the value of any therapeutic measures.

Acute hepatitis
There is no specific treatment for hepatitis due to viral infections. The patient should rest in bed until the jaundice has cleared. For amoebic liver abscesses and leptospirosis the administration of metronidazole and antibiotics respectively is indicated. For hepatitis due to poisoning with heavy metals, chelating agents such as penicillamine are of real value. In most cases good results can be expected from the well-tried programme of rest, abstinence from alcohol, and diet.

DIETETIC REGIMEN
In mild and moderately severe cases
Most patients suffer from nausea and lack of appetite. Hence meals should be well cooked and attractively served. Several small meals may be better tolerated than three large meals.

There is no evidence that the course of the disease is influenced by the fat content of the diet, but when jaundice is marked, fat and fatty foods are poorly tolerated. In addition, the absorption of fat from the intestine is impaired because of the lack of bile salts. Under these circumstances the intake of fat must be restricted temporarily to 20 to 50 g daily. Energy then has to be provided mainly from carbohydrate, but an ample intake of protein is indicated to prevent any possible adverse effect of protein malnutrition. Diets Nos. 10 and 11 are suitable. Fried foods and the articles of food likely to cause dyspepsia, listed in Diet No. 17, should be avoided. When the appetite has returned, milk and butter are usually well tolerated. Diet No. 1, with its high protein content, is suitable for convalescence.

Provided the patient is taking adequate amounts of fruit, vegetables and milk, there is no need to give supplements of any vitamin or mineral.

In severe cases
Loss of appetite and nausea are prominent features and may greatly complicate dietary treatment. When there is fever and intense distaste for food, it may only be possible to give the patient sweetened fruit drinks and to persuade him to eat small quantities of any food for which he has a fancy. For such patients, it is generally advisable to prescribe for a few days an entirely fluid diet of at least 2½ to 3 litres daily, given in small feeds at two-hourly intervals. If possible, 200 to 300 g of carbohydrate should be taken every day. Glucose polymers may be useful. If the condition of the patient is so grave that he can neither ingest nor retain sufficient fluid or nourishment, he should be treated by the measures described on page 417 for hepatic coma.

Prolonged cases
Recovery from the acute phase of an attack of hepatitis is usually rapid but sometimes there may be many weeks or even months before it is complete. The appetite during this stage often remains poor, particularly for fats and fried foods. The patient may be easily fatigued and the liver may remain enlarged and tender.

The same principles for dietary treatment as in the less severe forms of acute hepatitis apply: a generous diet high in energy and rich in protein and carbohydrate should be given. It is important to get the patient to eat. If he has been previously on a low fat diet, the fat intake should be gradually increased. Fried foods are best avoided until convalescence is complete. Well cooked and attractively served foods will do more to restore appetite than too great attention to the chemical composition of the diet. Diet No. 11 will be found satisfactory for the initial treatment of a case of moderate severity.

Alcohol tends to bring on attacks of nausea with abdominal discomfort and loss of appetite. For this reason physicians impose an absolute ban on alcohol during the acute and subacute stage and for 6 to 12 months after recovery.

Drugs
The value of corticosteroids is still uncertain, but in patients who show prolonged cholestasis prednisone, 30 mg/day, assists recovery.

Cirrhosis of the liver
Cirrhosis of the liver is a generic term applied to chronic diffuse liver disease of varied aetiology, characterised by destruction of liver cells, distortion of the normal lobular architecture with overgrowth of fibrous tissue and nodular regeneration of the cells. Three basic types have been described in the past:

1. Diffuse hepatic fibrosis (portal or Laennec's cirrhosis).

2. Postnecrotic scarring, which occurs in livers which have been the seat of massive necrosis.
3. Biliary cirrhosis, which occurs as a result of biliary obstruction and superimposed infection, i.e. cholangitis and cholangiohepatitis.

The modern tendency is to use a purely descriptive classification according to size of nodules, i.e. macronodular, micronodular and intermediate. This avoids any hypothesis of causation.

The epidemiology and aetiology have already been discussed. In portal cirrhosis, which is much the most common type, a fine fibrosis starts around the portal tract; a previous attack of acute hepatitis may or may not have been evident clinically. The condition passes imperceptibly into chronic cirrhosis of the liver. When cirrhosis of the liver has advanced to a late stage, there are associated signs of malnutrition—loss of flesh, a low plasma albumin, oedema and sodium retention. Obstruction of the portal veins leads to congestion of abdominal viscera and ascites, and spider naevi.

The dietetic treatment of patients with hepatic cirrhosis is much more likely to be successful if they have previously been taking a poor diet, as occurs frequently in underdeveloped countries, and in alcoholics, than when the disorder is the end result of infective or toxic agents and the patient has been eating well.

There is no specific treatment for hepatic cirrhosis except for the small minority of cases that are caused by an inborn error of metabolism, such as haemochromatosis, Wilson's disease and galactosaemia. A high energy, high protein intake is desirable. This may be difficult to achieve in the late stages of the disease on account of the poor appetite or when jaundice is present as the fat intake must then be reduced. The protein intake can be supplemented by 20 to 40 g of Casilan or Lonalac daily, which may be given in milk, soups or ice cream (p. 445). A high protein diet carries the risk of precipitating encephalopathy (p. 417). Vitamin supplements may be required for specific deficiencies, e.g. vitamin K for the bleeding tendency due to hypoprothrombinaemia. Alcohol should be forbidden entirely. If the patient can take and digest a high energy, high protein diet as indicated above, temporary improvement can be anticipated in most cases. When the condition is due to alcoholism, if the damage is not too far advanced, excellent therapeutic results can confidently be expected provided the patient accepts strict abstinence. The treatment of the principal complications, namely ascites, portal hypertension, and hepatic coma, requires to be considered separately.

Ascites. This is the accumulation of fluid in the peritoneal cavity. The three principal factors responsible are (1) portal hypertension and lymphatic obstruction secondary to intrahepatic fibrosis, (2) reduced osmotic pressure of the plasma due to a failure of the liver to synthesise plasma albumin and (3) increased retention of sodium. One cause of this is excessive renal tubular absorption of sodium consequent on an increased production of aldosterone and the reduced capacity of the liver to inactivate it.

The ascitic fluid often amounts to 10 litres and contains protein in concentrations of 10 to 20 g/1. Tapping the abdomen to remove the ascitic fluid (paracentesis) is not desirable except for diagnostic purposes. It depletes the body of plasma proteins and carries a risk of introducing infection. It is rarely necessary with modern treatment which consist of giving a diet rich in protein and low in sodium, and also diuretics to increase the urinary output of sodium and fluid. A wide variety of diuretics have been used with success. With all of them there is a danger of electrolyte imbalance. Overdosage may lead to sodium deficiency and also to potassium depletion. The latter can be prevented by giving a potassium supplement.

The construction of a high protein diet which is also low in sodium is difficult because the protein-rich foods (meat, eggs, dairy products) have a high sodium content. Diets No. 7 or 12 are suitable. The former provides a high protein intake from a variety of sources but contains more sodium than Diet No. 12. The latter can be increased in protein by adding a proprietary preparation of casein such as Casilan, which is practically free from sodium. Fluid need not be restricted. The assessment of control of ascites and oedema is best made by weighing the patient.

When the response to the above treatment is poor, spironolactone, which antagonises the action of aldosterone on the distal renal tubular cells, is worthy of trial. It is particularly effective when given with chlorothiazide, because spironolactone reduces the absorption of sodium from the distal and chlorothiazide from the proximal renal tubules. Another advantage of spironolactone is that it reduces the increased excretion of potassium caused by chlorothiazide.

As a result of these measures the accumulation of ascitic fluid decreases and may finally cease, and the level of plasma albumin usually increases. Thereafter the sodium intake can be gradually increased, but the patient should not add table salt to his food. Salt-rich foods should also be avoided (p. 566).

Portal hypertension. This frequently leads to the production of varicose veins in the lower end of the oesophagus and in the stomach. From these severe haemorrhage may arise, which often proves fatal. Portal hypertension may be reduced by the natural development of anastomotic communications between the portal and systemic circulations which enable the portal venous blood to short-circuit the liver. Surgical portacaval shunts may precipitate encephalopathy and may not lengthen the life of patients, who die from hepatocellular failure. This operation should thus be performed only in carefully selected cases. The dietetic treatment of portal hypertension is that of the underlying disorder of the liver as already described. Iron should be given for the hypochromic anaemia which results from haemorrhage from the oesophageal and gastric varices, and repeated blood transfusions when blood loss is large.

Hepatic encephalopathy

This may develop in acute or subacute hepatocellular failure or more frequently as a late feature of cirrhosis of the liver. The clinical features are disordered sleep rhythm, restlessness or drowsiness, as well as impaired intellectual function, confusion, stupor and, in severe cases, coma. A slow 'flapping' tremor and a characteristic odour to the breath (foetor hepaticus) are diagnostic signs.

The provision of adequate nutrition during this emergency may be very difficult because there is usually a marked loss of appetite, and nausea and vomiting readily occur. In addition the decision in regard to the degree and duration of restriction of protein is obviously a difficult one since too much protein precipitates hepatic coma, while too little may prolong the illness.

There has long been controversy of the cause, in metabolic terms, of the encephalopy in liver failure. Formerly the view was that ammonia and amines produced from dietary amino acids by intestinal bacteria were not adequately removed from the portal circulation; increased amounts reached the arterial circulation and so impaired the function of the brain. The concentration of NH_4 in arterial blood, and of glutamine in the CSF is often raised when there is liver failure, but it is unlikely that this is the sole cause of the cerebral disorders. The pattern of amino acids in the blood is altered. Concentrations of aromatic amino acids and methionine, normally metabolised in the liver, are raised and of branch chain amino acids, metabolised mainly in muscle, lowered. Entry of aromatic amino acids into brain cells may be facilitated. These amino acids are precursors of noradrenaline and 5-hydroxytryptamine, neurotransmitters in the central nervous system. The raised availability of these amino acid precursors may be responsible for the cerebral disorder (Munro et al., 1975).

Treatment

For energy needs it is necessary to rely on carbohydrates. It is important to avoid starvation as this involves a danger of hypoglycaemia because reserves of body fat and protein may not be adequately metabolised by the diseased liver. It is also necessary to provide ample fluids and to preserve electrolyte balance which may be gravely upset, especially if vomiting is severe.

All dietary protein is stopped and 6.2 MJ (1600 kcal) daily is given in the form of glucose or glucose polymer drinks flavoured with fruit juice by mouth in small feeds at one-hour or two-hour intervals. If the patient's level of consciousness does not permit this, intravenous feeding with glucose solutions must be given. Fructose causes severe acidosis and should not be used as an energy source

in these patients. The amount of saline used as carrier for the carbohydrate should be adjusted daily, taking into account the urinary output and the state of electrolyte balance. A preparation of B vitamins and ascorbic acid is added to the fluid or given by intramuscular injection. Even in the absence of dietary protein the bacteria in the gut appear to contribute to the clinical picture, probably by producing toxic nitrogenous compounds. Because of this, oral neomycin, 1.0 g six-hourly, is recommended to kill off the major intestinal bacterial flora. Lactulose, a non-absorbable sugar which is fermented in the colon producing lactic acid, has been used with success and may constitute the basis for the supposed value of yogurt. Both of these measures probably act by increasing lactobacilli in the colon at the expense of Gram-negative bacilli which possess urease and produce ammonia.

As soon as signs of recovery from hepatic failure are noted, e.g. a reduction in the degree of mental confusion or apathy 20 g of protein should be added to the diet. If there is no mental deterioration, further additions of protein to the diet may be tried; 500 ml of skimmed milk contains approximately 20 g of protein and this can be given in small feeds several times a day as a supplement to the glucose drinks. It may be possible to increase the consumption of skimmed milk to 1.5 l/day which provides about 60 g of protein. The ideal is for the patient to take a balanced convalescent diet with sufficient protein to prevent deterioration of hypoalbuminaemia. However, in the late stages of cirrhosis it is usually necessary to keep the patient indefinitely on a restricted protein intake (40 to 50 g), otherwise mental symptoms tend to recur.

Various methods are under trial for tiding the patient over the acute phase of hepatic failure when there seems to be a chance of quick liver regeneration. Exchange transfusion and temporary bypass through animal livers are in use in some special centres. The immediate results are sometimes quite remarkable but fatal relapse follows unless spontaneous liver regeneration occurs. The latter is difficult to predict.

Biliary cirrhosis

Disease of the liver may also be caused by damage to the cells which line biliary ductules within the hepatic lobules and the interlobular branches of the bile ducts. These small biliary vessels (cholangioles) may be damaged by stagnation of the bile due to obstruction lower down in the biliary passages; they may become infected with intestinal bacteria or damaged directly, either by drugs or as part of an autoimmune reaction. Cholangitis arising in these ways may progress after months or years to cholangiohepatitis and biliary cirrhosis. The autoimmune variety (primary biliary cirrhosis) occurs most commonly in middle-aged women. Pruritus may be intense and often precedes the jaundice.

Jaundice is a characteristic feature and depends on the

degree of biliary obstruction. The liver is usually uniformly enlarged and smooth and the spleen is seldom palpable. Flatulence and nausea may be present. The infection which may also involve the gall-bladder causes fever, often in recurrent attacks with rigors and prostration and associated with upper abdominal pain, fluctuating jaundice and leucocytosis. Months or years of infection and obstruction may elapse before biliary cirrhosis becomes established. Ascites and the features of portal hypertension may be absent throughout the whole course of the disease. In the late stages due to the absence of bile salts from the small bowel, the clinical picture is that of a severe form of the malabsorption syndrome with steatorrhoea.

Prevention and treatment

Biliary cirrhosis can be prevented in a proportion of cases by prompt surgical treatment of obstructive jaundice. When no obstruction to the extrahepatic bile ducts is found at operation, treatment is unsatisfactory and largely symptomatic. Patients usually die within five years from hepatic failure severe pruritus may be treated with the anion exchange resin, cholestyramine, which adsorbs bile salts in the intestine, thus eliminating these in the faeces and producing a fall in the level of bile salts in the plasma. The dose of cholestyramine should be the smallest which controls pruritus since it increases the amount of fat in the faeces. The principles of dietetic therapy recommended for portal cirrhosis should be followed, with the qualification that fat is usually less well tolerated. Medium chain triglycerides containing C_8 and C_{10} fatty acids are digested and absorbed quite well in the absence of bile salts.

If jaundice persists, fat soluble vitamins may not be absorbed from the intestine. Intramuscular injection of vitamin K_1 (10 mg), of vitamin A (30 mg) and vitamin D (2.5 mg) should be given every four weeks as maintenance therapy. If, however, hypoprothrombinaemia has developed as evidenced by bruising or bleeding or if signs of osteomalacia or xerophthalmia are present, daily or weekly supplements of the fat soluble vitamins must be given by intramuscular injection. Calcium supplements are essential. Bile salt therapy with sodium glycocholate and taurocholate or dehydrocholic acid are often prescribed to relieve the dyspepsia associated with steatorrhoea but the results are far from satisfactory.

DISEASES OF THE GALL-BLADDER AND BILE DUCTS

The function of the gall-bladder and bile ducts is to concentrate, store and deliver bile into the duodenum at appropriate times to assist in the process of digestion; hormonal and nervous factors play a part in this process. The stimulus for this activity is the entry of food into the small intestine; this causes the mucosa of the duodenum and jejunum to secrete a hormone, cholecystokinin, which is carried in the blood to the gall-bladder and causes it to contract. Fats and foods rich in fats are especially effective for this purpose. The gall-bladder and the sphincter of Oddi appear to be reciprocally innervated. Thus vagal stimulation causes contraction of the gall-bladder and relaxation of the sphincter, while stimulation of the sympathetic nerves produces the reverse effects. Disturbance of these reciprocal effects and of the hormonal mechanism may be responsible for initiating both organic disease and functional disorders of the biliary tract. The latter include biliary achalasia (failure in relaxation of the sphincter of Oddi), biliary dyskinesia (spasm of the sphincter of Oddi) and bilious vomiting associated with such conditions as migraine.

Gall-stones (cholelithiasis)

The bile is concentrated in the gall-bladder, and when it becomes supersaturated, gall-stones are likely to form. These are of various types. By far the most common are mixed stones composed of cholesterol, bile pigment and various calcium salts, including calcium palmitate (Sutor and Wooley, 1971). In the centre there is often a protein nidus from which bacteria may sometimes be isolated, suggesting an infective origin. They are always multiple and their surfaces are faceted. Much rarer are multiple small stones of almost pure bile pigment and very occasionally a single large stone is almost entirely cholesterol.

Gall-stones are found in about 20 per cent of autopsies and are more common in women than men and in fat people than in thin. Advancing age, repeated pregnancies and a sedentary life are claimed to be contributing factors. Prevalence is higher in some ethnic groups, notably the Pima Indians in Arizona; in nearly 50 per cent of adults stones can be detected by cholecystography (Sampliner *et al.*, 1970). A traditional mnemonic about the predisposition of fair women has not been confirmed and gall-stones are not associated with a high plasma cholesterol.

Formation of cholesterol gall-stones depends on the relative concentrations in the bile of cholesterol and its solubilising agents, lecithin (phospholipid) and conjugated bile salts; these keep cholesterol in a micellar soluble phase but, if the cholesterol concentration is too high, the bile is 'lithogenic.' The lithogenic tendency can be assessed by analysing samples of bile obtained by peroral duodenal intubation or at operation. Obese patients with gall-stones secrete bile with a high concentration of cholesterol (Grundy *et al.*, 1974). It is likely that dietary factors influence bile lipid composition in man as they are known to do in different ways in several animal species (Dam, 1971), but there are no consistent human data, apart from the findings in obesity.

It has been estimated that at a given point of time half the people who have gall-stones have no symptoms. As many of the patients with silent stones found accidentally eventually require treatment for either cholecystitis or obstructive jaundice, prophylactic surgery is often advisable.

Administration of the bile acid, chenodeoxycholic acid, dissolves the stones in many cases. It is useless if the stones are calcified and so radio-opaque, and it is contraindicated in women during their reproductive life. Chenodeoxycholic acid is given in gelatin-coated capsules in a dose of 1000 mg/day. It is absorbed in the distal ileum and enters the enterohepatic circulation. In the liver it may reduce secretion of cholesterol or increase secretion of bile salts, but its exact mode of action on the stones is not known. It may be six to 12 months before the stones are dissolved.

The fact that the composition of the bile can be altered by giving chenodeoxycholic acid suggests that it might also be changed beneficially by dietary fibre which also influences the enterohepatic circulation. Future work may provide a dietary means of preventing stones forming and of dissolving those already present.

Acute cholecystitis

Acute cholecystitis is rarely due primarily to infection of the gall-bladder but almost always occurs in association with obstruction to the cystic duct or neck of the gall-bladder, upon which infection is usually superimposed. In most cases gall-stones are the cause of obstruction.

Treatment

Cholelithiasis with accompanying cholecystitis is primarily the province of the surgeon who usually prefers to postpone operation until the acute infection has subsided. The treatment at the onset is that of any acute febrile illness. The patient should be in bed and given suitable analgesics and antibiotics. Heat should be applied to the gall-bladder region and ample fluids given intravenously if the patient is vomiting. So long as the gall-bladder is acutely inflamed, it is advisable to keep the organ at rest as far as possible. To this end fat, which causes contraction of the gall-bladder, should be excluded from the diet. For acute cases an entirely fluid diet of at least 2 to 3 litres daily, given in small feeds at hourly or two-hourly intervals is advisable for a few days.

When the condition settles down. as it usually does within two or three days, clear soups, beef tea, milk, fruit jellies, and cereals may be added, and the diet is rapidly built up to normal or to that recommended for chronic cholecystitis (see below). After recovery if radiographs of the abdomen or cholecystography show gall-stones or a non-functioning gall-bladder, cholecystectomy should be advised some weeks after the inflammation has subsided.

Chronic cholecystitis

Pending the decision to remove the gall-bladder or if for any reason operation is contraindicated, dietetic treatment along the following lines should be given. The principles are the same for the small minority of cases without stones as for the majority who have them.

Foods which precipitate or aggravate the symptoms should be avoided. These are likely to include cooked meats rich in fat and fried foods. Since biliary stasis predisposes to the formation of gall-stones, a moderate intake of uncooked fat, e.g. in milk, butter and cream cheese is permitted, and may promote drainage of the gall-bladder. Eggs may be permitted in moderation, if they do not cause symptoms. The diet should be bland and contain adequate protein.

Care should be taken to avoid large meals and indigestible articles of food because of the ease with which dyspepsia occurs, and ample quantities of fluids should be taken first thing in the morning, last thing at night and between meals. If, as is frequently the case, the patient is obese, Diet No. 3 should be prescribed.

Obstructive jaundice

When jaundice is due to obstruction of the main bile passages by stone, stricture or malignant disease, the liver cells are, at least for some time, relatively uninjured and hence if the obstruction is removed in time, no permanent cellular damage occurs. Nevertheless, it is advisable to ensure that the patient takes an ample supply of carbohydrate and protein of good quality in the form of skimmed milk and skimmed milk powder. This is particularly desirable as a preoperative measure to prevent the toxic effects of general anaesthesia. Since the flow of bile is reduced, a low intake of fat is indicated.

Laparotomy should be carried out in all cases if the jaundice does not subside within a few weeks, unless the history and biochemical tests strongly suggest that the patient has acute hepatocellular disease with superimposed intrahepatic obstruction.

Diet No. 10 is suitable for most cases of obstructive jaundice. When the patient's appetite improves Diet No. 11 can be used. If the obstruction is suddenly produced, as by impaction of a gall-stone, colic, vomiting and fever may temporarily necessitate a fluid diet, as for acute cholecystitis. If jaundice continues for more than a few days supplements of the fat-soluble vitamins A, D and K should be given parenterally. In long-continued obstructive jaundice there is a risk of osteomalacia developing and an oral supplement of calcium should be given. If the obstructive jaundice cannot be relieved and continues for many months or years, the condition terminates in hepatocellular failure.

DISEASES OF THE PANCREAS

The external secretion of the pancreas may be impaired by inflammatory disease and this leads to failure of digestion and absorption.

Pancreatic juice is an alkaline secretion containing sodium bicarbonate, other salts and the main digestive enzymes, lipase, amylase and trypsin. The flow of pancreatic juice reaches a maximum between one to two hours after a meal. Secretion is stimulated partly by nervous mechanisms acting through the vagus nerves but chiefly in response to the hormones, secretin and pancreozymin, which are formed when acid chyme comes into contact with the mucosal cells of the duodenum. The volume of pancreatic juice secreted daily is probably about 2 litres, which may contain 300 mmol of sodium and up to 40 g protein, most of which is absorbed.

Acute pancreatitis

This is a serious disorder which may lead to haemorrhagic necrosis of the pancreas, peritonitis and death. It usually occurs in middle-aged and elderly persons. Its aetiology is far from clear but in at least 60 per cent of cases there is an association with biliary tract disease. In some of these cases obstruction by gall-stones or oedema or spasm of the sphincter of Oddi causes a reflux of bile along the pancreatic duct. This activates the pancreatic enzymes which results in autodigestion of the cells and blood vessels of the pancreas. As a consequence a serosanguinous exudate is liberated into the peritoneal cavity with the production of peritonitis and hydrolysis of the fat in the omentum and mesentery. About a quarter of the cases give a history of alcoholism in Britain, but this proportion is much higher in some other countries.

The main symptom is the sudden onset of agonising pain in the epigastrium which may radiate to the back; it may follow a heavy meal or an excess of alcohol. Nausea and vomiting are frequently present. Moderate fever occurs and jaundice may develop. In addition there are signs of peritonitis and profound shock.

The plasma amylase rises and when activity is above 7500 Somogyi units/1 a diagnosis of acute pancreatitis is virtually certain.

Treatment

When the diagnosis of acute pancreatitis has been established, medical management consists of the relief of pain and the control of shock,. Continuous gastrointestinal suction is essential to reduce vomiting and distension and to rest the pancreas by preventing the initiation of pancreatic secretory mechanism by acid gastric secretion. Atropine and propanthaline bromide should also be given, Antibiotics should be administered to prevent secondary infection of damaged tissues.

When the acute stage has settled down, diet therapy as for chronic pancreatitis should be instituted and surgery considered.

Subacute recurrent pancreatitis

In some parts of the world recurrent attacks of subacute pancreatitis are common and are usually associated with intermittent heavy drinking. Unless the subject abstains completely these attacks, any one of which may be fatal if not properly treated, lead to a final picture of inanition, diabetes and malabsorption. With abstinence the prognosis is good. Relapsing subacute pancreatitis may sometimes be due to an undiagnosed stone in the common bile duct.

Chronic pancreatitis

This may follow repeated attacks of acute or subacute pancreatitis or be associated with chronic inflammation of the biliary tract or with the penetration of a chronic duodenal ulcer into the pancreas. In these conditions fibrosis is marked between the lobules of acinar tissue and destroys the epithelial cells. The islet cells are spared for a long time. In many cases the pathogenesis is not understood. The disease occurs most commonly in males in the fifth and sixth decades and is often associated with alcoholism.

Clinical features

The main features are recurrent attacks of mid-abdominal and lumbar pain, often relieved by a crouching position, lasting for three or four days and accompanied by nausea, vomiting and pyrexia. In milder cases there may be chronic diarrhoea with undigested fat and muscle fibres in the stools and loss of weight may be prominent. The association of these findings and a diabetic type of glucose tolerance curve is virtually diagnostic. Plain radiographs of the abdomen may show a fine stippled calcification of the pancreas. Plasma amylase estimations are of little value. There may be a slowly progressive and painless jaundice with enlargement of the liver, and a history of chronic cholecystitis and gall-stones is not uncommon. Ultimately the full picture of the malabsorption syndrome and diabetes may develop.

Treatment

Initially this is medical. If exacerbations of pain, colic and vomiting occur, the measures described under acute pancreatitis should be instituted. Alcohol must be prohibited. This is of the greatest therapeutic importance. The dietetic treatment of the diarrhoea and loss of weight may be difficult; defects in the digestion of carbohydrate and protein are usually present in addition to failure of fat digestion. Nevertheless it is mainly from carbohydrate and protein that the diet has to be constructed, because the principal defect is a failure of fat digestion. Fried and greasy food and foods rich in fats should be prohibited. Only skimmed milk should be given. Small helpings of chicken, white fish or very lean meat are allowed with any vegetable (except fried potatoes). Fruits (fresh or stewed), jams, jelly and sugar should be taken plentifully. Diet No. 11, which contains 45 g of fat daily, is suitable for the initial treatment of cases of moderate severity. If the patient is not able to take this diet it may be necessary to omit for a few days some of the solid foods and give extra protein; Casilan or Lonalac, preparations of dried milk proteins, can be added to the milk or other beverage. Medium-chain fatty acids may also be given. Supplements of the fat-soluble vitamins and calcium should be given to all cases with a long history of steatorrhoea.

The deficient secretion of the pancreas should be supplemented by active pancreatic extracts. These should be taken at each main meal sprinkled on the food, sipped in a liquid vehicle or as tablets. Response to substitution therapy is assessed by improvement in the character and frequency of the stools. Insulin or hypoglycaemia drugs may be necessary when diabetes mellitus supervenes.

Surgery may be required for the relief of obstructive jaundice.

48. The Anaemias

Anaemia is said to be present when the concentration of haemoglobin (Hb) in the blood falls. There are wide ranges of Hb concentrations in healthy persons and adult men have slightly higher values than adult women and children. Table 48.1 gives figures below which anaemia may be said to exist. Most persons who are only slightly anaemic by these necessarily arbitrary standards are free of symptoms and may appear in good health; it is a mistake to assume that minor symptoms arising in a person who is only mildly anaemic by the above standards are necessarily due to the anaemia. Yet their capacity for hard physical work may be reduced and they are at increased risk of serious consequences if they suffer a haemorrhage as a result of any accident, during childbirth or from any disease.

There are three main causes of anaemia.

1. Loss of blood from the circulation, i.e. external or internal haemorrhage.
2. Haemolysis, i.e. increased destruction of red blood cells (erythrocytes).
3. Reduced production of erythrocytes and haemoglobin—dyshaemopoisiesis.

The life of the erythrocyte is about 120 days. The bone marrow replaces them at a rate which enables their number to be maintained. Ingredients of the effete erythrocytes are used so that the call on haemopoietic nutrients in the diet is minimised. The nutritional anaemias are dyshaemopoietic anaemias in which marrow activity is limited by deficiency of erythrocyte and haemoglobin building blocks.

For the production of erythrocytes, a variety of nutrients are needed. The most important are iron, folic acid and vitamin B_{12}, but others are protein, pyridoxine, ascorbic acid, copper and vitamin E. It is unusual for anaemia to arise in an otherwise healthy person solely as a direct result of a poor diet. However the diet often contains insufficient of one or more of the essential nutrients to meet increased needs caused by chronic haemorrhage, infection and genetic defects affecting the red blood cell. Disorders of the alimentary tract often lead to impaired absorption of the essential nutrients and so to anaemia. Hence secondary anaemias are exceedingly common and treatment has to be aimed not only at removing the primary cause, but also at meeting increased demands of nutrients.

Reviews of nutritional anaemias by WHO (1972 and 1975) deal with the public health aspects.

HAEMATOLOGICAL FINDINGS

If there is an insufficiency of iron for the formation of haemoglobin, the red blood corpuscles are pale and small and the anaemia is said to be **hypochromic** and **microcytic.** If the maturation of the red blood corpuscles in the bone marrow is impaired by lack of folate or vitamin B_{12}, the cells which enter the blood stream are irregular in size and shape, but usually on average larger than normal, and contain their full complement of haemoglobin. Such anaemia is **orthochromic** and **macrocytic.**

However it is usually referred to as **megaloblastic**, after the typical immature precursor of the red blood corpuscles, the megaloblast, which is seen in the bone marrow. Samples of bone marrow are obtained by sternal or iliac puncture. This procedure is safe and carried out with a local anaesthetic.

Occasionally in Britain and very often in the tropics, the bone marrow lacks both iron and either folate or vitamin B_{12}. This gives rise to a hypochromic macrocytic or **dimorphic anaemia.**

A measurement of the Hb concentration in the blood does not distinguish between these types of anaemia. Two additional measurements made on peripheral blood are useful. The first is the haematocrit or packed cell volume (PCV) obtained by centrifuging blood under standard conditions and reading the height of the column of packed red cells. The second additional measurement is the red cell count (RBC).

Three ratios derived from these measurements help differentiate the types of anaemia. Hb/PCV gives the **mean corpuscular haemoglobin concentration** (MCHC), expressed in g/dl. If the value is below 30, the red cells are lacking in haemoglobin and the anaemia is hypochromic. This finding is an indication for iron therapy.

$Hb \times 10/RBC$ gives the **mean corpuscular haemog-**

Table 48.1 Haemoglobin levels below which anaemia is likely to be present at sea level (WHO, 1972)

	Age	Hb g/dl
Children	6 months to 6 years	11
	6 years to 14 years	12
Adults	Men	13
	Women	12
	Pregnant women	11

Table 48.2 Typical findings in peripheral blood in anaemia due to deficiencies of iron and folate

	Normal range in women	Deficiency Iron	Deficiency Folate
Basic measurements			
Haemoglobin (Hb) g/dl	12–16	7	7
Packed cell volume (PCV) per cent	36–47	28	22
Red blood cells (RBC) $\times 10^{-12}$/l	3.9–5.6	3.5	2.0
Derived values			
Mean corpuscular haemoglobin concentration (MCHC) per cent	30–36	25	32
Mean corpuscular haemoglobin (MCH) pg	27–32	20	35
Mean corpuscular volume (MCV) fl	75–95	80	110

lobin (MCH) in picograms (10^{-12} g). This is also low in hypochomic anaemia.

PCV/RBC gives the **mean corpuscular volume** (MCV) in femtolitres (10^{-15}l). A value of over 95 fl indicates that the erythrocytes are on average larger than normal. This suggests that there may be a deficiency of either folate or vitamin B_{12}.

The Hb content and PCV can be measured accurately with simple apparatus by persons with limited laboratory experience. The RBC count is a more difficult and time consuming procedure, and reliable results can be obtained only by persons with experience of the method. In many laboratories it is now mechanised (e.g. the Coulter counter). Table 48.2 gives the normal range of findings in women and typical values found in patients deficient in iron or folate.

An additional measurement in peripheral blood is the **reticulocyte count.** Reticulocytes are immature erythrocytes, which can be easily identified by the presence of small granules on staining with cresyl blue. Normally they are less than 1 per cent of the total number of erythrocytes, but they increase when the bone marrow is more than normally active. For example in a patient responding to vitamin B_{12} therapy, they may amount to 20 per cent or more.

CLINICAL FEATURES OF ANAEMIA

Anaemias give rise to the same general clinical features whatever the cause. As the partial pressure of oxygen in the blood is not reduced, symptoms only arise when the transport of oxygen by the blood is insufficient to meet the needs of the body. As the need for oxygen is related to physical activity, a person leading a sedentary life may have a moderate degree of anaemia and yet be entirely free of symptoms, though these develop if unaccustomed exercise is taken. Any significant degree of anaemia is always associated with an inability to make sustained physical effort. As anaemia often develops very slowly, the patient may gradually and unknowingly reduce her physical activity to a lower level. Thus it is not unusual to find a woman undertaking her normal housework with a haemoglobin level of less than 7.5 g/dl, but doing it slowly.

The severity of the clinical features is dependent not only on the degree of anaemia, but on the rapidity of its development. Common symptoms are general fatigue and lassitude, breathlessness on exertion, giddiness, dimness of vision, headache, insomnia, pallor of the skin, palpitation, anorexia and dyspepsia, tingling and 'pins and needles' in the fingers and toes (paraesthesiae). Angina pectoris (due to myocardial hypoxia) is sometimes present in elderly patients. Physical signs include pallor of mucous membranes and fingernails, tachycardia, functional systolic murmurs, evidence of cardiac dilation and, in severe cases oedema of the ankles and crepitations at the bases of the lungs. In addition to these general features of anaemia there may be signs of nutritional deficiency, particularly angular stomatitis, koilonychia and glossitis. Atrophy of the papillae and mucous membranes gives the tongue a smooth glazed appearance (chronic atrophic glossitis). The atrophy begins at the edges and later affects the whole tongue. As a result the tongue appears moist and exceptionally clean. Koilonychia is the name given to certain changes in the nails; first there is brittleness and dryness: later there is flattening and thinning and finally concavity (spoon-shaped nails).

HYPOCHROMIC ANAEMIA DUE TO IRON DEFICIENCY

This is by far the most common variety of anaemia throughout the world, affecting mainly women in their reproductive years, infants and children. Figure 48.1 shows the average haemoglobin concentrations in members of the poor families in Aberdeen during the economic depression in the 1930s. At that time the estimated iron intake of poor people in the city was 7.5 mg/day (Fullerton, 1936). Probably today in many cities of the world where there is much poverty, haemoglobin concentrations are similar to those in Aberdeen 45 years ago. In Britain today iron deficiency is still common, but much less severe than formerly. In South Wales Elwood (1968) found that 120 out of 1080 women had haemoglobin concentrations below 12 g/dl.

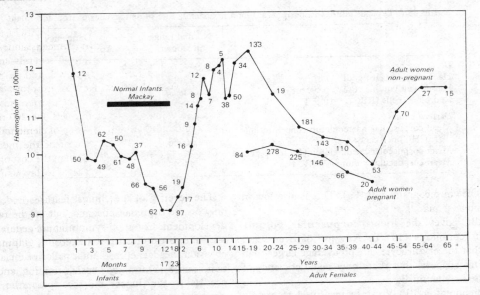

Fig. 48.1 Chart showing average haemoglobin levels among poor people of all ages (Davidson *et al.*, 1935).

In both rural and urban areas in the tropics this type of anaemia is extremely common. Losses of iron occur not only in menstruation and pregnancy but also as a result of infection with hookworms. Many tropical diets do not contain sufficient absorbable iron to make good these losses.

Iron deficiency anaemia is much less common in men than in women. When found in a male in Britain, it should not be assumed to be nutritional in origin unless all sources of pathological bleeding and organic disease have been excluded.

Even if a person is not anaemic, iron deficiency may still be present. It can be demonstrated by a low level of saturation of the total iron-binding capacity of the plasma (below 15 per cent), the absence of stainable iron in the bone marrow and a raised level of free protoporphyrin, the immediate precursor of haemoglobin, in the red cells (Heller *et al.*, 1971). The condition is known as **sideropenia**. It was found in 21 per cent of women in Glasgow (McFarlane *et al.*, 1967). It is analogous to hypovitaminosis C and hypovitaminosis D in that no features of deficiency of iron are present, but the person is at increased risk of developing anaemia.

Plasma ferritin, measured by immunoassay reflects iron stores in the tissues. Normal values for men and women are about 70 and 35 μg/l respectively and in patients with iron deficiency it is often as low as 10 μg/l (Jacobs *et al.*, 1972).

Women of child-bearing age

The main cause is the increased need for iron which is a direct consequence of menstruation and pregnancy. A secondary cause is a failure of iron absorption often associated with a diminished secretion of hydrochloric acid by the stomach.

Menstrual losses. The menstrual blood losses vary greatly (Jacobs and Butler, 1965). The amount of iron lost at each period is on average about 30 mg and to meet this 1.0 mg of iron has to be absorbed daily, in addition to an amount estimated at just below 1.0 mg/day to meet other losses. As no more than 20 per cent of dietary iron can normally be absorbed (p. 101) a dietary intake of 10 mg is only marginally adequate. Many women lose much more than this average figure. From measurements of menstrual flow Hallberg *et al.* (1966) estimated that if the menstrual loss is to be replaced in 90 per cent of women up to 1.4 mg of extra iron has to be absorbed daily, and to ensure safety for 95 per cent of women an extra 2 mg is needed. Few normal diets could meet these higher requirements.

Pregnancy and lactation. The loss of iron involved in a normal pregnancy (iron content of fetus, 400 mg), delivery (iron content of placenta, uterus and blood loss, 325 mg) and lactation (iron content of milk during six months of lactation, 175 mg) may total approximately 900 mg. This entails an extra demand for absorption of about 2 mg Fe/day for a period of 460 days. Even if we deduct an estimated saving from the omission of menstruation during pregnancy, the negative iron balance is still large.

It is obvious that menstruation and pregnancy greatly increase a woman's requirements for iron; it is not surprising that diet alone is often unable to meet the deficit.

Failure of absorption. The factors determining absorption of dietary iron are discussed on page 101. As haem-bound iron (in meats) is well absorbed and phytates and phosphates in coarse foods of vegetable origin impair iron absorption, it is easy to explain the high incidence of iron deficiency anaemia in women in poor tropical communities.

Clinical features

The anaemia is often well advanced, e.g. haemoglobin level 7.5 g/dl, before significant symptoms are apparent. These have been described on page 423. In addition dysphagia occurs occasionally in severe cases (p. 396) and sometimes koilonychia. While paraesthesiae are common, objective signs of disease of the central nervous system are never found in iron deficiency anaemia. If untreated the condition follows a chronic course. Then atrophic gastritis and a failure to secrete HCl are common; this may further impair iron absorption from a poor diet. The importance of the syndrome is not that it is dangerous to life but that it leads to a loss of efficiency and impaired general health and vitality.

Prophylaxis

For the prophylaxis of iron deficiency anaemia in women, the butcher and the greengrocer are of particular importance. Once anaemia has developed it is to the chemist that one should turn for help. Every doctor should have some knowledge of the iron content of foods (Table 11.5) so that he may give sensible advice on which foods are of value as cheap sources of iron. The most valuable dietary sources of iron are meats and liver; they should preferably be eaten once a day. Eggs also have a high iron content but this is poorly absorbed possibly because of phospholipid inhibitors in the yolk. Less expensive sources of iron are beans, especially soya beans, and nuts. Dark green vegetables, such as spinach and watercress and certain fruits, especially dried apricots, peaches, prunes and raisins, are useful sources of iron, but in general fresh fruits and vegetables are of greater value because of their ascorbic acid content, which facilitates iron absorption. Cereals cannot be relied upon to contribute greatly to the iron intake, since the phytates and phosphates reduce its absorption. Bread is enriched with iron in some countries. As already mentioned milk is a poor source of dietary iron. Women with heavy menstrual periods or who have repeated pregnancies usually require medicinal iron.

In addition to the dietetic measures discussed above, the following prophylactic measures for pregnant women are recommended: (1) routine estimation of the haemoglobin in all women at their first antenatal visit, (2) iron therapy for those with a haemoglobin below 12 g/dl and (3) routine administration of iron to all patients from the twenty-fourth week to term as mild anaemia is so common in the third trimester (Kerr and Davidson, 1958b). The recommended preparation is ferrous sulphate and the dose is one tablet of 200 mg thrice daily after food. In addition 300 μg of folic acid should be given daily during the last trimester. Only if intolerance to ferrous sulphate is clearly demonstrated should the more expensive proprietary preparations of iron be prescribed.

Treatment

Once anaemia has developed it is both unwise and uneconomic to try to correct it by dietary means alone. In 1935 Sir Stanley Davidson gave a group of severely anaemic poor women a diet rich in animal protein and other expensive foods known to be good sources of iron for a period of 30 days. The mean rise in Hb concentration was less than 1 g/dl. The women were then given one 200 mg tablet of ferrous sulphate containing 60 mg of elemental iron thrice daily for 30 days. The total cost of the medicinal iron therapy for this period was less than the cost of the dietary supplement of iron-rich foods for one day, while the mean rise in Hb concentration was 4 g/dl.

The administration of iron should lead to a rise of Hb concentration of at least 1 g/dl per week provided sepsis, toxaemia or haemorrhage are absent. Ferrous sulphate is the preparation of choice. The dose is 200 mg in tablets three times a day. A bottle of 100 tablets will last a month. Ferrous gluconate, ferrous succinate and ferrous fumarate are equally effective, but more expensive. For the exceptional patient who is unable to swallow tablets, a liquid preparation containing ferrous sulphate should be prescribed. The efficacy of ferrous salts is rapidly reduced if oxidation to the ferric state occurs. Accordingly they must not be prescribed in simple watery solutions but should be mixed with 50 per cent glucose and ascorbic acid which retard oxidation. The British Pharmacopoeia preparation, ferrous sulphate mixture (NF), is a suitable liquid preparation since it meets this requirement. One tablespoonful is equivalent to one 200 mg tablet of ferrous sulphate and should be given three times a day well diluted with water.

Gastrointestinal upsets and other indications of intolerance to iron have been commonly reported, but controlled trials (Kerr and Davidson, 1958a) have indicated that these are mainly psychological in origin.

Treatment should be continued for approximately two months after the haemoglobin level has returned to normal in order to restock the depleted body stores. In women past the menopause, recurrence is unlikely, but women who are still menstruating or who become pregnant may relapse and require regular checks on their haemoglobin.

Hydrochloric acid is of no value in improving absorption of iron. If the patient is taking a well-balanced diet, vitamin preparations are unnecessary and wasteful. The administration of trace elements (copper, cobalt, molybdenum, manganese) is also of no value.

Rarely oral iron therapy is unacceptable and then injections of a parenteral iron preparation should be given.

Infants and children

Aetiology

The following factors help to explain the frequency of anaemia in early life.

Prolonged milk feeding. Breast-fed and particularly

artificially fed infants may be kept too long on milk alone without supplements of iron-containing foods.

Low birth weight. At birth the full-term baby has a haemoglobin level of approximately 17 g/dl. After birth a haemolysis occurs and by the sixth to eighth week the haemoglobin falls to 11 g/dl. The iron set free is stored, principally in the liver, and utilised during the period of milk feeding. At the end of nine months the haemoglobin should have risen to 13 g/dl. Premature and full-term infants of low birth weight, for example twins, have a small blood volume and hence smaller stores of iron to tide them through the milk-feeding period. Moreover, their rate of growth is greater and hence the requirements for iron are increased.

Nutritional anaemia in the mother. When a mother is suffering from nutritional iron deficiency anaemia her child's antenatal stores of iron may be inadequate.

Infections. The common infections of infancy and childhood often depress the bone marrow.

Malabsorption. Gluten enteropathy is an occasional cause.

Clinical features

In infants the symptoms of anaemia are not so easily recognised as in adults, but there is always impairment of general health and vitality.

Prevention

The prophylactic measures may be summarised as follows:
1. The prevention and treatment of iron deficiency anaemia in pregnant women and those suffering with menorrhagia.
2. Efficient treatment of infections in infants.
3. The provision of supplementary feeds of broth, minced meat, vegetable purées and other easily digested sources of iron from the age of 4 to 6 months onwards.
4. The administration of prophylactic doses of iron to infants of low birth weight from the third month of life onwards.

Treatment

Once anaemia has developed, dietetic measures cannot be relied on to cure the anaemia and hence must be supplemented with medicinal iron in a dose of about 6 mg/kg. For this purpose the ferrous sulphate mixture for infants (BPC) is a suitable preparation. One to two teaspoonfuls well diluted with water three times a day is the usual dose depending on the age of the child.

Hypochromic anaemia due to haemorrhage

Acute haemorrhage. The sudden loss of a large volume of blood, 1 litre or more, from trauma or intestinal bleeding produces peripheral circulatory failure (shock).

The rapid loss of 2 to 3 litres of blood is usually fatal, whereas an even greater quantity may be lost without causing death if it is spread over a period of 24 to 48 hours. During this period restoration of the circulating blood volume is proceeding by the withdrawal into the blood of tissue fluid. This haemodilution, which takes some hours to develop, is reflected by a fall in the haemoglobin level and red cell count. Hence, immediately after a haemorrhage of 1 litre in a normal person, the haemoglobin may be 15 g/dl, but fall to 12 g some hours later when dilution has occurred. When the circulating blood volume is partially restored, the acute symptoms of shock subside. Treatment of acute haemorrhage, if large, requires blood transfusion.

Chronic haemorrhage. This results from persistent or repeated loss of small amounts of blood. The most frequent causes are menorrhagia, and bleeding from haemorrhoids, alimentary carcinoma, peptic ulcer and operations on the gastrointestinal tract. Alimentary bleeding from the taking of aspirin must be remembered. Such persistent blood loss causes a progressive fall in haemoglobin.

Diagnosis depends upon the finding of a blood picture of hypochromic anaemia and the discovery of a source of chronic haemorrhage. It is important to test the faeces for occult blood, look for haemorrhoids and sometimes to perform a radiographic examination of the alimentary tract.

Treatment involves the arrest of the haemorrhage by appropriate means where possible and the administration of iron and a good diet.

Hypochromic anaemia due to malabsorption of iron

Iron deficiency anaemia is common in the malabsorption syndrome and after gastrointestinal operations. As months or years may elapse before the anaemia becomes manifest, the patient will have left the charge of the surgical specialist and be under the care of the general practitioner, who should be on the lookout for this development.

ANAEMIAS DUE TO DEFICIENCIES OF VITAMIN B₁₂ AND FOLATE

Deficiency of these vitamins leads to megaloblastic anaemia. This may be due either to dietary lack or, much more commonly in Europe and North America, a defect in intestinal absorption. Pregnant women are especially liable to develop this type of anaemia. In all countries megaloblastic anaemia is much less common than iron-deficiency anaemia and, from the viewpoint of public health, is relatively less important.

Pernicious anaemia

The term pernicious anaemia should be limited to the group of megaloblastic anaemias which is due to a failure in secretion of intrinsic factor by the stomach other than from surgery. The history of the discovery of vitamin B_{12} is given on page 140.

Aetiology

There is failure to absorb dietary vitamin B_{12} owing to lack of production of intrinsic factor in the gastric mucosa. Antibodies against gastric mucosa can often be detected in the serum and are probably responsible for destroying the mechanism for producing intrinsic factor. The disease thus arises as an autoimmune disorder. It often has a family incidence.

Morbid anatomy

In the stage of relapse there is extension of red bone marrow into the shafts of the long bones. The marrow shows the presence of many megaloblasts and a great reduction in the number of normoblasts. There is evidence of increased blood destruction—enlargement of the spleen, hyperbilirubinaemia and increased deposition of iron (haemosiderin) in the liver, spleen, kidneys and bone marrow. The gastric mucosa is thin and atrophic. Gastric analysis invariably shows complete achlorhydria. In inadequately treated cases degenerative changes in the dorsal and lateral tracts of the spinal cord may be found (subacute combined degeneration).

Clinical features

This disease is rare before the age of 30 and affects females more than males between 45 and 65 years of age. The onset is insidious and the degree of anaemia is often great before the patient consults a doctor. The patient generally appears well nourished despite the fact that weight loss is a common feature. The skin and mucous membranes are pale, and in severely anaemic cases the skin may show a faint lemon-yellow tint. When the tongue is painful it often has a red, raw appearance; later the mucous membrane becomes smooth and atrophic. In about 80 per cent of cases in relapse paraesthesiae occur in fingers and toes—numbness, tingling, 'pins and needles'. Occasionally there are objective signs of involvement of the spinal cord (vitamin B_{12} neuropathy), which may rarely develop before the anaemia. Psychiatric symptoms may occur associated with low levels of vitamin B_{12} in the plasma, but in the absence of other signs of neuropathy and with no abnormality of the peripheral blood or marrow (Strachan and Henderson 1965).

Diagnosis

The differential diagnosis of pernicious anaemia from other forms of megaloblastic anaemia depends upon the age of the patient, the finding of histamine-fast or pentagastrin-fast achlorhydria, and upon the absence of pregnancy and the lack of evidence of malnutrition, malabsorption or structural change in the small intestine. Plasma vitamin B_{12} is below 160 ng/1 while plasma folate is usually normal. The Schilling test, with oral vitamin B_{12} labelled with radioactive cobalt, shows subnormal absorption which is corrected if intrinsic factor is given at the same time.

Treatment

General. The patient should be kept in bed until the haemoglobin is about 7 g/dl. The diet should be light, easily digested and rich in protein, iron and vitamin C. The decision to give a blood transfusion depends on the clinical state of the patient. When the haemoglobin level is so low as to endanger life. e.g. under 4 g/dl, it should always be given.

Specific. Hydroxocobalamin should be given in a dosage of 1000 μg intramuscularly twice during the first week, then 250 μg weekly until the blood count is normal. Folic acid should never be used alone in the treatment of pernicious anaemia as it does not prevent the development of neurological complications, and may precipitate them.

Within 48 hours of the first injection of a cobalamin the bone marrow shows a striking change from a megaloblastic to a normoblastic state. Within two to three days the reticulocyte count begins to rise, reaching a maximum about the fourth to seventh day.

In some cases the rapid regeneration of the blood depletes the iron reserves of the body so that the haemoglobin fails to rise above 10 to 11 g/dl. To prevent this, ferrous sulphate, 200 mg thrice daily, should be given.

When subacute combined degeneration of the cord is present the dose of a cobalamin should be 20 μg twice weekly and continued at this high level for at least six months.

Maintenance. The patient should continue to receive regular doses of a cobalamin for the rest of his life. The dose is so regulated that the haemoglobin level is maintained at the normal level. The dose of hydroxocobalamin recommended is 1000 μg given by intramuscular injection every four to six weeks. Regular blood counts are therefore essential every six months and the assessment should never be made solely on clinical impression or on the haemoglobin level alone. Only thus can the appearance of subacute combined degeneration of the cord be prevented.

Prognosis

If a case is properly treated with vitamin B_{12} the prognosis is excellent and the neurological complications are prevented, arrested or cured. Prior to the discovery of liver therapy the disease ran a progressive downhill course, death occurring usually within three years. Hence the title, pernicious.

Nutritional megaloblastic anaemia in adults

Folate deficiency. The classical studies of Wills (1931) in Bombay drew attention to this disease. Her patients were mainly pregnant women who had been living for long periods on poor diets consisting mainly of rice and lacking foods of animal origin and vegetables. They mostly responded well to Marmite, a yeast product.

Nutritional megaloblastic anaemia occurs commonly in underdeveloped countries and was formerly known as tropical macrocytic anaemia. It may occur at any age, but adult women, infants and young children are affected much more frequently than men. It is often made manifest by pregnancy. It is seldom important in a population which eats meat and green vegetables regularly. In Britain and other Western countries nutritional megaloblastic anaemia due to dietary deficiency is uncommon and then occurs most frequently in pregnancy (see below), but has been reported in Indian women (Britt et al., 1971). Very occasionally it occurs in housebound old people living alone and eating a very poor diet.

The disease also arises as a result of a failure to absorb folic acid in gastrointestinal disorders which lead to the malabsorption syndrome (p. 404). The condition may develop when the dietary folate is unable to meet demands for increased erythropoiesis caused by other diseases, e.g. the haemoglobinopathies (p. 430), and other haemolytic anaemias. After prolonged treatment with antiepileptic drugs plasma folate is often low and megaloblastic anaemia sometimes occurs. Oral contraceptives may impair folate absorption in some women (Streiff, 1970).

Clinical features and diagnosis
The disease progresses slowly and, if untreated, the haemoglobin concentration is likely to fall very low (2 to 4 g/dl). Loss of weight and signs of various vitamin deficiencies are frequently but not always observed. Glossitis is often present. Paraesthesia is a common complaint.

The peripheral blood shows a macrocytic anaemia and the bone marrow a megaloblastic reaction. Plasma folate is less than 3 ng/ml and red cell folate under 100 ng/ml. There is free hydrochloric acid in the gastric juice.

Treatment
Folic acid in a dose of 5 to 10 mg daily is effective. Patients who are seriously ill (haemoglobin level less than 5 g/dl) need blood transfusion to tide them over until the folic acid has acted. Iron is often required before a full haematological response can occur. The patient should be given a well-balanced diet, and continue on it. If poverty or custom makes this impossible the patient should be advised to change her habits so as to include some good sources of folate (Table 14.9) every day. Pregnant and lactating women have greater needs for folate than anyone else in the community. A follow-up clinic is invaluable for detecting relapses in their earliest stages and also for periodic dietetic advice which can help to prevent a return to the defective diet.

Vitamin B_{12} deficiency. Vitamin B_{12} is found only in animal foods so that strict vegetarians, or vegans, who regularly avoid eating dairy products and eggs as well as meat, are at risk of developing deficiency. Because liver stores of the vitamin are normally large, it takes several years for a previously well-nourished person to develop clinical manifestations on an inadequate diet. In Britain dietary vitamin B_{12} deficiency disease is very rare among Caucasians. In most vegans the plasma vitamin B_{12} is often moderately reduced and there may be a sore mouth and tongue but anaemia is unusual. Megaloblastic anaemia is more likely in Indian Hindu women who are strict vegetarians. Stewart et al. (1970) report 13 cases in London.

Because pure dietary deficiency is an uncommon cause of vitamin B_{12} deficiency anaemia, other conditions need to be ruled out before the diagnosis is established. Vitamin B_{12} absorption and gastric and intestinal function should be shown to be normal and the patients should not be on drugs such as biguanides which can impair vitamin B_{12} absorption. One of the cases reported by Stewart et al. (1970) showed a good reticulocyte response to only 1 μg cyanocobalamin daily by mouth. Other such patients have required larger oral or even parenteral doses at first, presumably because vitamin B_{12} deficiency can itself produce atrophic changes in the gastrointestinal mucosa.

Tapeworm anaemia
The tapeworm, Diphyllobothrium latum, absorbs vitamin B_{12} from the small intestine and so infection may lead to anaemia. Although the distribution of the worm in fishes is widespread, human infection has been studied mainly in Finland. There about 2 per cent of the adult population harbour the worm (Saarni et al., 1977). Only a small proportion of carriers develop megaloblastic anaemia, but many have low plasma concentrations of vitamin B_{12}.

Megaloblastic anaemia of pregnancy
A temporary macrocytic anaemia with megaloblastic reaction in the bone marrow sometimes occurs during pregnancy or the puerperium. The clinical features are the same as those of nutritional megaloblastic anaemias. The factors involved in its causation include increased demands and dietary deficiency, especially of folic acid and much more rarely of vitamin B_{12}.

Cases of megaloblastic anaemia of pregnancy usually respond dramatically to the oral ingestion of 10 mg of folic acid daily. If the anaemia is very severe and is not discovered until close to full term, blood transfusion is indicated. Megaloblastic anaemia may recur in subsequent pregnancies. A co-existing deficiency of iron is frequent, and this leads to a dimorphic blood picture. Iron therapy is indicated in such cases. Since there is biochemical evidence of folic acid depletion in about 20 per cent of pregnant women in Britain and because pernicious anaemia is rare in this age group, it is reasonable to give folic acid as a prophylactic. A dose of 300 μg daily is ample for this purpose and this may be given with iron in a suitable preparation during the last trimester of pregnancy. Since megaloblastic anaemia occurs more frequently in pregnant women in tropical underdeveloped countries, they have a special need for a folic acid/iron supplement.

Megaloblastic anaemia of infancy and childhood
Megaloblastic anaemia is not uncommon in association with protein-energy malnutrition and usually responds to folic acid. It is a rare disease in Britain and in other wealthy western countries. In the USA, Zuelzer and Ogden (1946) reported 25 cases. Most of the infants were severely anaemic and five had haemoglobin levels below 4 g/dl. Many had been fed on artificial infant foods which were unsatisfactory in their content of folic acid, protein and ascorbic acid. The disease can occur in premature infants (Hoffbrand, 1970). In Germany and in Italy megaloblastic anaemia in children has also been reported (Wintrobe, 1956), especially in infants fed exclusively on goat's milk, which has an exceptionally low folate content.

Clinical features
These do not differ from those of any other anaemia in childhood. The bone marrow is megaloblastic and the peripheral blood picture is macrocytic in some children. In others, however, the anaemia may be dimorphic. Plasma iron and transferrin together with plasma folate and vitamin B$_{12}$ and red cell folate should enable a provisional diagnosis to be made, which can be confirmed by the response to treatment. In difficult cases bone marrow biopsy is required. The disease generally responds to folic acid, but blood transfusions are sometimes needed.

Megaloblastic anaemia associated with the malabsorption syndrome
Megaloblastic anaemia is commonly seen in the malabsorption syndrome due to failure of absorption of folic acid, of vitamin B$_{12}$ or of both. It may also occur subsequent to resection or short-circuiting of a large segment of the small intestine.

The clinical features are those of the underlying alimentary disease together with the general symptoms of anaemia. Symptoms and signs of various vitamin and mineral deficiencies are also frequently present.

In gluten enteropathy and tropical sprue there is usually an excellent haematological response to folic acid, given intramuscularly for the first two or three days and orally in a dosage of 10 to 20 mg a day thereafter. It is wise to supplement this with 1000 μg of hydroxocobalamin by injection every four to six weeks, and, particularly in the tropics, iron by mouth may also be required. When megaloblastic anaemia is associated with blind or stagnant loops of the small intestine there is likely to be a response to cobalamin therapy, but surgical correction should be undertaken if possible.

OTHER NUTRITIONAL CAUSES OF ANAEMIA

The production of the protein portion of the framework of the red corpuscles and the synthesis of globin are affected by a diminished intake of amino acids. However, the deficiency must be severe and long continued because the protein requirement for the synthesis of haemoglobin takes precedence over that required for the manufacture of plasma proteins.

The role of protein-energy malnutrition in the causation of tropical nutritional anaemia has been extensively studied. In kwashiorkor the anaemia is usually moderate in degree. As there is often an associated dietary deficiency of iron, ascorbic acid, folic acid or, more rarely, vitamin B$_{12}$, and one or more of a variety of infections may be present, it is not surprising that no consistent haematological picture is found or that the anaemia is sometimes severe.

Patients who have lost weight from a simple insufficiency of food are often mildly anaemic. In the Minnesota experiment (Keys *et al.*, 1950) volunteers lived for 24 weeks on an inadequate diet and lost about 25 per cent of their body weight; the haemoglobin was reduced to an average of 11.7 g/dl. The cause of this anaemia is that all the organs of the body—with the exception of the skeleton and nervous system—shrink when the body is short of energy, yet the total volume of water in the body is little changed. The red cell population, or 'erythron', is no exception. So one effect of weight loss from lack of energy is a smaller red cell population in a normal plasma volume. If the patient has lost 25 per cent of his normal lean body weight, the haemoglobin concentration in his blood is likely to be 75 per cent of normal.

The anaemias of scurvy and pyridoxine deficiency are discussed on pages 296 and 148 respectively.

GENETIC DEFECTS OF RED BLOOD CELLS

There are hereditary defects of red blood corpuscles that make them more susceptible to haemolysis and persons who carry these genes are liable to become anaemic. Homozygotes are relatively uncommon and this is fortunate as in them anaemia is often severe and may be fatal. Heterozygotes are much more numerous and at least 100 million persons carry one or other of these genes which have become dispersed by migration all over the world. In them, anaemia, if present, is slight and there are usually no clinical features. Dietitians and nutritionists should know a little about these conditions because heterozygotes are at increased risk of becoming severely anaemic if exposed to nutritional or other haematological hazards. Brief notes are given below on the four commonest of these genetic defects.

Thalassaemia

The genotype originated in Mediterranean countries (Greek *thalassa*, sea) but has spread especially to the East across Asia. It is defined by a defect in synthesis of part of the polypeptide chain of haemoglobin A, which is partially compensated by persisting synthesis of fetal haemoglobin (Hb-F). There are also abnormalities of the red cell membrane. Homozygotes have thalassaemia major, a severe haemolytic anaemia and rarely survive into adult life. Heterozytes may or may not have a mild anaemia, thalassaemia minor.

Sickle cell trait

This is common in African Negroes and is due to an abnormal haemoglobin, haemoglobin S, differing only in having a single molecule of valine instead of one of glutamic acid in one of the polypeptide chains. The configuration of the molecules of Hb-S distort the red blood corpuscles into a characteristic sickle shape. Such corpuscles are abnormally sensitive to hypoxia, which can lead to haemolysis. Heterozygotes have the sickle cell trait and are only occasionally anaemic. Homozygotes have a severe anaemia, sickle cell disease.

Spherocytosis

This is the commonest congenital defect of red blood corpuscles in northern Europe. The abnormality lies in the cell membranes which are more than normally permeable to sodium ions. The cells assume the shape of spheres which are more easily trapped in the microcirculation of the spleen, where haemolysis takes place, than the normal biconcave discs. The defect is inherited as an autosomal dominant. In most cases the increased loss of cells by haemolysis is slight and can be made good by increased production in the bone marrow. When anaemia develops, removal of the spleen reduces haemolysis and cures the anaemia but does not change the underlying defect.

Glucose-6-phosphate deficiency

The genotype is found in all races and is present in up to 35 per cent of some Mediterranean populations and in 10 per cent of American Negroes. It is due to an incomplete dominant gene, and is fully expressed in males and in homozygous females. Glucose-6-phosphate is oxidised by a dehydrogenase linked to the conversion of NADP to NADPH$_2$ which in some way maintains the stability of red cell membranes. Persons with the defect are liable to develop anaemia when treated with oxidant drugs. More than 40 drugs are known to produce haemolysis and these include commonly used antimalarials, sulphonamides, antipyretics and analgesics. It is also produced by ingesting the broad bean, *Vicia faba*, or inhaling its pollen.

Continued ingestion leads to severe anaemia as was recognised many years ago in Mediterranean countries where it was known as **favism.**

A survey in Glasgow (Goel *et al.*, 1978) showed abnormal haemoglobins in the blood of 38 out of 380 children whose parents came from Africa, the Indian subcontinent and China, but none in 99 children of Scottish parents. However, the incidence of mild anaemia, usually due to iron deficiency, was only a little higher (20 per cent) in the children of immigrant parents than in those with Scottish parents (16 per cent). Thus these genetic defects are common in immigrant populations and, though they seldom affect health, their presence in a community is a potential cause of severe anaemia.

ANAEMIA IN TROPICAL COUNTRIES

In tropical countries the causes of the different types of anaemia, their clinical features and their treatment are similar to those occurring in temperate climates. There are, however, additional factors which are not present in temperate climates. Thus the demands for iron may be greatly increased by the loss of haemoglobin in the faeces and urine resulting from haemorrhage due to parasitic diseases such as hookworm and schistosomiasis. In addition significant amounts of iron may be lost in the sweat and shed epithelial skin cells during muscular work in hot climates. The role of malaria and hookworm in the production of anaemia requires special emphasis (see below). Other protozoal and helminthic infections as well as bacterial infections which are common in the tropics may be responsible for anaemia. When these additional factors operate in persons who live on diets deficient in iron and protein, it is not surprising that anaemia in tropical countries is both frequent and severe.

The nutritional megaloblastic anaemias of tropical climates are always associated with diets poor in animal protein and rich in carbohydrate, and hence low in vitamin B$_{12}$ and especially folate. Requirements of these substances are increased during periods of growth, in pregnancy, as a result of infections including malaria, and when increased red cell formation occurs as in haemolytic anaemias. It is therefore wise to add folic acid (up to 5 mg daily) to the therapeutic regime for infants and toddlers with protein-energy malnutrition and for all anaemic patients suffering from malnutrition, infections or haemolytic anaemias. Folic acid and iron should be given throughout pregnancy in tropical countries.

Malaria

An attack of malarial fever, especially when due to *Plasmodium falciparum,* is always accompanied by haemolysis, and in a severe or prolonged attack severe anaemia may ensue. During the stage of recovery anaemia may still be present although the evidence of haemolysis may be absent or minimal. When malarial infection is associated with pregnancy and malnutrition, the anaemia may present as megaloblastic anaemia due to folate deficiency, but is more usually hypochromic and microcytic because of iron deficiency. Since the blood destruction is intravascular, most of the iron liberated from the destroyed red cells is retained in the body and can be used again for synthesis of haemoglobin. If it were not for this conservation of iron, the incidence and severity of the anaemia would be much greater than it is. The treatment of malaria in the individual and its eradication from areas of low or moderate endemicity are thus prerequisites for the treatment and prevention of anaemia.

A vicious circle develops in communities suffering from chronic malaria—sickness, weakness and anaemia, economic inefficiency, poverty, malnutrition, bad housing and social conditions, reinfection. Experience has shown how effective malarial control can be in eradicating the disease from large areas and how remarkable are the benefits which ensue.

Hookworm infection

Infection with hookworm is a common cause of anaemia where there is 'wet' cultivation of the land. The clinical and haematological features are similar to those of chronic hypochromic anaemia. A heavy infection with hookworms is always associated with anaemia. Smaller loads may be carried without ill-effect. Haemorrhages occur at the site of the attachment of the worms to the intestinal mucous membrane. These are certainly in part responsible for the anaemia. It has been calculated that each worm may ingest from 0.03 to 0.15 ml of blood daily. A patient with a heavy infection, namely about 1000 worms (which would give a stool count of about 20 000 ova/g faeces) would sustain a heavy loss of blood and anaemia would quicly develop. Detailed studies of hookworm load, blood loss and anaemia have been made in Venezuela (Layrisse and Roche, 1964), in West Africa (Gillies *et al.*, 1964) and in Gambia (Topley, 1968).

Heavy hookworm infection usually occurs in populations whose dietary intake of iron is unsatisfactory. The hypochromic anaemia is then in part due to a poor diet and in part to the worms. This combination causes much ill-health; it may reduce greatly the working capacity of both men and women and is thus directly responsible for the poverty of many families in the tropics.

Experience has shown that in treating anaemia due to hookworm, whether in a single patient or in a large community, satisfactory results can only be obtained by the use of a combination of vermifuges, dietary improvement and the administration of medicinal iron.

Heavy infection may cause severe anaemia with haemoglobin levels below 4 g/dl. In such seriously ill patients, before administering a vermifuge, blood transfusions should be given and the general condition of the patient improved by bed rest, diet and medicinal iron.

OTHER CAUSES OF ANAEMIA

Anaemia may arise from a number of disorders where there is no satisfactory evidence that nutritional deficiency is of primary aetiological importance. They include the following:

Infection. A mild or moderate normochromic anaemia may develop secondary to chronic infection, particularly if fever is present. A mild degree of iron deficiency may be found. The response to iron therapy, both oral and parenteral, is usually unsatisfactory unless the primary cause of the anaemia is removed.

Uraemia. In chronic renal disease anaemia is common but the bone marrow remains cellular until renal damage is marked, when hypoplasia may be found. Deficiency of erythropoietin is a possible cause.

Hepatic cirrhosis. Here the anaemia is usually macrocytic or normocytic. If megaloblastic anaemia occurs this is probably due to primary malnutrition, and is found particularly in chronic alcoholics with cirrhosis. The occurrence of iron deficiency anaemia suggests gastric or oesophageal haemorrhage.

Malignant disease. The causes of anaemia in widespread malignant disease are numerous. They include impaired appetite, malabsorption or blood loss from the alimentary tract, multiple deposits in the bone marrow, and occasionally increased haemolysis.

Sideroblastic anaemia. Abnormal utilisation of iron by the marrow may cause a refractory anaemia. Some cases respond to pyridoxine therapy.

49. Diseases of the Nervous, Locomotor and Respiratory Systems and of the Skin

NERVOUS SYSTEM

The brain is responsible for about one-fifth of the basal metabolism and its need for glucose and oxygen has long been recognised. Nitrogenous and lipid material are also required for the growth and regeneration of myelin sheaths and axis cylinders and for the enzyme systems needed for cellular metabolism. Imbalances of sodium and potassium and other electrolytes affect the cerebrospinal fluid and the excitability of nerve cells. Vitamins, especially those belonging to the B complex, must be available in adequate amounts since they are essential for the utilisation of carbohydrate which plays such a predominant role in the metabolism of the nervous system. Neurological diseases in which malnutrition is of primary aetiological importance are the nutritional encephalopathies and neuropathies associated with pellagra (nicotinic acid deficiency), Wernicke's encephalopathy (thiamin deficiency), beriberi (thiamin deficiency), and subacute combined degeneration of the cord (vitamin B_{12} deficiency). The clinical features and treatment of these diseases and other primary nutritional disorders affecting the brain, spinal cord and peripheral nerves are described in Part III. Many of the inborn errors of metabolism (Chap. 39) also affect the nervous system. Severe undernutrition may follow a reduced intake of food due to psychiatric causes or neurological disease affecting the muscles and making feeding difficult. Anorexia nervosa (p. 241) is the classic example of the former and motor neurone disease of the latter.

The possible roles of nutrition in some of the major neurological and psychiatric disorders are now discussed.

NEUROLOGICAL DISORDERS

Cerebrovascular disease

This is numerically the most important of all diseases of the central nervous system. More people die or are disabled by a stroke than by coronary heart disease. Atherosclerosis of the cerebral vessels and hypertension are the main causes. Obesity (Gordon and Kannel, 1973) and a high salt intake as a cause of hypertension are predisposing factors. The Japanese, who consume more salt than any other nation, have a high incidence of cerebrovascular disease but low rates of coronary disease (Insull *et al.*, 1968). Blood lipids are not strongly correlated to cerebrovascular disease as they are to coronary disease (Greenhouse, 1971). Atherosclerosis affecting the cerebral vessels

differs from that affecting the coronary vessels in that the death rate associated with it is approximately the same in men and women, and has not increased significantly in the last 50 years (Table 49.1). The age incidence differs also. Cerebrovascular disease is much less common than coronary heart disease under the age of 45 years and more common over the age of 65 years. The reasons for these differences in the two diseases, both closely associated with atherosclerosis, remain unknown.

Nutrition has a role in the complex problems arising in the rehabilitation of patients after a stroke. Difficulties in feeding due to either physical or psychological disability may lead to undernutrition. On the other hand, many patients are overweight and a reducing diet might lower the blood pressure and so decrease the risk of a second stroke. A dietitian has therefore an important place in a rehabilitation team.

Table 49.1 Death rates per 100 000 in Ontario males and females aged 45 to 64 years from diseases of the circulation (Anderson, 1970)

	Males		Females	
	1925	1966	1925	1966
Heart disease	215	606	178	187
Cerebrovascular disease	59	68	65	60

Multiple sclerosis

This disease which affects about 1 in 2000 people in Britain usually starts early in adult life. It is characterised by relapses and remissions and leads to severe disability after a varying number of years. The symptoms are manifold and may include double vision, weakness of one or more limbs, sensations of numbness or pins and needles (paraesthesia), inco-ordination of movement (ataxia), nystagmus and loss of control of the bladder. The symptoms are caused by lesions disseminated in the central nervous system, consisting of areas of demyelination.

The cause of the disease remains unknown and there have been many theories. Current views are that it may be due to the action of an unidentified slow virus or that it is an immunological disorder related to an attack of measles in early life.

Two observations have suggested that nutritional factors might be responsible. First, there is a disease of lambs and sheep, characterised by areas of demyelination and known as swayback. It occurs when animals graze on pastures deficient in copper and can be prevented by administration of copper. There is no evidence of copper deficiency in human multiple sclerosis, but the possibility of a deficiency of another trace element is not excluded.

Secondly, there is an alteration in lipid metabolism. Not surprisingly, affected areas of brain show a loss of lecithin and other cerebral lipids, but the proportion of saturated to unsaturated fatty acids in cerebral lecithins is increased. Further, there is a reduction in plasma linoleate, and the phospholipids in both red blood corpuscles and platelets have a reduced proportion of linoleate. These findings have suggested the use of linoleic acid in treatment and in a controlled clinical trial involving 80 patients observed over two years, Millar et al. (1973) found that relapses were less severe and less prolonged in patients receiving daily a dose of a sunflower seed oil emulsion containing 8.6 g of linoleic acid than in those receiving an olive oil emulsion with only 0.2 g of linoleic acid. This finding has not be confirmed. In the past the hopes of patients have often been falsely raised by new remedies, which have subsequently been shown to be ineffective and it would be unwise to promise too much benefit from the ingestion of sunflower seed oil.

The final stages of the disease may be very distressing and intention tremor of the hands and severe tremor of the head may make feeding difficult.

Epilepsy

Epilepsy is a common disorder and about 1 in 200 people are affected. They are liable to periodic attacks usually associated with a disturbance of consciousness and commonly manifest as fits. In a small minority of cases a local lesion in the brain or a generalised metabolic disturbance is responsible. In the great majority of patients the cause is unknown and they are said to have idiopathic epilepsy.

Antiepileptic drugs are very effective in preventing the seizures. Before these were available many bizarre remedies were advocated to stop the fits, or, in the language of the past, to drive out the devils. A period of starvation was sometimes seen to reduce their frequency. Such benefit may have been due to a depression of the brain by the accompanying ketoacidosis. Ketogenic diets are advocated by Livingston (1972) when the fits cannot be controlled by drugs. Childhood myoclonic epilepsy is a rare form of the disease occurring in young children which is often resistant to drugs; it is usually associated with brain damage and patients have many attacks throughout the day. It is not good for a growing child to be ketoacidotic and a ketogenic diet should only be tried after thorough tests have shown that the fits cannot be controlled by drugs. Less than 1 in 100 epileptic children fail to respond to drugs. For this small minority a diet low in carbohydrate and high in fat may help to control the fits. Medium chain triglycerides are useful in designing such a diet.

Antiepileptic drugs induce changes in liver metabolism which may increase requirements of vitamin D and folic acid. Patients taking large doses over the years should be checked regularly for signs of anaemia and rickets or osteomalacia.

Patients with epilepsy should take normal well-balanced meals at regular intervals. Epileptic children should not be allowed to take very large meals as these may predispose them to fits.

Migraine

The headaches are characteristically periodic and unilateral, and are sometimes preceded by visual or other disturbances. They are due to vasomotor changes affecting intra- and extracranial vessels. Many different factors may bring about an attack and in some patients one is likely to follow consumption of a particular food, e.g. chocolates, cheese and wines, especially sherry and red wine. The substances in these foods responsible for the attacks have not been identified but, in the case of cheese, it is probably tyramine and in chocolate phenylethylamine. Alcohol, which is a vasodilator, precipitates attacks in some people and some wines contain histamine. Migraine is a common condition and those who suffer from it should note carefully whether their attacks follow consumption of any one food or drink. If they do, then this can be avoided. In mild attacks coffee is often helpful because of its content of caffeine.

PSYCHIATRIC DISORDERS

Deficiencies of thiamin, nicotinic acid and vitamin B_{12} may each be associated with psychological disorders, as described elsewhere. Occasionally the psychological symptoms are so marked and other symptoms and signs of the deficiency so slight that the correct diagnosis may be overlooked and the patient at first is treated as if he was a neurotic or had a psychotic disorder. Some of these patients appear to have requirements for a vitamin in excess of the recommended intake. Pauling's concept of orthomolecular medicine (p. 135) has appealed to some psychiatrists who have become enthusiastic advocates of megavitamin therapy for schizophrenia. Their claims were examined by the American Psychiatric Association (1973), who could find no evidence to justify them, but the Association's report, which represents the view of the 'establishment' has been challenged (Pauling, 1974).

Although schizophrenia may eventually be shown to be a metabolic disorder, or a collection of several differing ones, the nature of the underlying biochemical disturbances is at present largely unknown. There is no evidence from studies either of its chemical pathology or its epidemiology that dietary factors contribute in any way to its aetiology, or indeed that they are responsible for more than a small fraction of psychiatric disorders.

Psychiatric disorders may lead to abnormal feeding

behaviour and so to anorexia nervosa (Chap. 27) and obesity (Chap. 28).

LOCOMOTOR SYSTEM

Diseases of the bones, joints, muscles and ligaments include a variety of disorders, often loosely grouped together under the heading of 'rheumatism'. The cause of these disorders is seldom simple and often obscure. They differ from one another widely in their aetiology, pathology and clinical course. They are often chronic, painful, disabling illnesses from which there is frequently little relief except by palliative measures such as physiotherapy and the prescription of analgesic drugs and corticosteroids. It is not surprising that numerous patients and their doctors have resorted to every possible method of treatment, including special diets. Various dietary regimes have been prescribed in the past, but have been founded on false hopes and mistaken theory. For a time it was widely believed that 'rheumatism' was due to an accumulation of acids in the body; efforts were made to avoid 'acid' foods, or to prescribe a diet that would keep the urine permanently alkaline. However, there is no evidence to associate rheumatism with 'acidity', which is an outworn notion as explained on page 89. A diet low in meat was often recommended to maintain an alkaline urine and also because of the erroneous belief that rheumatism is due to disordered purine metabolism, which is only true of gout. Particular foods were often banned in the belief that they were the allergic cause of the disorder. Chapter 50 explains how tenuous the evidence is for attributing any disease to allergy unless a definite allergen has been demonstrated.

CHRONIC RHEUMATIC DISEASES

The principal members of this group are rheumatoid arthritis, osteoarthrosis and non-articular rheumatism. They account for a very important proportion of temporary or permanent disablement in temperate climates. The rheumatic group of diseases is second only to bronchitis in men and holds first place among women as a reason for seeking medical advice.

Rheumatoid arthritis

Rheumatoid arthritis occurs in people of all ages. The peak incidence in both men and women is approximately at the age of 40. It occurs in women at least three times as frequently as in men. It is mainly a disease of temperate climates which are associated with cold and damp. The principal tissue affected is the synovial membrane of joints, which becomes inflamed and thickened. A characteristic antibody, the rheumatoid factor is usually demonstrable in the plasma and the cause of the disease appears to be an autoimmune disorder.

The onset is usually insidious. Muscular stiffness develops first and is followed later by pain and swelling of many joints, starting frequently with the small joints of the hands and feet. During the active stage of the disease the patient suffers from general malaise and fatigue; fever is sometimes present and the appetite is poor. In such patients loss of weight usually occurs. There is frequently some degree of anaemia.

Treatment

Successful treatment depends on the co-ordinated efforts of the physician, orthopaedic surgeon, physiotherapist, occupational therapist and social worker. The programme of treatment should be carefully co-ordinated to meet the needs of each individual case. All factors likely to have an adverse influence on the patient should be dealt with, and recommendations as to future activity based on an accurate knowledge of functional capacity. These ends can best be achieved in special units devoted to the study and treatment of the chronic rheumatic diseases.

Although diet has no specific curative value, common sense dictates that an attempt should be made to correct anaemia and loss of weight by diet and other measures.

To improve the state of nutrition the whole art of the dietitian may be needed. Any foods that tempt the patient to eat may be tried, but in general those rich in protein, iron and ascorbic acid should be offered first. Additional vitamin and mineral concentrates are often prescribed, although their value is doubtful. In the acute stage, when loss of weight, anorexia and continued fever are present, the instructions for the dietetic treatment of pyrexia (p. 443) are indicated. Marked clinical improvement is often associated with a better state of nutrition.

Osteoarthrosis

Osteoarthrosis is characterised by degeneration of the articular cartilage and the formation of bony outgrowths at the edges of the joints. A generalised form of the disease occurs normally in middle-aged women in whom the small joints of the fingers, the carpometacarpal joint of the thumb and the interfaecetal joints of the spine are particularly affected. The more localised form, in which only one or two of the larger joints are involved, occurs amongst elderly people of both sexes. There is no impairment of general health.

Osteoarthrosis is an exaggeration of normal ageing in the joints. When one joint is particularly affected, there is frequently a history of an injury to that joint some years before. Malalignment following fractures of the long bones gives rise to osteoarthrosis in adjacent joints. Symptoms are prone to develop in the weight-bearing joints or those joints subjected to excessive strain at work. Obesity predisposes to osteoarthrosis of the weight-bearing joints in the lower half of the body.

The joints most frequently involved are those of the

spine, the hips, knees, elbows and the terminal joints of the fingers. The symptoms are gradual in onset. Pain is at first intermittent and of an aching character, appearing especially after the joint has been used, and relieved by rest. As the disease progresses, movement in the affected joints becomes increasingly limited, at first by muscular spasm and later by the loss of joint cartilage and the formation of osteophytes. General health is usually excellent.

Treatment

The pathological changes in osteoarthrosis are irreversible, but much can be done to alleviate the symptoms. For this purpose, rest, graduated physical exercises and physiotherapy, including hydrotherapy, are of particular value. Analgesics should be prescribed according to the patient's needs. In selected cases orthopaedic operations are indicated. Diet has a limited, though useful, part to play in treatment. There is no evidence that deficiency of any nutrient is responsible for the primary defect, the degeneration of the articular cartilage. On the other hand obesity, by placing an extra strain on the joints, may hasten the onset. In addition, once the disease is established, pain and joint deformity reduce the patient's capacity for physical exercise and this renders him more liable to become obese unless he takes the necessary dietary precautions. Hence the prevention and correction of obesity is a valuable aid in management.

A curious form of osteoarthrosis which affects children occurs in Siberia, China and Korea; it is called **Kaschin-Beck disease** after its discoverers (Nesterov, 1964). Degeneration of joint cartilage is probably due to toxins from a fungus *Fusaria sporotrichiella* which can contaminate cereal crops in the region.

Non-articular rheumatism

'Non-articular rheumatism', 'muscular rheumatism' and 'fibrositis' are terms which describe a number of conditions characterised by pain and stiffness, often of sudden onset, affecting mainly the neck, shoulders, back and gluteal regions. Usually no cause can be found but exposure to cold and damp, excessive or unaccustomed muscular activity, injury to muscles and tendons and poor posture may each be held responsible. Muscular pain and stiffness arise often as a result of strain or injury to ligamentous or articular structures. Thus most cases of brachial neuralgia, lumbago and sciatica may result from degenerative changes in the intervertebral discs, either from prolapse of the nucleus pulposus or from narrowing of the intervertebral foramina, leading to pressure on spinal nerve roots.

In the acute stage the patient may be severely incapacitated by pain and stiffness. In the more chronic stage pain is felt most often after rest and improves with moderate activity. Muscular spasm may be marked and movement limited.

Treatment.

In the acute attack of muscular rheumatism such as lumbago, rest in bed is essential, together with heat to the affected part and analgesics in ample amounts. At a later stage physiotherapy (heat, massage and graduated exercise) is essential. In cases with lesions of the intervertebral disc causing root pressure, operation should be considered.

Diet has no specific part to play in curative treatment but if the patient is obese, reduction in weight may be of value in the relief of symptoms.

RESPIRATORY SYSTEM

The main causes of disease in the respiratory system are (1) infection (2) inhaled irritants, (3) allergy, (4) vascular accidents, and (5) malignant disease.

Infection. This is by far the most important cause of disease in the respiratory tract. Infection may be caused by a virus, as in the case of coryza, influenza and virus pneumonia, or by bacteria, as in bronchitis, bronchopneumonia, lobar pneumonia and tuberculosis. The complex problems of the part which the state of nutrition plays in preventing infections are discussed in Chapter 59, and also the contribution which diet makes to helping the patient to overcome an infection once it has been acquired.

Irritants. Exposure to tobacco smoke, industrial pollution or other inhaled irritants over many years leads to chronic bronchitis. When severe and prolonged and complicated by heart failure, this may lead to severe undernutrition and a state of cachexia. This is probably due to anorexia caused by chronic hypoxaemia.

Allergy. Certain respiratory diseases are allergic in origin, the most obvious example being hay fever. Another disease in which allergy plays an important role is bronchial asthma. Besides inhaled dust or pollen, ingested foods such as eggs, milk, wheat, shellfish, etc. can be responsible for asthma. The detection of a food allergen and it subsequent exclusion from the diet may be an important factor in the treatment of asthma. The role of food allergy in the causation of disease is dicussed in Chapter 50.

Vascular accidents. The most common vascular accident in the lung is embolism from a thrombosis formed usually in the veins of the lower limb or pelvis. If this dislodges it travels through the right side of the heart and obstructs one of the pulmonary arteries. It occurs especially in elderly people confined to bed, e.g. after an operation. There is no good evidence that nutritional factors play a part in the aetiology.

Malignant disease. Malignant disease of the bronchial tree and lungs has greatly increased in frequency in recent years. Tobacco smoke and pollution of the atmosphere with smoke and fumes are of great aetiological importance. There is little evidence that nutritional factors play any part in the causation of bronchial carcinoma or that dietetic treatment influences the course of the disease.

SKIN DISEASES

The skin manifestations of scurvy and pellagra have already been described, and Chapter 37 gives an account of various conditions of the skin commonly found in malnourished communities. The skin manifestations of linoleic acid deficiency and Refsum's disease respond to appropriate nutritional therapy.

Since there are several skin diseases of which the cause is unknown and which persist for long periods and respond poorly to treatment, it is not surprising that both patients and doctors have sometimes attributed their origin to dietary errors and attempted to cure them by dietetic means. Krehl (1973) gives references going back to 1912 for claims of the therapeutic value of various low fat and low protein diets in the treatment of **psoriasis.** One which

received publicity in the lay press was for a reputedly low tryptophan diet based on turkey meat, but this has not stood up to critical evaluation (*Lancet,* 1971). Chronic psoriasis is a distressing condition and patients should not be asked to take on the additional burden of dietary restrictions, for which there is no scientific justification.

Acne vulgaris, so common in teenagers, is often attributed by their parents to eating excessive amounts of sweets and chocolates. There is no evidence to support this view or that dietary factors are in any way responsible for the disease. However, many of those with severe acne may benefit in health from general dietetic advice, which includes moderation in the consumption of chocolates.

The one chronic skin disorder that may be improved by dietary measures is **dermatitis herpetiformis.** Over 70 per cent of these patients have varying degrees of atrophy of the jejunal mucosa and are sensitive to gluten. They benefit greatly from a gluten-free diet, though it may take many months before the skin lesions clear up completely. Dermatitis herpetiformis appears to be one manifestation of coeliac disease and should be managed as such.

50. Diet and Allergy

The word 'allergy' means an altered or abnormal tissue reactivity after exposure to a foreign antigen. An allergic reaction may occur after contact between a foreign protein (an 'allergen') and tissues that are sensitive to it. The allergen may reach the tissues by direct contact with the skin or mucous membranes, or through the blood stream after absorption. A single allergen may cause reactions at several sites; thus a patient allergic to egg protein may suffer a local reaction in the gut and also an attack of asthma when the absorbed allergen is carried by the blood to the lungs. Ingested proteins do not usually enter the blood stream, for they are normally split into their component amino acids in the gut; these after absorption have no allergic properties. But sometimes small amounts of polypeptide may be absorbed and set up an allergic state.

An allergic reaction results from the combination of the antigenic allergen with a special type of antibody, an immunoglobulin IgE, within the tissues. Cell damage releases histamine and other vasoactive substances which produce the clinical effects. Normal immune reactions between antigen and antibody evoke no such effects. The abnormality depends on the property of IgE of combining with sites on cell membranes, notably those of mast cells, and so making them sensitive when subsequently exposed to an allergen. Some individuals are more liable to form IgE antibodies and this tends to be inherited. Previous exposure to the antigenic allergen in small sensitising amounts is sometimes a predisposing cause. If the initial dose of antigen is large, it provokes a large response of IgG antibody which circulates in the blood and is likely to take up the antigen before it can reach the small amounts of IgE in tissues. The clinical type of allergic reaction depends on the tissue in which the IgE antibodies are localised.

Allergic manifestations may occur within a few minutes of the patient coming in contact with the allergen, or be delayed for many hours or even for several days.

Allergic reactions may be trivial and local, e.g. a mild urticaria (nettle-rash), or may be general and so serious as to result in sudden death. Serious reactions are known as **anaphylactic shock.** The mechanism underlying this severe form is illustrated by the following experiment. A guinea-pig is made sensitive to the serum of another animal by a single small injection of the serum. This produces a specific antibody, but on an inadequate scale. Thereafter a second but larger dose of the serum is given, which results in profound and often fatal collapse of the animal. Anaphylactic shock is most frequently encountered in people who receive a therapeutic or prophylactic injection containing some foreign protein to which they have been made sensitive by a previous injection of the same material. It is very rare for it to occur after ingestion of a food.

Foods liable to give rise to allergic reactions

Food allergies are most common in infants and young children. Milk, eggs and wheat are frequently incriminated, presumably because they are the most important initial foods of the young. Sensitivity to the wheat protein, gliadin, is well known and responsible for coeliac disease; to what extent this is due to allergy is uncertain and is discussed on page 405. After the age of 5 there is a tendency to the spontaneous disappearance of food allergy, while allergy to inhaled substances such as pollens, dusts and animal hair and danders becomes increasingly frequent. The list of foods that have been claimed to cause allergic reactions is very large; in addition to those mentioned above it includes such diverse items as fish (especially shellfish), various meats, nuts, mustard, tomatoes, celery, chocolate and oranges.

Some food additives may be bound to protein and then can cause allergic reactions. An example is tartrazine, an azo dye, which is added to many foods and soft drinks, and may cause urticaria and asthma (Zlotlow and Settipane, 1977). The food preservatives sulphur dioxide and sodium benzoate, present in many orange drinks, have also been responsible for attacks of asthma (Freedman, 1977).

CLINICAL MANIFESTATIONS

Skin. Urticaria (nettle rash or hives) is a common allergic reaction at all ages. A less common but more severe giant form is known as angioneurotic oedema. Eczema is an allergic reaction usually due to sensitivity to an agent applied directly to the skin, but often in infants and young children and occasionally in adults to a food allergen.

Respiratory system. Asthma is an allergic disorder. Usually the allergen has been inhaled but sometimes in adults and often in young children the symptoms are due to a food allergen.

Gastrointestinal system. Dyspepsia, abdominal discomfort, vomiting and diarrhoea may all be the results of an allergic reaction. There are many causes of these common symptoms. When they persist or recur repeatedly for no obvious reason, a food allergy should be suspected.

Circulatory system. Anaphylactic shock is due to release of large amounts of histamine which causes widespread vasodilation and circulatory collapse. It is often fatal. It seldom occurs except when an allergen has been injected intravenously. When protein hydrolysates were used for intravenous feeding, an acute anaphylactic reaction was not uncommon. It remains a potential hazard of intravenous feeding but with preparations now available it is very rare.

DETECTION OF FOOD ALLERGIES

Dietary history

A careful dietary history must always be taken. In some cases of food allergy the symptoms develop so rapidly and dramatically, almost immediately after eating the offending food, that the patient is able to make his own diagnosis. More often it is not so easy to associate symptoms with any particular food, especially if there is a delay of some hours between the eating of the suspected food and the onset of illness. A particular food may be wrongly believed by the patient to be the cause of his allergy because it happened to be eaten immediately before an attack, which was in fact due to some other cause. In cases of doubt, the patient should be given a diary in which he records with great care and detail over a period of many days or even weeks all the foods which he eats and the times of his meals. He should note in the diary any disturbances which he believes may be due to food allergy, recording the nature and intensity of the symptoms and the time of their occurrence. If a careful study of the diary suggests a relationship between the intake of a certain food and the onset of allergic manifestations the following tests should be carried out.

Provocative food test

The patient should be given a small quantity of the suspected food in a made-up dish, so that he is unaware that he is eating the food that he suspects and dreads. If the patient notes in his diary his typical symptoms at the appropriate interval after the meal, this strongly suggests that the food is responsible. Owing to the variability of allergic responses, however, the test should be repeated two, or preferably three, times before either a positive or negative result is accepted. If a negative result is obtained on three occasions, it can be concluded that the symptoms are not due to the suspected food. If the tests are positive, then appropriate treatment must be undertaken as discussed below. Provocative food tests should not be made in patients who develop severe allergic reactions immediately after the ingestion of a recognised article of food; the test is unnecessary and may be dangerous.

Strict elimination diets

If the history, skin tests (see below) and trial and error with restricted diets fail to provide a clue to the diagnosis, strict elimination diets may be helpful. With infants and young children this is easier than with adults, because of the limited variety of foods which they eat. It is possible to eliminate from a child's diet separately, and in turn, the common causes of children's food allergy: milk, eggs and wheat. In adults the procedure is much more difficult because of the number of foods to which sensitivity may develop. Hence various types of elimination diets have been devised with the object of discovering the offending article. Patients may have to be fed on such diets for many weeks before the offending article of food is discovered and, as the diets are complicated, they are normally only suitable for the investigation of patients in a hospital with a dietetic department and by a physician experienced in the subject of allergy. As such elimination tests are tedious and time consuming for both patient and doctor, they should be undertaken only when symptoms believed to be due to food sensitivity are seriously inconveniencing the patient.

Skin tests

These have been much used in the past. A minute quantity of an extract of the suspected food is injected into the skin or rubbed into a scratch. If a weal develops and there is a surrounding red flare, this is sometimes taken as indicative of sensitivity to the food in question. The presence of pseudopodia extending out from the weal may be taken as confirmatory evidence. Yet because a patient is sensitive to a foreign protein introduced to the skin in this way, it does not necessarily follow that he is sensitive to the same protein when taken by mouth. Moreover, the skin test may be negative to a protein which is producing allergic reactions elsewhere, e.g. in the gut. Such apparently contradictory results are common. A possible explanation is that the cells in contact with the allergen are not necessarily the site of the appropriate antibody to it. It is only when the allergen combines with its specific antibody that symptoms arise.

The value of skin tests is limited by the frequency of these false positive and negative results. If, however, there is a well-marked reaction to one single article of food, while tests of other food extracts are negative, this may be of value in confirming a suspicious history.

TREATMENT

Elimination of the causative food

If a food can be identified and eliminated from the diet, then the symptoms will not recur. For example, if the responsible article of food is one which is not consumed regularly (e.g. shellfish), it can easily be avoided: it is far more difficult in the case of eggs, milk and wheat, which are present in so many foods—cakes, puddings, sauces gravies, soups, etc. Fontana and Strauss (1973) give a full list of articles of diet to be avoided if a patient is allergic to milk, eggs or wheat. In addition other methods must be tried in such a situation.

A clinical trial showed that the incidence of eczema in

infants whose mother or father had a history of allergy was greatly reduced by following an allergen-avoiding regimen for six months (Matthew *et al.*, 1977). The dietary aspects of the regimen were continuation of breast feeding for six months; if supplements were needed, a soya bean preparation, Velactin, was used and all cow's milk preparations, dairy products, fish and eggs were excluded from the diet. Older children with eczema have benefited from exclusion of eggs and cow's milk from their diet and substitution of a soya milk (Atherton *et al.*, 1978),

Denaturation of the protein. Sometimes if a protein is denatured by heat it ceases to act as an allergen. Thus a patient sensitive to raw milk or lightly boiled eggs may be able to take with impunity boiled milk or an egg which has been boiled for at least 10 minutes. Patients who are sensitive to eggs may be able to take the yolks, especially if well cooked, although the whites may continue to cause symptoms.

Desensitisation. Many attempts have been made to desensitise patients who suffer from food allergy by repeatedly injecting small quantities of the allergen or giving small amounts by mouth. This method is generally regarded as being of little or no value.

Effect of age. Patients tend to outgrow their sensitivity to food allergens. Foods known to have caused reactions in childhood may be tried months or years later when perhaps they can be taken with impunity.

Drugs. Antihistamines are often effective in controlling local forms of allergy such as urticaria and angioneurotic oedema. Somnolence is sometimes an inconvenience if they have to be taken regularly. Bronchodilator drugs are used to treat bronchial spasm in attacks of asthma. Corticosteroids are highly effective in preventing attacks, but their adverse effects limit their long-term use, especially in children. The prescription of tranquillisers and sedatives is often indicated because of the close connection between emotion and allergy, but no drug is capable of bringing about desensitisation.

General advice
Every patient proved to be allergic to a particular food should be advised to avoid it, at least for a time. Some years later he may try it cautiously, especially if it is an important article of diet. All people with a well-defined food allergy should know about it and inform their doctor; otherwise they may suffer a severe or even fatal reaction from a therapeutic injection given for the treatment of some other disease. For instance, a patient sensitive to eggs may react badly to immunising injections prepared on an egg medium, such as those for poliomyelitis, influenza or yellow fever. Similarly patients who are sensitive to pork may develop an allergic response to soluble or zinc protamine insulin (prepared from the pancreas of pigs), should they develop diabetes mellitus and require insulin injections. Insulin zinc suspensions are useful in this respect since they are uncontaminated by species-specific proteins. Injections of ACTH derived from cattle may cause shock in patients allergic to beef.

Maintaining the nutrition of the patient
Many intelligent allergic patients, knowing something of the nature of their disease, go to great lengths to avoid any food that may aggravate it. Some avoid so many kinds of food that they become severely undernourished. A similar result may follow from unwise advice from their doctors. This is particularly true in the case of growing children. It must be stressed that allergic patients should not be subjected to dietary restrictions without good evidence that their symptoms are due to a food allergen. In many cases this can only be determined in a clinic where the appropriate tests can be carried out.

51. Injury, Surgery and Fever

INJURY AND SURGERY

Severe injuries and many disorders requiring major surgical operations are frequently complicated by malnutrition. In the last 20 years an increasing number of surgeons have become interested in nutrition, a subject which now occupies an important place in surgical literature. The standard textbook on the subject is *Metabolic Care of the Surgical Patient* (Moore, 1959), a book which can be strongly recommended to all surgeons, and a symposium edited by Richards and Kinney (1977) gives an account of later work.

Malnutrition secondary to disease of the alimentary tract

This can arise secondary to a variety of conditions which reduce appetite or interfere with swallowing or with digestion and absorption. Carcinoma of the oesophagus and the stomach are typical examples and give rise to a cachexia which is indistinguishable from that of primary starvation. There is a rapid wasting of adipose tissue, muscle and other tissues. Weight may decline rapidly and in extreme cases may fall by as much as 0.5 kg a day. In such patients the loss of nitrogen may be as much as 10 g/day, equivalent to 62 g of protein. This will be associated with a loss of water of up to 200 g/day. There are also losses of potassium which may be as great as 30 mmol/day.

There is much experience to indicate that it is impossible either to prevent or to make good such losses as long as the surgical lesion persists. It is seldom justifiable to delay an operation whilst an attempt is made to improve the nutritional state of the patient. The immediate needs for protein can be met by giving adequate and repeated transfusions of plasma and whole blood. When the lesion is treated satisfactorily, and normal feeding becomes possible, then the nutritional state of the patient improves rapidly.

Malnutrition secondary to operation on the alimentary tract

Operations on the stomach for peptic ulcer are commonly performed and it is perhaps surprising that after a partial gastrectomy digestion and absorption are usually unimpaired. Postcibal syndromes are described on page 401. However, nutritional disorders may arise. Many patients are underweight before the operation, owing to anorexia caused by their symptoms. There is inevitably a loss of weight associated with the operation and the immediate postoperative period. It is common for these losses not to be made good completely and many patients remain thin, but few are seriously undernourished.

An iron-deficiency anaemia arises in about 40 per cent of patients. This is due to a failure in absorption of iron present in foods, perhaps due to loss of acid secretion, but medicinal iron is well absorbed. Much less commonly a megaloblastic anaemia arises due to failure to absorb vitamin B_{12} owing to loss of intrinsic factor. Owing to the store of the vitamin in the liver, this may not develop for several years. Sometimes, mainly in elderly patients, failure to absorb vitamin D and calcium leads to the development of osteomalacia.

Now that vagotomy and pyloroplasty are tending to replace partial gastrectomy in the surgical treatment of peptic ulcer, these nutritional changes are seen less frequently, but they may occur after any gastroduodenal operation. As they may be present in patients who profess to be satisfied with the result of operation, a satisfaction which may result from a loss of pain rather than a true return to health, it is essential that all patients after gastroduodenal operations should be examined by the family doctor at regular intervals (at least once a year) after operation. If anything untoward is found the patient should be referred to the operating surgeon for special investigation.

Catabolic response to injury

Any severe injury or major surgical operation leads to a generalised loss of tissue. Cuthbertson (1930) was the first to show that injury is followed by an increased excretion of urinary nitrogen due to a breakdown of proteins throughout the body, and he has again reviewed the effects of trauma (Cuthbertson, 1971). The resultant negative nitrogen balance is usually of the order of 12 to 15 g/day, corresponding to a loss of 350 to 450 g of muscle and other lean tissues. This rate of loss continues for two to three days and then decreases, provided convalescence is proceeding satisfactorily. A negative nitrogen balance may, however, persist for as long as a week, even in cases in which the operation has been entirely satisfactory. Potassium loss from the cells also occurs and is often higher than the corresponding nitrogen loss. Healthy muscles contain about 3 mmol of potassium/g of nitrogen. During the catabolic phase after injury the K/N ratio in the urine may be as high as 7.5 mmol/g.

This tissue breakdown in response to injury or surgery is partly due to an increased secretion of cortical hormones by the adrenal glands. This is part of the normal physiological response to stress and is mediated through the pituitary gland and increased secretion of ACTH. Other endocrine changes that follow injury are an increase in plasma catecholamines and in glucagon concentration (Lindsey *et al.*, 1974). Plasma insulin is low (Blackburn *et al.*, 1973).

These endocrine responses are often accompanied by a reduced dietary intake, and these together have an effect on the metabolic mixture. There is increased utilisation of amino acids for gluconeogenesis which maintains the blood glucose. Oxidation of fatty acids is increased and this may provide 70 to 80 per cent of the energy needs (Tweedle and Johnston, 1971). The mild ketosis that is often present may be beneficial as acetoacetic acid and β-hydroxybutyric acid are readily utilised by the tissues.

It is not possible to prevent this loss of tissue by dietary measures and, in so far as it seems to be a physiological response, there is little justification for attempting to do so. However, the loss must be made good when convalescence is established.

A typical example of the loss of tissue that may occur after gastrectomy is given by Wilkinson (1961), whose data are reproduced in Table 51.1. The losses of the patients are compared with those of healthy controls who underwent the same restrictions of food and water for a similar period of four days. During this period the patients' loss of weight was nearly 1 kg more than that of the controls; while the patients also lost 100 g more protein and twice as much potassium. The figures in Table 51.1 for the electrolyte losses in starving healthy persons, notably the large loss of sodium, suggest strongly that in simple starvation most of the water lost comes from the extracellular compartments. In contrast, when severe injuries or major surgical procedures cause malnutrition the large potassium loss indicates that most of the water lost comes from the intracellular compartment.

Table 51.1 Mean values for the loss of weight and other body substances by 15 patients after gastrectomy, and by four healthy controls during a period of 4 days. Both groups received no food for 4 days and no water for the first 2 days and limited water for the second 2 days (modified from Wilkinson, 1961)

	Patients after gastrectomy	Healthy controls
Weight loss (kg)	4.13	3.26
Protein loss (N × 6.25 g)	390	280
K loss (mmol)	312	154
Na loss (mmol)	167	264

(All values expressed per 65 kg body weight)

Sepsis and malnutriton

Malnutrition may develop in patients with chronic illnesses associated with sepsis. Large septic burns, infection of the site of a fracture, peritonitis or chronic abscesses in any part of the body are examples. The associated toxaemia may so impair appetite that little food is eaten. Further, the accompanying fever, by raising the metabolic rate, increases the needs for nutrients. Large negative balances of energy, proteins and other essential substances may result. Loss of weight may be rapid and can be as much as 1 kg/day. When a big area of skin is destroyed over a septic burn the direct loss of protein from the burnt surface may be as much as 50 g/day.

ASSESSMENT OF THE NUTRITIONAL STATE

Wasting, which may be severe, is commonly found in patients who have had to undergo major abdominal surgery, have extensive burns, or who are suffering from chronic sepsis. It is important to be able to assess the progress toward recovery and to judge the success or failure of treatment designed to restore the lost tissues. Changes in body weight may be a useful guide and weighing beds are available which enable patients who are seriously ill to be weighed with a minimum of disturbance. The interpretation of changes in weight is, however, often difficult. Patients who are wasted always have a relative increase in body water and are often oedematous. A recorded gain in weight may be due to an increase in oedema rather than a replacement of lost tissue. In wasted patients the aim is to build up the 'cell mass'. Methods of measuring the cell mass have been outlined in Chapter 2.

Wasting is always associated with depletion of protein and potassium. These are the most important nutritional deficiencies in surgical practice. The concentration of plasma albumin is a useful index of the state of protein repletion. The lower limit of normality is 35 g/1. Levels in severely wasted patients are often well below this figure. A rise or fall in plasma albumin is an index of progress provided there is no haemoconcentration or haemodilution.

Plasma potassium is not a reliable guide to the state of the potassium in the body. In the absence of diarrhoea it is not difficult to get a rough approximation of the potassium balance. The output in the urine can be easily measured. An assessment of the intake in the food can be made with the use of food tables. The amount of medicinal potassium given will be known. A good positive potassium balance strongly suggests that tissue regeneration is occurring. The measurement of the total exchangeable potassium provides a good indication of the state of potassium deficiency.

Vitamins

Vitamin K is the vitamin of particular interest to the surgeon because deficiency of this vitamin may be associated with a tendency to bleed consequent on hypoprothrombinaemia. Since vitamin K is fat soluble, a deficiency may occur when a failure in fat absorption develops from any cause. In surgical practice this most frequently arises in diseases of the biliary system associated with jaundice.

Vitamin C deficiency may develop in surgical patients. Operations, injuries and especially burns increase utilisation of ascorbic acid. This is part of the response to stress and is brought about by increased activity of the adrenal cortex. The needs of such patients for vitamin C are therefore augmented. It has long been known that when there is severe depletion of vitamin C in the tissues, the healing of wounds may be grossly impaired. In surgical practice in Britain and in other prosperous countries, frank scurvy is exceedingly rare, and it is very uncommon for depletion of reserves of the vitamin to be so severe as to prejudice the healing of wounds. The great majority of surgical patients do not require extra vitamin C in the form of synthetic ascorbic acid, provided they are given a well-balanced diet. However, in chronic illnesses, especially if sepsis is present, it is essential to make sure that the intake of the vitamin is adequate. In countries where the usual diet contains little, it is advisable to provide all patients, who have been severely injured or burnt or who have had major operations, with a good supply either in the form of fruit juice or as synthetic ascorbic acid.

DIETARY MANAGEMENT

Preoperative
As a surgical operation is a nutritional stress, the patient should be well nourished before undergoing one.

Weakness, loss of appetite due to anxiety and other causes may create difficulties and the care of a dietitian is often invaluable. Routine hospital diets are often monotonous, and should be adjusted to the needs and tastes of the individual patient. If the patient is undernourished it is advisable to attempt to correct this, provided the need for the operation is not urgent. A diet rich in energy and protein should be given. However, if the malnutrition is directly attributable to a disease or an injury it is wrong to postpone the operation, since it is difficult, if not impossible, to achieve dietary rehabilitation until the surgical condition has been corrected.

Obese patients are poor anaesthetic risks. If the need for an operation is not urgent, it is usually wise to postpone it until some reduction in weight has been achieved by dietetic treatment. This may help the surgeon and anaesthetist in their immediate technical tasks and perhaps improve the patient's ability to recover more quickly. The management of obese patients who are also diabetics and who require an operation is described on page 362.

While it is unwise to starve a patient before operation, it is also dangerous to anaesthetise a subject whose stomach is full of food. This risk can be obviated by making the patient fast overnight. If the operation is to take place in the afternoon, he may be given a very light breakfast. If for any reason the start of the operation has to be postponed, the patient should be given small quantities of sweetened fruit juices in water. This helps to maintain his reserves of energy and prevent dehydration.

Postoperative
Neither fluid nor food should be given until the patient is fully recovered from the anaesthetic. Otherwise there is a risk that they will be inhaled into the lungs with the subsequent danger of aspiration pneumonia. This risk is also present if attempts are made to give the patient food or fluids when recumbent. If the patient cannot sit up after recovery from the anaesthetic, or if he cannot eat and drink normally because he is seriously ill or for any other reason, e.g. continuous gastric suction after operations on the stomach and duodenum, he should be fed intravenously (Chapter 52).

With modern anaesthetics a patient is likely to be hungry and able to eat as soon as he has recovered consciousness fully. At first he should be given small frequent feeds. If postoperative convalescence proceeds normally and there are no complications, the patient's appetite is usually a reliable guide to requirements; there is no need to force food in the early stages of convalescence. As the patient has to make good the losses of K and N, the convalescent diet should contain ample fruit and milk, meat, pulses or other good sources of protein, but there is no need for a special diet.

FEVER

During fever basal metabolism increases by about 10 per cent for every degree centigrade rise in body temperature (Du Bois, 1948). Associated with the general increase of metabolism, there are increased nitrogen losses in the urine. For these reasons and because there is usually a loss of appetite and diminished food intake, a febrile patient loses weight and, if the fever is prolonged, may become severely emaciated.   The metabolic responses to fever have also been studied experimentally by inducing self-limiting infections in healthy human volunteers. Sandfly fever produces a sharp and uncomfortable fever lasting a few days but complete recovery is invariable. US army volunteers given the infection experimentally showed a negative nitrogen balance, decreased plasma concentrations of all amino acids except phenylalanine and decreased plasma iron and zinc (Wannemacher et al., 1972). Urinary riboflavin excretion increased (Beisel et al., 1972) and in another mild infection, the common cold, plasma ascorbic acid fell while urinary excretion increased (Hume and Weyers, 1973). These changes are presumably more marked in long-lasting fevers.

In a long-continued fever, therefore, an effort should be

made to prevent undue loss of body protein by the prescription of a diet in which the protein intake is in excess of the maintenance requirement in health. There is no ground for the old belief that a high protein intake increases the height of the fever.

Apart from these theoretical considerations, the arrangement of the diet is made difficult by the anorexia, present in most fevers, which may be complicated by nausea and vomiting. Much can be done to help by ensuring that the mouth is kept clean. If the tongue is furred and sordes are allowed to accumulate, it is not surprising that the patient has a distaste for food. The mouth should be washed or swabbed out with a weak solution of sodium bicarbonate or other mouthwash before and after every meal.

DIET IN FEVER

The introduction of antibiotics and chemotherapeutic agents has greatly reduced the length of most febrile illnesses. Formerly in diseases like enteric fever, pyrexia frequently persisted for three or four weeks, but now it is usually restricted to a few days as a result of treatment. Likewise, in the severe forms of pulmonary tuberculosis pyrexia was present for months or years prior to the introduction of chemotherapeutic agents which now bring it under control in days or weeks. In consequence the wasting and malnutriton that in the past were so frequently associated with long-continued fevers are fortunately seldom seen. Nevertheless there are still febrile illnesses in which the infection cannot be brought under control for a considerable time and in such cases the provision of an adequate diet is of great importance and often presents many difficulties. It is best to consider diet in fever under two headings: (1) fevers of short duration, e.g. influenza and pneumonia; (2) long-continued fevers, when the infection does not respond to antibiotics. Long periods of fever often occur in immunological disorders, in some forms of malignant tumour and in leukaemia and then loss of weight, malaise and anaemia are frequently present.

Short febrile illnesses

In fevers of short duration such as influenza and pneumonia, which last a matter of days, not weeks, the diet should be constructed with the chief object of saving the patient from all possible exertion in the taking of his food; the actual amount of nourishment given is of less importance.

For the first two or three days the diet should be fluid or semifluid and given in the form of small feeds at frequent intervals, usually every two to three hours. Milk is the mainstay of the diet and about 2 pints (1 litre) should be given daily. This provides about 40 g protein and about 3.0 MJ (700 kcal). Some of the milk feeds should be flavoured with cocoa, coffee or tea, or given as an egg switch. Two or three eggs may be given daily, switched in milk or an egg and fruit drink. Liquid cooked cereals such as a gruel or any of the proprietary preparations, served with cream, and cup custards may be given at some of the feeds to vary the diet. Fresh fruit juice should be given in ample amounts for its sugar content and also as a flavouring agent for the water, which should be supplied to the patient between feeds in liberal quantities. At least 2 to 3 litres of fluid should be taken daily. Diet No. 16 meets these requirements.

As soon as the temperature falls and the patient's appetite improves, a bland diet containing ample protein and energy should be given. Within another two or three days the patient should be taking a good well-balanced diet suitable for convalescence (Diet No. 1). Due attention should be given to the instructions in Diet No. 17 for the prevention and treatment of dyspepsia which is liable to occur in patients recovering from febrile illnesses and from the effects of chemotherapeutic agents on the gastrointestinal tract.

Long-continued fever

If in seven days a fever is not responding to antibiotics, it.is necessary to see that the dietary intake, and particularly the intake of protein and energy, is sufficient to meet the extra requirements imposed by the fever. The object of dietetic treatment is to reduce mortality by providing the nutrients required for the body's immune mechanisms, to prevent or curtail the weakness and loss of weight which is so noticeable in long-continued fevers, and to accelerate convalescence. The principles governing the construction of the diet in these circumstances are as follows.

1. The diet should have a high energy value—up to 50 per cent more than the normal maintenance intake for a person in bed. This means that the diet should yield at least 10 MJ (2400 kcal)/day.

2. A liberal protein quota is needed to make good the loss of body protein. Owing to the anorexia and the necessity for providing food in liquid or semisolid form, it may not be possible to give more than 70 to 90 g of protein daily, but this covers the protein loss except in the most severe fevers.

3. A large proportion of the food ingested should be in the form of carbohydrate. This prevents ketosis, which may arise if the patient is burning his own body fat in increased amounts owing to the raised metabolism. The protein sparing property of a high carbohydrate diet is also of practical importance.

4. Food should be served initially in liquid or semisolid form and must be easily digestible, well cooked and appetising. Large meals should be avoided and small feeds should be given every two or three hours.

5. Fluids should be given in abundance. Owing to the loss of fluid in sweat and the disinclination of patients to take fluids and food, dehydration may develop in fever. Fluids require to be given in greater amounts than are usually ingested, but excessive amounts should not be

forced on the patient. A daily total fluid intake of about 2½ to 3 litres is ample. If vomiting and diarrhoea are prominent features, parenteral treatment may be required.

Salt depletion occurs from sweating and this should be made good by adding sodium chloride to suitable feeds and to the glucose lemonade drinks. Diet No. 16 is a semifluid one, which may be used in the early stages of a long-continued fever.

As the patient improves and can take solid food, this diet should be modified by the addition of toast or bread with butter or margarine, milk puddings, custards and stewed or fresh fruit, puréed vegetables, eggs, cream of chicken and fish. It is advisable to supplement the diet with vitamins if the patient is eating poorly.

In convalescence the appetite is usually increased, but it is best to proceed slowly and not allow a food intake too great for the patient's power of digestion. The food should be easily digestible and rich in protein and vitamins. Foods such as pastries and cakes and highly seasoned and indigestible articles should be avoided. Diet No. 1 is suitable for use during convalescence.

Fever in infants and children

Children are more susceptible to the ill-effects of fever than adults. Feverish children should be nursed in a cool room, wear light clothing and have plenty of fresh air. The principles of the dietetic treatment of adults as described above are applicable for infants and children and are even more important since they are particularly susceptible to dehydration and protein malnutrition. This is especially the case in tropical countries where nutritional diseases are common. For example, a child with pre-kwashiorkor who contracts measles may become extremely ill in a short time and develop severe protein-energy malnutrition rapidly.

CONVALESCENCE

Diet has an important part to play in determining the speed with which a patient recovers from a surgical operation, fever or any serious illness, and hence in the length of time that he occupies a hospital bed. Ample amounts of protein are needed to make good the drain on the body's reserves of protein and, if the patient is underweight, plenty of energy to build him up. Routine hospital diets are often inadequate for these purposes. Furthermore, the patient's appetite may be fickle. Every art of the dietitian may be needed to tempt his jaded appetite.

Once normal feeding has been re-established, a regimen such as Diet No. 1 is satisfactory for most adult patients. Medicinal iron may be needed if the patient is still anaemic from previous bleeding.

Finally it should be remembered that many patients are necessarily confined to bed for long period during convalescence—e.g. those recovering from multiple injuries involving fractures of bone and those requiring repeated skin grafts for extensive burns. Prolonged immobilisation in bed often leads to extensive demineralisation of the bones. Physiotherapy and occupational therapy can do much to check this process by keeping the movable parts of the body active; at the same time a good calcium intake, provided by plenty of milk, is desirable, to assist remineralisation. The calcium lost from the bones is excreted in the urine and, if the flow or urine is sluggish, calcium stones may develop in the urinary tract. A high fluid intake (2 to 3 litres daily) should be encouraged, to ensure that the urine is sufficiently dilute to keep calcium salts in solution.

52. Special Feeding Methods and Food in Hospitals

Patients are often unable to take by mouth sufficient quantities of ordinary foods and fluids to supply their daily needs or to make good previous deficiencies. The circumstances under which this may arise are many and include the following.

1. Any severe illness such as a continued fever, prolonged sepsis, extensive burns or malignant disease: these may result in loss of appetite and leave the patient too weak to take sufficient food to meet his increased requirements. Some victims of famine are reduced to this condition.

2. Cancer or any other disease of the mouth, pharynx and oesophagus, which obstructs the passage of food and so makes normal feeding difficult, if not impossible.

3. Patients who are unconscious or delirious and so unable to feed themselves, e.g. with severe disease or injury of the brain, hepatic failure, diabetic coma or acute uraemia.

4. Similar problems have to be solved in cases where diseases of the lower intestine lead to diarrhoea or malabsorption. They may lead to anorexia, to impairment of absorption and to loss of fluids and nutrients per rectum. Such diseases include ulcerative colitis, regional enteritis and dysentery at all ages and gastroenteritis in infants and young children. In the latter group the intestinal disease is often associated with malnutrition—the familiar vicious circle of PEM.

The supply of energy and protein and of fluid and electrolytes presents different problems which are considered separately.

ENERGY AND PROTEINS

Five methods are available for giving extra energy and protein: (1) normal foods taken by mouth may be enriched by adding suitable supplements; (2) The use of **elemental diets** in which all the components are identifiable chemicals; protein may be replaced by amino acids, and carbohydrate is in easily assimilable forms; (3) food may be introduced into the stomach by a tube passed through the nose or mouth down the oesophagus; (4) food may be introduced into the stomach or jejunum through a tube inserted at an operation for gastrostomy or jejunostomy; (5) nutrients may be given intravenously.

It was the practice in days gone by to give foods of various kinds per rectum. Nutrient enemas have now been abandoned, because only small amounts of nutrients were absorbed and rectal irritation was frequently produced.

ORAL SUPPLEMENTS

Increased intakes of energy and protein can be obtained by enriching ordinary foods such as milk, proprietary milk preparations, soups, soufflés, jellies, cakes and ice-creams with casein, fat emulsions or sugars. Proprietary preparations of casein and of fat are on the market and can be incorporated readily into the other foods. Complan (Glaxo Ltd) is a powdered preparation of milk proteins: 100 g provides 31 g of protein, 44 g of carbohydrate and 16 g of fat, and it is also rich in minerals and vitamins, though low in sodium. Casilan (Glaxo Ltd) is a preparation of milk protein, almost devoid of fat, carbohydrate and sodium. Lonalac (Mead Johnson) is a milk protein preparation almost devoid of sodium.

These preparations can be mixed with sugar and vegetable oil in any proportion and a number of recipes made up. Flavouring agents—coffee, vanilla, strawberry, etc.—may be added. If cane sugar or glucose is used, this makes any mixture very sweet; hence patients may prefer dextrins as a source of carbohydrate. The components can be made up with varying quantities of water to different consistencies and served either as a hot drink or a cold ice-cream. If a little gelatin is added, the whole mixture can be made to set as a jelly.

With suitable encouragement it may be possible to persuade patients to take sufficient quantities of such concentrated foods to enable satisfactory progress to be made during convalescence from severe medical illnesses or from operations.

These considerations apply especially to patients with cancer and to those receiving radiotherapy. There is no good evidence that either effect nutrition directly, except when there is a neoplasm of the alimentary tract or liver, but patients are often depressed and have little appetite. The gross wasting that may occur in cancer patients, malignant cachexia, is usually preventable by providing appetising meals with a high energy density and coaxing the patient to eat.

NASOGASTRIC FEEDING

Advantages. Nasogastric feeding can supply all types of nutrients in adequate amounts. They can be—but are not always—in the form of natural foodstuffs. Large quantities of fluid can be given daily with safety; this is important in dehydrated patients. Food supplements and medicines, which may be distasteful to the patients, can be given down the tube. Feeds are easily prepared, stored and administered; they are usually well tolerated and can be readily modified. Both the hazards and the cost are much less than with intravenous feeding.

Contraindications. Diseases of the mouth, pharynx or oesophagus may make the passage of the tube difficult or impossible. If the patient already has a cuffed endotracheal tube or a tracheostomy, the presence of tubes in both trachea and oesophagus may cause necrosis of the intervening soft tissue. Diseases of the intestines which interfere with digestion and absorption may make tube feeding difficult, though diarrhoea may be the result of an unsuitable feed rather than organic disease in the gastrointestinal tract. If the patient is vomiting, tube feeding is dangerous and contraindicated.

Introduction of the tube

A soft plastic tube is used and should be lubricated with olive oil or liquid paraffin. While usually unnecessary, in nervous patients the nose may be sprayed with a surface anaesthetic. Generally one nostril is more patent than the other, and this side should be used for the initial passage of a tube. When about 20 cm of the tube have been inserted it has reached the pharynx , and the patient may cough or retch. At this point he should be encouraged to swallow, with the result that the tube enters the oesophagus; thereafter it can be pushed quickly down into the stomach with little or no discomfort to the patient. Little difficulty arises in patients who co-operate and who retain the swallowing reflex. When this reflex is lost, or when a patient is in coma or delirium, the tube may be directed manually behind the epiglottis into the entrance of the oesophagus. The insertion of a thin wire stylet inside the tube may facilitate its passage. It is essential in all cases to be sure that the tube has passed into the oesophagus and not into the trachea, since the introduction of fluid into the lungs causes intense discomfort to the patient, and may be fatal. If the tube is in the trachea or bronchus, dyspnoea and coughing occur, and air can be felt and heard issuing from the outlet of the tube.

Fluid should never be introduced into the tube unless a sample of gastric juice has first been aspirated. Having made certain that the tube is in the stomach, it is strapped to the forehead and connected with a gravity drip apparatus, fixed in position to a stand above the level of the patient. The rate of flow is controlled by a screw clamp. Delirious and insane patients may attempt to pull the tube from the nose, and this must be prevented by adequate sedation and, if necessary, by splinting the arms. Although a tube may be left in position in the same nostril for six days without any apparent harm it is better to withdraw it every 48 hours and, after washing and boiling, to reinsert it into the stomach through the other nostril. Once in position,

the patient complains of little or no discomfort, and no interference with sleep usually results. As the mouth is unobstructed, the patient can cough and spit in comfort, and can supplement the gastric feeds by oral ingestion if he is able and wishes to do so.

Feeding procedure

1. The first fluid down the tube should be about 50 ml of water. An hour later the stomach is aspirated to check that the water has been absorbed and thereafter feeds are worked up in volume and strength over one to two days.

2. Before each feed it is essential to check that the tube is still in the stomach. Regurgitation of gastric contents into the lungs is the most important hazard of tube feeding.

3. Feeds are usually given every four hours but the day's amount may be made up in bulk and stored in a refrigerator. If this is done, the feed should be warmed before it is administered. The usual volume of a feed is 250 ml, which should be followed by 50 ml of water to rinse the tube.

4. The most important component is water. Sufficient must be given to prevent dehydration and to allow the kidneys to excrete the solute load. For an adult 2 litres/24 hours is the usual amount, but more may be needed if the patient is dehydrated or has excessive fluid losses.

5. The feed used may be 'homemade' and a recipe for one day is as follows: milk 1500 ml, eggs 2, glucose 100 g and vegetable oil 100 g. This provides 9.0 MJ (2150 kcal), 66 g of protein and 1370 ml of water. Additional water is needed and for some patients the lactose content is too high. To meet this, part or most of the milk can be replaced by a thin porridge and the protein made up with casein or comminuted chicken.

6. Alternatively, proprietary foods may be used and a recipe for one day is a mixture of 250 g Complan, 100 ml Prosparol (a 50 per cent emulsion of peanut oil in water) and 100 g glucose or glucose polymer with water to 1800 ml. This provides 70 g protein, 50 g fat and 8.0 MJ (1900 kcal) plus all essential nutrients; as it is low in sodium (1.0 g or 40 mmol Na/day), extra salt is normally added. This feed can be easily modified to a high or low protein content by adjusting the amount of Complan or it can be thickened by replacing some of the glucose with a form of starch such as cornflour.

A list of suitable proprietary formulae is given in Appendix 3 (p. 573). Most of these are manufactured in the USA. Some are made from mixed foods, many are based on milk, and some are a combination of natural foods with chemically defined substances. A fourth group are entirely made up of chemically defined substances; in these elemental diets proteins are replaced by mixtures of pure amino acids, and they are residue-free. As they are more expensive than other formulae, they are indicated only for special conditions, e.g. after bowel surgery.

7. Tube feeds do not always meet requirements for

some minerals, e.g. iron, magnesium or zinc. Supplements may be necessary for patients on long-term treatment. Most of the complete formulae provide the requirements of the major vitamins, but this should be checked and supplements given if the patient was previously malnourished.

8. The patient's fluid balance should be charted and a watch kept for diarrhoea or vomiting. The blood urea, electrolytes and haemoglobin should be measured regularly.

9. Pitfalls are to give feeds unnecessarily rich in protein and not to provide enough water to allow the urea to be excreted. High sodium intakes may also increase the solute load for the kidneys. Temporary or chronic renal disease may be a cause of a rise in blood urea. Unless the patient is losing excessive amounts of protein there is no reason for giving more than 35 to 40 g of protein/4.2 MJ (1000 kcal). Some of the complete formulae should therefore be mixed with one of the carbohydrate or fat preparations.

10. Diarrhoea is common and often the result of giving too strong a feed to a patient who has not been eating for some days. High concentrations of sugar, and especially lactose, are liable to cause diarrhoea, and dextrins and glucose polymers are better tolerated. If a patient has steatorrhoea, medium chain triglycerides may be substituted for vegetable oil emulsions.

Day and Buckell (1971) have written a helpful paper on tube feeding of unconscious patients.

GASTROSTOMY AND JEJUNOSTOMY FEEDING

Feeds can be given through tubes inserted at operation into the stomach or jejunum. Feeding by either route often enables weight to be maintained, but lost tissue is seldom replaced. A mixture similar to that recommended for nasogastric feeding can be used. Resort to gastrostomy and jejunostomy feeding is necessary only when it is impossible to pass an intragastric tube or, in the case of jejunostomy, when there is gross disease of the stomach.

INTRAVENOUS FEEDING

Intravenous feeding, also known as parenteral nutrition, bypasses the processes of digestion and absorption in the gut. Indications for its use are conditions which prevent or make difficult or undesirable either oral feeding or the passing of a nasogastric tube. These arise after injuries or operations involving the face, mouth, oesophagus, stomach and small intestine. Usually it is required to help to tide the patient over a crisis lasting only a few days. However, the technique can be used to provide complete nutrition for many weeks or even years; this may be necessary in a patient who has had a large part of the small bowel resected and, very rarely, for other conditions, such as prolonged coma after a head injury. It should not be used to prolong the life of patients for whom there is no hope of recovery.

Effective intravenous feeding has only been possible since about 1965. Intravenous glucose solutions had been in regular use for many years before this. However, because of the tendency for glucose to irritate veins and cause thrombophlebitis, it was undesirable to infuse solutions of glucose at a concentration higher than 5 or at most 10 per cent into a peripheral vein. Using only a 5 per cent solution, it is impossible to give sufficient glucose to meet even half the requirements of basal metabolism. The introduction of inert polythene catheters, which could be inserted subcutaneously and manipulated into a central vein, greatly reduced the risk involved in using concentrated glucose solutions, e.g. 40 per cent.

Many preparations of amino acid solutions and emulsions of lipid were tried and discarded because the danger of febrile reactions which they provoked outweighed any nutritional benefit from their use. The technical problems of removing pyrogenic substances and of preparing stable emulsions of lipids have been overcome, and now a number of preparations of nutrients suitable for intravenous use are available commercially.

Nutrient solutions

Table 52.1 lists some solutions available in Britain, made up and sterilised in bottles containing 500 ml. Choice of solution obviously depends on the nature of the patient's illness. Glucose tolerance is often impaired in patients who are seriously ill and large infusions may induce a state of diabetes. For this reason fructose or sorbitol which are not dependent on insulin for their metabolism may be preferred. However, rapid infusions (>0.5 g/kg hourly) can cause abdominal pain and lactic acidosis. Invert sugar, a mixture of equal parts of glucose and fructose is sometimes used. Sorbitol is converted in the body into fructose and its loss in the urine is higher than with glucose or fructose; there seems to be no advantage in using it.

Casein or fibrin hydrolysates contain only the natural L-amino acids; their preparation involves dialysis to separate remaining peptides which may be antigenic or pyrogenic. Synthetic amino acids are at first a mixture of the D and L forms; the former cannot be used for protein synthesis; they are deaminated or excreted by the kidneys. Trophysan is a racemic mixture of the essential amino acids but contains only glycine of the non-essential acids. Vamin contains only the L-amino acids which have been separated by chemical means and is therefore expensive. In practice the synthetic amino acids appear to have little or no advantage over casein hydrolysates. However, attention has been drawn to the high content of ammonia in protein hydrolysates, which makes them unsuitable for newborn babies (Ghadimi *et al.*, 1971).

Emulsions of soya-bean oil and cotton seed oil are now prepared in isotonic media in which the droplets are less than 1 μm in diameter. These enable energy to be supplied in a more concentrated form than solutions of carbohydrate or amino acids and hence the water load is less. The

Table 52.1 Some nutrient solutions available for intravenous use. Amounts of nutrients are those present in a bottle containing 500 ml of solution

Carbohydrate solution	Concentration per cent	Energy MJ	kcal
Glucose or fructose	5	0.4	94
	10	0.8	187
	20	1.6	375
	50	4.0	940

Amino acid solutions	Protein equivalent (g)	Additional sources of energy (g)	Total energy kJ	kcal	Sodium (mmol)	Potassium (mmol)
Casein hydrolysates						
Aminosol-glucose*	16	glucose, 25	630	150	25	—
Aminosol-fructose-ethanol*	16	fructose, 75 ethanol, 12	1760	425	25	—
Aminosol 10%*	50	—	690	165	80	—
Amigen 5%	20	—	360	85	17	10
Synthetic amino acids						
Trophysan 5%	18	sorbitol	750	180	3	4
Trophysan 10%	36	sorbitol	1500	360	5	4
Vamin	35	fructose	1360	325	25	10

Fat emulsions	Lipid (g)	Glycerol (g)	Sorbitol (g)	Energy MJ	kcal
Intralipid 10% (soya-bean oil + egg lecithin)	50	12.5	—	2.3	550
Intralipid 20%	100	12.5	—	4.2	1000
Lipiphysan 10% cotton seed + soya lecithin)	50	—	25	2.6	620

* This is the Aminosol made by Vitrum in Sweden. It should not be confused with Aminosol, Abbott, used in the USA which is prepared by enzymic hydrolysis of beef fibrin.

fat is metabolised in the same way as that absorbed after oral ingestion. As the liver plays a major role in fat metabolism, emulsions should not be given to patients with impaired liver function. Also they should not be given to patients with coronary heart disease.

Ethyl alcohol is rapidly metabolised by the liver and is used as a source of energy (p. 59). Up to 25 ml may be added to a bottle of carbohydrate solution and, provided it is given slowly, this dose has a sedative effect and is not intoxicating.

Hazards. Peripheral veins readily develop thrombophlebitis as a reaction to the cannula or to the irritant effects of glucose, a low pH or other constituent of the solution, or to bacterial infection. For this reason if parenteral nutrition is to be maintained for more than a few days, it is essential to pass a catheter into a central vein. Thromboembolism and septicaemia are serious complications but fortunately rare.

Dosage

After an operation on the upper alimentary tract when it is expected that the patient will be able to take food in two or three days, three to four bottles of an amino acid solution and a 5 or 10 per cent glucose or fructose solution can be given over 24 hours via a peripheral vein. This does not meet full requirements for either energy or protein, but goes some way to preventing the metabolic effects of starvation and relieves the patient of an uncomfortable sense of hunger. In some surgical clinics after operations for peptic ulcer, it is usual to keep the stomach empty by the use of continuous suction for two or three days; then the above dosage is satisfactory.

If it is intended to meet energy and protein requirements or to exceed them, so as to build up tissue lost as a result of disease, then more bottles and more concentrated solutions must be used. For this purpose and in all cases where intravenous feeding is to be continued for several days, it is essential to infuse the fluid into a central vein. Table 52.2 shows how it is possible to give a patient 12.5 MJ (3000 kcal) of energy and 64 g of protein in 24 hours using in all seven bottles of three different solutions. The number and nature of the bottles used can be varied according to the amount of nutrients deemed necessary.

Intravenous feeding necessitates careful monitoring of

Table 52.2 Solutions for parenteral nutrition for 24 hours

Solution	Number of bottles	Volume (ml)	Energy MJ	Energy kcal	Protein (g)
Glucose 20%	1	500	1.6	375	—
Intralipid 10%	2	1000	4.6	1100	—
Aminosol+fructose+ethanol	4	2000	7.0	1700	64
Total	7	3500	13.2	3175	64

water and electrolyte balances. The amount of fluid infused and the urinary volumes should be recorded daily. Concentrations of plasma electrolytes and blood urea should be measured at first daily, and thereafter at frequent intervals. All patients require a vitamin supplement and iron medication may be needed. Blood has often been lost around the time of the injury or at the operation. The amount of blood removed for analyses can be an additional loss, especially in children, and patients may need parenteral iron therapy. If intravenous feeding is continued for weeks, it is essential to ensure that the patient receives all the nutrients listed in Table 15.3. Patients have now lived for over four years solely on intravenous feeding and this can be given in the home. For further information an article by Lee (1977) and a monograph by Greep et al. (1977) may be consulted.

WATER AND ELECTROLYTES

Deficiencies of water and electrolytes are most easily corrected by the oral route including nasogastric feeding, but this may be difficult or impossible under the circumstances listed at the beginning of this chapter and then parenteral replacement is essential. Intravenous infusion is the method of choice. Only in this way is it possible to be certain that absorption is rapid and complete. Fluid may also be given subcutaneously, intraperitoneally or per rectum. These routes should only be used when for some technical reason intravenous infusion cannot be given.

It is beyond the scope of this book to deal fully with the many problems presented by fluid replacement therapy. There are several excellent monographs on the subject, notably that by Wilkinson (1972). Here only a brief outline of some general principles is given. Parenteral therapy may be used either for replacement of losses that have already taken place or for maintenance when oral intake is impossible. When the intake by mouth ceases or is insufficient, water continues to be lost in the urine and by the insensible loss from the lungs and skin. Some electrolytes are lost but the main deficiency is of water. A frequent cause of deficiency of both water and sodium is loss of gastrointestinal secretions from diarrhoea or vomiting. Potassium deficiency may develop under similar circumstances and whenever there is marked wasting of tissues.

Before starting parenteral therapy a decision is necessary on what solution should be used and how much should be given. This is based on a careful history of the nature, amount and duration of the fluid and electrolyte losses and upon an estimation of the amount needed for maintenance. Rapid changes in weight may occur as a consequence of either loss or administration of fluid, and weighing the patient daily is the best means of both assessment and control but is not always practical. A careful record of fluid intake and output should be kept for all patients who receive parenteral fluids, and this balance chart should include a space in which can be written instructions on the quantities of fluid and electrolytes which are to be given.

Parenteral therapy has potential hazards both local and general. Any solution can irritate the wall of the vein and glucose is particularly prone to do so; the aseptic phlebitis produced is not dangerous, unless bacterial invasion of the clot occurs; then septicaemia may result. This is particularly liable to happen if a polythene catheter is passed into one of the great veins.

A general hazard is that of overloading the body with fluids. Two types of such overloading may occur; on the one hand an excess of water with sodium retention produces oedema usually first manifest as crepitations at the lung bases; on the other hand overloading with water alone may cause a state of water intoxication with a low plasma sodium concentration and an increase in intracellular water, leading to general symptoms of apathy and lethargy; coma and convulsions may follow.

PARENTERAL ADMINISTRATION OF WATER AND GLUCOSE

Water without electrolytes is usually required to correct insensible losses of fluid from the skin and lungs, when for any reason the patient is unable to drink sufficient fluid. For this purpose glucose is the best non-ionic substance with which to make an infusion isotonic with the blood. A concentration of 5 per cent (280 mM) is recommended, as this solution is both isotonic and relatively non-irritant to the vein.

PARENTERAL ADMINISTRATION OF WATER AND SODIUM

This is required when the extracellular fluid is reduced as a result of the loss of both sodium and water. Sodium depletion arises as a result of excessive losses either from the gastrointestinal tract or in the urine. Gastrointestinal causes include vomiting, all types of diarrhoea, and also fistulae. Urine losses arise from excessive diuretic therapy, in diabetes, owing to the large urine output caused by the osmotic effect of the sugar, and in salt-losing nephritis. The clinical picture is that of dehydration in which the skin is dry and inelastic, the eyes sunken, and often the tongue dry and the peripheral circulation inadequate. Isotonic sodium chloride is the principal fluid required for replacement. When clinical evidence of dehydration is present at least 4 litres are likely to be required to replace the deficit in extracellular fluid. In urgent situations the first 2 to 3 litres can advantageously be given within three hours; if the pulse is weak and the blood pressure low, the first litre of saline may be replaced by a litre of plasma or plasma substitute in order to expand selectively the reduced and inadequate plasma volume.

Occasionally a greater deficit of sodium than water is present. For example, in heat exhaustion large quantities of sodium and water are lost in the sweat, but the patient may have replaced only the latter by drinking water alone. Such deficits which are accompanied by low levels of sodium in the plasma can be made good by the intravenous infusion of small quantities of 5 per cent saline solution. Hypertonic saline should be used only under careful clinical and biochemical control.

TREATMENT OF A DISTURBED ACID–BASE BALANCE

Acidosis is frequently associated with a deficiency in the volume of extracellular fluid. This is also the case in alkalosis which occurs in severe vomiting. If the dehydration is treated with isotonic saline, the kidneys, provided they are healthy, can usually correct the disturbance of the acid–base balance by the secretion of the appropriate alkaline or acid urine. In severe acidosis they can be assisted in this task, if sodium bicarbonate is given in addition to isotonic saline. The two solutions may be given in a ratio of 1 to 2 and need not be mixed. A moderately severe case of diabetic coma might require 1 to 2 litres of isotonic sodium bicarbonate and 3 to 4 litres of isotonic saline.

CORRECTION OF POTASSIUM DEFICIENCIES

Potassium deficiency arises from alimentary losses due to acute or chronic diarrhoea or vomiting. It also occurs in acute wasting conditions, i.e. ketoacidosis in diabetes. It may also arise from a variety of renal causes.

Potassium depletion is normally made good by giving a potassium salt by mouth. When this is impossible or the depletion is severe, it may be given intravenously. However, severe toxic manifestations with cardiac irregularity and arrest occur if the level in the plasma is suddenly raised more than slightly above normal. Giving potassium by the intravenous route therefore carries a risk. However, the amount of potassium administered parenterally is usually small in comparison with total body potassium with which the additional ions are rapidly eliminated by this route. Thus the need for caution should not lead to the adminis-

tration of homoeopathic amounts in the doubtful expectation of correcting a large deficit. When clinical signs of potassium loss are present, or when the plasma potassium is low, or when the history suggests that a long-continued uncompensated loss of potassium has been taking place, the net reduction in total body potassium is rarely less than 300 to 400 mmol and may be in excess of 1000 mmol (total body potassium is between 3500 and 4000 mmol, p. 84). In starving patients, losses of this magnitude may make a significant contribution to the mental apathy and gastrointestinal atony which are factors in the failure to secure an adequate oral intake of food.

With this knowledge in mind it is possible to plan the intravenous administration of potassium on rational lines. Potassium chloride is available in sterile solutions, in ampoules containing 1 or 2 g of the salt. If an ampoule is added to a 500 ml bottle of normal saline or glucose saline, the resultant solution contains 26 or 52 mmol/1. One litre of this solution (52 mmol) can be given intravenously during a period of about four hours. If the plasma potassium remains low, an additional litre of fluid containing 4 g of potassium chloride (52 mmol) can be given.

FOOD IN HOSPITALS

The preparation and serving of food for a hospital community is a large operation involving many people and much equipment. In 1963 a report (Platt *et al.*, 1963) described an investigation into the feeding arrangements and nutritional value of the meals served in 152 hospitals in England and Wales. These were selected by random sampling and were visited with a minimum of warning to the Matron and administrative staff. It is distressing to read the tale of the deficiencies uncovered. It is our impression that there has been little improvement since the Platt report was published, and this is confirmed by some observations in London hospitals by Evans (1978). Similar deficiencies probably occur to a greater or lesser extent in all countries.

Hospitals are often handicapped by having old kitchens, many of those still in use were built more than 100 years ago. They may lack equipment and staff. Cooks, kitchen maids and cleaners are not easy to find. But the most important handicap is a lack of adequate supervision of meals served to individual patients.

Good food, well served is more likely to be found in the small hospitals with less than 60 beds. In the large hospitals, especially those serving the chronic sick and mental patients, serious deficiencies are most likely to be met. The requirements for ordinary diets are seldom estimated in relation to the nutritional needs of patients. Formerly a large number of hospital patients were suffering from infections which are wasting conditions and traditionally such patients needed 'feeding up'. Today a considerable proportion, perhaps as many as one-third of adult patients, are overweight and this factor has at least contributed to their illness. Such patients may be overfed in hospital. Elderly people in particular often enter hospital significantly underweight or overweight and their diet needs to be adjusted accordingly. In less than 10 per cent of the hospitals were the dietary scales related to the nutritive value of the food, and only 40 per cent made use of the admirable instructions in *General Hospital Diets* (King Edward's Hospital Fund for London, 1956).

The survey showed that the waste of food in hospital is excessive. Less than 60 per cent of the food sent to the wards was eaten by the patients. Waste was greater in the large hospitals. The cost of this waste must be enormous. The report is silent about the disposal of the swill. Lack of variety and a poor quality of food were common. Many patients resorted to their own provisions as an alternative to hospital food, which they did not like. Most received some outside food which was often needed to fill a long interval between an early supper and the next day's breakfast. In some hospitals it is regarded as 'an unhappy state of affairs to be in hospital with no food of one's own'. Analysis of sample diets did not reveal any gross deficiencies of nutrients, but very low values of vitamin C in samples of potatoes and vegetables taken from patients' plates reflected poor cooking and service. The serving of food is often unsatisfactory, partly because of a poor liaison between the kitchen and the ward and sometimes, but less excusably, because of the lack of rapport between the server of the food and the patient. In only 15 per cent of hospitals was the presentation of food graded as good. The chapter on Kitchens and Hygiene is a sorry record of dirt and disorder.

The state of affairs revealed in this report was not so bad as to cause malnutrition or undernutrition. However, meals of poor quality are likely to depress patients' morale and perhaps slow down recovery. The disorder in the meal service in some hospitals raises the question as to whether patients for whom special diets have been ordered as part of their therapeutic regime always receive these diets.

In some of the small hospitals the feeding of the patients is excellent. This is generally due to the Matron taking a personal interest in the patients' food and supervising the cooks and the service in the wards. Such Matrons are following in the Nightingale tradition. Florence Nightingale wrote in her *Notes on Nursing,* published in 1859; 'Remember that sick cookery should half do the work of your patient's weak digestion. But if you further impair it with your bad articles, I know not what is to become of him or it. If the nurse is an intelligent being, and not a mere carrier of diets to and from the patient, let her exercise her intelligence in these things.' The patients' food should certainly be the responsibility of the nursing staff. Some nurses and ward sisters are poorly informed about normal nutrition and the therapeutic role of a good diet suited to the individual patient's needs. In some hospitals the food

of the nurses may be worse than that of the patients. When no trouble is taken to provide the nurses with good meals it is not surprising if the patients are poorly served and fed. A study sponsored by the Royal College of Nursing (Jones, 1975) of the nasogastric feeds being given to unconscious patients in 12 hospitals showed that in many cases there was no medical prescription for the feeds which were made up by junior nurses with little knowledge of nutrition. Analyses of samples of feeds indicated that many would not meet the nutritional needs of the patients.

In most large hospitals there is a catering officer. The report is clear that many of these are extremely competent and well informed about nutritional problems and dietetics, but others are ill-fitted to their task. Catering officers lack status in the hospital hierarchy and their minimal training requirements are probably too low. A good caterer is a most important member of the staff. A bad one can cause much dissatisfaction amongst the patients.

Although dietitians are well qualified and competent, there are seldom enough of them. In general they have not the time to interest themselves in the diets of ordinary patients. Their attention should be directed to inspecting regularly the meals served in the wards and to weighing occasional samples.

In a hospital the responsibilities of the catering officer, the nursing staff and the dietitians may not be well defined. There are then ample opportunities for personal disagreements and consequent poor service. One of the main recommendations of Platt and his colleagues, which we strongly endorse, is that in every hospital one person should be made responsible for all aspects of hospital catering and for the supervision and control of all staff concerned with the preparation, cooking and service of food to the patient. The assignment of this responsibility depends on circumstances. It might be given to the catering officer, Matron or senior administrative nurse, the senior dietitian or even to a doctor or administrative officer. In army hospitals this duty is firmly placed on the Commanding Officer. Many of them take this task seriously, with great benefit to both sick and wounded soldiers. It does not seem to us to matter who is made responsible, provided a single person is given authority to supervise in detail all the stages in the service.

Another recommendation made by Platt is that attempts should be made to draw up dietary scales in each hospital, which would meet the probable different nutritional needs of various types of patients. The report also gives some detailed recommendations about the design of new kitchens and the equipment which is most suitable for them.

There is no doubt that many hospitals will continue to find difficulties in serving food of good quality to their patients as long as they occupy ancient buildings and sufficient staff is not available. Even with these handicaps much could be done to provide better feeding for patients if more people were aware of the possibilities for improvement, if extra thought was applied to the problem and if better administration was available. Every hospital should have a copy of the Platt report which should be studied carefully by the house physicians, the catering officers, the dietitians and the ward sisters.

PRE-COOKED FROZEN FOODS

These offer a possibility of overcoming many of the difficulties of preparing and distributing meals in large hospitals. Both palatability and nutritional value are retained in food which have been cooked, frozen rapidly and stored at -18^0C. Such foods are prepared as an industrial process in premises either in the hospital or in an outside factory by a staff working a 40-hour week. Cold storage space for two to three weeks supply is needed. The food is distributed in the frozen state to the wards which are provided with convector ovens. The cooking in the kitchen or factory is so adjusted that after a set time (e.g. 25 minutes) in the ward oven, all food is fully cooked and ready to serve. A bell on the convector heater is set to ring and continues ringing when this time for reheating is up. Thus reheating presents no problem to the ward staff, whose responsibility is limited to serving the food straight from the oven.

A hospital in Leeds has now used this method of feeding both patients and nursing staff for many years with satisfactory results. The research and development work was carried out by the Department of Food Science of Leeds University. The method is now used in many other hospitals elsewhere.

As yet the cost of the method has not been compared accurately with that of conventional cooking in hospitals, but it is likely to prove economical both in the use of staff time and in outlay on equipment. If, as appears likely, this method comes into widespread use, a code of practice governing production, storage, distribution and reheating of the frozen foods for hospitals would be necessary. The supervision required to ensure that bacteriological and nutritional standards were maintained would be similar to that required for conventional cooking.

STERILE DIETS

Patients undergoing treatment with cytotoxic or immuno-suppressive drugs have a greatly reduced natural resistance to infection. In some cases it may be desirable to provide them with sterile diets for a short period. It is impractical to provide attractive meals with food sterilised by orthodox methods, but irradiation (p. 207) is satisfactory and permissible for this purpose. A limited service is available and enquiries can be made to The Director, UK Atomic Energy Authority, Wantage Research Laboratory, AERE Wantage, Berkshire.

PART V

Public Health

53. Community Nutrition

A nutritionist may be consulted about the diet of institutions such as orphanages and prisons, about the feeding of special groups of a population such as mothers and young children or old people, about the feeding of various occupational groups such as night shift workers in industry, plantation labourers or members of the armed services. He may also be asked to advise on the food supply of small, local communities, for example a remote island, or a district or whole province, a country or through the United Nations and other international agencies of a whole continent or even the world.

Whatever the size or nature of a problem in community nutrition there are three aspects to be considered: (1) the causes that lead to its arising, (2) assessment of its extent and severity, and (3) the means of prevention. These are the subjects of the next three chapters. These correspond to the sections on aetiology, diagnosis and prevention in textbooks of clinical medicine.

Aetiology is the study of causes. The cause of a poor food supply may be a failure of agricultural production or a failure of distribution. The latter may be due to social, economic or political factors and ignorance and poverty are the most important.

Assessment is based on the findings of surveys. These may consist of clinical examinations, laboratory investigations of blood, urine and other tissues, anthropometric measurements, vital statistics which include birth and death rates and the incidence or prevalence of specific diseases and diet surveys in which the actual amounts of food consumed are recorded. A single survey can only give information about the state of nutrition of a group of people at a particular period of time. Much more valuable information is obtained by a series of continuing surveys, which go on over the years, a process known as **surveillance.**

Prevention may depend on changes in agricultural methods, in the introduction of new crops or improvements in animal husbandry. It may require changes in economic policy and in budgeting, new developments in industry and new wage policies. Always it necessitates a large educational programme.

From the nature of these problems a nutritionist does not work alone. He has to co-operate with people in many walks of life. He must be able to converse with agriculturalists, economists, sociologists, politicians, members of the medical and educational professions, works managers and many other people. A nutritional policy, whether for a small institution or a large country, is always based on collective decisions, formed after considering many factors. A nutritionist can only give advice; he does not make the final decisions.

Nutrition policies always depend on the climate of political opinion. In every country there are people who believe that social and economic problems, including the food supply, are primarily the responsibilities of governments, and others who believe that these problems are best left to the free enterprise of private individuals. In practice a compromise is always reached, though the point of compromise differs markedly in various countries. There is no doubt that excessive government action stifles initiative, for example in Russian agriculture after the revolution, and also that all problems cannot be resolved by free enterprise, however capable and well-intended individuals may be. In the nutrition field famine relief is an example where, since the time of Joseph and Pharoah, government action has always been necessary.

A nutritionist should also remember that in any society there are both rich and poor and that they have very different nutritional problems, all of which are important. In the affluent cities of North America and Western Europe, there is a small minority of very poor people. Many of these have nutritional problems, unknown to the majority, which are difficult to resolve. In Africa, Asia and Latin America, beside the poor peasant agriculturalists and urban slum dwellers there are many rich families, who have the same nutritional problems as wealthy North Americans and Europeans. Experience shows that the rich, like the poor, are not very good at looking after themselves nutritionally. Any nutritional programme should cover all sections of a community and pay particular attention to minority groups. Small minorities are easily overlooked by enthusiasts studying masses of statistics obtained from large populations.

Much good work can be done locally in community nutrition by harnessing and directing the enthusiasms of men and women of good will. Indeed, nutrition programmes, like all health programmes, are successful only if they receive the support of enthusiastic leaders of the local community. It is a task of nutritionists to seek out and direct such leaders.

In most countries, including the United Kingdom today, nutrition suffers from the lack of clear government policy. This is attributable to the fact that decisions affecting national nutrition are made in several different ministries. Ministries of Agriculture, Health, Education and Trade and above all the Treasury each determine nutrition policy in various ways. Some of these have nutritional advisers. Ministerial decisions are based on many sectional interests and not infrequently conflict with nutritional policies. Innumerable schemes to co-ordinate nutrition policy by means of interdepartmental government committees have been put on paper, and many have been tried out in practice in different countries. In general, it can be said that their successes have been small and limited. The role of governments in promoting good nutrition is discussed in the final section of Chapter 56 (p. 486). Prime ministers and other men of power are in general ignorant of the importance of nutrition in relation to health, and of individual health to the well-being and effectiveness of the community as a whole. That the educated section of a community is in general very poorly informed about human nutrition is attributable to its low prestige in the academic world. It is a subject neglected in most medical faculties and taught mainly as part of Domestic Science or Home Economics. Most science and arts graduates of the leading universities of the world have acquired no knowledge of the fundamentals of nutrition.

Experience shows that programmes aimed solely at raising the nutritional status of a community are seldom successful. All nutrition work should be part of a broader programme aimed at raising the general well-being of a community. The larger programme may include control of infectious diseases, better education, better housing, improved agriculture or better wages and higher production in industry. A nutritionist has to work with experts in these fields and should learn to communicate with them and understand their problems.

Anyone contemplating going into nutritional work should be warned to expect frustration. Their good advice will often be neglected or misinterpreted. They are more likely to get satisfaction from work in a small community and, if they move up to national and international fields, their sense of frustration is likely to increase. But the challenge is there. Every community, large or small, needs a nutrition programme although in most cases its members do not appreciate the need.

Nutritionists in the trials of their career may take comfort from considering three attributes of *Homo sapiens* which greatly influence the effectiveness of their work.

First, he is charitable and many men by giving their services and money to a community, either their own or in a foreign country, find the opportunity to follow the injunction of the evangelist, 'Beloved, let us love one another; for love is of God' (I John 4. 7). It is a great experience to work with such people.

Secondly, man is susceptible to bureaucracy. The classical description of this disease is the account of the Circumlocution Office in *Little Dorrit*. 'Whatever was required to be done, the Circumlocution Office was beforehand with all the public departments in the art of perceiving—how not to do it.' If Charles Dickens were alive today, he would find many circumlocution offices in Whitehall and other national government headquarters and especially in the various United Nations agencies.

Thirdly, man is corrupt. Sir Robert Walpole, a practical and successful British Prime Minister, is now best remembered for his saying in 1739: 'All those men have their price.' Many nutrition programmes depend on food contracts and it should be no surprise that money and goods, collected by the charitable to aid the needy, often go into venal hands. This is a factor which has often mitigated the hopes of those engaged in international aid to poor people in many countries.

Nowadays, people often appear surprised when they hear of charitable, bureaucratic or corrupt behaviour, but they are of the essence of human nature. The effectiveness of many community nutrition programmes depend on the blend of these essences in the men and women responsible for carrying them out.

54. Aetiology of Nutritional Disorders

Good health depends on an adequate food supply and this in turn on a sound agricultural policy and a good system of food distribution. The social, economic and agricultural factors that determine the food supply also determine the state of health and the incidence of disease amongst a population. These are the basic aetiological factors causing nutritional disease and they are closely linked with the dangers which arise from failure to control an excessive increase in the population. Even a good food supply and distribution system may fail if there is not proper selection and preparation of food in the home. Lack of health education is responsible for much malnutrition, especially in poor rural areas and urban slums.

The medical profession should help to shape public opinion so that people demand sensible nutritional programmes—both national and international. The doctor, who is respected by all sections of the people either as a man of magic or science, has an important role to play as an educator. Only by the wide propagation of a sound knowledge of basic health principles is it possible to create the demand for proper health policies. For these reasons the medical and dietetic professions should be familiar with the broad outlines of the social, economic and agricultural factors which determine food supply.

INSUFFICIENT FOOD PRODUCTION

The fundamental dependence of a satisfactory food supply upon a flourishing and sound agriculture is self-evident. It is a fact which has been realised from the earliest times, and has formed the basis of policy for innumerable wise rulers and leaders of mankind throughout history. Nevertheless the importance of a sound agricultural economy was generally overlooked throughout the 150 years before World War I. During this period the energies of the ablest of mankind had been mainly involved in exploiting the incredible riches provided by the industrial revolution. Throughout the Americas, Africa, Asia and Oceania an apparently inexhaustible supply of land, fresh to agriculture, became available for producing the foods necessary for the industrial populations. Although much underfeeding and malnutrition was present in the poorer sections both of industrial and agricultural communities throughout the world, the wealth and prosperity of the successful or privileged minority at the top prevented all

but a few of the clear-sighted from realising the extent and severity of underfeeding among the masses at the bottom of the economic scale. The world wars, with their interference first with food distribution and then with food production, gradually awakened the people of most countries to the importance of the relationships between food, agriculture and population.

Many factors have affected the world's food supply in the last 40 years. At the end of the fighting in World War II, many countries had serious deficiencies in their food supply and some were on the verge of famine. Both agriculture and the international food trade recovered rapidly. By 1955 throughout the world food supplies were at least as good as before the war. Yet in many countries this level was far below estimates of physiological needs. In these countries malnutrition and undernutrition were still widespread, but it was hoped that the pace of agricultural development could be increased and that levels of nutrition would soon be raised.

This hope has not been fulfilled because of the staggering increase in population. The Food and Agricultural Organisation of the United Nations publishes annually estimates of national food production related to population and expressed as an index, the mean value for the years 1961–65 being taken as 100. Indices for 1975 averaged 100 for countries in Africa, the Near East, the Far East and Latin America, 114 for countries in Western Europe, North America and Oceania (FAO, 1977). Thus in general in those countries where the vast majority of the poor and malnourished live, agriculture has been barely keeping up with the growth of population; the overall food supply is only marginally better than it was 20 years ago. In contrast, in many wealthy countries the disposal of agricultural surpluses continues to pose difficult problems, e.g. the 'butter mountain' in Europe.

In most of the poor countries of the world, agricultural production has risen, although to a lesser extent than in the rich countries, and death rates have fallen, often markedly, but there has been as yet little fall in birth rates. As a result the growth of agriculture is barely keeping up with the growth of population, and there has been little change in the amount of food available per head. Undernutrition and malnutrition remain widespread. While in some areas production has increased due to the green revolution (p. 481), the situation generally remains today similar to the picture presented in 1946 by Low. His cartoon illustrates the

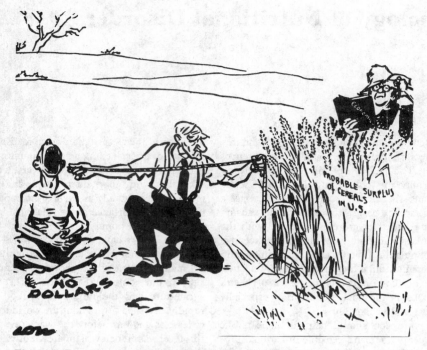

Fig. 54.1 'From land to mouth.' Lord Boyd Orr, first Director-General of FAO. (With acknowledgements to the *Evening Standard*, 26 August 1946.)

difficulty experienced by a prosperous and obese American in getting his surplus crops to the thin and hungry Asian (Fig. 54.1). He is studying a book on economics. For 30 years a whole generation of economists, sustained by much goodwill and humanitarianism, have attended innumerable conferences, but the 'surplus of cereals' remains and there are still 'no dollars'. In fact it now appears that any economic solution is unlikely. The poor countries have in the past obtained much of the foreign exchange by exporting agricultural products. Rich countries are now less dependent on these exports; since synthetic substitutes are being increasingly used in place of rubber, natural fibres and drugs of plant origin. The prices of agricultural products are in general less well maintained than those of industrial goods. It is thus becoming increasingly difficult for poor countries to purchase food from the rich. Gifts of food tend to disrupt the economy of both donor and recipient. In the recipient country, large entries of free food discourage local agricultural enterprise. Gifts of food have proved to immense value to many countries when a sudden emergency has arisen. This is a proper use of a surplus. However, in normal times the rich countries cannot be expected to feed the poor.

In many poor countries the nutritional state of the people can only be improved by three things, all of which are equally necessary: an improvement in the standard of education, a slowing down in the growth of population and an increase in agricultural production. The population

problems are discussed in Chapter 57. In this chapter some of the causes of agricultural unproductiveness are discussed and also other factors which contribute to nutritional disorders by preventing the proper distribution and use of the food available in a country. The only basis for continuing improvement in the nutritional status of a country is a satisfactory rise in its overall economic development.

The chief causes of agricultural unproductiveness may be discussed briefly under four heads:

Climatic irregularities and catastrophes
Soil erosion
War
Inefficient farming.

Climatic irregularities

It is a curious anomaly of nature that in Britain, where the daily variations in the weather are so marked and unpredictable as to colour general conversation and social planning, the seasonal variations from year to year are small. British farmers may have good or bad harvests, but their 'bad years' bear no relationship to the catastrophes which regularly afflict farmers in the large continents as a result of variations in rainfall. In parts of Africa, the Americas, Australia, India and China there are areas many hundreds of miles in extent subject to periodic failure of the annual rain supply. In years of failure the total rainfall may be less than 20 per cent of the average seasonal supply. Such years

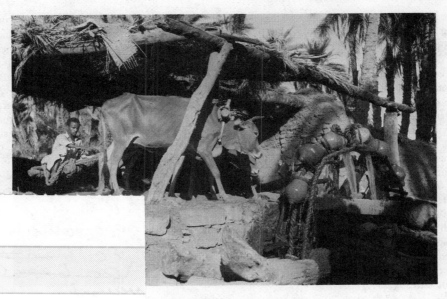

..., one of the most ancient types of water-wheels, can still be seen
... FAO photo by P. Morin.)

...mmoth contin-
...he mountains
...nd so destroy
...ortant part in
...husbanding of
...lled distribu-
...nagement and
...problems, the
...bound up with

...ds upon the
...vices like the
...eme there are
...ects involving
...pounds which
...improve the
...le. A modern
...d the produc-
...ar magnitude
...reat rivers of
...the continued
...asing popula-
tion of the world must rely for future food and health.

Soil erosion

The next most important problem in food production is the prevention of soil erosion and the recovery of land previously degraded by bad agriculture. The immediate agencies of erosion are wind and water, following removal or damage to the pre-existing plant cover. The cause of this damage is usually the improper exploitation of the land in grazing, ploughing, firing, felling or the collection of domestic fuel. This improper or too violent exploitation itself results from pressures—financial or biological.

A common sequence of events in many districts now barren has been as follows. Originally forest existed. Men came, exploited the forest wealth too rapidly and cut down too many trees. Small areas of arable land were interspersed with areas of waste, broken by large tree stumps. At this stage or earlier, goats were introduced. These beasts are the antithesis of good animal husbandry. Goats differ from cattle and sheep in their ability to grub up the roots of plants and consume them. Goats also eat the leaves and bark of trees and so kill them. Thus the soil is loosened and in succeeding rains washed away, leaving an arid desert or a barren hillside. One of the most striking examples of this process is to be seen in the deserts of North Africa. This barren and hostile land was once the glory of the Roman Empire; rich and fertile—a main source of grain and olive oil to metropolitan Rome. After the collapse of the Roman Empire, instead of a numerous peasant population who understood the land and tilled it industriously, nomads wandered through the desert with their flocks of goats, sheep and camels. It is not that the climate had changed, though it may have done a little, but in destroying the Roman Empire in North Africa the Berber and Arab tribes nearly destroyed the land itself. The dams and reservoirs in which the Romans had hoarded the precious water were broken or filled with sand. As a result the winter rains poured down the wadis and into the sea, taking with them much of the fertile top soil. And by recklessly grazing their flocks the nomads destroyed the natural forest and vegetation so that the sun and wind and rain stripped the earth from the hills. With nothing to stop it the desert, which can move like an army, slowly crept down to the coast.

Similarly, in a region that is now part of Iraq and Iran, huge irrigation schemes, fed by the Tigris, Euphrates and Karun, once supported a large and vigorous population whose civilised arts of writing and sculpture record the earliest history of mankind. Today the proud city of Cyrus and Darius is a mound of earth in the middle of a desert, over which nomads graze their starveling flocks. The last of the dykes on which its agriculture depended was finally destroyed by Timur (Tamerlane) in the fifteenth century.

There are few countries in the world where land degradation in one form or another is not of major importance for the health of future generations. South Africa, Australia, Pakistan, India and many of the new African states are all afflicted. Vigorous counter-measures have begun in the USA, the country of pioneers both in land spoilage and eventual costly cures.

War

War has always been a potent cause of nutritional diseases. It acts by interfering with food distribution, by taking away many of the young men from their normal task of agriculture, and sometimes by destruction of crops and livestock on a large scale. Civil wars have wrought the most havoc in this respect. The Thirty Years War in Europe, the Mahratta Wars in India, the wars that set up the Communist regime in Russia and the civil wars in China have all led to disruption of agriculture and so to famine. It should now be abundantly clear that these are the inevitable concomitants of all wars. The deliberate destruction of rice crops by herbicides carried out by the US armed forces in Vietnam (Mayer and Sidel, 1966) is one of the novel horrors of war. Militarily such action is not likely to be effective; when there are food shortages, fighting men are usually able to get food for themselves and they have seldom been starved into submission. It is the women, the children and the old people who die.

Inefficient farming

Ideally, farmers throughout the world should have enough basic education and capital to profit from the enormous developments of scientific knowledge. As yet the majority of the world's farmers possess neither of these essentials to reap the benefits of such knowledge. In underdeveloped countries new methods and techniques have been introduced much more readily into medical than into agricultural practice.

The great majority of the peoples of the world live in underdeveloped agricultural countries. Here they take part in a struggle for existence under conditions that have changed but little for thousands of years. More than half of the world's people still face the elemental problem of getting enough to eat. Those readers who have not had opportunities for travel can get a good picture of farming conditions at present existing in large parts of the world from a study of the Old Testament. In many countries conditions have changed but little from the time of the Pharaohs. Cairo is a fine modern city; yet within a few miles of the Mohamet Ali Mosque there are villages in which one can see all the simple features of primitive agriculture, which are familiar to the reader of the Bible: the threshing floor, the oxen ploughing, the old men, the asses, the camels—all remain unchanged. A similar picture can be painted in many parts of the world—India, the East and West Indies, South America and parts of Southern Europe, and an even more primitive one, without wheel or plough, in most countries of tropical Africa. What can be done has been demonstrated by European farmers. In the United Kingdom farm production has been increasing by 6 per cent per year. This is an achievement in productivity equalled only by the chemical industry.

UNEQUAL DISTRIBUTION OF FOOD

Poverty

As a cause of underfeeding and malnutrition, the unequal distribution of food caused by poverty is by far the most important factor. This is illustrated first by two studies in Britain during the industrial depression in the period 1930–40 and secondly by a study of national diets in 1960–70.

Food, health and income. Orr (1936) published a book with this title which had a great influence on the development of nutrition policies in Britain. It contained the results of a survey of 1152 families, in each of which the total food consumption was weighed for one week and a correlation made between food consumption per head and available income in each family. Those in the lowest economic group, which was believed to comprise 4½ million people (10 per cent of the total population), were living on diets which failed to reach proper standards in almost every respect, especially in energy, proteins, vitamins A and C, and the minerals, iron and calcium. In the next two economic groups, 40 per cent of the population, although the energy and protein intakes were satisfactory, intakes of vitamins and minerals were below standard. No serious student of nutrition has contradicted Orr's principal conclusion that between 1930 and 1935, 10 per cent of the population of Britain had insufficient money to purchase sufficient food for themselves; these people were underfed.

The other striking example of the complex relations between poverty, nutrition and public health was recorded by M'Gonigle and Kirby (1936). Their observations were made at Stockton-on-Tees on social groups at the bottom of the economic scale, a large proportion of the wage-

Table 54.1 Mortality in Stockton-on-tees
(Standardised quinquennial death rate: deaths per 10000 population)

	Total for the borough	Housewife Lane population	Riverside population
1923–27	12	23 (in a slum)	26 (in a slum)
1928–32	12	34 (in a housing estate)	23 (in a slum)

earners concerned being unemployed. In 1927 an unhealthy slum (Housewife Lane) was demolished and the population was moved into a modern housing estate. It was possible to keep separate figures for mortality rates for this population both before and after the move and to compare them with a control population remaining in a slum (Riverside) area. Table 54.1 shows that the move from the unhygienic slum into the apparently healthy environment of the new housing estate did not result in an improvement in health, but was unexpectedly followed by an increase in the death rate of the people above both their former level and the level of their neighbours who remained in the Riverside slum. The estate itself could not be blamed for the higher mortality, the houses being well constructed and possessing good sanitary arrangements. The deterioration in health was directly attributed to an increase in the rents in the new estate. This of necessity caused a corresponding reduction in the amount of money available for buying food. The amount of money spent on food fell and was considerably less than that spent by the controls in the slums. The benefits to health, which might have resulted from the improved hygiene of the external environment, were more than neutralised by the higher rents, which reduced the money available for the purchase of food.

These brief summaries of the main conclusions from the books by Orr, and M'Gonigle and Kirby serve to show in outline the striking effect of poverty on health. It is important to remember that at this time the overall food supply of Great Britain was satisfactory. Estimates agree that the total available food, as retailed in the shops, was equivalent to 12.6 MJ (3000 kcal)/head daily which was ample for the people if it had been properly distributed.

The system of distribution was so unsound that 1 in 10 of the people were underfed; this is a major indictment of the economic structure of our society between the two world wars. Only when the imagination has grasped the full implications of this failure upon individual families and homes is it possible to appreciate the new quality of British society. During the long period of food shortages, which occurred during and after World War II, successive Ministers of Food regulated by means of rationing, subsidies and controls, the distribution of food according to human needs and thereby reduced the effects of economic misfortune on health and well-being.

In other parts of the world the relationships between poverty, nutrition and health are even more striking and are often such a feature of everyday life that both the people and government become accustomed to the facts and blind to the consequences. This is well illustrated in two surveys by Mitra (1941), carried out in urban and rural India which demonstrate with detailed figures the close connection between income and food consumption.

Income and the structure of national diets
Figure 54.3 shows an analysis of the sources of dietary energy based on agricultural and trade statistics correlated with economic estimates of the value of gross domestic products per head. It shows that in all countries, rich and poor alike, protein provides just over 10 per cent of the dietary energy, but the proportion of animal origin rises with income. Whereas in the poorest countries carbohydrate provides over 75 per cent of the energy, in the richest the figure is only 50 per cent and nearly 20 per cent comes from sugar. As income rises, the consumption of cereals falls and of sugar rises. Whereas the poorest countries get little more than 10 per cent of their energy from fat, mostly as unseparated vegetable fat, wealthy countries get 40 per cent. Neither of the two extremes is to be recommended dietetically. Even if there is enough to eat in the poorest countries, which is unlikely, the supplies of vitamins A, C and D are almost certainly insufficient and, if most of the protein comes from a single vegetable source, the supply of one or more amino acids is probably insufficient to meet the needs of the growing children. The diets in the wealthiest countries are likely to contain saturated fatty acids and sucrose in amounts which predispose to atherosclerosis and also to dental caries and diabetes. Perhaps the countries with incomes in the middle of the scale feed best, but these figures represent national averages and in most countries the distribution of food is according to social class.

Lack of leisure
A secondary cause of inadequate nutrition may be lack of leisure. Proper nutrition demands time for the preparation of meals and for their consumption. The housewife who is doing a full day's work outside the home may lack time for shopping and for preparing meals. The increasing employment of women in industry in large towns in the tropics is an important contributory cause of malnutrition in young children. People who live far away from their place of work may leave home at an early hour without a proper

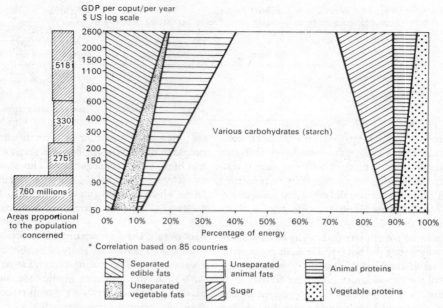

Fig. 54.3 Dietary energy derived from fats, carbohydrate and protein as percentage of total energy related to the incomes or gross domestic products (GDP) of countries. The figures in the shaded area show the population living in countries within each range of GDP. (Périssé *et al.*, 1969.)

breakfast. Many workers are still not provided with adequate breaks for their meals and suitable places for eating them. Restaurants and canteens may be so inadequately staffed that they are unable to provide meals in the time available to their patrons.

Lack of transport
Large numbers of the world's population live far from the land producing their food; food has to be taken to them in ships, in trains, in lorries and in carts. In times of peace, transport is usually available in sufficient quantity, but a major natural disaster such as fire, flood or earthquake can cut off the food supply of a large group of people; then the most urgent measure needed may be the collection and marshalling of sufficient transport to bring in food from outside. Similarly, the havoc of war may separate a large community from its usual source of food. In 1945, for instance, 5 million people in the mountains of Yugoslavia were isolated from the rich food-producing plains by the wartime destruction of road and railway bridges, lorries and rolling stock. Only by the construction of temporary bridges and the assembly of transport of every kind was a major famine averted.

Ignorance
In most agricultural communities the people are usually adequately nourished provided the harvest has not failed, disease has not destroyed their livestock, the farms have not been plundered by soldiers or rapacious landlords and

money lenders have not forced them to sell their crops. Experience of what constitutes a good diet is passed from one generation to another.

The situation is very different when a family moves into a city. Many customary foods are not available. New and strange foods are present in the markets and shops. The housewife may receive false or misleading information from advertisements and shopkeepers. Ignorance of the nutritional value of foods is widespread especially in the rapidly growing urban populations in developing countries. This is responsible for much nutritional disease especially in young children.

Important points on which education is frequently needed include proper methods of cooking vegetables, the nutritional value of fish, the deleterious effects of over-milled cereals, the value of vegetable gardens, and the special needs of children for milk, fruit juices and sunlight.

In prosperous countries ignorance leads to faulty habits, which certainly contribute to the onset of obesity and diabetes and probably to degenerative disorders. The need for nutritional education is discussed on page 477.

Religious customs
The effect of these on food habits may be important. In simple rural communities, all religions commemorate important events in the lives of saints and prophets, and the ceremonies associated with marriage and death are celebrated either by feasts or fasts. The feasts often provide

an excuse for the slaughter of an animal and the consumption of much extra animal protein. A variety of other delicacies may be set aside for use on these occasions only. Feasts are of value in supplementing a monotonous and inadequate day-to-day diet and in many communities dietary surveys, which omit such occasions, may be misleading. Fasts are generally fewer in number, and there is no evidence that an occasional day's fast ever did a healthy individual any harm. They may be of benefit to the richer members of community, but impair the health of people whose day-to-day food consumption is limited by inadequate supplies or low purchasing power. During Ramadan, which lasts for one lunar month in every year, many orthodox Muslims neither eat food nor drink water between sunrise and sundown. Even if the food intake during the hours of darkness is satisfactory, lack of sleep by night and lack of water by day make it difficult for a man to maintain working efficiency throughout a long and hot day, for four weeks, under these conditions. In Khartoum blood concentrations of uric acid and triglycerides rise during Ramadan (Gumaa et al., 1978), but the water balance is maintained and there is no change in plasma osmolality (Mustafa et al., 1978). Whatever the religious and spiritual significance of the fast may be, most people who have had to work with Muslims during Ramadan will agree that it causes loss of stamina and working efficiency. In most Christian communities fasting is limited to replacing a meat dish by fish on Fridays and giving up one item of food in Lent. However, in Ethiopia there are over 100 fast days during the year, in which the intake of energy, protein and other nutrients falls in vulnerable groups (Knutsson and Selinus, 1970).

Religions also enforce many food taboos. Jews and Muslims are forbidden the flesh of the pig, but more important is the Hindu prohibition of the consumption of beef and of the slaughter of cattle. In India the health of the cattle is the crux of the whole economic system. They plough the land, fertilise the soil, carry the crops to market, provide milk for the family and fuel for the hearth. A well-fed, healthy cattle population is a *sine qua non* of a well-fed and prosperous human community. The exact origin of the taboo on the slaughter of cattle is uncertain, but it was not a part of the Dravidian and earliest Hindu cultures. No doubt the prohibition arose as a practical expediency under certain acute local circumstances and thereafter received general sanction. A ban on slaughtering cattle might have little effect if abundant cattle fodder were available, enabling the community to pension off and preserve the older animals no longer useful to man. In modern India such conditions do not exist. The pressure on the land by both man and beast is great; sufficient food is at present grown for neither. It has been estimated that half of India's enormous number of cattle have no economic value. They can neither provide milk nor pull the plough, but use up land needed for the production of human food.

In tribal Africa (Trant, 1954) and in Polynesia (Jelliffe and Jelliffe, 1964) many food taboos have been described which are often strict during pregnancy and lactation. These taboos may reduce the nutritional value of a mother's diet and so affect her health and that of her child. Jelliffe (1957) describes how religious customs in West Bengal may delay the onset of mixed feeding and so be a factor in the causation of protein-energy malnutrition. Irrational views and prejudices about food are not confined to underdeveloped countries and food myths, fads and fallacies are held tenaciously in all communities (Jelliffe, 1967; Fox, 1970; Pyke, 1970).

55. Assessment of Nutritional Status

The nutritional status of an individual, such as an infant or a patient in hospital, is assessed from information of four types which are elicited along with other clinical data from a careful history and a systematic clinical examination. The history may indicate that the diet has been inadequate in total amount or in one or more nutrients. Anthropometry may show that the individual is underweight, too thin or, in the case of a child, has not been growing at the normal rate. Clinical examination may reveal signs of one of the qualitative forms of malnutrition described in other chapters, such as anaemia or a goitre. Lastly, biochemical tests may show low concentrations of one or more nutrients in blood or urine. Interpretation of this data requires clinical judgment in the same way as in the rest of medical diagnosis. A short stature has many possible causes, of which undernutrition is only one, and the same applies to anaemia and goitre. A low concentration of a nutrient in one of the body fluids may not be biologically important; it may only reflect a low intake for the preceding few days—too short a time to have affected the individual's health.

The same principles apply in assessing the nutritional status of whole populations or special groups or communities but there are two important differences. First, the task can only be done by a team, which may include physicians, dietitians, nutritionists, statisticians, biochemists, food analysts, agriculturalists and economists. Secondly, the purpose of assessing the nutrition of a population or group is to provide a basis for decisions, usually by government, on food policy and planning. Recognition of subclinical malnutrition in a sample of people examined therefore has implications which it does not have in an individual. If some people in the sample examined have, say, low intakes of iron or low plasma iron, then the community is at increased risk of iron deficiency anaemia, either in vulnerable segments of the population or if there should be any reduction of food supplies or increase in their price.

The nutritional status of a population is assessed in two different ways. First, there are large-scale, indirect indices, which are used for surveillance. These include food balance sheets, food prices, heights and weights of schoolchildren, hospital admissions and mortality figures for diseases related to nutrition. Different morbidity and mortality statistics are appropriate in different populations, depending on the weak points of the national diet and the problems of vulnerable groups. Berry (1972) discusses the principles of nutritional surveillance, as illustrated by the system used in Britain, and a WHO (1976) monograph discusses methodology.

The surveillance indices may point the need to focus attention on a particular group of the population or to search for deficiency of a particular nutrient. A team should then be organised to examine a sample of the population directly and assess their nutritional status. This involves a dietary survey, where necessary supplemented by chemical analysis of foods, together with a standardised clinical examination, anthropometry and selected biochemical tests on blood or urine. Sometimes other special investigations are required, e.g. radiography to detect evidence of rickets. An example of a survey of this kind, which investigated the nutrition of elderly people in Britain, is described on page 535. It is important that the sample surveyed should be as statistically representative of the population as possible. If a survey is carried out at only one time of the year in a country with marked seasonal fluctuations in food supply, the results can be very misleading. Even if an intensive study gives reassuring results, surveillance should continue. The standard manual on methods for nutrition surveys is the WHO monograph by Jellife (1966); it is particularly good on clinical methods. A chapter by Robson et al. (1972) also has a good discussion of the subject.

CLINICAL EXAMINATIONS

The most valuable of all the signs are the weight, height and skinfold thicknesses, as the measurements can be carried out quickly and do not require medical staff; they are discussed on page 468. In addition a sample of the population is clinically examined to detect signs listed in Table 55.1. It is not practicable to look for all the signs even in group 1.

It is better to select some of the signs which seem most relevant on the basis of background medical and dietary information in the area. All the medical staff should be trained in recognising the signs and grading them consistently. Some observer variability is inevitable and there should be more than one medical examiner in the team. They should compare notes frequently at the planning stage and during the examinations.

It is wrong and not practical to confine clinical attention solely to detection of signs of malnutrition. The presence of other diseases, e.g. malaria and tuberculosis, should be noted. They affect interpretation of the survey, and in a remote community the people expect treatment for these and sometimes for minor ailments as well.

Before starting a survey, it is useful to make out a form on which the information on each subject will be recorded. This information may include age, sex, number of pregnancies, social class and family income, anthropometric data, e.g. height, weight, skinfold thicknesses, arm circumference, etc. and results of clinical examinations of the hair, eyes, mouth and lips, teeth, skin, skeleton and nervous system; disorders known to be common in the population, e.g. angular stomatitis, glossitis, folicular keratosis or goitre, may be included and ticked if present. Space may be left for a record of examinations of blood, urine and faeces. Details vary and are obviously very different for a survey of preschool children in Africa and for one on old people in Britain. If the survey is large, a statistician should be consulted at the planning stage and the data recorded in a manner suitable for analysis by computer.

A trap into which an inexperienced team can fall in an unfamiliar country without regular streets and house numbers is to examine a sample of the people who are accessible, e.g. those who first crowd round the Land Rover when it arrives at the village centre. These are usually teenage boys and middle-aged men, the section of the community least likely to be malnourished. Sickly babies, pregnant women and frail old people are not apparent at first. But the survey will be of little value unless the team establishes sufficient rapport with the village to be allowed to examine its womenfolk and infants. In times of severe food shortage the clinical state of the people walking about in the streets may be no guide to the real situation. Those weak with undernutrition may be unable to leave their homes. This source of error misled some of those who accompanied the liberating armies into Holland in 1945 into underestimating the extent of the famine.

Clinical examination for signs of malnutrition is relatively cheap and easy to organise. It does not require elaborate apparatus and reagents. However, there are important limitations. The problem of observer error has already been referred to. Secondly, only a few of the signs are pathognomonic. Changes in the conjunctiva, lips, and skin can be caused by non-nutritional factors like cold, wet, dryness, heat, irritation, infections, habits, smoke, dust, pressure and insect bites. Even if a sign like angular stomatitis can be established as of nutritional origin there are several deficiencies that can cause it (Chap. 37). Thirdly, these clinical signs have diminishing frequency as the state of nutrition improves. In a well-nourished community signs of malnutrition will be infrequent and so more easily overlooked or misinterpreted. It is in such communities that biochemical tests are of special value.

The most valuable of the signs of malnutrition are those which are most specific. In general these include oedema,

the surface changes of mild kwashiorkor and pellagra, anaemia, goitre, signs of rickets and fluorotic mottling of the teeth.

LABORATORY INVESTIGATIONS

BIOCHEMICAL TESTS

Modern hospital medicine depends on biochemical tests for the diagnosis of subclinical disease, e.g. non-symptomatic uraemia and diabetes, and for monitoring the treatment of many common diseases, e.g. myocardial infarction, hepatitis and electrolyte disturbances. Without a clinical biochemistry service early and accurate diagnosis of many conditions would be difficult. Ideally nutritional deficiencies should be diagnosed in the same way. Thus subclinical protein deficiency can be diagnosed by a reduced plasma albumin concentration before oedema or skin changes appear. The cause of nutritional anaemia can be established by measuring iron, vitamin B_{12}, and folate in the plasma. In a nutrition survey in the field, however, there are great practical difficulties to be overcome before biochemical tests can be used. Either a field laboratory has to be set up or arrangements made to preserve plasma and urine specimens during transit to a central laboratory. Apparently healthy people may not be willing to have their blood taken. Uneducated people may believe that they can be bewitched if they allow a stranger to take a specimen of blood. To collect 24-hour specimens of urine is difficult in the field and timed specimens have limited diagnostic value. In addition, normal standards are not well established for those biochemical tests that are used only in nutrition surveys and not in general hospitals, e.g. urinary N'-methylnicotinamide and erythrocyte transketolase.

When an individual consumes less of a nutrient than his requirement, his nutritional state goes through three stages.

1. Reduced intake with adaptation. Urinary excretion of the nutrient or its metabolites is low and sometimes plasma concentration of the nutrient is reduced but there are no laboratory signs of disturbed function and no clinical signs.

2. Disturbed function but no definite illness. In addition to the above, biochemical tests may show subnormal function of an enzyme which responds to the specific addition of the nutrient. Erythrocyte transketolase with response to thiamin pyrophosphate is a good example. Alternatively, tissue concentrations of a nutrient may be low, e.g. reduced ascorbic acid in leucocytes. In this stage any clinical symptoms or signs are mild, non-specific or unrelated to nutrition.

3. Deficiency disease. The patient shows clinical features of a disease like pellagra or rickets, in which there are structural abnormalities which can be recognised clinically and the patient usually feels ill.

Clinical signs are not detectable until the beginning of

Table 55.1 Classified list of signs used in nutrition surveys (modified from Jelliffe, 1966)

	Group 1: Signs known to be of value in nutrition surveys	Group 2: Signs that need further investigation	Group 3: Some signs not related to nutrition
Hair	Lack of lustre Thinness and sparseness Straightness (in Negroes) Dyspigmentation Flag sign Easy pluckability		Alopecia Artificial discoloration
Face	Diffuse depigmentation Nasolabial dyssebacea Moon-face	Malar and supraorbital pigmentation	Acne vulgaris Acne rosacea Chloasma
Eyes	Pale conjunctiva Bitôt's spots Conjunctival xerosis Corneal xerosis Keratomalacia Angular palpebritis	Conjunctival injection Conjunctival and scleral pigmentation Corneal vascularisation Circumcorneal injection Corneal opacities and scars	Follicular conjunctivitis Blepharitis Pingueculae Pterygium Pannus
Lips	Angular stomatitis Angular scars Cheilosis	Chronic depigmentation of lower lip	Chapping from exposure to harsh climates
Tongue	Abnormally smooth or red Oedema Atropic papillae	Hyperaemic and hypertrophic papillae Fissures Geographic tongue Pigmented tongue	Aphthous ulcer Leucoplakia
Teeth	Mottled enamel	Caries Attrition Enamel hypoplasia Enamel erosion	Malocclusion
Gums	Spongy, bleeding gums	Recession of gum	Pyorrhoea
Glands	Thyroid enlargement Parotid enlargement	Gynaecomastia	Allergic or inflammatory enlargement of thyroid or parotid
Skin	Xerosis Follicular hyperkeratosis Petechiae Pellagrous dermatosis Flaky-paint dermatosis Scrotal and vulval dermatitis	Mosaic dermatosis Thickening and pigmentation of pressure points Intertriginous lesions	Ichthyosis Acneiform eruptions Miliaria Epidermophytoses Sunburn Onchocercal dermatosis
Nails	Koilonychia	Brittle, ridged nails	
Subcutaneous tissue	Oedema Amount of subcutaneous fat		
Skeletal system	Craniotabes Frontal and parietal bossing Epiphyseal enlargement (tender or painless) Beading of ribs Persistently open anterior fontanelle Deformities of thorax		Funnel chest
Muscles and nervous system	Muscle wasting Motor weakness Sensory loss Loss of ankle and knee jerks Loss of position sense Loss of vibration sense Calf tenderness	Winged scapulae Condition of ocular fundus	

Table 55.1—*continued*

	Group 1: Signs known to be of value in nutrition surveys	Group 2: Signs that need further investigation	Group 3: Some signs not related to nutrition
Gastrointestinal	Hepatomegaly		Splenomegaly
Cardiovascular	Cardiac enlargement Tachycardia	Blood pressure	
Psychological	Listlessness and apathy Mental confusion		

Group 1   *Signs that are considered to be of value in nutritional assessment,* as, according to present evidence, they indicate with considerable probability deficiency of one or more nutrients in the tissues in the recent past.

Group 2   *Signs that need further investigation,* but in whose causation malnutrition, sometimes of a chronic nature, may play some part, together with other factors. They are found more commonly in people with low standards of living than among more privileged groups.

Group 3   *Signs not related to nutrition,* according to present knowledge, but which, in some instances, have to be differentiated from signs of known nutritional value (Group 1).

Table 55.2 Biochemical methods for assessing nutritional status

Nutrient	Principal methods		Supplementary methods
	Indicating reduced intake	Indicating impaired function (IF) or cell depletion (CD)	
Protein	Urinary N	Plasma albumin (IF)	Fasting plasma amino acid pattern
Vitamin A	Plasma retinol Plasma carotene		
Thiamin	Urinary thiamin	RBC transketolase and TPP effect (IF)	Plasma pyruvate and lactate
Riboflavin	Urinary riboflavin	RBC glutathione reductase and FAD effect (IF)	RBC riboflavin
Nicotinamide	Urinary N'-methylnicotin- amide and 2-pyridone		Fasting plasma free tryptophan
Pyridoxine	Urinary 4-pyridoxic acid	RBC glutamic oxalacetic transaminase and PP effect (IF)	Urinary xanthurenic acid after tryptophan load
Folic acid	Plasma folate (*Lactobacillus casei*)	RBC folate (CD) Haemoglobin, PCV and smear (IF)	Urinary FIGLU after histidine load. Bone marrow morphology
Vitamin B_{12}	Plasma vitamin B_{12} (*Euglena gracilis*)	Haemoglobin, PCV and smear (IF)	Schilling test. Bone marrow morphology
Ascorbic acid	Plasma ascorbic acid	Leucocyte ascorbic acid (CD)	Urinary ascorbic acid
Vitamin D	Plasma 25-hydroxy- cholecalciferol	Plasma alkaline phosphatase (IF)	Plasma calcium and inorganic phosphorus
Vitamin E	Plasma tocopherol	RBC haemolysis with H_2O_2 *in vitro*	
Vitamin K		Plasma prothrombin (IF)	
Sodium	Urinary sodium	Plasma sodium	
Potassium		Plasma potassium	
Iron	Plasma iron and TIBC	Haemoglobin, PCV and smear	Bone marrow morphology and stainable iron
Calcium		Plasma calcium	
Iodine	Urinary (stable) iodine	Plasma thyroxine and T_3	

Table 55.3 Plasma concentrations and urinary outputs which may be useful in assessing the nutritional state of a patient. Values below those given in the table suggest an inadequate intake or a failure of absorption or an increased requirement (mainly from Stanstead *et al.*, 1969)

Plasma; all values/litre		Urine; all values/g urinary creatinine	
Albumin	35 g	Iodine	50 μg
Iron	700 μg	N'-Methylnicotinamide	1.6 mg
Retinol	200 μg	Riboflavin	80 μg
Carotene	800 μg	Thiamin	66 μg
25-OH vitamin D	3.5 μg		
Ascorbic acid	3 mg	*In children under six years*	
Vitamin B$_{12}$	70 ng	Riboflavin	300 μg
Folic acid	7 μg	Thiamin	120 μg

In addition, a serum alkaline phosphatase level in a child above 4 Bodansky (25 King–Armstrong) units suggests subclinical vitamin D deficiency. Higher values are, however, not infrequently found in children with no radiographic evidence of rickets.

stage 3 but biochemical dysfunction can usually be detected earlier. The principal biochemical tests for evaluation of nutritional status are shown in Table 55.2. Those in the left-hand column indicate reduced intake, i.e. stage 1, and may not be of biological significance in an individual. The tests in the middle column indicate some disturbed function and, if one of them is abnormal in a person without clinical signs, it can usually be taken to indicate subclinical nutritional deficiency. Some of these tests are difficult to carry out in the field. Those involving enzymes require a fresh specimen of whole blood. Suggested cut-off levels, between normal and possibly deficient, for some of the tests are shown in Table 55.3.

As with other biochemical tests, those used for nutritional diagnosis can be falsely negative or falsely positive. They cannot be properly used without a good chemical method, well standardised, backed up by experience of the pitfalls in interpretation. Most of the tests are discussed in the relevant chapters in this book; a fuller account of available methods and of interpretations of tests is given in a book by Sauberlich *et al.* (1974).

PHYSIOLOGICAL TESTS

The discovery that night blindness was a common feature of vitamin A deficiency led to the elaboration of tests for night vision. Many of these fell into disuse when it was found that they were profoundly affected by emotional and other factors. However, the apparatus designed by Wald (1941) and modified by Dow and Steven (1941) has overcome these difficulties and can be recommended as a practical and reliable test for the diagnosis of vitamin A deficiency.

Much time has been spent in attempting to measure the properties of human muscle and to correlate the results with nutritional status. Large numbers of measurements have been made of the power, speed, endurance and co-ordination of various muscular movements. Unfortu-

nately, in such tests the influence of psychological and emotional factors is so great, and impossible to control adequately, that the methods have fallen into disuse.

RADIOGRAPHY

Rickets and osteomalacia can be diagnosed in the early stage by radiography, but its use in nutritional surveys on young children and on pregnant women is contraindicated because it leads to an increased risk of developing leukaemia and other neoplasms.

EXAMINATION OF HAIR

The impaired growth of hair can be used in the diagnosis of malnutrition. In surveys it is easy to pull out with forceps a few hairs from the occipital region and to examine them later under the microscope. Changes in the structure of the hair root, such as a reduced diameter of the bulb, provide an index of the nutritional state which may be useful in populations at risk of protein-energy malnutrition (Bradfield, 1972, 1974).

ANTHROPOMETRY

HEIGHTS AND WEIGHTS

If children do not get sufficient food, they fail to grow properly. Similarly, adults without enough to eat lose weight and those who overeat gain weight. The weighing machine is a useful and accurate tool for investigating nutritional status. Measurements of weights of adults and of large groups of children at various ages are a valuable index of nutritional status, when correctly interpreted. The weighing machine has been widely used at child health clinics and in school medical services to detect those who may be undernourished. Children underweight should then be subjected to detailed medical examination and, if necessary, provided with extra food.

Other environmental factors besides the food intake and the genetic constitution determine the height and weight of individual children. In group surveys the effect of racial and ethnic differences is small compared to that of the environment (Habicht *et al.*, 1974). Hence the standards in the tables and charts given below are applicable internationally with very few exceptions.

There are certain difficulties involved in the use of such a simple piece of apparatus as a weighing machine. Every balance needs regular checking and, if necessary, recalibration. Lever balances made by firms of repute are very reliable and a yearly check is all that is necessary. Spring balances are unreliable and, if used regularly, need repeated checks. Indeed they cannot be recommended for accurate work. It is seldom practical to weigh people naked; a correction is usually needed for the articles of clothing worn. They may vary greatly from season to season and according to fashion. Men usually wear heavier underclothing than women. A rough estimate of a man's clothes in Britain without shoes or jacket is about 6 lb. Shoes and jacket usually weigh about 4 lb more. Women's shoes and clothes usually weigh about 6 lb. In comparing individual weights with standards, it is important to make certain the standards were obtained in the subjects wearing comparable clothing.

Height should be measured against a flat, vertical surface and the subject must stand as upright as possible on firm level ground without raising the heels from the ground. A sliding headpiece is necessary for accurate work. It is impossible to record standing height in infants and very young children and an apparatus can be made for measuring their length, lying down (Jelliffe, 1966). In older children and adults the measurement is subject to considerable daily variation, and is usually greater in the morning than in the afternoon (Whitehouse *et al.*, 1974) due to effects arising from fatigue and faulty posture. For these reasons measurements of recumbent length are better, especially for children up to 2 years of age. Over the range 110 to 180 cm (42 to 71 in) recumbent length exceeds height by an average of 0.5 cm (0.20 in) for boys and 1.1 cm (0.42 in) for girls.

In children it is necessary to record age accurately. In some parts of the world, children and their parents have no recollection of their age and no easy way round this difficulty has been found. However, serial records of weight can still be a useful check as to whether the child is gaining weight.

As in all other methods of nutritional assessment accurate sampling is necessary. Most children attend schools and it is usually easy to get a fair sample of the child population. But it is always difficult to get a random sample of an adult population. For instance during the food shortages in some central European cities after World War II, the occupying military authorities thought that a regular sample of the weights of the civilian population would provide an index of the adequacy of civilian food supplies and thus be a measure of the success of food policies. In this they were probably right. But they proceeded to station a sergeant and a military orderly with a weighing machine at vantage points in the cities with instruction to weigh every tenth passer-by. These records, on examination, were found to produce data heavily biased numerically in favour of the female sex and the age group 15 to 25 years. If these technical details can be overcome, as is usually possible, there remains the much more fundamental difficulty of the choice of proper standards for comparative purposes. Table 55.4 and Figure 55.1 gives values for the median or 50th centile of height and weight of boys and girls up to the age of 18. These are USA figures and known as the Boston standards (Nelson, 1971). Measurements made in Edinburgh (Thomson, 1954, 1955; Provis and Ellis, 1955) and in London (Tanner *et al.*, 1966) give almost identical data. There is little doubt that the Boston standards are physiological values for well-fed Caucasian children. Many studies of groups of children belonging to prosperous African and Asian communities indicate that they apply to most children. A new growth chart recommended for international use (WHO, 1978) is very similar to the Boston Standards.

Records of heights and weights of children are of no use unless they are carefully interpreted. It is often useful to plot the height against the weight, either of single children or average figures of small groups, on to a piece of graph paper on which standard heights against standard weights have previously been plotted. Children with a deficit in height-for-age may be said to be stunted and those with a deficit in weight-for-height are wasted. An excess in weight-for-height is an indication of obesity. Waterlow (1973) discusses the value of these ratios and shows that a weight-for-height index, the Dugdale (1971) index $(W/H^{1.6} \times 10^4)$, is independent of age over the years 1 to 4. This index has been shown to have a value of almost exactly 100 in groups of children in USA, Holland, Ghana and Uganda and of about 93 in Jamaican and upper social class Indian children. Thus it is little affected by race. Weight-for-height ratios are useful in assessing the nutrition of children in primitive communities where age is not accurately known.

Many British cities have records for the past 60 years of heights and weights of their school children at selected ages. Some data for Glasgow are shown in Figures 55.2 and 55.3. The genetic make-up of the population has been unchanged and there can be little doubt that the figures record a progressive increase in the growth rates of individual children in the first half of the century. There is no doubt that the changes are due to better diets and the control of infectious diseases. There has been no significant increase in the last 15 years and it is probable that Glasgow children now grow at rates determined primarily by their genetic make-up and not by inadequate diets.

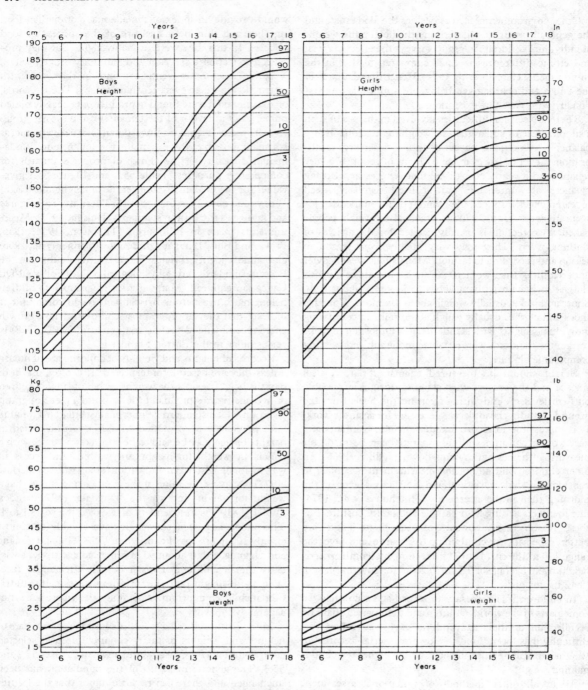

Fig. 55.1 Standard heights and weights of boys and girls 5–18 years old.

Table 55.5 gives desirable weights for adults. It was constructed by the Metropolitan Life Insurance Company (1959). The figures combine the experience of 26 life insurance companies in the USA and Canada with nearly 5 million insured persons between 1934 and 1954. Desirable weights are those associated with the lowest mortality. They are subdivided into those for persons with small, medium and large frames. This division was based on various anthropometric measurements, including width and depth of chest and hip width, but the exact criteria

Table 55.4 Weights for age, birth to 5 years, sexes combined (Jelliffe, 1966)

Age (Months)	Weight (kg) Standard*	80% Standard	60% Standard	Age (months)	Weight (kg) Standard*	80% Standard	60% Standard
0	3.4	2.7	2.0	31	13.7	11.0	8.2
				32	13.8	11.0	8.2
1	4.3	3.4	2.5	33	14.0	11.2	8.4
2	5.0	4.0	2.9				
3	5.7	4.5	3.4	34	14.2	11.3	8.5
				35	14.4	11.5	8.6
4	6.3	5.0	3.8	36	14.5	11.6	8.7
5	6.9	5.5	4.2				
6	7.4	5.9	4.5	37	14.7	11.8	8.8
				38	14.85	11.9	8.9
7	8.0	6.3	4.9	39	15.0	12.05	9.0
8	8.4	6.7	5.1				
9	8.9	7.1	5.3	40	15.2	12.2	9.1
				41	15.35	12.3	9.2
10	9.3	7.4	5.5	42	15.5	12.4	9.3
11	9.6	7.7	5.8				
12	9.9	7.9	6.0	43	15.7	12.6	9.4
				44	15.85	12.7	9.5
13	10.2	8.1	6.2	45	16.0	12.9	9.6
14	10.4	8.3	6.3				
15	10.6	8.5	6.4	46	16.2	12.95	9.7
				47	16.35	13.1	9.8
16	10.8	8.7	6.6	48	16.5	13.2	9.9
17	11.0	8.9	6.7				
18	11.3	9.0	6.8	49	16.65	13.35	10.0
				50	16.8	13.5	10.1
19	11.5	9.2	7.0	51	16.95	13.65	10.2
20	11.7	9.4	7.1				
21	11.9	9.6	7.2	52	17.1	13.8	10.3
				53	17.25	13.9	10.4
22	12.05	9.7	7.3	54	17.4	14.0	10.5
23	12.2	9.8	7.4				
24	12.4	9.9	7.5	55	17.6	14.2	10.6
				56	17.7	14.3	10.7
25	12.6	10.1	7.6	57	17.9	14.4	10.75
26	12.7	10.3	7.7				
27	12.9	10.5	7.8	58	18.05	14.5	10.8
				59	18.25	14.6	10.9
28	13.1	10.6	7.9	60	18.4	14.7	11.0
29	13.3	10.7	8.0				
30	13.5	10.8	8.1				

*Means of the Boston standards for boys and girls (Stuart and Stevenson, 1959). Means for boys are 0.05 to 0.15 kg heavier and for girls 0.05 to 0.15 kg lighter.

used have not been published. When a patient's weight is compared against the desirable weights for height in the table a decision has to be made about which reference frame size to use and there is no method for doing this accurately. In prevalence studies on obesity it has been recommended that the reference should be the upper end of large frame size (Bray, 1973). Obesity could then be defined as a bodyweight 20 per cent above this. The table allows no increase of weight with age, and it is stated that 'as a rule of thumb, if persons of any particular build keep their weight down to the average in the early 20's it would be fairly close to the desirable weight at ages over 25'. Observed weight expressed as a percentage of desirable weight for height is much used as an index of the degree of obesity.

OTHER ANTHROPOMETRIC DATA

The use of skinfold calipers to determine subcutaneous fat has already been described (p.244). The muscle mass in a limb can be assessed radiographically (Garn. 1963), but the radiological hazard precludes its use in surveys on children.

Measures of the circumference of the head, chest and arm are used in paediatric practice. Jelliffe (1966) describes the methods and gives normal values. Experiences with the use of the arm circumference in several

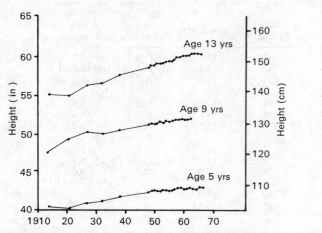

Fig. 55.2 Secular changes in growth of Glasgow schoolboys. Average values of height of age groups 5, 9 and 13 years for the periods indicated.

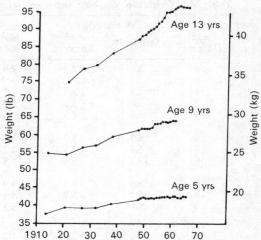

Fig. 55.3 Secular changes in growth of Glasgow schoolboys. Average values of weight of age groups 5, 9 and 13 years for the periods indicated.

Table 55.5 Desirable weights for men and women according to height and frame, based on measurements made in indoor clothing without shoes. Ages 25 years and over (modified from *Statistical Bulletin,* Metropolitan Life Insurance Company, 1959)

Height (metres)	Weight in kg		
	Small frame	Medium frame	Large frame
Men			
1.550	51–54	54–59	57–64
1.575	52–56	55–60	59–65
1.600	53–57	56–62	60–67
1.625	55–58	58–63	61–69
1.650	56–60	59–65	63–71
1.675	58–62	61–67	64–73
1.700	60–64	63–69	67–75
1.725	62–66	64–71	68–77
1.750	64–68	66–73	70–79
1.775	65–70	68–75	72–81
1.800	67–72	70–77	74–84
1.825	69–74	72–79	76–86
1.850	71–76	74–82	78–88
1.875	73–78	76–84	81–90
1.900	74–79	78–86	83–93
Women			
1.425	42–44	44–49	47–54
1.450	53–46	45–50	48–55
1.475	44–48	46–51	49–57
1.500	45–49	47–53	51–58
1.525	46–50	49–54	52–59
1.550	48–51	50–55	53–61
1.575	49–53	51–57	55–63
1.600	50–54	53–59	57–64
1.625	52–56	54–61	59–66
1.650	54–58	56–63	60–68
1.675	55–59	58–65	62–70
1.700	57–61	60–67	64–72
1.725	59–63	62–69	66–74
1.750	61–65	63–70	68–76
1.775	63–67	65–72	69–79

developing countries as an index of protein-energy malnutrition in early childhood were reported in a symposium edited by Jelliffe and Jelliffe (1969).

The QUAC stick was introduced by a Quaker Service Team for rapid screening of undernourished children during the Biafran war (Arnhold, 1969). It has a height-measuring stick, which is marked off in expected (80 or 85 per cent standard) measurements. Arm circumference measurements may be used instead of height measurements. If the arm circumference is less than it should be the child is probably undernourished. About 250 children an hour can be screened with this technique in a famine.

Midarm circumference changes very little between 12 and 60 months, and its measurement is a quick and inexpensive way of estimating thinness in large numbers of children when scales are not available. Shakir and Morley (1974) recommend the use of an inexpensive strip marked in three colours which are attached to the child. Green (13.5 to 17.5 cm) is normal, yellow (12.5 to 13.5 cm) indicates possible mild malnutrition and red (7 to 12.5 cm) definite malnutrition. These colours, like those on traffic signals, alert the staff.

Much ingenuity has been expended on attempts to construct formulae based on anthropometric measurements which provide an index of nutritional status. The essential difficulty is, of course, that size and shape is determined in part by genetic make-up and in part by environmental factors, of which the nature of the diet is only one, albeit usually the most important one. Early editions of this book gave references to several indices or formulae which had been tried out and, under certain circumstances, had proved useful as an aid to nutritional diagnosis. In the hands of the enthusiastic inventors, they provided useful information, but others found them less satisfactory and they are now seldom used. Height and weight accurately recorded and properly compared against suitable standards, are generally sufficient in surveys designed to assess the nutritional status of a community. The devising of anthropometric formulae and the testing of their usefulness is an occupation that has fascinated many able minds. If the results have proved disappointing, this does not mean that the problem is insoluble—only that it is very difficult.

VITAL STATISTICS

Most countries keep at least some vital statistics and from them it is usually possible to draw certain inferences about the nutrition of the people. The most used for this purpose has been the **infant mortality rate** (the number of babies dying in the first year of life per 1000 live births). In the period 1901–05 the rate for Scotland was 120 and most of the other countries had similar or even higher rates at that time. Since then there has been a fall in most countries,

partly attributable to improvements in infant feeding. However, there are still parts of the world where rates range from 75 to 100. In most prosperous countries the rate lies between 10 and 20 and is determined by the quality of the paediatric services and not by nutrition.

It has been suggested that the **perinatal mortality rate** (deaths of infants under 1 month and stillbirths per 1000 total births) may give an index of maternal nutrition. Many factors determine survival or death just before and after birth, e.g. the nutritional status of the mother, the genetic or constitutional make-up of both mother and child, the degree of exposure to infections and the standard of medical care available. Baird's (1960, 1974) analysis of trends in perinatal mortality in Britain is now a classic. He concluded that the war-time fall in the rates was due to the special supplementary rations which pregnant women received.

The manifestations and effects of malnutrition are well known to be severe in toddlers (children aged 1 to 4 years). Whereas in Europe and North America the death rate in this age group is usually around 1 per 1000, in many poor countries the figure is over 20. It may even rise to 100 and then only half the children born may survive to reach the age of 5. Although death certificates may record gastro-enteritis or respiratory infections, malnutrition contributes to many of the deaths. Thus, while infant mortality rates in underdeveloped countries are 5 to 10 times those in industrial countries, **1 to 4 years mortality rates** are 20 to 50 times as great.

Before the introduction of antibiotics, infectious diseases, such as measles, whooping-cough and pulmonary tuberculosis, were major causes of death. Chances of survival from these diseases were certainly reduced if the nutritional state of the patient was poor. Death rates from these infectious diseases have been used in the past as indications of the nutritional status of a population. They are, however, of little practical value in most countries at the present time, because of the use of specific remedies either against the diseases or their complications.

If in any community the perinatal, infant and toddler mortality rates are all falling, then it can be inferred that the general level of nutrition of the people is improving. On the other hand, a rise in any one of these rates should suggest the possibility that there has been a serious decline in standards of child care and probably nutrition.

In times of food scarcity, daily, weekly and monthly crude death rates may give valuable information about changes from conditions of hardship to conditions of famine. During World War II the Dutch had four years of food shortage and scarcity. These were very unpleasant but did not constitue a major hazard to health. They were followed from December 1944 to April 1945 by five months of real famine. Table 55.6, shows the effect of these changes on crude death-rates in some of the principal cities of Holland. In Amsterdam, Rotterdam and The Hague

Table 55.6 Number of deaths in four cities in Western Holland (Burger *et al.*, 1948)

City	Population	Number of deaths in the first 6 months of			Number of deaths per 1000 inhabitants calculated as mortality in 1 year		
		1939	1944	1945	1939	1944	1945
Amsterdam	800 000	3655	4393	9735	9.2	11.3	25.2
Rotterdam	640 000	2616	3260	7827	8.5	10.7	25.8
The Hague	520 000	2419	2940	6458	9.7	13.0	28.7
Utrecht	170 000	776	1120	2065	9.3	13.0	24.3

during the worst week of the famine, crude death-rates of about 40 per 1000 (calculated on a yearly basis) were recorded. Such figures are useful to famine administrators in gauging the extent of the disaster and the success of relief measures.

Had similar crude death-rates been available from rural Bengal early in 1943, the extent of the famine there would have been realised sooner, relief organisations would have started earlier and the mortality figure of 1½ million from starvation might have been much less.

DIETARY SURVEYS

Quantitative information about the food eaten by a people or a community, if compared with physiological standards of human needs, has enabled assessments of nutrition to be made that have been widely used and proved both useful and practical. Data can be collected covering a whole nation, from families of different economic classes or from individuals of special age-groups or occupations. Each type of survey can provide valuable information. For sound government planning, nationwide data covering all socioeconomic groups and age groups are required. In all cases the technique demands care and is time-consuming and exacting. Before describing the different methods and their difficulties, certain considerations common to all dietary studies require discussion.

A comparison can be made between the amounts of food consumed and a chosen physiological standard only when the data collected have been converted into quantities of energy, carbohydrate, protein, fat, minerals and vitamins. This involves the use of food tables and here errors are inevitably introduced (Chap. 16).

Another difficulty is to reach agreement on the physiological or other standards with which to compare the results of dietary surveys. If repeated dietary surveys are carried out systematically in a country, it is possible to tell whether the quantity or quality of the food consumed is improving or declining. This information is often more useful than a comparison with a physiological standard, which must always be arbitrary.

National studies. These are attempts to assess the total food supply of a whole nation or other large community. The basic data are the statistics of agricultural production and the statistics of the imports and exports of food. In this way it is possible to estimate total food supplies and, with a knowledge of the population, to calculate the average daily supply of the principal nutrients.

FAO collects national data on these lines and publishes them at regular intervals. The errors involved in such surveys may be very great. In some countries figures both for agricultural production and population can be nothing more than intelligent guesses. This applies to almost all of Africa and to many Asian and South American countries. On the other hand in a small, well-organised country such as Denmark, the degree of accuracy of such statistics is high.

Another important error that arises in the use of such data is that they give no accurate measure of wastage of food (p. 210). FAO usually makes allowances for losses in the wholesale trade and its figures are intended to describe the food available at the 'retail' or shop level. It is, of course, important not to attempt to match such figures directly against a standard of physiological 'requirements'. Some further wastage after purchase is inevitable.

The value of national estimates of food consumption has often been called in question: the errors involved are obvious. Nevertheless, an intelligent study of the figures can reveal much that is important about the nutritional status of many countries. Successive World Food Surveys have brought out valuable trends. FAO has done a great service in producing this information.

Family surveys. Most surveys have the family as the basic unit. A trained investigator with the co-operation of the housewife attempts to measure all the food consumed by a family over a period of time, usually a week. A log-book is kept for each family. The investigator visits the housewife at the start of the survey and weighs all the food in her stores. Each day, either the investigator or the housewife weighs all the food purchased and enters this in the log-book. The food wasted is also weighed and entered. At the end of the survey period all food remaining in the store is weighed. Thus all the food eaten in the household is recorded. The age, sex and occupation of members are also noted. The number of visitors eating occasional meals and number of meals eaten outside the home by members of the family are also noted and arbitrary corrections made for them. Measured intakes of nutrients can then be compared with recommended standards.

It must be emphasised that to conduct an accurate family dietary survey demands an exacting technique and experience on the part of the investigators. Here only a brief outline of the principles has been given. Further details of technique can be found in a monograph by Emma Reh (1962) and in a report from FAO (1964).

The family survey is useful for determining the food consumed by different economic and social groups. Experience has shown that it is usually sufficient to survey between 20 and 30 families in a group. As far as possible the families should be chosen by random selection, and every effort should be made to get a representative sample. Success depends on the tact and social skill of the organisers and investigators. Some housewives will never co-operate, but with care it should be possible to get the goodwill and help of at least four out of five.

A survey should cover 4 to 7 days and include the weekend when in most countries families change their daily dietary habits. To prolong a survey more than a week is irksome to the housewife.

In some countries there are marked seasonal variations in food intake and hence it may be necessary to repeat surveys at different times of the year. This is less necessary in towns than in country districts, for in the former the diet often changes little throughout the year.

There are two major sources of error in a family survey. The housewife may, through ignorance or carelessness, fail to record or report all her purchases. Alternatively the housewife may put on a show for the survey and feed her family better than usual. With good investigators the second error is the more probable and so surveys tend to overestimate normal consumption. A skilful investigator can often check up on these points and the record of any unreliable housewife should be discarded.

A valuable adjunct to a family dietary survey is often provided by an enquiry into the housewife's budget and the amount of money that she has available to spend on food. A comparison between this and local food prices serves as a check on the dietary assessment and sometimes provides clear evidence that the family concerned cannot possibly afford to purchase an adequate diet.

Institutional surveys are carried out on similar lines and usually are relatively easy.

An inherent drawback to family surveys is that no information is provided about how the food is distributed within the family. It does not distinguish between the food consumed by the housewife, the breadwinner, the children and other dependants.

Individual surveys. The principle is the same as that of family surveys. The selected individuals, assisted and supervised by investigators, weigh and measure everything consumed at each meal. This is a much more exacting task than a family survey, for a great deal of co-operation and a modest degree of intelligence on the part of the subject is needed. Nevertheless, many excellent individual surveys have been undertaken. Children of different age groups, old people, miners, soldiers, housewives and people in various occupations have been studied. A properly conducted series of individual dietary surveys gives a good assessment of nutritional status. However, it should never be assumed that an individual is deficient in a nutrient on the basis of a short dietary study. Clinical and biochemical examination are required to confirm any suspicions raised by the intake data.

Short-cut methods of estimating dietary intake by recall have been devised. The subject is asked either what he ate the day before or what he eats on a typical day. These methods are subject to many inaccuracies but are useful to compare different groups and, when repeated, may indicate important trends. The techniques of making individual dietary surveys are described in detail in a long review by Marr (1971), who has also given a brief summary of the subject (Marr, 1973).

NUTRITIONAL ASSESSMENT IN HOSPITAL

A good clinician has always assessed his patients' energy stores by non-instrumental appraisal of subcutaneous fat; he has noted subcutaneous and other general signs that suggest deficiency disease and has considered nutritional causes of low haemoglobin or plasma albumin concentrations. In acute illness the critical nutrient deficiencies tend to be different from those seen in apparently healthy people. Potassium deficiency is very important and folate deficiency common.

Medical nutritionists, working in some larger hospitals in North America, have realised that a proportion of medical and surgical patients have features of protein-energy malnutrition. This is not an inevitable accompaniment of the disease but can be largely prevented or treated by giving more attention to the patient's nutrition, including parenteral feeding where indicated. The techniques for assessing protein and energy status have been worked out and tested mostly in children in the Third World. There is no reason why they should not be used for adults with complicated medical and surgical diseases in hospital in affluent countries, though adaptations of techniques and of normal standards are sometimes called for. Measurements that may be useful include height and weight, skinfolds, mid-arm circumference, urinary creatinine and nitrogen balance (Bistrian et al., 1977). Concentrations of several plasma proteins are sensitive to nutritional state in surgical patients, e.g. albumin, transferrin, retinol-binding protein and pre-albumin (Young et al., 1978). All of these can be used to indicate poor nutrition before surgery or its deterioration post-operatively. We believe that diagnostic methods like these deserve standardisation and wider use in hospital practice.

COMMENT

The methods of nutritional assessment described above are of great value in poor communities where evidence of undernutrition and malnutrition is obvious. Dietary and clinical surveys supplemented by a few anthropometric and biochemical measurements, sufficient to indicate the main order of priorities in a nutritional programme, can be carried out by a small trained staff and at no great expense. Their value has been proven in many countries in Africa, Asia, Central and South America where the need for their continuing use remains great.

In prosperous countries it is much more difficult to identify and assess small minority groups in whom under-nutrition exists. In Britain material for nutritional surveillance is provided by the results of the National Food Survey, the records of School Medical Services and the tables of mortality given by the Registrar General. The National Food Survey records food consumption in large numbers of homes throughout the country each year. As it has been in operation since 1940, it provides material for monitoring changes in patterns of food consumption (Greaves and Hollingsworth, 1966; Marr and Berry, 1974). However, it is not planned primarily to detect the incidence of malnutrition in minority groups. The Department of Health and Social Security has carried out nutritional surveys on young children and old people on a large scale. These are two groups in which some malnutrition is known to exist, but the surveys have shown that the incidence in both groups is small. In order to detect cases large numbers of healthy well-fed individuals have to be surveyed and large numbers of laboratory tests are required. In consequence the expense is high. The prob-lem of how to assess quickly the effects on health, if any, of a change in national food policy, e.g. the reduction in school milk in 1971, remains unsolved.

In the USA, the federal government in 1967 sanctioned a National Nutrition Survey 'to determine the prevalence of malnutrition and related health problems among low income populations in the United States'. Some 40 000 individuals were examined in 10 states and the sample was weighted to include more of the age, income and ethnic groups believed to be at risk of malnutrition. Clinical examination revealed few signs of malnutrition. Anthropometry showed that Negro children were in general taller than whites. Sizeable minorities of children and teenagers were underweight and many adults were obese. The most common positive findings were in the laboratory tests, especially low haemoglobin, which correlated with low dietary or plasma iron, and low plasma vitamin A in Spanish-Americans; some groups showed biochemical evidence of low intakes of protein, riboflavin and vitamin C. The findings are set out in a 940-page report extending to five books (US Department of Health, Education and Welfare, 1972). This is by far the largest nutrition survey ever carried out.

A similar Canadian study was reported in 1974 (Sabry et al., 1974). Samples of all the different groups of people throughout the country were included, totalling 19 000. The commonest type of malnutrition appeared to be iron deficiency. There was also biochemical evidence of low folate reserves; some cases of goitre and scurvy were found, especially in Eskimos; biochemical evidence of insufficient riboflavin was unusual; obesity and high plasma cholesterol concentrations were common.

56. Prevention of Nutritional Disorders

Nutritional disorders do not arise when there is ample food production, when the people know how to make the best use of available foods and when steps are taken to ensure that the needs of the very poor and of mothers and young children and others who may be specially liable to malnutrition (vulnerable groups) are met. Agriculture, nutrition education and nutritional support are considered in three separate sections of this chapter. Each of these depends on governments' policies for food and nutrition, or the lack of them, and the chapter ends with a general discussion of the role of governments.

NUTRITION EDUCATION

The question is sometimes asked, what is the need for education in nutrition? Do we not know instinctively what is good food and so eat well and wisely, unless prevented by poverty or other circumstance? This is only a half truth. Our food habits are dependent on attitudes, prejudices and taboos acquired early in life and form a pattern of behaviour which is characteristic of a group. This is as true for prosperous urban communities as for poor rural agriculturalists. Nutrition is, amongst other things, a behavioural science. Further, both the nature of the foods produced and their processing and distribution are changing rapidly owing to the scientific revolutions taking place in agriculture and food technology. Everywhere new food habits are being formed. If these changes are to be for the better, widespread knowledge of the principles of nutrition is required. A monograph which covers many aspects of education in nutrition by Jean Ritchie (1971) and a manual on education in primary schools (FAO, 1971) are recommended. Here we discuss the subject under four heads: (1) general education, (2) education in mothercraft, (3) community education (applied nutrition programmes), and (4) professional training.

GENERAL EDUCATION

This includes the teaching of children in schools and adult education. In general, we do not recommend courses specifically on nutrition, but rather that nutrition should have a prominent part in courses on biology and in health education. Elementary biology, with a large emphasis on human physiology, provides a good introduction to science, for a child has a natural curiosity about how his body works. It is unfortunate that physiology is often considered as a subject suitable only for medical students, whereas it can be taught to young children, even those with limited intelligence; also many teachers specialising in biology are poorly informed on human physiology.

There is a general agreement that health education is an important subject, but dispute about how it should be taught and who should teach it. Much can be done by example. A school which provides good meals and has clean toilets and washing facilities and in which the teachers do not smoke in public may do more to teach children healthy habits than one which gives elaborate formal instruction. Visual aids on nutrition, including films and film strips, are available and many of them are excellent, but they are no substitute for an enthusiastic teacher.

There are numerous elementary textbooks on nutrition, not all of them by writers who are well informed. In Britain the Ministry of Agriculture, Fisheries and Food's handbook, *The Manual of Nutrition,* written in 1945 by Dr Magnus Pyke and since revised many times, is recommended. *Human Nutrition in Tropical Africa* by Dr Michael Latham and published by FAO is an excellent book for teachers in Africa.

Newspapers, radio and television are also important vehicles of nutrition education. The women's magazines have an enormous circulation in prosperous countries and are beginning to circulate widely in African and Asian cities. They frequently contain articles on food and nutrition, which are well written and informative. In most countries the big firms in the food industry have enormous advertising programmes which have a large educational role, often beneficial, but sometimes misleading. In Britain advertisements on commercial television are regulated by a code of practice drawn up by the advertising agencies and by government regulations, designed to prevent false and misleading claims for foods. Unfortunately many commercials keep to the letter rather than the spirit of the law, and the majority are for confectionery and alcoholic drinks.

So far we have discussed elementary education, which is concerned only with the role of the different nutrients in the economy of the human body, the nutritive value of common foods and how these can be selected to make a balanced diet. There is also a need for nutrition in higher education, which provides the material which informed public opinion needs if it is to support sound food policies in a country. There is little education related to nutrition in the sixth forms of schools or in most university classes outside the medical faculty. Three books (Salaman, 1948; McCance and Widdowson, 1956; Masefield, 1963) dealing with historical, social and economic aspects of bread, potatoes and famine respectively, can be recommended for study courses in any liberal arts.

EDUCATION IN MOTHERCRAFT

A mother has dual responsibilities for feeding the young infant and for preparing food for older children and adult members of the family. Education in the former is the task of the Maternity and Child Health services. The latter falls within the scope of Home Economics, which is now realised to be increasingly important especially in underdeveloped countries.

Maternity and child health (MCH) centres

These are designed to supervise the health of normal pregnant women and their babies and pre-school children. They are an established part of the medical services, although in many countries their number is far below that necessary to cover even a fraction of the population. The centres ideally should be associated with a hospital to which patients can be sent. All babies and young children are liable to minor ailments and injuries for which they need treatment. At a visit to a clinic a few words of advice from a doctor or nurse, who has treated the ailment, is more likely to be effective than most attempts at instruction through other educational channels. In the words of Dr Cicely Williams a centre 'should give individual patients whatever treatment is necessary and whatever prevention they can take'. The public health nurses on the staff of MCH centres visit the homes of the people. This enables them to see the family background, appreciate special difficulties and to tailor instruction to the needs of individual circumstances. The extension of the MCH services is an urgent problem for the medical services in all countries where malnutrition is widespread. In all but the largest centres the best arrangement is to have a trained nursing sister in charge, backed up by a doctor who makes periodic visits and can be consulted by telephone or radio. The sister is assisted by health workers or assistant nurses who should be recruited from the local population. Morley (1973) gives practical advice on how to set up and run an 'Under Fives clinic'.

In prosperous countries, where most of the infants and young children are well fed there are feckless and ignorant mothers: it is amongst their children that cases of rickets and scurvy are still occasionally seen. The MCH services probably are the best means of influencing this group.

The MCH services are the proper channel for the education of mothers in the feeding of infants and preschool children. They have the professional competence and the means of getting the goodwill and respect of the people. However, at the moment and for some time to come they are not sufficiently developed in many countries to meet the need. The assistance of other organisations is needed. These include community centres, women's clubs, youth clubs, rural service centres, etc. These have the advantages of being in touch with the people and of being able to use the enthusiasm of voluntary workers. Much valuable education comes from such organisations and the case for their extension is argued strongly. When there is urgent need for a job to be done, it does not matter greatly who does it. However, there are dangers. All the above organisations need financial help—for training local workers, for administrative assistance and for some full-time trained staff. For this they depend on national and international aid. Too many competing organisations do not lead to efficiency. Indeed at the village level a series of rival organisations, each giving different advice to mothers (as has been known to happen), is worse than useless.

Home economics. We support the views of Autret, given in an introduction to a report on home economics centres (Haglund and Magnusson, 1967), in which he states: 'The moral, economic, social and civic responsibilities of women are great: management of the home; the moral and emotional climate of the family and community; the practical aspects of family life including child care, catering, cooking and household budgeting; all these depend in great part on the skill, tact, knowledge and ability of the mother. This knowledge, passed from mother to daughter, by word of mouth, was for a long time sufficient in a slowly developing and almost static world. Today such traditional knowledge has proved to be rudimentary and out of date in a world in the process of rapid development.'

FAO helps national governments with a large number of field projects in home economics, for many of which experienced teachers and consultants are provided. The subject of home economics is having to adapt to revolutionary concepts of the role of women in society. Its horizons can no longer be confined to needlework and cookery. Mistakes have been made in the past by teaching domestic kitchen technology suitable for New York in the African bush. Food preparation traditions of peasant communities need to be understood and adapted to modern conditions but not replaced.

COMMUNITY EDUCATION

In many countries the subject of nutrition can be fitted into the various parts of a complex educational system which already exists. In primitive rural communities, educational facilities, if they exist at all, are often limited to an elementary school. In these circumstances new methods and organisations have to be developed. Means have to be found to teach farmers to improve yields of traditional crops and to grow new ones. New methods of sorting, processing and marketing of foods may be required. There is ignorance of mothercraft and elementary hygiene. Education on these matters is best undertaken on a communal basis, which includes all aspects of the health and welfare of the people. For this purpose the UN agencies have developed Applied Nutrition Programmes (ANP) defined as 'a comprehensive type of interrelated educational activities aimed at the improvement of local food production, consumption and distribution in favour of local communities, particularly mothers and children in rural areas, in which the guiding principles are co-ordination among different agencies and institutions, and the active participation of the people themselves' (FAO/WHO, 1966).

Over 100 such programmes have been assisted by FAO, and their failures and successes reviewed by McNaughton (1975). A common mistake on the part of the international agencies has been not to recognise the futility of introducing a programme into a country where there were not sufficient resources and staff to continue to run it. Outsiders can provide a community with a stimulus and with material and expert help at the start but only local enterprise can maintain it. The programmes have, however, been the means of interesting a number of national governments in nutrition and have motivated large numbers of local staff. Future programmes should be related to economic realities and be flexible; they should take in other aspects of health, especially the control of infectious diseases, besides nutrition.

Such programmes are not the monopoly of the UN. If this were so, progress would indeed be on a very small scale. Initiative can come from central or local governments, from large foundations or from private individuals. We ourselves know something of the work of the Valley Trust, which runs a sociomedical project at Botha's Hill in Natal, South Africa, designed to promote the health and well-being of the local Zulu community, in which great emphasis is placed on nutritional problems related to agriculture and the educational needs of the people. The trust is run by a few energetic helpers led by Dr H. H. Stott, from whom the annual report can be obtained. The government provides the medical staff and expenses of the Health Centre at the settlement.

Any scheme for community education is bound to fail unless it has the enthusiastic support of the leaders of the community. These are almost inevitably conservatives, often with little conception of the need for change. The first task of the organisers, and often the most difficult one, is to persuade such leaders that the scheme is worth while. Until this has been done agriculturalists, nutritionists, MCH workers, home economists and health educators begin their work under grave difficulties. In some circumstances there is need for the services of an expert in social anthropology to study and report on the community before any work begins.

Community education is expensive in the use of the time of skilled people and also in money. It is therefore essential to have a continuous evaluation of the results which are being achieved in any programme. Indeed the initial planning of a scheme must include ways and means of evaluation (Ritchie, 1971).

Local circumstances make it inevitable that each programme is different from others. It is impossible to draw up a general blueprint. The headquarters staff of the Nutrition Division of FAO in Rome has now a wide experience of community education and the factors which make for success or failure. They are able and willing to advise on the details of any proposal for a new subject, and have published a monograph on planning and evaluation (Latham, 1972).

PROFESSIONAL TRAINING

Medical schools

Nutrition is not a clinical speciality in the way that cardiology or endocrinology is. In medical schools some nutrition is taught as part of the undergraduate courses in biochemistry, physiology, pharmacology, pathology, medicine, paediatrics, obstetrics, surgery, community medicine and dentistry. Teaching is generally diffuse and uneven, and physicians are weak at translating the science into practical answers to patients' questions (White, 1973). Others have put the position more strongly. *Time* magazine (1972) considered that 'the field of nutrition is terra incognita for the average doctor. Courses are not widely taught in medical schools, and even among specialists there are substantive disagreements.' Doctors need a good theoretical and practical understanding of nutrition in their daily work, in situations ranging from intensive care of an unconscious patient to answering the questions about preventive dietetics that healthy people bring to their general practitioner. Anyone who has worked through the preceding pages of this book will probably agree that, while parts of the material could be considered in courses on biochemistry, paediatrics and internal medicine, yet there is a scientific core to nutrition which is unlikely to be covered elsewhere in a medical course. This includes such topics as the assessment of nutritional status, interactions of nutrients with one another and with diseases, recommended intakes of nutrients, food composition, food technology, world food problems and psychological and sociological aspects of food habits.

A conference on guidelines for nutrition education in medical schools, held at Williamsburg, Virginia (White *et al.*, 1972), agreed that medical schools should be encouraged to develop and require as part of the main curriculum a basic nutrition course and, in addition, attractive, competitive elective courses should be available to undergraduates. It is equally important that during his clinical experience, the medical student should learn that applied nutrition is an intrinsic part of the clinical assessment and management of patients. The International Union of Nutritional Sciences (IUNS) Committee on Nutrition Education in Medical Faculties (1971) recommends that each medical school should have a committee to advise on a programme in nutrition which should cover teaching in various preclinical and clinical departments. In this way it should be possible to see that important parts of the subject are not omitted and that unnecessary repetition is avoided. There can be no hard and fast rules as to which department teaches particular aspects; this should depend on the interest and expertise of individual lecturers in different departments.

The IUNS committee considers that ideally each medical school should have a Chair in Nutrition. We do not think that this is necessary for every medical school but there would be great advantages if professorial departments of nutrition were seeded among the medical schools of each country as centres of research, training and information. Most Swedish medical schools now have a professor of nutrition and several schools in the USA are making efforts to co-ordinate their teaching of the subject and to introduce students to practical and research aspects of human nutrition (Christakis *et al*, 1972). In some cases this has been requested by the medical students themselves.

Nursing. Nurses should have a sound elementary knowledge of nutrition and dietetics because of their responsibilities in the feeding of patients. Judging by the Platt report (p. 450) this is not always the case.

Dietitians. In Britain there have been different ways of training which are approved for State Registration by the Council for Professions Supplementary to Medicine and for membership of the British Dietetic Association. Today most students do a BSc course in a polytechnic. A four-year 'sandwich' course for an honours BSc Nutrition with State Registration in Dietetics is available at Surrey University and at Queen Elizabeth College, London. All courses include some six months training in the dietetic department of a recognised hospital. Details can be obtained from the Secretary, British Dietetic Association, 305 Daimler House, Paradise Street, Birmingham.

A Working Party of the Dietitians Board took evidence from the profession and produced a report, *Dietitians of the Future*. They consider that in Britain dietitians should be far less concerned with the preparation and service of individual diets and must be willing to act as consultants, exercising their own judgment and making their own decisions. They must not regard themselves as technicians waiting for instructions. The report makes interesting reading but we consider it politically unwise for the dietetic profession to lose control of food service management in hospital (Truswell, 1977).

In the USA and Canada all dietitians must have a Bachelor's degree from an accredited college. Courses for such degrees are based on a syllabus which divides the period of study between chemistry, biochemistry and physiology and the practical work of hospital and public health dietetic departments. Senior dietitians have been at great pains to ensure that standards of professional training are high. The American Dietetic Association (1972) has examined carefully what dietitians do and how their work is likely to change. It makes recommendations for their training.

Nutritionists. A few years ago an acceptable explanation of the difference between a nutritionist and a dietitian might have been that a nutritionist deals with the science of nutrition for health while a dietitian applies this in the treatment of sick people, usually in hospital. The distinction has become blurred now that some dietitians are specialising in community preventive work and some nutritional scientists are doing research on the effect of infections or nutritional metabolism. We welcome this and consider that BSc graduates in nutrition should as a rule take dietetics as part of their training. At Sydney University the postgraduate course which one of us teaches is an integrated Diploma in Nutrition and Dietetics.

Many of those who call themselves nutritionists have come to the subject after undergraduate study in another discipline—chemistry, biochemistry, agriculture, medicine or, more recently, the social sciences. Dr W. R. Aykroyd in 1935, at the Nutrition Research Laboratories in South India, started informal courses on nutrition lasting for two to three months: the courses were at first

Table 56.1 Yields of cereals in various countries in 100 kg per hectare (data from FAO, 1971)

Wheat		Rice	
Netherlands	46.0	Spain	60.2
United Kingdom	42.1	Japan	54.8
United Arab Republic	26.5	USA	50.4
USA	21.4	Italy	49.8
Canada	18.2	Malaysia	27.9
USSR	13.8	Sri Lanka	26.3
India	12.3	Indonesia	20.9
Pakistan	11.1	Thailand	19.6
Iraq	5.6	India and Pakistan	17.0
Libya	2.3	Uganda	8.0

intended primarily for doctors, but people with different backgrounds soon began to attend. The courses continue at the laboratories, now moved to Hyderabad as the National Institute of Nutrition. Similar courses are now run in many parts of the world and are an established part of FAO and WHO programmes. They have proved especially valuable in French-speaking Africa, the Middle East and the Far East. The emphasis is on field work and they are a means of training numbers of people in the practical approach to nutritional problems. In Britain London University gives an MSc degree in nutrition to graduates in various disciplines from other universities, after attending a one-year course at Queen Elizabeth College or at the London School of Hygiene and Tropical Medicine. Cambridge University has a course in nutrition lasting for nine months, to which graduates with very varying backgrounds are admitted. A diploma is given. These three courses are well attended by students from many parts of the world.

Several American universities run excellent postgraduate courses in nutrition. A course started by Dr F. Stare at the Harvard School of Public Health has run for many years and acquired a world-wide reputation. Briggs *et al.* (1974) have prepared a list of degree courses in nutrition throughout the world.

AGRICULTURE

There are three ways in which the food supply of the world could be increased. First, there are enormous areas of land which are not used for food production or only for rough grazing or shifting cultivation. There are millions of acres of desert or semi-desert, tropical jungle, tundra and moorland which could be made to produce food. The Israelis have given the world a striking example of how to make the desert bloom. However, the difficulties and expense of utilising such lands are very great and in the most densely populated parts of the world almost all the potentially good land is already under cultivation. The second way is to improve methods of farming on lands already in use. There are possibilities for large increases in food supplies in this way by the use of agricultural methods already established. Thirdly, it is possible to produce nutrients which could be used as foods, on a large scale, by the methods of chemical engineering. These are briefly discussed on page 482.

Table 56.1 shows yields of wheat and rice in selected countries. In the countries at the bottom of the league table, farmers for the most part have as good land as those at the top. With the proper use of modern farming techniques most wheat-growing countries could produce yields of the same order as those obtained in the Netherlands and in Britain. Indian and Bangladesh rice farmers could grow crops as big as Spanish and Japanese farmers

do. Whether they will be able to develop the necessary skills before being overtaken by the growth of population is more doubtful. Intensive agriculture is also limited by the heavy input of energy (diesel fuel) which it requires.

A major development is the production of high-yielding seeds, as a result of trials at the International Maize and Wheat Improvement Center in Mexico and at the International Rice Center in the Philippines. These are each supported largely by the Rockefeller and Ford Foundations. Dwarf varieties of wheat Sonora 64 and Lerma Roja 64 each commonly yield 4 tons per hectare and sometimes 5 to 8 tons, in conditions where the standard variety yields 1 to 3 tons. Similarly with IR 8 rice, yields can be increased up to fourfold.

Improved varieties were sown on a large scale in the underdeveloped countries for the first time for the 1967 harvest. Some 500 000 hectares in Pakistan and 800 000 hectares in India were sown with improved wheats. Many other countries including Afghanistan, Iran, Iraq, Kenya, Lebanon, Libya, Morocco, Rhodesia, South Africa, Tunisia and Turkey began to use them at that time. In the Tanjore district of South India some 200 000 farmers raised the yield of their 1967 rice harvest by 450 000 tons as a result of the use of improved seeds. In 1967 for the first time for a decade in many underdeveloped countries agricultural production increased significantly more than the growth of population. The 1970–71 harvest of food grains in India was sufficient for the first time for many years to meet the country's needs and an optimistic Minister of Food is reported to have said: 'We will have to go out in search of foreign markets in a big way in 1974.' However, in 1974 India was importing cereals to meet famine conditions in large areas of Maharastra. The minister had overlooked the vagaries of the monsoon rainfall and the fact that improved seeds can give high yields only if they are properly cultivated. They make heavy demands on fertilisers; weeds, insects and plant diseases must be controlled.

For peasant farmers all this is new and they are naturally conservative and reluctant to spend money on seeds and chemicals, unless they have seen results. Further, owing to agricultural indebtedness such money usually has to be borrowed. A feature of modern agriculture is that it needs a much smaller labour force than traditional farming and so creates rural unemployment. Unless jobs can be found in the towns, it is likely to lead to social unrest. The new varieties of cereals provide hope for agriculture in many countries, but they bring also a multitude of technical, economic and social problems.

New techniques in agriculture are exploited much more effectively by large international corporations than by peasant farmers. Underdeveloped land in poor countries is used too often to grow cattle food and raise stock to provide steaks for New Yorkers, Londoners and Parisians. This

agribusiness (George, 1976; Moore Lappé and Collins, 1977) may benefit a few landowners and entrepreneurs in the poor countries but not the peasants. It promotes rural unemployment since modern agricultural methods require a much smaller labour force than traditional farming. Economic factors divert the use of land from the production of beans, which the poor need, to the production of food for export to wealthy countries for consumption by people who are already overfed. The gross national income of the country in which the extra food is grown may rise but this is a paper statistic which does not feed the poor. Indeed the poor are often worse off and suffer more malnutrition.

The indictment of agribusiness by Susan George, Francis Moore Lappé and Collins is well presented and convincing. It raises political questions about the organisation of society. American capitalists have failed to help the poor in Latin America, Africa and Asia to utilise the new agricultural knowledge to grow the foods they need, but they have been able to export huge quantities of grain to make good the deficiencies caused by the failure of Russian Communists to organise agriculture in their country. It is easy to condemn those responsible for these failures, but well to remember that among the men who sit on the boards of the giant corporations and on the Soviet committees there is probably a mixture of altruism and roguery similar to that familiar to most of us in our little committees.

CHEMICAL ENGINEERING

Food production ultimately depends on the fixation of solar energy by photosynthesis and the subsequent formation of organic compounds. The essential ingredients are sunlight, carbon dioxide, water, inorganic nitrogen and phosphorus. There is an abundance of unused sunlight in most parts of the world. The supply of CO_2 is being continually made available locally by the respiration of plants and animals. There is plenty of water, nitrogen and phosphorus in the world. These ingredients could be put together by chemical engineers to make carbohydrates, fats and proteins on a scale far larger than farmers achieve at the present time. Schmitt (1965), an enthusiast from the University of California, foretells that '30 billion people may ultimately lead fairly free and enriched lives on this planet. The physical resources of the earth for the production of food are many times greater than man's needs as far ahead as one can see.' All this may be technically possible, and there seems no reason why any of mankind should starve now or in the foreseeable future. Personally we have no regrets that we shall not be alive to be numbered among the 30 billion. To us it seems a better choice, and choice there is, for mankind to plan his reproduction so that the numbers are limited to those who can be fed by food supplied by scientific agriculture. At the present time equal effort should be applied to teaching the new techniques in family planning and in farming.

NUTRITIONAL SUPPORT

FOOD SUBSIDIES

The importance of poverty in preventing the equitable distribution of foods has already been stressed (p. 460). Artifically lowering the price of foods by means of government subsidies helps families with low incomes to purchase an adequate diet. During World War II the British Government lowered and controlled the prices of beef, mutton, bacon, bread, sugar, milk, potatoes, margarine, butter, cheese and eggs by means of subsidies. These varied from 20 to 50 per cent of the true cost of the food. There is little doubt that this policy contributed to the improvement in the nutrition of the nation that occurred during the war.

Subsequently these subsidies on consumer goods were reduced and by 1954 all had gone except that on Welfare milk. Direct subsidies on bread and milk were introduced in 1974 to keep the cost of living down at a time when big wage claims were being made. There are still large subsidies to agriculture and the British housewife does not pay the full economic prices for all the food she buys. Agricultural subsidies and farm prices are important subjects of contention in the European Economic Community, where the British and the French seldom see eye to eye.

RATIONING SCHEMES

Rationing is simple in principle and applicable to any food which may be available only in limited amounts. In Britain, during World War II, it was considered necessary to ration the following foods: butcher's meat, bacon, milk, cheese, sugar, fats, and in addition during 1946–48 bread and in 1947–48 potatoes. Such elaborate controls are only possible when the people have the necessary discipline and administrative aptitude. In countries with a simpler dietary pattern and a limited administrative machinery, it is unnecessary and impractical to attempt so much. For instance, during threats of famine in India, it is usual to ration only the staple grain of the district. This has proved for the most part to be practical, that is within the scope of the administration, and yet effective in preventing serious deterioration of health in threatened areas. By contrast, in Germany after the war schemes for rationing of bread, cereals, potatoes, fats, sugar, meat, cheese, milk, fish and dried fruits were drawn up and put into operation. The German authorities were unable to enforce these regulations and large black markets thrived. Any rationing scheme should be related to the normal dietary habits of the population, their probable reaction to discipline and the efficiency of the administration.

Black markets. A proportion of goods supposed to be rationed always reaches consumers by channels independent of government control. Such distribution of rationed goods through illegal channels is known throughout the world as a 'black market'. The size of black markets is a measure of the efficiency of the administration and the extent to which the government represents the will of the people. Human nature necessitates that in time of scarcity some exchange of primary products and services must occur without the use of the medium of money and outside any state control. Experience has shown that, as long as this barter of services and products is limited to exchanges between principals for their personal use, it has little effect on the efficient working of a rationing system. No government can hope to prevent such exchanges. Once, however, such exchanges become organised by intermediaries, who themselves produce no goods and perform no essential services, then chaos results. The control of the activities of such men is a most important task. Bengal and Germany have known the evils that result from black marketeers. Such offenders against food regulations should receive the severest penalties of the law.

FOOD ENRICHMENT

Foods may be enriched or fortified by the addition of nutrients. Such additions may be statutory under the law or made voluntarily by food manufacturers, and many examples have been given in previous pages. The addition of vitamins A and D to an artificial food, margarine, to make it comparable with the natural food, butter, was a major advance in nutrition. The addition of thiamin to white flour to replace loss of the vitamin in milling is sensible and a widespread practice. The additions of iodine to salt or bread and of iron to flour are examples of mass medication. The value of the former in preventing goitre is proven, but there is as yet no satisfactory evidence that the latter is of any benefit in preventing anaemia. Many dried and concentrated preparations of milk have vitamins added and this certainly helps to prevent rickets, although there is a danger from excess of vitamin D. Enrichment is now an established practice in wealthy countries with a good food industry and there is little doubt of its value in appropriate cases. Whether or not the benefit of some additions made or advocated, e.g. those of iron, calcium and lysine to wheat flour, are worth the cost is doubtful.

Enrichment is used much less in underdeveloped countries, where the need for it is potentially greater. Although it is possible to enrich rice with thiamin and other vitamins this is seldom done, and with the marked decline in the prevalence of beriberi the need for it is now much less. There is a strong case for enriching maize with nicotinamide in areas where pellagra is endemic; this is done in the USA but would be of much more benefit in southern Africa. As with rice the big problem is that much of the maize is grown by subsistence farmers. There is the possibility that addition of excess of a vitamin to a diet already unbalanced may uncover a deficiency of another nutrient. Enrichment policies should always be accompanied by general measures to improve the diet. Guidelines for those responsible for advising food manufacturers or governments have been prepared by the American Medical Association's Council on Food and Nutrition (1973).

WELFARE FOODS

The growing child needs protein, calcium and iron, and vitamins A and D in larger proportions than does the adult. Children and expectant and nursing women constitute a 'vulnerable group', particularly prone to develop nutritional disorders. Welfare foods and school meals are two established methods whereby the extra needs of this vulnerable group are met.

Old people also form a vulnerable group in which nutritional disorders are liable to occur. This is not because they have any extra need for nutrients but is due to the fact that for social and medical reasons they may be unable to obtain or prepare an adequate diet.

Since time immemorial religious people have felt themselves under obligation to help to feed the children of the poor. Such help has usually been sporadic and not always well directed to physiological needs. Historically the experiments carried out by Auden (1923) in Birmingham and by Corry Mann (1926) were of great importance in showing that even a comparatively good diet might not supply all the specific needs of growing children. Corry Mann carried out experiments on groups of boys in institutions near London. The basic diet was considered satisfactory at the time, though we now know that it was far from ideal; there was no evidence of any nutritional disorders among the boys. A group aged 7 to 11 years were given a supplementary ration of a pint (600 ml) of milk a day; these boys grew 0.8 in taller and 3.13 lb heavier in a year than a control group receiving no supplement of milk. Supplements of sugar, butter, watercress and other foods did not produce the same beneficial effects. In the opinion of the schoolmasters the milk improved the general alertness and vitality of the children. Similar experiments have now been carried out in many parts of the world and draw the attention of health authorites and the public to the special needs of children.

In 1940 when the food situation in Britain caused grave anxiety, an extensive system of Welfare Foods was introduced to protect the vulnerable group of women and children. In the next five years the health of children of all ages and of mothers improved markedly. Growth rates increased and mortality rates were decreased. This improvement occurred despite a marked decline in the standards of housing and the hazards of health associated with the evacuation of large numbers of children and the disruption of families. The wartime Welfare Food Services were a notable contribution to child health, but such an elaborate scheme could only be carried out in a well-disciplined country with an exceptional aptitude for administration.

Since the war, with the rise in prosperity, Welfare Food Services have been curtailed. The Cohen report (1957) recommended the discontinuation of Welfare orange juice after the age of 2 years, as the more varied diet after this age was considered to provide sufficient ascorbic acid. The provisions of the service were re-enacted in the Welfare Foods Order (1968). This described the beneficiaries (expectant and nursing mothers, children under 5 and handicapped children) and the welfare foods (liquid or dried milk, concentrated orange juice, cod-liver oil or vitamin tablets) to which each was entitled. Under the Welfare food order (1971) milk ceased to be available free for all expectant mothers and young children, but continues to be provided for needy families. Those on supplementary benefit qualify automatically, but families in which the father or mother is in full-time work can also qualify on financial grounds. They can also receive free a liquid preparation of vitamins A, D and C, known as vitamin drops. Vitamin preparations can be bought at special prices by families not entitled to a free supply.

Welfare Food Services have an especially important role in poor communities throughout the world where the vulnerable groups have a great need for extra protein and vitamins. International organisations, such as UNICEF and many voluntary organisations, have distributed large amounts of skimmed-milk powder—the surplus of the butter industry in North America, Australia and New Zealand—but this source of protein is only available in limited amounts. In some underdeveloped countries it is possible to increase the local production of milk and also facilities for processing it. FAO and UNICEF have helped governments greatly in these respects. In others, where pasture is extremely limited or the tsetse fly prohibits the existence of dairy herds, such an increase will be impossible for many years.

Mixtures of vegetable proteins can replace satisfactorily the animal protein in the diet of the young child. The production of suitable mixtures of vegetable proteins from plants which can be grown locally is essentially a problem of regional research.

SCHOOL MEALS

There are few, if any, countries which do not have some school meal services although, on account of the high cost of running them, many are but little more than demonstrations. Great Britain has a large and comprehensive system of school meals which, like many of our social services, has its roots in history. As in most European countries, our present centralised services are almost entirely financed by public money, but evolved out of small private charities. Thus in 1864 the Destitute Children's Dinner Society was founded and, five years later, had 58 dining-rooms open in London. Other charities, notably the London School Dinner Association, followed and spread to other big industrial cities. Elementary school teachers and others soon realised that the work of these charities was not sufficiently extensive to meet the needs of the great number of children in nineteenth-century Britain, who got too little food at home to derive full benefit from their education. The extent of malnutrition amongs the population, disclosed during the recruiting drives for the South African War, disturbed the social conscience and prepared public opinion for an Act of Parliament in 1906, which permitted local authorities to provide free meals for certain pupils from public funds. At first only destitute children received help, but the service gradually expanded (with many ups and downs) and by 1939 about a quarter of a million children were having midday meals at school.

The outbreak of war in 1939 saw a complete transformation of policy. It was realised that growing children needed foods rich in protein, minerals and vitamins above the normal ration of the adult community and increased employment of women in industry prevented many mothers from finding the time to prepare their children's meals. Bombing and the subsequent movements of population led to the establishment of canteens all over the country and especially in the schools. At the end of 1946, 2¼ million children in England and Wales were receiving school meals. After the war this policy did not change; the aim of the British Government was to provide a midday meal for every school child.

In 1976 in England and Wales 4.8 million children were eating school meals, 57 per cent of the number present. About 10 per cent of the children in school received them free of charge; for all the other children the charge is less than a comparable meal would cost even at home. The School Meals Service is the largest catering organisation in the country. The nutritional standards (Department of Education and Science, 1975) aim to provide one-third of the recommended daily energy and between a third and a half (42 per cent) of the recommended daily protein intake. The usual meal has two courses and children can ask for extra helpings. Regular amounts of meat and milk are included so that a child whose school lunch is the main meal of the day is well provided for. A survey in twelve London schools (Bender et al., 1977) showed that the average protein and energy content of the meals fell below the standards for all age groups. This was due to inadequate purchases of food, poor planning of menus and general problems of management. The response to a questionnaire indicated that 5 per cent of the children had poor diets. The proportion of children having no breakfast rose from 4 per cent in infant schools to 21 per cent in senior schools. How far any of these findings are representative of the country as a whole is unknown.

School meals should be more than a refueling exercise and are an opportunity for introducing healthy eating habits.

Similar arrangements now exist in many industrial countries. Norway was a pioneer in school meals with the 'Oslo breakfast'. School feeding in Norway is described by Eeg-Larsen (1969) and in Sweden by Skerfring (1969).

Arrangements in Eastern Europe are discussed by Tarján (1973) and the programme in Japan by Shimazono (1973). As in Britain the aim is to provide one-third of the daily energy need and three-eighths of the recommended daily protein intake. In the USA less than half the children in school are served a full meal. The White House Conference recommended that the National School Lunch Program should be further extended (Perryman, 1973).

School milk. Formerly every child in Britain got one-third of a pint (200 ml) of free milk at school. This was withdrawn from secondary schools in 1968 and from primary schools in 1971. A child may, however, still receive free milk at school if the school medical officer certifies that this is necessary for his health. This decision was taken by the government not because they considered that children do not need milk, but because in their opinion parents rather than the taxpayers should pay for it. Nutrition surveys in prosperous communities are difficult to interpret and it will be some time before it is possible to say whether the loss of the free milk has had a significant adverse effect on child-health. A report by the Department of Health and Social Security (1973) describes how the effects of changes in the Welfare Milk Scheme and the provision of school milk are being studied.

Even if there were no adverse effects, in our opinion free school milk is justified on educational grounds. A child needs a richer diet than does an adult and milk is the most effective means of enrichment and free school milk was incorporated as one of the fundamental preventive measures of our public health service. Its distribution provided a lesson which all could learn, including, it may be added, the teaching profession. Although in the past teachers have been in the forefront of advocating public health measures, the medical officer of health for Edinburgh in his 1971 report made a bitter complaint about lack of support from the education authorities for his programme of health education and he is not alone in this complaint. As the government's reason for stopping the free school milk was primarily one of cost, it may be pointed out that the £14 million of taxpayers' money which was saved could have been raised by a tax on sweets, which would probably lead to an improvement in children's teeth.

School meals in tropical countries. An elaborate school meals service is only possible in a country in which the people are prepared to pay to provide health services for children. In many countries school meal services often have to be cut to a much smaller pattern. A committee from the rice-eating countries of Asia (FAO, 1948) recommended the following type of free meal.

	oz	g
1. Cereals (cereals available, such as lightly milled rice, high extraction wheat, millets or other cereals)	2½	75
2. A pulse (e.g. peas or beans)	½	15
3. Small fish of which the whole body is eaten (such fish provide calcium)	¼	7
4. Vegetable (green leafy vegetables preferred)	1	30
5. Oil (preferably an oil containing carotene)	¼	7
6. Salt	⅙	5

The committee added: 'A meal of this kind will provide about 400 kcal (1.7 MJ) and will contain all the essential nutrients. It should be regarded as illustrating the general pattern of a cheap school meal, and may of course be modified in various ways in accordance with local conditions and the availability of various foods. For example, a greater amount of vegetables might be included, or fruits might be supplied as an alternative to vegetables. When facilities are not available for the distribution of full meals, specially prepared buns, cakes, *chapattis* made from flour, food yeast, and other ingredients such as powdered small fish may be found satisfactory,' Such meals provide a valuable supplement of protein, vitamins and minerals.

INDUSTRIAL CANTEENS

Those who perform heavy physical work must of necessity consume large amounts of foods of high energy value, Workers in heavy industry, if a choice is available, often prefer to take a proportion of this extra energy in the form of animal protein, although there is no evidence that this is a physiological necessity. In many industrial firms the managers have for long realised the importance of satisfactory midday meals to the working man's efficiency and have provided canteens and restaurants for their employees. On the outbreak of World War II and the introduction of rationing in Great Britain, what had previously been the policy of a few enlightened firms was made compulsory by law. In 1945 there were 18 900 industrial canteens of various types and these were serving 8 million meals a day.

Throughout the world, progressive firms are providing canteens for their workers. Reviews of the situation in European countries (FAO, 1965) and in tropical countries (Lloyd Davies, 1964) are available. The more enlightened managements realise the importance of providing their workmen with proper accommodation for meals and rest. In many firms the canteen is a real source of pride and great trouble is taken to make the meals attractive. Managements often subsidise canteens by bearing part of the wages of the catering staff, and the provision and replacement of equipment. In consequence, they usually provide meals which are cheaper than those served in commercial restaurants. In some countries the government itself runs popular restaurants, providing nutritious meals for workers at low prices. Special problems may arise in industry in the feeding of night-shift workers, adolescents and others.

ROLE OF GOVERNMENTS

HISTORICAL PERSPECTIVE

Food and Nutrition Strategies in National Development is the title of a United Nations report (FAO/WHO, 1976) that reflects discussions now common in ministries, universities and research institutes. The idea that governments have a responsibility for planning and distribution of food supplies, now widespread, only arose in the present century, although governments have always had an effect on food supplies through taxes on agriculture.

Land taxes were a main source of government revenue in many early civilisations. Tithe, a tax on agricultural production, was in use in Palestine and neighbouring countries in Biblical times. Jesus in castigating the Pharisees (St Matthew 23.23) said, 'Woe unto you...for ye pay tithe of mint and anise and cummin.' Tithe was a main source of income for the Christian Churches; it became part of ecclesiastical law in the sixth century and was made obligatory under secular law in the eighth century. The tax, a tenth part of all agricultural production, was paid either in cash or in crops or livestock. It remained a major tax for centuries, but was not taken to America by the early settlers.

When American wheat became a major source of the bread eaten by the growing populations of European industrial cities, this depressed the price of home-grown wheat. To protect farmers the British Government introduced in 1815 the Corn Law, a tax on imported wheat. The price of bread rose, causing much industrial unrest and contributing to malnutrition in the cities. The Corn Law was at the centre of British political argument until it was repealed in 1846. Governments, however, were not relieved of the responsibility for holding a balance between the interests of agriculturists and consumers. Today agricultural prices are the main cause of contention between member countries of the European Common Market, and the agricultural lobby is one of the most powerful pressure groups influencing US governments. In the nineteenth century and even today nutritional considerations have played only a small part in government bargaining with farmers.

Since the time of the Pharoahs, most governments have accepted responsibility for providing and distributing food to the people in times of famine and other disasters, but in normal times there has been no food strategy related to nutritional needs. The laws of economics set the limits on the food supply of each family. The relief of the poor and needy depended on charity, and in Europe mainly on the Church. In England under the Tudors the State began to accept some responsibility and a series of Poor Laws were enacted. These were aimed mainly at providing work for the indigent so that they could get money to buy food for their families.

Human rights

The conception that charity is not enough and that every individual has a right to receive food sufficient in both quantity and quality to maintain health has developed slowly and is not yet accepted everywhere. However, it was incorporated in the United Nations' *Universal Declaration of Human Rights,* issued in 1948, Article 25 of which reads:

1. Everyone has the right to a standard of living adequate for the health and well-being of himself and of his family, including food, clothing, housing and medical care and necessary services, and the right to security in the event of unemployment, sickness, disability, widowhood, old age or other lack of livelihood in circumstances beyond his control.
2. Motherhood and childhood are entitled to special care and assistance. All children, whether born in or out of wedlock, shall enjoy the same social protection.

Article 25 sets out in writing the ideas which are the basis of the work of the World Health Organisation (WHO). Like Magna Carta in 1215, the Virginia Declaration of Rights in 1771 and the Declaration of the Rights of Man and of the Citizen adopted in Paris in 1789, the Declaration of the United Nations is an expression of hope. Noble ideas are not easily converted into legal codes that are enforceable. Even slavery, now universally condemned, continues to exist.

Development of government interest in health and nutrition

Governments' interest in health was stimulated by the outbreaks of cholera in Europe and North America which first occurred in 1832 and continued for the next forty years. These led to the appointment by local authorities of medical officers of health, and the effective separation of the systems for water supply and sewage disposal. The work of Pasteur (1822–95) and Koch (1843–1910) led to the discovery of the bacterial origin of tuberculosis and many other infectious diseases. The problems of preventing the spread of these infections became the main preoccupation of health authorities and diverted attention from the problems of malnutrition. The discovery of vitamins and the general recognition of the importance of the quality of the foods in the diet followed a generation later.

The first of many International Sanitary Conferences was held in Paris in 1851 and was concerned mainly with cholera. There was no international establishment of health workers until 1907, when the Office International d'Hygiène Publique was set up. This was followed in 1921 by the establishment of the Health Committee of the League of Nations with a small full-time staff. The organisation became actively interested in nutrition, and a report on the physiological bases of nutrition (League of Nations, 1935) was a landmark in stimulating the interests of national governments in nutrition.

A member of the staff of the health division of the League of Nations and a main author of their nutrition report, Dr W. R. Aykroyd, was appointed Director of the Nutrition Laboratory of the Government of India in 1935; at the same time a distinguished agriculturalist, the Marquess of Linlithgow, was appointed Viceroy. There were high hopes of a 'marriage between Health and Agriculture', but the marriage did not take place; the agricultural partner's interest and energy were diverted by the political problems arising from nationalists fighting for independence. But nutritionists in India were the first to collect systematically the data necessary for a national food strategy. They continue to do so, but their effect on agriculture is still piecemeal and uncoordinated.

In 1943 the National Research Council of the USA published a report on Recommended Dietary Allowances, now in its ninth edition. The report dealt with vitamins and minerals quantitatively, whereas the League of Nations' report had been able to give only general qualitative statements about protective foods. The US report was intended 'as a measure in planning diets and food supplies.' At once it had, and continues to have, a great influence in the USA and also in other countries. Much legislation providing nutritional support for vulnerable groups is based on it. Its effect on agriculture has been small. Food production in North America continues to be determined more by the interests of 'agribusiness'(p. 482) rather than by nutritional considerations.

Two success stories
Nutrition planning has had two outstanding successes, both in emergency situations. The first was the feeding of the people of Britain during World War II, and the second the prevention of famine arising in Europe after the end of World War II by the United Nations Relief and Rehabilitation Administration (UNRAA).

Feeding Britain in World War II
Mortality and morbidity statistics and the records of the growth and development of children indicate that the health and nutrition of the people of Britain improved between 1939 and 1945. Yet during this period of war much of the necessary imports of food from North America was sunk by German submarines in the continuous battle of the Atlantic; large numbers of the population of the industrial cities were evacuated from their homes as a result of air raids; the civilian health services were depleted by doctors, nurses and others who joined the armed services.

That the food supply of the people was maintained and its nutritive value improved was due to the setting up of a Ministry of Food at the start of hostilities in September 1939. The country was fortunate in that the Minister, Lord Woolton, an industrialist, and his chief scientific adviser, Sir Jack Drummond, a former professor of biochemistry,

were two men of exceptional ability who served throughout the war. Churchill was also fully aware of the importance of nutrition, as is shown by his statement in a speech in 1943 in the House of Commons: 'There is no finer investment for any community than putting milk into babies.' The Ministry of Food was responsible for an elaborate scheme of rationing and also for a great expansion of the welfare food services for mothers and children, of school meals and of community feeding in industrial and other canteens, as already described in this chapter. Administrative action was also taken to improve the quality of bread and flour (p. 170) and to fortify margarine with vitamins A and D. The food supply was maintained by the planning of agriculture and the control of imports; the administrative means by which this was done are admirably described in a small book by Fenelon (1952).

Many of these measures, especially the rationing, called for marked changes in food habits and were therefore unpopular. They succeeded because the people realised that they were fair and had the discipline and administrative ability needed for their enforcement.

UNRRA
The United Nations Relief and Rehabilitation Administration was set up when the tide of World War II began to turn against the Axis Powers. Plans for bringing immediate relief to the invaded countries awaiting liberation were drawn up by representatives of 44 nations, who met in the White House, at the invitation of President Roosevelt. The countries that had not been invaded agreed to contribute 2 per cent of their annual income to the resources of UNRRA. The largest contributions were from the USA, £675 million; Britain, £155 million; and Canada, £35 million. With these vast resources—three times more than was spent on relief after the first world war—UNRRA poured supplies into Albania, Austria, Byelorussia, China, Czechoslovakia, Italy, Greece, Poland, the Ukraine and Yugoslavia. Limited aid was also given to seven other countries. Beginning in March 1945, 25 million tons of goods costing £750 million were shipped overseas by UNRRA in more than 6000 ships. The goods included locomotives, trucks and freight cars, more than 300000 farm animals, thousands of tractors and ploughs and many tons of seed grains, all necessary for restarting agriculture in devastated areas; in addition, UNRRA provided fully equipped hospitals, and much-needed medical supplies and personnel. But agriculture could not be set on its feet overnight and the people had to be fed; the most vital part of UNRRA's work was therefore the provision of food; the foodstuffs were of every kind including hundreds of tons of dried milk for children, and vast quantities of cereals. In all, UNRRA shipped enough grain to make about 12000 million 1 lb loaves, enough to give five such loaves to every man woman and child in the world. The result was that at least three famines were prevented and untold misery,

hardship and underfeeding among many millions of people were alleviated. It was a condition of UNRRA aid that the supplies sent in should be distributed without regard to politics, race or religion. It is a pleasure to recall that these conditions were effectively observed.

UNRRA was wound up when its immediate task was done, but its story is a reminder of what effective international cooperation can do.

The position today

All countries have laws and regulations which affect nutrition. In Britain, the USA and other countries with large government departments, ministries of health, agriculture, industry, education and others each pass legislation that affects nutrition, but there is no overall policy. Only a few countries now have a ministry of food and, where there is one, it is usually of limited influence and the minister is low down in the pecking order of his government colleagues. Many countries now have tables of recommended allowances or intakes of nutrients (p. 152) which are officially recognised and these are used in drafting regulations, e.g. for school meals and the enrichment of foods. Departments of health and medical organisations lay down guidelines for the diet of the general population (p. 163) and these are aimed mainly at reducing the incidence of coronary heart disease. They influence government departments, but except in Norway (see below) are not a formal basis for a national food and nutrition policy.

The United Kingdom

After World War II the Ministry of Food was merged with the Ministry of Agriculture. Successive ministers have had an impossible task in representing the legitimate interests of both farmers and consumers, inevitably often at variance. There is an alliance between the Ministry of Agriculture and the nutrition division of the Department of Health which, although always amicable, is uneasy, wasteful of time and has not led to an overall policy. A good case can be made out for a separate Ministry of Food and Nutrition that could give coherence to planning and legislation, but it is unlikely that one will be created. There is no popular demand and it would increase bureaucracy in a country where there is already an excess of central government. In its absence there is a need for a small body of men and women with wisdom and the knowledge of nutrition to provide policies for ensuring that our food supply is adequate, of good quality and obtainable by all sections of the population. The case for a food policy has been well put by Whitehead (1978) in a lecture to the Royal Society for the Encouragement of Arts.

The United States

In the USA there is much more popular concern with food and nutrition than in Britain. A large White House Con-

ference on Food, Nutrition and Health was assembled in 1969 and its deliberations have been summarised and published (Mayer, 1973). They are set out under four headings: (1) improving the nutrition of those most vulnerable to hunger and malnutrition, (2) monitoring the wholesomeness and nutritional value of our foods, (3) improving education concerning nutrition and (4) improving large-scale programmes and agencies. The conference led to the appointment of a Senate Select Committee of Nutrition and Human Needs. Their report, *Dietary Goals for the United States*, was issued in 1977. Known as the McGovern report, after the prestigious chairman of the committee, it provoked widespread comment, both favourable and unfavourable. Those who liked the report attempted to get the goals established as national nutrition policy, but the Senate did not concur. The McGovern committee was disbanded in December 1977 and has not been replaced.

The McGovern report was reproduced in full in *Nutrition Today* together with lengthy comments from twenty leading authorities on health and nutrition (*Nutrition Today* 1977, volume 12, parts 5 and 6). Criticisms are also summarised by Harper (1978). Its main recommendations are given on page 532. While large parts of the report received general approval, the recommendations to reduce cholesterol consumption to 300 mg a day and a salt consumption to 3 g a day were criticised as impractical and insufficiently supported by scientific evidence. Such recommendations may provide good advice for patients with various types of heart disease, but were unacceptable for the whole population because they appeared unnecessarily restrictive. It is unfortunate that misplaced enthusiasms made the McGovern report, with its many excellent recommendations, not generally acceptable, which leaves the USA still without an official statement of its food policies.

Norway

Norway has a smaller population than the USA and the UK and so has fewer nutrition 'experts'. This may be the explanation of why the Norwegian Government has been the first to set out a national food and nutrition policy (Ministry of Agriculture, Government of Norway, 1975). This appears as a model for other governments to study and an outline of the report prepared by Rigen (1977) is given.

The proposal has four major goals:

1. To stimulate the consumption of healthy foodstuffs;
2. To develop guidelines for food production in accordance with the recommendation of the World Food Council;
3. To increase domestic independence from the importation of food supplies by encouraging increases in the production and consumption of domestic foodstuffs that both satisfy health requirements in terms of nutritional value and agricultural requirements in terms of the specific natural conditions delimiting the potential for food production;

4. In response to the general economic aim of strengthening outlying districts, agricultural production is to be promoted in districts and regions with otherwise poor industrial bases.

The more specific objectives of the Government's policy are:

1. To maintain the existing advantageous nutritional aspects of current agricultural production and patterns of consumption. It is recognised that taste cannot be altered significantly through policy, and it is also recognised that variations in consumption patterns differ both regionally and with regard to different population groups. It is the aim of the policy to work within the limitations imposed by those differences;
2. To improve the nutritional quality of the overall national diet, it is the aim to reduce the overall intake of fats as a source of energy. The reduction in fats should eventually be to about 35 per cent of the total diet;
3. To substitute for the decline in fat consumption, it is the aim to increase the intake of foodstuffs with heavy concentrations of starches, especially grains and potatoes. Sugar as a source of energy ought to be reduced.
4. In terms of total fat consumption it is the aim to increase the proportion of polyunsaturated fats and decrease the proportion of saturated fats.

United Nations

Adequate food is on the United Nations list of human rights for everyone (p. 486) and its **Food and Agricultural Organisation** (FAO) was one of the first of UN special agencies and set up in 1945 on the following premises.

The world has never had enough to eat. At least two-thirds of its people are ill-nourished in spite of the fact that two-thirds of the world's people are farmers.

The modern science of production shows that it is entirely possible to produce enough of the right kinds of foods.

The modern science of nutrition proves beyond doubt that if all people could get enough of the right kinds of foods, the average level of health and well-being could be raised much higher than it is now.

But production alone is not enough. Foods must be so distributed that the levels of consumption of those who do not have enough are progressively raised.

This implies an expanding world economy, in which each nation will play its own part, but all will act together. FAO owes much to the first Director-General, Lord Boyd Orr, who brought to his office the traditions of an Aberdeen farmer and the experience of a lifetime of work in medical and agricultural research, these being mixed and leavened by a spirit and eloquence characteristic of an ancient Hebrew prophet.

In the early days of FAO many people, including the Director-General, hoped that the organisation would become an effective executive agency; they wanted FAO to acquire the surplus food from the crops of the richer agricultural countries and to distribute these, as need arose, amongst countries afflicted with grave food deficiencies or famine. However, under its original constitution such power was not given. FAO could not order the adoption of particular policies nor embark on 'the executive functions of purchase and procurement in order to stimulate output and equalise distribution.' It can only recommend, demonstrate and discuss, and in all countries its work has to be channelled through the ministries of national government.

The **World Health Organisation** (WHO) was established in 1948 and its nutrition division cooperates closely with FAO. A joint FAO/WHO Expert Committee on nutrition first met in 1949 and has now produced nine reports. These lay down the broad policy of both organisations; they recommend and encourage work on assessment of nutritional status, standards of requirements for nutrients, protein-energy malnutrition, nutritional anaemia, endemic goitre, xerophthalmia, food technology and toxicology.

Any reader of this book who looks at the list of references will see how much we owe to FAO and WHO. The bringing together of experts of repute and the preparation of international reports does much to facilitate the use of new knowledge.

The nutrition divisions of FAO and WHO, whose headquarters are in Rome and Geneva respectively, have established reputations as educationalists. Besides producing technical reports, they arrange conferences in many countries and have selected and financed many hundreds of men and women from underdeveloped countries for fellowships that enable them to study for long periods abroad. They have also sent almost as many consultants to aid national nutrition programmes in many countries. Many of the consultants and fellows, after their return home, have been able to influence governments to initiate and carry out nutrition programmes. Thanks largely to FAO and WHO there are now throughout the underdeveloped parts of the world a large number of people with a sound professional knowledge of nutrition.

The work of FAO and WHO has been, and continues to be, assisted by the United Nations Children's Fund (UNICEF), which was set up in 1947 when UNRRA had completed its immediate tasks (p. 487) and closed down. UNICEF aids governments to provide essential needs for children. Food, medicines, trained children's nurses, diapers, shoes, etc. have been made available in many parts of the world. At first the greater portion of the resources of the Fund was devoted to the provision of children's meals. For long periods, some four million children were receiving each day a meal partly provided by UNICEF. This effective organisation of material aid of every sort for needy children and their mothers led the UN to establish it on a more permanent basis. UNICEF remains a nontechnical organisation and works in conjunction with FAO, WHO and other UN agencies, including the Bureau of Social Affairs and the Educational Scientific and

Cultural Organisation (UNESCO). Many joint projects for the control of diseases such as malaria, tuberculosis and yaws have been successfully carried out. UNICEF continues to undertake the purchase and free distribution of milk powder to needy children and others throughout the world and cooperates with FAO in the development of milk-processing plants and dairies. Any UNICEF contribution to a country has to be matched in value by a contribution from the government of the assisted country.

FAO and WHO can only improve food production and distribution indirectly by influencing national governments. They cannot do things themselves, but they can suggest what needs to be done. In all countries where malnutrition is common this needs money which the government has not got. Financial aid is available from the World Bank, the United Nations Development Programme (UNDP), the International Fund for Agricultural Development (IFAD), national overseas funds and private foundations. A World Food Council, which meets periodically, after a session in Manila issued a communiqué setting out how available money could be used to eradicate malnutrition (FAO, 1977). The communiqué estimates that to achieve and maintain an annual 4 per cent rate of growth of food production in developing countries requires 8.3 thousand million dollars of international aid annually. This 'minimum package of inputs' should be used to supply 'fertilisers, pesticides, high-yield varieties of seeds which are pest- and disease-resistant, improved breeds of livestock, credit to small farmers, irrigation equipment and selective and appropriate implements for mechanisation'.

This appears to assume that the techniques which have revolutionised agriculture in Europe and North America in the last thirty years can be exported to peasant farmers in Africa, Asia and Latin America, provided sufficient money is made available. There are critics who doubt this assumption. They point out that much of the money that has already been given for agriculture development has benefited mainly importers, merchants, landowners and corrupt government officials, and that too little has gone to benefit peasant farmers. It is also claimed that the existence of international aid on a large scale stifles local enterprise and initiative.

An analogous situation exists in medicine. There are few large cities in the developing countries which do not have a modern hospital with a competent staff, trained abroad, and adequate equipment, provided by international aid. Yet in these countries most of the people live in villages with no safe water supply and almost no access to trained health workers and essential drugs. WHO has now begun to direct its resources in underdeveloped countries to primary health care in the villages. This policy is set out in an article entitled 'Blueprint for Health for All' (Mahler 1977). This includes the passage:

Malnutrition is probably the single most important health problem in developing countries. The national and international health sectors must now come to grips with their responsibilities in nutrition, identify their proper political strategies, define realistic policies and strategies, generate appropriate techologies, and formulate applicable programmes. If we do not succeed in making effective and realistic nutritional activities a cornerstone of primary health care, we are hardly worth our salt as health managers. Once more we seem to have the knowledge but neither the political will nor the social imagination to apply it.

Mahler, the present Director-General of WHO, like Boyd Orr, has flair and enthusiasm. We hope that his enthusiasm will be infectious and spread ideas for food and nutrition policies and strategies throughout the world, in rich and poor countries alike. In this way a true marriage of nutrition and agriculture will be possible. Agribusiness does not even flirt with nutrition.

DECISION-MAKING

The prelude to action in a national food programme is the definition of remedial possibilities and their arrangement in order of importance and feasibility. This requires not only knowledge but wisdom and judgment. Decisions have to be made and they are not easy. The United Nations agencies FAO, WHO and UNICEF can help with gathering of facts and opinions and can give advice, but the decisions have to be taken and implemented by national governments. Often a programme requires outside help and wealthier countries have to decide what they can offer to a less prosperous one.

Cost benefit analysis

The government of a developing nation with a problem of malnutrition and an estimated £x million to devote to its correction needs a method of comparing the costs of different courses of action, such as food subsidies, food enrichment, meals supplied to vulnerable groups, in relation to expected benefit or value to the community. How does it determine the cost and value of such courses of action and compare them with other public health measures such as better housing, sanitation and hygiene? Public health and nutrition authorities have recently started to adapt the methods of economists. The technique consists in putting a monetary value to every benefit or utility.

Such an assessment is open to criticism of its accuracy but an attempt does open the way to discussion and is likely, after revision, to yield figures which are at least as accurate as intelligent guesswork, and more easily compared with monetary expenditure (Kiker, 1971). Extremes of opinion are clearly brought out and range from 'impossible' and even 'immoral' to 'possible' and 'desirable'.

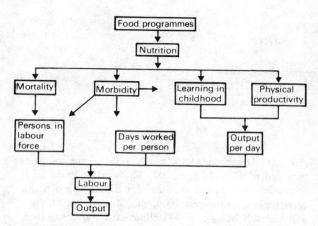

Fig. 56.1 Food programmes as an investment. The outputs to which improvements in nutrition should aim should be appropriate and not necessarily an increase in national income. The effect on education may give numerous benefits and that on morbidity and morality in early childhood may lead to a fall in the birth rate.

Figure 56.1 shows a planner's view of a food programme as an investment. It comes from an international conference on Nutrition, National Development and Planning (Berg *et al.*, 1973), which we recommend to those who wish to read more about the techniques of nutrition planning and programming. It seems likely that they are going to have much more influence on preventive nutrition in the near future. At the same time we can anticipate new problems. Examples have occurred in recent years in which economic development has been accompanied by a deterioration in nutrition. This can happen when subsistence farmers, eating a mixed diet that they grow themselves, change to a cash crop which takes up most of their land and labour (Vahlquist, 1972). Weighting of alternative plans depends on uncertain data so that in places either

no values can be put into the equations or subjective estimates must be used. It has been said that the planning process is like the love-making of elephants. It takes a year to learn the technique, the event can be painful and hazardous and one has to wait 18 months for the result. If planners become too obsessed in searching for the perfect model plan, action is delayed, and in one of the large development agencies the lengthy and cumbersome planning procedures prompted one food programmer to retort, 'let them eat plans!'

Benefits which follow the use of improvements in methods of food production have to be set off against the risk of adverse effects. Thus pesticides, herbicides and fertilisers improve the yield of crops but are potential toxic hazards. In animal husbandry, antibiotics and oestrogens promote growth but have other biological effects which are adverse. In food technology, the use of food additives is essential, but many are potentially dangerous. Suitable yardsticks are becoming available to measure the ratio of benefit to risk.

Politics in decision-making
Most of the decisions which have to be made by governments in the field of nutrition involve financial benefit or loss to sections of the community. Farmers' lobbies want subsidies and higher prices; consumers want cheaper and better food. Industrial lobbies press for additives in food products; the public fear the word additive. The choice is usually determined by those politicians who have the loudest or biggest lobby. In our fallible world this kind of judgment (or misjudgment) will continue to be a feature of all systems of government. Enlightened decisions on programmes for health and nutrition require an educated people and just, forward-looking leaders. The 'keys to the solutions of problems' of health and nutrition throughout the world lie in education.

57. The Population Problem

Every second of the day and night—somewhere in the world—four babies are born. Every 24 hours there are 20 000 more births than deaths (FAO, 1974).

HISTORICAL PERSPECTIVES

Malthus

In 1798 Malthus published his famous *Essay on the Principles of Population as it Affects the Future Improvements of Society with Remarks on the Speculation of Mr Godwin, Mr Condorcet and other Writers.* Mr Godwin achieved some fame as the father-in-law of the poet Shelley, over whom he had considerable influence. At the end of the eighteenth century Godwin had seen the results of the great improvements that had recently taken place in British agriculture and had a prophetic glimpse of the possibilities for wealth that the Industrial Revolution was to bring forth. He considered that with these material aids the perfecting of human society was a practical proposition. Malthus' father, a Surrey squire, was a disciple of Godwin and the essay on the principles of population is perhaps a reaction against excessive paternal optimism. The main argument is that any temporary or local improvement in human living conditions will increase a population faster than corresponding agricultural developments can increase the food supply. Hunger and starvation with their associated war and pestilence will then automatically set back the advance and check the population growth: these disasters are inescapable features of human society, which by its very nature can never be stable. Such, in brief, is the Malthusian dilemma. It is today a major problem in most countries and has a large literature. Monographs by Ehrlich (1971) and Loraine (1972) with the appropriate titles *The Population Bomb* and *The Death of Tomorrow* are recommended.

Death, births and population growth

Table 57.1 gives population data for the world in 1978. It was drawn up by the Population Reference Bureau, Inc., 1337 Connecticut Avenue NW, Washington DC, USA. The data come from national statistics, and their accuracy depends on the reliability of the census and of the notification of births and deaths in the various countries. For countries in Europe, North America and Oceania the order of accuracy is high, but the figures for most countries in Africa and for many in Asia are little more than intelligent guesses. China and India contain about two-fifths of the inhabitants of the world.

In some countries birth rates still lie between 40 and 50 per 1000. Death rates vary widely, but in some countries have fallen below 10 per 1000. The world population is increasing by 70 million a year and in the absence of major catastrophes, by the year 2000, only 20 years ahead, there will probably be up to 3000 million extra mouths to feed.

It has been pointed out in Chapter 55 that agricultural expansion in many countries is barely keeping pace with the present growth of population. If the above forecast is accepted, the agricultural problem becomes extremely serious. To what extent is it possible to control the numbers of the world population by active social and health policies? To what limits can agricultural production be increased? Before attempting to answer these very important questions, it is necessary to consider briefly some of the factors affecting death rates and birth rates.

Populations with high death rates and high birth rates

For about a thousand years—from the beginning of the Middle Ages to the middle of the eighteenth century—the population of Europe probably remained more or less constant. There is also no evidence of any important permanent changes in the number of inhabitants of Asia during this period. This stability existed because birth rates in all countries were probably over 40 per 1000 of the population yearly. This rate of reproduction probably represents the maximum of which the human species is capable. Yet it was only just sufficient to make up the losses due to war, famine and disease. For the biological survival of man, it was necessary that every adult woman should be as fertile as possible. The organisation of society in all countries, both in the East and in the West, was such as to encourage fertility. In this, all the great religions of the world, Confucianism, Hinduism, Judaism, Christianity and Mohammedanism, have co-operated. An early marriage and a large family was the avowed aim for every girl. Those who achieved this aim received both social and religious approval. The infertile woman was an object of scorn and derision. This attitude to women was all but universal until 200 years ago. Under the circumstances it was sensible—indeed essential—if mankind was to survive. However, now under very different circumstances, it still persists to some extent in all countries and in many it wrongly remains the dominant concept of woman's role in society.

Fall of death rates in Europe in the eighteenth century

In the middle of the eighteenth century the death rate in most European countries began to fall and has for the most part fallen steadily ever since. The reasons for the start of this fall are uncertain. Popular opinion, and even eminent historians such as Trevelyan (1942), often ascribed it to the benefits of the new medical science. In fact therapeutics only advanced sufficiently to have a significant effect on death rates within the last 50 years. Indeed it is only in the last three decades, with the widespread use of antibiotics and insecticides, that medical science has seriously affected demographic processes and so caused renewed interest in the Malthusian dilemma. The fall in death rates in Europe in the eighteenth century can be attributed in part to the spread of religious toleration. Toleration put an end to the lethal civil wars of religions in the previous centuries. Then law and order could be more easily maintained and so roads and communications opened up. In addition, new improved agricultural methods and the introduction of the potato from America markedly reduced the effects of bad agricultural seasons and virtually abolished European famines which had hitherto caused heavy losses of life in most countries (Salaman, 1948). Further, both bubonic plague and smallpox, which caused so many deaths in the sixteenth and seventeenth centuries, declined in Europe and were no longer such important factors in the population equilibrium. The effect of a natural decline in the virulence of smallpox was increased by the discovery of vaccination by Jenner.

Fall of death rates in Asia and Africa

In Asia a similar fall began in the middle of the nineteenth century, often following a period of colonial rule. Law and order gradually replaced civil war; there were enormous increases in transport facilities and by the end of the nineteenth century famine, plague, smallpox and cholera were in large measure controlled. These factors all operated most markedly in the countries which became subjugated to European or Japanese metropolitan powers. Whatever the demerits of colonialism, it was always associated with a fall in the death rate and a rise in the numbers of the colonial peoples.

In most underdeveloped countries, including Africa, death rates fell slowly during the first half of this century but a dramatic drop in many countries first occurred after World War II (United Nations, 1954), brought about by the increased economic prosperity, and the widespread use of insecticides and antibiotics.

POPULATION PROBLEMS 1980–2000

In nearly all countries of the world, birth rate exceeds death rate and the population is expanding. In many poor and underdeveloped countries, already overpopulated, agricultural production is barely increasing sufficiently to keep pace with the growth of population. Low standards of nutrition are likely to fall lower, unless radical changes occur soon. Disastrous famines and the accompanying chaos appear probable. More food and fewer new mouths are equally urgent problems.

The population is also increasing in the rich and prosperous countries, in some of which the birth rates are double the death rates. In the United States the number of women of child-bearing age was 32 million in 1940; it rose slowly to 34 million in 1950 and 43 million in 1970. It will be 54 million in 1980. The girls are here now and their potential fertility could raise the population of the United States to 420 million by 2065. A feature of the population increase in all prosperous countries, which is consequent upon the fall in the death rate, is the greater number of old people. This is very marked in the United Kingdom. Whereas in 1941 men over 65 and women over 60 formed just over one-tenth of the population, by 1975 they were about one-fifth. In North America and most European countries the population increases have been more than met by increased food production. Prosperous countries with an agriculture based on modern science are sometimes faced with difficult economic and social problems caused by agricultural surpluses. There are, however, other problems caused by the increasing number of people—the provision of houses, schools, hospitals and medical services, traffic facilities and opportunities for recreation.

The increase in the population in both rich and poor countries alike is not due to an increase in human fertility and only occasionally is it associated with a rise in the birth rate. It is always caused almost entirely by a decrease in the death rate. In recent years this has resulted from advances in medical and ancillary sciences and in the medical and social services which make this new knowledge available. Since medical science is largely responsible for creating the problems of overpopulation, it should assume responsibility for solving them. This it could do if it were not for the fact that modern methods of family planning and contraception are not generally or easily applicable in underdeveloped countries. Even in prosperous countries such as the United States and the United Kingdom, birth control has only recently become part of the 'establishment' and formerly received little support either from goverment or organised medical bodies. However, times are changing. The year 1974 was noteworthy for being nominated World Population Year by the UN and for the holding of a World Population Conference in Bucharest. In the UK it saw provision made for family planning within the National Health Service and the appointment of a Minister of Population Affairs.

Attitudes only change slowly. In Western medicine, the treatment of an individual patient continues to attract more prestige and money than has attention to the health of the population as a whole. The control of the birth rate

Table 57.1 World population 1978 (from Data Sheet of the Population Reference Bureau, Washington DC, USA).

Region or country	Population estimate mid-1978 (millions)	Birth rate	Death rate	Rate of natural increase (annual, %)	Number of years to double population	Population projection to 2000 (millions)	Infant mortality rate	Population under 15 years (%)	Population over 64 years (%)	Life expectancy at birth (years)	Urban population (%)	Projected labour force increase 1978–2000 (millions)	Per capita gross national product (US$)
WORLD	4219	29	12	1.7	41	6233	99	36	6	60	39	811	1650
AFRICA	436	46	19	2.7	26	813	147	44	3	46	25	121	440
NORTHERN AFRICA	103	43	14	2.9	24	184	128	44	3	52	40	25	650
Algeria	18.4	48	14	3.4	20	36.4	145	48	3	53	52	4.7	990
Egypt	39.6	38	12	2.5	28	63.5	108	41	3	53	44	7.4	280
Libya	2.8	48	9	3.9	18	5.3	130	49	3	53	30	0.6	6310
Morocco	18.9	45	14	3.1	22	35.4	133	46	4	53	38	5.3	540
Sudan	17.1	48	16	3.1	22	33.3	141	45	2	49	20	5.8	290
Tunisia	6.0	36	13	2.3	30	10.5	135	45	4	55	50	1.3	840
WESTERN AFRICA	128	49	22	2.7	26	243	158	45	3	42	19	36	350
Benin	3.4	49	22	2.7	26	6.0	149	46	4	41	14	1.1	130
Cape Verde	0.3	28	9	1.8	38	0.4	105	48	5	50	8	*	260
Gambia	0.6	43	23	2.0	35	0.9	165	41	2	40	16	0.1	180
Ghana	10.9	49	20	2.9	24	21.4	115	47	4	49	31	3.5	580
Guinea	4.8	46	21	2.5	28	8.4	175	43	3	41	20	1.3	150
Guinea-Bissau	0.6	41	24	1.7	41	0.8	208	37	4	39	23	0.1	140
Ivory Coast	7.2	45	19	2.6	27	13.2	154	43	3	44	20	1.7	610
Liberia	1.7	50	21	2.9	24	3.0	159	42	3	45	28	0.4	450
Mali	6.3	50	25	2.5	28	11.5	188	49	2	38	13	2.2	100
Mauritania	1.5	45	24	2.1	33	2.6	187	42	6	39	23	0.2	340
Niger	5.0	52	24	2.7	26	9.6	200	43	3	39	9	1.3	160
Nigeria	68.4	49	21	2.8	25	134.8	157	45	2	41	18	19.4	380
Senegal	5.4	47	23	2.4	29	9.2	159	43	3	40	32	1.1	390
Sierra Leone	3.3	44	19	2.5	28	5.8	136	43	3	44	15	0.7	200
Togo	2.4	50	22	2.8	25	4.5	163	46	3	41	15	0.7	260
Upper Volta	6.5	48	25	2.3	30	11.1	182	43	3	38	4	2.0	110
EASTERN AFRICA	124	47	20	2.7	26	238	146	45	3	45	12	39	210
Burundi	4.0	48	22	2.5	28	7.2	150	44	2	42	2	1.2	120
Comoros	0.3	45	20	2.5	28	0.5	160	43	3	46	10	0.1	180
Djibouti	0.1	48	24	2.4	29	0.2	—	—	—	70	*	1940	
Ethiopia	30.2	49	25	2.4	29	53.9	162	44	3	42	12	8.0	100
Kenya	14.8	48	15	3.3	21	31.3	119	46	3	50	10	5.0	240
Madagascar	8.0	47	22	2.5	28	16.3	102	45	3	44	16	3.5	200

Malawi	5.4	50	26	2.4	29	9.8	142	45	3	43	10	1.5	140
Mauritius	0.9	26	8	1.8	38	1.2	40	38	4	63	44	0.2	680
Mozambique	9.9	42	19	2.3	30	17.7	140	43	3	44	6	2.1	170
Reunion	0.5	28	7	2.1	33	0.7	44	43	4	63	51	0.1	1920
Rhodesia (Zimbabwe)	7.0	48	13	3.5	20	15.2	122	48	2	52	19	2.2	550
Rwanda	4.5	51	22	2.8	25	8.6	133	44	3	41	4	2.0	110
Seychelles	0.1	28	8	2.0	35	0.1	35	43	6	65	26	*	580
Somalia	3.4	48	21	2.7	26	6.5	177	45	2	41	28	0.9	110
Tanzania, United Rep. of	16.5	47	22	2.5	28	33.1	167	47	2	44	7	5.7	180
Uganda	12.7	45	15	3.0	23	24.8	160	44	3	50	7	4.1	240
Zambia	5.5	50	19	3.1	22	11.5	159	46	3	44	36	1.7	440
MIDDLE AFRICA	50	44	20	2.4	29	90	164	43	3	42	27	12	230
Angola	6.4	47	23	2.4	29	11.7	203	42	3	38	18	1.3	330
Cameroon, United Rep. of	8.0	41	21	2.0	35	13.7	137	40	3	41	29	1.5	290
Central African Empire	1.9	43	21	2.2	32	3.4	190	42	3	41	36	0.6	230
Chad	4.3	44	23	2.1	33	6.9	160	40	3	38	14	0.8	120
Congo, People's Rep. of	1.5	45	19	2.6	27	2.8	180	42	3	44	40	0.4	520
Equatorial Guinea	0.3	36	18	1.7	41	0.5	165	37	3	44	45	0.1	330
Gabon	0.5	29	21	0.8	87	0.7	178	32	3	41	32	*	2590
Sao Tome and Principe	0.1	40	13	2.7	26	0.1	75	—	—	53	16	*	490
Zaire	26.7	45	18	2.7	26	49.9	160	44	3	44	29	7.1	140
SOUTHERN AFRICA	31	41	16	2.5	28	57	119	42	4	52	44	10	1240
Botswana	0.7	47	21	2.6	27	1.4	97	48	6	56	12	0.3	410
Lesotho	1.3	40	18	2.1	33	2.1	114	46	4	46	3	0.3	170
Namibia	1.0	45	16	2.9	24	1.9	177	41	4	49	32	0.2	980
South Africa	27.5	40	15	2.5	28	51.0	117	41	4	52	48	8.5	1340
Swaziland	0.5	49	20	2.9	24	1.0	168	48	3	44	8	0.2	470
ASIA	2433	30	12	1.9	36	3656	105	38	4	58	26	509	610
SOUTHWEST ASIA	92	40	13	2.7	26	166	117	43	4	55	45	25	1730
Bahrain	0.3	43	8	3.5	20	0.6	78	44	3	63	78	—	2410
Cyprus	0.6	20	10	1.0	69	0.8	27	28	10	71	42	0.1	1480
Gaza	0.4	49	16	3.3	21	0.9	—	53	5	52	87	—	—
Iraq	12.2	48	14	3.4	20	24.2	104	48	5	53	65	3.1	1390
Israel	3.7	28	7	2.1	33	5,6	20	33	8	73	86	0.9	3920
Jordan	2.9	48	13	3.4	20	5,8	97	48	2	53	42	0.7	610
Kuwait	1.1	43	5	3.9	18	2.8	44	44	2	69	56	0.4	15480
Lebanon	2.9	40	9	3.1	22	5.6	59	41	5	64	60	0.9	—
Oman	0.8	49	18	3.2	22	1.6	138	—	—	—	5	—	2680
Qatar	0.1	44	14	3.0	23	0.2	138	—	—	—	69	*	11400
Saudi Arabia	7.8	49	19	3.0	23	14.9	152	45	3	45	21	2.1	4480
Syria	8.1	45	14	3.1	22	16.0	114	48	3	57	47	2.1	780
Turkey	42.2	34	11	2.3	30	71.1	119	40	4	57	45	12.3	990
United Arab Emirates	0.8	44	14	3.0	23	1.6	138	40	—	—	52	*	13990
Yemen	5.8	49	19	3.0	23	10.9	155	45	3	45	9	1.7	250
Yemen, Democratic	1.9	49	19	3.0	23	3.5	155	48	4	45	33	0.4	280
MIDDLE SOUTH ASIA	879	37	15	2.2	32	1459	133	41	3	49	21	222	220
Afghanistan	17.8	48	22	2.6	27	31.2	190	44	3	40	15	5.4	160
Bangladesh	85.0	47	20	2.7	26	153.5	153	43	3	46	9	22.8	110

Table 57.1—*continued*

Region or country	Population estimate mid-1978 (millions)	Birth rate	Death rate	Rate of natural increase (annual, %)	Number of years to double population	Population projection to 2000 (millions)	Infant mortality rate	Population under 15 years (%)	Population over 64 years (%)	Life expectancy at birth (years)	Urban population (%)	Projected labour force increase 1978-2000 (millions)	Per capita gross national product (US$)
Bhutan	1.3	43	19	2.4	29	2.1	—	42	3	44	3	0.4	70
India	634.7	34	14	2.0	35	1017.7	129	40	3	49	21	155.6	150
Iran	35.5	45	14	3.1	22	65.4	104	47	2	57	47	9.8	1930
Maldives	0.1	50	23	2.7	26	0.2	—	44	3	—	11	*	110
Nepal	13.4	44	20	2.3	30	23.0	152	40	3	44	4	4.4	120
Pakistan	76.8	44	14	3.0	23	145.1	139	46	3	51	26	20.4	170
Sri Lanka	14.2	26	9	1.7	41	20.4	47	39	4	68	22	3.0	200
SOUTHEAST ASIA	341	37	13	2.4	29	574	118	43	3	52	21	94	330
Burma	32.2	38	15	2.4	29	52.7	140	40	4	50	22	7.6	120
Dem. Kampuchea (Cambodia)	8.2	47	18	2.9	24	14.7	150	45	3	45	12	2.6	—
East Timor	0.8	44	22	2.3	30	1.2	175	42	3	40	11	0.1	
Indonesia	140.2	38	14	2.4	29	226.4	137	44	3	48	18	33.7	240
Lao People's Dem. Rep.	3.6	44	21	2.4	29	5.8	175	42	3	40	15	0.9	90
Malaysia	13.0	31	6	2.5	28	21.7	41	43	3	68	27	4.1	860
Philippines	46.3	35	10	2.5	28	84.7	80	43	3	58	32	15.7	410
Singapore	2.3	19	5	1.4	50	3.1	12	32	4	71	100	0.4	2700
Thailand	45.1	33	10	2.3	30	83.3	89	45	3	61	13	17.8	380
Vietnam	49.2	41	19	2.2	32	80.3	115	41	4	48	22	11.4	
EAST ASIA	1122	22	8	1.4	50	1457	59	33	6	66	31	167	900
China, People's Rep. of	930	22	8	1.4	50	1213	65	33	6	65	24	136.9	410
Hong Kong	4.5	18	5	1.3	53	5.8	14	30	6	72	92	0.7	2110
Japan	114.4	16	6	1.0	69	132.1	9	24	8	74	76	12.0	4910
Korea, Dem. People's Rep. of	17.1	34	9	2.5	28	27.4	70	42	4	61	43	6.1	470
Korea, Rep. of	37.1	24	7	1.7	41	53.5	47	39	4	65	48	8.3	670
Macao	0.3	25	7	1.8	38	0.4	78	38	5	—	97	*	780
Mongolia	1.6	35	8	2.7	26	2.7	70	44	3	61	46	0.5	860
Taiwan (Rep. of China)	16.9	26	5	2.1	33	22.1	25	35	4	70	63	2.7	1070
NORTH AMERICA	242	15	9	0.6	116	292	15	25	10	73	74	30	7850
Canada	23.6	16	7	0.9	77	31.3	14	26	8	73	76	3.7	7510
United States	218.4	15	9	0.6	116	260.4	15	24	11	73	74	26.6	7890
LATIN AMERICA	343	36	9	2.7	26	606	84	42	4	62	61	96	1100
MIDDLE AMERICA	87	42	8	3.3	21	174	68	46	3	63	58	28	1000
Costa Rica	2.1	29	5	2.4	29	3.6	38	44	4	68	41	0.6	1040

	1	2	3	4	5	6	7	8	9	10	11	12	13
El Salvador	4.4	40	8	3.3	21	8.5	55	46	3	58	39	1.5	490
Guatemala	6.6	43	12	3.1	22	12.2	75	45	3	53	36	1.8	630
Honduras	3.0	47	13	3.5	20	6.1	103	47	2	55	31	1.1	390
Mexico	66.9	42	8	3.4	20	135.2	66	46	3	65	64	21.4	1090
Nicaragua	2.4	47	13	3.4	20	4.8	110	48	3	53	49	0.9	750
Panama	1.8	32	7	2.6	27	3.2	47	43	4	66	50	0.5	1310
CARIBBEAN	28	29	8	2.0	35	44	64	41	5	64	48	6	1060
Bahamas	0.2	20	5	1.4	50	0.3	35	44	3	66	58	*	3310
Barbados	0.3	19	9	0.9	77	0.3	28	34	9	69	44	*	1550
Cuba	9.7	21	5	1.5	46	14.7	27	37	6	70	60	2.1	860
Dominican Republic	5.1	39	9	3.0	23	10.6	96	48	6	58	47	1.7	780
Grenada	0.1	27	6	2.2	32	0.1	24	—	—	63	16	*	420
Guadeloupe	0.3	28	7	2.1	33	0.4	35	40	5	65	48	0.1	1500
Haiti	4.8	39	17	2.2	32	7.1	115	42	4	50	23	1.0	200
Jamaica	2.1	30	7	2.3	30	2.8	20	46	6	68	41	0.5	1070
Martinique	0.3	22	7	1.6	43	0.4	32	41	5	65	50	0.1	2350
Netherlands Antilles	0.3	28	7	2.1	33	0.4	28	38	5	62	48	*	1680
Puerto Rico	3.4	24	6	1.7	41	4.2	21	35	7	72	62	0.4	2430
Trinidad and Tobago	1.1	23	6	1.6	43	1.4	31	39	4	66	49	0.2	2240
TROPICAL SOUTH AMERICA	188	37	9	2.8	25	337	93	43	3	61	60	57	1090
Bolivia	4.9	47	18	2.9	24	8.7	157	42	4	48	34	1.5	390
Brazil	115.4	36	8	2.8	25	205.2	109	42	3	61	60	33.5	1140
Colombia	25.2	33	9	2.4	29	46.7	90	44	3	61	64	8.7	630
Ecuador	7.8	40	9	3.2	22	14.8	66	45	4	60	41	2.7	640
Guyana	0.8	27	7	2.0	35	1.2	50	44	3	68	40	0.2	540
Paraguay	2.9	39	8	3.1	22	5.3	65	45	3	62	37	019	640
Peru	17.1	40	11	2.9	24	31.2	80	45	3	56	55	5.1	800
Surinam	0.5	37	7	3.0	23	0.9	30	50	4	66	50	0.2	1370
Venezuela	13.1	36	7	3.0	23	23.2	49	45	3	65	75	4.1	2570
TEMPERATE SOUTH AMERICA	40	23	9	1.4	50	52	57	30	7	66	80	5	1400
Argentina	26.4	23	9	1.3	53	32.9	59	29	8	68	80	2.7	1550
Chile	10.8	25	7	1.8	38	15.4	56	35	5	63	79	2.1	1050
Uruguay	2.8	21	10	1.1	63	3.4	49	28	9	69	83	0.3	1390
EUROPE	480	15	10	0.4	173	538	20	24	12	71	65	30	4420
NORTHERN EUROPE	82	13	12	0.1	693	90	13	23	14	72	73	5	4910
Denmark	5.1	13	11	0.2	347	5.4	10	23	13	74	67	0.2	7450
Finland	4.8	14	9	0.5	139	4.8	10	22	10	71	59	0.1	5620
Iceland	0.2	19	6	1.3	53	0.3	8	30	9	75	87	*	6100
Ireland	3.2	22	10	1.1	63	4.0	15	31	11	71	52	0.4	2560
Norway	4.1	13	10	0.3	231	4.5	10	24	14	75	45	0.3	7420
Sweden	8.3	12	11	0.1	693	9.2	9	21	15	75	83	0.6	8670
United Kingdom	56.0	12	12	0.0	—	61.6	14	23	14	72	76	3.5	4020
WESTERN EUROPE	153	12	11	0.1	693	169	14	23	14	72	79	9	6900
Austria	7.5	12	13	-0.1	—	8.0	18	23	15	71	52	0.5	5330
Belgium	9.9	12	12	0.0	—	10.7	14	23	14	71	87	0.4	6780
France	53.4	14	10	0.3	231	61.2	13	24	14	73	70	4.9	6550
Germany, Federal Rep. of	61.3	10	12	-0.2	—	65.6	17	21	15	71	92	2.1	7380

Table 57.1—continued

Region or country	Population estimate mid-1978 (millions)	Birth rate	Death rate	Rate of natural increase (annual, %)	Number of years to double population	Population projection to 2000 (millions)	Infant mortality rate	Population under 15 years (%)	Population over 64 years (%)	Life expectancy at birth (years)	Urban population (%)	Projected labour force increase 1978-2000 (millions)	Per capita gross national product (US$)
Luxembourg	0.4	11	13	-0.2	—	0.4	18	20	13	70	69	*	6460
Netherlands	13.9	13	8	0.5	139	16.0	11	25	11	74	75	1.0	6200
Switzerland	6.2	12	9	0.3	231	6.9	11	22	13	73	55	0.4	8880
EASTERN EUROPE	108	18	11	0.7	99	122	25	23	11	70	58	8	2820
Bulgaria	8.8	16	10	0.6	116	9.9	23	22	11	71	58	0.3	2310
Czechoslovakia	15.2	19	11	0.8	87	17.0	21	23	12	70	67	1.0	3840
German Democratic Rep.	16.7	12	14	-0.2	—	17.4	14	21	16	72	76	0.9	4220
Hungary	10.7	18	12	0.5	139	11.1	30	20	13	69	50	0.2	2280
Poland	35.1	20	9	1.1	63	40.2	24	24	9	71	55	3.5	2860
Romania	21.9	20	10	1.0	69	26.0	31	25	10	70	48	1.9	1450
SOUTHERN EUROPE	137	17	9	0.8	87	158	24	26	11	71	51	8	2620
Albania	2.6	32	8	2.4	29	4.1	87	40	5	68	34	0.9	540
Greece	9.3	16	8	0.8	87	9.9	23	24	12	72	65	0.2	2590
Italy	56.7	14	10	0.4	173	61.8	19	24	12	72	53	2.1	3050
Malta	0.3	19	10	0.9	77	0.3	14	26	9	70	94	*	1390
Portugal	9.7	19	10	0.9	77	10.8	39	27	10	69	26	0.4	1690
Spain	36.8	18	8	1.0	69	45.3	11	28	10	72	61	2.8	2920
Yugoslavia	22.0	18	8	1.0	69	25.6	36	26	8	68	39	1.7	1680
USSR	261	18	9	0.9	77	313	28	25	9	69	62	20	2760
OCEANIA	22	21	9	1.2	58	32	41	32	7	68	71	5	4730
Australia	14.3	17	8	0.8	87	19.9	14	28	8	72	86	2.7	6100
Fiji	0.6	29	7	2.2	32	0.8	41	39	3	70	38	0.1	1150
New Zealand	3.2	18	8	1.0	69	4.3	16	30	9	72	81	0.5	4250
Papua New Guinea	3.0	41	16	2.5	28	5.1	106	44	4	48	13	0.9	490
Samoa, Western	0.2	37	7	3.0	23	0.3	40	50	3	63	21	*	350
Solomon Islands	0.2	36	13	2.3	30	0.4	52	44	3	—	9	*	250

*A labour force increase of less than 50000.—Data not available.

by family planning is considered a far less urgent medical problem than heart disease or cancer.

The official Roman Catholic Church still considers contraception to be morally wrong and forbids research and teaching in contraception and the sale of contraceptives, though many of its members dissent from this view. This attitude is responsible for much ill health in poor families in many countries, especially in Latin America. In our opinion the widespread distribution of modern contraceptive knowledge is an urgent necessity and this presents a major public health problem.

Community health approach

Exhortation to uneducated women to limit their families is unlikely to be effective. Particularly in areas where the infant mortality rates are high, it is quite useless to preach birth control. It is natural for men and women to desire healthy children to take their place in life and to provide for their parents in old age. In societies where the women are ignorant of the elementary laws of hygiene and cannot manage either to raise their children properly or to protect them against the common infectious diseases associated with dirt and squalor, a woman must produce many children if she is to expect to rear even two or three up to adult life. Children are often considered to be a source of social security. In most countries, both in the East and in the West, it is probable that most women who have successfully produced two, three or four healthy children seek ways and means to prevent the arrival of more. If women can be shown how to raise a small healthy family, then many of them will actively seek advice as to how to prevent more arrivals. It is easy to teach people who desire knowledge.

If this reasoning is accepted, it follows that a first step in any attack on the birth rates must be through the Maternity and Child Health Centres. In these Centres women can be taught mothercraft; nutritional education is, of course, a most important part of such teaching. When the Public Health Nurses have successfully educated the majority of the women in a community how to rear healthy children, then the demand for advice on contraception will inevitably and automatically follow. As in the case of so many other aspects of preventitive medicine, the Maternity and Child Health Centres can provide centres from which new ideas must spread out amongst a people. A practical way in which Family Planning can be linked with Child Health Services is by explaining to the mother how a longer birth interval improves the prospects for the present baby and by planning the time to start and discontinue contraceptive measures on the present baby's growth chart (Morley and Cutting, 1974). However, the women have to win their husbands over to new ideas; in many communities failure of arrival of another child after two years is regarded as evidence of lack of virility in the husband.

A most important factor, which restricts the birth rate, is the delay in the age of marriage. A girl who is married at 13 or 14 is likely to have more children than one whose marriage is delayed until after she is 20 years of age. The extension of higher education to women has already had an important effect on birth rates in many countries and this influence is spreading. Family Planning and nutrition services are each part of community health. Many women need help from both. Nutritionists should be aware of the Family Planning Service and be ready to work with its members in their community.

Modern contraceptive techniques

Methods of contraception such as the rhythm method and coitus interruptus have been employed since time immemorial. Unfortunately such simple methods have proved either unsatisfactory or ineffective. More modern methods involving the placing of some kind of barrier, either mechanical or chemical, between the sperm and the ovum have not proved suitable for use on a large scale by people who are both poor and ignorant. Now oral contraceptives, intrauterine devices (IUD) and voluntary male sterilisation by vasectomy are being extensively tried in underdeveloped countries. Female sterilisation by tubectomy is also used. The merits of the different methods and the problems arising in their use in Family Planning programmes in several countries are discussed by Mills (1974).

COMMENT

Comparison of Table 56.1, which is mainly 1976 data, with the similar table in our last edition, mainly 1969 data, shows that estimated world population has gone up in the seven years by 668 million, an annual rate of increase of over 2 per cent. High rates of increase in countries in Africa, Asia and Latin America have not changed greatly, though in India the rate has fallen from 2.5 to 2.0 per cent. This was due to a fall in the birth rate from 43 to 34 and indicates that the family planning campaign has had some effect. However, in these regions, if agriculture production does not continue to increase by at least 2 per cent annually, available food supplies cannot be maintained.

In Europe, North America and Oceania the annual rates of increase have continued to decline. In North America the fall has been from 1.1 per cent to 0.6 per cent. It has been more marked in Europe where in six countries the population has now ceased to rise. There are 18 other countries in these regions, and also Japan and Singapore in Asia, that are approaching zero growth and should reach it within the lifetimes of our younger readers. This is good news, but only for some 20 per cent of the world population who live in rich countries. We believe that only if both contraception and scientific agriculture are practised on a worldwide scale can disasters be avoided.

58. Famine and Disasters

As far back as history records, mankind has suffered at irregular intervals from great famines. In many the disaster has been so great that a million or more people have perished. Enormous advances in agriculture and in methods of transport, notably the introduction of potatoes to Europe in the seventeenth century and of railways to India in the nineteenth century, made the prevention and relief of famine technically very much easier. During the first half of the twentieth century great famines appeared to belong to the past and there was little interest in famine relief. This optimism was rudely shattered in 1943 when at least a million people died in the Bengal famine. Severe famine conditions arose again in Bihar in India in 1965–66 and in the civil wars that preceded the establishment of the states of Zaire and Bangladesh and kept Nigeria politically intact. In 1974 there were famines in countries south of the Sahara where the desert is spreading, in Ethiopia and in Maharastra in India. The problems of famine are very much alive today.

The worst disasters have occurred when the famine has not been foreseen and the government has lacked the administrative experience to organise relief. On the other hand there are many examples of foresight which have enabled relief measures to be planned ahead. A well-planned and organised relief service can help a people to survive a period of famine, not without hardship and suffering but at least with no great increase in the number of deaths. Although there are many books giving excellent historical accounts of particular famines, there are few devoted primarily to the scientific aspects of the prevention and relief of famine. The monographs by Masefield (1963, 1967), the Swedish Nutrition Foundation (1971) and Aykroyd (1974) are recommended.

This chapter attempts to give only a broad outline of conditions and to set out a few general principles. Based on experience of famine in India (Passmore, 1951) it has been changed little since the first edition. Throughout the nineteenth century governments of Indian provinces had a series of severe famines to deal with and a Famine Code was evolved. It has on many occasions been the means of preventing excess mortality, if not hardship. The success of the relief measures in the Bihar famine (Ramalingaswami et al., 1971) followed the application of its principles. The administrative organisation needed for international famine relief today is given by Ifekwunigwe (1977). If a Punjab civil servant of 100 years ago could have read his

paper, he would have appreciated its clarity but not have been surprised.

CAUSES OF FAMINE

Drought
In tropical and subtropical countries large numbers of people have lived and continued to live under the yearly threat of drought. Failure of the rains, often in successive seasons, has been a frequent cause of famine. The importance of the science of irrigation in the husbanding and control of natural water has been discussed on page 459. In Asia and in Africa irrigation schemes, often on a vast scale, have made large areas of land practically independent of yearly variations in rainfall. Yet much remains to be done and in many districts throughout the tropics and subtropics failure of the rains can bring the people to the verge of disaster.

Crop diseases and pests
The great Irish famines of the nineteenth century were caused by the destruction of the potato crops by a fungus, which produces a disease known as 'the blight'. A good account of this famine has been given by Woodham-Smith (1962). Whenever people are largely dependent on a single crop for their main source of food, there is always the risk that the crop may be destroyed by disease, and famine conditions follow. Plagues of locusts can cause great destruction of all crops and, in some parts of the world, these greedy insects are a potential cause of famine.

Great natural disturbances
Floods and earthquakes are a constant natural threat to man in many parts of the world. They can destroy crops, food stores and communications and so cause famine.

Man-made causes: war, civil commotion and economic factors
Wars and especially civil wars have been directly responsible for many famines throughout history. Food shortages are an inevitable result of all wars and these can readily lead to famine conditions. Nuclear warfare on a large scale in an industrial country might quickly lead to famine amongst the survivors, through destruction of transport, docks and warehouses. Poor social organisation, poverty and lack of transport can prevent the proper distribution of a food

supply which is potentially adequate, and so bring about famine.

Each of these four primary causes is still operative. It is reasonable to suppose that on occasions—and probably unexpectedly—each may again give rise to famine.

EFFECTS OF FAMINE

Literature contains many moving accounts of human suffering during famines. Two of these are given below. The first is a letter from Ireland addressed to the Duke of Wellington on 17 December 1846 (Edwards and Williams, 1956).

Having for many years been intimately connected with the western portion of the county of Cork, and possessing some small property there, I thought it right, personally, to investigate the truth of the several lamentable accounts which had reached me of the appalling state of misery to which that part of the country was reduced....Being aware that I should have to witness scenes of frightful hunger, I provided myself with as much bread as five men could carry, and on reaching the spot I was surprised to find the wretched hamlet deserted. I entered some of the hovels to ascertain the cause, and the scenes that presented themselves were such as no tongue or pen can convey the slightest idea of. In the first, six famished and ghastly skeletons, to all appearance dead, were huddled in a corner on some filthy straw, their sole covering what seemed a ragged horse-cloth and their wretched legs hanging about, naked above the knees. I approached in horror, and found by a low moaning they were alive, they were in fever—four children, a woman, and what once had been a man. It is impossible to go through the details, suffice to say, that in a few minutes I was surrounded by at least 200 of such phantoms, such frightful spectres as no words can describe. By far the greater number were delirious either from famine or from fever. Their demoniac yells are still ringing in my ears, and their horrible images are fixed upon my brain...the same morning the police opened a house on the adjoining lands, which was observed shut for many days, and two frozen corpses were found lying upon the mud floor *half devoured by the rats*. A mother, herself in fever, was seen the same day to drag out the corpse of her child, a girl about 12, perfectly naked; and leave it half covered with stones. In another house...the dispensary doctor found seven wretches lying, unable to move, under the same cloak—one had been dead for many hours but the others were unable to move either themselves or the corpse. To what purpose should I multiply such cases? If these be not sufficient, neither would they hear who have the power to send relief and do not, even though "one came from the dead".

The second (Hunter, 1868) describes from contemporary letters the scene in Western Bengal in 1770, when it is estimated that 10 million people—or a third of the population—died.

All through the stifling summer the people went on dying. The husbandmen sold their cattle; they sold their implements of agriculture; they devoured their seed grain; they sold their sons and daughters, till at length no buyer of children could be found; they ate the leaves of trees and the grass of the field; and in June 1770, the Resident at the Durbar affirmed that the living were feeding on the dead. Day and night a torrent of famished and disease-stricken wretches poured into the great cities. At an early period of the year pestilence had broken-out. In March we find smallpox at Moossheda-bad, where it glided through the vice-regal mutes, and cut off the Prince Syfut in his palace. The streets were blocked with promiscuous heaps of the dying and the dead. Interment could not do its work quick enough; even the dogs and jackals, the public scavengers of the East, became unable to accomplish their revolting work, and the multitude of mangled and festering corpses at length threatened the existence of the citizens.

Of the many effects of famine, it is practical for the purposes of administrating relief to keep three constantly in mind.

Deaths from starvation
It is of prime importance to procure and distribute sufficient food to prevent such deaths. Their number is the measure of the severity of the famine and the effectiveness of the relief organisation. Old people and young children are particularly liable to die of starvation. Adolescents often manage to survive. Women usually survive better than men.

Panic and social disruption
It is natural for starving people, if there is no food in their immediate neighbourhood, to leave home and go in search of something to eat. If such wandering takes place on a large scale, social chaos is inevitable and all relief work becomes many times more difficult. Families are easily disrupted and only with great difficulty later reunited. If parents die, infants and young children may be found helpless with no knowledge of their family name or the whereabouts of their home or of other relations. Adolescents, if separated from their families, readily form gangs, which are actively opposed to all forces of law and order. Such gangs may be a source of much mischief and the subsequent rehabilitation of the members very difficult.

Spread of epidemics
Louse-borne typhus was the great famine disease in Europe, and cholera and smallpox in Asia. But large epidemics of relapsing fever, influenza, tuberculosis,

enteric fever—or indeed of any infectious disease—may be associated with famine. In malarious countries famine usually occurs in times of drought and so conditions are unsuitable for the mosquitoes which transmit the disease. When the rains do come, often in excessive amounts, malaria may spread rapidly among the enfeebled survivors of the famine. On some occasions there have been more deaths in the malaria epidemic subsequent to a famine than in the famine itself.

It is unusual to find epidemics of any of the diseases attributable to vitamin deficiencies in a famine, though scurvy may afflict the inhabitants of a besieged city or a desert people.

The rapid spread of infectious diseases among a starving people is attributable to the ease with which the infecting organisms can pass from person to person as a result of overcrowding and the breakdown of normal sanitary arrangements. It is the absence of all hygienic precautions that is responsible for epidemics rather than an increased susceptibility of the starving body to infective micro-organisms. In many famines far more people have died of infectious diseases than of starvation.

These three effects of famine, deaths from starvation, social disruption and the spread of epidemics, should be constantly in the mind of relief workers. It is important to repeat and emphasise this; for in a famine there is always more to do than can be done. The time and energy of the workers must be disciplined, for it is easy to be distracted by a charitable heart to a task which may be very worthy yet of secondary importance.

FAMINE RELIEF

Procurement and distribution of food

Transport problems. Fortunately for mankind the causes of famine are local. A district, a province or even occasionally a whole country may be involved, but never a whole continent. Stores of surplus food have always been available—somewhere. How to get the food to the right place fast enough is always the fundamental problem. Modern methods of transport have greatly mitigated the effects of famine. The rapid development of railways throughout India in the middle of the nineteenth century facilitated the organisation of relief and was the means of saving many lives.

Ships, trains, aeroplanes, lorries and sometimes bullock carts, camels and other pack animals may be needed. The procurement and organisation of these is the first and most important problem of a relief organisation.

Quantities of food required. The urgent need is for energy foods; the correction of vitamin and mineral deficiencies in the diet may have to wait until the peak of the famine is past. For infants and children a source of good protein is desirable and can sometimes be provided by dried skimmed milk. The minimum amount of food necessary to preserve human life has been much debated in

the past. FAO in 1946 set out recommendations for subsistence and maintenance levels of energy intake, which are given in Table 58.1. These figures represent a compromise between physiological needs and practical difficulties. Nutritionists must warn governments that unless food is available at this emergency subsistence level, deaths from starvation and civil unrest are likely. The figures in Table 58.1 have to be converted into tons of cereal grain. One ton of cereals provides about 15 million MJ. This will suffice for about 1850 sedentary males for a day at the emergency subsistence level. To calculate the total food that must be imported into a famine area, it is also necessary to know or estimate (1) the number of people in the area, (2) the amount of physical labour that is required of them, (3) the proportions of women and children, (4) the stores of food already in the area, and (5) the probable duration of the emergency. With these data, tables of physiological needs can be converted into statements of cargo space required.

Such estimates can be nothing more than intelligent guesses unless a recent and reliable census is available. The importance of a census can never be overestimated.

Public works. The growth of the British Empire throughout the eighteenth century compelled civil servants to consider ways and means of distributing food to famine victims. They were greatly influenced by two principles. The first was that trade was the natural and proper means for the distribution of all goods, including food, and that governments should interfere with trading operations as little as possible. The second was that charity ultimately degrades the recipient, who should if possible pay for the relief which he receives. In the formulation of these principles the influence of Adam Smith was great.

Table 58.1 Scales of energy allowances suitable for use in time of famine (megajoules/day)

Category	Emergency subsistence level*	Temporary maintenance level†
0–2	4.2	4.2
3–5 years	5.3	6.3
6–9 years	6.3	7.4
10–17 years	8.4	10.5
Pregnant and nursing women	8.4	10.5
Normal consumers (sedentary)		
Male	8.0	9.5
Female	6.8	9.2
Moderate workers	8.4	10.5
Heavy workers	10.5	12.5
Very heavy workers	12.5	14.6

Emergency subsistence level needed to prevent the most serious undernutrition leading to disease and the danger of civil unrest.

† *Temporary maintenance level* sufficiently high to maintain populations in fairly good health but not sufficient for rapid and complete recovery.

His book *The Wealth of Nations* was published in 1776 and his laissez-faire economic doctrines were widely accepted at the beginning of the nineteenth century. They greatly affected the organisation of famine relief. It was concluded that the real need of the famine victim was for money. If he was provided with money, food would become available through the channels of normal trade, which would be developed to meet his needs. He could get money if he had the opportunity to work. The solution to the problem was thus the setting up of public works. There has been much experience of the public works system of relief, but it is difficult either to condemn or approve the system whole-heartedly.

In Ireland in 1846–47 and in Bengal in 1943, the system failed to prevent the deaths of hundreds of thousands. It must be added that in both these countries it was administered by local civil servants who were without experience of famine and who were not adequately forewarned. Time and experience are needed to plan and organise public works.

On the other hand, in several parts of India where famine conditions arise owing to failure of the rains, relief works have frequently been the means of helping people through an emergency period without loss of life, but not without hardship and suffering. Here there has been the advantage that the probability of famine was usually foreseen, and experienced local staff available to plan ahead and administer relief work.

Even under the best conditions the system has its disadvantages. The food requirements of the people are increased by the physical work involved and also by the walk from their homes to the work sites. Even with the best planning, it is impossible to organise work for all the immediate neighbourhood. Furthermore, the old and those physically handicapped may be unable to work and so get no relief. Pride may prevent members of the middle classes from undertaking manual labour. Often the work itself is of little value. Road-making has been commonly undertaken and many of the roads have led from 'nowhere in particular to nowhere at all', in the words of Salaman (1948), an historian of the Irish famine. Useless physical work may be demoralising. Well-planned public works have their place in famine relief under many circumstances, but it is unwise to rely too heavily on them, especially if an experienced supervisory staff is not available.

Public kitchens. Cooked food may be distributed from public kitchens. This is usually essential in a severe famine. Only in this way is it possible to ensure that food reaches those too old, too young or so severely handicapped that they cannot work. Further, it is often impossible to bring into a famine area the foods to which the people are accustomed. The introduction of strange foods, which the people may not know how to cook or prepare, has presented great difficulties in the past. This can be overcome in part by the distribution of meals at special centres.

Price control. It is essential that the prices of such foods as are available be kept within the means of the famine victims. There are always some merchants who are willing to exploit the sufferings of others to their own financial gain. Legislation to prevent any excessive rise in prices is essential, and direct subsidies on cereal grains and other foods may be desirable. The extent to which prices are kept down is a measure of the efficiency of the government.

ORGANISATION OF FOREIGN AID

A threat of famine evokes much public sympathy and people wish to give aid to the victims through private charities, their national government and the UN agencies. Two factors operate to prevent this goodwill being turned into effective relief.

First the number of agencies seeking to help may be large and their efforts lack coordination. Administrators and field workers of different agencies may differ in their opinions as to how best to give relief. As famine rouses the emotions, it is not surprising that there are stories of personal animosity between relief workers. Government officials in the country receiving relief have had to deal with many foreign helpers who are at loggerheads. Famine conditions are going to continue to recur in the world and there is need for international planning to channel all foreign aid through a single administrative machinery in the country receiving the aid.

Secondly famine conditions often arise in times of war and especially of civil war. It is a common view that it is possible to win a war by starving the enemy out and military policy has often been directed to this aim. Such a policy has seldom been successful and Mayer (1971) gives many examples of its ineffectiveness. When food is scarce, the young men in the armed forces get enough to keep them an effective fighting force and they still have to be defeated in battle before a war is won. It is civilians who suffer from such a policy and the children and old people who starve to death. There is a widespread move amongst governments to outlaw all chemical and bacteriological means of waging war. Such a ban should be extended to include starvation. Notably in the Nigerian civil war relief work for the civilian population was much hindered by the military authorities on both sides. In times of war the Geneva Convention permits the International Red Cross to care for the wounded and sick of both sides and this has been the means of saving much suffering and countless lives. There is need for a similar international organisation for the care of victims of starvation. The practicability of this important idea has been discussed by the Swedish Nutrition Foundation (1971) and merits serious study.

Foreign aid depends on local organisations. Governments in countries where famine is recurrent should have civil servants permanently employed in keeping plans for famine relief up to date.

MEDICINE IN A FAMINE

The problem before every member of the medical services engaged in famine relief is not 'What is there for me to do?' but rather 'Of the many jobs to be done, which will save most lives?' In a famine there are never enough doctors or nurses; hospital beds and equipment are insufficient; drugs and vaccines are scarce.

Assessment of the state of the famine

The efficient organisation of relief depends upon accurate assessments of the course of the famine. The number of people likely to be in need of relief in the near future must be forecast. This is never an easy matter and there are always those who, for political reasons, seek either to minimise or exaggerate the extent of the distress. Great disasters seldom arise suddenly and without warning. A Public Health Service that can give week-by-week reports on the numbers of deaths and the numbers seeking admission to hospital is invaluable. If possible, the causes of death and the nature of the diseases requiring hospital treatment should be stated; even if the diagnosis cannot always be precise and accurate, the information is still useful, especially as an indication of the appearance of a new infectious disease. The organisation of accurate medical statistics is thus of first importance.

Observation of the state of nutrition of the people is also valuable. As discussed in Chapter 55, there is no single simple method of assessing nutritional status. Nevertheless an observant medical staff, who can move freely over the whole of a famine area, will be able to detect quickly any signs of deterioration in the health of the people.

Prevention of epidemics

An adequate supply of sanitary stores, including vaccines, insecticides and disinfectants, should be available, with sufficient reserves kept in medical stores to meet any further emergency. Most epidemic diseases can be readily controlled by prompt action in the first few days after their appearance; once they are established, control may become impossible before a large toll of mortality has been taken.

The Public Health Service must be maintained and, as far as possible, expanded, even at the expense of the clinical staff. Any breakdown in this service can be the direct cause of innumerable deaths.

Organisation of famine hospitals

Small hospitals widely dispersed amongst the people are more valuable than large institutions. A nearby hospital will help to maintain confidence and so prevent wandering and social disruption. In such hospitals elaborate diagnostic equipment is of secondary importance. Sufficient blankets, kitchen and sanitary equipment, simple drugs and enough staff to allow rapid expansion in an emergency, are essential. Relief workers, if healthy and intelligent, can be rapidly trained to perform hospital duties, even if previously quite inexperienced in hospital work. At Belsen, medical students made excellent workers and their energy, enthusiasm and common sense more than compensated for any deficiencies in technical training. It is the first duty of a medical superintendent to recruit and train a staff sufficiently large to meet any foreseen emergency. In selecting recruits enthusiasm, intelligence and health are the essentials: deficiencies in technical knowledge can rapidly be made good.

Treatment in a famine hospital

The treatment of starvation has been described in Chapter 27. In the early stages rapid recovery frequently follows a few days feeding and attention to minor ailments. If treatment is neglected at this stage the condition of the patient may deteriorate rapidly. Once appetite is lost and strength is so feeble that he cannot support his weight upright, the prognosis is uncertain, and recovery always slow, even with the best medical and nursing care. It is therefore very important to give the best medical care to the minor sick.

Feeding arrangements must be simple and there is no place for elaborate dietary regimes. In a famine hospital the first essential is the preparation of simple, well-cooked meals. The provision of suitable kitchen and dining-room accommodation and equipment may be difficult and should command the doctors' attention. A large staff of nurses and orderlies are necessary when many patients are too weak to go to the dining rooms.

Experience has shown that even a small medical service, if well run, will have a beneficial effect in maintaining public confidence. A shortage of doctors, nurses and orderlies is inevitable and every individual doctor must train his assistants to accept the work delegated to them. His chief task is thus administration and supervision. The ability to foresee needs for simple remedies and equipment is essential, and for success it is necessary to be a master of improvisation.

CONCLUSION

Famine relief inevitably presents many and diverse problems. It is often difficult for a worker on the spot to sort out what is essential from what is only desirable. It is hoped that this chapter will stimulate thought on the principles of relief, for in famine forethought is the best antidote to disaster.

59. Nutrition and Infection

The recorded history of mankind demonstrates repeatedly the close association between war, pestilence, famine and death. They are represented as the four horsemen of the apocalypse in St John's allegory (Revelation, Chap. 6). Fevers, poverty and poor nutrition went together in the slums of industrial cities. Famines have been associated with outbreaks of disease such as typhus, relapsing fever, smallpox and cholera. The great tropical diseases, especially malaria, dysentery and ankylostomiasis were most prevalent among the poverty-stricken. Eighty years ago in the cities of Europe fatal respiratory infections were common in poor children with rickets in the overcrowded slums. Rheumatic fever following streptococcal infection was more frequently found in the children of the poor than of the well-to-do. Wherever in the world there has been hunger and poverty, victims of pulmonary tuberculosis have been numerous. However, poverty is also associated with inadequate houses, overcrowding and insufficient sanitary services. Overcrowding facilitates the passage of micro-organisms from person to person (cross-infection). This is so whether a disease is spread as an airborne infection or by food or water, or transmitted by insects.

There is no doubt that severe or repeated infections are a common cause of malnutrition. The extent to which malnutrition itself contributes to the incidence and severity of infections is much more difficult to assess.

INFECTIONS AS A CAUSE OF MALNUTRITION

Infections increase the rate of metabolism and the breakdown of tissues (p. 442) and so create a need for extra nutrients. Accompanying fever usually reduces appetite, and when the infection affects the function of the gastrointestinal tract, as is frequent, absorption of nutrients is impaired. In these ways an infection increases requirements of nutrients and at the same time may reduce their supply. These effects may be of trivial significance, if the infection lasts only a few days and the patient was previously well-nourished. If the infection is prolonged or there are repeated attacks or the patient's previous diet was only just adequate, severe malnutrition may arise. How attacks of gastroenteritis, measles and whooping cough frequently precipitate severe and fatal protein-energy malnutrition is described in Chapter 29. These three diseases are ubiquitous and few children escape attacks. In prosperous countries where the children are well fed, the illness is only occasionally serious; in countries where many children have a poor diet these infections carry a high mortality rate (Table 59.1). Most of these deaths would be ascribed more accurately as due to malnutrition than to the infections. Similar high mortality rates have been found in the Caribbean islands and in West Africa (McGregor et al., 1961; Ashworth and Waterlow, 1974). Less seriously, infections slow down the growth, and in a Gambian village a close association was found between attacks of gastroenteritis and of malaria with weight gain in children under 3 years of age (Rowland et al., 1977). Further information about how infections may impair the nutrition of young children can be found in two reviews (Scrimshaw et al., 1968; Scrimshaw, 1975).

Attacks of the classical deficiency diseases have often

Table 59.1 Mortality from gastroenteritis, measles and whooping cough, in children under 5 years (from National and WHO reports by Dr J. M. Bengoa)

	Gastroenteritis, 1964		Measles, average 1963–64		Whooping cough, 1964	
	under 1 year (rate per 100000 liveborn)	1–4 years (rate per 100000 population)	under 1 year (rate per 100000 liveborn)	1–4 years (rate per 10000 population)	under 1 year (rate per 100000 liveborn)	1–4 years (rate per 100000 population)
Austria	139.0	6.8	4.5	2.2	2.2	1.0
Denmark	40.8	1.7		1.0	2.4	0.3
England and Wales	42.0	3.5	2.1	1.5	3.7	0.3
Chile	1588.0	69.3	413.2	137.6	68.3	8.1
Guatemala	1275.9	704.2	248.0	310.0	589.4	309.2
Mexico	1224.0	267.4	71.0	103.7	112.7	75.8
Phillipines	521.0	149.6	58.4	25.6	12.3	2.6

been precipitated by an infection, e.g. keratomalacia by pneumonia (Oomen, 1958) and beriberi by dysentery (Smith and Woodruff, 1951).

Infectious diseases also contribute to malnutrition by reducing the working capacity of individuals. This is illustrated by malaria. The peasant farmer afflicted with it has an attack of fever when the rains come, and so cannot sow his seed at the right time. His family suffer the next winter from his incapacity, and nutritional troubles result. In a more general way, whenever the breadwinner is struck down by a prolonged infection nutritional failure is likely to affect his dependants.

NUTRITIONAL STATE AND RESISTANCE TO INFECTION
That the natural immunological mechanisms which protect the body against invasion by pathogenic parasites may be impaired by malnutrition is beyond doubt. Reduced immunity to infections in severe cases of protein-energy malnutrition have been described in Chapter 29. Yet both epidemiological findings and laboratory studies indicate that immunity may be little impaired by malnutrition unless it is severe.

Observations of human epidemics
Many times in history infections have spread like wildfire among men and women stricken with poverty. This was usually because the insanitary state of their environment has provided ideal circumstances for pathogenic organisms to pass easily from one host to another. Opportunities to study infectious diseases in a malnourished community living under good sanitary conditions seldom arise.

Infectious diseases in Europe in 1939–45
Although there was a marked increase in tuberculosis during World War II, in general the widespread scarcity of food was not associated with epidemics of infectious diseases. In Greece in 1942 and in Holland in 1944–45 there were famine conditions. After the war in Germany there was a marked deterioration in the food supplies. Yet in none of these countries did epidemics of common infectious diseases arise. The unsatisfactory food intakes did not lead to outbreaks of diseases such as influenza, meningitis and diphtheria.

Suppression of infections in malnutrition
Some infections, notably malaria, have appeared to be less virulent in malnourished populations. The severe form of malaria caused by *Plasmodium falciparum* is often fatal due to large numbers of red blood cells containing the parasites becoming sludged and blocking capillaries in the cerebral cortex. Malaria is endemic in the Sahel area of Africa and observations have been made on its manifestations under famine conditions by Murray *et al.* (1978). They observed that during the height of the famine the severe form of the disease was suppressed and cerebral malaria was not seen.

After the famine cerebral malaria reappeared especially in settled communities where the diet of the children was mainly cereal grain; its incidence was much less in normal communities where milk was available. The authors discuss their findings in relation to observations of experimental malaria in animals. They suggest that the sludging of the blood may be part of the immune responses of the tissues and does not take place where these are impaired by malnutrition; on the other hand, the malarial parasites themselves are dependent on nutrients and their multiplication may be reduced when the supply, which is dependent on the host's diet, is impaired. In Tanzania patients with iron-deficiency anaemia were found to have fewer bacterial infections, but not less malaria, than patients with other forms of anaemia (Masáwe *et al.*, 1974). It is suggested that iron deficiency may increase resistance to bacterial infections.

Infectious disease in well-nourished people
It is well known that good nutrition does not necessarily protect against infection. Fit and healthy young men and women frequently contract typhus, malaria, smallpox, cholera, infective hepatitis, poliomyelitis, pneumonia and other infections. This is particularly likely when their duties as doctors, nurses, soldiers or missionaries take them into areas where an epidemic is present. They are also susceptible to sporadic infections in the course of their ordinary work. Good nutrition provides no safeguard against influenza, the last great plague against which man has so far no means of protection (Beveridge, 1977). The pandemic of 1918–19 was responsible for 15–25 million deaths. In the USA and many other countries the incidence was highest in healthy young adults, many of whom died. The mortality rate was, however, highest in the very old. In epidemics today with less virulent strains of the virus incidence continues to be high in young adults who are well nourished

Pulmonary tuberculosis
This infectious disease has been closely associated with poverty and it was held that malnutrition increases susceptibility In the first edition of this book instances were given in which the deaths from tuberculosis increased when nutritional standards fell, but without any obvious corresponding decline in their general hygiene. Since then, observations in the Madras among an urban population living in very poor houses on deficient diets have shown that the disease can be arrested and its spread from 'open' cases to their families and other close contacts can be controlled if the infection is adequately treated with chemotherapeutic drugs (Andrews *et al.*, 1960; Fox, 1962). In Madras this was found to be effective without the necessity of isolating the patients in sanatoria and with no change in the poor diet, housing and other hygienic circumstances of the community.

Controlled field studies

There have been two field trials in which the effects of improvements in nutrition, medical care and sanitation have been studied independently in separate villages in the tropics. In the one in Guatemala, which was on a small scale, the results were inconclusive (Ascoli *et al.*, 1967). In a much larger trial in the Punjab four groups of children aged 0 to 3 years were studied. One group received nutritional care, another medical care with emphasis on the treatment and prevention of infectious diseases, a third group received both nutritional and medical care, and a fourth group acted as a control. Each group consisted of all the children (200 to 380) in two or three villages. Analyses of the growth rates, morbidity and mortality rates at different ages shows the benefits derived from both the nutritional and the medical care, but does not show clearly which was the greater (Kielmann *et al.*, 1978; Taylor *et al.*, 1978). In this trial the methods and health staff used were those that could be made available throughout India and Pakistan. The results indicate the practical possibilities of combined attacks on malnutrition and infectious diseases.

Laboratory studies

Most bacteriologists would agree that the previous diet of an experimental animal in general makes little difference to its susceptibility to infection. Unless the diet has been grossly defective either in quantity or quality for a long time, response to experimental infection is unaltered. Yet there are experiments in which it has been unequivocally shown that a poor diet has increased the susceptibility of laboratory animals to an infection, owing to a failure of one or other of these protective mechanisms. The evidence has been reviewed by Schneider (1946), Howie (1949) and Axelrod (1971).

Immunity depends on two types of responses by the tissues. **Humoral responses** are the production of antibodies in response to the stimulus of foreign proteins in the invading organisms (antigens). Antibodies are immunoglobulins which may circulate in the blood where they may be detected about a week after injection of an antigen. Antibodies react specifically with antigens of the invader and thereby may destroy it. Antibody may also be formed in response to stimulation by a bacterial toxin; such antibody may neutralise the effect of the toxin. After many specific infectious diseases antibodies persist in the blood for years and prevent or mitigate a second infection. **Cellular responses** are responsible for the mobilisation and production of macrophages, polymorphs and other connective tissue cells. These accumulate at local sites of infection were they may ingest and destroy invading microorganisms (phagocytosis). Different types of cell are evoked by different microorganisms: polymorphs by staphylococci and other pyogenic bacteria, lymphocytes by viruses and tubercle bacilli, and eosinophils by helminths. They may also form a fibrinous exudate which may seal off a local infection and prevent the invader spreading by entering blood or lymph vessels.

Many studies on men have shown that even severe malnutrition may not alter humoral responses to injected antigens (Balch, 1950; Gell, 1951; Larsen and Tomlinson, 1952). In tropical countries where malnutrition and chronic infections and infestations so frequently co-exist, deficiency of protein in the diet may lead to a marked fall in the concentrations of albumin in the plasma, while those of immunoglobulins remain high. On the other hand, in malnourished children in Thailand serum concentrations of proteins which made up the complement system, necessary for the interaction of many antibodies with antigen, were found to be low (Sinsinha *et al.*, 1973). Defects in cell immunity have also been found in children in protein-energy malnutrition (p.262).

The cells responsible for producing immune responses, both humoral and cellular, arise in the thymus, spleen and lymph nodes, the lymphoreticular organs. Their function, like that of neurones in the central nervous system, is very immature at birth and develops rapidly in the first two years of life. Lymphoreticular organs and the brain are probably both very susceptible to lack of nutrients during this period. Once they have become mature they may be less susceptible than other organs and tissues to malnutrition, perhaps because they receive priority in supply when amounts of essential nutrients are limited. There is a large literature on the effects of inanition in man and experimental animals on the morphology of the lymphoreticular organs which is reviewed and summarised by Jackson (1925). In the young, atrophy of the thymus is marked and often greater than that of other organs. Lymph nodes and the spleen certainly atrophy when inanition is severe and prolonged. In less severe cases the findings are very variable and they have sometimes been reported to be enlarged.

CONCLUSION

Fortunately the uncertainties of the precise relation of nutrition to infection do not affect public health policy. In countries where severe malnutrition is uncommon, resistance to infection or recovery from infection is probably little influenced by nutritional and dietetic factors. In other countries where malnutrition is common and often severe, nutritional factors are of great importance in both the prevention and the treatment of infections.

Much practical experience has shown that one-sided public health programmes, aimed solely at improving diets or eradicating a single infectious disease, are relatively unsuccessful in raising the health of a community. This can best be improved by an attack on a broad front against all the factors that contribute to disease. Public health programmes must be well balanced and the activities of individual health workers integrated. Isolated programmes may do more harm than good by diverting money and distracting attention from other more important problems. Nutrition workers must always be in active collaboration with those whose duty it is to control infectious diseases and must make themselves acquainted with the problems and difficulties of other health workers.

Similarly all the staff of a public health department, especially those concerned with the control of infectious diseases, must appreciate the ill-effects of a poor diet on health and know something of the methods available for improving the nutrition of a community.

60. Food, Nutrition and Cancer

Cancer is a term used by both laymen and the medical profession to refer to malignant neoplasms or tumours. However, the term has no precise meaning and is not used by pathologists. Neoplasia or new growth is said to occur when cells in a tissue or organ proliferate without the normal controls on growth. In malignant neoplasms the cells spread to adjacent tissues by direct invasion or to distant organs by passage through blood or lymph vessels. Then a secondary tumour or metastasis forms. In benign neoplasms growth is limited to the organ of origin, and the tumour may have a well-defined capsule. Benign neoplasms usually cause symptoms only as a result of increasing size and the pressure which they may exert on other tissues. The distinction between benign and malignant neoplasms is usually, but not always, clear cut. Some benign neoplasms have a tendency to become malignant and there are certain hyperplastic states in which neoplasia is liable to arise; these are known as precancerous states. Many neoplasms are called by the name of the tissue together with the suffix '-oma'.

A malignant tumour arising in an epithelial tissue is known as a carcinoma and one arising in connective issue as a sarcoma. Leukaemia is a malignant condition in which the abnormal cells are in the blood and bone marrow.

The Greek word for a tumour is *onkos* and the study of neoplasia is known as oncology. Substances known to produce tumours are said to be carcinogenic or oncogenic.

Neoplasms occur in all animal species and can be studied in common laboratory animals. Irradiation, some viruses and chemical agents are proven oncogenic factors, and there is a well-defined genetic factor for some tumours. There are thus several known causes of cancer. However, in the great majority of cases of human cancer there is no obvious cause. Probably more than one factor is responsible in most cases.

The rate at which malignant neoplasms grow and their liability to form metastatic tumours varies from one type of neoplasm to another, and also in different individuals with the same neoplasm. For instance, one patient may be dead with metastases all over the body within a few weeks of the discovery of a neoplasm; another patient with an apparently similar tumour may be alive and well many years later. In many neoplasms there are intervals in which growth ceases or is very slow. Although it is most unusual, there are many well documented cases of spontaneous cure. There are immunological processes which may protect a patient against the spread of cancer but their nature is not well understood. Nutritional factors may contribute to this protection.

Neoplastic tissue may be removed by surgery or destroyed by radiation or chemotherapeutic agents. The effectiveness of these methods varies greatly depending on the site and nature of the tumour. Thus, provided the diagnosis is made early, the outlook for a patient with carcinoma of the colon or cervix uteri is good; it is at best very uncertain for a patient with carcinoma of the lung or stomach.

There are four separate nutritional problems related to cancer. First, diet may influence the incidence of tumours in a community; secondly, diet may influence the rate of growth of tumours; thirdly, malignancy almost always leads to undernutrition or malnutrition; and fourthly, many patients need special dietary therapy.

DIETARY FACTORS AND THE INCIDENCE OF CANCER

EPIDEMIOLOGY

The geographical distribution of cancer has been studied for many years, but has been beset by difficulties in standardising diagnostic criteria and methods of reporting. Partly as a result of the work of the International Union against Cancer, a reliable picture of the situation throughout the world is emerging. This is sketched out in an article by Doll (1972) and in a symposium which he introduced (Doll, 1973).

In brief, there is a variation in the incidence of cancer at all sites throughout the world. The incidence at many sites differs in some countries by factors which range from × 10 to × 400. Only a small part of this variation can be attributed to genetic factors; it is estimated that 80 per cent of human cancers are environmentally determined and so, in theory, preventable.

There is little to suggest that the incidence of cancer at such common sites in the body as the lung or the cervix uteri is in any way related to dietary habits. On the other hand, there is much to suggest that the wide variation in incidence of cancer at various sites in the alimentary canal and in the liver may be due to oncogenic factors in the diet. The segments of the gastrointestinal tract where cancer usually occurs are those in which the passage of contents down the lumen is slowed. These are the lower end of the oesophagus, the pyloric end of the stomach, the region of the ileocaecal valve and the left side of the large intestine. At these places there is more time for contact between an oncogenic agent derived from food and the mucous membrane. Once absorbed, an oncogenic agent passes to the liver, which is exposed to higher concentrations of it than other tissues. The agent or a water-soluble metabolite may be excreted by the kidneys and then comes in prolonged contact with the mucosa of the urinary bladder. The above are sites where repeated and prolonged chemical irritation may be oncogenic.

ONCOGENIC AGENTS

Many years ago chimney sweeps, cotton spinners and shale oil workers were known to have a high incidence of skin cancer attributed to prolonged exposure to soot or oil. In 1928 Kennaway first showed that a pure chemical, dibenzanthracene, when repeatedly applied to the skin, produced a squamous carcinoma. Many chemicals applied to the skin, inhaled or taken by mouth, are now known to be potentially oncogenic. In many instances exposure has to continue for a long period, sometimes up to 20 years, before a tumour develops. Oncogenic agents in foods may be natural substances or they can be chemicals deliberately added to food.

Tobacco

Tobacco smoke is a proven cause of carcinoma of the lung. Tobacco chewing may also be responsible for carcinoma of the buccal cavity and of the oesophagus (see below).

Aflatoxins

These are a group of complex difuranocoumarins formed by some strains of the mould *Aspergillus flavus*, which may grow on groundnuts and other foods when stored in damp warm conditions after harvesting. In animals a single dose of aflatoxin causes acute poisoning with severe liver damage; and aflatoxin B_1 is the most potent hepatic carcinogen known. Only 0.2 μg/day in the diet for 470 days induces liver tumours in 100 per cent of rats. In some parts of the world human foods have been found to be contaminated with small amounts of alfatoxins and this may contribute to a high incidence of hepatoma in some areas (see below).

Pyrrolizidine alkaloids

These substances are present in many species of the herbs *Senecio* and *Crotalaria* and they have been shown to produce hepatoma in rats. These herbs are sometimes used for making bush teas and this practice may be responsible for some human cases of hepatoma.

Cycad nuts

Cycads are an ancient family of tree-ferns grown in many parts of the tropics. Their nuts, which have been much used both as food and medicine in some countries, contain the glycoside, cycasin, which causes tumours of the liver in rats and guinea pigs, but is not known to do so in man.

Nitrosamines

Nitrites may react with secondary amines in the gut to form a class of compounds known as nitrosamines. Some of these, e.g. dimethylnitrosamine, have been shown to be oncogenic in experimental animals. Nitrates are widespread in the soil and present in small amounts in plant and animal tissues, where they may be reduced to nitrites. Nitrates and nitrites are added to foods for their preservative action, especially against clostridial infections of meats. Nitrosamines have been found in several foods in concentrations of the order of 0.1 to 5 μg/kg and also in gastric juice. It is not certain to what extent they arise from added or naturally occurring nitrites. Although there is evidence consistent with the view that ingested nitrate could be a contributary cause of carcinoma of the stomach (see below), nitrates are permitted food additives. The FAO/WHO acceptable daily intake is up to 125 mg/kg body weight.

Food additives

The dye, butter yellow, and the sweetener, cyclamate, were formerly added to foods, but are no longer permitted since they have been shown to produce tumours in experimental animals. All food additives have to undergo rigorous tests for oncogenic activity in animals before they are permitted to be used in foods.

The above observations show that oncogenic agents may be present in the food of all classes of people. Primitive rural and industrialised urban communities may each be at risk. However, the risks, except in a few well known cases, appear to be small. The possible role of dietary oncogenic agents in the aetiology of specific tumours is now discussed.

TUMOURS OF THE ALIMENTARY TRACT AND LIVER

Tongue, buccal mucosa and pharynx

These are the commonest sites for tumours in Bombay and such tumours are also common in many parts of south-east Asia, south-east Africa and Puerto Rico; they are uncommon in Europe and the USA. The relative incidence may differ by a factor of 30. Many more males than females are affected in Bombay where the tumours are associated with chewing *pan,* a green vine leaf in which are rolled sliced betel nut, tobacco, slaked lime and some small amounts of other spices. No specific oncogenic agent has been identified.

Oesophagus

Incidence varies greatly. Standardised rates per 100 000 persons aged 35 to 64 years are low (below 6) in most European countries, in the white population of the USA and South Africa, in Australia, in Nigeria and in Uganda. They are moderately high (from 15 to 30) in Switzerland, France, the non-white population of the USA, India and Japan, and very high (over 60) in the African population of southern and eastern Africa. Rates over 100 have been reported in some USSR and Iranian towns bordering on the Caspian Sea.

Carcinoma of the oesophagus is frequently associated with alcoholism and excessive smoking or chewing of tobacco, but this does not explain the wide variations in incidence. In Africa it is associated with drinking beer made from maize (Cook, 1971). Incidence varies greatly in towns round the Caspian Sea, and very high rates are found in the south-east corner, where the soil is dry and salty (Joint Iran/IARC Study Group, 1977). The people are Muslim and do not take alcohol or tobacco. Their diet is monotonous and consists of coarse wheat bread, tea, milk and a little meat; fruit and vegetables are lacking; oncogens have not been found in local foods. Urinary metabolites of morphine were found and it appears that opium is eaten. The area of high incidence extends over the border of Iran to south central USSR and right across Asia to parts of northern China. The high incidence in northern Iran appears to go back to antiquity, but in southern Africa carcinoma of the oesophagus was rare 40 years ago.

Stomach
Standardised incidence rates for carcinoma of the stomach vary from over 160 per 100 000 in Japan to less than 10 in some African countries. Other areas with high rates are Iceland, Costa Rico, Chile and parts of Colombia and Eastern Europe. In most parts of Europe it ranges from 30 to 60. In the USA it is 36 in the non-white population, but only 15 in the whites. In India it is 17 and in Australia 23. In South Africa the rate is a little lower in the African than in the white population, a marked contrast to the rates for carcinoma of the oesophagus. In general, the rate falls from east to west as one goes from the USSR to the USA. Rates in immigrant groups tend to correspond more closely to those of the host country than to their country of origin; this particularly applies to Japanese. Clearly, an environmental factor plays a major part in aetiology and it is a reasonable guess that this enters the body with the diet.

The incidence of carcinoma of the stomach is highest in the lower socioeconomic classes but has been falling for the last 20 years or more in most industrial countries, including the USA and Japan. There is a slightly greater incidence in people of blood group A, which reflects the genetic contribution, and an increased risk in patients with chronic atrophic gastritis.

Dietary studies show positive associations of carcinoma of the stomach with salted or pickled foods, e.g. dried salted fish or cured meats and with environmental nitrate (in well water, soil fertilisers, etc.). But negative associations have been found with salad vegetables, citrus fruit and milk consumption (Haenszel and Correa, 1975). The most plausible hypothesis at present to link all these features is that dietary nitrates may be reduced to nitrites and react in the stomach with secondary amines (from fermented foods) to form nitrosamines. Conditions are suitable for nitrosamine formation in patients with atrophic gastritis (Ruddell et al., 1978). But vitamin C inhibits the nitrosation reaction and refrigeration probably reduces production of secondary amines.

Small intestine
Tumours of the small intestine are rare in all countries. This might be because the contents are not in contact with the mucous membrane for as long as in the stomach and the large intestine.

Large intestine
Standardised incidence rates for carcinoma of the colon are low (0 to 5 per 100 000) in most African countries, higher (5 to 15) in Asian countries, including Japan, and much higher (15 to 35) in Europe, North America and Australia. Japanese migrants to the USA acquire the higher incidence in the first generation. The disease is associated with affluence and coronary heart disease. Comparisons between countries show a positive correlation ($r = + 0.6$) between incidence and both total fat and meat consumption (Armstrong and Doll, 1975a). Three hypotheses, not mutually exclusive, may help to explain these dietary associations.

High fat intake. This is accompanied by increased secretion of bile acids. Some of their desaturated metabolites present in the faeces are oncogenic when tested on animals. These are formed by the action of some of the bacterial flora of the colon and there may be more such bacteria in populations where incidence of the disease is high (Hill, 1975). Cholesterol is also formed from bile acids in the gut but, surprisingly, in six prospective studies of coronary heart disease, plasma cholesterols in those subjects who later developed carcinoma of the colon were lower than the standard values (Rose et al., 1974).

High meat intakes. Meat and total fat intakes are usually correlated, but in Copenhagen meat intake is higher and fat consumption lower than in rural Finland; and yet incidence of carcinoma of the colon is four times higher in Copenhagen (International Agency for Research on Cancer, 1977). Meat itself is unlikely to contain oncogens but they might be formed during roasting and grilling.

Low fibre intakes. Burkitt (1971) pointed out that increasing the dietary fibre shortens the transit time of food in the gut and makes the contents of the colon more watery; therefore, if any exogenous or endogenous oncogen is present, the mucosa is exposed to it for a shorter time and at a lower concentration. The weights of the stools, an index of the fibre content of the diet, were found to be higher in rural Finland than in Copenhagen and are in general much higher in African than in European populations. In this way a high fibre diet may protect against carcinoma of the colon.

Carcinoma is less common in the rectum than in the colon but, as the site is not always correctly recorded, there is some confusion in the figures. Carcinoma of the rectum is commoner in men than women and may be correlated with beer consumption (Breslow and Enstrom, 1974), but not so closely as to cause the authors to change their habits.

Liver

Whereas primary carcinoma of the liver is rare in Europe and North America, it is commonly seen in many parts of Africa. The work of Peers and Linsell (1973) suggested that aflatoxins were in part responsible, at least in Kenya. After measuring the aflatoxin content of 2400 samples of food in one district, they concluded that dietary intakes ranged from 1 to 21 μg/kg body weight daily. Carcinoma of the liver accounted for about half of the total number of cases of malignant disease in the community. Carcinoma of the liver was rarely found in areas where dietary intakes of aflatoxins were less than 5 μg/kg body weight daily. Similar geographical association of aflatoxins in food and primary carcinoma of the liver is found in Mozambique, which has the highest incidence in the world, and in Thailand (Wogan, 1975). The risk of exposure to aflatoxins is much less in industrialised countries.

TUMOURS AT OTHER SITES

Breast

Carcinoma of the breast has a similar geographic distribution to carcinoma of the colon. A high incidence (100 or more per 100000) is found in the USA, Canada, northwest Europe, Australasia and the white population of South Africa. It is commoner in the higher socioeconomic classes and in unmarried and nulliparous women. The protective effect of pregnancy is greater when it has occurred before the age of 25 years. Lactation has only a small protective effect, but oophorectomy and an early artificial menopause reduces the risk. Migrants from Japan, where the incidence is low, to the USA develop a high rate but only after two generations. The environmental factors responsible for the differences between countries therefore appear to operate early in life. Obesity is a little more common in patients with the disease than in control groups. Comparisons between countries show that the dietary component with the strongest correlation with incidence of the disease is total fat intake (Armstrong and Doll, 1975a). It is the commoner post-menopausal type of the disease which differs between countries and appears to show partial relationship to the diet. It has been suggested that high fat intakes lead to patterns of hormone secretion, more oestradiol and oestrone, less oestriol, which favour oncogenesis. Differences in the patterns of urinary oes-

trogens of Japanese and Caucasian women are in keeping with this view (Dickinson et al., 1974) Alternatively, animal experiments suggest that prolactin could be the intermediary hormone in the promotion by dietary fat of mammary tumours in rats given a chemical oncogen (Chan and Cohen, 1975). Berg (1975) even speculates that 'the present affluent diet from childhood onward may overstimulate the endocrine system, producing the same effects that one would obtain running a diesel engine on high-octane airplane fuel.' In well-nourished populations the onset of menstruation is earlier and there is a higher incidence not only of neoplasms of the breast but also of the ovary (British Medical Journal, 1978) and endometrium of the uterus (Geisler et al., 1969), organs which depend on sex hormones for their normal function.

Urinary bladder

The artificial sweeteners cyclamate and saccharin have induced bladder tumours in animals when given in very high dosage. The human population who have taken relatively large amounts of saccharin are diabetics but in Britain they have not shown any excess of deaths from bladder cancer (Armstrong and Doll, 1975b).

The relationship between diet and cancer is an important and growing field of research. Components of food or drink may contain exogenous oncogens or stimulate production of endogenous oncogens or hormones that favour oncogenesis. Further, a dietary factor may be protective (e.g. fibre) or a dietary deficiency may predispose to cancer. Although the cause of most human cancers is unknown, many oncogenic agents have been identified and their actions are known to be affected by genetic factors and by environmental factors, which include the diet. Methods for recording the food intake of populations for studies on the epidemiology of cancer need to be different from those for investigating the prevalence of malnutrition. Up to now they have mostly been inadequate or inappropriate but they are improving as there is more dialogue between epidemiologists and nutritional scientists (Sixth Marabou Symposium, 1979).

DIET AND TUMOUR GROWTH

Tumours, like the tissues of the body, need nutrients which are derived ultimately from the diet. In theory, it might be possible to devise a diet on which the tissues could survive and a tumour cease to grow. There are many reports describing how reducing the energy content of a diet or the amount of an essential nutrient inhibited the growth of tumours in experimental animals (Shils, 1973; Alcantara and Speckmann, 1975). Unfortunately, in humans, malignant tumours often grow rapidly in an emaciated and malnourished body.

Two attempts to interfere with the nutrition of a tumour have met with some success. A folic acid antagonist, methotrexate, which reduces production of RNA and DNA, has an established place in the treatment of chorion carcinoma and leukaemia. The amino acid asparagine can be synthesised by mammalian cells, but not by some malignant cells. A preparation of the enzyme, asparaginase, produced by bacteria *Escherichia coli* has been reported to produce remissions in some types of leukaemia. Finally, there is a preliminary report of the regression of some human malignant tumours when magnesium and potassium deficiency has been induced by diet and haemodialysis (Parsons *et al.*, 1974).

MALIGNANT DISEASE AS A CAUSE OF MALNUTRITION

Severe emaciation and malnutrition follow an untreated malignant tumour of the alimentary tract at any site from the lips down to the pyloric sphincter. This is readily explainable by mechanical interference with eating, swallowing or the passage of food from stomach to duodenum.

With neoplasms at other sites, some patients do not lose weight and appear well nourished despite the presence of a large tumour and sometimes numerous secondaries. However, a cancer patient usually loses some weight and may become extremely emaciated. This is sometimes due to secondary bacterial infection or pressure on a vital structure, but often there is no obvious cause. When a middle-aged or elderly person loses weight for no apparent reason, he should have a thorough clinical and radiological examination for the presence of a neoplasm.

The loss of weight in patients with malignant neoplasm may sometimes be explained by loss of appetite. Anorexia is often marked, but why this should be so is far from clear. Possibly severe cachexia may be the result of metabolic disturbances brought about by the tumour. Some neoplasms are known to produce kinins and hormones, which have marked effects on other tissues of the body. The best-known example is the Zollinger–Ellison syndrome in which there are multiple peptic ulcers arising from excess secretion of gastrin by a carcinoma in the pancreas or duodenal wall. There may be a loss of tissue amino acids due to the catabolic action of a neoplasm. It is also possible that some neoplasms produce a lipid-mobilising factor. It is seldom humane to ask a patient with severe malignant cachexia to undergo the inconveniences and discomforts of an elaborate metabolic investigation, from which there is little hope that he himself will derive benefit. This is why so little is known about malignant cachexia. The extent of our ignorance is shown in a report by DeWys (1970) on a conference of the American Cancer Society.

DIETARY THERAPY

Doctors and dietitians should be constantly aware of the diagnostic significance of loss of weight, anorexia and food aversions as early signs of malignant disease. When the diagnosis has been made and a programme of ablative surgery, radiation or treatment with cytotoxic drugs laid down, a supportive diet should be carefully drawn up. This should be higher than normal in energy and nutrient content, and in a form which is acceptable and appetising to the patient while avoiding any food aversions he may have. Should there be uncorrectable obstruction to the functions of eating, mastication, swallowing or digestion these must be bypassed by dividing the day's diet into smaller and more frequent feedings or by parenteral feeding. Some applicable special feeding methods are discussed in Chapter 52. These include nasogastric tube feeds, parenteral alimentation and feeding by gastrostomy or jejunostomy. Dietary modifications may be necessary as a result of ileostomy and colostomy. There is no evidence that a good diet can cure any type of cancer, but there is no doubt that it can add greatly to the comfort of the patient. Since the ultimate hope for the patient may lie in a strong immune reaction to the invading tumour cells, and since there is evidence that a good diet supports the immune system, a rational basis for diet therapy is at least dimly perceptible.

For the most part, however, good diet therapy supports the patient's morale; it provides normal pleasurable gratifications of the body and mind when these are being restricted by advancing disease. Great care should therefore be taken about the aesthetic aspects of the diet, such as arrangement, appearance, odour or bouquet, and taste of the foods. Wine and other alcoholic liquors in moderation may be of great help, although occasionally, as in a few cases of Hodgkin's disease, they may bring on pain.

When a patient is going downhill with an apparently incurable disease, he and his relatives may catch at any straw. Innumerable cancer nostrums have been promoted by well-meaning enthusiasts and by rogues wanting to make a fast buck. Laetrile, which has caused a legal furore in the USA, is a cycanogenic glucoside obtained from apricot pips. Its promoters claim that it is a vitamin which is untrue and the evidence that it cures cancer is only anecdotal (Jukes, 1977). The legal and other problems posed by 'laetrileomania' are discussed by Ingelfinger (1977).

Finally, there comes a time when the battle is lost. Henceforth there is no point in prolonging life by fussy and uncomfortable attentions. The dietitian should accept the verdict of the doctor and feed the patient in whatever way is most comfortable and least distasteful to him. His nutrition no longer matters; what matters is to keep up as far as possible his morale and whatever enjoyment remains in the sight and taste of food.

PART VI

Diet and Physiological Status

61. Pregnancy, Lactation, Infancy, Childhood and Adolescence

PREGNANCY

Despite our ignorance of many aspects of nutrition in pregnancy and lactation, there is much sound empirical knowledge gained in medical practice in favour of the view that the expectant mother needs a good mixed diet. When assessing the relation of diet to pregnancy the following problems require consideration:
1. What is the effect of diet on fertility?
2. What is the effect on the outcome of pregnancy of the diet eaten in the years prior to a woman becoming pregnant?
3. What is the effect on the outcome of pregnancy of the diet eaten during pregnancy?

An admirable monograph *The Physiology of Human Pregnancy* by Hytten and Leitch (1971) gives a full account of the relation of diet to pregnancy. A WHO report (1965) on *Nutrition in Pregnancy and Lactation* is also recommended.

DIET AND REPRODUCTIVE EFFICIENCY

Diet and fertility
The very high birth rate in poor women in Asia, Africa and other underdeveloped countries in which the diet is notoriously defective in many nutrients, suggests that it is very unlikely that undernutrition or malnutrition plays a significant role in fertility.

During and after the occupation of Singapore by the Japanese in World War II, food was very scarce and there was also a great increase in prices. Despite the poor nutrition of large numbers of women (Chinese, Malays and Indians), fertility was not impaired. The pre-war and immediate post-war figures for the birth rate were both between 45 and 50 per 1000 of the population (Millis, 1952).

In Europe and North America, the much lower birth rates are not due to reduced fertility consequent on overnutrition, but to the knowledge of contraception and to family planning. Reduced conception rates were, however, reported in Holland in 1944 when there was an acute food shortage for six months, and in Russia during the siege of Leningrad in 1942. The dietary deficiencies and emotional stresses were greater and more prolonged in the siege of Leningrad than in Holland. It is probable that the amenorrhoea which occurred so frequently in Dutch and

Russian women during these times of stress was due both to psychological and nutritional causes.

Diet prior to pregnancy
The likelihood of a normal labour is better in women brought up in good circumstances, who have eaten a satisfactory diet from birth to maturity, who have received good medical care and who continue to have these advantages during pregnancy, than in women of the poorer socioeconomic classes. The chances of such a woman producing a healthy baby are also better (British Perinatal Survey, 1969). This is not surprising since the size of the pelvis is closely correlated with height, and in well-nourished women the shape of the pelvic brim is round. In women who have had rickets in childhood the pelvic brim may be very much flattened and even kidney shaped owing to the extent of the projection of the promontory of the sacrum downwards. Such severe deformities of the pelvis are rare nowadays, but flattening of the posterior segment of the brim is still found in short stunted women.

Other factors influencing a satisfactory outcome of pregnancy are fetal size and presentation. The introduction of antibiotics and better hygiene, housing and general medical care have all helped to reduce the hazards of labour. The outcome of pregnancy may be influenced more by these factors and by the diet prior to conception than by the diet eaten during pregnancy.

Diet during pregnancy
Birth weight of infants. The diet of pregnant women of the upper socioeconomic class in Aberdeen contains more energy, protein, calcium and vitamins than the diet of women in the lower socioeconomic class (Thomson, 1958). The average weight of full-term babies in the former class is higher than those in the lower socioeconomic class. There is good statistical evidence to show that a high energy intake during pregnancy is associated with a birth weight which is above the average (Thomson, 1959). In India 29 per cent of babies of women from the lower socioeconomic classes, but only 14 per cent of those from the higher socioeconomic classes had birth weights below 2.5 kg (Belavady, 1969).

During periods of severe malnutrition, birth weights fall. In contrast to the unchanged fertility rate, Millis (1952) found that the average birth weights of Indian and

Chinese babies in Singapore was significantly lower in 1947 than in 1950, when the nutritional situation had considerably improved but was still far from satisfactory.

At various periods between 1940 and 1945 in Holland, France, Austria, Germany and Russia, there was a grave shortage of food. Ample evidence from these countries shows that when the mothers were severely undernourished there was a decrease in the birth weight of their infants and that this could be correlated with the degree of undernourishment.

In a trial in Taiwan women were given daily throughout pregnancy either of two supplements. One provided 20 g protein, 1700 kJ of energy, minerals and vitamins; the other only 170 kJ, no protein and the same minerals and vitamins. In a second pregnancy the same mothers were given the alternative supplement. While the increases in mean birth weights were very small in babies of mothers who had taken the protein and energy supplement, there were significantly fewer babies below 2500 g (Blackwell *et al.*, 1973). A supplementation trial in four rural villages in Guatemala similarly showed fewer babies with low birth weight were born to mothers who took larger amounts of either of two supplements (a gruel or a refreshing drink), only one of which contained protein. Extra energy thus appeared to increase the birth weight, but not extra protein, under the conditions of this experiment (Lechtig *et al.*, 1975).

Low birth weights from whatever cause are associated with increased death rates. More than half the babies born weighing less than 1.5 kg do not survive one week. However, if the baby weighs 2 kg the chances of survival are good, provided proper care is available.

Weight gain in pregnancy. It is normal for a woman to gain 3.5 kg (8 lb) in weight by the end of the first 20 weeks of pregnancy and thereafter to gain about 0.5 kg or 1 lb a week until term, when the total gain is 12.5 kg (28 lb). Table 61.1 gives an analysis of how these weight gains are made up. Besides the products of conception and increased size of the reproductive organs, blood volume expands; as the plasma increases a little more than the red cells, it is normal for the haemoglobin concentration in the blood to fall slightly by the end of the pregnancy. In the last 10 weeks there is an increase in the extracellular water, additional to the increase in plasma. The extra fat deposited is about 4 kg. This is an energy store of 150 MJ (36 000 kcal), enough to supply the needs of the body for two to three weeks in an emergency. This fat is deposited throughout pregnancy, but especially in the period between 10 and 20 weeks.

These are average figures and wide variations are compatible with health. If the weight gain is less than half that anticipated, a careful search for the cause should be made. This may be either an inadequate dietary intake or excessive physical activity. If these two are excluded, the possibility of a major physical disorder should be considered. An excessive gain in weight, more than 50 per cent above the figure given, may be due to accumulation of oedema fluid as well as fat.

When obesity is present, pregnancy is more likely to be attended by pregnancy hypertension, and other undesirable complications. Emerson (1962) reviews the literature and gives the findings in his studies of 1145 cases. An average gain in weight of a little less than 0.5 kg per week during the second half of pregnancy is associated with the lowest overall rates for pregnancy hypertension, prematurity and perinatal mortality. With higher rates of gain, the chances of developing pregnancy hypertension are increased, whereas with lower rates there is an increase of prematurity (Thomson and Billewicz, 1957). Yet there is no satisfactory evidence that overnutrition is the primary cause of pregnancy hypertension.

Some women, mainly in the USA, have been led by fashion to restrict their diets so as to reduce their gain in weight to less than 7 kg. This practice may lead to the delivery of babies of low birth weight with increased risk of perinatal death.

Stillbirth rates, perinatal mortality rates and maternal morbidity rates. The policy of food rationing in Britain during World War II and the placing of pregnant women in a priority group which received extra rations of milk, cod-liver oil and fruit juice, greatly improved the diet of women belonging to the lower socioeconomic class. This measure was undoubtedly a factor in causing a fall in the stillbirth rate from about 38 to

Table 61.1 Analysis of the weight gain in pregnancy (modified from Hytten and Leitch, 1971)

		Increase in weight		
		Up to 10 weeks (g)	20 weeks (g)	30 weeks (g)	40 weeks (g)
Fetus, placenta and liquor		55	720	2530	4750
Uterus and breasts		170	765	1170	1300
Blood		100	600	1300	1250
Extracellular water		—	—	—	1200
Fat (by difference)		325	1915	3500	4000
	Total gain	650	4000	8500	12500

28 per 1000. The fall was greatest in South Wales where unemployment had been high before the war started. This decrease appears less impressive when it is restated as follows: after the institution of priority rationing during the war, 97 per cent of pregnant women in Britain had a live child, compared with 96 per cent before the war. In Singapore between 1947 and 1950 a decrease in maternal mortality, neonatal and infant mortality rates may have resulted from better nutrition of the mother and child (Millis, 1952). However, during this period, there was not only an improvement in the diet, but health services were re-established. It is always difficult to determine the extent to which diet, as distinct from other environmental factors, including medical care, influences beneficially or adversely the outcome of pregnancy.

In Hong Kong, the stillbirth rate is low when one takes into account that a high proportion of the Chinese families are of refugee origin and live in grossly overcrowded conditions. However, the nutritional state of the women and children in these families is good. This is because of the industry and efficiency of the people. A joint investigation by the University Departments of Obstetrics in Hong Kong and Aberdeen (Thomson et al., 1963) showed that the incidence of most causes of stillbirths, including pregnancy hypertension, and of fetal malformation was lower in Hong Kong than in Aberdeen.

DIETARY REQUIREMENTS IN PREGNANCY

There are no 'special diets' for pregnancy, nor are there any particular foods that must be taken or avoided. Nevertheless, most pregnant women require some dietary advice as to how best to modify their usual diet so as to supply the extra needs for nutrients. The nature of this advice depends on the economic status of the family and the foods available. The recommended extra intakes for nutrients during pregnancy are on pages 153 and 154.

To account for the fact that pregnant women living on poor diets have often been observed to show surprisingly little evidence of malnutrition, Beaton (1961) suggested that 'adaptive changes take place in the pregnant woman to minimise the requirements for protein, iron and calcium'. This is a sensible idea.

Protein. Naismith and Ritchie (1975) have shown that rats store protein in the maternal tissues in early pregnancy and transfer it in late pregnancy to the rapidly growing fetus and that with these changes there are changes in activities of several enzymes controlling amino acid metabolism. In this way the protein cost of pregnancy is distributed over the whole period of gestation. The scope of metabolic experiments in pregnant women is greatly limited by ethical considerations. However, low concentrations of blood urea have been known for many years (Peters and van Slyke, 1932) and this indicates that a greater proportion of dietary amino acids are used for protein storage and less for gluconeogenesis and use as a fuel. Protein metabolism during pregnancy and its relation to maternal diet is reviewed by Naismith (1977).

The increased need for protein is met by half a litre of milk daily, which provides 18 to 20 g. In many countries poor women have to depend on cereals for their main source of protein. A good mixture of plant proteins should be taken and can be an effective substitute for milk.

Iron. Anaemia is common in pregnant women because of the increased demands for iron by the mother and fetus. Of 1071 patients seen in Edinburgh in the first 11 weeks of pregnancy (Kerr and Davidson, 1958), 32 per cent were mildly anaemic (haemoglobin level less than 12.6 g/dl). The reduction in haemoglobin levels was due to anaemia and not to physiological dilution of the blood as this is minimal during the first trimester of pregnancy. Incidence of iron deficiency anaemia in pregnancy is much higher in many parts of the world. Even women with high initial levels often have a large fall in the second or third trimester. For these reasons we recommend: (1) a liberal diet with a good supply of meat, fruit and vegetables; (2) routine haemoglobin estimation at the first visit to an antenatal clinic; (3) iron therapy for all patients with an initial haemoglobin level of less than 12.0 g/dl; (4) iron therapy from the twenty-fourth week to term. This can be taken in the form of one pill containing 180 mg of ferrous sulphate three times a day, which provides a total of 180 mg of elemental iron daily. This raises the haemoglobin in most women, and is a valuable prophylaxis against anaemia.

Calcium. The extra needs for calcium to make the bones of the fetus are best met by increasing the milk intake. Half a litre of milk supplies about 600 mg of calcium, half of the recommended intake.

Vitamins. Milk, fruit and vegetables in adequate amounts can supply all the necessary vitamins. If a good mixed diet is eaten there is no need to prescribe any vitamin supplements. When there is any doubt about the quality of the diet, a concentrated fruit juice and vitamin A and D tablets or a fish-liver oil should be given.

We also advise a small daily supplement of synthetic folic acid (300 μg) for all women during the last trimester to prevent megaloblastic anaemia. Although megaloblastic anaemia of pregnancy is not common in Britain, it is potentially severe and dangerous. In countries, where the diet and medical services are inadequate, a supplement of folic acid in the last trimester of pregnancy is clearly indicated.

Energy. Extra energy is required for the growth of the fetus and also to meet the increased physiological needs of the mother (p. 24); in some social circumstances it is likely to become available through a restriction in physical activities, in which case there is no necessity for an increase in the quantity of the diet. This is important, for there is no doubt that an excessive intake of energy (as judged by the weighing machine) is harmful. Measured energy expenditure and consumption in American pregnant women are reported by Blackburn and Calloway (1976). Mean energy intakes averaged around 8.4 MJ (2000 kcal)/day, less than the calculated need, and varied greatly between individuals, all of whom put on weight adequately. A proper balance between energy intake and energy output is necessary. Many women, especially those responsible for the care of young children, lead a very active life when pregnant. Others, particularly primigravidas who live in towns, may reduce their normal physical recreations. For such it is better to continue their recreations rather than to reduce the intake of food. Many hobbies and sports can be continued in a modified form until the last trimester of pregnancy, and this is to be recommended provided very strenuous activity is avoided. In the last few weeks walking is the most satisfactory form of exercise.

Any marked departure from the normal rate of gain demands attention. A pregnant woman should be weighed monthly up to the 20th week of pregnancy; thereafter she should be weighed and examined once every one or two weeks. If she has gained no weight at all, or if she has gained too much weight she should be given a full medical examination; if no pathological explanation can be found, she should be advised either to increase or reduce her diet. All obstetricians are agreed on the undesirability of excessive gain in weight during pregnancy. This weight may not be lost after delivery and with successive pregnancies frank obesity may develop.

General advice

Some women have a greatly increased appetite and this may lead to gross obesity with all its ill-effects. In others there may be a longing for some unusual article of food. Such bizarre appetites (pica) appear much less common than formerly. The explanation for these whims is uncertain. Pregnant women should be told frankly that such behaviour and cravings are not a normal accompaniment of pregnancy but are not serious. An effort should be made to correct them by simple explanation and encouragement. Heartburn and other symptoms of indigestion are common and sometimes troublesome, especially in the last trimester, when pressure from the enlarged uterus on the stomach may be responsible. Often there is no obvious cause and no treatment is necessary beyond advising the patient to avoid foods commonly associated with indigestion (see Diet No. 17), to take frequent small meals, to use insoluble antacids as required and to avoid bending or lying flat. Constipation and also haemorrhoids are common minor complications of pregnancy. To minimise this, women should be advised to eat plenty of wheat fibre as wholemeal bread or bran products as well as the fruit and vegetables recommended above.

With regard to the need for fluid, milk has already been recommended. A glass of water immediately on rising in the morning and at each main meal is desirable; tea and coffee may be taken in moderation.

The dangers of excess alcohol in pregnancy are now established. A **fetal alcohol syndrome** found in children of alcoholic mothers consisting of low birth weight, low intelligence and congenital defects, especially of the face, is recognised as a public health problem in several countries (Kessell, 1977). In Boston the incidence of congenital anomalies in children whose mothers were alcoholics was four times as great as in children whose mothers were abstainers (Oulette et al., 1977). In a survey of middle-class mothers in Washington Little (1977) found a negative correlation between daily alcohol consumption and birth weight, but the effect was small and there were no other adverse consequences of moderate drinking. It is thus necessary to warn mothers, in appropriate cases, of the serious effects that heavy drinking may have on their child, but there are not grounds for a total prohibition of alcohol during pregnancy for all women.

There is no need to restrict the intake of salt provided it is taken in moderation unless oedema is present. The evidence supporting the view that salt restriction reduces the incidence of pregnancy hypertension and hydramnios is far from convincing. Indeed, there is some evidence to the contrary (Robinson, 1958).

DISORDERS OF PREGNANCY

Morning sickness

In the early weeks of pregnancy most women suffer a little from nausea, especially in the early morning, and there may be vomiting. The cause of this is not known. 'Morning sickness' is certainly not psychological in origin, although psychological factors often aggravate the symptoms. It may be presumed that these arise from some metabolic or endocrine change brought about by the presence of the fetus or placenta, to which adjustment is usually quickly made.

There are innumerable 'old wives' remedies for morning sickness, but unfortunately no scientific treatment. The patient should be reassured that the condition will shortly disappear. Occasional morning sickness in early pregnancy may be relieved by taking a light snack before rising. Psychological disturbances may require treatment. If the vomiting persists, an antiemetic drug, e.g. cyclizine 50 mg/day by mouth, may be given.

In some women, both primigravidas and multigravidas, morning sickness and nausea become progressively worse. The cause is not known but a psychological element is certainly a contributory factor. Vomiting may persist throughout the day so that neither fluid nor food is retained. The resulting metabolic changes may be severe and then she should be admitted to hospital; in many cases this measure alone stops the vomiting. It is necessary to correct the dehydration, ketosis, haemoconcentration and the electrolyte imbalance which are the consequence of vomiting and nausea; the patient should receive ample amounts of fluid, carbohydrates, electrolytes and water-soluble vitamins, especially thiamin and pyridoxine. These can be given by mouth in mild cases, or intravenously in severe cases. With improvement of the patient's condition, which usually occurs within a day or two of admission to hospital, the diet can be gradually increased.

Pregnancy hypertension

The terms 'toxaemia of pregnancy' and pre-eclampsia were formerly used to describe a group of disorders characterised by a raised blood pressure, oedema and albuminuria which develops for the first time during pregnancy. As no toxin has been identified and the condition seldom leads to eclampsia, these terms are unsuitable and the condition is best referred to as pregnancy hypertension. It is convenient to describe two forms.

Mild pregnancy hypertension. The patient feels well but the blood pressure is slightly raised, i.e. over 140/90 mmHg. There may be slight oedema of the ankles and a trace of albumin in the urine. The urinary output is well maintained and the specific gravity is normal. The condition is common and was found in 24 per cent of primigravida and 10 per cent of multigravida in a survey in Scotland. With good antenatal care the prognosis is excellent.

Severe pregnancy hypertension. The blood pressure is over 160/100 mmHg. In addition the oedema is increased in degree and may extend to the hands, face and abdominal wall. Albuminuria exceeds 250 mg/24 hours. In very severe cases other serious features are headache, disturbances of vision, vomiting and oliguria. This condition is relatively rare, occurring in the Scottish survey in 5 per cent of primigravidas and 1 per cent of multigravidas, but is associated with greatly increased risk to both the mother and fetus.

Treatment

For mild cases modified rest, i.e. two hours rest in bed in the afternoon, and adequate sleep, achieved if necessary by the use of a sedative or hypnotic drug, are of prime importance. It is unnecessary to restrict fluids or protein foods, since renal function is satisfactory.

Severe cases and mild cases which do not respond to the above treatment should be admitted to hospital. In addition to complete bed rest, and the administration of adequate amounts of sedative and hypnotic drugs, the protein intake should be reduced. Antihypertensive drugs should seldom be used as they may reduce uteroplacental blood flow and so jeopardise the fetus. If vomiting is a marked feature, the patient may be able to take only small amounts of milk and diluted fruit juice at two-hourly intervals until improvement occurs. If as is usual, the patient improves in hospital, she may be allowed home, but should be kept under close observation. When there is

no improvement, it is best for the mother if the pregnancy is terminated.

Eclampsia

This condition may follow severe pregnancy hypertension and is recognised by the development of epileptiform convulsions. Medical treatment is the same as that described for severe pregnancy hypertension and in addition, the fits should be treated by suitable sedative drugs such as intravenous magnesium sulphate. If severe oliguria (less than 200 ml/day) or anuria occurs, the output of nitrogen in the urine diminishes and correspondingly the blood urea rises. Then treatment consists in giving glucose 100 to 300 g daily and fluid in limited quantities (500 to 1000 ml daily) intravenously or by intragastric drip. Delivery by Caesarian section is advisable in most cases.

LACTATION

Peasant women, like all mammals, lactate 'with nae bother at all', to use a common Scottish term of speech. For them it is a part of life and a natural experience which gives emotional satisfaction. Urban life and the acquisition of wealth each bring distractions and for many women make lactation difficult and sometimes distasteful. The decline in breast feeding was marked. In the decade 1960–70 no more than 15 per cent of infants in Scotland got a significant amount of breast milk (Arneil, 1967), and this figure probably applied to most European and North American communities (Fomon, 1971), and to the wealthy in Africa and Asia. In some countries this decline has stopped and is being reversed. Thus in 1975 in England and Wales 51 per cent of babies were put to the breast at birth, 24 per cent were being breast fed at 6 weeks and 13 per cent at 4 months; a baby's chance of being breast fed was higher the higher the social class of its mother and the longer her period of full-time education (DHSS, 1978; Martin, 1978).

Paid employment and a full social life are obstacles to lactation. Fashion, advertisements for artificial milks and, regretfully, often the convenience for staff of obstetrical wards each operate against natural feeding. The European visitor to India may be surprised to see women contentedly suckling their babies under the shade of a wayside tree or on the platform of a railway station. He may never have seen a baby at the breast before, since in most parts of Europe there is a taboo against suckling, except in strictest privacy. This taboo is an important factor against breast feeding. However, the main reason given by British mothers who had started feeding their baby and given it up at 6 weeks, was that they thought that the baby was not getting sufficient milk (Martin, 1978). If this was indeed true, the failure of lactation was probably due to psychological causes. Experience in other societies is that it is unusual for a healthy woman with no local disease of the breast to fail to produce enough milk for her baby.

ARGUMENTS FOR AND AGAINST BREAST FEEDING

It is of course common knowledge that many millions of babies have been reared successfully on cow's milk or on preparations based on it. The majority appear none the worse for the experience. Nevertheless the consensus of medical opinion is that mothers' milk is the best food for babies at least in the first weeks of life. The arguments in favour of breast feeding are very different in a poor urban community and a wealthy society.

Artificial feeding in a community is satisfactory only if three conditions are met. First, there must be a food industry capable of producing infant feeds of high quality in large amounts. Secondly, mothers must have sufficient money to purchase them in sufficient amounts. Thirdly, mothers must have the space and equipment to prepare each feed in an hygienic manner. In many of the rapidly growing towns of the world all of these are absent. As a result infants are given insufficient amounts of over-diluted feeds, frequently contaminated with pathogenic micro-organisms. This is an ideal prescription for the development of gastroenteritis and of protein-energy malnutrition, and inevitably leads to a large infant mortal-ity. In many communities it is unrealistic to hope that conditions for satisfactory artificial feeding will become available to the majority of mothers in the near future. In such circumstances the reversal of the present trend away from breast feeding is essential for reducing a high infant mortality. To re-establish the custom of breast feeding is a main task of many public health authorities. It requires not only a full use of all the techniques of health education, but also social and economic changes to permit women who work to have the time to feed their babies.

In prosperous communities the arguments in favour of breast feeding are less strong. Thus in a study in Sweden (Mellander et al., 1959), there was little difference in the health records over the first year of life between babies breast fed and those given cow's milk. In a study in Kuala Lumpur of 250 Malay and Chinese mothers attending Maternity and Child Health clinics, 30 per cent gave their babies no breast milk; these babies suffered no more respiratory or alimentary illnesses than those breast fed and their growth rates were satisfactory (Dugdale, 1971).

Human milk contains immunoglobulin A, lactoferrin and lysozyme (Table 61.2). The antimicrobial actions of these substances probably help to protect breast-fed infants against infection. The output of IgA falls rapidly as lactation becomes established, although the total amount of IgA transferred in the milk remains substantial. Nevertheless, since the infant's own intestine starts to produce IgA after one or two weeks, the protection given by milk IgA probably has greatest importance in very young infants. Immunoglobulins G and M and small amounts of complement components are also present in milk, but in very much smaller concentrations than IgA. IgE is rarely detectable in milk. Colostrum and early milk also contain substantial numbers of viable macrophages and lymphocytes, but it is not known whether these cells are of any benefit to the infant.

Samples of colostrum and milk from healthy mothers in the Baragwanath Hospital, Johannesburg, did not contain antibodies against rotavirus (Schoub et al., 1978). In Johannesburg gastroenteritis is common in bottle-fed infants but breast-fed infants are less susceptible. The authors attribute this to increased opportunity for rotavi-rus to spread with bottle feeding rather than to the presence of specific protective antibody in maternal milk.

Breast-fed babies are at reduced risk of neonatal tetany, hypertonic dehydration, infantile obesity, allergy to cow's milk and certain other hazards. Artificially fed babies are often bigger than breast fed babies, but whether this is disadvantageous is uncertain. The many differences in the

Table 61.2 Antimicrobial factors in human milk (from McClelland, et al., 1978)

	Day of lactation	Concentration (mg/dl)	Output (mg/24h)
IgA	2	4400	3516
	5	250	1369
	8–28	137	1061
	50–200	73	668
Lactoferrin	2	1741	1351
	5	673	3173
	8–28	294	2407
	50–200	112	1094
Lysozyme	2	39	37
	5	14	75
	8–28	14	48
	50–200	11	113

nutrient composition of human and cow's milk are described in Chapter 20 and in Tables 61.3, 61.4 and 61.5. One may speculate that adaptations to an unnatural food in the first months of life may sow seeds which appear later as chronic disorders such as allergies, atherosclerosis, hypertension and diabetes.

An additional argument is that not to breast feed deprives both mother and infant of a natural part of their life cycle, which may be a comforting and satisfying experience. Lastly, continued lactation tends to delay the resumption of ovulation and so increase birth spacing in populations. It is not, however, a reliable method of contraception.

In Britain and in other countries there are recommendations that 'all mothers be encouraged to breast feed their babies for a minimum of two weeks and preferably for the first 4 to 6 months of life' (DHSS, 1974).

A small minority of women are unable to breast feed; they do not produce a sufficient volume of milk. More rarely breast feeding is contraindicated by illness in the mother.

Doctors and nurses have a duty to advise mothers of the advantages of breast feeding and to encourage them to do so. However, the choice is hers. If she is unable or unwilling to do so, she should not be made to feel guilty. In our society kindly persuasion is more likely to promote the cause of breast feeding than militant advocacy.

Diet during lactation

Similar dietary principles apply as during pregnancy. The recommended intakes for nutrients are given in Chapter 15. The mother who is breast feeding her baby requires a good all round diet, especially if she is doing active work in the house, shop or factory; otherwise she will lose weight and become easily tired. If she is providing all the needs of a 5 kg infant, she must produce about 800 ml milk daily, which increases her need for energy by about 2.5 MJ (600 kcal). Dietary surveys in Aberdeen (Thomson et al., 1970) and in London (Whichelow, 1975; Naismith and Ritchie, 1975) indicate that lactating mothers increase their energy intake by this amount or more. They can also draw upon stores of fat laid down during pregnancy for additional energy. The weighing machine provides evidence as to whether the mother and her baby are getting too little or too much nourishment. The extra calcium and protein required are most conveniently provided by milk. If possible, at least 500 ml a day should be drunk and preferably more. Since a lactating woman may be producing 800 ml of milk daily it is obvious that she should take adequate amounts of fluid. Neither the quantity of the milk is increased nor its quality improved by forcing her to take large amounts of fluid (Illingworth and Kilpatrick, 1953). Tea and coffee, as well as beers and wines, may be drunk in moderation and do not alter the quality of the milk. Most drugs in common use are excreted in the milk,

but usually in such small amounts as to cause no ill-effects to the infant. However, all drugs and chemicals are potentially dangerous if given in large amounts. Arena (1970) advises against the use of the following drugs whilst breast feeding: diuretics, oral contraceptives, atropine, reserpine, steroids, radioactive preparations, morphine and its derivatives, anticoagulants, antithyroid drugs. Breast feeding should usually be discontinued by a mother who requires large doses of a drug to control epilepsy.

It is well known that the supply of milk is usually maintained even if the mother's diet is inadequate. Her own stores of nutrients are drawn upon and evidence of malnutrition appears in the mother before it does in her child. An excellent study of lactation in poor Indian communities made by Gopalan (1962) shows the remarkable ability of poor women to breast-feed their infants for long periods.

A mother's diet determines the pattern of fatty acids and concentrations of water-soluble vitamins in her milk. Fat-soluble vitamins are influenced to a lesser extent (Gebre-Medhin et al., 1976) while protein concentration is usually maintained in poorly nourished mothers (Strasberg et al., 1977); however, volume and fat (hence energy) content are sometimes suboptimal (Jelliffe and Jelliffe, 1978). The adequacy of breast milk as the sole food for the baby depends not only on the mother's diet while she is lactating but also on her nutritional status during pregnancy, when fetal stores of iron and vitamin A and maternal stores of energy in subcutaneous fat are laid down. Thus in Teheran urban women of low socioeconomic class were more often unsuccessful in lactating than middle-class women, and adequacy of lactation was related to postpartum weight (Geissler et al., 1978).

Even for a healthy woman with a good diet, the provision of sufficient milk to meet all the needs of a vigorous infant weighing 5.5 kg or more is a physiological strain. Supplementary feeding, i.e. the substitution of a bottle feed for one or more breast feeds, may be indicated. The introduction of solid foods, weaning, is discussed below. It is important that the mother's haemoglobin should be checked in the puerperium. Iron deficiency anaemia is common, especially if blood loss was excessive at or after delivery, and folate deficiency anaemia can present in the puerperium. For further reading a Ciba Symposium, Breast-feeding and the Mother (1976) is recommended.

INFANCY

Lactation is not fully established for two or three days, and during this short period of partial starvation an infant derives much of his energy from a large store of glycogen in the liver. The glycogen content of the liver in a full-term infant at birth is about 100 g/kg and falls to the normal adult value of about 20 g/kg by the end of the first week.

Whether feeding is by the breast or by bottle, there has in the past been much dispute as to whether it should take place according to a rigid time-table or 'on demand'. Nowadays a flexible time-table is recommended. Most infants adjust well to a regime of five daily feeds at four-hourly intervals, the first at 6 a.m. and the last at 10 p.m. Others seem to get unduly hungry if left so long without food, and these may be fed three-hourly at first. Regular meal times are good for an infant and convenient for mother, but a meal can always be put forward if he seems hungry. If for any reason his meal is delayed for an hour or so, he may well show his annoyance but comes to no harm. The amount given at each meal is also determined by experience. If he is not given enough, he is hungry and cries. If he is offered too much, he may take it and vomit soon after. Confirmation that he is getting enough and not too much can be obtained by weighing him at weekly intervals. If there is doubt about the amount of a mother's milk supply, this can be checked by test weighing him before and after a series of feeds without changing his napkin between the two weighings. A healthy infant needs about 160 ml/kg daily of breast milk, but there are wide variations.

COMPARISON OF HUMAN AND COW'S MILK

Cow's milk and preparations made from it can substitute for human milk and much effort is directed to manufacturing products that resemble human milk as closely as possible. Figures for the amounts of most of the known nutrients in a pooled mixture of human milks obtained from 96 mothers in five centres in Britain are available (DHSS, 1977) and provide a standard at which manufacturers can aim. Human milk is often stated to be the ideal food for infants. This may be true but it is an emotional rather than a scientific judgment. There are circumstances where man can improve upon nature.

Energy, protein, fat and carbohydrate. Table 61.3 shows that cow's milk contains much more protein and much less carbohydrate than human milk. There is a little less fat and about the same amount of energy. The simplest modification is therefore dilution and the addition of carbohydrate.

Variations of up to ± 10 per cent of the figures in the table are common and of up to ± 25 per cent not unusual. The composition of milk from the two breasts is not always

Table 61.3 Energy, protein, fat and carbohydrate in human and cow's milk (typical values in 1 dl when lactation is well established)

	Human milk	Cow's milk
Energy (kJ)	290	290
(kcal)	70	70
Protein (g)	1.0	3.5
Fat (g)	4.0	3.8
Carbohydrate (g)	7.4	4.5

Table 61.4 Fatty acids g/100 g of total fatty acids in human and cow's milk (Paul and Southgate, 1978)

Fatty acids	Human milk	Cow's milk
Saturated		
$C_{4:0}$	0	3.2
$C_{8:0}$	0	2.0
$C_{10:0}$	trace	1.2
$C_{10:0}$	1.4	2.8
$C_{12:0}$	5.4	3.5
$C_{14:0}$	7.3	11.2
$C_{15:0}$	26.5	26.0
$C_{18:0}$	9.5	11.2
Monounsaturated		
$C_{16:1}$	4.0	2.7
$C_{18:1}$	35.4	27.8
Polyunsaturated		
$C_{18:2}$	7.2	1.4
$C_{18:3}$	0.8	1.5

identical, and for the first 5 to 10 minutes of a feed the milk from each breast may be thin and watery (Hall, 1975).

Protein. About 20 per cent of the energy in cow's milk comes from protein, but a little less than 7 per cent in human milk. Thus human milk is not a rich source of protein, but the amino acid mixture which it provides contains ample quantities of all the amino acids essential for growth (p. 42).

Fatty acids. Table 61.4 gives typical values for the main fatty acids present in the two milks. Cow's milk also contains about 150 mg/dl of short-chain fatty acids, of which only traces are found in human milk. Over 50 fatty acids have been identified in human milk (Egge *et al.*, 1972), but the total amount present of those not in the table is less than 500 mg/dl.

The main difference is the much greater amount of linoleic acid present in human milk. Cow's milk can be made to resemble human milk more closely by removing the cream and replacing it with vegetable oils rich in linoleic acid. The benefit from this is uncertain. Premature infants thrived on a formula in which linoleic acid provided only 0.5 per cent of the energy (Combes *et al.*, 1962), a little less than the proportion provided in human milk.

Carbohydrates. Lactose is the main carbohydrate in both human and cow's milk. Sucrose rather than lactose was formerly added to most cow's milk preparations because it was much cheaper but now lactose is generally used. Two groups of babies with low birth weights fed on a cow's milk formula, one with added lactose and the other with added sucrose, did equally well (Fosbrooke and Wharton, 1975). Whether in the long term the use of sucrose has any adverse metabolic effects is unknown, but in this way a 'sweet tooth' may be acquired very early in life.

Minerals and electrolytes. Concentrations of sodium and potassium are much higher in cow's milk than in

Table 61.5 Normal values for the electrolyte and mineral content of human and cow's milk

	Human milk	Cow's milk
Sodium (mmol/litre)	7	25
Potassium (mmol/litre)	15	35
Calcium (mg/dl)	34	120
Magnesium (mg/dl)	3	12
Phosphorus (mg/dl)	14	95
Iron (μg/dl)	70	50
Copper (μg/dl)	40	20
Zinc (μg/dl)	28	35

human milk (Table 61.5). Unmodified cow's milk, if given to very young children, would lead to an osmolar load greater than the excretary capacity of their immature kidneys. Cow's milk also contains much more calcium and phosphorus than human milk, but has a much lower Ca/P ratio. The relatively high phosphorus content may reduce calcium absorption for the intestine and produce hypocalcaemia (p. 92). All recommended formulae prepared from cow's milk have, when reconstituted with water, much lower concentrations of Na, K, Ca and P than the original milk.

Vitamins. Both human and cow's milk are normally good sources of all the vitamins, except vitamin D. However, amounts depend on the maternal diet and, reflecting plasma concentrations, are very variable.

The normal amount of ascorbic acid in human milk is about 3 to 4 mg/dl. Even if a mother's diet is very poor her milk provides enough to prevent scurvy, which is practically unknown in breast-fed infants. As the vitamin is readily destroyed by heat, preparations of cow's milk are a poor source unless it is added artificially and infantile scurvy was formerly a common hazard of bottle feeding.

Amounts of thiamin normally range between 10 and 20 μg/dl in human milk, but values below 6 μg/dl have been reported in Malaya (Simpson and Chow, 1956) and in Vietnam (Plagnol and Dutrenit, 1956). Infantile beriberi is common in areas where the adult form of the disease is present.

All milks are a poor and uncertain source of vitamin D. However, human milk contains some 8 μg/dl, nearly all as the water-soluble sulphate, and five times more than cow's milk (Lakdawala and Widdowson, 1977).

Human milk contains about 30 μg/dl of riboflavin, adequate for infants. Cow's milk contains much more, up to 230 μg/litre, and so is very effective in preventing riboflavin deficiency in older infants and young children. However, the vitamin is rapidly destroyed in milk exposed to sunlight in glass bottles.

Bottle feeding

In prosperous countries liquid cow's milk has been almost entirely replaced for infant feeding by preparations of dried milk powders and evaporated milks. In poorer countries liquid cow's milk may still be used in rural areas, but the increasing urban populations depend more and more on manufactured preparations.

Liquid milk

Cow's milk cannot be given to very young infants until it has been processed. First it has to be diluted to reduce the protein concentration. About one part of water should be added to two parts of milk. Then as the carbohydrate content is lower than that of human milk, sugar is added. If 3.5 g of sugar is added to 100 ml of diluted feed (one level teaspoonful to just over 3 oz), then 100 ml of the feed contains about 2.2 g protein, 2.5 g fat and 7.0 g carbohydrate and has an energy value of 300 kJ (76 kcal). An infant's normal requirement of such a feed is the same as for breast milk namely 160 ml/kg daily. Finally, irrespective of whether the original milk was pasteurised, the mixture is boiled. After boiling it is covered to protect it from pathogens in the atmosphere and from flies. It is kept until use in as cool a place as possible.

Dried milk powders

Many commercial preparations of cow's milk have been made. Table 61.6 gives a list of those available and recommended in Britain, together with the composition of the milks when the dried powders are made up with water according to instructions. In all of them the content of protein and sodium is much less than in natural cow's milk and approaches that in human milk; calcium and phosphorus content is also reduced. All have added sugar, lactose except in one case. In some the animal fat has been replaced by vegetable oils. All are fortified with vitamin D to much higher concentrations than those found in either cow's or human milks.

These preparations have the advantage of convenience, since a mother can buy and carry away two or three weeks' supply, which can easily be stored. As bacteria cannot grow on dry powders, these are much safer than liquid preparations.

Instructions for making up the feeds are given with each tin, which includes a scoop for measuring out the powder. Mothers often make up feeds incorrectly and excessive amounts of powder may be used (Wilkinson et al., 1973). Overconcentrated feeds carry the risks of hypernatraemia and obesity. Mistakes may be made because scoops are not standardised, but of various sizes. When bottle-feeding was usually with liquid milk, doctors, nurses and midwives made a point of instructing mothers carefully in how to prepare feeds. Preparation is much easier with milk powders and this instruction appears to be often omitted. There are many mothers who cannot or do not follow the written instructions accurately.

Evaporated milk

This is defined on page 195. Like dried milk powders, it is

Table 61.6 Dried milk powders recommended for infant feeding in Britain: constituents per 100 ml reconstituted feed (from Wharton and Berger, 1976)

Brand	Type	Protein (g)	Fat (g)	Carbohydrate Lactose (g)	Carbohydrate Other (g)	Energy (kJ)	Sodium (mmol)	Calcium (mg)	Phosphorus (mg)	Vitamin D (µg)	Vitamin C (mg)
Cow and Gate Baby Milk Plus	Added carbohydrate	1.8	3.3	6.6		263	1.3	62	50	1.1	5.3
Cow and Gate Premium	Demineralised whey	1.8	3.3	6.9		263	1.0	55	40	1.1	5.0
Cow and Gate V Formula	Substituted fat	1.8	3.0	7.0		259	1.4	63	50	1.1	5.3
Ostermilk Complete Formula	Added carbohydrate	1.7	2.7	2.8	5.8	271	1.3	56	46	1.0	6.4
SMA	Substituted fat	1.5	3.5	7.0		271	1.1	53	43	1.1	5.3
SMA Concentrated Liquid	Substituted fat	1.5	3.5	7.0		271	1.1	53	43	1.1	5.3
Gold Cap SMA S26	Demineralised whey	1.5	3.6	7.2		280	0.6	42	33	1.1	5.3

convenient, readily available and sterile. Instructions for adding water are provided. Most evaporated milks are fortified with vitamin D but not with ascorbic acid, a supplement of which is necessary.

Ready-to-feed milks
These are preparations of milk powders or evaporated milks which have been diluted. Hence they can be given to a baby without further preparation. At present in Britain they are only in use in hospitals.

Hazards of bottle feeding
Protein-energy malnutrition and keratomalacia. These are the main hazards of infants prematurely deprived of their mother's milk and fed on inadequate substitutes under unhygienic conditions. They have already been described.

Neonatal tetany. This consists of twitches and spasms occurring between the third and fourteenth day of life. It is very rare in breast fed infants. The plasma concentration of calcium is usually low and sometimes also that of magnesium. Alimentary absorption of these elements may be impaired by the high phosphate content of the feeds or by steatorrhoea, owing to inability to absorb fully the fatty acids present in cow's milk. Immaturity of the parathyroid glands is probably a contributory factor and the spasms cease spontaneously by about the fourteenth day or earlier. Treatment by giving calcium gluconate (10 ml of a 10 per cent solution) by mouth with each feed is usually effective. Whether or not there is hypomagnesaemia, magnesium sulphate (50 per cent solution) given intramuscularly in a dose of 0.2 mg/kg of body weight is equally effective and may be the treatment of choice.

Hypertonic dehydration. Sodium concentration in human milk is 7 mmol/l. It is between 20 and 25 mmol/l in natural cow's milk and 10 to 15 mmol/l in most preparations of cow's milk which have been reconstituted according to the instructions. Healthy infants can excrete this extra load of sodium, but have to secrete a more concentrated urine. Taitz and Byers (1972) found the mean osmolalities of the urine were 105 and 380 mosmol/kg in breast fed and bottle fed babies. Three common circumstances may prevent them excreting the load and lead to a rise in plasma sodium. These are an attack of diarrhoea, fever or a failure of the mother to make up the feed according to the instructions. Diarrhoea and fever increase water losses from the gut and from the skin and lungs, and so reduce the amount available for excreting solutes in the urine. Taitz and Byers measured the sodium concentration of 32 feeds obtained from mothers attending their clinic in Sheffield. In 21 of the samples it was over 30 mosmol/l and in 4 over 40. Many mothers give their babies overconcentrated feeds by not levelling the powder in the scoop as the instructions indicate.

The clinical features of hypertonic dehydration are anorexia and irritability; there may be convulsions. If the condition is allowed to continue, permanent damage to the brain may follow. The diagnosis is made by finding a plasma sodium concentration above 150 mmol/l. Treatment is effected by attending to the underlying cause and, if the condition is severe, by giving dextrose and water or hypotonic saline intravenously. The nature and dosage of the intravenous fluids required is determined by careful monitoring of plasma electrolytes.

Although preparations of cow's milk with a reduced content of sodium can be made, their cost is high and it is possible that the demineralisation would remove essential trace elements. Hence they cannot be recommended. This condition could be prevented by improving the manufacturer's instructions, and designing scoops less likely to be misused. Doctors and nurses have a duty to see that all mothers using artificial milks understand how to make up feeds accurately. A novel method of trying to ensure that such instruction is given is being tried in Papua, New Guinea. Here a mother cannot buy an infant feeding bottle without a doctor's prescription.

Obesity. Babies on artificial feeding on average grow faster than breast fed babies; they are also likely to become obese. This may be due in part to mothers making up too concentrated feeds. Probably more important is the too early introduction of solid foods providing concentrated sources of energy. Infantile obesity is discussed below.

The infant food industry

Most infant milk preparations are manufactured by large companies which trade internationally. Competition between them is keen and this has ensured that, when a customer buys a preparation bearing the brand name of one of the well-known firms, she is getting a good and reliable product. The firms are, however, not only competing with themselves but with manufacturers of breast milk. The promotion and advertising of their products has been an important factor in the decline of breast feeding. The consequences have been disastrous for poor mothers in many countries who have neither the money to buy sufficient quantities for their babies nor a home environment where the milk can be reconstituted with safety. Firms have been castigated as 'baby killers' by enthusiastic proponents of breast feeding. This led to a long legal action for libel in a Swiss court, and in the USA firms have been sued for improper practices. There is substance in many of the criticisms of the sales techniques of some firms but the fault is not all theirs. Apathy and lack of knowledge among doctors, nurses and nutritionists have also been responsible for large numbers of mothers using artificial milks unnecessarily and without adequate facilities. Breast feeding versus bottle feeding is a controversy which arouses strong emotions, but the issues are not simple. Social, psychological, educational and economic factors determine the sales of infant milk preparations. All of these and the nutritional factors are discussed in a large book (Jelliffe and Jelliffe, 1978). The authors have an unrivalled experience of infant feeding practice in many parts of the world and set out the case for breast feeding with enthusiasm.

A visitor to a small town in a poor country who goes into a chemist shop to buy some toothpaste is likely to see on the shelves large stocks of imported infants food and also of vitamin preparations and many drugs which are of little or no value and which the country cannot afford. Manufacturers by skilful advertising create a 'want' where there is no 'need'. On the credit side the infant food industry has been the means of saving the lives of those infants whose mothers have died or who cannot lactate because of some physical disease. It has also enabled mothers who, for good reasons, do not wish to lactate to rear healthy babies, provided they have the knowledge and sufficient means. These are no mean achievements.

WEANING

Weaning is the process whereby feeding from the breast or a bottle is replaced by the use of unmodified cow's milk and solid foods. Except in an emergency it should take place gradually. The dangers that may arise in peasant communities and in urban slums from weaning on to inadequate diets have been discussed in the chapter on protein-energy malnutrition. Here the concern is with weaning in affluent societies.

Baby foods

In affluent societies most babies are weaned on to foods prepared not by their mothers but by food manufacturers. They are usually precooked and sold in tins and are perhaps the best examples of convenience foods.

These foods are at present in Britain subject only to normal labelling legislation which does not include a statement of content of nutrients. Those made by reputable firms are well suited to the needs of infants after they have reached the age of 4 months. However, many mothers give them to their babies at a much earlier age. Thus in a survey in Worcestershire Shukla *et al.* (1972) showed that among 300 babies 40 per cent were receiving solid foods at the age of 4 weeks and 90 per cent by the age of 4 months. It is probable that these babies are representative of babies in general in Britain. There is no doubt that the introduction of solid foods at these early ages is unnecessary, and there are good reasons for considering that it is undesirable.

Infantile obesity. The baby foods used in the first four months are mainly cereal preparations and rusks. They may be sweetened with sugar to make them appetising. Babies like these pleasant foods and it is easy to understand why a mother may offer them in excessive quantities and how with their high energy content they may lead to obesity.

Paediatricians are agreed that they see more cases of infantile obesity than formerly. However, its prevalence is uncertain because, as for adult obesity, there is no accepted definition. Using a weight for age chart (p. 471), infants over the 97th percentile or more than 20 per cent over the median values have been defined as obese; those lying between the 90th and 97th percentile or between 10 and 20 per cent above the median value have been termed overweight. In an infant a measurement of triceps skinfold over 12 mm suggests obesity and one over 14 mm strongly indicates the diagnosis. By these or similar criteria, there are several reports indicating that about one-fifth of all infants in Britain are obese. Most mothers would regard such an infant as chubby rather than obese. He appears as a healthy and cheerful member of the family and enjoys his food.

While there is no doubt that some obese infants and young children go on to become obese adolescents and adults, there is increasing evidence that obesity early in life is usually only temporary (Mellbin and Vuille, 1973; Poskitt and Cole, 1977; Hawk and Brook, 1979).

Hirsch and Knittle (1970) and Brook (1972) have counted the number of adipocytes in biopsy samples of adipose tissue obtained from obese children and from controls. Brook puts forward the view that the adipose tissue organ in man has a sensitive period in the first year of life during which its basic complement of cells is determined. Overfeeding in infancy may lead to an increased number of adipocytes which persists into childhood and later life. Widdowson and Shaw (1973) and Jung et al. (1978) are cautious in accepting this hypothesis, pointing out the technical difficulties in counting adipocytes, the uncertainty as to whether the small biopsy sample is representative and in assessment of the total amount of adipose tissue in a child. They also point out that young pigs that are kept severely undernourished for the first year of life become extremely fat, when later they are given a plentiful supply of food. Marasmic infants also may become fat after rehabilitation.

Other hazards. When a baby is taking solids food regularly, he can be given the same pasteurised cow's milk as the rest of the family. After the changeover from a dried milk powder, it is important to see that he does not become thirsty, and he may need more water to excrete the larger intake of electrolytes. Baby foods, like all other manufactured foods, may contain added salt. Manufacturers believe that, if they did not make this addition, they would not sell their products which must taste good to the mother as well as to the infant. Except in very early life, a healthy infant has no difficulty in excreting this extra sodium load but, if Dahl's hypothesis (p. 341) of a role for dietary salt in the aetiology of hypertension is correct, it may be preparing the ground for the development of this disease several decades later.

Similarly sweetened baby foods may give an infant early in life too 'sweet a tooth'. This may lead later to excessive consumption of sugar, predisposing him to dental caries and obesity.

It is possible that early introduction of cereals containing gluten may make a predisposed infant more likely to develop coeliac disease, a condition which appears to be becoming more prevalent in some countries.

Spinach purée is a popular infant food which infants like and mothers believe is good for them, as indeed it may well be. However, spinach often contains large amounts of nitrate which is reduced to nitrite during storage of the vegetable. Fetal haemoglobin is much more readily oxidised by nitrite to methaemoglobin than adult haemoglobin. Infants given too much spinach too early in life are at risk of methaemoglobinaemia.

Innumerable babies have now been given solid foods very early in life and come to no harm. But the practice is unnecessary. Milk and milk preparations are adequate sources of nourishment for the first 6 months of life. There is no need to give other foods earlier, and to start them before the age of 5 months adds unnecessary risks.

When it is decided to wean an infant, solid foods such as cereal gruels, minces, boiled vegetables and stewed fruits may be given at first. It is not necessary to sieve the food, but hard particles should be removed. On the first day solid food should be substituted for one feed from the breast or the bottle, and at the same time the infant should be encouraged to drink milk from a cup. Weaning should be gradual, but should be completed within 7 to 14 days.

After weaning and in the latter half of infancy, milk should still form a major part of the diet. Initially specially cooked baby foods or commercial preparations are used, but the infant gradually shares more and more in the family meals. Meal times are mainly a matter of convenience. He may be fed with the family at breakfast, the midday and evening meal, but many mothers prefer to feed a young infant and put him to rest before serving the family. Three meals a day usually suffice, with snacks in between. During the day he should not normally go more than four hours without food, but during the night can be allowed to go 12 hours.

There are many books that give details of practical aspects of infant feeding. Those by Gunther (1973) and by Cameron and Hofvander (1971) can be strongly recommended. The former is suited for mothers in affluent societies and the latter to those in underdeveloped communities.

CHILDHOOD

After his first birthday a child is able to share in most of the dishes served to a family, but requires relatively more protein of good quality than adults. This is best provided by milk.

Milk. A child at the age of 1 year needs about 4.2 MJ (1000 kcal) daily. If he is getting about 0.5 litre of cow's milk daily (a satisfactory allowance) then about 35 per cent of the energy is derived from milk. The remainder of the energy is provided by a mixed diet—in practice usually of the same quality as that of the rest of the family. As the child grows and the need for energy increases, the proportion provided by milk falls and the diet gradually approaches the adult pattern.

The value of milk as a food for children has been established by practical experience and put on a scientific basis by Corry Mann (p. 483) and many others in controlled field trials. It is desirable that every child up to the age of 5 should have 500 ml daily, and after 5 until growth ceases at least 250 ml. Milk is chiefly valuable as a source of good-quality protein and of calcium needed for growth. In practice, growth and development are usually slow in children who receive poor diets containing little or no milk. This need not be so, for McCance and Widdowson (p. 000) showed that if a good mixture of vegetable proteins is provided excellent growth rates are obtained, despite the virtual absence of milk from the diet.

Larger amounts of milk are sometimes recommended. These may accelerate growth further and, less certainly, increase the adult size, but there is no evidence that either is desirable or contributes to health and well-being.

Vitamins. Requirements for vitamins are relatively increased in childhood and it is well known that children are more liable than adults to many deficiency diseases. If the family diet is not satisfactory, then it is desirable to provide daily for the child extra vitamins C, A and D, either as a special supplement or in the form of fruit juice and a fish-liver oil. The beneficial effect of these Welfare Foods has been repeatedly demonstrated and a great increase in their use is needed in many countries. After the age of 2 years, provided the child is healthy and eats a good mixed diet including fruit and vegetables, there is no necessity for these extra vitamins, except in northern countries where there is little sunshine in winter. In these circumstances a supplement of vitamin D should be continued up to the age of 5 years or longer if cases of rickets have occurred in older children in the community.

Energy. The recommended intakes for nutrients given on pages 153 and 154 are a useful guide for those responsible for feeding large numbers of children in schools and orphanages. They form a basis on which practical ration scales can be drawn up. However, they are no guide to the needs of an individual child. Children vary greatly in their needs and a healthy child may ingest only half, or more than double, the allowance. If given the opportunity, many children and most adolescents of both sexes have an enormous capacity for games and physical recreations. Their food requirements are then much greater than is indicated in the tables. Conversely, if they become accustomed to watching television or engage in other sedentary recreations they require less.

Appetite is normally a sound guide to requirements. Children's feeding behaviour is far less a matter of habit than adults. A child may eat voraciously for a day or two and then lose all interest in his food for a while. This is natural and there is no necessity to restrict his meals in one phase or to attempt to force food during another. Many children occasionally develop specific appetites for one food. This may make the diet temporarily quite unbalanced. This again will do no harm for it will soon be rectified naturally, and so need not be checked unless it offends against good manners.

The best guide that the food intake is satisfactory is provided by the weighing machine. It is sound practice to weigh and measure the height of a child every three months. Provided the increase in weight and height is satisfactory (the charts on p. 470, are useful guides) there is no need to worry about a child's diet.

MANAGEMENT OF CHILDREN'S DIETS
A child's diet is best taken equally divided between three main meals. Breakfast is usually taken with the family. It is a meal which is frequently skimped by adults, who may indeed do well with very little food in the morning. It is, however, important for children to go to school with a good breakfast inside them. The midday meal may be taken either at home or, more often, at school. If the school does not provide a satisfactory meal, a good packed lunch is needed. Young children under 5 should go to bed early and it is best for them to have their evening meal separately before the rest of the family. If the main family evening meal is taken after 7 o'clock, children under 10 will also need a meal earlier.

In many countries it is customary to give schoolchildren a glass of milk at the mid-morning break and this is sound practice. If the evening meal is late, children want something in the middle of the afternoon. This is permissible. Otherwise children are best without snacks between meals.

Some children readily become obese and there is need to watch that weight gain is not excessive.

Sweets and candies. An excessive consumption of these spoils the appetite for the main meal and predisposes to dental caries. Nevertheless, taken in moderation, especially after meals, they do no harm and are a legitmate pleasure of childhood. The danger of excessive consumption is always present and there is need for discipline.

ADOLESCENCE

The nutritional requirements of the adolescent are conditioned primarily by the 'spurt' in growth which occurs at puberty. In boys this is responsible for a gain in height of about 20 cm (8 in) and in weight of 19 kg (40 lb). In girls the gains are usually less. The additional food requirements are indicated to the adolescent by his increased appetite and are usually met by the mother providing sufficient of the necessary foods at mealtimes. If this is not done the adolescent satisfies his appetite by snacks between meals, as is clearly indicated by investigations of the energy consumption of boys at boarding schools. Not only may this habit lead to an unbalanced diet, but it is also liable to play an important role in the promotion of dental caries.

There is little scientific information on nutrient requirements during adolescence. Recommended intakes are almost entirely based on extrapolation. This is a time of life when youngsters are breaking away from the family pattern of eating and become very susceptible to peer group and advertising pressures. There is not enough information on the range and variation of food intakes of adolescents, especially those living in permissive affluent societies. The proceedings of a symposium on *Nutrient Requirements in Adolescence* are available (McKigney and Munro, 1976).

Obesity, anorexia nervosa and, in girls, iron-deficiency anaemia, are the important nutritional disorders in adolescence and have been discussed on pages 252, 241 and 424 respectively. In parts of the world where goitre is endemic, adolescent girls are most likely to be affected (p. 268). In some parts of the world adolescents are at special risk of deficiency of iodine (p. 267) and zinc (p. 105).

62. Adult Man and the Aged

ADULT MAN

In prosperous communities, mean values for plasma cholesterol, blood pressure and body weight rise with age. Books set out normal values related to age with the implication that the rises are physiological. Yet many studies show that in communities of hunter-gatherers and primitive peasants such rises do not occur. They are the result of a way of life. Although the changes do not become marked until middle age, they begin early; values at the age of 25 are usually slightly but significantly higher than at the age of 20 years.

These early changes predispose to the development of obesity, diabetes, coronary heart disease and hypertension. Increasing prevalence of these diseases in many countries has prevented the decline in general mortality rates between the ages of 35 to 70 years that would be expected to have followed the new effective methods for the prevention and treatment of infectious diseases.

Many factors, dietary and others, have been suggested as responsible for these diseases, but it is certain that no single one has a role comparable to those of the tubercle bacillus, the pneumococcus and the other microorganisms formerly responsible for so many deaths in the prime of life. These diseases arise from a combination of causes and are said to be multifactorial.

Of non-dietary factors, the increase in the use of tobacco has been shown beyond any reasonable doubt to be mainly responsible for the increased prevalence of not only lung cancer, but also partly for that of coronary heart disease. Most people who have studied the literature consider that diminished physical activity is in part responsible for increased prevalence of obesity and coronary heart disease. The extent to which stress arising from psychological causes has increased and contributed to higher prevalence rates of organic disease is uncertain. Hunter-gatherers and peasants also have to adapt to numerous stresses which are qualitatively different from those arising in more complex environments.

Of dietary factors which may contribute to the increased prevalence of non-communicable diseases in adults, excessive intake of saturated fatty acids and sugar appear important; less certain is a low intake of polyunsaturated fatty acids. Excessive intakes of sodium chloride appear to predispose to hypertension. Whether or not there is deficiency or excess of any trace element is a matter for speculation and research.

In the practice of public health, it is wrong to give dietary advice specifically related to one particular non-communicable disease. For healthy people advice aimed at reducing risk of CHD, hypertension, obesity and diabetes is essentially the same. The advice also applies to both sexes. Women are relatively immune to CHD before the menopause, but in some countries there has been a significant rise in female mortality rates in the 50 to 70 age group.

RECOMMENDATIONS

Committees in 18 countries have issued reports setting out details of suggested changes in national diets, which are considered likely to reduce the prevalence of CHD and related diseases. Extracts of four, from Scandinavia, the USA and the UK, are given below. They show substantial agreement on many points, but there are important differences in emphasis of what is desirable or practical.

Scandinavia

The Medical Boards of Finland, Norway and Sweden (1968) made the following recommendations, aimed at reducing the prevalence of obesity, CHD and other disorders of an industrial country.

The supply of calories in the diet should in many cases be reduced to prevent overweight.

The total consumption of fat should be reduced from 40 per cent—the present figure—to between 25 and 35 per cent of the total number of calories.

The use of saturated fat should be reduced and the consumption of polyunsaturated fats be increased simultaneously.

The consumption of sugar and products containing sugar should be reduced.

The consumption of vegetables, fruit, potatoes, skimmed milk, fish, lean meat and cereal products should be increased.

From the medical and nutritional standpoint the importance of taking regular exercise from an early age for all those who have mainly sedentary occupations should also be emphasised.

To carry out the above programme, we require the co-operation not only of doctors but of all those who give instruction on questions of nutrition or who are responsible for catering on a large scale, particularly in schools, the military forces, hospitals and similar institutions and other eating places.

It is of pressing importance that the food industry pay attention to the recommendations made here in their choice of raw products and in the manufacture of cooked meats and provisions, other semi-prepared foods and ready-cooked food. The industry ought to specify the contents used in their products in a better way than before.

Proposed menus and the composition of recipes for large-scale catering should meet the requirements of nutritional physiology and the food value should be calculated. Consumer information on questions of nutrition should be circulated in the press and on the radio and TV on the basis of the points made above.

United States

The contentious McGovern report prepared by a Select Committee of the Senate (1977) has already been discussed (p. 488). A second edition of the report, in which the main change is that the daily intake of salt is raised from 3 to 5 g, sets out seven dietary goals.

1. To avoid overweight, consume only as much energy (calories) as is expended; if overweight, decrease energy intake and increase energy expenditure.
2. Increase the consumption of complex carbohydrates and 'naturally occurring' sugars from about 28 per cent of energy intake to about 48 per cent of energy intake.
3. Reduce the consumption of refined and processed sugars by about 45 per cent to account for about 10 per cent of total energy intake.
4. Reduce overall fat consumption from approximately 40 per cent to about 30 per cent of energy intake.
5. Reduce saturated fat consumption to about 10 per cent of total energy intake and balance that with polyunsaturated and monounsaturated fats, which should account for about 10 per cent of energy intake each.
6. Reduce cholesterol consumption to about 300 mg a day.
7. Limit the intake of sodium by reducing the intake of salt to about 5 g a day.

The goals suggest the following changes in food selection and preparation:

(i) Increase consumption of fruits and vegetables and whole grains.
(ii) Decrease consumption of foods high in total fat, and partially replace saturated fats, whether obtained from animal or vegetable sources, with polyunsaturated fats.
(iv) Decrease consumption of animal fat, and choose meats, poultry and fish which will reduce saturated fat intake.

(v) Except for young children, substitute low-fat and non-fat milk for whole milk, and low-fat dairy products for high-fat dairy products.
(vi) Decrease consumption of butterfat, eggs and other high cholesterol sources. Some consideration should be given to easing the cholesterol goal for pre-menopausal women, young children and the elderly in order to obtain the nutritional benefits of eggs in the diet.
(vii) Decrease consumption of salt and foods high in salt content.

United Kingdom

A report of an advisory panel of the Committee on Medical Aspects of Food Policy of the Department of Health and Social Security (1974) made the following recommendations.

1. Obesity should be avoided both in the child and the adult. The Panel recommend that those individuals who are already obese should so reduce their food intake in relation to their physical activity that they are no longer obese.
2. The majority of the members of the Panel recommend that the amount of fat in the United Kingdom diet, especially saturated fat from both animal and plant sources, should be reduced.
3. The Panel unanimously agree that they cannot recommend an increase in the intake of polyunsaturated fatty acids in the diet as a measure intended to reduce the risk of the development of ischaemic heart disease. In their opinion the available evidence that such a dietary alteration would reduce that risk in the United Kingdom at the present time is not convincing.
4. The Panel recommend that the consumption of sucrose, as such or in foods and drinks, should be reduced, if only to diminish the risk of obesity and its possible sequelae.

A joint Working Party of the Royal College of Physicians and the British Cardiac Society (1976) made the following recommendations.

Diet

1. Dietary recommendations for the whole community involve a reduction in the amount of saturated fats and partial substitution by polyunsaturated fats.
2. Where plasma lipid concentrations indicate particularly high risk or where other risk factors are concurrently present, the dietary recommendations should be followed more strictly.
3. Widespread screening for plasma lipid levels is not recommended but estimations should be carried out in certain groups known to be at high risk for CHD.
4. Maintenance of a desirable weight is important as obesity is commonly associated with other more potent

risk factors for CHD. Weight reduction should be based on a decrease in all the dietary components; sugar and alcohol are recognised as common sources of excess energy intake. A combination of exercise and diet is strongly recommended.

It can be seen that there is complete agreement on the importance of preventing obesity and reducing intake of sugar, and almost complete agreement on the desirability of reducing the proportion of the dietary energy derived from saturated fatty acids of animal origin.

One British group did not share the view that significant benefit would follow increased consumption of polyunsaturated acids. The American report is the only one to recommend a reduction in cholesterol intakes.

The implementation of these recommendations involves national policies directed toward health education, agriculture and the food industry, as discussed in Chapter 56.

In health education, emphasis on moderation in all things, including diet, is important. The advice that doctors have been giving to their patients for over two thousand years on how to live sensibly, which we have summarised on p. 340, needs continuing repetition to the healthy, as well as to the sick. In prosperous communities vast numbers of people have dietary habits which do not conduce to health, and which they should be advised to modify. They do not need special diets. Rigid dietary regimens are required by only a small minority of sick persons, who should always be under strict medical supervision. Most diets which have acquired a vogue of popularity also have inherent dangers, e.g. the Atkins diet (p. 250).

In agriculture, the modern trend to produce lean rather than fat meats is to be commended. So also are the attempts to reduce the proportion of saturated fatty acids in carcass fat by modifications in animal feeding. An American suggestion that egg production should cease, so as to reduce dietary cholesterol, is absurd. The human race has thousands of years of experience to show that eggs are a good and safe food for persons of all ages. Provided consumption is modest, the extra dietary cholesterol inhibits endogenous production and the body's total supply may be unchanged. Butter is not a dangerous food for healthy persons provided it is eaten in small amounts.

The modern food industry has a great responsibility to the public, when it manufactures and puts on the market a new food. The classic example is margarine. When first produced it was inferior to butter in every respect; now the best margarines provide vitamins A and D and their fatty acids have a high P/S ratio. Collaboration between food technologists and nutritionists has here given excellent results. Similar collaboration is needed in launching any new food.

The labelling and advertising of new foods are of great importance. Consumers should be fully informed about the ingredients in all manufactured foods and the amounts present of the main nutrients. They should not be misled into thinking that any food by itself prevents the development of disease. Foods are good or bad in relation to their contribution to a diet. Just as there are no slimming foods, so there are no heart foods, but many natural and manufactured foods can be valuable items in diets which limit the risk of developing either obesity or heart disease. Misleading claims are to be avoided.

THE AGED

It is often said that a man is as old as his arteries and there is much justification for this saying. People with advanced degenerative arterial disease at the age of 60 may have the stigmata of old age, while others with healthy arteries and a normal blood pressure continue to lead an active physical and mental life till 80 years and more. Age in years does not necessarily coincide with biological age.

PROBLEMS OF LONGEVITY

The decline in death rates in children and young people in the last 50 years has changed the structure of the population. Table 62.1 shows that the percentage of elderly people in the population has more than doubled. This increase has lead to many economic and other problems (Office of Health Economics, 1968). The majority of elderly people in Britain live in private households and only 6 per cent are in hospitals and institutions. However, they occupy over 30 per cent of hospital beds and make a heavy demand on health and welfare services. Atherosclerosis involving the coronary and cerebral blood vessels and malignant neoplasms are responsible for most of the deaths in old people.

It is inevitable that many elderly people are ill and sick and regrettable that the facilities for looking after them are not always adequate. Many individual tragedies come to light in which society has failed to care for an old person. Yet there is another side to the picture, which is fortunately more common. While inevitably with increasing years the pace of life must be slowed down, many people remain healthy and active both in body and mind, even up to the age of 100 years or more. After the age of 90 life can still be enjoyed and many of the very old are charming in

Table 62.1 The changes in the population of Scotland and in the numbers of elderly people (Cohen, 1965)

Year	Total population	Numbers 65 years or over	Percentage 65 years or over
1861	3 069 000	150 000	4.9
1901	4 536 000	217 000	4.8
1951	5 169 000	512 000	9.9
1961	5 226 000	545 000	10.5
1981 (estimate)	5 641 000	711 000	12.6

their manners and capable of retaining and also making friendships.

Prevention of senescence

It is probable that once biological old age has been reached the condition is irreversible, but it seems reasonable to assume that various measures may be available which might at least slow down the ageing process. There are two main groups of factors which influence the life span, namely genetic and environmental factors, and the former are probably the more important. If we could make a judicious choice of our parents, our chance of living to a ripe and healthy old age would be greatly increased. There is also no doubt that physical and mental activity after retiral play an important part in postponing the onset of morbid old age. Likewise, it is always important to prevent and treat infections with modern drugs and antibiotics, and nutritional disorders by appropriate dietetic measures. At first thought it might appear obvious that the better diet which has been eaten by the majority of the people in Britain, Western Europe and the USA has played an important role in increasing the life span so spectacularly in the last 30 years, but many other factors, including better sanitation, better housing and modern chemotherapy, have all been operating simultaneously. Coincidental with this improvement in nutrition there has occurred a remarkable increase in the height and weight of children and adolescents of the working classes. Whether these children will survive to an older age accompanied by increased mental and physical well-being is a question which cannot be answered for many years to come.

Shangri-la

There are about 6600 centenarians in the USA or about 3 in 100 000 of the population. In the Hunza province of Pakistan, in parts of Georgia and Azerbaijan in southern USSR and in Vilcabamba in Ecuador high in the Andes centenarians are much more prevalent. They have been reported to number from 30 to 60 per 100 000 of the populations, although these figures are suspect as they cannot be supported by birth certificates, except in Vilcabamba where there are baptismal records, but these are unreliable. However, a professor of medicine at Harvard (Leaf, 1973) has visited all of these areas and found large numbers of active and healthy old people in each. The one factor common to all of them, men and women alike, was that they had led and continued to lead a hard life in the fields as peasant agriculturalists, usually in a harsh environment. The remarkable absence of chronic degenerative disease might perhaps be attributed to a simple diet, but some of them, particularly in Georgia, lived well and ate meat, dairy products and sugar and were not averse to feasts, alcohol and tobacco. Dr Leaf obviously enjoyed his visit and was well entertained. If there is any message for us from these people, perhaps it is that the secret of a long

and healthy old age is not a life of abstinence but one of hard physical labour. After studying ten Russian publications Medvedev (1974) is doubtful whether very old people are more numerous in Georgia than elsewhere; he suggests that there is a cult of old people there and they may be used for State propaganda.

Experiments on animals

There has been much study of the effects of diet on the length of life of experimental animals (Ross, 1976). In this work McCay (1949, 1955) at Cornell was a pioneer. Many carefully controlled investigations into the effects of giving to insects, fish and mammals a diet which leads to a rapid increase of growth and weight, have actually shown a reduction in life span. In addition such a diet has been shown to produce in rats and mice an increased liability to degenerative diseases and various tumours, including carcinoma. The reverse was found to occur when the energy intake was below the optimum for rapid growth. Rats, whose growth has been retarded by restricting their food intake, have lived much longer than controls fed unlimited amounts of food. Much more information must be available before it should be justifiable to accept these results from animal experiments as being necessarily applicable to man; they certainly draw attention to the question whether maximum growth rates are desirable.

Dietetic requirements

The majority of old people remain physically active and eat a varied diet in amounts which differ little from that of the rest of the population, as many surveys in Britain have shown (Durnin et al., 1961; Exton-Smith et al., 1965; Department of Health and Social Security, 1970; Lonergen et al., 1975). As activity declines, the need for energy falls but the need for minerals and vitamins remains unchanged, as the metabolism of the tissues is unaltered, except for a small fall in resting metabolism due to a reduced cell mass. Provided activities are sufficient to require an energy intake of 8.4 MJ (2000 kcal), the usual mixed diet is likely to contain sufficient of all the essential nutrients. When activities are reduced, the proportion of energy-rich foods should be reduced and that of protective foods, e.g. milk, fruit and vegetables, increased to prevent the risk of deficiencies of nutrients arising. Anyone who becomes inactive requires a smaller diet with a higher nutrient density than when active.

Nutritional disorders in the elderly

A low blood concentration of a nutrient or other evidence of low tissue reserves has been found in many surveys of selected groups of old people, e.g. deficiency of iron (McLennan et al., 1973), of folate (Girdwood et al., 1967), of ascorbic acid (Milne et al., 1971; Burr et al., 1974), of thiamin (Griffith et al., 1976) and of pyridoxine (Rose et al., 1976).

Anaemia usually due to iron deficiency is common in old people but perhaps not more so than in other age groups. Any geriatrician is likely to see occasionally cases of megaloblastic anaemia, scurvy and osteomalacia; when as a result of any disease or general infirmity, an old person cannot go out, a supplement of vitamin D is needed. The digestive and absorptive power of the gut is normally well maintained in old people. Dental disease or lack of suitable dentures may prevent an adequate food intake, as may alcoholism.

Mainly because of economic and psychological factors, old people are at increased risk of deficiency diseases. Early detection, the responsibility of the health services, is important and allows the social services to take steps to ensure that the patient gets adequate food, e.g. the 'meals on wheels' service (see below).

Nutritional assessment

Methods which may be used are illustrated by summarising the findings in a large survey in Britain (Department of Health and Social Security, 1972). The survey covered 879 men and women aged 65 or over in six different areas. The subjects were selected from the registers of the local executive councils of the National Health Service and formed a representative sample of all aged people in the country. The survey consisted of four parts, (1) a clinical examination, (2) a dietary study lasting one week, (3) analyses of a sample of blood, and (4) skeletal status.

Clinical examination. Only 27 subjects (3.2 per cent) were diagnosed as malnourished. Of these two had frank scurvy and eight angular stomatitis, and the reason given for the diagnosis was in most cases excessive thinness. In 12 of the subjects there were major medical disorders which may have contributed to the malnutrition and in seven cases there were socioeconomic causes. In eight cases there was no clear reason for the finding.

The great majority of the subjects appeared well fed. Obesity is probably the commonest nutritional disorder in the elderly, at least in women.

Diet survey. The dietary energy intake is shown in Table 62.2. For men the mean intakes are almost exactly the recommended intakes, but for women they are 13 and

Table 62.6 Mean daily energy intake

	MJ/day		kcal/day	
	age 65–74	age 75+	age 65–74	age 75+
Men	9.7	8.8	2340	2100
Women	7.5	6.8	1790	1630

14 per cent below the recommendation. However the fact that most of the subjects appeared well fed suggests that the latter may be too high.

The survey showed that the diets contained foods and nutrients in the same proportion as they are consumed by the population as a whole. There was no evidence that the quality of the diet changes as age advances. However as old people eat less, intakes of nutrients fall and the risk of a deficiency arising must increase.

Blood findings. Table 62.3 shows the percentage of subjects in whom the concentrations of various components of the blood was lower than values considered satisfactory. A low value does not necessarily mean that the subject is suffering from any deficiency disease, but does suggest that his diet is lacking in quality and that he may be at increased risk of developing malnutrition, should his diet deteriorate or any disease develop which impairs alimentary absorption of nutrients or increases requirements.

Skeletal status. From radiographs of the second metacarpal bone, the ratio of the areas of cortical bone surface to total bone surface was calculated by the method of Exton-Smith et al. (1969). This ratio correlates well with the ash content of bone and can be used as an index of bone mass. In those of the subjects in whom the bone ratio was low, the prevalence of high values for plasma alkaline phosphatase and low values for plasma calcium was greater than in the remainder. This suggests that the diminished cortical thickness of the bone in this group might be due to early osteomalacia. The finding that in this group the proportion with low intakes of dietary vitamin D was the same as in the remainder, while the proportion who were housebound was higher suggests that in old people the skin is a more important source of the vitamin than the diet.

Table 62.3 Percentage of subjects with concentrations of various components of the blood below values considered to be satisfactory

Component	Lower limit considered satisfactory	Men		Women	
		age 65–74	age 75+	age 65–74	age 75+
Haemoglobin	13 g/dl	5.5	9.6	—	—
	12 g/dl	—	—	8.1	5.3
Serum albumin	35 µg/l	10.7	15.3	10.2	13.6
Serum iron	600 µg/l	15.9	16.9	20.5	24.6
Serum vitamin B$_{12}$	100 pg/ml	0.5	2.6	1.2	0.7
Serum folate	3 ng/ml	14.8	14.5	10.6	18.0
Leucocyte ascorbic acid	7 µg/10^8 cells	6.3	15.9	2.6	5.7

The numbers involved here are small, but are consistent with the view that subclinical osteomalacia may be not uncommon.

There was no correlation between the dietary calcium and the bone ratio in any of the groups of subjects in the survey.

Supply of foods. 'Meals on wheels' provides a valuable service for those old people who for one reason or another find difficulty in buying and preparing food. Of the subjects in the survey about 3 per cent received from one to five meals in a week from the service, but a further 4 per cent said that they would like the meals if they were available. Clearly the service is appreciated and should be extended.

In a survey of the nutritional value of 'meals on wheels' in one town, Davies *et al.* (1973, 1974) found the average meal provided 3.5 MJ of energy, but little ascorbic acid because of the prolonged time that cooked vegetables were kept warm. Menus should be designed to obviate this, e.g. by including fresh fruit.

Old people like foods which can be purchased easily, store well and are readily prepared. The egg is the prototype 'convenience food' and is popular; old people eat on average just over five a week, rather more than the general population. If the food industry can produce inexpensive and nutritious convenience foods, there is a large potential market amongst old people.

There does not appear to be a case for a general provision of free or cheap milk for old people. The average intake in the survey was 350 ml/day, but individual variation was very wide. However, in view of the low intake of vitamin D and the limited exposure of old people to sunlight, there is a case for a trial of milk fortified with vitamin D.

Comment

The good state of nutrition of the great majority of old people is a cause for satisfaction. However, although the proportion of old people who were clinically malnourished is only 3 per cent, as there are now about seven million old people in Britain, the total number of malnourished old people might be about 200 000. This is a sizeable social and medical problem.

The survey showed that in many of those malnourished remediable medical or social conditions contributed. If the health authorities had been aware of the condition of these patients, malnutrition in many cases could have been prevented and in almost all alleviated. Old people may allow their health to deteriorate without consulting their doctor. Early detection is the key to this problem.

This would be greatly facilitated by a register of all persons over 65 years of age on the list of each general practitioner. This would enable each old person to be visited regularly at intervals determined by their age and state of health. The visits could be made either by public health nurses or by specially trained geriatric visitors, who could be attached to general practitioners.

For further reading a report of a Swedish Nutrition Foundation Symposium (Carlson, 1972) is recommended.

MEDICAL CARE OF THE AGED

It was once a common view that the disorders and disabilities of old age are incurable. Such an outlook must be energetically opposed. The primary requirement of the aged sick is accurate diagnosis, followed by medical treatment based on modern scientific principles. Much can be done to alleviate the infirmities of the aged by seeing that they get a good mixed diet in sufficient quantities, by obtaining for them suitable dentures, spectacles and hearing aids, and by ensuring that their corns are treated regularly by a chiropodist. Antibiotics and other drugs are just as valuable in the aged as in the young. With modern anaesthesia, the surgical treatment of piles, a hernia, a prolapsed uterus or enlarged prostate is usually possible and the results well worth while.

Many of the disabilities and frailties of age are the result of emotional causes leading to a failure of morale and a lack of interest in living. This attitude of mind develops as a result of isolation, immobility, loneliness and poverty; the doctor should make every attempt to deal with these problems with the help of voluntary organisations and local and national health authorities. He should have first-hand knowledge of the personnel and services provided by the health authorities in his district, e.g. home nurses, home helps, 'meals on wheels', special laundry facilities, residential accommodation in welfare homes and geriatric hospitals and financial aid from government and other agencies.

Lastly, some of the problems and disabilities of old age would be lessened if persons about to retire gave thought to this matter in good time, as by this means functional activity, mental and physical, could be better maintained for many years after retiral. This important subject is dealt with in a book called *Facing Retirement* (Country Doctor, 1960) which contains much information and advice on the social, medical and financial aspects of old age and is a valuable guide to those facing retirement.

63. Athletics

Only a minority of athletic records are 10 years old. In all classes of athletics, and indeed in sports generally, there has been a sharp rise in the standards of performance. These new standards have been made possible by newer methods of training. Most important, the top class athlete trains far harder than his predecessors. The extra physical activity in training involves extra energy.

In the past there was no sphere of dietetics in which faddism and ignorance had been more conspicuous than in the field of athletics, and many fantastic diets have been recommended. Mayer and Bullen (1960, 1964) have provided two good reviews which separate the few established facts from the large volume of fiction which is still widespread about diet and athletics. It is now known that the dietetic requirements for the athlete in training are based on the same fundamental principles which govern the nutrition of human beings in general, as already outlined. These principles have been generally applied to athletes in training and this no doubt has contributed to some extent to the general improvement in athletic performances in recent years.

It can be stated categorically: (1) that none of the ordinary foods eaten by man are either of special value or contraindicated in athletic training; (2) that preparations of vitamins and minerals, given in addition to a good mixed diet, do not improve athletic performance; (3) that alcoholic drinks taken in small quantities by people accustomed to them have no effect on training.

Athletic training nearly always involves a large expenditure of physical energy and this energy must be provided in the diet. Many athletes in training consume diets providing up to 20 MJ (5000 kcal)/daily, though lower intakes are probably more usual. It is essential that adequate amounts of protein be provided and this is ensured if 10 per cent of the energy is provided by protein. Surveys have shown that many athletes take by choice more protein than this (Steel, 1970), but there is no evidence that this extra protein is beneficial: nor does it do harm. Many first-class athletes have been vegetarians, and provided the protein intake is adequate, vegetarian diets are suitable for hard training. High energy diets should contain large quantities of fat, unless they are to become very bulky. Physical activity prevents the disturbances in blood lipids which commonly arise in sedentary people on high fat diets, and large quantities of fat in the diet will do no harm to men and women undergoing physical training. Provided the requirements for protein, carbohydrate, fat, minerals and vitamins are properly satisfied, the diet for the athlete in training differs only from the ordinary well-balanced diet in that it must provide extra sources of energy. The quantity of food required can usually be assessed by the individual's natural appetite, and no food schedules are required. At the beginning of a period of training, if the subject has previously been taking little physical exercise, there may be some loss of weight due to the using up of excess fat. Subsequently there is often a gain in weight, attributable to hypertrophy of muscles.

Many types of sport and athletics involve large losses of fluid in the sweat. Losses up to 1 litre in an hour are not uncommon. It is important that these losses are promptly made good by the necessary fluid intake. Even a very minor degree of dehydration may impair the efficiency of muscles. The restrictions on fluid intake often imposed by trainers of a previous generation must have done nothing but harm.

There is usually no need to alter the training diet in the days immediately before an event, but the pattern of the meals should be adjusted to allow an interval of two to three hours between the end of a main meal and the start of the event.

Physiologists have shown that the glycogen stores in muscles can be raised above the normal level by dietary means. The main fuel for heavy exercise is carbohydrate (p. 74) and if an event requires continuous work at near maximum capacity for more than 30 minutes, depletion of muscle glycogen may become a factor limiting performance. These discoveries followed the introduction of a punch technique for taking samples of deep muscle for analysis and depended on a supply of athletes willing to provide repeated samples of their quadriceps femoris, the great extensor muscle of the legs which covers the front and sides of the femur.

Normally the glycogen content of this muscle is about 15 g/kg. During running to exhaustion it fell to about 7.5 g after 30 minutes and to about 1 g after an hour, when the subjects had to reduce their work rate. The initial glycogen content of muscle was shown to be of decisive importance in determining how long an individual can sustain heavy exercise (Hermansen et al., 1967). That the glycogen content of muscle could be raised above the usual value was shown in an experiment in which two men worked to exhaustion on the same bicycle ergometer, one using his right leg and one his left leg; their other two legs were resting. At the start of the experiment the glycogen content of the muscles of all four legs was about 25 g/kg; at the end of the exercise it was about 1 g/kg in the exercised legs and little changed in the rested pair. The subjects were then given a high carbohydrate diet for three days during which the glycogen in the muscles of the exercised legs rose up to 35g/kg but there were only very small rises in the two rested legs (Bergström and Hultman, 1966).

The unusually high store of glycogen depends on giving a high carbohydrate diet after the store has been completely depleted by exercise, and the highest values, up to 50 g/kg, were obtained when the depleted state had been maintained by a diet of protein and fat only for three days, followed by carbohydrate for three days (Saltin and Hermansen, 1967).

Such a regimen is quite unnecessary for the great majority of athletes, but might be useful for some long distance races whether running, swimming, cycling or skiing. It also has one drawback: 1 g of glycogen is stored with 2.7 g of water and body weight would be increased perhaps up to 1 kilogram. This would increase the work done in lifting the body during running. Some athletes may also be upset psychologically by taking an artificial diet for several days.

In top-class athletics and other sporting events the difference in performance between the winner and the second is small and more likely to be the result of psychological than physiological factors. Many distinguished athletes are more than normally sensitive people. A wise trainer humours their dietary fancies and sees that they have the food that they like and they think suits them best. He should not impose his or any other dietary theories and remember that individual requirements vary greatly.

A book edited by Pařízkova and Rogozkin (1978) with contributors from 16 countries reflects contempory interest in nutrition, sport and health and gives many viewpoints.

64. Climate; Diets for Expeditions; Survival Rations

CLIMATE

Much has been written about the modification of dietary habits considered to be necessary in different climates. Most of this has little scientific background. The effects of climate on the need for nutrients have often been exaggerated. The extra need for water and salt in hot weather is of great importance but, apart from this, climate imposes no important change in the physiological needs.

WATER AND SALT

In hot climates the body can only be maintained at an even temperature by sweating. The amount of sweat lost will be determined by the environmental temperature, the humidity and the air movement, and also by the amount of physical work done. A man engaged in physical labour in the tropics may readily lose 4 litres of sweat a day and under exceptional circumstances double this amount. Sweat contains from 20 to 80 mmol NaCl/litre, the concentration being lower in the acclimatised and trained subject. The body may lose about 240 mmol of NaCl each day or about 14 g of salt on a hot day in the tropics and much more if heavy work is done. It is essential that these losses of water and salt should be made good by increased intakes.

Effects of heat

In mild cases fainting, or **heat syncope,** occurs. This is due to vasodilation in the skin expanding the vascular bed. When the compensatory mechanisms are inadequate, blood flow to the brain diminishes and causes fainting. This is not due to the direct effect of sunlight on the head and neck, a myth which gave rise to the use of pith helments or topees.

Three syndromes are responsible for the severe cases. The first is caused directly by **salt and water depletion.** As in mild cases there is evidence of circulatory shock, but low blood·pressure and tachycardia persist; loss of appetite, nausea, headache and emotional changes are common. The muscle cramps characteristic of salt deficiency may occur. The output of urine is always greatly diminished and it is of high specific gravity. The diagnostic test is the absence of salt from the urine; there is no white precipitate of silver chloride on the addition of silver nitrate after acidification with nitric acid.

Anhidrotic heat exhaustion is attributable to failure of the sweat glands to secrete, due to fatigue. This loss of ability to sweat may follow many weeks or months in excessive heat. The principal clinical features are dizziness, palpitation, breathlessness and lack of sleep. It has often been preceded by prickly heat, in which the sweat glands get blocked and inflamed.

The dangerous state is **heat hyperpyrexia.** Coma, convulsions or delirium are very likely to occur at a body temperature over 41°C (106°F) and may do so at temperatures between 39.5 and 41°C (103 and 106°F). Even with the·best medical care renal failure and other fatal complications may occur.

Prevention

It is important to reduce exposure as far as possible. Shade and shelter against the sun are obviously desirable. It is also important to arrange that no unnecessary physical work is carried out and that, as far as possible, men do not have to work in the midday heat. However, even with the best of management, men will always be exposed to excessive heat and its consequent risks.

It is essential that all exposed men should know these risks and how they can best be avoided. All newcomers to the tropics need such education and should be taught to respect the heat. They should learn that thirst is not always a reliable guide to water requirements, nor is the natural appetite for salt always reliable. Liberal amounts of drinking water must be available not only in canteens, but in places of work. It is important to see that this water is cool. While men readily drink cool water, they may neglect to drink tepid water, even if there is a physiological need. Each individual can judge whether he is taking enough water by his urine output. If there is not a good flow of urine at least four times in the 24 hours, he is not taking enough. Ample salt should be available on the table at all meals and people told to use it. Cooks should be instructed to salt the food well. As much as 30 g of NaCl may be necessary to make good the losses in the sweat, i.e. at least double a normal intake. It may be desirable to add salt to the drinking water. Amounts up to 0.1 per cent are barely perceptible. This is provided by the addition of ½ oz (2 teaspoonsful) to one gallon. There is a risk that men may not drink water in which they can taste salt; provided adequate table salt is available and the men use it, there should be little need to add salt to the drinking water.

OTHER NUTRIENTS

The effects of climate on the need for the remaining

nutrients are small and unimportant in comparison with the extra need for salt and water in the tropics. They are briefly set out below.

Energy. As discussed in Chapter 3, the chief factor determining energy needs is the amount of physical activity undertaken. This is generally little affected by climate except by extremes of heat or excessive cold. Both of these restrict activity, especially by making active physical recreations unpleasant or impossible.

There is some indication that the energy cost of performing a standard task of physical work falls with the rise of environmental temperature, but the evidence is conflicting and the effect, if it exists, is small and probably negligible. In cold climates, the cost of physical work may be increased by up to 5 per cent by the 'hobbling' effect of the protective clothing. This may weigh 6 kg or more and of necessity restricts the ease of movement, besides involving extra energy for carrying it about.

Fat. When undertaking hard work such as sledging in very cold climates, up to 20 MJ (5000 kcal)/day may be needed. If the diet is not to be very bulky, large quantities of fat (up to 250 g or even more) are required and can be digested and absorbed. A high intake of fat is probably essential if hard physical exercise is to be undertaken in any climate.

Protein. Reduction in protein intake in hot climates has been stated to be desirable, owing to the extra heat liberated by the specific dynamic action of protein. A liberal intake of protein does not disturb the heat balance or cause discomfort and there is no good reason to reduce the intake of meat or other protein-rich foods below what is customary in a mixed diet.

Minerals. The sweat contains very small amounts of minerals, but the losses of iron may be significant; it has been suggested that this may contribute to the causation of anaemia, which is so common in many countries with hot climates.

Vitamins. No significant losses occur in the sweat. There is no evidence that the recommended intakes for vitamins need be in any way altered on account of climate, except perhaps in the case of vitamin C. Lind (1753) reported that scurvy was much more common and severe in winter than in summer, and in ships going to Greenland and the Baltic than in those going to Southern latitudes. On the other hand, Eskimos appear to have managed with their traditional diets, which contained few sources of ascorbic acid in the long winter months. In cold climates it is certainly important to see that intakes of vitamin C in the food are satisfactory.

Alcohol. Europeans and Americans working in the tropics are much more prone to alcoholism than at home. Alcohol is readily used as an escape from the annoyances and discomforts caused by excessive heat, insects, the absence of family and friends, the lack of customary recreations and the necessity to work with strange people, whose way of life is not fully appreciated. The expatriate man or woman in the tropics who is unable to make adjustments and to develop new interests, readily falls a victim to alcoholism. Nevertheless, despite its dangers, we would not be without alcohol in the tropics. Taken in moderation, it is a valuable sedative and helps to distract from obsessional attention to duty, and to promote social life. Midday drinking is especially dangerous and the old adage, 'never drink before sunset', is to be recommended. It is also necessary to have the strength of mind to withstand the pressure to have rounds of drinks when in convivial and congenial company.

GENERAL CONSIDERATIONS

An adverse climate, whether very hot or very cold, imposes considerable strains, both physical and psychological, on an individual. If the diet is not satisfactory he is less able to stand these strains. The provision of a satisfactory diet is made difficult by the fact that good supplies of fresh fruit and vegetables are generally not available locally in very cold climates and are usually very limited in very hot dry climates. Modern transport, refrigeration and food technology have made it possible to overcome this difficulty, although often at considerable expense.

The importance of good catering and good cooking for men and women who have to live and work in a harsh climate cannot be overstressed. Apart from their effect on physical health, they sustain morale. The changes imposed by climate in the physiological requirements of nutrients are negligible (except for the increased requirements for salt and water in hot climates), compared with the need to provide a good mixed diet and to ensure that it is well cooked and attractively served.

DIETS FOR EXPEDITIONS

Explorers and others often go to parts of the world where the opportunities for obtaining food are either limited or altogether absent. In such circumstances the expedition has to take with it sufficient food for its members. The planning and provision of the rations may make all the difference between the success or failure of the expedition or military operation. A symposium of the Nutrition Society (1954) on *The Provisioning of Expeditions in the Field* sets out the nutritional principles on which this is based and these have changed little, but there are now many improvements in the preparation and packaging of the dietary items.

Members of expeditions are usually active young men. Their requirements for nutrients when on the expedition are essentially the same as the daily allowances appropriate for men of their class (p. 153). The circumstances of an expedition do not raise physiological requirements above these liberal allowances. A practical point is the assessment of probable physical activity and the consequent need for energy. Climbers usually expend between 1.7 and 2.5 MJ (400 and 600 kcal)/h with surprisingly little variation (Pugh, 1958). Similar hourly rates of energy expenditure have been found in sledging parties (Masterton *et al.*, 1957). The organisers of any expedition have to estimate the daily energy expenditure of the members when in the field and provide food accordingly.

It is important to see that all members of an expedition have been well fed before the expedition sets out. This ensures the presence of sufficient stores of the nutrients normally carried by the body. While these enable a man to survive for a long time with intakes of nutrients far below the daily recommended intakes, this is only at the expense of some loss of physical fitness.

Further, there is no evidence that any period of previous training prevents such physiological deterioration. In particular no previous training can prevent the dehydration and consequent deterioration that follow rapidly upon a reduction in the fluid intake below the physiological losses. It is impossible to train oneself to do without water. Nevertheless, in some circumstances it may be a valuable experience for members of an expedition to live for a few days on an inadequate diet and with a reduced fluid intake, for it will provide an opportunity for the men to feel the adverse effects on themselves of such deprivations. This experience may enable them to adjust their plans sensibly in a crisis. Fit young men frequently overestimate their 'toughness' and ability to carry on in a crisis. Such overconfidence may be disastrous both for themselves and those for whom they may be responsible. The importance of an adequate water supply for expeditions cannot be overstressed. On Sir John Hunt's first successful assault on Everest great care was taken to see that all members of the expedition drank sufficient water. This may have been one of the factors responsible for their success.

After assessing the physiological needs for nutrients the organisers of an expedition have to translate these into terms of food and then to arrange for the supply of the food. A first consideration is an estimate of the extent to which an expedition can 'live off the country'. In practice, this is negligible on high mountains and near the North or South Poles, and very limited in deserts and sub-Arctic regions. But in tropical and subtropical regions there is usually game which can be trapped or shot, and often natives from whom grain can be purchased. It is always a wise precaution to see that members of an expedition have the necessary equipment for fishing, trapping or shooting and the skill to use them in an emergency. Arctic expeditions have perished for lack of such equipment and skill under conditions in which the Eskimos have survived.

In most expeditions the major portion of the food has to be carried with the party. It is clearly important to reduce the load to be carried—no matter whether the means of transport are aeroplanes, trucks, pack animals, porters or members of the expedition. Modern food technology has contributed enormously to this problem. Meat, fruit and vegetables can be prepared so that only the edible portions are packed and no waste is carried. Great improvements have been made in the quality of dehydrated foods. Packing materials and methods have also improved, so that packages can be made which withstand damage, rough handling and long storage in any climate without deterioration of the contents. In these ways it has been possible to reduce the weight of stores. It is also important to arrange the packing so that the food can be easily distributed and, if necessary, divided up into smaller units for small parties.

The food should be provided in a form so that meals can be prepared with a minimum of cooking and served as attractively as possible. As many members of an expedition as possible should have some training in cookery.

SURVIVAL RATIONS

Lifeboats have long been provided with rations for those who survive the immediate disaster of shipwreck. Many civilian and military aeroplanes also carry emergency rations for use in the event of a forced landing in an isolated place. In some military planes the pilot can, in an emergency, eject himself and his seat from the plane and descend by parachute. Attached to the undersurface of the seat are rations and equipment for survival. There has been much study of the most suitable type of emergency ration for these and other purposes (Hervey and McCance, 1954).

Castaways are usually rescued, if at all, within a period of 14 days. It is not generally considered practical to plan for any longer period of survival. Rescue equipment must provide many other things besides food and, in selecting what articles to include, it is necessary to keep the total bulk of the supplies to a minimum. Food, in fact, receives a very low priority: for no healthy man will die of starvation in 14 days; nor will he suffer any permanent adverse effect from the experience, although his physical efficiency will be somewhat reduced at the time. However, within 14 days he can readily die of lack of water or from exposure to extremes of heat or cold. Water and protection against the environment, including mosquitos, have, therefore, priority over food, as also has radio equipment which enables the survivor to get in touch with rescue parties. Nevertheless all emergency equipment contains some food which will, in part, prevent the physical deterioration consequent upon total fasting and, perhaps more important, sustain the morale of the survivors. Before discussing these rations it is proper to discuss the more essential problem of water supply.

Minimal water requirements

A man at rest in an equable climate loses at least 800 ml of water daily by evaporation from the skin and lungs. This may be increased fourfold or more by the necessity to do hard physical work or in a hot environment. The minimum amount of water that his kidneys must pass is a little less than 500 ml daily. Against these essential losses may be offset the metabolic water produced by the oxidation of carbohydrate, protein and fat in the tissues. Under conditions of fasting and rest this amounts to about 200 ml daily. Thus to prevent a loss of body water the minimum daily intake must be 1 litre, but much more is needed if physical work is undertaken or the weather hot. As stated in Chapter 2, the body of a healthy man contains about 40 litres of water. A loss of 2 litres or more will usually cause discomfort and inefficiency, a loss of 4 litres is disabling and a loss of 8 litres will rapidly lead to death. Thus even with everything else in their favour, few men would survive 10 days without water.

It is rarely possible to provide emergency water which would be sufficient to cover the losses that might arise under very hot conditions. Small solar stills have been designed which can meet in part the extra needs of castaways on a tropical sea. In such conditions it is essential to attempt to minimise water losses by the provision of tents or other material which give shade; survivors must be warned of the adverse effects of unnecessary physical activity. In great heat, sea water can be used to keep the body cool.

The danger of drinking sea water. Sea water has a concentration of sodium ions of 420 mmol/l and 470 mmol/l of chloride ions. The corresponding concentrations in the blood plasma are about 142 and 104. Sea water is thus much more concentrated than the body fluids. Moreover, the human kidney is not normally able to concentrate either sodium or chloride to as high a level as in the sea (Hervey and McCance, 1952). Experiments in which small quantities of sea water have been drunk have given equivocal results. There may be some temporary retention of water, but this is associated with an increased tonicity of the body fluids. This may be expected to give rise to an osmotic diuresis in a short time in which the water retained will be lost. In experimental studies on man, it has proved difficult to demonstrate either a beneficial or an adverse effect of drinking small quantities up to 250 ml of sea water. The heroic experiments of Bombard

(1953) showed only that one man could drink a lot of sea water and survive. Critchley (1943), however, studied carefully the records of castaways during World War II and showed that the drinking of large amounts of sea water was usually fatal. It is wise to forbid the drinking of any sea water.

COMPOSITION OF SURVIVAL RATIONS

The first consideration is that the salt intake should be as low as possible, for the necessity to excrete salt will increase the need for water. Proteins also produce nitrogenous end-products which require water for their elimination and so it is desirable that the protein intake should not be high. Deprivation of protein for a temporary period of 14 days will cause no harm, nor will a similar temporary restriction of the intake of minerals and vitamins. Survival rations have been devised in which the foods are restricted to a mixture of carbohydrate and fats which can be made up in sweets and toffees. Fat has the advantage over carbohydrate that it provides over twice the amount of energy for a given unit of weight. The more fat in the rations, the less is their bulk. On the other hand, dietary carbohydrate is more effective than fat in 'sparing' endogenous nitrogen metabolism and so will reduce the loss of body protein and also the urine volume. Carbohydrate also prevents the ketosis that arises when an excess of fat is metabolised. Johnson and Sargent (1958) carried out on a large scale realistic field trials of various emergency rations in different climates for periods of 14 days. In many of these trials the daily water intake was limited to 900 ml. Their results indicated that men survived best if provided with an emergency ration in which the proteins, carbohydrates and fats were distributed in the normal manner (15 per cent of energy from protein, 52 per cent from carbohydrate and 33 per cent from fat).

Whatever the nature of the ration, it is essential that it be provided in a compact form, that requires no cooking or other preparation and that it does not deteriorate on storage even under adverse conditions. Various forms of boiled sweets, candies, toffees and meat bar can be used for this purpose.

Appendix 1. Glossary of Foods

Abalone. A mollusc resembling a large scallop which may be served in a salad or soup or fried; other names are **muttonfish** (Australia) and **ormer** (Channel Is.).

Ackee (*Blighia sapida*). Popular in Jamaica, about 3 cm long, red in colour and opens naturally when ripe to expose the edible portion of fleshy, cream-coloured aril which surrounds each of the three seeds. The other tissues, of the fruit are poisonous (p. 220), as is under- or over-ripe fruit. The aril is usually eaten fried or boiled.

Almond (*Prunus dulcis var dulcis*). A close relative of the peach and plum, grown in southern Europe and California, mainly for confectionery, notably marzipan. Also eaten as a nut.

Angelcake (N. Am.). A light, spongy, fat-free cake, leavened by air by stiffly beating a large number of egg-whites.

Aubergine (*Solanum melongena*). A glossy, firm fruit, oval or oblong in shape from 10 to 50 cm in length, white or deep purple in colour; other names are **egg plant** and **brinjal** (India); eaten as a cooked vegetable, sliced and fried, or incorporated into curries and other dishes.

Bannock (Scot.). A flat, round cake made from oatmeal, rye, barley or wheat: may take the place of bread in the diet.

Bap (Scot.). A soft breakfast roll, similar in appearance to an American hamburger bun.

Barbecue. A method of grilling (broiling) food on a grid over a flameless heat from charcoal briquettes to produce a distinctive flavour; popular in North America.

Barcelona nut (*Corylus* spp.). A Spanish variety of hazelnut.

Bass. Fresh- and salt-water fish similar in shape and colouring to the salmon; the flesh is firm, lean and delicately flavoured.

Beetroot (*Beta vulgaris*). A crimson spherical root, which is boiled and eaten fresh or pickled; known simply as **beet** in North America.

Betty (N. Am.). A simple pudding: consists of layers of sliced fruit and breadcrumbs baked in a deep, buttered dish, e.g. apple betty.

Bilberry (*Vaccinium myrtillus*). Also known as **blaeberry** and **whortleberry**, a small fruit, blue in colour similar in appearance to a small American blueberry, used mainly for jam or tarts.

Biscuit (N. Am.). A small, soft unsweetened cake, similar in composition to a scone; leavened with baking powder and frequently served as a hot bread in the southern USA.

Biscuit (UK). A crisp, semisweet cracker or a sweetened, flat cookie which is shaped and flavoured. A much wider term than in North America.

Blackberry (*Rubus ulmifolius*). Found wild in most parts of the British Isles; bears a black, seedy berry, eaten fresh or, with apples, stewed or made into jam; also known as **bramble** (Scot.) and **thimbleberry** (N. Am.).

Blackbun (Scot.). A rich fruitcake, enclosed in a pastry case.

Black pudding (blood sausage). A sausage made with pig's blood, ground pork, fat, onions, herbs and oatmeal; different versions are found throughout Europe and North America.

Blueberry (*Vaccinium corymbosum*). Native of North America, where blueberry pie is a traditional dessert; a delicious, bluish-black fruit, 7 mm across with a smooth skin. Larger than a bilberry.

Boiled sweets (UK). Any type of hard sugar candy, made without fat.

Bologna. A large round cooked sausage with a mild flavour.

Boston brown bread (N. Am.). A moist, dark bread made from a variety of cereal flours including cornmeal, mixed with butter-milk, molasses, raisins, and steamed; an excellent accompaniment to 'Boston baked beans'.

Boxty (Eire). A type of Irish potato pancake.

Brawn. A cold aspic, made with the trimmings of a pig and may include parts of the head, gristle and feet; cooked with onions and herbs. **Head cheese** is a type of brawn.

Brazil nut (*Bertholletia excelsa*). As the name implies, these nuts flourish in the tropical forests of Brazil; following harvest, the nuts have to be 'humoured' carefully so that they dry slowly and arrive in overseas shops in fine condition just before Christmas.

Breadfruit (*Artocarpus communis*). A starchy fruit, up to 20 cm in diameter, with a thick warty skin; usually eaten roasted and an important item of diet in many parts of the tropics.

Brinjal. See Aubergine.

Broad beans (*Vicia faba*). Consumed in Britain as the freshly shelled bean, also called **fava bean** (N. Am.). A hardy crop, it has been suggested as a substitute for soybeans, in areas where the latter do not grow well (see favism, p. 220).

Brownie (N. Am.). A rich chocolate cake, dense and chewy; usually containing walnuts.

Bubble and squeak (UK). A dish of leftover potatoes and cabbage, cooked and fried together; the name derives from the cooking noises.

Bun. In Britain the term refers to a sweetened, light yeast roll, often containing currants; varieties include Bath bun, Chelsea bun and the hot cross-bun (to symbolise the crucifixion, and eaten on Good Friday). In America, a variety of soft, plain rolls such as, the hamburger bun; also several types of sweet rolls.

Butter beans (*Phaseolus lunatus*). Large white, mature seeds also known as **lima beans** (N. Am.); most commonly eaten boiled as a vegetable, or in soups and stews.

Buttermilk. A cultured milk, made by adding *Streptococcus lactis* to pasteurised milk (usually skim milk in North America) until the lactic acid content is 0.9 per cent; it has a characteristic tangy flavour and smooth rich body.

Canadian bacon (N. Am.). Also known as **back bacon**, a lean oval-shaped cut from the back of the pig.

Candy (N. Am.). Generic name for any type of concentrated sweets; may refer to a range of confections from chocolate to boiled sweets. In UK, has a more limited meaning.

Cape gooseberry (*Physalis peruviana*). Similar in appearance but less sweet than the ground cherry, found in South Africa and elsewhere and also known as **goldenberries**.

Caramel. A product of indefinite composition, formed when sugars of any kind are partially broken down by heat; its brown colour, slightly burnt flavour and sticky consistency make it a valuable adjunct to the art of the good cook.

Cashew nut (*Anacardium occidentale*). A South American nut with a unique and delicious flavour, spread by the Portuguese to other parts of their former Empire; India is now a major producer of these popular dessert nuts.

Catfish. In Europe includes a number of fish such as the **seawolf** and **dogfish**. The American 'catfish' refers to members of the *Letalarus* family, which is widespread and includes varieties from 1 to 150 lb in weight. The small members of the species are particularly popular in the southern states where catfish and hushpuppies (fried cornmeal puffs) are traditional.

Catsup. (N. Am.). Also known as **ketchup**; a mildly seasoned tomato purée, used as table condiment.

Celeriac (*Apium graveolens* var *repaceum*). An irregular-shaped root resembling a turnip; the flavour is similar to that of celery.

Chapatti (India). A thin cake of unleavened bread.

Char (N. Am.). Member of the salmon family; a medium-fat fish, cooked like trout.

Chard (*Beta vulgaris*). Sometimes known as the **seakale beet** and **spinach beet**; grown mainly for its leaves which are similar to but less acid than spinach; the broad white stalk may also be eaten.

Cheesecake. More common in North America than elsewhere, a rich dessert consisting of a sweetened cream cheese custard over a biscuit or pastry base; sometimes topped with fruit or preserves.

Chick pea (*Cicer arietinum*). A hard, round yellow-white legume used extensively in India and also popular in Spain and Mexico, where it is given the name **garbanazo**; may be used in a variety of soups and curries or served as a vegetable.

Chicory (*Cichorium intybus*). A compact head of large leaves; most frequently used as a salad vegetable in the same way as endive; it may also be served as a cooked vegetable. The roots of some varieties may be dried, roasted and blended with coffee.

Chinese water chestnut (*Eleocharis tuberosa*). A tuber, valued for its crisp texture; eaten in the East Indies and China and Japan and canned for export to Europe and North America.

Chips (potato) (UK). Long, square-section pieces of potato, deep fried. Very popular in Britain. Traditionally eaten with fish fried in batter, but some British enthusiasts like chips with everything (the title of a play by Arnold Wesker).

Chipolata (Italy). A very small sausage, often seasoned with chives.

Chipped beef (N. Am.). Lean top round which has been corned, dried and sliced very thin.

Chitterlings. Small intestines of any animal but usually the pig, sometimes used as sausage casings; also the trimmings from a freshly killed pig; popular in southern USA.

Chowder. A thick soup, often with a milk base, made with a variety of foods, frequently fish, e.g. clam chowder (N. Am.) and bouillabaise (Fr.); from the French word *chaudiere*—a large, heavy soup pot.

Clam. A bivalve mollusc, common on the Atlantic coast of North America; may be fried, pickled, steamed, or made into a thick soup or chowder.

Clementine. A variety of tangerine or an orange-tangerine hybrid; intermediate between the two in size and colour, peels easily.

Clod (UK). Often 'clod and sticking'; **clod** is the front chest cut of beef and **sticking** the coarse part of the neck; these are cheaper cuts, which contain much gristle and fat, mainly used for stews. Clod is known as **chuck** in North America.

Cloudberry (*Rubus chamaemorus*). A golden berry similar to a raspberry which grows in the northern regions of Canada and Europe.

Cockles (UK). A small mollusc with a delicate flavour, boiled and eaten with a variety of condiments.

Coffeecake (N. Am.). A scone-like cake covered with a crumbly mixture of sugar, flour, and butter, often containing fruit.

Collard (*Brassica oleracea*) (N. Am.). A smooth-leaf variety of cabbage, the leaves of which may be boiled and served like spinach.

Collop. A piece of meat made tender by beating.

Cookie (N. Am.). Any sweetened, flat biscuit; made in a variety of shapes and flavours.

Corn. The North American term for maize (*Zea mays*). In Britain, it may refer to a variety of cereal grains, usually wheat but also oats and maize.

Cornbread (N. Am., especially southern states). A large number of breads made with maize meal, including corn pone, johnny cake, shortening bread, and hoecake. Egg bread and spoon bread are baked from a cornmeal, milk and egg batter and served as a main meal accompaniment.

Cornflour (UK). British for **cornstarch.**

Corn-on-the-cob (N. Am.). The cooked, freshly picked maize cob; when in season, a popular adjunct to the main meal throughout North America.

Cornish pasty (UK). A small, pastry-enclosed pie, containing meat, potato and vegetables; a portable meal which may be eaten hot or cold.

Courgette (*Cucurbita pepo*). A French marrow developed for early cutting, like the Italian **zucchini**, when only a few inches long. The mature courgette is no different from other vegetable marrows. Cooking methods include steaming or frying with garlic and tomato.

Cowpea (*Vigna unguiculata*). An annual legume, used as the dried white seeds; mostly grown in Africa and the United States; it is also an important animal feed.

Cracker (N. Am.). A crisp, flaky, non-sweet biscuit; low-fat varieties include **saltines** and **soda crackers**, which are usually sprinkled with course salt but are otherwise similar to the British cream cracker or water biscuit. Other types may be flavoured, contain more fat and be made from an assortment of cereal flours, e.g. **Graham crackers** which are made from wholemeal flour.

Crackling. The scored skin or rind of a roast of pork after it has been baked crisp.

Cream. A milk product containing at least 18% fat.* Single cream (UK), light cream, table or coffee cream (N. Am.). is 18–30% fat; double cream (UK) or heavy cream (N. Am.) contains 36–48% milk fat; whipping cream is 30–36% fat; half cream (N. Am.) is 12% fat; Devonshire cream (UK) is 60% fat and plastic cream (N. Am.) 65-83% milk fat. Dairy sour cream (N. Am.) is a thick, tangy-flavoured cream made by adding a bacterial culture to cream which contains 18% or more of fat.

* Figures are approximate only; legal requirements vary in different states and countries.

Cream cracker (UK). A round unsweetened biscuit, the equivalent of an unsalted soda cracker.

Cream of wheat (N. Am.). Coarsely ground particles of refined, hard wheat; usually served as a hot breakfast cereal.

Crisps (potato) (UK). See **Potato chips.**

Crispbreads. The original Swedish crispbreads are made with rye flour but now many varieties are made with wheat. As the water content is lower and the energy correspondingly higher than in ordinary bread, they have no advantage in reducing diets but are pleasant and convenient alternatives to ordinary bread.

Crumpet (UK). A round, flat breadlike teacake, studded with holes, similar to, but spongier than what Americans term an **English muffin**; toasted and served hot with butter and jam.

Custard (UK). A sweet sauce prepared from milk and eggs, flavoured with sugar and vanilla and served with a variety of desserts; eggs may be replaced by custard powder, which consists largely of cornflour.

Damson (*Prunus damascena*). Soft purple fruit with a rich, sour flavour; smaller than plum, native in Britain.

Dandelion greens (*Taraxacum officinale*). Leaves of the common dandelion; sometimes used as a salad vegetable like endive or chicory in North America; however in Britain the dandelion is regarded only as a noxious weed.

Dripping. Beef fat extracted as the meat is cooked; formerly much used for baking and frying.

Dumplings. A main-meal accompaniment, in Britain, made from a stiff dough of flour and suet, often boiled in beef broth. The American variety is made with flour, milk and baking powder and contains less fat.

Eccles cake (UK). A flat, oval pastry with a filling of spiced currants. Related forms include Banbury cakes and Chorley cakes; also known as 'flies' graveyards' to English schoolboys.

Egg plant. See **Aubergine.**

Endive (*Cichorium endivia*). A salad plant with leaves which are characteristically divided and curled. As the green leaves are bitter, they may be blanched to a pale yellow colour by covering to exclude the light for 5 to 10 days before cutting. Sometimes termed **chicory** or **Belgian endive** in America.

Escarole (*Cichorium endivia*). A variety of endive.

Faggots (N. Eng.). Also known as **savoury ducks**, a spiced mixture of ground offal, pork, breadcrumbs and herbs, which are baked and eaten hot or cold.

Fat back (S. USA). The fatty, cheaper scraps of bacon, used to flavour stews and vegetable or cereal dishes.

Filbert (*Corylus maxima*). A robust variety of hazelnut.

Filled milk. Milk in which the cream has been replaced by a vegetable fat; those containing polyunsaturated oils are useful in cholesterol-lowering diets.

Finnan haddie (Scot.). Smoked haddock, cooked in a milk sauce.

Flan (UK). A shallow shell of pastry or sponge, usually filled with jellied fruits or custard. Savoury flans contain various mixtures of cheese, onions and tomatoes.

Fool (UK). A thick, chilled pudding, made with fruit and sugar, mixed with cream or custard, e.g. gooseberry fool.

Fortified milk (N. Am.). Whole or skim milk to which has been added one or more of the nutrients normally present in milk, usually vitamins A, D or skim-milk solids.

Frankfurter. A long thin cooked sausage often served in a roll as a **hot dog**; also known as a wiener.

French beans (*Phaseolus vulgaris*). The immature medium-length soft green pods are popular as a boiled vegetable. If allowed to mature the seeds vary in colour and shape from the purple **kidney bean** to the white or multicoloured **haricot bean**, which is used for the ubiquitous 'baked beans'.

French fries (N. Am.). The American word for deep-fried potato sticks, which are familiar to the British as **chips.**

French toast (N. Am.). Bread which is dipped in a mixture of beaten egg and milk and fried until crisp on the outside; may be served with sugar, syrup or bacon.

Gammon (UK). A cut from the hind leg of a pig, cured in the same manner as bacon, while still on the side of the animal.

Gelatin desserts (N. Am.). Commonly referred to by trade names such as 'Jell-O', these are fat-free puddings made from gelatin, sugar and fruit flavouring; known as **jellies** in Britain.

Ghee (Indian). Butter-fat clarified by heating.

Gigot (Scot., Fr.). Leg of mutton.

Golden syrup (UK). A light refined treacle similar to American **corn syrup.**

Gooseberry (*Ribes grossularia*). The European gooseberry bears large yellowish-green or red berries, with a downy skin and a tart but distinctive flavour. Usually made into jam; when mature, many varieties are sweet and excellent to eat raw. The American gooseberry (*R. divaricatum*) is similar but smaller. In England, gooseberry pie is traditional fare for Whitsuntide.

Graham flour (N. Am.). Another name for wholemeal flour.

Granadilla. See **Passion fruit.**

Greengage (*Prunus italica*). Several varieties of soft, yellow-green plums, grown in Europe and North America.

Griskin (UK). Lean bacon from the loin of pork.

Ground beef (N. Am.). See **Hamburger.**

Ground cherry (*Physalis pruinosa*). A native of parts of Europe and North America, a yellow, round berry, 2 cm in diameter, enclosed within a lantern-like calyx; flavour is sweet and slightly acid.

Guava (*Psidium guajava*). Light-yellow fruit of the tropics and subtropics; has a sharp flavour, is often stewed or made into jam or jelly; a particularly rich source of vitamin C.

Gumbo (S. USA). A dish or soup thickened with okra; often contains seafood, other ingredients vary.

Haggis (Scot.). The ground liver, heart and lungs of a sheep mixed with suet, oatmeal and herbs, encased in a sheep's stomach; steamed and traditionally accompanied by Scotch whisky.

Hake (UK). A large, round fish caught off the west coast of Britain; cooked in same way as cod or haddock.

Hamburg(er) (N. Am.). Raw, ground meat, usually beef, which may be incorporated into numerous dishes; also a cooked patty of ground meat which is served on a split roll with various garnishes. In Britain, hamburger or ground beef is known as **mince.**

Hazelnut (*Corylus avellana*). Ovoid nut in a hard, brown shell; grows in the hedges in Britain; eaten as a dessert nut and used in confectionery; also known as the **cobnut.**

Head cheese. See **Brawn.**

Herring, Fish with oily flesh, trawled round the shores of Britain and USA; may be served fried, grilled, smoked or pickled. See **Kippers.**

Hominy (N. Am.). The starchy portion of the endosperm of maize, left after the whole grain is softened by steaming and the bran and germ removed, popular in some parts of the USA. **Grits** are a coarsely ground form.

Hot dog. A hot frankfurter sausage in a long, split roll.

Hot pot (UK). An oven-baked casserole, consisting of layers of meat and vegetables topped with sliced potatoes; popular in Lancashire.

Hough (Scot., N. Eng.). Shin and foreleg of beef; gelatinous cuts, which require a long cooking time, also sometimes used for ground beef. The same portion of beef is termed **shank** in North America.

Hovis (UK). Bread made from wheat flour, to which extra germ has been added; a good source of the B-vitamins.

Huckleberry (*Solanum intrusum*). A black, smooth-skinned berry, rather flavourless, used in pies and preserves in North America.

Humble pie (UK). Originally 'umble pie', umbles being the offal of a deer which were traditionally huntsman's fare (this type of deer haggis is now rated much higher).

Ice cream. A range of milk-based frozen desserts. The fat may be of milk or vegetable origin but is usually saturated. An exception is **Mellorine,** an American product, which contains a substantial amount of polyunsaturated fat. Ice cream may contain 8–20% fat by weight and 5–12% milk solids. **Ice milk** is a low-fat product containing 2–5% fat.

Ices (water ices). A frozen confection made from water, sugar and fruit juice or flavouring; known to children in America as **popsicles** and in Britain as **ice lollies.**

Jambalaya (S. USA). A traditional Creole dish, consisting of rice, with tomatoes, meat, fish or shell-fish to give it a characteristic flavour.

Jelly (UK). Usually a gelatin dessert (*q.v.*), less often made by boiling cuts of meat rich in collagen, e.g. calve's foot jelly.

Joint (UK). In Britain, this term refers to a portion of the carcass of an animal, such as a roast of meat. Traditional for main course of Sunday dinner.

Kale (*Brassica oleracea*). A large-leaved vegetable sometimes crimped and curled; used as **winter-greens** in Britain.

Kasha. The Russian name for buckwheat (*Polygonum* spp.); seeds hulled and cracked for quick preparation, usually as a side dish with meat or in stews and casseroles; has a distinctive hearty flavour.

Kedgeree (UK). Derives from an Indian recipe **Khichri** which consisted of rice, lentils, onion and spices. The English added fish (often smoked), parsley and eggs to produce a famous dish.

Kippers (UK). Split, salted and smoked herring.

Kohlrabi (*Brassica oleracea*). The turnip-like swollen base is green or purple in colour; usually served as a boiled vegetable.

Kumquat (*Fortunella* spp.). Similar in appearance to a small orange, has an acid taste and is used mainly for preserves or pickled whole.

Lard. A soft, animal fat from the pig, a non-ruminant; used in home-baking.

Leek (*Allium ampeloprasum* var *porrum*). A member of the onion family, the blanched, elongated bulb is used in soups and stews or as a separate vegetable. National emblem of Wales.

Lemon curd (UK). A smooth, thickened mixture of sugar, eggs, lemon juice and butter; used as a spread or as a filling for tarts. Also called **lemon cheese.**

Lentils (*Lens culinaris*). One of the oldest leguminous crops, the orange-coloured seeds are usually sold split and decorticated; may be used in a variety of dishes.

Loganberry (*Rubus loganobaccus*). A dull-red, acid fruit, developed in California by a cross between the blackberry and the raspberry; named after its originator; grown commercially for canning. The **boysenberry** is a similar hybrid.

Lotus root (*Nelembium nuciferum*). The sacred lotus of India and China, a water plant used more in times of food scarcity; the rhizomes may be roasted or steamed and when young have a flavour similar to that of artichokes.

Macadamia nut (*Macadamia ternifolia*). A crisp, sweet nut, white in colour, with a high fat content, native to Australia where it is sometimes known as the **Queensland nut;** also cultivated in Hawaii.

Malted milk. Whole or partly skimmed milk, combined with the liquid extract from a mash of barley and wheat, and dried. This is combined with sugar to form the basis of a number of commercial beverages, such as Ovaltine and Horlicks.

Mango (*Mangifera indica*). A native of India, oval-shaped fruit with greenish-yellow skin and a delicious, sweet-sour, orange-coloured pulp.

Maple syrup (N. Am.). A uniquely flavoured syrup made by concentrating the sap of the sugar maple; delicious on pancakes and waffles and also used to flavour confectionery and ice-cream; now, many commercial brands consist of sucrose syrup with maple flavouring.

Marzipan. Confectionery made from powdered almonds, and eggs.

Matzo. A Jewish unleavened, unsalted bread, made from flour and water; eaten especially during Passover.

Medlar (*Mespilus germanica*). A fruit the size of a small apple, with brown, firm skin; edible only when 'bletted', i.e. aged until soft and brown. Its chief use in Britain is for making jam.

Melba toast (N. Am.). Very thin slices of bread baked in an oven until crisp.

Melon (*Cucumis melo*). Includes several varieties of medium to large-sized fruit: **musk** melon has a netted, yellow-green skin with aromatic flesh and grows in Britain and other temperate regions; **cantaloupe** is a round, rough-skinned variety with sweet, orange flesh; **winter melons** require a longer ripening season but store well and are grown mainly in Mediterranean countries and southern USA; the **honeydew,** a light, smoothed-skinned variety, with sweet, greenish flesh, belonging to this class; **watermelon** is a large melon, commonly cultivated in hot countries and very refreshing.

Mince (UK). See **Hamburger.**

Mincemeat (UK). A spiced preserve, consisting of chopped apples, dried fruit and peel, eggs, sugar and suet; used as a filling for pies and tarts; in America it usually contains cooked ground meat; may be matured in rum or brandy.

Mince pies (Eng.). Pies of short or flaky pastry filled with mincemeat, and traditionally eaten at Christmas.

Mince pies (Scot.). Raised pastry filled with minced beef or mutton. Also known as **Scotch pies.**

Miso (Japan). A paste, made from soybeans, salt, wheat or barley and water; may be used as a spread or condiment.

Molasses (N. Am.). A dark syrup, drained from sugar during refining; known as **black treacle** in Britain.

Muesli (Switz.). A mixture of dry cereals, notably oat or wheat flakes, combined with dried fruit and nuts; a popular and nutritious breakfast cereal, taken with milk.

Muffin. A British muffin is a light, spongy, unsweetened yeast-cake, toasted, and served hot. The American varieties are more numerous and are a type of small, quick bread, leavened with baking powder. Favourites are bran-, corn-, and blueberry muffins.

Mulberry (*Morus nigra*). A native of Europe and Asia, bears a delicate, purple-red fruit, which is delicious when eaten fresh and fully-ripe; easily damaged; also used for making wine and jam. Silkworms are reared on the leaves.

Mullet (UK). A small, round fish with a white flesh.

Mush (N. Am.). A cornmeal porridge served with milk and brown sugar.

Nectarine (*Prunus persica* var *nectarina*). A smooth-skinned peach with a rich flavour, smaller and more brightly coloured than other varieties of peaches.

Oatcakes (UK). The true variety originated in Scotland and consists of a crisp flat, unsweetened biscuit made with oatmeal.

Offal (UK). The word derives from 'off-fall', the parts of an animal removed in the dressing process; offal includes the brains, sweetbreads, stomach and intestines of an animal as well as the organ meats.

Okra (*Hibiscus esculentus*). Immature pods, also known as **lady's fingers** or **gumbo**; mucilaginous in texture, are often used in tropical cookery to thicken soups and stews.

Palm kernel oil. A pale fat from the inner kernel of the oil palm; more expensive than red-palm oil; used for margarine.

Palm oil. An orange oil extracted from the fibrous pulp of the fruit of the oil palm (*Elaeis guineensis*); used in West Africa as food; exported for industrial purposes, used for margarine after refining to remove carotene.

Papaya (*Carica papaya*). Also known as **paw paw**, tropical fruit the shape of a small elongated melon, usually yellow-orange in colour; the flesh is succulent, orange to pink, with a mass of seeds in the central cavity. The plant is the source of the enzyme, papain.

Parkin (UK). A flat cake made from oatmeal, ginger, syrup and treacle in the north of England.

Passion fruit (*Passiflora edulis*). A purple, egg-shaped fruit of the tropics and subtropics; the sweet juicy pulp may be eaten fresh or the juice extracted and bottled; also known as **granadilla**.

Pasta (Ital.). Now popular all over the world in several forms including macaroni, spaghetti, vermicelli and noodles; made from a variety of hard wheat (*Triticum durum*) which is high in gluten.

Pecan (*Carya illinoensis*). Similar to the walnut with a mild sweet flavour; popular in North America where they are sometimes called **hickory nuts**; little known in Britain.

Persimmon (*Diospyros* spp.). The Japanese varieties are 5 to 7 cm in diameter, yellow-red in colour and similar in appearance to a tomato. American varieties are smaller and dark red in colour. The ripe fruit is very sweet and often eaten fresh with lemon or used in sauces, jams or compotes.

Pie (UK). A broad term which refers to (1) a deep dish filled with fruit or meat and vegetables, covered with a pastry top, (2) pork, fruit or custard surrounded by pastry and eaten cold in individual-size pies, (3) **Shepherd's pie**, a meat and vegetable dish covered with mashed potato which has been lightly browned.

Pie (N. Am.). A shallow fruit and pastry tart; the British 'pie' is termed a 'deep-dish' pie.

Pigeon pea (*Cajanus cajan*). A tropical legume; widely grown in India where it is known as **red gram**; also popular in the West Indies.

Pilchards. Fully grown sardines, smaller than herrings; usually canned in oil, brine or tomato sauce.

Pistachio (*Pistacia vera*). Nuts cultivated in Asia, the Mediterranean countries, and southern United States, green kernels with a pleasant, mild flavour; commonly eaten salted or used in confectionery and ice cream.

Plaice (UK). A flat fish low in fat, usually served fried.

Plantain (*Musa* spp). Green plantains are a type of banana used for cooking. Higher in starch and lower in sugar than dessert bananas, they are picked when the flesh is too hard to be eaten raw; dietary staple in parts of East Africa.

Polenta (Ital.). A maize porridge, to which cheese, barley and chestnuts may be added.

Pomegranate (*Punica granatum*). A yellow-purple fruit about the size of an orange, with thick leathery skin; the seeds are enclosed in a pulpy flesh which is bright red, delicious and juicy.

Popcorn (N. Am.). A variety of maize which is heated in a covered pan until the starch granules swell to four times their size and the kernels burst; may be served salted and buttered. The traditional movie-theatre snack.

Popover (N. Am.). Somewhat similar to a Yorkshire pudding; baked from a flour, milk, and egg batter in lightly greased, individual dishes in a hot oven until the mixture puffs and becomes crisp on the outside.

Porgy. Several species of salt-water fish, in Europe, members of the Pagrus family; in the United States 'porgy' includes the **scup** and **menhaden** fishes. Porgy is prepared and cooked like catfish.

Potato chips (N. Am.). The American term for thinly sliced potatoes, which have been fried, dried and salted before packaging. They are known as **potato crisps** in Britain.

Prawn. A small crustacean, similar to but larger than a shrimp.

Pressed beef. Boned, salted and pressed brisket.

Pretzel. Rings of a flour and water paste, baked in a very hot oven and then glazed and sprinkled with coarse salt; popular as a snack in Germany and North America.

Pudding (UK). Usually used to refer to the sweet or dessert course of a meal; also encompasses a variety of dishes made from a flour base or enclosed in pastry; these contain anything from custard and fruit to meat and vegetables. There are hundreds of English puddings, among the more famous are 'steak and kidney pudding' and the traditional Christmas pudding.

Puris (India). Made by rolling a small flat piece of dough and then frying it in deep butter fat. As butter is expensive, puris are regular food for the rich only and are reserved for festive occasions by other classes.

Quince (*Cydonia vulgaris*). A hard, acid fruit, similar in appearance to a pear or apple; is used mainly for jams and jellies in Britain.

Ragoût. A spicy stew made with meat, fish or poultry, with or without vegetables; from the French *ragoûter*, to awaken the taste.

Rasher (UK). A slice especially of bacon.

Red snapper. An important food fish caught off the eastern seaboard of the United States. The flesh is white, delicate and low in fat.

Rissole (Fr.). A patty of ground meat or fish coated in breadcrumbs and fried; the American equivalent is a **croquette**.

Roe. Refers to both the **milt** (soft roe) of the male fish and the eggs (hard roe) of the female, usually from cod or herring; caviar is the roe of the sturgeon. Roes are rich in nucleic acids and cholesterol.

Romaine (*Lactuca sativa*) (N. Am.). Long-leaved lettuce corresponding to cos lettuce in Britain.

(Scarlet) runner bean (*Phaseolus coccineus*). A popular green bean or **string bean** in Britain; grows up to 10 feet in height and produces long, wide pods, often over a foot in length. Scarlet refers to the colour of the flower. An exceptionally tall plant featured in the fairy story 'Jack and the Beanstalk'.

Rutabaga (*Brassica* spp.). A variety of turnip.

Sago. A starch extracted from the sago palm tree (*Metroxylon sagu*), used to thicken soups and puddings.

Saltine. See **Cracker**.

Salsify (*Tragopogon porrifolius*). A white, elongated root eaten as a winter vegetable, boiled, baked, or in soups; the young leaves may be used for salad.

Satsuma. This name, which originates from a cream-coloured Japanese pottery, is now applied to a particular type of tangerine (*Citrus reticulata*) and also to some types of plum.

Sausage. Ground meat, often mixed with cereal, which is enclosed in a thin skin, varieties are numerous and may be raw, cooked or smoked; often highly seasoned. Spicier varieties include **salami** (Ital.) and **bratwurst** (Ger.). See **Bologna** and **Frankfurter**.

Savoury duck. See **Faggot**.

Scampi. A very large prawn.

Scone (UK). A teacake similar in composition to the American baking-powder biscuit.

Scotch collop. Minced meat garnished with tomatoes.

Scrag (end) (UK). The bony part of an animal's carcass; usually refers to the neck of mutton.

Scrapple (N. Am.). Made with the cooked scraps of meat from the head of a pig, combined with salt, spices and cornmeal, cooked and pressed into tins; termed **ponhaws** by Pennsylvania German settlers.

Seakale (*Crambe maritima*). Native to the coasts of Western Europe, the blanched leaf-stalks are boiled like asparagus and are noted for their nutty, slightly bitter flavour.

Semolina. Coarsely ground particles of refined durum wheat, used to make sweetened puddings or to thicken soups; also the basis of several pastas including macaroni.

Seville orange (*Citrus aurantium*). A bitter-flavoured orange used for making marmalade; popular in Britain.

Shallot (*Allium* spp.). A variety of onion, which produces several lateral bulbs, used fresh or for pickling.

Sherbet. A frozen dessert made from a mixture of fruit juice, milk and sugar; fat content is low ranging from 1.2% in North American varieties to 3% in British products; word of Arabic origin.

Shortbread (Scot.). A brittle dry cake, made from flour, and much butter and sugar; may contain 30% fat.

Sillabub (syllabub) (UK). A light, frothy dessert, consisting of whipped cream, wine, spices and sugar.

Silverside (UK). The outer part of the round of beef, usually salted and boiled.

Snap beans. See **French beans.**

Soda bread (Eire). An Irish bread leavened with baking soda.

Sole, Dover (UK). A flat white fish with dark rough skin, also known as **black sole**; noted for the excellency of its fine firm flesh.

Sole, Lemon (UK). Distinguishable from Dover sole as it is more oval and has smooth sandy-brown skin; flesh is good but inferior to that of the Dover sole.

Squab pie (UK). Neck of mutton with thinly sliced apples, baked in a casserole.

Squash (drink) (UK). A fruit-flavoured, sweetened liquid concentrate to which about 3 parts of water or soda water are added, e.g. orange squash, lemon squash.

Squash, Summer (*Cucurbita pepo*). Several varieties which include the warty, orange-coloured **summer crookneck** and the **zucchini**, a long, thin, green marrow.

Squash, Winter (*Cucurbita maxima*). Popular in North America; require a longer ripening season than do the summer squashes. Familiar varieties are the green, warty, **Hubbard squash** and the green, smooth-skinned **acorn squash**; they keep well, the texture being firm and floury and the water content lower than that of summer squashes, they are also a rich source of vitamin A.

Streaky bacon (UK). Term for fatty bacon, similar to **side bacon** in America.

Suet. Shredded beef fat used in steamed puddings.

Sugar. Sucrose, chiefly derived from the sugar cane (*Saccharum officinarum*) and the sugar beet (*Beta vulgaris* subsp. *cicla*). Less refined products contain traces of other sugars and have a flavour and texture which may be preferred for certain purposes. The terminology in Britain differs from that used in North America; **caster sugar** (UK) is superfine white (N. Am.); **icing sugar** (UK) is confectioner's; **Demerara** is crystallised light brown sugar and **Barbados** is soft, moist, brown sugar.

Sultana (*Vitis vinifera*). A seedless, golden raisin, made by drying a variety of wine grapes with a firm flesh and high sugar content.

Swede (*Brassica napus* var *napobrassica*). Resembles a turnip and is similarly used in stews or mashed and served as a separate vegetable.

Sweetbreads. The pancreas and thymus glands of an animal, usually a calf.

Sweet chestnut (*Castanea sativa*). A glossy, brown nut 2 to 5 cm wide and enclosed in a spiny, green capsule; may be eaten whole, after boiling or roasting or ground into flour for use in stuffings and other dishes; native to southern Europe; also known as **Spanish chestnuts.**

Tangelo. Sweet-tart hybrid of the tangerine and grapefruit; an example is the **ugli** which resembles a sweet, easily peeled grapefruit.

Tart (UK). A shallow, round pastry shell of any diameter with a sweet, usually fruit filling; known as **pie** in North America.

Tenderloin (N. Am.). Fillet of beef or pork, the tenderest part of an animal.

Timbale (Fr.). A small pastry shell with a variety of sweet or savoury fillings.

Toad in the hole (UK). Pieces of meat or sausages baked in a batter.

Tofu (Japan). A curd or cheese, made from fresh soybeans, rich in protein, has a soft texture and bland flavour and may be incorporated into a number of recipes.

Topside (UK). The top of the round of beef, this is a lean, boneless fine-grained cut, suitable for roasting.

Tortilla (Mex.). A thin, flat pancake made from ground maize; the grains are softened by heating in limewater and then ground directly into a dough and cooked on a hot, iron plate. The lime may provide an important contribution to the calcium intake. A **taco** is a tortilla filled with a mixture of meat, beans and chilli and is a popular snack in the southwest USA.

Tripe. The first and second stomachs of a ruminant, more familiar in Europe and Britain than in North America. Tripe is cooked with milk and onions and requires a long cooking time to tenderise.

Turbot. A large white fish, low in fat; ranks with sole in culinary excellence.

Vanaspatti (India). A vegetable substitute for ghee.

Vegetable marrow (*Cucurbita pepo*) (UK). Same species as many pumpkins and summer squash; the fruit is green, white or striped; the varieties most common in Britain produce large oval or cylindrical fruits, eaten as a boiled vegetable or stuffed with a savoury mixture of meat, onions and tomatoes.

Waffle (N. Am.). Made from a light, spongy batter, which contains more fat than a pancake batter, cooked on an iron grid until it puffs up crisp and golden brown; served hot with syrup.

Walnut (*Juglans regia*). Known to the classical Greek and Hebrew writers and now grown in many parts of Europe and America; used extensively in biscuits and cakes. Its fat is the most polyunsaturated of the dessert nuts.

Water chestnut (*Trapa natans*). Also known as **caltrops**, the edible seed is eaten raw, roasted or baked in Central Europe and Asia; floury in texture with an agreeable flavour. See **Chinese water chestnut.**

Wax beans (*Phaseolus vulgaris*). Yellow podded, stringless beans which may be eaten like French beans, when young and tender. The mature black seeds, which have earned it the name **Mexican black,** are also eaten and have a mushroom-like flavour.

Whitebait (UK). The young of herring, sprats or pilchard, small silver fish caught in the estuaries of rivers around the coast of Britain; usually served fried whole.

White currant (*Ribes sativum*). Variety of redcurrant lacking the pigment; less acid than the red kind.

Whiting (UK). A light, low-fat fish of the cod family. In North America, the name applies to a number of other small fish.

Wineberry (*Rubus phoenicolasius*). A variety of raspberry originating in North China; the fruit is golden orange and pleasantly flavoured.

Yeast extract. A salty preparation used as a savoury spread or to flavour meat dishes; rich in B vitamins and salt but only used in small amounts; often referred to by trade names, e.g. 'Marmite' (UK).

Yorkshire pudding (UK). Made from a batter of flour, milk and eggs, cooked in meat drippings or other fat and traditionally served hot with roast beef. In Yorkshire eaten on its own with gravy as a first course.

Zucchini (*Cucurbita pepo*). A long, thin, Italian marrow developed for cutting while immature.

Zwieback (Germ.). A type of rusk, German in origin, the word literally means 'twice-baked'.

Appendix 2. Diet Sheets

DIETS

The diet sheets that follow have been constructed to illustrate the quantitative and qualitative aspects of diets required for the treatment of various diseases. The quantities given may require modification in relation to the size, age, sex and occupation of the patient. In the dietetic treatment of most diseases it is unnecessary to weigh accurately the amounts of the different foods eaten. Under these circumstances sufficient accuracy will be secured by the use of the terms 'small', 'medium' or 'large helping'. A small helping weighs approximately 30 to 60 g, a medium helping 60 to 90 g and a large helping 120 g or more.

Some diet sheets can best be described as dietary regimens. They are confined to elucidating principles in the selection, preparation and consumption of the meals for a day. Quantities may be left to the patient's choice.

The main meal is usually shown at midday, with a lighter meal in the evening. These can, however, be interchanged.

To facilitate reference to the diets a summary table is given.

SUMMARY OF DIET SHEETS

No.	Titles	Purpose
1	High energy, well balanced	Convalescence and underweight
2	Moderate energy, well balanced	A normal diet
3	Low energy, well balanced	Weight reduction, including diabetes
4	Very low protein, low-to-moderate energy	Acute glomerulonephritis or hepatic encephalopathy
5	Very low protein, moderate energy (modified Giovannetti)	Severe chronic renal failure
6	Low protein	Moderate chronic renal failure, subacute hepatic encephalopathy
7	High protein, restricted sodium	Nephrotic syndrome, hypoalbuminaemia
8	Diabetic diets	Diabetes mellitus
9	Diabetic diets in the USA	Diabetes mellitus
10	Very low fat, high carbohydrate	Nausea, hepatitis, type I hyperlipidaemia
11	Low fat, high energy	For malabsorption and steatorrhoea
12	Low sodium, moderate energy	Intractable oedema, e.g. in chronic heart failure, cirrhosis and hypertension
13	Restricted sodium, low energy	Acute cardiac failure
14	Reduced saturated, increased polyunsaturated fat	To lower plasma cholesterol, e.g. type IIA hyperlipidaemia
15	Gluten-free	Coeliac disease
16	Semi-liquid	Upper gastrointestinal obstruction and irritable states
17	Bland regimen	Dyspepsia and peptic ulcer
18	High fibre (roughage)	Atonic constipation and diverticulosis

Diet No. 1   HIGH ENERGY, WELL BALANCED

Indications   For convalescent patients (medical and surgical) and those with wasting diseases, or who are undernourished

Nutrients   Energy 12.6–14.7 MJ (3000–3500 kcal); protein 100–120 g; adequate in all other nutrients.

Food for the day

Milk	750–1000 ml	Fruit	2–4 servings
Meat and 'protein'	3–5 servings	Fat	90 g
Bread and cereal	8–12 servings	Desserts	1–2 servings

Sample daily menu

Early morning   Tea or coffee with sugar, and biscuits.

Breakfast   Fruit *or* fruit juice.
Cereal with milk and sugar.
1 or 2 eggs.
Bacon or sausage.
Toast or roll with 30 g butter and jam, jelly, marmalade or honey.
Beverage with cream.

Mid-morning   Milky beverage or fruit juice with snack.

Midday meal   Soup *or* fruit.
120 g meat, fish or poultry.
Potato or substitute.
Vegetable, and salad with dressing if desired.
Dessert or pudding.
Biscuits or roll with butter and cheese.
Beverage with milk.

Mid-afternoon   Sandwiches with filling.
Cake or biscuit.
Tea with milk and sugar.

Evening meal   Fruit juice *or* soup.
90 g meat, fish or cheese *or* 1–2 eggs.
Vegetable, and salad with dressing if desired.
Bread or roll with butter.
Dessert or pudding.
Beverage with milk.

Bedtime   Milk drink or eggnog *and* biscuits or sandwich.

Management

Appetite and food tolerance are often poor, requiring extra consideration and individual attention. Wavering appetites may respond best to small servings at first; amounts may then gradually be increased.

Between meal snacks. Fruit or fruit drinks which may be taken with milk or ice cream; milk drinks (flavoured milks, eggnog, malted milk, yogurt, milk shake, hot milk); biscuits (crackers), sandwiches (filled with egg, cheese, meat, sardines, dates, banana, meat or yeast extract, honey, jam or peanut butter), toast; nuts; desserts containing milk and eggs.

Diet No. 2   MODERATE ENERGY, WELL BALANCED

Indications   A normal diet suitable for a patient in bed.

Nutrients   Energy 8.4–10.5 MJ (2000–2500 kcal); protein 75–100 g; adequate in all other nutrients.

Food for the day

Milk	450–680 ml	Fruit	2–3 servings
Meat and 'protein'	3–4 servings	Fat	60–75 g
Bread and cereal	6–10 servings	Desserts	1–2 servings

Sample daily menu

Breakfast

Fruit *or* fruit juice.
Cereal with milk and sugar.
1 or 2 eggs.
Bacon or sausage.
Toast or roll with 20 g butter.
Marmalade, jelly or honey.
Beverage with milk.

Midday meal

120 g meat, fish or poultry.
Potato or substitute.
Vegetable.
Salad with dressing if desired.
Bread or roll with 30 g butter or biscuits and cheese.
Dessert or pudding.
Beverage with milk.

Mid-afternoon

1 serving of fruit.

Evening meal

Fruit juice *or* soup.
60–90 g cheese, fish or meat *or* an egg.
Vegetable.
Salad, with dressing if desired.
Bread or roll with butter.
Dessert or fruit.
Beverage with milk.

Management

The energy intake may need to be adjusted. It is too much for a small female and may not be enough for a patient who is febrile or undernourished.

Diet No. 3	LOW ENERGY, WELL BALANCED

Indications For patients with obesity, with or without maturity onset diabetes.

Nutrients Energy 4.2 MJ (1000 kcal), protein 60 g, fat 35 g; adequate in all other nutrients.

Sample daily menu

Breakfast 20 g bread (with butter from allowance) *or* 120 ml orange juice *or* ½ grapefruit.
1 boiled egg, *or* 20 g breakfast cereal or 120 g porridge with milk from allowance.
Coffee or tea (no sugar) with milk from allowance.

Mid-morning Coffee or tea (no sugar) with milk from allowance.

Midday meal Bouillon or clear soup.
Sandwiches made from 2 thin slices of bread, 60 g chicken or tuna
or 30 g cheese, and butter from allowance.
Small salad (see vegetable list).
1 serving of fruit.

Mid-afternoon Tea or coffee (no sugar) with milk from allowance.

Evening meal 120 ml tomato juice.
60 g chicken or lean meat *or* 90 g steamed or grilled white fish.
Salad or boiled vegetable (see list).
1 small boiled potato.
2 wafers of crispbread with butter from allowance.
1 serving of fruit.
Coffee (no sugar) and milk from allowance.

Allowance for day 300 ml skim milk *or* whole milk allowed to stand with the cream poured off.
15 g butter or margarine.

Management

Foods which may be taken as desired

Vegetables: Asparagus, aubergine (egg plant), French, runner or string beans, broccoli, Brussels sprouts, cabbage, cauliflower, celery, chicory, courgettes, cucumber, kale, leeks, lettuce, mustard and cress, mushrooms, okra, onion, parsley, peppers, pumpkin, radishes, sauerkraut, seakale, spinach, summer squash, swede, tomatoes, turnips, turnip tops, watercress.

Drinks: Water, soda water, tea, coffee (ground or instant), sugar-free lemonade, sugar-free carbonated drinks, diabetic fruit drinks, meat and yeast extracts.

Miscellaneous: Saccharine preparations, salt, pepper, vinegar, mustard, herbs, spices, gelatine, pickles, relish and soy sauce, unthickened gravy.

Foods to be avoided

Sugar (white or brown), glucose, sorbitol. Sweets, toffees, chocolates, candies, cornflour, custard powder. Jam, marmalade, jelly, lemon curd, honey, syrup, molasses. Canned or frozen fruits (unless preserved without sugar).

Dried fruits, e.g. dates, figs, apricots, raisins. Cakes, pastries, puddings and rich desserts. Sweet or chocolate biscuits.

Ice cream and gelatine dessert (table jelly). Condensed or evaporated milk, cream. Peas, parsnips, beetroot, sweetcorn, haricot, lima and navy beans, broad beans, lentils. Nuts.

Salad dressing and mayonnaise. Thick and cream sauces. Fatty meats, sausages and fatty fish. All fried foods. Sweetened fruit juices, fruit squashes. Carbonated beverages. Beer, wine, sherry, spirits—all alcoholic drinks.

The items in the sample daily menu can be exchanged in the same way as diabetic exchanges. People who need to take this diet should be advised where to find low energy recipes and to build up a file of these. There are several suitable books on the market, e.g. Good Housekeeping *Slimmers' Cook Book* (London: Ebury Press).

It is usually wise not to get too hungry. Sometimes a snack between meals saves overdoing it at a meal. No meal should be missed.

Diet No. 4   VERY LOW PROTEIN, LOW-TO-MODERATE ENERGY

Indications   For patients with acute glomerulonephritis or with hepatic encephalopathy.

Nutrients   Protein 20 g, fluids 1200 ml, energy 6.7 MJ (1600 kcal), sodium restricted.

Food for the day

Double cream	60 ml
with water	150 ml
Unsalted butter	35 g
Sugar and glucose	60 g
Jam, jelly, marmalade or honey	45 g
Bread (salt-free may be required)	90 g
Fruit	300 g

Sample daily menu

Breakfast
150 g fruit juice with glucose.
20 g cornflakes or similar breakfast cereal and sugar.
Cream mixture.
30 g bread, toast or roll.
Unsalted butter.
250 ml tea or weak coffee.

Mid-morning
125 ml tea or coffee.
Sugar and cream mixture.
2 biscuits or cookies.

Midday meal
30 g meat *or* 1 egg.
90 g potato, mashed (no salt) with butter *or* 60 g boiled rice.
60 g grilled tomato or other vegetable
Fruit—fresh, stewed or canned.
125 ml tea or carbonated beverage.

Mid-afternoon
30 g bread and unsalted butter.
Jam, jelly or honey.
125 ml tea with cream mixture.

Evening meal
30 g bread toasted or low salt crackers with unsalted butter.
Vegetable salad with oil dressing, if desired.
Water ice or fruit.
125 ml coffee with cream mixture and sugar.

Bedtime
125 ml tea with cream mixture and sugar.
Biscuit or cookie.

Management
Fluid intake may need to be adjusted depending on fluid balance.

Fruits and potatoes are relatively rich in potassium; if plasma K is rising, potassium intake can be restricted by replacing natural fruit juice by a proprietary fruit squash, by using rice instead of potato and by using only fruits relatively low in potassium, especially pears and apples. (This is not necessary in hepatic encephalopathy.)

Table salt should not be used (no salt on tray). Biscuits and cookies should be low in salt and baking soda. To restrict the sodium further salt-free bread may be used.

Diet No. 5   VERY LOW PROTEIN, MODERATE ENERGY
(Modified GIOVANNETTI)

Indications   For patients with severe chronic renal failure.

Nutrients   Protein 17 g (of high biological value), energy approx. 9.2 MJ (2200 kcal), fluid about 500 ml, Na 12 mmol and K 15 mmol/day. This diet is low in B vitamins, iron and calcium.

Sample daily menu

Breakfast   Oatmeal porridge (5 g oats, 50 ml double cream, 40 ml water).
Glucose or sugar.
30 g salt-free protein-free bread, toasted.
Salt-free butter.
Jam, jelly, marmalade or honey.
80 ml tea with glucose and 10 ml milk.

Mid-morning   50 ml liquid glucose polymer.

Midday meal   25 g chicken (dry weight).
30 g boiled rice (dry weight).
Salt-free butter.
30 g very low protein vegetable.
30 g very low protein fruit and cream.

Mid-afternoon   40 ml grapefruit juice and glucose.
10 g salt-free, protein-free biscuit or rusk.

Evening meal   1 egg, scrambled on toasted, salt-free, protein-free bread with salt-free butter.
Plain ice cream*.
30 g very low protein fruit.

Bedtime   90 ml milk with glucose or sugar.
10 g salt-free, protein-free biscuit.

Management

Salt-free, protein-free bread, biscuits and rusks are baked from wheatstarch flour and obtainable in the UK from Welfare Foods, Stockport.

Proprietary preparations of liquid glucose polymer are Hycal, Caloreen and Controlyte; they are very low in electrolytes.

Very low protein vegetables are tomatoes, egg plant, pumpkins, carrots, onions and green beans.

Very low protein fruits are pears, apples, pineapple, mandarins and grapefruit.

The diet does not meet requirement for the B vitamins, iron and calcium and supplements of these should be given; 500 mg of methionine should also be given daily (250 mg tablet twice daily with meals).

Extra fluid, e.g. tea with cream and a little milk or a liquid glucose drink or a little beer or wine, may be given depending on the urine output.

This diet is modified from a three-day cycle of menus given by Berlyne *et al.* (1967).

* Made from 25 ml cream, 25 ml oil, 25 g glucose, 10 ml water, colour and flavour.

Diet No. 6   LOW PROTEIN

Indications   For patients with chronic renal failure of moderate severity or with subacute hepatic
                           encephalopathy.

Nutrients   Protein 40 g/day, energy 7.6–8.4 MJ (1800–2000 kcal), Na 40 mmol and
                           K 60 mmol/day. Adequate in other nutrients but iron and calcium need to be
                           supplemented, if used for a long time.

Food for the day

	Protein (g)
Milk: 120 ml	4
Meat, protein foods: 90 g	21
Fruit or juice: 5 to 6 servings	5
Low protein vegetables: 2 servings	4
Bread, cereals: 3 to 4 servings	6

Cream, fat, sugar, jelly, syrup, hard candy, water ice, tea,
coffee and seasonings except salt, as desired.

Sample daily menu

Breakfast   Fruit or fruit juice.
                           Breakfast cereal with milk.
                           1 slice of toast with butter and jelly or marmalade.
                           Coffee with sugar and cream.

Mid-morning   Fruit juice with sugar.

Midday meal   60 g meat, poultry or fish.
                           Vegetable salad with oil dressing.
                           1 slice of toast.
                           Butter, jam or jelly.
                           Water ice or fruit.
                           Coffee or tea with sugar and cream.

Mid-afternoon   Tea with sugar and cream, *or* carbonated beverage.

Evening meal   1 egg *or* 30 g meat.
                           Potato or rice with butter.
                           Cooked low protein vegetable with butter.
                           Fruit.
                           Coffee or tea with sugar and cream.

Bedtime   Fruit juice with sugar *or* tea with cream.

Management

A variety of cakes and cookies containing 2 g protein can be substituted for 1 slice of bread.

Suitable low protein vegetables and salads are green beans, beetroot, cabbage, carrots, cauliflower, celery,
cucumber, egg plant, lettuce, mushrooms, onions, pumpkin, radishes, summer squash, tomatoes and turnips.

Most fruits are suitable except dried fruits.

Diet No. 7   HIGH PROTEIN, RESTRICTED SODIUM

Indications   For patients with nephrotic syndrome or hypoalbuminaemia.

Nutrients   Protein 90–120 g, energy 10 MJ (2400 kcal), Na 80–120 mmol/day; adequate in other
                           nutrients.

Sample daily menu
Breakfast   Fruit or fruit juice.
                           Breakfast cereal.
                           2 eggs (poached, boiled or scrambled).
                           1 slice of bread or toast.
                           Butter and marmalade, jelly or jam.
                           Tea or coffee with milk and sugar.

Mid-morning   Tea or coffee, with milk and sugar.

Miday meal   90–120 g chicken, unsalted meat or fish *or* 2 eggs as omelet.
                           Vegetable.
                           Salad.
                           Milk dessert.
                           Fruit.

Mid-afternoon   2 slices of bread as sandwiches filled with egg, minced meat or chicken.
                           Tea with milk and sugar.

Evening meal   150–180 g meat, poultry or fish.
                           Roll with butter.
                           Potato.
                           Vegetable.
                           Dessert made with milk and fruit.
                           Coffee with milk and sugar.

Bedtime   Drink of malted milk.

Allowance for day   600 ml milk or more.
                           45 g butter or margarine.

Management
Sodium intake is restricted by using no table salt and avoiding all highly salted foods, e.g. ham, bacon, sausages,
corned beef, smoked fish, cheese, most ketchups and commercial sauces, canned and convenience foods. Some
patients may find difficulty in eating so much meat with little salt for flavour. Extra protein may be given by
incorporating Casilan or a similar product into various dishes. 30 g Casilan provides 26 g protein.

DIABETIC DIETS

Diabetic diets aim to restrict carbohydrate intake while meeting normal needs for protein and providing just sufficient energy to maintain normal weight in adults and to allow for growth in children. Diets are made up from lists of exchanges, quantitatively defined. Different systems of exchanges are used by the British and American Dietetic and Diabetic Associations. The British Associations use carbohydrate exchanges, and some clinics, as in Edinburgh, use protein and fat exchanges as well. The American Associations use bread, meat, milk, fruit and vegetable exchanges.

The planning of diabetic diets is illustrated below in the following stages.

1. A method is given for calculating the nature and number of the exchanges required to make up a diet in which amounts of energy, carbohydrate, protein and fat have been prescribed. The sample calculation is based on the system used at the Western General Hospital, Edinburgh.
2. A diet plan sets out how these exchanges may be apportioned among each of the day's meals (p. 557).
3. The British exchange system is described (pages 558 to 559).
4. A diet (No. 8a) based on the above plan is drawn up.
5. An unmeasured diabetic regimen (No. 8b) suitable for mild diabetics who are unable or unwilling to weigh out their foods is described.
6. Diabetic diets based on the American exchange system are summarised (p. 563).

CONSTRUCTING THE DIET

Nutrients   Energy 7.5 MJ (1800 kcal), carbohydrate 180 g, protein 80 g, fat 80 g.

Each **carbohydrate exchange** contains approximately 10 g carbohydrate, 1.5 g protein and 0.3 g fat. Energy value is about 210 KJ (50 kcal) (equivalent to ⅔ oz bread).

Each **protein exchange** contains approximately 7 g protein and 5 g fat. Energy value is about 290 kJ (70 kcal) (equivalent to 1 oz meat).

Each **fat exchange** contains approximately 12 g fat and almost no carbohydrate or protein. Energy value is about 460 KJ (110 kcal) (equivalent to ½ oz butter).

One pint of milk contains approximately 30 g carbohydrate, 18 g protein and 24 g fat. Energy value is about 1.73 MJ (410 kcal).

In practice, for quick construction of a diabetic diet it is usually only necessary to work in terms of grams of carbohydrate and total energy. For this purpose the energy value of the exchanges can be rounded to the nearest 10, i.e.

1 carbohydrate exchange	= 210 kJ (50 kcal)	1 fat exchange	= 460 kJ (110 kcal)
1 protein exchange	= 290 kJ (70 kcal)	1 pint of milk	= 1720 kJ (410 kcal)

Thus, a diet prescription for 180 g carbohydrate, 7.5 MJ would be calculated as follows:

1. The daily intake of carbohydrate (180 g) represents 18 carbohydrate exchanges.
2. The daily allowance of milk is decided either on the basis of the patient's food habits or on his special requirements. In this example it is 1 pint, which contains 3 carbohydrate exchanges, leaving 15 for distribution throughout the day.
3. The daily allowance of protein is then decided. Six protein exchanges provide 1.74 MJ (420 kcal) and 42 g of protein (in addition to 20 g from the milk and approximately another 20 g in 15 carbohydrate units).
4. The energy allocated so far amounts to 6.6 MJ (1580 kcal); a further 920 kJ (220 kcal) are needed to bring the total up to 7.5 MJ (1800 kcal). This must be provided by fat. As one fat exchange provides 460 kJ (110 kcal), two are needed.

Exchanges	Grams of carbohydrate	Energy MJ	kcal
1 pint milk = 3 carbohydrate exchanges	30	1.72	410
15 carbohydrate exchanges	150	3.15	750
6 protein exchanges	–	1.74	420
Total	180	6.61	1580
2 fat exchanges		0.92	220
Grand total	180	7.50	1800

5. Finally the exchanges (15 carbohydrate, 6 protein and 2 fat) are distributed throughout the day according to the eating habits and daily routine of the patient, and the insulin regime.

PLAN OF DISTRIBUTION into meals

Exchanges provide

Energy 7.5 MJ (1800 kcal), carbohydrate 180 g, protein 80 g, fat 80 g.

Breakfast

1 protein exchange.
4 carbohydrate exchanges.
Butter and milk from allowance.
Tea or coffee (no sugar).

Mid-morning

1 carbohydrate exchange.
Butter and milk from allowance.
Tea or coffee (no sugar).

Midday meal

Clear soup if desired.
3 protein exchanges.
4 carbohydrate exchanges.
Vegetables if desired (permitted list, p. 559).
Butter and milk from allowance.

Mid-afternoon

1 carbohydrate exchange.
Butter and milk from allowance.
Tea (no sugar).

Evening meal

2 protein exchanges.
4 carbohydrate exchanges.
Vegetables if desired (permitted list, p. 559).
Tea or coffee (no sugar).

Bedtime

1 carbohydrate exchange.
Remainder of butter and milk from allowance.

Allowance for day

1 pint (500 ml) whole milk.
30 g butter or margarine.

BRITISH DIETARY EXCHANGES

1. CARBOHYDRATE EXCHANGES

These are the recommendations of the British Diabetic Association. All the literature prepared for patients by the Association is based on these exchanges.

Each item on this list = 1 carbohydrate exchange (10 g CHO).
The energy value is approximately 210 kJ (50 kcal)

	Raw or cooked	Measure	oz	g
Bread				
White or brown	Plain or toasted	½ slice of thick cut sliced large loaf	⅔	20
		⅔ slice of a thin cut sliced large loaf	⅔	20
		1 slice of a small sliced loaf	⅔	20
Cereal Foods				
All Bran		3 level tablespoons	⅔	20
Biscuits	Plain or semi-sweet	2 biscuits	½	15
Chapattis		made with fat	⅔	20
Cornflakes or other un-sweetened breakfast cereal		3 heaped tablespoons	½	15
Cornflour	Before cooking	2 heaped teaspoons	½	15
Cornmeal		1 level tablespoon	½	15
Custard powder	Before cooking	2 heaped teaspoons	½	15
Flour		1 level tablespoon	½	15
Macaroni	Before cooking	1 heaped tablespoon	½	15
Noodles	Before cooking	1 heaped tablespoon	½	15
Oatcakes			⅔	20
Porridge	Cooked with water	4 level tablespoons	4	120
Rice	Before cooking	2 heaped teaspoons	½	15
Rye crispbread		1½ biscuits	½	15
Sago	Before cooking	2 heaped teaspoons	½	15
Semolina	Before cooking	2 heaped teaspoons	½	15
Spaghetti	Before cooking	1 heaped tablespoon	½	15
Tapioca	Before cooking	2 heaped teaspoons	½	15
Miscellaneous				
Cocoa powder		5 heaped teaspoons	1	30
Horlicks and Ovaltine		2 heaped teaspoons	½	15
Coca Cola or Pepsi Cola			3 fl oz	90 ml
Milk	Fresh		7 fl oz	210 ml
Milk	Evaporated	6 tablespoons	3 fl oz	90 ml
Milk	Sweetened, condensed	1½ tablespoons	⅔	20 ml
Ice cream	Plain		2	60
Sausages			3	90

Carbohydrate exchanges—*continued*

	Raw		Stewed (without sugar)	
	oz	g	oz	g
Dried Fruits				
Apricots	1	30	2½	75
Figs	⅔	20	1½	45
Prunes (with stones)	1	30	2	60
Dates (without stones) ⎫				
Currants ⎪				
Sultanas ⎬	½	15		
Raisins ⎭				
*Fresh Fruits**				
Apples (with skin)	4	120	5	150
Bananas (with skin)	2	60		
Cherries	3	90	4	120
Damsons	4	120	6	180
Grapes	2	60		
Greengages	3	90	4	120
Oranges and tangerines				
—with skin	6	180		
—without skin	4	120		
Orange juice	4	120		
Peaches (with stones)	4	120		
Pears	4	120	5	150
Pineapple (fresh)	3	90		
Plums (dessert)	4	120	7	210
Raspberries	6	180	7	210
Strawberries	6	180		
Vegetables †				
Potatoes (raw or boiled)	2	60		
Potatoes (roast or chipped)	1	30		
Potato crisps	⅔	20		
Baked beans ⎫				
Butter beans ⎪				
Haricot beans ⎬	2	60		
Sweet corn ⎪				
Tinned peas ⎭				
Fresh or frozen peas ⎫	4	120		
Beetroot (boiled) ⎬				
Parsnips ⎭	3	90		

The following contain only a small quantity of carbohydrates and may be eaten in moderate quantity (if unsweetened) without being counted in the diet.

* *Fruits*: Avocado pear, blackberries (brambles), blackcurrants, grapefruit, gooseberries, lemons, loganberries, redcurrants and whitecurrants.

† *Vegetables*: Asparagus, Brussels sprouts, cabbage, carrots, cauliflower, celery, cucumber, French beans, leeks, lettuce, marrow, mushrooms, mustard and cress, onions, parsley, runner beans, spinach, swede, tomatoes, turnips and watercress.

2. PROTEIN EXCHANGES (Western General Hospital, Edinburgh)

Each item on this list = 1 protein exchange.
The energy value is approximately 290 kJ (70 kcal)

	Amount		Remarks
	oz	g	
Beef, mutton, lamb, pork, veal, bacon, ham, venison, chicken, duck, goose, turkey, pigeon, rabbit, hare, liver, kidney, heart, sweetbreads, tongue, mince, stew	1	30	Cooked weight
Corned beef, corned mutton, tinned meat	1	30	—
Meat paste and pâté	1½	45	—
Egg (1)	2	60	—
Cheese	1	30	—
Tripe. Fish—white, smoked, cured, oily shell or tinned	1½	45	Cooked weight
Sausages (include 1 carbohydrate exchange)	2	60	Cooked weight

Gravies should not contain proprietary thickening, cornflour or flour. Frying should be avoided as much as possible.

3. FAT EXCHANGES (Western General Hospital, Edinburgh)

Each exchange contains approximately 12 g fat and almost no carbohydrate or protein.
Energy value is approximately 460 kJ (110 kcal)

	Amount	
	oz	g
Butter, margarine, lard, dripping, cooking fat, olive oil, vegetable oil	½	15
Cream (single)	2	60
Cream (double)	1	30
Salad cream or mayonnaise	1	30

Group A: foods which may be taken in any quantity

Tea, coffee (milk from allowance, no sugar), meat and yeast extracts.
Tomato juice, lemon juice.
Diabetic fruit squashes.
Saccharine preparations.
Clear soup.
Herbs, seasonings and spices.
Low carbohydrate vegetables and fruits (see p.559).

Group B: to be taken in strict moderation in consultation with the doctor
Spirits, dry wines, dry sherries.

Group C: foods not allowed
Sugar, glucose, sweets, chocolate, honey, syrup, treacle, jam, marmalade, cakes, biscuits (except those specified), pies, fruit tinned in syrup, fruit squash, lemonade, or similar aerated drinks.

Diet No. 8a   A DIABETIC DIET BASED ON THE DISTRIBUTION OF EXCHANGES IN THE PLAN ON page 556 .

Nutrients   Protein 80 g, carbohydrate 180 g, fat 80 g, energy 7.5 MJ (1800 kcal).

Sample daily menu

Breakfast   120 g porridge with milk from allowance. 1 egg.
60 g bread with butter from allowance. Tea or coffee with milk from allowance.

Mid-morning   15 g low sugar biscuit(s) or crispbread.
Tea or coffee with milk from allowance.

Midday meal   Clear soup with shredded vegetables.
90 g lean meat.
120 g boiled potatoes.
60 g canned peas.
Salad or other unrestricted vegetables if desired.
120 g orange (peeled weight).
Milk from allowance with coffee or as curds.

Mid-afternoon   15 g wheatmeal biscuits.
Tea or coffee with milk from allowance.

Evening meal   90 g fish.
Tomato or other unrestricted vegetables from Group A if desired.
60 g bread with butter from allowance.
120 g raw apple.
Tea or coffee with milk from allowance.

Bedtime   Remainder of milk from allowance and 15 g Ovaltine.
or
20 g bread and butter from allowance.

Allowance for day   500 ml milk.
30 g butter or margarine.

Note—Most 'Diabetic' foodstuffs on sale at Chemists and Health Food Stores *do* contain some carbohydrate and must therefore *not* be taken without consulting your doctor or dietitian.

A cookery book for diabetics, *Measure for Measure,* and carbohydrate values of proprietary foods, *Carbohydrate Countdown,* are obtainable from The British Diabetic Association, 3/6 Alfred Place, London WC1E 7EE.

Diabetic diet sheets used in Britain are surveyed by Thomas *et al.* (1974).

Diet No. 8b   UNMEASURED DIABETIC REGIMEN

Indications   Elderly mild diabetics, who are not obese and patients who are unable to weigh their
diet may be given a list of foods which are grouped into three categories.

I. *Foods to be avoided*

1. Sugar, glucose, jam, marmalade, honey, syrup, treacle, tinned fruits, sweets, chocolate, lemonade, glucose drinks, proprietary milk preparations and similar foods which are sweetened with sugar.
2. Cakes, sweet biscuits, chocolate biscuits, pastries, pies, puddings, thick sauces.
3. Alcoholic drinks unless permission has been given by the doctor.

II. *Foods to be eaten in moderation only*

1. Breads of all kinds (including so-called 'slimming' and 'starch-reduced' breads, brown or white, plain or toasted).
2. Rolls, scones, biscuits and crispbreads.
3. Potatoes, peas and baked beans.
4. Breakfast cereals and porridge.
5. All fresh or dried fruit.
6. Macaroni, spaghetti, custard and foods with much flour.
7. Thick soups.
8. Diabetic foods.
9. Milk.

III. *Foods to be eaten as desired*

1. All meat, fish, eggs.
2. Cheese.
3. Clear soups or meat extracts, tomato or lemon juice.
4. Tea or coffee.
5. Cabbage, Brussels sprouts, broccoli, cauliflower, spinach, turnip, runner or French beans, onions, leeks, mushrooms, lettuce, cucumber, tomatoes, spring onions, radishes, mustard and cress, asparagus, parsley, rhubarb.
6. Herbs, spices, salt, pepper and mustard.
7. Saccharine preparations for sweetening.

For mild diabetics who are obese Diet No. 3 or a similar regimen is used.

Diet No. 9   DIABETIC DIETS IN THE USA

The American Diabetes and Dietetic Associations have nine standard meal plans, which are widely used throughout the USA. The system uses six food exchange groups.

Unlike the British Diabetic Association, which now uses a 10 g carbohydrate exchange unit, the American Diabetes Association uses a 15 g bread exchange.

FOOD EXCHANGES PER DAY IN SAMPLE MEAL PLANS

Diet	Milk	Vegetables	Fruits	Bread exchanges	Meat exchanges	Fat exchanges	Energy MJ	kcal
1	455 ml	1	3	4	5	1	5.0	1200
2	455 ml	1	3	6	6	4	6.3	1500
3	455 ml	1	3	8	7	5	7.5	1800
4	455 ml	1	4	10	8	8	9.2	2200
5	910 ml	1	3	6	5	3	7.5	1800
6	910 ml	1	4	10	7	11	10.9	2600
7	910 ml	1	6	17	10	15	14.7	3500
8	455 ml	1	4	12	10	12	10.9	2600
9	455 ml	1	4	15	10	15	12.6	3000

Whole milk 455 ml = 1 US pint and 910 ml = US quart.

In fat-controlled diabetic diets, this fat is polyunsaturated and the milk is skim milk.

These diets contain more milk and are especially suitable for children.

Milk includes yogurt. *Vegetables* include most vegetables, but starchy vegetables (legumes, potatoes, etc.) are put among *bread exchanges* while lettuce, parsley, radishes and watercress may be taken ad lib. *Fruits* cover all fruits as long as no sugar is added. *Meat exchanges* include fish and cheese, also peanut butter. *Fat exchanges* include avocados, olives and some fat-rich nuts as well as butter, margarine, cooking oils, cream and salad dressings.

COMPOSITION OF FOOD EXCHANGES

Food	Household measures	Weight g	CHO g	Protein g	Fat g	Energy kJ	kcal
Milk exchanges	½ pint (8 oz)	240	12	8	10	710	170
Vegetable exchanges	½ standard cup	100	5	2		105	25
Fruit exchanges	Varies		10			168	40
Bread exchanges	Varies		15	2		285	68
Meat exchanges	1 oz	30		7	5	305	73
Fat exchanges	1 tsp.	5			5	190	45

Standard cup has a volume of 8 oz (see Appendix 4).

Further information may be obtained from The American Diabetes Association, 1 West 48th Street, New York, NY 10020, USA.

Diet No. 10   VERY LOW FAT, HIGH CARBOHYDRATE

Indications   For patients with nausea due to hepatitis or obstructive jaundice and for
                       Type I hyperlipidaemia.

Nutrients   Fat 20–25 g, protein 80–90 g, carbohydrate 400 g, energy 8.4–9 MJ (2000–2300 kcal);
                       other nutrients adequate with possible exception of iron.

Food for the day

Milk, skim	750 ml
Lean meat, poultry and fish	two 90 g portions
Bread and cereal	8–12 slices or equivalent
Vegetables, salad	2–3 servings
Fruit and juice	4–7 servings
Fat	0
Sweets and dessert	Any with no fat

Sample daily menu

Early morning   Glass of fruit juice with glucose or sugar.

Breakfast   Strained porridge or breakfast cereal with skim milk.
                       Fruit.
                       Bread or toast with marmalade, jelly or jam.
                       Coffee or tea with skim milk and sugar.

Mid-morning   Coffee or tea with skim milk and sugar *or* fruit juice.

Midday meal   Clear soup or fruit juice.
                       60 g very lean meat, poultry, kidney or white fish (steamed or boiled).
                       Potato or rice (boiled).
                       Vegetable or salad.
                       Slice of bread or a roll.
                       Pudding made with cereal or gelatine and skim milk and sugar.
                       Fruit and sugar.
                       Coffee or tea with skim milk and sugar.

Mid-afternoon   2 thin slices of bread with jam or jelly *or* plain biscuits (low fat).
                       Tea with skim milk and sugar *or* carbonated beverage.

Evening meal   Similar to midday meal but with items varied.

Management

No butter, margarine or cream should be taken. No cooking fat or oil should be used and the following foods should be avoided: whole milk, egg yolk, cheese, ice cream, cakes, potato crisps, pastries and cookies; sweets containing fat, e.g. fudge and milk chocolate; bacon, organ meat, fatty fish, e.g. herrings, mackerel, sardines and salmon; and all canned meat.

Diet No. 11   LOW FAT, HIGH ENERGY

Indications   For patients with malabsorption and steatorrhoea.
Nutrients   Fat 45–50 g, protein 120 g, energy approx. 11.7 MJ (2800 kcal); adequate in all
                         nutrients.

Food for the day

Milk, skim	680–1360 ml
Lean meat, poultry, fish	200–230 g
Bread, cereal	8–12 slices or equivalent
Vegetables	2–3 servings
Fruit	4–8 servings
Fat	20 g
Sweets and desserts	Any with no fat

Sample daily menu

Breakfast
Fruit *or* fruit juice.
Cereal or porridge with skim milk.
1 egg.
Toast or rolls with jelly, jam or marmalade.
7 g margarine.
Coffee or tea with skim milk and sugar.

Mid-morning
Fruit juice.

Midday meal
Fruit juice *or* meat soup.
90 g lean meat or fish.
Potatoes and vegetables or salad.
Bread or roll.
15 ml salad dressing.
Fruit *or* fat-free dessert made from cereal, skim milk and sugar.
Coffee or tea with skim milk and sugar.

Mid-afternoon
Tea with skim milk and sugar.

Evening meal
Same as midday but omit salad and salad dressing.

Bedtime
Skim milk (flavoured) with crackers and jelly.

Management
The following foods should be avoided: all fried foods, pork, organ meats, whole milk, cheese, cream and cream substitutes, ice cream, milk chocolate, cream soup, gravies, commercial cakes, pies and cookies.

Medium-chain triglycerides can be used to increase energy intake without causing steatorrhoea. Proprietary preparations are Portagen (Mead Johnson) and MCT Oil (Cow and Gate). Recipes for incorporating these into food are obtainable from the manufacturers.

Diet No. 12	LOW SODIUM, MODERATE ENERGY

Indications   For patients with oedema from congestive heart failure, nephrotic syndrome, chronic glomerulonephritis and cirrhosis of the liver with ascites; may also be used for hypertension.

Nutrients   Sodium 40 mmol, protein 60–90 g, energy 6.7–8.4 MJ (1600–2000 kcal); adequate in other nutrients.

Sample daily menu

Breakfast   Fruit or fruit juice, sweetened as desired.
Low-salt cereal (e.g. Puffed Wheat, Shredded Wheat).
Milk from allowance and sugar.
1 egg (unsalted).
Low sodium bread or toast.
Butter from allowance.
Jelly or marmalade.
Coffee or tea with milk from allowance.

Midday meal   Fruit or fruit juice.
90 g unsalted meat, poultry or fresh white fish, which may be grilled or fried in oil.
Potato *or* rice *or* pasta.
Permitted fresh or frozen vegetable.
Salad with low sodium dressing.
Low sodium bread with butter from allowance.
Fruit and sugar.
Tea or coffee with milk from allowance.

Evening meal   Fruit or fruit juice.
60 g unsalted meat or fish *or* 1 egg.
Permitted vegetable and salad if desired.
Low sodium bread or roll with butter from allowance.
Tea or coffee with milk from allowance.

Bedtime   Cup of milk.

Allowance for day   250 ml milk.
30 g low salt butter or margarine.

Management

No salt to be used in cooking or at table.

Avoid all cured meat and fish, e.g. bacon, ham, tongue, pickled brisket and silverside, smoked haddock, kippers, sardines, pilchards, smoked salmon; all canned meats, fish and vegetables and soups; cheeses, bottled sauces, pickles, sausages, and all foods made with bicarbonate of soda or baking powder, e.g. cakes and biscuits; seasoned salts. Check labels of processed foods carefully to see if salt, sodium bicarbonate, sodium benzoate or monosodium glutamate are mentioned among the contents.

To increase the energy intake the following may be added: sugar, fruit, jam, marmalade and boiled sweets and pastilles.

The sodium intake can be reduced further to about 20 mmol/day by the use of low sodium milk, e.g. Lonalac, Loso or Edosol.

A low sodium diet is unappetising and many patients can only take it for a short period. If the low sodium bread and salt-free butter is replaced by normal bread and butter, sodium intake is increased to 60–80 mmol/day. For many patients such a restricted sodium diet is tolerable and therapeutically useful.

Diet No. 13   RESTRICTED SODIUM, LOW ENERGY

Indication   For patients with severe, acute heart failure.

Nutrients   Sodium 40 mmol, protein 40 g, energy 3.8 MJ (900 kcal).

Sample daily menu
Breakfast   1 thin slice of crisp toast.
                                   Butter and milk from allowance.
                                   Weak tea.

Mid-morning   Small glass of fruit juice.

Midday meal   Small helping of white fish, chicken or sweetbreads.
                                   1 tablespoonful of sieved vegetable.
                                   Small helping of milk pudding made with milk from allowance.

Mid-afternoon   1 thin slice of very crisp toast.
                                   Butter and milk from allowance.
                                   Weak tea.

Evening meal   Egg custard made with milk from allowance.
                                   Small helping of sieved fruit.

Bedtime   Milk drink made with remainder of milk from allowance.

Allowance for day   500 ml milk.
                                   15 g butter.

Management
No salt to be used in cooking or at table.

Diet No. 14   REDUCED SATURATED, INCREASED POLYUNSATURATED FAT

Indications   To lower plasma cholesterol, as in Type IIA hyperlipidaemia.

Nutrients   Reduced saturated fats and cholesterol; increased polyunsaturated fats.
Adequate in nutrients, with possible exception of iron. Energy
and protein determined by individual needs.

Sample daily menu

Breakfast   Fruit or fruit juice.
Cereal or porridge with skim milk and sugar.
Toast.
Polyunsaturated margarine and marmalade or jelly.
Coffee or tea with skim milk and sugar.

Mid-morning   Coffee or tea with skim milk and sugar.

Midday meal   Sandwiches made from bread and polyunsaturated margarine and filled with
sardines or tuna.
Salad.
Fruit *or* allowed dessert.
Tea with skim milk and sugar.

Mid-afternoon   Fruit.

Evening meal   Cooked poultry, fish or lean meat, which may be fried in polyunsaturated oil.
Potatoes *or* rice *or* pasta.
Vegetables, raw or cooked.
Bread or plain roll and polyunsaturated margarine.
Fruit *or* allowed dessert.
Coffee with skim milk and sugar.

Bedtime   Tea with skim milk *or* juice.
Crackers with a little peanut butter.

Management

Foods to be avoided: Butter and hydrogenated margarine. Lard, suet and shortenings; cakes, biscuits and pastries made with these. Fatty and marbled meat and visible fat on meat; meat pies, sausages and luncheon meats. Whole milk and cream and commercial cream toppings. Chocolate and ice cream. Cheese, except low fat cottage cheese. Coconut, coconut oil and Coffee Mate. Eggs: no more than 2 eggs per week, including those used in cooking. Organ meats: liver, kidneys and brain. Fish roes, caviar and shrimps. Fried foods, unless fried in polyunsaturated oil. Potato chips (crisps) and most nuts. Gravy, unless made with polyunsaturated oil, and canned soups. Salad dressing unless made with polyunsaturated oil.

Foods allowed: Bread, white and wholemeal, toast, crispbreads and plain biscuits. Breakfast cereals and porridge. Pasta, potatoes and rice. All vegetables and pulses, salads and fruit (fresh, canned and dried). Fish, white and fatty, which may be baked or fried in polyunsaturated oil. Lean meat, preferably chicken or veal. Jam*, jelly, marmalade*, honey*, sugar*, boiled sweets*, pure sugar candy*, gum drops, marshmallow*. Condiments and spices and clear soups. Tea, coffee and fruit drinks. Polyunsaturated oils, e.g. sunflower, maize, cottonseed and soya. Polyunsaturated margarines. Walnuts and pecans. Skim milk, low fat yogurt. Cottage cheese and skim milk cheese. Meringues* and cakes* and biscuits made with egg white, skim milk and polyunsaturated fat. Alcohol with discretion.

Beef, lamb, ham and pork should be limited to three (90 g) helpings a week, and all visible fat removed by trimming.

For baking only polyunsaturated fats or oils, egg whites and skim milk may be used.

If the patient is obese, it is important to adjust the energy intake so that the body weight is reduced, and then maintained at the normal level or a little below.

* For Type IIB hyperlipidaemia concentrated sweets should be avoided.

Diet No. 15   GLUTEN-FREE

Indications   For patients with coeliac disease or gluten-induced enteropathy.

Nutrients   Energy and protein intake adjusted according to age and activity. All cereals containing gluten (gliadin), i.e. wheat, oats, rye, barley and buckwheat must be omitted.

Sample daily menu

Breakfast   Fruit *or* fruit juice.
Cornflakes or puffed rice with milk and sugar.
Egg and bacon.
Gluten-free bread (toasted) with butter and marmalade or jelly.
Coffee or tea with milk and sugar.

Midday meal   Soup made with meat or vegetable stock and thickened with gluten-free flour; rice, peas or lentils may be added.

Meat *or* fish; any gravy is thickened with cornflour or other gluten-free flour.
Potato *or* rice.
Vegetables, avoiding those prepared with mayonnaise or sauce (e.g. canned baked beans). Salad with dressing made without flour.
Fruit or permitted dessert/pudding; special brands of ice cream.
Coffee or tea, with milk and sugar.

Evening meal   Fruit *or* fruit juice.
Main dish with an egg, cheese, fish or meat.
Potato *or* rice.
Vegetables.
Gluten-free bread or roll with butter.
Fruit *or* permitted dessert.
Tea with milk and sugar.

Management

Forbidden foods: Bread, biscuits, cakes, cookies, crackers, crispbreads, doughnuts, flour (white or wholemeal), muffins, pancakes, pastry, pies, pretzels, rolls, rusks, scones, toast and waffles. Breakfast cereals made with wheat or oatmeal, e.g. All Bran, Wheat Flakes, Puffed Wheat, Shredded Wheat, Weetabix, Shreddies, Sugar Smacks, Grapenuts, oatmeal, wheat germ. Macaroni, noodles, spaghetti, semolina, vermicelli and other pasta. Meat pie, luncheon meat, canned meat, meat loaf, commercial hamburgers, sausages, bologna and frankfurters. Canned soups and soup mixes. Vegetables with cream sauces or crumbs, e.g. baked beans. Proprietary sauces and ketchups, gravies, commercial salad dressings. Packet and pudding mixtures, pastry mixtures, patent infant foods. Malted milk, Ovaltine, postum and beer, commercial milk flavouring. Baking powder. Cheese spreads. Most ice creams (except those listed below). Commercial chocolates and liquorice sweets.

Foods that may be used freely: Milk (all kinds) and yogurt; may be flavoured with home-made syrup or unprocessed cocoa. Fresh meats and poultry and bacon, fish (fresh or canned), shellfish, organ meats. Gravies made with cornstarch or rice flour. Cheese and egg (boiled, poached, scrambled, omelet and in mixed dishes). Vegetables (fresh, frozen, canned), raw or cooked. Potatoes and rice. Nuts. All fruits and fruit juices. Bread and flour made from wheatstarch, arrowroot, cornmeal, soyabean, rice or potato flour. Breakfast cereals made from rice and maize. Cream, butter, margarine, peanut butter, cooking fats and oils. Sugar, jam, jelly, marmalade, honey, syrup, boiled sweets, hard candies, home-made candy, plain chocolate. Desserts and puddings made with gelatine, tapicoa, sago, rice and cornstarch. Cakes and cookies made with gluten-free flour. Coffee, tea and carbonated beverages. Salt, pepper, mustard, spices, garlic and vinegar. Ice cream (in UK made by Wall's, Lyons, Eldorado or Hoods).

Successful treatment depends on not eating wheat starch containing more than 0.3 per cent protein. Many mixed and manufactured foods contain small amounts of wheat flour, and lists of forbidden and permissible foods should be continuously checked and brought up to date. A current list of gluten-free foods and recipes can be obtained from the Coeliac Society, P.O. Box No. 181, London NW2 2QY.

Diet No. 16   SEMI-LIQUID

Indications   For patients with difficulty in chewing or swallowing or who are severely ill with
                             ulcerative or malignant disease of the gastrointestinal tract.
Nutrients   Energy 6.3–8.4 MJ (1500–2000 kcal), protein 50–75 g.

Sample daily feeds
Early morning   Fruit juice with sugar.

Breakfast   Cereal gruel (strained porridge) with cream and sugar. Milk flavoured with tea or
                             coffee and sugar.

Mid-morning   Eggnog (commercial mix) *or* milk.

Midday meal   Strained cream soup *or* broth.
                             Savoury custard, using cheese *or* scrambled egg *or* omelet.
                             Milk, flavoured with tea or coffee, and sugar.

Mid-afternoon   Strained fruit juice and ice cream *or* milk desserts.

Evening meal   Savoury custard, using finely minced chicken, ham or fish.
                             Gelatine and milk dessert and cream.
                             Milk flavoured with tea or coffee.

Bedtime   Eggnog *or* malted milk drink.

Allowance for day   500–1500 ml milk.
                             2 to 4 eggs.
                             150–250 ml fruit juice.

Management

  Foods that may be used: Milk in all forms, including chocolate- and other-flavoured milks, eggnog, yogurt,
malted milk and cream. Meat, strained in broth or cream soups; finely minced poultry, meat and fish. Eggs in
eggnog and soft-cooked eggs (boiled, poached, scrambled or omelet). Vegetables strained in cream soups. Fruit
juices. Cereal gruels. Dessert: flavoured gelatine, junket, custard, ice cream, sherbet and simple puddings. Milk,
tea, coffee and cocoa. Sugar and syrups and glucose.

  This diet may be inadequate in energy, iron, vitamin A, thiamin and nicotinamide. It is a transition diet used
until more adequate oral feeding is possible and may need to be supplemented by parenteral feeding.

  Energy can be increased by using more cream, butter and glucose; some patients may not tolerate large intakes
of milk and for them the cereal gruel and cream can be increased, and combinations of a glucose polymer (e.g.
Hycal), Casilan and cream used.

Diet No. 17   BLAND REGIMEN

Indications   The advice given below is likely to relieve symptoms in patients with peptic ulcers, gastritis and some other gastrointestinal disorders. How many points in the advice are used depends on the physician's judgment and on the patient's individual sensitivity to particular food items.

General Advice
1. Take four meals a day.
2. Take your meals at regular times each day.
3. Eat your meals slowly and chew your food carefully.
4. Avoid rush and hurry before and after meals; if possible rest for a few minutes before and after eating.
5. Do not smoke or drink alcohol before meals, when the stomach is empty.
6. Avoid large, heavy meals and any articles of food which you find disagree with you.
7. Remember that anxiety and worry can upset digestion.
8. See that you get sufficient sleep at night.
9. Consult your dentist at regular intervals.

The following foods should be avoided during the acute stage of dyspepsia or peptic ulcer, and taken sparingly during intermissions by those liable to frequent attacks. By trial and error the patient can find out which of the articles listed below should be avoided thereafter.
1. Alcohol, strong tea and coffee, cola beverages, gravies and soups made from meat extracts.
2. Pickles, spices, curries and condiments.
3. All fried foods.
4. Tough, twice-cooked or highly seasoned meats, sausages, bacon and pork.
5. Salted fish and some fatty fish such as herring, mackerel and sardines.
6. New bread and scones, wholemeal bread, crispbreads, pastry and cakes containing dried fruit or peel.
7. Rich, heavy puddings.
8. Excess sugar and sweets.
9. Raw and unripe fruit and dried fruits, nuts and the pips, skins and peel of all fruits.
10. Raw vegetables, celery, cucumber, onions, radishes and tomatoes.

The following foods are recommended.
1. Dairy products, i.e. milk, cream, butter, mild cheese and eggs (not fried).
2. White fish, steamed, baked or grilled.
3. Bland meats—chicken, tender beef and lamb, sweetbreads, and tripe.
4. White bread and toast, macaroni and rice.
5. Butter and margarine on bread and in cookery.
6. Plain biscuits and cakes; honey, syrup and jellies.
7. Refined and well-cooked cereals, e.g. cornflour, semolina, ground rice and oatflour porridge.
8. Puddings—junket, jellies, custards, blancmange, soufflé, mousse and plain ice cream.
9. Vegetables—potatoes, creamed or mashed, and green and yellow vegetables which may be sieved and puréed with butter.
10. Fruits, stewed and preferably sieved and served as purées or fools and ripe raw bananas.
11. Weak tea, decaffeinated coffee and malted milk drinks.

The use of a bland diet in the treatment of chronic duodenal ulcer is discussed in a position paper by the American Dietetic Association (1971).

Diet No. 18   HIGH FIBRE (ROUGHAGE)

Indications   For patients with diverticulosis and constipation.

Nutrients   Energy and protein according to individual needs; increased fibre.

Sample daily menu
Early morning   Fruit juice, tea or coffee.

Breakfast   Orange juice *or* ½ grapefruit.
                       Oatmeal porridge or bran cereal (e.g. All Bran) or muesli (oatmeal, chopped fruit and
                           nuts) with milk.
                       Egg and bacon.
                       Wholemeal bread (may be toasted), oatcakes or crispbread.
                       Chunky marmalade or jam.
                       Coffee or tea with milk (and sugar).

Midday meal   Vegetable soup, including plenty of chopped fresh vegetables, dried peas, lentils and
                       barley. Sandwiches made from wholemeal bread and filled with salad, including raw
                           carrots or celery and cheese.
                       Tea or coffee with milk and sugar.

Mid-afternoon   Oatcakes, wholemeal wheat biscuits or crispbread.
                       Tea or coffee with milk (and sugar).

Evening meal   Serving of any kind of meat or fish.
                       Baked potatoes (in jackets).
                       Green beans.
                       Salad with dressing.
                       Wholemeal bread or bran muffins and butter.
                       Fruit.
                       Coffee or tea with milk and sugar.

Management

Liberal use should be made of unrefined cereals, e.g. wholemeal bread and flour, of fresh fruit, fibrous
vegetables and nuts. One teaspoonful of an unprocessed bran may be taken morning and evening. Refined cereals
and flours, e.g. white bread, rice, pasta, cakes and pastries, should be avoided.

   People vary in their response to a high fibre diet, and in some individuals amounts of foods high in fibre should
be small at first and increased gradually. The selection of foods for high fibre diets is discussed by Adamson *et al.*
(1973).

Appendix 3. Oral or Tube Feeds

Table A.1 Commercially available oral or tube feeding formulae

Ingredients		Composition per 1000 kcal (4.2 MJ)					
		Protein (g)	Fat (g)	CHO (g)	Na (mmol)	K (mmol)	Mg (mmol)
I. Mixed foods							
Compleat B (liquid) (Doyle)	Deionised water, beef purée, malto-dextrin, green bean purée, pea purée, skim milk powder, corn oil, sucrose, peach purée, orange juice, 6M, 9V*	40	40	120	68	34	9
Gerber MBF (Gerber)	Beef heart, water, sucrose, sesame oil, modified tapioca starch, 13M, 8V	50	57	72	14	19	3
Formula 2 (Cutter)	Skim milk, beef, corn oil, egg yolks, sucrose, orange juice, farina, dextrose	37	40	122	26	45	4
II. Milk-based							
Complan (Glaxo)	Skim milk powder, peanut oil, caseinate, malto dextrin, sucrose, whey solids, 7M, 13V	70	37	100	20	100	5
Instant Breakfast (Carnation) — in water	Skim milk powder, sucrose, glucose syrup solids, lactose, 1M, 5V	65	28	124	37	63	17
Meritene—liquid (Doyle)	Skim milk conc., corn syrup solids, vegetable oil, caseinate, sucrose, 7M, 11V	60	33	115	40	43	12
Nutrament (Mead Johnson)	Whole milk, sucrose, skim milk, soya flour, corn syrup, 3M, 6V	50	33	125	22	58	11
Nutri-1000 (Syntex)	Skim milk, corn oil, sucrose, corn syrup solids, 8M, 13V	34	52	96	22	36	8
Sustacal—liquid (Mead Johnson)	Skim milk conc., sucrose, corn syrup solids, soya oil, caseinate, soya protein, 8M, 12V	60	23	138	40	53	6
Sustagen (Mead Johnson)	Whole and non-fat dried milk, caseinate, maltose, dextrins, dextrose, 5M, 11V	60	9	171	30	51	9
Clinifeed 400 (Roussel)	Milk, corn syrup solids, whey proteins sucrose, egg yolks, maize oil, soya oil, glyceryl stearate, alginate, carageenan, 12V, 6M	38	33	138	26	31	5
III. Partially chemically defined							
Ensure (Ross)	Water, corn syrup solids, sucrose, corn oil, caseinate, soya protein, 10M, 11V	35	35	137	30	31	8
Flexical (Mead Johnson)	Sucrose, corn syrup solids, hydrolysed casein, soya oil, tapioca starch, MCT oil, 3 AA, 9M 15V	22	34	155	15	32	8
Isocal (Mead Johnson)	Corn syrup solids, soya oil, caseinate, MCT oil, soya protein, 9M, 13V	33	42	125	22	32	8

Table A1—*continued*

Ingredients		Composition per 1000 kcal (4.2 MJ)					
		Protein (g)	Fat (g)	CHO (g)	Na (mmol)	K (mmol)	Mg (mmol)
Precision LR	Maltodextrin, egg white solids, sucrose, vegetable oil, 7M, 12V	22	0.7	226	27	20	8
Precision HN (Doyle)	Maltodextrin, egg white solids, sucrose, vegetable oil, 7M, 12V	42	0.5	207	41	22	5
W-T Protein L4 (Warren Teed)	Dextrose, oligosaccharide, skim milk powder, caseinate, methionine, vegetable oil, 11M, 14V	25	1.1	222	42	33	9
IV. Chemically defined Vivonex Standard (Eaton)	Glucose, oligosaccharide, 17 L-amino acids, safflower oil, 10M, 15V	20.6	1.4	226	37	30	8
Vivonex HN (Eaton)	Glucose, oligosaccharide, 17 L-amino acids, safflower oil, 10M, 15V	41	0.9	202	34	18	4
V. Lactose-free milk substitutes Nutramigen (Mead Johnson)	Casein hydrolysate, dextrimaltose, corn oil	32	39	130	21	25	5
ProSobee (Mead Johnson)	Soya flour, corn syrup solids, soya and coconut oils	37	50	100	27	28	5
Velactin (Wander)	Full-fat soya flour, dextrose, corn dextrin, cornstarch, peanut oil, methionine, 4M, 12V	51	42	114	15	14	-
VI. Supplements containing MCT oil (for malabsorption syndromes) Portagen (Mead Johnson)	Corn syrup solids, sucrose, MCT, caseinate, corn oil	35	48	115	20	32	9
Pregestimil (Mead Johnson)	Glucose, MCT, casein hydrolysate	32	41	130	21	25	5

★ M = minerals, V = vitamins, AA = amino acids.

Table A.2 Oral or tube feeding supplements

Description	Energy		Composition per 100 g				
	KJ	kcal	Protein (g)	Fat (g)	CHO (g)	Na (mmol)	K (mmol)
I. High carbohydrate							
Caloreen (Roussel) — Low osmolar glucose polymer	1680	400	0	0	96	<0.1	<0.1
Gastro-Caloreen (Roussel) — Low osmolar glucose polymer	1680	400	0	0	100	5.2	0.12
Controlyte (Doyle) — Low osmolar, corn starch hydrolysate	2117	504	tr	24	72	0.66	0.1
Hycal (Beechams) — Flavoured liquid glucose syrup	1033	246	0.02	0	60	0.6	0.02
Calonutrin (Geistlich) — Glucose polymer and glucose	1726	410	0	0	94	4.0	0.3
II. High fat							
Lipomul (Upjohn) — Flavoured corn oil emulsion	2520	600	0	67	0.7	1.7	0.05
Prosparol (British Drug House) — Peanut oil/water emulsion	1890	450	0	50	0	0.7	0
MCT Oil (Mead Johnson) — Medium chain triglycerides	3486	830	0	100	0	0	0
III. High protein							
Aminutrin (Geistlich) — Powdered L-amino acids	1306	311	78	0	0	0	0
Casilan (Glaxo) — Hydrolysed casein	1512	360	90	1.8	tr	4.3	na
Comminuted chicken meat (Cow & Gate) — Finely ground chicken meat in water	250	60	8	3	0	0.4	1.3
Forceval Protein (Unigreg) — Low sodium protein powder	1537	366	53	tr	30	5.2	1.3
Lonalac (Mead Johnson) — Low sodium milk product	2124	510	27	28	38	0.9	24
Edosol (Cow & Gate) — Unhydrogenated coconut and maize oil, lactose and partially demineralized casein	2125	506	28	28	38	1.3	18
Albumaid (Scientific Hospital Supplies) — Hydrolysed bovine serum proteins	1499	357	75	0	0	43	5

Note: The list is not exhaustive; new products are developed and replace old ones from time to time. The composition may change and should be checked with the manufacturer where it needs to be known exactly.

Appendix 4. Weights and Measures

Weights   *Approximate equivalents*

1 ounce (oz)	= 28.35 g	30 g
1 pound (lb)	= 453.6 g	
1 stone (14 lb)	= 6.35 kg	
1 gram (g)	= 0.0353 oz	
1 kilogram (kg)	= 2.205 lb	2.2 lb

Fluid measures

1 fluid ounce (fl oz) (Imperial)	= 28.41 ml	30 ml
1 fluid ounce (fl oz) US	= 29.57 ml	
1 Imperial pint (20 fl oz)	= 568.3 ml	600 ml
1 US pint (16 fl oz)	= 473.0 ml	
1 Imperial gallon (160 fl oz)	= 4.546 litres	
1 US gallon (128 fl oz)	= 3.785 litres	
1 millilitre (ml)	= 0.0352 fl oz (Imperial)	
1 litre (l)	= 1.760 Imperial pints	2 pints
	= 2.11 American pints	

Length

1 inch (in)	= 2.54 cm	
1 foot	= 30.48 cm	30 cm
1 mile	= 1.609 km	
1 centimetre (cm)	= 0.394 in	
1 kilometre (km)	= 0.621 miles	

Kitchen measures

*In Britain**

1 teaspoonful	= $\frac{1}{8}$ fl oz = about 4 ml
1 dessertspoonful	= $\frac{1}{4}$ fl oz = about 10 ml
1 tablespoonful	= $\frac{1}{2}$ fl oz = about 18 ml

In North America

1 teaspoonful = 4.7 ml

1 tablespoonful = 3 teaspoonsful = 14 ml
1 standard cup = 8 fl oz = 237 ml

* Teaspoons, dessertspoons and tablespoons vary greatly in Britain (Lockwood *et al.,* 1968).

References

Aaron, J. E., Gallagher, J. C., Anderson, J., Stasiak, L., Longton, E. B., Nordin, B. E. C. & Nicholson, M. (1974). *Lancet* **1**, 229.

Abdellatif, A. M. M. & Vles, R. O. (1973). *Nutr. Metabol.* **15**, 219.

Abdulla, Y. H. & Adams, C. W. M. (1965). *J. Atheroscler. Res.* **5**, 504.

Abedin, Z., Hussain, M. A. & Ahmad, K. (1976). *Bangladesh med. res. Counc. Bull.* **2**, 42.

Abell, L. L., Levy, B. B., Brodie, B. B. & Kendall, F. E. (1952). *J. biol. Chem.* **195**, 357.

Ablett, J. G. & McCance, R. A. (1971). *Lancet* **2**, 517.

Adams, E. B., Scragg, J. N., Naidoo, B. T., Liljestrand, S. K. & Cockram, V. I. (1967). *Br. med. J.* **3**, 451.

Adamson, C., Brown, A. & Truswell, A. S. (1973). *Nutrition, Lond.* **27**, 159.

Addis, T., Poo, L. J. & Lew, W. (1936). *J. biol. Chem.* **116**, 343.

Adelaide Obesity Study Group (1978). *Med. J. Aust.* **2**, 58.

Agarwal, A. K. (1975). *New Scientist* 30 Jan., 260.

Agate, J. N. & 12 others (1949). *Medical Research Council,* Memo. no. 22.

Aherne, W. & Hull, D. (1964). *Proc. R. Soc. Med.* **57**, 1172.

Ahlborg, G., Felig, P., Hagenfeldt, L., Hendler, R. & Wahren, J. (1974). *J. clin. Invest.* **53**, 1080.

Ahlman, K. L., Eränko, C., Karvonen, M. J. & Lepänen, V. (1952). *J. appl. Physiol.* **4**, 911.

Ahrens, E. H., Jr, Hirsch, J., Oetta, A., Farquahar, J. W. & Stein, Y. (1961). *Trans. Ass. Am. Physns* **74**, 134.

Ahrens, E. H., Jr, Insull, W., Jr, Hirsch, J., Stoffel, W., Peterson, M. L., Farquahar, J. W., Miller, T. & Thomasson, H. J. (1959). *Lancet* **1**, 115.

Aitken, J. M., Hart, D. M. & Lindsay, R. (1973). *Br. med. J.* **3**, 515.

Alberti, K. G. M. M. (1973). *Postgrad. med. J.* **49** (Dec. suppl.), 955.

Albutt, E. C. & Chance, G. W. (1969). *J. clin. Invest,* **48**, 139.

Alcantara, E. M. & Speckmann, E. W. (1975). *Am. J. clin. Nutr.* **29**, 1035.

Alfin-Slater, R. B. & Aftergood, L. (1968). *Physiol. Rev.* **48**, 758.

Alfrey, A. C., LeGendre, G. R. & Kaehny, W. D. (1976). *New Engl. J. Med.* **294**, 184.

Allbrink, M. J. & Meigs, J. W. (1964). *Am. J. clin. Nutr.* **15**, 255.

Allbrink, M. J. & Meigs, J. W. (1965). *Ann. N.Y. Acad. Sci.* **131**, 673

Alleyne, G. A. O. (1970). *Br. J. Nutr.* **24**, 205.

Alleyne, G. A. O., Halliday, D. & Waterlow, J. C. (1969). *Br. J. Nutr.* **23**, 783.

Alleyne, G. A. O., Hay, R. W., Picou, D. I., Stansfield, J. P. & Whitehead, R. G. (1977). *Protein-Energy Malnutrition.* London: Arnold.

Alleyne, G. A. O., Viteri, F. & Alvarado, J. (1970). *Am. J. clin. Nutr.* **23**, 875.

Alleyne, G. A. O. & Young, V. H. (1967). *Clin. Sci.* **33**, 189.

Allison, J. B. (1964). In *Mammalian Protein Metabolism,* vol. 2, pl 41, ed. Munro, H. N. & Allison, J. B. New York: Academic Press.

Al Rashid, R. A. & Spangler, J. (1971). *New Engl. J. Med.* **285**, 841.

Al Samarrae, W., Ma, M. C. F. & Truswell, A. S. (1975). *Proc. nutr. Soc.* **34**, 18A.

Alvarez, W. C. (1943). *Nervousness, Indigestion and Pain,* New York: Hoeber.

Al-Witry, H., Shaby, J. A. & Kantarjian, A. D. (1950). *J. Fac. Med. Iraq,* **14**, 143.

American Dietetic Association (1972). *The Profession of Dietetics.* The Report of the Study Commission on Dietetics. Chicago: American Dietetic Association.

American Heart Association (1969). *Mass Field Trials of the Diet-Heart Question.* Monograph No. 28.

American Heart Association (1973). Monograph 38. In *Circulation* (March, suppl. 1), **47**.

American Medical Association, Council on Foods and Nutrition (1973a). *J. Am. med. Ass.* **224**, 1415.

American Medical Association, Council on Foods and Nutrition (1973b). *J. Am. med. Ass.* **225**, 1118.

American Psychiatric Association (1973). Megavitamin and Orthomolecular Medicine in Psychiatry. Task Force Report no. 87. Washington D.C.

Anderson, G. H. (1977). In *Advances in Nutritional Research,* ed. Draper, H. H., vol. 1, p. 145. New York & London: Plenum Press.

Anderson, H. & Gillberg, R. (1977). *Lancet* **2**, 677.

Anderson, J., Campbell, A. E. R., Dunn, A. & Runciman, J. B. M. (1966). *Scott. med. J.* **11**, 429.

Anderson, J. T., Grande, F. & Keys, A. (1971). *Am. J. clin. Nutr.* **24**, 524.

Anderson, T. W. (1970). *Lancet* **2**, 753.

Anderson, T. W:, Suranyi, G. & Beaton, G. H. (1974). *Can. med. Ass. J.* **111**, 31.

Andres, R., Cader, G. & Zierler, K. L. (1956). *J. clin. Invest.* **35**, 681.

Anitschkow, H. (1933). In *Arteriosclerosis*, ed. Cowdry, E. V., p. 271. New York: Macmillan.

Ansell, J. E., Kumar, R., Deykin, D. (1977). *J. Am. med. Ass.* **238**, 40.

Antar, M. A., Ohlson, M. A. & Hodges, R. E. (1964). *Am. J. clin. Nutr.* **14**, 169.

Antoniou, L. D., Shalhoub, R. J., Subhakar, T. & Smith, C. J., Jr. (1977). *Lancet* **2**, 895.

Antonis, A. & Bersohn, I. (1961). *Lancet* **1**, 3.

Aoki, T. T., Brennan, M. F., Muller, W. A., Soeldner, J. A., Saltz, S. B., Kaufmann, R. L., Tan, M. H. & Cahill, G. F. (1976). *Am. J. clin. Nutr.* **29**, 340.

Aoki, T. T., Teows, C. J., Rossini, A. A., Ruderman, N. B. & Cahill, G. F. (1975). *Adv. Enz. Req.* **13**, 329.

Arakawa, T. (1970). *Am. J. Med.* **48**, 594.

Archer, H. E., Dormer, A. E., Scowen, E. F. & Watt, R. W. E. (1957). *Lancet* **2**, 320.

Arena, J. M. (1970). *Nutrition Today* **4**, 2.

Arimoto, K. (1957). Personal communication.

Armstrong, B. & Doll, R. (1975a). *Int. J. Cancer.* **15**, 617

Armstrong, B. & Doll, R. (1975b). *Br. J. prevent. soc. Med.* **29**, 73.

Armstrong, B., Lea, A. J., Adelstein, A. M., Donovan, J. W., White, G. C. & Rittle, S. (1976). *Br. J. prev. soc. Med.* **30**, 151.

Arneil, G. C. (1967). *Dietary Studies of 4365 Scottish Infants*. Scottish Health Services Studies No. 6.

Arneil, G. C. (1973). *Practitioner*, **210**, 331.

Arneil, G. C. (1975). *Proc. nutr. Soc.* **34**, 101.

Arnhold, R. (1969). *J. trop. Pediat.* **15**, 243.

Artman, N. R. & Smith, D. E. (1972). *J. Am. oil Chemists' Soc.* **49**, 318.

Aschoff, L. & Koch, W. (1919). *Scorbut: eine Pathologisch-Anatomische Studie*. Jena: Fischer.

Ascoli, W., Guzman, M. A., Scrimshaw, N. S. & Gordon, J. E. (1967). *Archs environl Hlth* **15**, 439.

Ashby, W. R., Humphreys, J. & Smith, S. J. (1965). *Br. med. J.* **2**, 1409.

Ashley, B. C. E. & Whyte, H. M. (1961). *Aust. Ann. Med.* **10**, 92.

Ashwell, M. & Garrow, J. S. (1975). *Nutrition, Lond.* **29**, 347.

Ashworth, A. (1969). *Br. J. Nutr.* **23**, 835.

Ashworth, A., Bell, R., James, W. P. T. & Waterlow, J. C. (1968). *Lancet* **2**, 600.

Ashworth, A. & Harrower, A. D. B. (1967). *Br. J. Nutr.* **21**, 833.

Ashworth, A., Milner, P. F., Waterlow, J. C. & Walker, R. B. (1973). *Br. J. Nutr.* **29**, 269.

Ashworth, A. & Waterlow, J. C. (1974). *Nutrition in Jamaica 1969-70.* Univ. West Indies.

Atherton, D. J., Sewell, M., Soothill, J. F. & Wells, R. S. (1978). *Lancet* **1**, 401.

Atwater, W. O. & Benedict, F. G. (1899). *Experiments on the Metabolism of Matter and Energy in the Human Body.* Bulletin no. 69, p. 76. Washington D.C.: US Department of Agriculture.

Atwater, W. O. & Benedict, F. G. (1902). *Mem. natn. Acad. Sci.* **8**, 231.

Atwater, W. O. & Woods, C. D. (1896). *The Chemical Composition of American Food Materials.* US Office of Experiment Stations Bulletin 28.

Auden, G. A. (1923). *Jl R. sanit. Inst.* **44**, 236.

Avery, M. E. & 6 others (1967). *Pediatrics* **39**, 378.

Axelrod, A. E. (1971). *Am. J. clin. Nutr.* **24**, 265.

Aykroyd, W. R. (1930). *J. Hyg., Camb.* **30**, 357.

Aykroyd, W. R. (1957). *Ann. Nutr. Aliment.* **11**, 171.

Aykroyd, W. R. (1967). *Sweet Malefactor: Sugar, Slavery and Human Society.* London: Heinemann.

Aykroyd, W. R. (1974). *The Conquest of Famine.* London: Chatto and Windus.

Aykroyd, W. R. & Doughty, J. (1964). In *FAO Nutritional Studies* no. 19. Rome: FAO.

Aykroyd, W. R. & Doughty, J. (1970). *Wheat in Human Nutrition.* FAO Nutritional Studies, no. 23. Rome: FAO.

Aykroyd, W. R., Krishnan, B. G., Passmore, R. & Sundararajan, A. R. (1940). *Indian med. Res. Mem.* no. 32.

Aykroyd, W. R. & Swaminathan, M. (1940). *Indian J. med. Res.* **27**, 667.

Bagnis, R., Berglund, F., Elias, P. S., van Esch, G. J., Halstead, B. W. & Kojima, K. (1970). *Bull. Wld Hlth Org.* **42**, 69.

Baird, D. (1960). *Lancet* **2**, 557.

Baird, J. D. (1972). *Acta diabetologica Latina,* **9** (suppl. 1), 621.

Baird, J. D. (1973). In *Symposia: Anorexia Nervosa,* ed. Robertson, R. F. & Proudfoot, A. T., no. 42, p. 83.

Baird, J. D. (1974). In *Companion to Medical Studies,* ed. Passmore, R. & Robson, J. S., vol. 3, chap. 44. Oxford: Blackwell.

Baird, J. D., Hunter, W. M. & Smith, A. W. M. (1973). *Postgrad. med. J.* **49** (Feb. suppl.), 132.

Baker, E. M., Halver, J. E., Johnson, D. O., Joyce, B. E., Knight, M. K. & Tolbert, B. M. (1975). *Ann. N.Y. Acad. Sci.* **258**, 72.

Baker, E. M., Hodges, R. E., Hood, J., Sauberlich, H. E., March, S. C. & Carnham, J. E. (1971). *Am. J. clin. Nutr.* **24**, 444.

Bakin, F. & 10 others (1973). *Science, N.Y.* **181**, 230.

Balch, H. H. (1950). *J. Immunol.* **64**, 397.

Ball, K. & Turner, R. (1974). *Lancet* **2**, 822.

Balogh, M., Kahn, H. A. & Medalie, J. H. (1971). *Am. J. clin. Nutr.* **24**, 304.

Barbezat, G. O. & Hansen, J. D. L. (1968). *Pediatrics* **42**, 77.

Barboriak, J. J. & Meade, R. C. (1971). *Atherosclerosis* **13**, 199.

Barger, G. (1931). *Ergot and Ergotism.* London: Gurney & Jackson.

Barkhan, P. & Shearer, M. J. (1977). *Proc. R. Soc. Med.* **70**, 93.

Barnes, D. E., Adkins, B. L. & Schamschula, R. G. (1970). *Bull. Wld Hlth Org.* **43**, 769.

Barnes, J. M., Austwick, P. K. C., Carter, R. L., Flynn, F. V., Peristianis, G. C. & Aldridge, W. N. (1977). *Lancet* **1**, 671.

Barnes, M. J. (1975). *Ann. N.Y. Acad. Sci.* **258**, 264.

Barnes, N. D., Hull, D., Balgobin, L. & Gompertz, D. (1970). *Lancet* **2**, 244.

Barness, L. A. (1975). *Ann. N.Y. Acad. Sci.* **258**, 523.

Baron, D. N., Dent, C. E. Harris, H., Hart, E. W. & Jepson, J. B. (1956). *Lancet* **2**, 421.

Barry, R. E., Baker, P. & Read, A. E. (1974). *Clins Gastroenterol.* **3**, 55.

Bartley, W., Krebs, H. A. & O'Brien, J. R. P. (1953). *Spec. Ser. med. Res. Coun., Lond.* no. 280.

Basu, K. P. (1946). *Indian Res. Fund. Ass. spec. Rep.* no. 15.

Bateson, M. C. & Lant, A. E. (1973). *Lancet* **2**, 381.

Baugh, C. M., Malone, J. M. & Butterworth, C. E. (1968). *Am. J. clin. Nutr.* **21**, 173.

Baumann, E. (1895). *Hoppe-Seyler's Z. physiol. Chem.* **21**, 319.

Beadle, G. W. (1948). *A. Rev. Physiol.* **10**, 17.

Beaton, G. H. (1961). *Fedn Proc. Fedn Am. Socs exp. Biol.* **20**, suppl. 7; 196.

Beattie, J., Herbert, P. H. & Bell, D. J. (1948). *Br. J. Nutr.* **2**, 47.

Beaumont, J. L., Carlson, L. A., Cooper, G. R., Feifar, Z., Fredrickson, D. S. & Strasser, T. (1970). *Bull. Wld Hlth Org.* **43**, 891.

Begum, A. & Pereira, S. M. (1969). *Br. J. Nutr.* **23**, 905.

Behar, M. (1969). *Am. J. Dis. Child.* **117**, 114.

Behnke, A. R., Feen, B. G. & Welham, W. C. (1942). *J. Am. med. Ass.* **118**, 495.

Beisel, W. R., Herman, Y. F., Sauberlich, H. E., Herman, R. H., Bartelloni, P. J. & Canham, J. E. (1972). *Am. J. clin. Nutr.* **25**, 1165.

Belavady, B. (1969). *Indian J. med. Res.* **57**, Suppl. p. 63.

Belavady, B., Srikantia, S. G. & Gopalan, C. (1963). *Biochem. J.* **87**, 652.

Belchetz, P. E., Lloyd, M. H., Johns, R. G. S. & Cohen, R. D. (1973). *Br. med. J.* **2**, 510.

Bell, H. & Nordhagen, R. (1978). *Br. med. J.* **1**, 822.

Bender, A. E. (1977). In *Physical, Chemical and Biological Changes in Food Caused by Thermal Processing,* ed. Høyem, T. & Kvåle, O., p. 360. London: Applied Science.

Bender, A. E., Harris, M. C. & Getreuer, A. (1977). *Br. med. J.* **1**, 757.

Bender, A. E. & Zia, M. (1976). *J. Food Technol.* **11**, 495.

Bengoa, J. M. (1973). In *Man Food and Nutrition,* ed. Rechcigl, M., Jr., p. 1. Cleveland, Ohio: Chemical Rubber Co.

Bengoa, J. M. & Donoso, G. (1974). *PAG Bulletin,* **4**, 24.

Bennett, P. H., Burch, T. A. & Miller, M. (1971). *Lancet,* **2**, 125.

Benterud, A. (1977). In *Physical, Chemical and Biological Changes caused by Thermal Processing,* ed. Høyem, T. & Kvåle, O. London: Applied Science.

Berg, A., Scrimshaw, N. S. & Call, D. L. (eds.) (1973). *Nutrition, National Development and Planning.* Proceedings of an International Conference. Cambridge, Mass: MIT Press.

Berg, B. & Johansson, B. G. (1973). *Acta med. scand.* **194**, suppl. 552, 13.

Berg, J. W. (1975). *Cancer Res.* **35**, 3345.

Bergeson, F. T. & Hipsley, E. H. (1970). *J. gen. Microbiol.* **60**, 61.

Bergström, J. & Hultman, E. (1966). *Nature, Lond.* **210**, 309.

Berlin, R. (1948). *Acta med. scand.* **129**, 560.

Berlyne, G. M., Bazzard, F. J., Booth, E. M., Janabi, K. & Shaw, A. B. (1967). *Q. Jl Med.* **36**, 59.

Berlyne, G. M., Yagil, R., Ben Ari, J., Weinberger, G., Knopf, E. & Danovitch, G. M. (1972). *Lancet* **1**, 564.

Bernard, C. (1850). *C.r. hebd. Séanc. Acad. Sci., Paris* **31**, 571.

Bernstein, D. S., Sadowsky, M., Hegsted, D. M., Guni, C. D. & Stare, F. J. (1966). *J. Am. med. Ass.* **198**, 499.

Berry, W. T. C. (1972). *Nutr. Rev.* **30**, 127.

Bertram, G. C. L. (1954). *Proc. Nutr. Soc.* **13**, 69.

Best, C. H., Lucas, C. C. & Ridout, J. H. (1956). *Br. med. Bull.* **12**, 9.

Best, C. H. & Taylor, N. B. (1961). *The Physiological Basis of Medical Practice,* 7th edn, p. 850. London: Baillière.

Beveridge, W. I. D. (1977). *Influenza, the Last Great Plague.* London: Heinemann.

Bibile, S. W., Lionel, N. D. W., Dunuwille, R. & Perera, G. (1957). *Br. J. Nutr.* **11**, 434.

Bierenbaum, M. L., Fleischman, A. I. & Raichelson, R. I. (1972). *Lipids* **7**, 202.

Bierman, E. L. & 6 others (1971). *Diabetes* **20**, 633.

Billings, F. L. (1970). *Biotin: An Annotated Bibliography.* Montreal: Hoffman La Roche.

Billings, F. L. (1975). *Biotin: An Annotated Bibliography. Supplement.* Montreal: Hoffman La Roche.

Bing, R. J. & Tillmanns, H. (1976). In *Metabolic Aspects of Alcoholism,* ed. Lieber, C. S., p. 117. Lancaster: MTP Pres.

Bingham, S., McNeil, N. I. & Cummings, J. H. (1977). *J. hum. Nutr.* **31,** 367.

Birch, T. W. & György, P. (1936). *Biochem. J.* **30,** 304.

Bistrian, B. R., Blackburn, G. L., Vitale, J., Cockran, D. & Naylor, J. (1976). *J. Am. med. Ass.* **235,** 1567.

Black, D. A. K. (1968). *Essentials of Fluid Balance,* 4th edn. Oxford: Blackwell.

Black, W. A. P. (1953). *Proc. Nutr. Soc.* **12,** 32.

Blackburn, G. L., Flatt, J. P., Clowes, G. H. A. & O'Donnell, T. E. (1973). *Am. J. Surg.* **125,** 447.

Blackburn, M. W. & Calloway, D. H. (1976). *J. Am. diet. Ass.* **69,** 29.

Blacket, R. B. & Palmer, A. J. (1960). *Br. Heart J.* **22,** 483.

Blackwell, R. Q., Chow, B. F., Chinn, K. S. K., Blackwell, B. N. & Hsu, S. C. (1973). *Nutr. Rep. Internat.* **7,** 517.

Blankenhorn, D. H., Freiman, D. G. & Knowles, H. C. (1956). *Circulation* **4,** 912.

Bloch, C. E. (1921). *J. Hyg., Camb.* **19,** 283.

Bloch, C. E. (1924a). *Am. J. Dis. Child.* **27,** 139.

Bloch, C. E. (1924b). *Am. J. Dis. Child.* **28,** 659.

Blood, F. R. & Rudolph, G. G. (1966). In *Toxicants Occurring Naturally in Foods,* p. 62. Washington, D.C.: National Academy of Sciences/National Research Council.

Bloom, A., Hayes, T. M. & Gamble, D. R. (1975). *Br. med. J.* **3,** 580.

Bloom, S. R., Adrian, T. E., Mitchell, S. J., Barnes, A. J. & Polak, J. M. (1976). *Gut* **17,** 817.

Bloom, S. R. & Polak, J. M. (1978). *Proc. Nutr. Soc.* **37,** 259.

Bloom, W. L. (1959). *Metabolism,* **8,** 214.

Boass, A., Toverud, S. U., McCain, T. A., Pike, J. W. & Haussler, M. R. (1977). *Nature, Lond.* **267,** 630.

Böddeker, H. & Mishkin, A. R. (1963). *Analyt. Chem.* **35,** 1662.

Bombard, A. (1953). *The Bombard Story.* London: André Deutsch.

Bondy, P. K. & Rosenberg, L. E. (1974). *Duncan's Diseases of Metabolism,* 7th edn. Philadelphia: Saunders.

Bonnet, R. and 5 others (1955). *Nature, Lond.* **176,** 328.

Booth, C. C. (1970). *Br. med. J.* **3,** 725 and **4,** 15.

Boston Collaborative Drug Surveillance Program (1972). *Lancet* **2,** 1278.

Bothwell, T. H. & Bradlow, B. A. (1960). *Archs Path.* **70,** 279.

Bothwell, T. H., Bradlow, B. A., Jacobs, P., Keeley, K. J., Kramer, S., Seftel, H. C. & Zail, S. (1964). *Br. J. Haematol.* **10,** 50.

Böttcher, C. J. F., Boelsma-van Houte, E., ter Haar, Romeny-Wachter, C. Ch., Woodford, F. P. & van Gent, C. M. (1960). *Lancet* **2,** 1162.

Bowman, F. (1973). *J. Am. diet. Ass.* **62,** 180.

Bozian, R. C., Ferguson, J. L., Heyssel, R. M., Meneely, G. R. & Darby, W. J. (1963). *Am. J. clin. Nutr.* **12,** 117.

Bradfield, R. B. (1972). *Am. J. clin. Nutr.* **25,** 720.

Bradfield, R. B. (1974). *J. Pediat.* **84,** 294.

Bradfield, R. B. & Jelliffe, D. B. (1974). *Lancet* **1,** 461.

Bradfield, R. B. & Jourdan, M. H. (1973). *Lancet* **2,** 640.

Branch, W. J., Southgate, D.A.T. & James, W. P. T. (1975). *Proc. Nutr. Soc.* **34,** 120A.

Bras, G. & Hill, K. R. (1956). *Lancet* **2,** 161.

Bray, G. A. (ed.) (1975). *Obesity in Perspective,* vol. 2, part 1, p. 72. Washington D.C.: DHEW Publication.

Brenton, D. P. & Cusworth, D. C. (1971). In *Inherited Disorders of Sulphur Metabolism,* ed. Carson, N. A. & Raine, D. N., p. 264. Edinburgh: Livingstone.

Breslow, N. & Enstrom, J. E. (1974). *J. nat. Cancer Inst.* **53,** 631.

Bridgforth, E. B. (1962). *Am. J. clin. Nutr.* **11,** 433.

Briggs, G. M., Bender, A. E., Engel, R. W., den Hartog, C., Olson, J. A., Oyenuga, V. A. Tashev, T. & Tejada, C. (1974). *Voeding* **35,** 376.

Briggs, M. H. (1974). *Lancet* **1,** 220.

Briggs, M. H., Garcia-Webb, P. & Davies, P. (1973). *Lancet* **2,** 201.

Brin, M. (1962). *Ann. N.Y. Acad. Sci.* **98,** 528.

Brink, A. J., Lewis, C. M. & Weber, H. W. (1965). *S. Afr. med. J.* **39,** 108.

Brinton, D. (1946). *Proc. R. Soc. Med.* **39,** 173.

Bristowe, W. S. (1953). *Proc. Nutr. Soc.* **12,** 44.

British Dental Association (1969). *Fluoridation of Water Supplies: Questions and Answers.* London.

British Medical Association (1950). *Report of the Committee on Nutrition.* London: B.M.A.

British Medical Journal (1969). Editorial, **3,** 729.

British Medical Journal (1970). Editorial, **1,** 188.

British Medical Journal (1972). Editorial, **4,** 746.

British Medical Journal (1978). Editorial, **1,** 198.

British Nutrition Foundation (1977). *Why Additives?* London: Forbes.

British Paediatric Association (1964). *Br. med. J.* **1,** 1661.

British Perinatal Survey (1969). *Perinatal Problems.* Edinburgh: Livingstone.

Britt, R. P., Harper, C. & Spray, G. H. (1971). *Q. Jl Med.* **40,** 499.

Brobeck, J. R. (1957). *Yale J. Biol. Med.* **29,** 565.

Brock, J. F. (1964). In *Proceedings of the Sixth International Congress of Nutrition,* ed. Mills, C. F. & Passmore, R., p. 115. Edinburgh: Livingstone.

Brock, J. F. (1972a). *Lancet* **1,** 701.

Brock, J. F. (1972b). *S. Afr. med. J.* **46**, 1109.

Brock, J. F. & Autret, M. (1952). *Kwashiorkor in Africa.* WHO Monograph Series no. 8. Geneva: WHO.

Bronte-Stewart, B. (1953). *Q. Jl Med.* **22**, 309.

Bronte-Stewart, B. (1958). *Br. med. Bull.* **14**, 243.

Bronte-Stewart, B., Antonis, A., Eales, L. & Brock, J. F. (1956). *Lancet* **1**, 521.

Bronte-Stewart, B., Botha, M. C. & Krut, L. H. (1962). *Br. med. J.* **1**, 1646.

Brook, C. G. D. (1972). *Lancet* **2**, 624.

Brooke, O. G. & Ashworth, A. (1972). *Br. J. Nutr.* **27**, 407.

Brown, J. & 18 others (1970). *World Review of Nutrition and Dietetics* **12**, 34.

Brown, R. G. (1973). *J. Am. med. Ass.* **224**, 1529.

Brown, S. S., Forrest, J. A. H. & Roscoe, P. (1972). *Lancet* **2**, 898.

Brown, W. R., Hansen, A. E., Burr, G. O. & McQuarrie, I. (1938). *J. Nutr.* **16**, 511.

Brozek, J., Grande, F., Taylor, H. L., Anderson, E. R., Buskirk, E. R. & Keys, A. (1957). *J. appl. Physiol.* **10**, 412.

Bruch, H. (1974). *Eating Disorders, Obesity, Anorexia Nervosa and the Person Within.* London: Routledge & Kegan Paul.

Bruch, H. (1978). *The Golden Cage, the Enigma of Anorexia Nervosa.* London: Open Books.

Brunette, M. G., Delvin, E., Hazel, B. & Scriver, C. R. (1972). *Pediatrics* **50**, 702.

Brunzell, J. D., Lerner, R. L., Hazzard, W. R., Porte, D. & Bierman, E. L. (1971). *New Engl. J. Med.* **284**, 521.

Brusis, O. A. & McGandy, R. B. (1971). *Fedn Proc. Fedn Am. Socs exp. Biol.* **30**, 1417.

Buchanan, N. & van der Walt, L. A. (1977). *Br. J. Anat.* **49**, 247.

Buchanan, N., van der Walt, L. A. & Strickwold, B. (1976). *J. Pharmaceut. Sci.* **65**, 915.

Bullen, J. J., Rogers, H. J. & Leigh, L. (1972). *Br. med. J.* **1**, 69.

Bunnell, R. H., Keating, J., Quaresimo, A. & Parman, G. K. (1965). *Am. J. clin. Nutr.* **17**, 1.

Burch, G. E. (1972). *Am. Heart J.* **83**, 285.

Burger, J. C. E., Drummond, J. C. & Sandstead, H. R. (1948). *Malnutrition and Starvation in Western Netherlands, September 1944 to July 1945.* The Hague: General State Printing Office.

Burkitt, D. P. (1969). *Lancet* **2**, 1229.

Burkitt, D. P. (1971a). *Cancer* **28**, 2.

Burkitt, D. P. (1971b). *Br. J. Surg.* **58**, 695.

Burkitt, D. P. (1972). *Br. med. J.* **2**, 556.

Burkitt, D. P. (1973). *Br. med. J.* **1**, 274.

Burkitt, D. P. & Trowell, H. C. (1975). *Refined Carbohydrate Foods and Disease. Some Implications of Dietary Fibre.* London: Academic Press.

Burnett, W. & 5 others (1976). *Lancet* **1**, 1084.

Burr, G. O. & Burr, M. M. (1929). *J. biol. Chem* **82**, 345.

Burr, M. L., Sweetnam, P. M., Hurley, R. J. & Powell, G. H. (1974). *Lancet* **1**, 163.

Butson, A. R. C. (1950). *Lancet* **1**, 993.

Butterfield, W. J. H. & Whichelow, M. J. (1968). *Lancet* **2**, 785.

Butterworth, C. E., Jr, Baugh, C. M. & Krumdieck, C. (1969). *J. clin. Invest.* **48**, 1131.

Buttery, P. J. & Annison, E. F. (1973). In *The Biological Efficiency of Protein Production,* ed. Jones, J. G. W., p. 141. Cambridge Univ. Press.

Buttfield, I. H., Black, M. L., Hoffman, M. J., Mason, E. K. & Hetzel, B. S. (1965). *Lancet* **2**, 767.

Cabanac, M. (1971). *Science, N.Y.* **173**, 1103.

Cahill, G. F., Jr (1970). *New Engl. J. Med.* **282**, 668.

Cahill, G. F. (1975). In *Obesity in Perspective,* ed. Bray, G. A. DHEW Publ. no. (NIH) 75-708, p. 58. Washington D.C.: Superintendent of Documents.

Cahill G. F. (1976). *Clinics Endocr. Metab.* **5**, 397.

Caird, F. I. (1971). *Acta diabetologica Latina,* **8** (suppl. 1), 394.

Caldwell, M. D., Jousson, H. T. & Othersen, H. B. (1972). *J. Pediat.* **81**, 894.

Callender, S. T., Marney, S. R. Jr & Warner, G. T. (1970). *Br. J. Haematol.* **19**, 657.

Callender, S. T. & Warner, G. T. (1968). *J. clin. Nutr.* **21**, 1170.

Calloway, D. H. & Margen, S. (1971). *J. Nutr.* **101**, 205.

Cameron, D. P. (1966). *Pfizer Medical Monographs I: Diabetes, Mellitus,* ed. Duncan, L. J. P., p. 145. Edinburgh Univ. Press.

Cameron, M. & Hofvander, Y. (1976). *Manual on Feeding Infants and Young Children,* 2nd edn. Protein-Calorie Advisory Group of the United Nations System.

Campbell, G. D. (1963). *S. Afr. med. J.* **37**, 1195.

Campbell, T. C. & Stoloff, L. (1974). *J. agric. Fd Chem.* **22**, 1007.

Carlisle, E. M. (1973). *Fedn Proc. Fedn Am. Socs exp. Biol.* **32**, 930.

Carlisle, E. M. (1976). In *Nutrition Reviews' Present Knowledge in Nutrition,* p. 337. New York: Nutrition Foundation.

Carlson, L. A. (ed.) (1972). *Nutrition in Old Age.* Symposia of the Swedish Nutrition X. Uppsala: Almqvist & Wicksell.

Carlson, L. A., Boberg, J. & Hogstedt, B. (1965). In *Adipose Tissue,* ed. Renold, A. E. & Cahill, G. F. p. 625, Washington: American Physiological Society.

Carlson, L. A. & Böttiger, L. E. (1972). *Lancet* **1**, 865.

Carlson, L. A. & Lindstedt, S. (1968). *Acta med. scand.* suppl. 493.

Carlson, L. A., Olsson, A. G., Orö, L. & Rossner, S. (1971). *Atherosclerosis* **14**, 391.

Carmel, R. & Herbert, V. (1969). *Blood* **33**, 1.

Carroll, K. K. & Hamilton, R. M. G. (1975). *J. Fd Sci.* **40**, 18.

Castelli, W. P. & 7 others (1977). *Lancet* **2**, 153.

Castle, W. B. (1929). *Am. J. med. Sci.* **178**, 748.

Castle, W. B. (1955). *New Engl. J. Med.* **249**, 603.

Catto, G. R. D., MacLeod, M., Pelc, B. & Kodicek, E. (1975). *Br. med. J.* **1**, 12.

Caughey, J. E. (1973). *N.Z. med. J.* **77**, 98.

Cavell, P. A. & Widdowson, E. M. (1964). *Archs Dis. Childh.* **39**, 496.

Chait, A., Mancini, M., February, A. & Lewis, B. (1972). *Lancet* **2**, 62.

Chalmers, J., Conacher, W. D. H., Gardner, D. L. & Scott, P. J. (1967). *J. Bone Jt Surg.* **49B**, 403.

Chan, H. (1968). *Br. J. Nutr.* **22**, 315.

Chan, P.-C. & Cohen, L. A. (1975). *Cancer Res.* **35**, 3384.

Chanarin, I. & Perry, J. (1969). *Lancet* **2**, 776.

Chanarin, I. & Perry, J. (1977). In *Folic Acid. Proceedings of a Workshop on Human Folate Requirements* (June 1975), p. 156. Washington D.C.: National Academy of Sciences.

Chandra, H., Venkatachalam, P. S., Belavadi, B., Reddy, V. & Gopalan, C. (1960). *Indian J. Child Hlth* **9**, 589.

Chandra, R. K. (1970). *Lancet* **1**, 537.

Chapman, J. A. Grant, I. S., Taylor, G., Mahmud, K., Sardur-ul-Mulk & Shahid, M. A. (1972). *Phil. Trans. R. Soc.* B **263**, 459.

Chatterjee, K. K. & Mukherjee, K. L. (1968). *Br. J. Nutr.* **22**, 145.

Chaudhuri, R. N., Chhetri, M. K., Saha, T. K. & Mitra, P. P. (1963). *J. Indian med. Ass.* **41**, 169.

Chaves-Carballo, E., Ellefson, R. D. & Gomez, M. R. (1976). *Mayo Clin. Proc.* **51**, 48.

Chesney, A. M., Clawson, T. A. & Webster, B. (1928). *Bull. Johns Hopkins Hosp.* **43**, 261.

Chick, H. (1942). *Lancet* **1**, 405.

Chick, H. (1951). *Nutr. Abstr. Rev.* **20**, 523.

Chick, H. (1976). *Med. Hist.* **20**, 41.

Chick, H. & 5 others (1923). *Spec. Rep. Ser. med. Res. Coun. Lond.* No. **77**.

Chick, H., Macrae, T. F., Martin, A. J. P. & Martin, C. J. (1938). *Biochem. J.* **32**, 12.

Chittenden, R. H. (1909). *The Nutrition of Man.* London: Heinemann.

Chong, Y. H. & Ho, G. S. (1970). *Am. J. clin. Nutr.* **23**, 260.

Chowdury, S. R., Rapagopal, K. & Chakrabarty, A. N. (1954). *Indian med. Gaz.* **89**, 283.

Christakis, G., Frankle, R., Brown, R. E., Jeffers, R., Walter, J. & Deutschele, K. (1972). *Am. J. clin. Nutr.* **25**, 997.

Christensen, E. H. (1953). In *Ergonomics Society Symposium on Fatigue,* ed. Floyd, W. F. & Welford, A. T. p. 93, London: Lewis.

Christensen, E. H. & Hansen, O. (1939). *Acta physiol. scand.* **81**, 157.

Chu, J. Y., Margen, S. & Costa, F. M. (1975). *Am. J. clin. Nutr.* **28**, 1028.

CIMMYT – Purdue (1975). *Symposium: High Quality Maize.* Stroudsberg, Pa: Dowden, Hutchinson & Ross.

Clark, H. E., Allen, P. E., Meyers, S. M., Tuckett, S. E. & Yamamura, Y. (1967). *Am. J. clin. Nutr.* **20**, 825.

Clark, H. E., Howe, J. M. & Lee, C. J. (1971). *Am. J. clin. Nutr.* **24**, 324.

Clark, R. B. (1968). *Lancet* **2**, 770.

Clarke, C. A. & Sircus, W. (1952). *Lancet* **2**, 113.

Clarkson, E. M. & 8 others (1972). *Clin. Sci* **43**, 519.

Clements, F. W., Gibson, H. B. & Howeler-Coy, J. F. (1970). *Lancet* **1**, 489.

Clements, F. W. & Wishart, J. W. (1956). *Metabolism* **5**, 623.

Coelingh Bennink, H. J. L. & Schreurs, W. H. P. (1975). *Br. med. J.* **3**, 13.

Cohen, A. M., Bavley, S. & Poznanski, R. (1961). *Lancet* **2**, 1939.

Cohen, H. (1957). *Report of the Joint Sub-Committee on Welfare Foods.* London: HMSO.

Collins, E. J. T. (1976). In *History of Breakfast Cereals,* ed. Oddy, D. & Miller, D., p. 26. London: Croom Helm; Totowa, N.J.: Rowman & Littlefield.

Collins, F. D., Sinclair, A. J., Royle, J. P., Coats, D. A., Maynard, A. T. & Leonard, R. J. (1971). *Nutr. Metab.* **13**, 150.

Colvin, B. T. & Lloyd, M. J. (1977). *J. clin. Path.* **30**, 1147.

Combes, M. A., Pratt, E. L. & Wiese, H. F. (1962). *Pediatrics,* **30**, 136.

Committee on Food Protection, Food and Nutrition Board, National Research Council (1973). *Toxicants Occurring Naturally in Foods,* 2nd edn. Washington, D. C.: National Academy of Sciences.

Committee on International Dietary Allowances of the International Union of Nutritional Sciences (1975). *Nutr. Abstr. Revs* **45**, 89.

Committee on Nutrition, American Academy of Pediatrics (1974). *Pediatrics* **53**, 115.

Connor, W. E. (1970). In *Atherosclerosis, Proceedings of the 2nd International Symposium,* ed. Jones, R. J., p. 253. Berlin: Springer-Verlag.

Consolazio, C. F., Johnson, R. E. & Pecora, E. (1963). *Physiological Measurements of Metabolic Functions in Man.* New York: McGraw-Hill.

Consolazio, C. F., Matoush, L. O., Nelson, R. A., Hackler, L. R. & Preston, E. E. (1962). *J. Nutr.* **78**, 78.

Cook, G. C. (1973). In *Intestinal Enzyme Deficiencies*, ed. Borgström, B., Dahlquist, A. & Hambreus, L. Uppsala: Almqvist & Wiksell.

Cook, G. C. (1974). *Trans. R. Soc. trop. Med. Hyg.* **68**, 419.

Cook, G. C. (1977). *Annual Report of the London School of Hygiene and Tropical Medicine 1976-7*, p. 65.

Cook, G. C. & Hutt, M. S. R. (1967). *Br. med. J.* **2**, 454.

Cook, G. C. & Lee, F. D. (1966). *Lancet* **2**, 1263.

Cook, J. (1777). *A Voyage towards the South Pole and round the World*, vol. 2, p. 112. London: Printed for W. Strahan and T. Cadell.

Cook, P. (1971). *Br. J. Cancer*, **25**, 853.

Corry Mann, H. C. (1926). *Spec. Rep. Ser. med. Res. Coun. Lond.* No. **106**.

Coulehan, J. L., Reisinger, K. S., Rogers, K. D. & Bradley, D. W. (1974). *New Engl. J. Med.* **290**, 6.

Country Doctor (1960). *Facing Retirement*. London: Allen & Unwin.

Coursin, D. B. (1954). *J. Am. med Ass.* **154**, 406.

Coursin, D. B. (1964). *Vitams Horm.* **22**, 755.

Cowan, D. W., Diehl, H. S. & Baker, A. B. (1942). *J. Am. med. Ass.* **120**, 1267.

Coward, W. A., Whitehead, R. G. & Lunn, P. G. (1977). *Br. J. Nutr.* **38**, 115.

Craddock, D. (1975). In *Recent Advances in Obesity Research: Proceedings of the First International Congress on Obesity*, ed. Howard, A., p. 220. London: Newman.

Craig, I. H., Bell, F. P., Goldsmith, C. H. & Schwartz, C. J. (1973). *Atherosclerosis* **18**, 277.

Cramp, D. G., Moorhead, J. F. & Willis, M. R. (1975). *Lancet* **1**, 672.

Crandon, J. H., Lund, C. C. & Dill, D. B. (1940). *New Engl. J. Med.* **223**, 353.

Crandon, J. H., Mikal, S. & Landau, B. R. (1953). *Proc. Nutr. Soc.* **12**, 273.

Crawford, M. A. (1962). *Lancet* **1**, 352.

Crawford, M. A. (1968). *Lancet* **1**, 1329.

Crawford, M. A., Gale, M. M., Somers, K. & Hansen, I. L. (1970). *Br. J. Nutr.* **24**, 393.

Crawford, M. D., Gardner, M. J. & Morris, J. N. (1968). *Lancet* **1**, 827.

Crawford, M. D., Gardner, M. J. & Morris, J. N. (1971). *Lancet* **2**, 327.

Crawhall, J. C., Scowen, E. F. & Watts, R. W. E. (1959). *Lancet* **2**, 806.

Crisp, A. H. (1977a). *Proc. R. Soc. Med.* **70**, 464.

Crisp, A. H. (1977b). *Proc. R. Soc. Med.* **70**, 686.

Critchley, M. (1943). *The Shipwreck Survivor—A Medical Study*. London: Churchill.

Cruickshank, E. K. (1952). *Vitams Horm.* **10**, 1.

Cruickshank, E. K. (1962). *Mod. Trends Neurol.* **3**, 200.

Cruickshank, E. W. H., Duckworth, J., Kosterlitz, H. W. & Warnock, G. M. (1945). *J. Physiol.* **104**, 41.

Cummings, J. H. (1973). *Gut* **14**, 69.

Cummings, J. H., Southgate, D. A. T., Branch, W., Houston, H., Jenkins, D. J. A. & James, W. P. T. (1978). *Lancet* **1**, 5.

Cuthbertson, D. P. (1930). *Biochem. J.* **24**, 1245.

Cuthbertson, D. P. (1971). *Proc. Nutr. Soc.* **30**, 150.

Dahl, L. K. (1972). *Am. J. clin. Nutr.* **25**, 231.

Dahlquist, A. B. & Asp, N.-G. (1975). *Biochem. Soc. Trans.* **3**, 227.

Dakin, H. D. (1913). *J. biol. Chem.* **14**, 321.

Dalderup, L. M. & van Haard, W. B. (1971). *Voeding* **32**, 439.

Dalyell, E. J. & Chick, H. (1921). *Lancet* **2**, 842.

Dam, H. (1935). *Biochem. J.* **29**, 1273.

Dam, H. (1971). *Am. J. Med.* **51**, 596.

Dam, H. & Schönheyder, F. (1934). *Biochem. J.* **28**, 1355.

Danks, D. M., Stevens, B. J., Campbell, P. E., Gillespie, J. M., Walker-Smith, J., Blomfield, J. & Turner, B. (1972). *Lancet* **1**, 1100.

Darby, W. J., Ghalioungui, P. & Grivetti, L. (1976). *Food: The Gift of Osiris*. New York: Academic Press.

Darby, W. J. & 5 others (1960). *Publ. Hlth Rep., Wash.* **75**, 738.

Darke, S. J. (1960). *Br. J. Nutr.* **14**, 115.

Darke, S. J. & Stephen, J. M. L. (1976). *Vitamin D Deficiency and Osteomalacia*. London: HMSO.

Davidson, J. D., Waldmann, T. A., Goodman, D. S. & Gordon, R. S. (1961). *Lancet* **1**, 899.

Davidson, L. S. P. & Fullerton, H. W. (1938). *Edinb. med. J.* **45**, 1.

Davidson, L. S. P., Fullerton, H. W. & Campbell, R. M. (1935). *Br. med. J.* **2**, 193.

Davidson, L. S. P. & Girdwood, R. H. (1947). *Br. med. J.* **1**, 587.

Davidson, L. S. P. & Gulland, G. L. (1930). *Pernicious Anaemia*. London: Kimpton.

Davies, D. F., Johnson, A. P., Rees, B. W. G., Elwood, P. C. & Abernethy, M. (1974). *Lancet* **1**, 1012.

Davies, J. N. P. (1964). *Lancet* **2**, 195.

Davies, L., Hastrop, K. & Bender, A. E. (1973). *Mod. Geriatr.* **3**, 390.

Davies, L., Hastrop, K. & Bender, A. E. (1974). *Mod. Geriatr.* **4**, 220.

Davis, A. E. & Badenoch, J. (1962). *Lancet* **2**, 6.

Davis, R. H., Morgan, D. B. & Rivlin, R. S. (1970). *Clin. Sci.* **39**, 1.

Dawber, T. R., Moore, F. E. & Mann, G. V. (1957). *Am. J. publ. Hlth* **47** (April suppl.), 4.

Day, S. (1974). *Nutrition, Lond.* **28**, 289.

Day, S. & Buckell, M. (1971). *Proc. Nutr. Soc.* **30**, 184.

Dayton, S. (1971). *Fedn Proc. Fedn Am. Socs exp. Biol.* **30**, 850.

Dayton, S., Pearce, M. L., Hashimoto, S., Dixon, W. J. & Tomiyasu, U. (1969). *American Heart Association Monograph.* no. 25.

de Lange, D. J. & Joubert, P. (1964). *Am. J. clin. Nutr.* **15**, 169.

Delange, F., Hershman, J. M. & Ermans, A. M. (1971). *J. clin. Endocr.* **33**, 261.

Delange, F., Thilly, C., Pourbaix, P. & Ermans, A. M. (1969). In *Endemic Goitre,* ed. Stanbury, J. B., p. 118. Pan American Health Organisation Scientific Publication no. 193. Washington, D.C.

DeLuca, H. F. (1976). *Ann. intern. Med.* **85**, 367.

DeLuca, L., Schumacher, M. & Nelson, D. P. (1971). *J. biol. Chem.* **246**, 5762.

DeLuca, L., Maestri, M., Rosso, G. & Wolf, G. (1973). *J. biol. Chem.* **248**, 641.

Demakis, J. E. & 7 others (1974). *Ann. intern. Med.* **80**, 293.

Denny-Brown, D. (1947). *Medicine* **26**, 41.

Denson, K. W. & Bowers, E. F. (1961). *Clin. Sci.* **21**, 157.

Dent, C. E. (1969). *Proc. R. Soc. Med.* **63**, 401.

Dent, C. E. & Gupta, M. M. (1975). *Lancet* **2**, 1057.

Dent, C. E. & Sutor, D. J. (1971). *Lancet* **2**, 775.

Deo, M. G., Dayal, Y. & Ramalingaswami, V. (1970). *J. Path. Bact.* **101**, 47.

Deosthale, Y. G. & Gopalan, C. (1974). *Br. J. Nutr.* **31**, 351.

Department of Education and Science Welsh Office (1975). *Nutrition in Schools.* Report of the Working Party on the Nutritional Aspects of School Meals. London: HMSO.

Department of Experimental Medicine, Cambridge (1951). *Spec. Rep. Ser. med. Res. Coun. Lond.* no. 275.

Department of Health and Social Security (1969a). *Rep. publ. Hlth med. Subj. Lond.* no. 120.

Department of Health and Social Security (1969b). *Rep. publ. Hlth med. Subj. Lond.* no. 122.

Department of Health and Social Security (1970). *Rep. publ. Hlth med. Subj. Lond.* no. 123.

Department of Health and Social Security (1972). *Rep. Hlth soc. Subj.* no. 3.

Department of Health and Social Security (1973). *Rep. Hlth soc. Subj.* no. 6.

Department of Health and Social Security (1974a). *Rep. Hlth soc. Subj.* no. 7.

Department of Health and Social Security (1974b). *Rep. Hlth soc. Subj.* no. 9.

Department of Health and Social Security (1977). *The Composition of Mature Human Milk.* Report on Health and Health Subjects no. 12.

Department of Health and Social Security (1977). DHSS Subjects no. 17.

Department of Health and Social Security (1978). *Breast Feeding.* London: DHSS.

Deutsche Gesellschaft für Ernährung (1975). *Empfehlungen für die Nahrstoffzufuhr.* Frankfurt: Umschau.

De Wardener, H. E. & Lennox, B. (1947). *Lancet* **1**, 11.

De Wolfe, M. S. & Whyte, H. M. (1958). *Aust. Ann. Med.* **7**, 47.

De Wys, W. (1970). *Cancer Res.* **30**, 2816.

Dicke, W. K. (1950). *Thesis.* University of Utrecht.

Dickens, C. (1867). *Little Dorrit,* chap. 31. London: Chapman & Hall.

Dickinson, L. E., MacMahon, B., Cole, P. & Brown, J. B. (1974). *New Engl. J. Med.* **291**, 1211.

Dietitians Board (1975). *Dietitians of the Future.* A Report by a Working Party. London: Council for Professions Supplementary to Medicine.

Dietschy, J. M. & Wilson, J. D. (1970). *New Engl. J. Med.* **282**, 1128, 1179, 1241.

Dister, P. *et al.* (1975). *Gut* **16**, 193.

Dobbing, J. & Sands, J. (1973). *Archs Dis. Childh.* **48**, 757.

Dole, V. P. (1958). In *Chemistry of Lipids in Relation to Atherosclerosis,* ed. Page, I, p. 189. Springfield, Thomas.

Dole, V. P. (1965). In *Handbook of Physiology,* section 5. *Adipose Tissue,* ed. Renold, A. E. & Cahill, G. F., p. 13. Wastington, D. C.: American Physiological Society.

Doll, R. (1972). *Proc. R. Soc. Med.* **65**, 49.

Doll, R. (1973). *Proc. R. Soc. Med.* **66**, 307.

Doll, R. & Hill, A. B. (1964). *Br. med. J.* **1**, 1399.

Doll, R., Hill, I. D. & Hutton, C. F. (1965). *Gut* **6**, 19.

Dong, F. M. & Oace, S. M. (1973). *J. Am. diet. Ass.* **62**, 162.

Donnell, G. N. & Lieberman, E. (1970). In *Current Pediatric Therapy,* no. 4, ed. Gellis, S. S. & Kagen, B. M. Philadelphia: Saunders.

Donovan, D. (1848). *Dublin med. Press* **19**, 67.

Dorris, R. J. & Stunkard, A. J. (1957). *Am. J. med. Sci.* **233**, 622.

Dow, D. J. & Steven, D. M. (1941). *J. Physiol., Lond.* **100**, 256.

Dowler, E. A. (1977). *J. hum. Nutr.* **31**, 171.

Drug and Therapeutics Bulletin (1974). **12**, 73.

Drug and Therapeutics Bulletin (1975). **13**, 64.

Drummond, J. C. (1939). *Chemy Ind.* **57**, 808, 827, 914.

Drummond, J. C. & Wilbraham, A. (1939). *The Englishman's Food.* Revised Hollingsworth, D. (1958). London: Cape.

Drury, A. N. & Jones, N. W. (1927). *Heart* **14**, 55.

Du Bois, E. F. (1948). *Fever and the Regulation of Body Temperature.* Springfield: Thomas.

Dugdale, A. E. (1971a). *Am. J. clin. Nutr.* **24**, 174.

Dugdale, A. E. (1971b). *Br. J. Nutr.* **26**, 423.

Duguid, J. B. (1954). *Lancet* **1**, 891.

Dumont, J. E., Delange, F. & Ernans, A. M. (1969). In *Endemic Goitre*, ed. Stanbury, J. B., p. 91. Pan American Health Organisation Scientific Publication No. 193. Washington, D.C.

Duncan, W. R. H., Ørskov, E. R. & Garton, G. A. (1974). *Proc. Nutr. Soc.* **33**, 81A.

Dunlap, W. M., James, G. W. & Hume, D. M. (1974). *Ann. intern. Med.* **80**, 470.

Dunnigan, M. G., Fyfe, T., McKiddie, M. T. & Crosbie, S. M. (1970). *Cli. Sci.* **38**, 1.

Durnin, J. V. G. A. (1961a). *J. Physiol.* **156**, 294–306.

Durnin, J. V. G. A. (1961b). *Geront. clin. (Basel)* **4**, 128.

Durnin, J. V. G. A. (1970). In *Proc. 8th Int. Congr. Nutr. Excerpta med. int. Congr. Ser.* No. 213, p. 321.

Durnin, J. V. G. A., Blake, E. C., Brockway, J. M. & Drury, E. A. (1961). *Br. J. Nutr.* **15**, 499.

Durnin, J. V. G. A. & Passmore, R. (1967). *Energy, Work and Leisure.* London: Heinemann.

Durnin, J. V. G. A. & Womersley, J. (1974). *Br. J. Nutr.* **32**, 77.

Dziewiatskowski, D. D. (1962). In *Mineral Metabolism,* ed. Comar, C. L. & Bronner, F., vol. 2, part B., p. 175. New York: Academic Press.

Eastwood, M. A. & Mitchell, W. D. (1976). In *Fiber in Human Nutrition,* ed. Spiller, G. A. & Amen, R. J., p. 109. New York: Plenum Press.

Easty, D. L. (1970). *Br. J. Nutr.* **24**, 307.

Eddy, T. P., Stock, A. L. & Wheeler, E. F. (1971). *Br. J. ind. Med.* **28**, 342.

Ederer, F., Leren, P., Turpeinen, O. & Frantz, I. D. Jr (1971). *Lancet* **2**, 203.

Edwards, O. M.(1977). *Proc. R. Soc. Med.* **70**, 690.

Edwards, R. D. & Williams, T. D. (1956). *The Great Famine,* p. 274. Dublin: Brown & Nolan.

Eeg-Larsen, N. (1969). In *Nutrition in Preschool and School Age,* ed. Blix, G. Symposia of the Swedish Nutrition Foundation, VII, p. 131. Uppsala: Almqvist & Wiksell.

Eekhof-Stork, N. (1976). *The World Atlas of Cheese.* London: Paddington Press.

Egan, H. (1966). *Proc. Nutr. Soc.* **25**, 44.

Egan, H. & Weston, R. E. (1977). *Pesticide Sci.* **8**, 110.

Egge, H., Murawski, U., Ryhage, R., György, P., Chatranon, W. & Zilliken, F. (1972). *Chem. Phys. Lipids* **8**, 42.

Ehrlich, P. R. (1971). *The Population Bomb.* London: Pan Books.

Eijkman, C. (1897). *Virchows Arch. path. Anat. Physiol.* **149**, 187.

Eldjarn, L., Try, K., Stokke, O., Munthe-Kaas, A. W., Refsum, S., Steinberg, D., Avigan, J. & Mize, C. (1966). *Lancet* **1**, 691.

Eley, C., Goldsmith, R., Layman, D., Tan, G. L. E. & Walker, E. (1978). *Ergonomics* **21**, 153.

Elliott, W., Hall, M., Kerr, D. N. S., Rolland, C. S., Smart, G. A. & Swinney, J. (1961). *Lancet* **2**, 630.

Ellis, H. (1969). *A History of Bladder Stone.* Oxford: Blackwell.

Elvehjem, C. A., Madden, R. J., Strong, F. M. & Wooley, D. W. (1937). *J. Am. chem. Soc.* **59**, 1767.

Elwood, P. C. (1968). *Proc. Nutr. Soc.* **27**, 14.

Elwood, P. C., Mahler, R., Sweetnam, P., Moore, F. & Welsby, E. (1970). *Lancet* **1**, 589.

Elwood, P. C., Waters, W. G. & Sweetnam, P. (1971). *Clin. Sci.* **40**, 31.

Emerson, K., Saxena, B. N. & Poindexter, E. L. (1972). *Obstet. Gynec., N.Y.* **40**, 726.

Emerson, R. G. (1962). *Br. med. J.* **2**, 516.

English, R. M. & Hitchcock, N. E. (1968). *Br. J. Nutr.* **22**, 615.

Epstein, F. H. (1973). *Circulation* **48**, 185.

Ernest, I., Linner, E. & Svanborg, A. (1965). *Am. J. Med.* **39**, 594.

Estrich, D., Ravnik, A., Schierf, G., Fukayama, G. & Kinsell, L. (1967). *Diabetes* **16**, 232.

Evans, D. J. & Patey, A. L. (1974). *Clins Gastroenterol.* **3**, 199.

Evans, E. (1978). *Proc. Nutr. Soc.* **37**, 71.

Evans, H. M. & Bishop, K. S. (1923). *J. Am. med. Ass.* **81**, 889.

Exton-Smith, A. N., Hodkinson, H. M. & Stanton, B. R. (1966). *Lancet* **3**, 999.

Exton-Smith, A. N., Millard, P. H., Payne, P. R. & Wheeler, E. F. (1969). *Lancet* **2**, 1154.

Exton-Smith, A. N., Stanton, B. R., Newman, M. & Ramsey, M. (1965). *Report on an Investigation into the Dietary Habits of Elderly Women Living Alone.* London: King Edward's Hospital.

Eyberg, C., Moodley, G. P. & Buchanan, N. (1974). *S. Afr. med. J.* **48**, 2564.

Fabry, P. (1967). In *Handbook of Physiology. Section 6: Alimentary Canal,* vol. 1, p. 31. Washington: American Physiological Society.

Fabry, P., Fodor, J., Hejl, Z., Braun, T. & Zvolankova, K. (1964). *Lancet* **2**, 614.

Fabry, P., Petrasek, R., Horakova, E., Konopasek, E. & Brawn, T. (1963). *Br. J. Nutr.* **17**, 295.

Fain, J. N. (1973). *Pharmac. Rev.* **25**, 67.

Faires, J. S. & McCarty, D. J. (1962). *Lancet* **2**, 682.

Falaiye, J. M. (1971). *Br. med. J.* **4**, 454.

Farquhar, J. W. & Sokolow, M. (1958). *Circulation* **17**, 890.

Farquharson, J. & Adams, J. F. (1976). *Br. J. Nutr.* **36**, 127.

Farrell, P. M., Bieni, J. G., Fratantoni, J. F., Wood, R. E. & di Sant'Agnese, P. A. (1977). *J. clin. Invest.* **60**, 233.

Farrell, P. M., Levine, S. I. Murphy, M. D. & Adams, A. J. (1978). *Am. J. clin. Nutr.* **31,** 1720.

Feeley, R. M., Criner, P. E. & Watt, B. K. (1972). *J. Am. diet. Ass.* **61,** 134.

Felig, P. & Wahren, J. (1975). *New Engl. J. Med.* **293,** 1078.

Felig, P., Wahren, J., Sherwin, R. & Hendler, R. (1976). *Diabetes* **25,** 1091.

Fell, G. S., Fleck, A., Cuthbertson, D. P., Queen, K., Morrison, C., Bessent, R. G. & Husain, S. L. (1973). *Lancet* **1,** 280.

Fenelon, K. G. (1952). *Britain's Food Supplies.* London: Methuen.

Ferguson, J. (1975). *Learning to Eat: Leader Manual and Students Manual.* Palo Alto, Calif.: Bull Publ. Co.

Fierro-Benitez, R., Raminez, I., Garces, J., Jaramillo, C., Moncayo, F. & Stanbury, J. B. (1974). *Am. J. clin. Nutr.* **27,** 531.

Findlay, J. M., Smith, A. N., Mitchell, W. D., Anderson, A. J. B. & Eastwood, M. A. (1974). *Lancet* **1,** 146.

Fisher, R. B. (1954). *Protein Metabolism.* London: Methuen.

Fitzgerald, G., McCarthy, D. & O'Connell, L. G. (1976). *Br. med. J.* **1,** 1149.

Fitzgerald Moore, D. G. (1937). *W. Afr. med. J.* **9,** 35.

Fitzsimmons, J. T. (1972). *Physiol. Rev.* **52,** 468.

Flatz, G. & Rotthauwe, H. W. (1973). *Lancet* **2,** 76.

Fleisch, A. (1951). *Helv. med. Acta* **18,** 23.

Flendrig, Kruis, H. & Das, H. A. (1976). *Dialysis, Transplantation Nephrology,* vol. 13, pp. 355–361. London: Pitman.

Fletcher, A. P. (1959). *Q. Jl Med.* **23,** 331.

Fletcher, W. (1907). *Lancet* **1,** 1776.

Florey, C. Du V., McDonald, H., Miall, W. E. & Milner, R. D. G. (1973). *J. chron. Dis.* **26,** 85.

Florey, H. W. (1955). *Proc. R. Soc.* B **143,** 147.

Flynn, T. F., Beirn, S. F. O. & Burkitt, D. F. (1977). *Irish J. med. Sci.* **146,** 285.

Fohlin, H. (1977). *Acta paediat., Stockh.* suppl. 268.

Follis, R. H. (1958). *Deficiency Diseases.* Springfield: Thomas.

Fomon, S. J. (1971). *Bull. N.Y. Acad. Med.* **47,** 569.

Fomon, S. J. & Owen, G. M. (1964). In *Proceedings of the Sixth International Congress of Nutrition,* ed. Mills, C. F. & Passmore, R., p. 66. Edinburgh: Livingstone.

Fontana, V. J. & Strauss, M. B. (1973). In *Modern Nutrition in Health and Disease,* ed. Goodhart, R. S. & Shils, M. E., p. 924. Philadelphia: Lea & Febiger.

Food Additives and Contaminants Committee (1970). *Report on Emulsifiers and Stabilisers* London: HMSO.

Food Additives and Contaminants Committee (1970). *Report on Packaging.* London: HMSO.

Food Additives and Contaminants Committee (1972). *Report on Preservatives.* London: HMSO.

Food Additives and Contaminants Committee (1974). *Report on Solvents.* London: HMSO.

Food Additives and Contaminants Committee (1975). *Report on Antioxidants.* London: HMSO.

Food Additives and Contaminants Committee (1975). *Report on Lead.* London: HMSO.

Food Additives and Contaminants Committee (1976). *Report on Flavourings.* London: HMSO.

Food Additives and Contaminants Committee (1978). *Report on Additives and Processing Aids in Beer.* London: HMSO.

Food and Agriculture Organisation (1948). *FAO Nutr. Mtg Rep. Ser.* no. 2.

Food and Agriculture Organisation (1953). *School Feeding.* Nutritional Studies no. 10. Rome: FAO.

Food and Agriculture Organisation (1954a). *Rice and Rice Diets.* Nutritional Studies no. 1. Rome: FAO.

Food and Agriculture Organisation (1954b). *Rice Enrichment in the Philippines.* Nutritional Studies no. 12. Rome: FAO.

Food and Agriculture Organisation (1957a). *Calorie Requirements.* Nutritional Studies no. 15. Rome: FAO.

Food and Agriculture Organisation (1957b). *Protein Requirements.* Nutritional Studies no. 16. Rome: FAO.

Food and Agriculture Organisation (1962). *The State of Food and Agriculture, 1962.* Rome: FAO.

Food and Agriculture Organisation (1964). *Program of Food Consumption Surveys.* Rome: FAO.

Food and Agriculture Organisation (1965). *The State of Food and Agriculture, 1965.* Rome: FAO.

Food and Agriculture Organisation (1971a). *The State of Food and Agriculture, 1971.* Rome: FAO.

Food and Agriculture Organisation (1971b). *Food and Nutrition Education in the Primary School.* Nutritional Studies no. 25. Rome: FAO.

Food and Agriculture Organisation/World Health Organisation (1976). Food and Nutrition Strategies in National Development. *Tech. Rep. Ser. Wld Hlth Org.* no. 584.

Food and Agriculture Organisation/World Health Organisation (1977). *Wholesomeness of Irradiated Food.* Food and Nutrition no. 6. Rome: FAO.

Food and Agriculture Organisation (1977). Manila Communiqué of the World Food Council. *Fd Nutr.* **3,** 22.

Food and Agriculture Organisation (1977). *The State of Food and Agriculture, 1976.* Rome: FAO.

Food and Agriculture Organisation/World Health Organisation (1959). *Nutrition Seminar. Belgian Congo, 1959.* Rome: FAO.

Food and Agriculture Organisation/World Health Organisation (1962). *Tech. Rep. Ser. Wld Hlth Org.* no. 230; *FAO Nutr. Mtg Rep. Ser.* no. 30.

Food and Agriculture Organisation/World Health Organisation (1965). *FAO Nutr. Meetings Rep. Ser.* no. 37.

Food and Agriculture Organisation/World Health Organisation (1966). *Tech. Rep. Ser. Wld Hlth Org.* no. 340; *FAO Nutr. Mtg Rep. Ser.* no. 39.

Food and Agriculture Organisation/World Health Organisation (1967). *Tech. Rep. Ser. Wld Hlth Org.* no. 362.

Food and Agriculture Organisation/World Health Organisation (1968). *Amino Acid Content of Foods and Biological Data on Proteins.* Rome: FAO.

Food and Agriculture Organisation/World Health Organisation (1970a). *Tech. Rep. Ser. Wld Hlth Org.* no. 452.

Food and Agriculture Organisation/World Health Organisation (1970b). *FAO Nutr. Meetings. Rep. Ser.* no. 47.

Food and Agriculture Organisation/World Health Organisation (1973). *Tech. Rep. Ser. Wld Hlth Org.* no. 522.

Food and Agriculture Organisation/World Health Organisation Expert Committee on Nutrition (1971). *Tech. Rep. Ser. Wld Hlth Org.* no. 477.

Food and Agriculture Organisation/World Health Organisation Mission (1965). *Nutrition Education in Six Western European Countries.* Rome: FAO.

Food and Nutrition Board (1974). *Recommended Dietary Allowances.* National Research Council Publication no. 1694. Washington, D.C.: National Academy of Sciences.

Food Standards Committee (1964). *Report on Labelling.* London: HMSO.

Food Standards Committee (1966). *Report on Claims and Misleading Descriptions.* London: HMSO.

Food Standards Committee (1974a). *Report on Bread and Flour.* London: HMSO.

Food Standards Committee (1974b). *Report on Novel Proteins.* London, HMSO.

Food Standards Committee (1975). *Report on Yogurt.* London: HMSO.

Food Standards Committee (1976). *Report on Soft Drinks.* London: HMSO.

Food Standards Committee (1977). *Report on Beer.* London: HMSO.

Food Standards Committee. (1978). *Report on Water in Food.*

Ford, J. A., Colhoun, E. M., McIntosh, W. B. & Dunnigan, M. G. (1972). *Br. med. J.* **3**, 446.

Ford, J. A., Colhoun, E. M., McIntosh, W. B. & Dunnigan, M. G. (1972). *Br. med. J.* **3**, 677.

Forfar, J. O. & Tompsett, S. L. (1959). *Adv. clin. Chem.* **2**, 167.

Fosbrooke, A. S. & Wharton, B. A. (1975). *Archs Dis. Childh.* **50**, 409.

Fourman, P. & Royer, P. (1968). *Calcium Metabolism and the Bone.* Oxford: Blackwell.

Fox, F. W. (1970). *S. Afr. med. J.* **44**, 736.

Fox, W. (1962). *Lancet* **2**, 413, 473.

Foy, J. M. & Parratt, J. R. (1962). *Lancet* **1**, 942.

Francis, D. E. M. (1975). *Diets for Sick Children.* Oxford: Blackwell.

Fraser, D. R. & Kodicek, E. (1970). *Nature, Lond.* **228**, 764.

Fredrickson, D. S. & Levy, R. I. (1973). In *The Metabolic Basis of Inherited Disease,* 3rd edn, ed. Stanbury, J. B., Wyngaarden, J. B. & Fredrickson, D. S. New York: McGraw-Hill.

Fredrickson, D. S., Levy, R. I., Bonnell, M. & Ernst, N. (1973). *Dietary Management of Hyperlipoproteinemia. A Handbook for Physicians and Dietitians.* Department of Health, Education and Welfare Publication No. (NIH) 73-110, National Heart and Lung Institute, Bethesda, Md.

Fredrickson, D. S., Levy, R. I. & Lees, R. S. (1967). *New Engl. J. Med.* **276**, 34, 94, 148, 215, 273.

Freedman, B. J. (1977). *Clin. Allergy* **7**, 407.

Freinkel, N. & 7 others (1972). *Israel J. med. Sci.* **8**, 426.

Friedman, C. J., Sherry, S. K. & Ralli, E. P. (1940). *J. clin. Invest.* **19**, 685.

Friedman, G. D., Kannel, W. B. & Dawber, T. R. (1966). *J. chron. Dis.* **19**, 273.

Friedman, M. & Rosenman, R. H. (1969). *J. Am. med. Ass.* **169**, 1286.

Frimpton, G. W. (1966). In *The Metabolic Basis of Inherited Disease,* 2nd edn, ed. Stanbury, J. B., Wyngaarden, J. B. & Fredrickson, D. S., p. 409. New York: Blakiston.

Frisch, R. E. & McArthur, J. W. (1974). *Science, N.Y.* **185**, 949.

Fullerton, H. W. (1936). *Br. med. J.* **2**, 577.

Funk, C. (1913). *J. Physiol., Lond.* **46**, 173.

Gallery, E. D. M., Bloomfield, J. & Dixon, S. R. (1972). *Br. med. J.* **4**, 331.

Galton, J. D. & Wilson, J. P. D. (1970). *Br. med. J.* **2**, 444.

Gariboldi, F. (1974). *Rice Parboiling.* Rome: FAO.

Garn, S. M. (1963). *Ann. N.Y. Acad. Sci.* **110**, 429.

Garn, S. M. (1972). *Orthop. Clin. N. Am.* **3**, 503.

Garrod, Sir Archibald (1908). *Lancet* **2**, 1, 73, 142, 214.

Garrow, J. S. (1974). *Proc. Nutr. Soc.* **33**, 29$_\mathrm{A}$.

Garrow, J. S. (1978). *Energy Balance and Obesity in Man.,* 2nd edn. Amsterdam, London & New York: North Holland/American Elsevier.

Garrow, J. S., Fletcher, K. & Halliday, D. (1965). *J. clin. Invest.* **44**, 417.

Garrow, J. S. & Hawes, S. F. (1972). *Br. J. Nutr.* **27**, 211.

Garrow, J. S. & Pike, M. C. (1967). *Br. J. Nutr.* **21**, 155.

Garry, R. C., Passmore, R., Warnock, G. M. & Durnin, J. V. G. A. (1955). *Spec. Rep. Ser. med. Res. Coun. Lond.* No. **289**.

Gastineau, C. F. (1976). *Mayo Clin. Proc.* **51**, 88.

Gear, J. C. S., Ware, A. C., Nolan, D. J., Fursdon, P. S., Brodribb, A. J. M. & Mann, J. I. (1978). *Proc. Nutr. Soc.* **37**, 13A.

Gebre-Medhin, M., Vahlquist, A., Hofvander, Y., Uppsäll, L. & Vahlquist, B. (1976). *Am. J. clin. Nutr.* **29**, 441.

Geisler, H. E., Huber, C. P. & Rogers, S. (1969). *Am. J. Obstet. Gynaec.* **104**, 657.

Geissler, C., Calloway, D. H. & Margen, S. (1978). *Am. J. clin. Nutr.* **31**, 341.

Gelfand, M. (1967). *S. Afr. med. J.* **41**, 490.

Gell, P. H. G. (1951). *Spec. Rep. Ser. med. Res. Coun. Lond.* No. 275, p. 193.

Gelzayd, E. A., Breuer, R. I. & Kirsner, J. B. (1968). *Am. J. digest. Dis.* **13**, 1027.

Gemmil, J. S. & Manderson, W. G. (1960). *Lancet* **2**, 307.

George, S. (1976). *How the Other Half Dies.* London: Penguin Books.

Gey, K. F. & Carlson, L. A. (1971). *Metabolic Effects of Nicotinic Acid and its Derivatives,* Berne: Hans Huber.

Ghadimi, H., Abaci, F., Kumar, S. & Rathi, M. (1971). *Pediatrics* **48**, 955.

Ghafoorunissa, Rao, B. S. N. (1975). *Am. J. clin. Nutr.* **28**, 325.

Gilat, T., Russo, S., Gelman-Malachi, E. & Aldor, T. A. M. (1972). *Gastroenterology,* **62**, 1125.

Gilbert, R. J. & Roberts, D. (1977). *Proc. Nutr. Soc.* **36**, 97.

Gillanders, A. D. (1951). *Br. Heart J.* **13**, 177.

Gillies, H. M., Watson Williams, E. J. & Ball, P. A. J. (1964). *Q. Jl Med.* **33**, 1.

Ginsberg, H., Olefsky, J. & Farquhar, J. W. (1974). *Ann. intern. Med.* **80**, 143.

Giovannetti, S. & Maggiore, Q. (1964). *Lancet* **1**, 1000.

Girdwood, R. H., Thomson, A. D. & Williamson, J. (1967). *Br. med. J.* **2**, 670.

Glass, R. L. & Fleisch, S. (1974) *J. Am. dent. Ass.* **88**, 807.

Glass, R. L., Rothman, K. J. Espinal, F., Velaz, H. & Smith, N. J. (1973). *Archs oral Biol.* **18**, 1099.

Glazebrook, A. J. & Thomson, S. (1942). *J. Hyg., Camb.* **42**, 1.

Gleibermann, L. (1973). *Ecol. Fd Nutr.* **2**, 143.

Glomset, J. A., Norum, E. R., Nichols, A. V., Forte, T., King, W. C., Albers, J., Mitchell, C. D., Applegate, K. J. & Gjone, E. (1974). *Scand. J. Clin. Lab. Invest.* **33**, suppl. 137, 165.

Glorieux, F. H., Scriver, C. R., Reade, T. M., Goldman, H. & Rosenborough, A. (1972). *New Engl. J. Med.* **287**, 481.

Glueck, C. J., Levy, R. I. & Fredrickson, D. S. (1969). *Diabetes* **18**, 739.

Glueck, C. J., Tsang, R., Fallat, R., Buncher, C. R., Evans, G. & Steiner, P. (1973). *Metabolism* **22**, 1287.

Godden, W. & Thomson, W. (1939). *J. Soc. chem. Ind., Lond.* **58**, 81.

Godwin, H. A. & Rosenberg, I. H. (1975). *Gastroenterology,* **69**, 364.

Goel, K. M., Logan, R. W., Arneil, G. C., Sweet, E. M., Warren, J. M. & Shanks, R. A. (1976). *Lancet* **1**, 1141.

Goel, K. M., Logan, R. W., House, F., Connell, M. D., Stevens, E., Watson, W. H. & Bulloch, C. B. (1978). *Hlth Bull.* **36**, 176.

Goldberg, A. (1963). *Q. Jl Med.* **32**, 51.

Goldberger, J., Wheeler, G. A., Lillie, R. D. & Rogers, L. M. (1928). *Publ. Hlth Rep. Wash.* **43**, 1385.

Goldblatt, L. A. (ed.) (1969). *Aflatoxin.* New York: Academic Press.

Goodwin, T. W. (1954). *Caretenoids.* New York: Chemical Publishing Co.

Gopalan, C. (1946). *Indian med. Gaz.* **81**, 22.

Gopalan, C. (1962). *Bull. Wld Hlth Org.* **26**, 203.

Gopalan, C. (1969). *Lancet* **1**, 197.

Gordon, E. S. & Goldberg, M. (1964). *Metabolism,* **13**, 775.

Gordon, E. S., Goldberg, E. M., Brandabur, J. J., Gee, J. B. L. & Rankin, J. (1962). *Trans. Ass. Am. Physns* **75**, 118.

Gordon, J. E., Chitkara, I. D. & Wyon, I. B. (1963). *Am. J. med. Sci.* **245**, 129.

Gordon, T. & Kannel, W. B. (1973). *Geriatrics,* **28**, 80.

Gordon, T. & Thom, T. (1975). *Prevent. Med.* **4**, 115.

Graeber, J. E., Williams, M. L. & Oski, F. A. (1977). *J. Pediat.* **90**, 282.

Grafe, E. (1933). *Metabolic Diseases and Their Treatment.* Philadelphia: Lea & Febiger.

Grafe, E. & Graham, D. (1911). *Hoppe-Seylers Z. physiol. Chem.* **73**, 1.

Graham, G. G., Baertl, J. M., Claeyssen, G., Suskind, R., Greenberg, A. H., Thompson, R. G. & Blizzard, R. M. (1973). *J. Pediat.* **83**, 321.

Graham, G. G. & Cordano, A. (1969). *Johns Hopkins med. Jl* **124**, 139.

Grande, F. (1964). In *Adaptation to the Environment,* ed. Dell, D. B. Washington, D.C.: American Physiological Society.

Grande, F., Anderson, J. T. & Keys, A. (1965). *J. Nutr.* **86**, 313.

Grande, F., Anderson, J. T. & Keys, A. (1972). *Am. J. clin. Nutr.* **25**, 53.

Greaves, J. P. & Hollingsworth, D. F. (1966). *Wld Rev. Nutr. Diet.* **6**, 34.

Green, R. G., Carlson, W. E. & Evans, C. A. (1942). *J. Nutr.* **23**, 165.

Green, R., van Tonder, S. V., Oettle, G. J., Cole, G. & Metz, J. (1975). *Nature, Lond.* **254**, 148.

Greenhouse, A. H. (1971). *J. chron. Dis.* **23**, 823.

Greep, J. M., Soeters, P. B., Wesdorp, R. I. C., Phaf, C. W. R. & Fischer, J. E. (1977). *Current Concepts in Parenteral Nutrition.* The Hague: Martinus Nijhoff.

Greer, M. A. & Deeney, J. M. (1959). *J. clin. Invest.* **38**, 1465.

Grey, N. J., Karl, I. & Kipnis, D. M. (1975). *Diabetes* **24**, 10.

Grey, N. & Kipnis, D. M. (1971). *New Engl. J. Med.* **285**, 827.

Griffiths, L. L., Brocklehurst, J. C., Scott, D. L., Marks, J. & Blackley, J. (1967). *Geront. clin.* **9**, 1.

Gross, J. & Pitt-Rivers, R. (1952). *Lancet* **1**, 439.

Grundy, S. M., Duane, W. C., Adler, R. D., Aron, J. M. & Metzger, A. L. (1974). *Metabolism* **23**, 67.

Guggenheim, F. G. (1977). *Med. Clins N. Am.* **61**, 781.

Gull, W. W. (1874). *Trans. clin. Soc., Lond.* **7**, 22.

Gumaa, K, A., Mustafa, K. Y., Mahmoud, N. A. & Gader, A. M. A. (1978). *Br. J. Nutr.* **40**, 573.

Gunther, M. (1973). *Infant Feeding.* Harmondsworth: Penguin Handbooks.

Gurevic, G. P. (1966). Cited *Nutrition Abstracts and Reviews* no. 2206, 367.

Gurr, M. I. & James, A. T. (1975). *Lipid Biochemistry. An Introduction.* London: Chapman & Hall.

Gustafsson, B. E. & 6 others (1954). *Acta odont. scand.* **11**, 232.

Guthrie, B. E., & Robinson, M. F. (1977). *Br. J. Nutr.* **38**, 55.

Guyton, A. C., Harris, J. G. & Taylor, A. E. (1971). *Physiol. Rev.* **51**, 527.

Gwinup, G. (1975). *Archs intern. Med.* **135**, 676.

Gwinup, G., Byron, R. C., Roush, W. H., Kruger, F. A. & Hawmi, G. J. (1963). *Am. J. clin. Nutr.* **13**, 209.

György, P. (1971). *Am. J. clin. Nutr.* **24**, 1250.

Haber, G. B., Heaton, K. W., Murphy, D. & Burroughs, L. F. (1977). *Lancet* **2**, 679.

Habicht, J. P., Martorell, R., Yorbrough, C., Malina, R. M. & Klein, R. E. (1974). *Lancet* **1**, 611.

Haddad, J. G. & Hahn, T. J. (1973). *Nature, Lond.* **244**, 515.

Hadden, D. R., Montgomery, D. A. D., Skelly, R. J., Trimble, E. R., Weaver, E. A. & Buchanan, K. D. (1975). *Br. med. J.* **3**, 276.

Haenszel, W. & Correa, P. (1975). *Cancer Res.* **35**, 3452.

Haglund, E. & Magnusson, L. E. (1967). *Planning, Building and Equipping Home Economic Centres.* Rome: FAO.

Hakami, N., Neiman, P., Canellos, G. P. & Lazerson, J. (1971). *New Engl. J. Med.* **285**, 1163.

Hall, A. P., Barry, P. E., Dawler, T. R. & McNamara, P. M. (1967). *Am. J. Med.* **42**, 27.

Hall, B. (1975). *Lancet* **1**, 779.

Hallberg, L., Björn-Rasmussen, E., Rossander, L. & Suwanik, R. (1977). *Am. J. clin. Nutr.* **30**, 539.

Hallberg, L., Harworth, H.-G. & Vannotti, (ed.) (1970). *Iron Deficiency.* London: Academic Press.

Hallberg, L., Hogdahl, A.-M., Nilsson, L. & Rybo, G. (1966). *Acta obstet. gynec. scand.* **45**, 320.

Halliday, D. (1967). *Clin. Sci.* **33**, 365.

Halliday, D. (1971). *Br. J. Nutr.* **26**, 147.

Halperin, M., Cornfield, J. & Mitchell, S. C. (1973). *Lancet* **2**, 439.

Halstead, J. A. & Smith, J. C. (1970). *Lancet* **1**, 322.

Halstead, J. A., Ronaghy, H. A., Abadi, P., Haghshenass, M., Amirhakemi, G. H., Barakat, R. M. & Reinhold, J. G. (1972). *Am. J. Med.* **53**, 277.

Halstead, S. B. & Valyasevi, A. (1967). *Am. J. clin. Nutr.* **20**, 1312.

Hambidge, K. M., (1974). *Am. J. clin. Nutr.* **27**, 505.

Hambidge, K. M., Hambidge, C., Jacobs, M. & Barum, J. D. (1972). *Pediatric Res.* **6**, 868.

Hanni, R., Bigler, F., Meister, W. & Englert, G. (1976). *Helv. chim. Acta* **59**, 2221.

Hansen, A. E., Haggard, M. E., Boelsche, A. N., Adam, D. J. D. & Wiese, H. F. (1958). *J. Nutr.* **66**, 565.

Hansen, Aa. P. & Johansen, K. (1970). *Diabetologia* **6**, 27.

Hansen, J. D. L. (1956). *S. Afr. J. Lab. clin. Med* **2**, 206.

Hansen, J. D. L., Brinkman, G. L. & Bowie, M. D. (1965). *S. Afr. med. J.* **39**, 491.

Hansen, J. D. L., Howe, E. E. & Brock, J. F. (1956). *Lancet* **2**, 911.

Hansen, J. D. L. & Lehmann, B. H. (1969). *S. Afr. med. J.* **43**, 1248.

Harington, C. R. (1926). *Biochem. J.* **20**, 293.

Harington, C. R. & Barger, G. (1927). *Biochem. J.* **21**, 169.

Harkins, R. W. & Sarrett, H. P. (1968). *J. Am. Med. Ass.* **203**, 272.

Harper, A. E. (1978). *Am. J. clin. Nutr.* **31**, 310.

Harries, J. M., Hubbard, A. W., Aldo, F. E., Kay, M. & Williams, D. R. (1968). *Br. J. Nutr.* **22**, 21.

Harris, J. W. & Horrigan, D. L. (1964). *Vitams Horm.* **22**, 721.

Harris, L. J., Passmore, R. & Pagel, W. (1937). *Lancet* **2**, 183.

Harrison, G. G., Rathje, W. L. & Hughes, W. W. (1975). *J. Nutr. Educ.* **7**, 13.

Harrison, M. T., McFarlane, S., Harden, R. M. & Wayne, E. (1965). *Am. J. clin. Nutr.* **17**, 73.

Havel, R. J. (1965). In *Adipose Tissue*, ed. Renold, A. E. & Cahill, G. F., p. 575. Washington: American Physiological Society.

Hawk, L. J. & Brook, C. G. D. (1979). *Br. med. J.* 1, 151.

Hawthorn, J. (1959). *Proc. Nutr. Soc.* 18, 44.

Heady, J. A. (1974). *Br. med. J.* 1, 115.

Health and Welfare Canada (1976). *Dietary Standards for Canada*. Ottawa: Printing and Publishing Services.

Heaton, K. W. (1973). *Plant Foods for Man* 1, 33.

Heffernan, A. G. A. (1964). *Am. J. clin. Nutr.* 15, 5.

Hegsted, D. M. (1975). *J. Am. diet. Ass.* 66, 13.

Hegsted, D. M. Moscoso, I. & Collazos, C. (1952). *J. Nutr.* 46, 181.

Hehir, P. (1922). *Br. med. J.* 1, 865.

Hejda, S. (1978). Fifth Marabou Symposium: Why Obesity? *Näringsforskning* 22, suppl. no. 15, 46.

Hellendoorn, E. W., Noordhoff, M. G. & Slagman, J. (1975). *J. Sci. Fd Agric.* 26, 1461.

Heller, S. R. Labbe, R. F. & Nutter, J. (1971). *Clin. Chem.* 17, 525.

Helmkamp, G. M., Jr, Wilmore, D. W., Johnson, A. A. & Pruitt, B. A., Jr (1973). *Am. J. clin. Nutr.* 26, 1331.

Helweg-Larsen, P. & 6 others (1952). *Acta med. scand.* suppl. 274.

Hempner, G. W., Booth, C. C., Cowan, J., Hoffbrand, A. V. & Mollin, D. L. (1968). *Lancet* 2, 302.

Herbert, V. (1973). In *Modern Nutrition in Health and Disease*, 5th edn, ed. Goodhart, R. S. & Shils, M. E., p. 242, Philadelphia: Lea & Febinger.

Herbert, V. (1976). In *Nutrition Reviews' Present Knowledge in Nutrition*, 4th edn, p. 191. New York: The Nutrition Foundation.

Herbert, V. (1968). *Vitams Horm.* 26, 525.

Herbert, V. & Zalusky, Z. (1962). *J. clin. Invest.* 41, 1263.

Hercus, C. E. & Purves, H. D. (1936). *J. Hyg., Camb.* 36, 182.

Hermansen, L., Hultman, E.K. & Saltin, B. (1967). *Acta physiol. scand.* 71, 129.

Hertzig, M. E., Birch, H. G., Richardson, S. A. & Tizard, J. (1972). *Pediatrics* 49, 814.

Hervey, G. R. (1969). *Nature, Lond.* 222, 629.

Hervey, G. R. (1971). *Proc. Nutr. Soc.* 30, 109.

Hervey, G. R. & McCance, R. A. (1952). *Proc. R. Soc.* B 139, 527.

Hervey, G. R. & McCance, R. A. (1954). *Proc. Nutr. Soc.* 13, 41.

Heyden, S. (1976). *J. chron. Dis.* 29, 149.

Hilditch, T. P. & Williams, P. N. (1964). *The Chemical Constitution of Natural Fats*, 4th edn. London: Chapman & Hall.

Hill, K. R. (1952). *W. Indian med. J.* 1, 243.

Hill, M. J. (1975). *Cancer Res.* 35, 3398.

Hillman, R. W. *et al.* (1963). *Am. J. clin. Nutr.* 12, 427.

Hills, O. W., Liebert, E., Steinberg, P. L. & Horwitt, M. K. (1951). *Archs intern. Med.* 87, 682.

Himsworth, H. P. (1935). *Clin. Sci.* 2, 117.

Himsworth, H. P. (1949). *Proc. R. Soc. Med.* 42, 323.

Himsworth, H. P. (1950). *The Liver and Its Diseases*, 2nd edn. Oxford: Blackwell.

Hindhede, M. (1913). *Skand. Arch. Physiol.* 30 97.

Hinton, J. J. C. (1948a) *Br. J. Nutr.* 2, 237.

Hinton, J. J. C. (1948b). *Nature, Lond.* 112, 913.

Hirsch, J. (1975). In *Handbook of Physiology*, section 5, p. 148. American Physiology Society.

Hirsch, J. & Knittle, J. L. (1970). *Fedn Proc. Fedn Am. Socs exp. Biol.* 29, 1518.

Hobbs, B. C. & Gilbert, R. J. (1978). *Food Poisoning and Food Hygiene*, 4th edn. London: Arnold.

Hockaday, T. D. R., Hockaday, J. M., Mann, J. I. & Turner, R. C. (1978). *Br. J. Nutr.* 39, 357.

Hodge, H. C. (1964). In *Mineral Metabolism*, vol. 2, part A, ed. Comar, C. L. & Bronner, F. p. 573, New York: Academic Press.

Hodges, R. E. (1971). *Am. J. clin. Nutr.* 24, 383.

Hodges, R. E. (1973). In *Modern Nutrition in Health and Disease*, ed. Goodhart, R. & Shils, M. Philadelphia: Lea & Febiger.

Hodges, R. E., Hood, J., Canham, J. E., Sauberlich, H. E. & Baker, E. M. (1971). *Am. J. clin. Nutr.* 24, 432.

Hodges, R. E., Ohlson, M. A. & Bean, W. B. (1958). *J. clin. Invest.* 37, 1642.

Hodgkin, D. C., Pickworth, J., Robertson, J. H., Trueblood, K. N. & Prosen, R. J. (1955). *Nature, Lond.* 176, 325.

Hodgkinson, A. (1962). *Clin. Sci.* 23, 203.

Hoekstra, W. G. (1975). *Fedn Proc. Fedn Am. Socs exp. Biol.* 34, 2083.

Hoffbrand, A. V. (1970). *Archs Dis. Childh.* 45, 441.

Hollingsworth, D. F. & Greaves, J. P. (1967). *Am. J. clin. Nutr.* 20, 65.

Holloszy, J. O., Skinner, J. S., Toro, G. & Cureton, T. K. (1964). *Am. J. Cardiol.* 14, 753.

Holloway, P. J., James, P. M. C. & Slack, G. L. (1963). *Br. dent. J.* 115, 19.

Holmes, A. M., Enoch, B. A., Taylor, J. L. & Jones, M. E. (1973). *Q. Jl Med.* 42, 125.

Holt, C. von, Chang, J., Holt, M. von & Bohm, H. (1964). *Biochim. biophys. Acta* 90, 611.

Holt, L. E., György, P., Pratt, E. L., Snyderman, S. E. & Wallace, W. M. (1960). *Protein and Amino Acid Requirements in Early Life*. New York: New York Univ. Press.

Holt, L. E., Halac, E. & Kajdi, C. N. (1962). *J. Am. med. Ass.* 181, 699.

Holt, L. E., Snyderman, S. E., Norton, P. M., Roïtman, E. & Finch, J. (1963). *Lancet* **2**, 1343.

Hope, T. C. (1798). *Trans. R. Soc. Edinb.* **4**, part 2, 3.

Hopkins, F. G. (1912). *J. Physiol., Lond.* **44**, 425.

Hopkins, F. G. (1942). *Proc. R. Soc.* B **130**, 359.

Hoppner, K., Lampi, B. & Perrin D. E. (1972). *J. Inst. Can. Sci. Technol. Aliment.* **5**, 60.

Hoppner, K., Phillips, W. E. J., Murray, T. K. & Campbell, J. (1968). *Can. med. Ass. J.* **99**, 983.

Horne, C. H. W. & McCluskie, J. A. W. (1963). *Scott. med. J.* **8**, 489.

Hornstra, G. (1971). *Nutr. Metabol.* **13**, 140.

Hornstra, G. (1975). In *The Role of Fats in Human Nutrition*, ed. Vergroesen, A. J., p. 303. London: Academic Press.

Hornstra, G., Lewis, B., Chait, A., Turpeinen, O., Karvonen, M. J. & Vergroesen, A. J. (1973). *Lancet* **1**, 1155.

Horwitt, M. K. (1960). *Am. J. clin. Nutr.* **8**, 451.

Horwitt, M. K., Harvey, C. C. & Dahm, C. H. Jr (1975). *Am. J. clin. Nutr.* **28**, 403.

Horwitt, M. K., Harvey, C. C., Rothwell, W. S., Cutler, J. L. & Haffron, D. (1956). *J. Nutr.* **60**, suppl. 1.

Howie, J. W. (1949). *Br. J. Nutr.* **2**, 331.

Huque, T. & Truswell, A. S. (1979) *Proc. nutr. Soc.* In press.

Hull, D. & Segall, M. M. (1965). *J. Physiol., Lond.* **181**, 449.

Hume, E. M. & Krebs, H. A. (1949). *Spec. Rep. Ser. med. Res. Coun. Lond.* no. 264.

Hume, R. & Weyers, E. (1973). *Scott. med. J.* **18**, 3.

Hunt, J. N., Cash, R. & Newland, P. (1975). *Lancet* **2**, 905.

Hunt, S. P., O'Riordan, J. L. H., Windo, J. & Truswell, A. S. (1976). *Br. med. J.* **2**, 1351.

Hunter, D. (1955). *The Diseases of Occupation.* London: English Universities Press.

Hunter, W. M., Fonseka, C. C. & Passmore, R. (1965a). *Q. Jl exp. Physiol.* **50**, 406.

Hunter, W. M., Fonseka, C. C. & Passmore, R. (1965b). *Science, N.Y.* **150**, 1051.

Hunter, W. W. (1868). *Annals of Rural Bengal*, p. 26. London.

Hurrell, R. F. & Carpenter, K. J. (1975). *Br. J. Nutr.* **33**, 101.

Hurrell, R. F. & Carpenter, K. J. (1977). In *Physical, Chemical and Biological Changes in Food Caused by Thermal Processing*, ed. Høyem, T. & Kvåle, O., p. 168. London: Applied Science.

Hutchison, J. B., Moran, T. & Pace, J. (1956). *Proc. R. Soc.* B. **145**, 270.

Hutner, S. H. & McLaughlin, J. J. A. (1958). *Scient. Am.* **199**, 92.

Hytten, F. E. (1954). *Br. med. J.* **1**, 249.

Hytten, F. E. & Leitch, I. (1971). *The Physiology of Pregnancy*, 2nd ed. Oxford: Blackwell.

Hytten, F. E., Taylor, K. & Taggart, N. (1966). *Clin. Sci.* **31**, 111.

Ibels, L. S., Simons, L. A., King, J. O., Williams, P. F., Neale, F. C. & Stewart, J. H. (1975). *Q. Jl Med.* **44**, 601.

Ikefwunigwe, A. E. (1977). *Ann. N. Y. Acad. Sci.* **300**, 87.

Illingworth, R. S. & Kilpatrick, B. (1953). *Lancet* **2**, 1175.

Indian National Institute of Nutrition (1976). *Annual Report*, p. 25. Hyderabad.

Indian National Institute of Nutrition (1977). *Annual Report*, p. 27.

Ingelfinger, F. J. (1977). *New Engl. J. Med.* **296**, 1167.

Inglett, G. E. & May, J. F. (1969). *J. Food Sci.* **34**, 408.

Insull, W., Osia, T. & Tsuchiya, K. (1968). *Am. J. clin. Nutr.* **21**, 753.

International Agency for Research on Cancer (1977). *Lancet* **2**, 207.

International Union of Nutritional Sciences Committee (V-I) on Nutrition Education in Medical Faculties (1971). *Proc. Nutr. Soc.* **30**, 191.

Irvin, M. S. & Hegsted, D. M. (1971). *J. Nutr.* **101**, 1.

Irvine, W. J. Cullen, D. R., Ewart, R. B. L., Baird, J. D. & Webster, J. N. H. (1974). *In Companion to Medical Studies*, ed. Passmore, R. & Robson, J. S., vol. 3, p. 23.74. Oxford: Blackwell.

Irvine, W. J., Davies, S. H., Delamore, I. W. & Wynn Williams, A. (1962). *Br. med. J.* **2**, 454.

Ismail-Beigi, F., Faraji, B. & Reinhold, J. G. (1977). *Am. J. clin. Nutr.* **30**, 1721.

Itoh, T., Tamura, T. & Matsumoto, T. (1973). *J. Am. Oil Chem. Soc.* **50**, 122.

Jackson, C. M. (1925). *The Effects of Inanition and Malnutrition upon Growth and Structure.* London: Churchill.

Jackson, R. L., Morrisett, J. D. & Gotto, A. M (1976). *Physiol. Rev.* **56**, 259.

Jackson, W. P. U. (1972). *Postgrad. med. J.* **48**, 391.

Jacobs, A. & Butler, E. B. (1965). *Lancet* **2**, 407.

Jacobs, A., Milla, F., Worwood, M., Beamish, M. R. & Wardrop, C. A. (1972). *Br. med. J.* **4**, 206.

Jacobs, A. & Worwood, M. (ed.) (1974). *Iron in Biochemistry and Medicine.* London: Academic Press.

Jacobs, P., Bothwell, T. & Charlton, R. W. (1964). *J. appl. Physiol.* **19**, 187.

Jager, F. C. (1975). In *The Role of Fats in Human Nutrition,* ed. Vergroesen, A. J., p. 381. London: Academic Press.

James, W. P. T. (1968). *Lancet* **1,** 333.

James, W. P. T. (1971). *Ann. N.Y. Acad. Sci.* **176,** 244.

James, W. P. T. (ed.) (1976). *Research on Obesity.* A DHSS/MRC Report. London: HMSO.

James, W. P. T., Branch, W. J. & Southgate, D.A.T. (1978). *Lancet* **1,** 628.

James, W. P. T., Davies, H. L., Bailes, J. & Dauncey, M. J. (1978). *Lancet* **1,** 1122.

James, W. P. T. & Trayhurn, P. (1976). *Lancet* **2,** 770.

Jansen, B. C. P. & Donath, W. F. (1926). *Verh. Akad. Wet. Amst.* **29,** 1390.

Janus, E. D. & Sharman, J. R. (1972). *N.Z. med. J.* **75,** 339.

Jardin, C. (1972). *Organo-minerals and Ciguatera,* FAO Nutrition Newsletter, vol. 10, part 3, p. 14.

Jeejeebhoy, K. N., Chu, R. C., Marliss, E. B., Greenberg, G. R. & Bruce-Robertson, A. (1977). *Am. J. clin Nutr.* **30,** 531.

Jeffrey, F. E. & Abelmann, W. H. (1971). *Am. J. Med.* **50,** 123.

Jelliffe, D. B. (1957). *Pediatrics, N.Y.* **20,** 128.

Jelliffe, D. B. (1959). *J. Pediat.* **54,** 227.

Jelliffe, D. B. (1966). *The Assessment of the Nutritional Status of the Community.* Geneva: WHO.

Jelliffe, D. B. (1967). *Am. J. clin. Nutr.* **20,** 279.

Jelliffe, E. F. P. & Jelliffe, D. B. (1964). *Clin. Pediat.* **3,** 604.

Jelliffe, E. F. P. & Jelliffe, D. B. (1969). *J. trop. Pediat.* **15,** 177–260.

Jelliffe, E. F. P. & Jelliffe, D. B. (ed.) (1973). Deciduous Dental Eruption, Nutrition and Age Assessment. Monograph no. 28. *J. trop. Pediat. Envir. Child Hlth* **19,** 193–248.

Jelliffe, D. B. & Jelliffe, E. F. P. (1978). *Human Milk in the Modern World.* Oxford Univ. Press.

Jelliffe, D. B. & Stuart, K. L. (1954). *Br. med. J.* **1,** 75.

Jenkins, D. J. A. & 7 others (1977). *Lancet* **2,** 779.

Jepson, J. B. (1966). In *The Metabolic Basis of Inherited Disease,* 2nd edn, ed. Stanbury, J. B., Wyngaarden, J. B. & Fredrickson, D. S., p. 1283. New York: Blakiston.

Jick, H., Miettinen, O. S., Neff, R. K., Shapiro, S., Heinonen, O. P. & Slone, D. (1973). *New Engl. J. Med.* **284,** 63.

Joffe, N. (1961). *Br. J. Radiol.* **34,** 429.

Johnson, H. (1971). *The World Atlas of Wine.* London: Mitchell Beazlev.

Johnson, M. L., Burke, B. S. & Mayer, J. (1956). *Am. J. clin. Nutr.* **4,** 37.

Johnson, R. E. & Passmore, R. (1962). *Metabolism* **107,** 43.

Johnson, R. E. & Sargent, F. (1958). *Proc. Nutr. Soc.* **17,** 179.

Joint Iran-IARC Study Group (1977). *J. nat. cancer Inst.* **59,** 1127.

Joint Working Party of the Royal College of Physicians (London) and the British Cardiac Society (1976). *Jl R. Coll. Physns* **10,** 213.

Jolly, S. S., Singh, B. M. & Mathur, O. C. (1969). *Am. J. Med.* **47,** 553.

Jones, D. C. (1975). *Food for Thought.* London: Royal College of Nursing.

Jones, F. Avery (1957). *Br. med. J* **1,** 719, 786.

Jones, F. Avery, Gummer, J. W. P. & Lennard-Jones, J. E. (1968). *Clinical Gastroenterology,* 2nd edn. Oxford: Blackwell.

Jordan, H. A. (1973). In *Obesity in Perspective.* Fogarty International Center Series, vol. 2, part 2, ed. Bray, G. A., p. 35. DHEW Publ. NIH 75–708. Washington. D. C.

Joslin, E. P. (1928). *The Treatment of Diabetes Mellitus,* 4th edn. Philadelphia: Lea & Febiger.

Jourdan, M., Glock, C., Margen, S. & Bradfield, R. B. (1979). *Am. J. clin. Nutr.* In press.

Jowsey, J., Riggs, B. L., Kelley, P. J. & Hoffman, D. L. (1972). *Am. J. Med.* **53,** 43.

Jukes, T. H. (1977). *Nutrition Today* **12,** 12.

Jung, R. T., Gunn, M. I., Robinson, M. P. & James, W. P. T. (1978). *Br. med. J.* **2,** 319.

Kamel, K. & 8 others (1972). *Am. J. clin. Nutr.* **25,** 152.

Kanagaratnam, K., Boon, W. K. & Hoh, T. K. (1960). *Lancet* **1,** 538.

Kannel, W. B., Brand, N., Skinner, J. J., Jr, Dawber, T. R. & McNamara, P. M. (1967). *Ann. intern. Med.* **67,** 48.

Kannel, W. B. & Gordon, T. (1970). *The Framingham Diet Study. Diet and the Regulation of Serum Cholesterol.* Public Health Service Monograph no. 24, Washington, D.C.: US Government Printing Office.

Kapp, J. P., Duckert, F. & Hartman, G. (1971). *Nutr. Metab.* **13,** 92.

Kapur, K. K., Glass, R. L., Loftus, E. R., Alman, J. E. & Feller, R. P. (1972). *Aging hum. Devel.* **3,** 125.

Karam, J. H., Grodsky, G. M. & Forsham, P. H. (1963). *Diabetes,* **12,** 197.

Karmarkar, M. G., Deo, M. G., Kochupillai, N. & Ramalingaswami, V. (1974). *Am. J. clin. Nutr.* **27,** 96.

Kaser, M. M., Steinkamp, R. C., Robinson, W. D., Patton, E. W. & Youmans, J. B. (1947). *Am. J. Hyg.* **46,** 297.

Kaunitz, H. (1956). *Nature, Lond.* **178,** 1141.

Kay, R. G. & Tasman-Jones, C. (1975). *Aust. N.Z. Jl Surg.* **45,** 325.

Kay, R. M. & Truswell, A. S. (1977a). *Am. J. clin. Nutr.* **30**, 171.

Kay, R. M. & Truswell, A. S. (1977b). *Br. J. Nutr.* **37**, 227.

Kay, Ruth M. (1974). *Nutrition, Lond.* **28**, 97.

Kekwick, A. & Pawan, G. L. S. (1956). *Lancet* **2**, 155.

Kekwick, A., Pawan, G. L. S. & Chalmers, T. M. (1959). *Lancet* **2**, 1157.

Kempner, W. (1945). *N. Carol. med. J.* **6**, 117.

Kendall, E. C. & Osterberg, A. E. (1919). *J. biol. Chem.* **40**, 265.

Kennedy, G. C. (1953). *Proc. R. Soc.* B **140**, 78

Kerr, D. N. S. & Davidson, L. S. P. (1958a). *Lancet* **2**, 489.

Kerr, D. N. S. & Davidson, L. S. P. (1958b). *Lancet* **2**, 483.

Kerr, N. (1977). *Proc. R. Soc. Edinb.* B. **75**, 263.

Kessel, N. (1977). *Hlth Trends* **9**, 86.

Keys, A., (1952). *Circulation* **5**, 115.

Keys, A. (1953). *J. Mt Sinai Hosp.* **20**, 118.

Keys, A. (1955). In *Weight Control*, ed. Eppright, E. S. Swanson, P. & Iverson, C. A. Iowa: Iowa State College Press.

Keys, A. (ed.) (1970). *Circulation,* **41**, suppl. 1, 199.

Keys, A. (1973). *Atherosclerosis* **18**, 352.

Keys, A., Anderson, J. T. & Grande, F. (1958a). *Proc. Soc. exp. Biol. Med.* **98**, 387.

Keys, A., Anderson, J. T. & Grande, F. (1965). *Metabolism* **14**, 759.

Keys, A., Anderson, J. T., Mickelsen, O., Adelson, S. F. & Fidanza, F. (1956). *J. Nutr.* **59**, 39.

Keys, A., Brozek, J., Henschel, A., Mickelsen, O. & Taylor, H. L. (1950). *The Biology of Human Starvation*, vol. 1, p. 497. Univ. Minnesota and Oxford Univ. Press.

Keys, A., Grande, F. & Anderson, J. T. (1974). *Am. J. clin. Nutr.* **27**, 188.

Keys, A., Henschel, A., Taylor, H. L., Michelsen, O. & Brozek, J. (1945). *Am. J. Physiol.* **144**, 5.

Keys, A., Karvonen, M. J. & Fidanza, F. (1958b). *Lancet* **2**, 175.

Keys, A., Kimura, K., Kusukawa, A., Bronte-Stewart, B., Larsen, N. & Keys, M. H. (1958c). *Ann. intern. Med.* **48**, 83.

Keys, A. & 5 others (1957). *Fedn Proc. Fedn Am. Socs exp. Biol.* **16**, 204.

Keys, A. & 10 others (1972). *Ann. intern. Med.* **77**, 15.

Khachadurian, A. K. & Uthman, S. M. (1973). *Nutr. Metabol.* **15**, 132.

Kiehm, T. G., Anderson, J. W. & Ward, K. (1976). *Am. J. clin. Nutr.* **29**, 895.

Kielmann, A. A., Taylor, C. E. & Parker, R. L. (1978). *Am. J. clin. Nutr.* **31**, 2040.

Kiker, B. F. (ed.) (1971). *Investment in Human Capital.* Columbia: Univ. S. Carolina.

King Edward's Hospital Fund for London (1956). *General Hospital Diet,* 2nd edn. London: KEHF.

King, J. D., Mellanby, M., Stones, H. M. & Green, H. N. (1955). *Spec. Rep. Ser. med. Res. Coun.* no. 288. London: HMSO.

Kingsbury, K. J. (1971). *Lancet* **1**, 199.

Kinsell, L. W., Partridge, J., Boling, L., Margen, S. & Michaels, G. (1952). *J. clin. Endocr.* **12**, 909.

Kinsey, B. E. (1947). *Am. J. Ophthalmol.* **30**, 1262.

Kirklin, J. K., Watson, M., Bondoc, C. C. & Burke, J. F. (1976). *New Engl. J. Med.* **294**, 938.

Kirwan, W. O., Smith, A. N. McConnell, A. A., Mitchell, W. D., Eastwood, M. A. (1974). *Br. med. J.* **2**, 187.

Kissebah, A. K., Adams, P. W. & Wynn, V. (1974). *Clin. Sci.* **47**, 459.

Kitabachi, A. E. & Duckworth, W. C. (1970). *Am. J. clin. Nutr.* **23**, 1012.

Kitabachi, A. E. & West, W. H. (1975). *Ann. N.Y. Acad. Sci.* **258**, 422.

Knight, R. A., Christie, A. A., Orton, C. R. & Robertson, J. (1973). *Br. J. Nutr.* **30**, 181.

Knutson, K. E. & Selinius, R. (1970). *Am. J. clin. Nutr.* **23**, 956.

Kodicek, E. (1962). *Bibl. Nutritio Dieta,* **4**, 109.

Kodicek, E. (1967). *Proc. Nutr. Soc.* **26**, 67.

Kodicek, E. (1974). *Lancet* **1**, 325.

Kodicek, E., Ashby, D. R., Muller, M. & Carpenter, K. J. (1974). *Proc. Nutr. Soc.* **33**, 105 A.

Kofrányi, E., Jekat, F. & Müller-Wecker, H. (1970). *Hoppe-Seyler's Z. physiol. Chem.* **351**, 1485.

Komrower, G. M., Wilson, V., Clamp, J. R. & Westall, R. G. (1964). *Archs Dis. Childh.* **39**, 250.

Kon, S. K. (1972). *Milk and Milk Production in Human Nutrition.* FAO Nutritional Status no. 27.

Kooh, S. W., Fraser, D., Reilly, B. J., Hamilton, J. R., Gall, D. G. & Bell, L. (1977). *New Engl. J. Med.* **297**, 1264.

Koppert, J. (1977). *Nutrition Rehabilitation. Its Practical Application.* London: Tri-Med Books.

Kopple, J. D. & Swenseid, M. E. (1975). *J. clin. Invest.* **55**, 881.

Korns, R. F. (1972): *Nutrition Today* **7**, 21.

Kottke, B. A. (1969). *Circulation* **40**, 13.

Kouwenhoven, T. & Drijver, A. A. (1973). *Voeding* **34**, 180.

Krall, L. P. (1969). *Proceedings of the Eighth International Nutrition Congress*, ed. Masek, J., Osancova, M. & Cuthbertson, D.P., p. 376. Amsterdam: Excerpta Medica.

Krebs, H. A. (1964). In *Mammalian Protein Metabolism*, ed. Munroe, H. N. & Allison, J. B., vol. 1, p. 125. New York: Academic Press.

Krehl, W. A. (1970). *Nutrition Today* **5**, 26.

Krehl, W. A. (1973). In *Modern Nutrition in Health and Disease*, 5th edn, ed. Goodhart, R. S. & Shils, M. E. Philadelphia: Lea & Febiger.

Kretchmer, N. (1972). *Scient. Am.* Oct., p.71.

Kretchmer, N., Ransome-Kuti, O., Hurwitz, R., Dungy, C. & Alakija, W. (1971). *Lancet* **2**, 392.

Krikler, D. M. & Schrire, V. (1958). *Lancet* **1**, 510.

Krishnamachari, K. A. V. R., Bhat, R. V., Nagarajan, V. & Tilak, T. B. G. (1975). *Lancet* **1**, 1061.

Krishnamachari, K. A. V. R. & Krishnaswamy, K. (1973). *Lancet* **2**, 877.

Krishnaswamy, K. & Ramana Murthy, P. S. V. (1970). *Clin. chim. Acta,* **27**, 301.

Krishnaswamy, K., Rao, S. B., Raghum, T. C. & Srikantia, S. G. (1976). *Am. J. clin. Nutr.* **29**, 177.

Kruger, R. H. (1969). *Lancet* **2**, 514.

Kuhn, R., György, P. & Wagner-Jauregg, T. (1933). *Ber. dt. chem. Ges.* **66**, 1034.

Kumar, P. J., Oliver, R. T. D., O'Donoghue, D. P., Ngahfoong, L. & Pillai, A. (1978). *Gut* **19**, 438.

Kurland, L. T. (1972). *Fedn Proc. Fedn Am. Socs exp. Biol.* **31**, 1540.

Kwiterovich, P.O., Jr, Levy, R. I. & Fredrickson, D. S. (1973). *Lancet* **1**, 118.

Kwok, R. H. M. (1968). *New Engl. J. Med.* **278**, 796.

Laguna, J. & Carpenter, K. J. (1951). *J. Nutr.* **45**, 21.

Lai, C. S. & Ransome, G. A. (1970). *Br. med. J.* **2**, 151.

Lakdawala, D. R. & Widdowson, E. M. (1977). *Lancet* **1**, 167.

Lal, R. B., Mukherji, S. P., Das Gupta, A. C. & Chatterji, S. R. (1940). *Indian J. med. Res.* **28**, 163.

Lal, R. B. & Roy, S. C. (1937). *Indian J. med. Res.* **25**, 163.

Lambertsen, C. J., Kough, R. H., Cooper, D. Y., Emmel, G. L., Loeschek, H. H. & Schmidt, C. F. (1953). *J. appl. Physiol.* **5**, 471.

Lancet (1961). **2**, 1391.

Lancet (1964). **1**, 540.

Lancet (1971a). Editorial, 2, 475.

Lancet (1971b). Editorial, 2, 1407.

Lancet (1971c). Annotation, 2, 1410.

Lancet (1971d). Editorial, 1, 382.

Lancet (1972a). Editorial. 1, 193.

Lancet (1972b). Editorial (Death cap poisoning). 1, 1320.

Lancet (1973a). 1, 1041.

Lancet (1976). Editorial 2, 1230.

Landor, J. V. & Pallister, R. A. (1935). *Trans. R. Soc. trop. Med. Hyg.* **29**, 121.

Lang, P. D. & Insull, W., Jr. (1970). *J. clin. Invest.* **49**, 1479.

Langman, M. J. S. (1974). In *Gastroenterology,* ed. Bockus, H. L. Philadelphia: Saunders.

Lanzkowsky, P. (1970). *Am. J. Med.* **48**, 580.

Larsen, D. L. & Tomlinson, L. J. (1952). *J. Lab. clin. Med.* **39**, 129.

Lathan, M. C. (1972). *Planning and Evaluation of Applied Nutrition Programmes.* FAO Nutritional Studies no. 26. Rome: FAO.

Lawes, J. B. & Gilbert, J. H. (1853). *Report of the 22nd Meeting of the British Association for the Advancement of Science,* p. 323.

Lawrie, R. A. (1974). *Meat Science,* 2nd edn. Oxford: Pergamon Press.

Lawrie, T. D. V., McAlpine, S. G., Rifkind, B. M., Dunnigan, M. & Cockburn, J. (1964). *Clin. Sci.* **27**, 89.

Lawson, D. E. M., Fraser, D. R., Kodicek, E., Morris, H. R. & Williams, D. H. (1971). *Nature, Lond.* **230**, 228.

Layrisse, M. & Roche, M. (1964). *Am. J. Hyg.* **79**, 279.

Leaf, A. (1973). *Nutrition Today,* **8**, 4.

League of Nations, Technical Commission of the Health Committee (1935). *Report on the Physiological Bases of Nutrition.* Series of League of Nations Publications III. Health III. 6. Geneva.

League of Nations, Technical Commission of the Health Committee (1936). *The Problem of Nutrition, Vol. II. Report on the Physiological Basis of Nutrition.* Series of League of Nations Publications II. Economic and Financial II B.4. Geneva.

Lechtig, A., Delgado, H., Lasky, R. E., Klein, R. E., Engle, P. L. Yarborough, C. & Habicht, J. P. (1975). *Am. J. dis. Child.* **129**, 434.

Lee, H. A. (1977). In *Nutrition in the Clinical Management of Disease,* ed. Dickerson, J. W. T. & Lee, H. A. London: Arnold.

Lee, R. B. (1967). *What Hunters Do for a Living: A Comparative Study in Man the Hunter,* ed. Lee, R. B. & De Vore, p. 41. Chicago: Aldine.

Leeds, A. R. & 7 others (1978). *Proc. Nutr. Soc.* **37**, 23A.

Lehmann, G., Müller, E. A. & Spitzer, H. (1950). *Arbeitsphysiologie,* **14**, 166.

Lehringer, A. L. (1975). *Biochemistry,* 2nd edn. New York: Worth.

Leibowitz, S. F. (1976). In *Hunger: Basic Mechanisms and Clinical Implications,* ed. Novin, D., Syrwicka, W. & Bray, G. A., p. 1.

Leichenger, H., Eisenberg, G. & Carlson, A. J. (1948). *J. Am. med. Ass.* **136**, 388.

Leitch, I. (1964). In *Nutrition,* vol. 1, ed. Beaton, G. M. & McHenry, E. W. New York: Academic Press.

Leitner, Z. A., Moore, T. & Sharman, I. M. (1952). *Br. J. Nutr.* **6**, x.

Lelbach, W. K. (1968). *Germ. med. Mon.* **13**, 31.

Lendrum, R., Walker, G. Cudworth, A. G., Theophanides, C., Pyke, D. A., Bloom, A. & Gamble, D. R. (1976). *Lancet* **2**, 1273.

Leonard, P. J. & Losowsky, M. S. (1971). *Am. J. clin. Nutr.* **24**, 388.

Leone, N. C. & 6 others (1955). *Publ. Hlth Rep. Wash.* **69**, 925.

Leren, P. (1966). *Acta med. scand.* suppl. 466.

Lesch, M. & Nyhan, W. L. (1964). *Am. J. Med.* **36**, 561.

Levene, C. J. & Bates, C. J. (1975). *Ann. N.Y. Acad. Sci.* **258**, 288.

Leverton, R. M., Johnson, N., Pazur, J. & Ellison, J. (1956). *J. Nutr.* **58**, 219.

Levitz, L. S. & Stunkard, A. J. (1974). *Am. J. Psychiat.* **131**, 423.

Levy, A. M. (1907). The Physiology of Metabolism. In *Metabolism and Practical Medicine,* ed. von Norden, C., vol. 1. London: Heinemann.

Levy, R. I., Bilheimer, D. W. & Eisenberg, S. (1971a). In *Plasma Lipoproteins.* Biochemical Society, Symposium, ed. Smellie, R. M. S. no. 33, p. 3. London: Academic Press.

Levy, R. I., Bonnell, M. & Ernst, N. D. (1971b). *J. Am. diet. Ass.* **58**, 406.

Lewis, B. (1976). *The Hyperlipidaemias. Clinical and Laboratory Practice.* Oxford: Blackwell.

Lieber, C. S. (ed.) (1977). *Metabolic Aspects of Alcoholism.* Lancaster: MTP Press.

Lieber, C. S. & Rubin, E. (1968). *Am. J. Med.* **44**, 200.

Liener, I. E. (1966). In *Toxicants Occurring Naturally in Foods,* p. 40. Washington, D.C.: National Academy of Sciences/National Research Council.

Liener, I. E. (ed.) (1969). *Toxic Constituents in Plant Foodstuffs.* New York: Academic Press.

Liener, I. E. (ed.) (1974). *Toxic Constituents of Animal Foodstuffs.* New York: Academic Press.

Lightwood, R. (1952). *Proc. R. Soc. Med.* **45**, 401.

Lind, J. (1753). *A Treatise of the Scurvy.* Reprinted by Edinburgh Univ. Press, 1953.

Linden, V. (1974). *Br. med. J.* **3**, 647.

Lindsey, C., Santeusanio, F., Braaten, J., Faloona, G. R. & Unger, R. H. (1974). *J. Am. med. Ass.* **227**, 757.

Link, K. P. (1944). *Fedn Proc. Fedn Am. Socs exp. Biol.* **4**, 176.

Linkswiler, H. M. (1976). In *Nutrition Reviews' Present Knowledge in Nutrition,* 4th edn, p. 232. New York: Nutrition Foundation.

Little, R. E. (1977). *Am. J. pub. Hlth* **67**, 1154.

Livingston, S. (1972). *Comprehensive Management of Epilepsy.* Springfield: Thomas.

Lloyd Davies, T. A. (1964). In *Proceedings of the Sixth International Congress of Nutrition,* ed. Mills, C. F. & Passmore, R., p. 24. Edinburgh: Livingstone.

Lloyd, J. K. & Muller, D. P. R. (1971). In *Protides of the Biological Fluids.* 19th Colloquium, ed. Peters, H., p. 331. Oxford: Pergamon Press.

Lloyd-Still, J. D. (1976). *Malnutrition and Intellectual Development.* Lancaster: MTP.

Lockwood, M. J., Riding, K. H. & Keen, H. (1968). *Nutrition, Lond.* **12**, 7.

Logan, R. L. & 11 others (1978). *Lancet* **1**, 949.

Loomis, W. F. (1967). *Science, N.Y.* **157**, 501.

Lonergan, M. E., Milne, J. S., Mauk, M. M. & Williamson, J. (1975). *Br. J. Nutr.* **34**, 517.

Loraine, J. A. (1972). *The Death of Tomorrow.* London: Heinemann.

Lovland, J., Harper, J. M. & Frey, A. L. (1976). *Lebensmittel-Wissenschaft und Technologie* **9**, 131.

Lowenstein, M. S., Balows, A. & Gangarosa, E. J. (1973). *Lancet* **1**, 529.

Lucasse, C. (1952). *Ann. Soc. belge Méd. trop.* **32**, 391.

Lumeng, L., Cleary, R. E., Wagner, R., Yu, P.-L. & Li, T.-K. (1976). *Am. J. clin.* **29**, 1376.

Lunn, P. G., Whitehead, R. G., Hay, R. W. & Baker, B. A. (1973). *Br. J. Nutr.* **29**, 399.

Lunven, P., Le Clement de St Marcq, C., Carnovale, E. & Fratoni, A. (1973). *Br. J. Nutr.* **30**, 189.

Lusk, G. (1928). *The Science of Nutrition,* 4th edn. Philadelphia: Saunders.

Lyon, T. P., Yankley, A., Gofman, J. W. & Strisower, B. (1956). *Calif. Med.* **85**, 325.

Lysons, A. (1975). In *Reports on the Progress of Applied Chemistry,* p. 457. London: Academic Press.

McCance, R. A. (1936). *Lancet* **1**, 823.

McCance, R. A. (1946). *Lancet* **1**, 77.

McCance, R. A. (1951). *Spec. Rep. Ser. med. Res. Coun. Lond.* no. 275, 83.

McCance, R. A. & Barrett, A. M. (1951). *Spec. Rep. Ser. med. Res. Coun. Lond.* No. 275, 83.

McCance, R. A. El Neil, H., El Din, N., Widdowson, E. M., Southgate, D. A. T., Passmore, R., Shirling, D. & Wilkinson, R. T. (1971). *Phil. Trans. R. Soc.* **259**, 533.

McCance, R. A., Ford, E. H. R. & Brown, W. A. B. (1961). *Br. J. Nutr.* **15**, 213.

McCance, R. A. & Widdowson, E. M. (1937). *Lancet* **2**, 680.

McCance, R. A. & Widdowson, E. M. (1942). *J. Physiol. Lond.* **101**, 44, 304.

McCance, R. A. & Widdowson, E. M. (1951). *Proc. R. Soc.* B **138**, 115.

McCance, R. A. & Widdowson, E. M. (1956). *Breads White and Brown.* London: Pitman.

McCance, R. A. & Widdowson, E. M. (1967). *Spec. Rep. Ser. med. Res. Coun. Lond.* no. **297.**

McCance, R. A. & Widdowson, E. M. (1974). *Proc. R. Soc* B **185**, 1.

McCance, R. A. Widdowson, E. M. & Lehmann, H. (1942). *Biochem. J.* **36**, 686.

McCance, R. A., Widdowson, E. M., Moran, T., Pringle, W. J. S. & Macrae, T. F. (1945). *Biochem. J.* **39**, 213.

McCarrison, R. (1908a). *Lancet* **2**, 1275.

McCarrison, R. (1908b). *Indian med. Gaz.* **43**, 441.

McCarrison, R. (1936). *Nutrition and Health.* Cantor Lectures republished (1953). London: Faber.

McCarrison, R. (1919). *Studies of Deficiency Disease.* Oxford: Medical Publications, 1921.

McCay, C. M. (1949). *Vitams Horm.* **7**, 147.

McCay, C. M. (1955). In *Colloquia on Ageing,* vol. 1, ed. Wolstenholme, G. E. W. & Cameron, M. P. Ciba Foundation. London: Churchill.

McClellan, W. S. & Du Bois, E. F. (1930). *J. biol. Chem.* **87**, 651.

McClelland, D. B. L., McGrath, J. and Samson, R. R. (1978). *Acta paed. scand.* suppl. 271, 1–20.

McCollum, E. V. & Davis, M. (1913). *J. biol. Chem.* **15**, 167.

McCollum, J. P. K., Pearson, R. C. M., Ingham, H. R., Wood, P. C. & Dewar, H. A. (1968). *Lancet* **2**, 767.

McConnell, A. A., Eastwood, M. A. & Mitchell, W. D. (1974). *J. Sci. Fd Agric.* **25**, 1457.

McCrae, W. M., Eastwood, M., Martin, M. R. & Sircus, W. (1975). *Lancet* **1**, 187.

McFarlane, D. B., Pinkerton, P. H., Dagg, J. H. & Goldberg, A. (1967). *Br. J. Haemat.* **13**, 790.

McGandy, R. B., Hegsted, D. M. & Meyers, M. L. (1970), *Am. J. clin. Nutr.* **23**, 1288.

McGarry, J. D. & Foster, D. W. (1977). *Archs intern. Med.* **137**, 495.

McGregor, I. A., Billewicz, W. Z. & Thomson, A. M. (1961). *Br. med. J.* **2**, 1661.

McIntyre, N. & Stanley, N. N. (1971). *Br. med. J.* **3**, 567.

McIntyre, O. R., Sullivan, L. W. & Jeffries, G. H. (1965). *New Engl. J. Med.* **272**, 981.

McKigney, J. I. & Munro, H. N. (ed.) (1976). *Nutrient Requirements in Adolescence.* Cambridge, Mass.: MIT Press.

McLaren, D. S. (1963). *Malnutrition and the Eye.* New York: Academic Press.

McLaren, D. S. (1966a), *Lancet,* **2**, 485.

McLaren, D. S. (1966b). *Trans. R. Soc. trop. Med. Hyg.* **60**, 436.

McLaren, D. S. (1980). *Nutritional Ophthalmology.* London and New York: Academic Press.

McLaren, D. S., Oomen, H. A. P. C. & Escapini, H. (1966). *Bull. Wld Hlth Org.* **34**, 357.

McLaren, D. S. & Zekian, B. (1971). *Am. J. Dis. Child,* **121**, 78.

McLennan, W. J., Andrews, G. R., Macleod, C. & Caird, F. I. (1973). *Q. Jl Med.* **42**, 1.

McLester, J. S. & Darby, W. J. (1952). *Nutrition and Diet in Health and Disease,* p. 263. Philadelphia: Saunders.

McMichael, H. B. (1975). *Biochem. Soc. Trans.* **3**, 223.

McMichael, H. B. (1971). *Proc. Nutr. Soc.* **30**, 248.

McNaughton, J. (1975). *Fd Nutr.* **1**, 17.

Macdonald, I. (1967). *Am. J. clin. Nutr.* **20**, 185.

Macdonald, I. & Braithwaite, D. M. (1964). *Clin. Sci.* **27**, 23.

MacDonald, R. A. (1964). *Hemochromatosis and Hemosiderosis.* Springfield, Illinois: Thomas.

MacDonald, W. C., Dobbins, W. O. & Rubin, C. E. (1965). *New Engl. J. Med.* **272**, 448.

Mackenzie, I. L., Donaldson, R. M., Jr, Trier, J. S. & Mathan, V. I. (1972). *New Engl. J. Med.* **286**, 1021.

Mackinnon, A. E. & Bancewicz, J. (1973). *Br. med. J.* **2**, 277.

MacLachlan, M. J. & Rodnan, G. P. (1967). *Am. J. Med.* **42**, 38.

MacLennan, R., Gaitan, E. & Miller, M. C. (1969). In *Endemic Goitre,* ed. Stanbury, J. B., p. 67. Pan American Health Organisation Scientific Publication No. 193. Washington, D.C.

MacMillan, M. G., Reid, C. M., Shirling, D. & Passmore, R. (1965). *Lancet,* **1**, 728.

Mahadeva, K., Seneviratne, D. R., Jayatilleke, D. B., Serthe Shanmuganathan, S., Premachandra, P. & Nagarajah, M. (1968). *Br. J. Nutr.* **22**, 527.

Mahler, R. (1972). *Acta Diabetologica Latina,* **9**, Suppl. 1, 449.

Mahoney, M. J. & Rosenberg, L. E. (1970). *Am. J. Med.* **48**, 584.

Majoor, C. L. H. (1978). *Jl R. Coll. Physns, Lond.* **12**, 143.

Makene, W. J. & Wilson, J. (1972). *J. Neurol., Neurosurg., Psychiat.* **35**, 31.

Malm, O. J. (1953). *Scand. J. clin. Lab. Invest.* **5**, 75.

Malm, O. J. (1958). *Scand. J. clin. Lab. Invest.* **10**, suppl. 36.

Man, E. B. & Gildea, E. F. (1932). *J. biol. Chem* **99**, 61.

Man, Y. K. & Wadsworth, G. R. (1969). *Clin. Sci.* **36**, 479.

Mancini, M., Mattock, M., Rabaya, E., Chait, A. & Lewis, B. (1973). *Atherosclerosis* **17**, 445.

Mann, G. V. (1977). *Atherosclerosis* **26**, 335.

Mann, J. I., Hockaday, T. D. R., Hockaday, J. M. & Turner, R. C. (1976). *Proc. Nutr. Soc.* **35**, 72A.

Mann, J. I. & Truswell, A. S. (1972). *Br. J. Nutr.* **27**, 395.

Mann, J. I. & Truswell, A. S. (1974). *Proc. Nutr. Soc.* **33**, 2A.

Mann, J. I., Truswell, A. S. & Pimstone, B. L. (1971). *Clin. Sci.* **41**, 123.

Mansford, K. R. L. (1967). *Proc. Nutr. Soc.* **26**, 27.

Manson, J. A. & Carpenter, K. J. (1974). *Proc. Nutr. Soc.* **33**, 103A.

Mariam, T. W. & Sterky, G. (1973). *J. Pediat*, **82**, 876.

Marine, D. (1924). *Medicine*, **3**, 453.

Marine, D. & Kimball, O. P. (1920). *Archs intern. Med.* **25**, 661.

Marine, D. & Lenhart, C. H. (1911). *J. exp. Med.* **13**, 455.

Marks, I. N. & Banks, S. (1965). In *Modern Treatment*, ed. Knight, W. A., vol. 2, p. 326. New York: Harper & Row.

Marliss, E. B., Aoki, T. T., Unger, R. H., Soeldner, J. S. & Cahill, G. F., Jr (1970). *J. clin. Invest.*, **49**, 2265.

Marr, J. W. (1971). *Wld Rev. Nutr. Diet.* **13**, 105.

Marr, J. W. (1973). *Proc. R. Soc. Med.* **66**, 639.

Marr, J. W. & Berry, W. T. C. (1974). *Nutrition, Lond.* **28**, 39.

Marrison, L. W. (1957). *Wines and Spirits*. Pelican Book A383. London: Penguin Books.

Marshall, D. H., Nordin, B. E. C. & Speed, R. (1976). *Proc. Nutr. Soc.* **35**, 163.

Marshall, W. A. (1977). *Human Growth and Its Disorders*. London: Academic Press.

Martin, C. J. & Robson, R. (1922). *Biochem. J.* **16**, 407.

Martin, J. (1978). *Infant Feeding 1975: Attitudes and Practices in England and Wales*. Office of Population Censuses and Surveys. HMSO.

Martinez-Torres, C. & Layrisse, M. (1971). *Am. J. clin. Nutr.* **25**, 531.

Masawe, A. E., Muindi, J. M. & Swai, G. B. R. (1974). *Lancet* **2**, 314.

Masefield, G. B. (1963). *Famine. Its Prevention and Relief*. Oxford Univ. Press.

Masefield, G. B. (1967). *FAO Nutrition Study* no. 21.

Masironi, R. (1970). *Bull. Wld Hlth Org.* **42**, 103.

Masironi, R., Miesch, A. T., Crawford, M. D. & Hamilton, E. I. (1973). *Bull. Pan Am. Hlth Org.* **7**, 53.

Mason, D. Y. & Emmerson, P. M. (1973). *Br. med. J.* **1**, 389.

Mason, E. D., Jacob, M. K. & Munkur, V. (1965). *Indian J. med. Res.* **53**, 309.

Mason, J. B., Gibson, N. & Kodicek, E. (1973). *Br. J. Nutr.* **30**, 297.

Mason, J. B., Hay, R. W., Leresche, J., Peel, S. & Darley, S. (1974). *Lancet* **1**, 332.

Masterton, T. P., Lewis, H. E. & Widdowson, E. M. (1957). *Br. J. Nutr.* **11**, 346.

Mathan, V. I. & Baker, S. J. (1968). *Am. J. clin. Nutr.* **21**, 1077.

Mathew, R., Rizvi, S. N. A., Rao, M. B. & Vaishnava, R. (1975). *J. Ass. Physns India* **23**, 871.

Matthew, D. J., Norman, A. P., Taylor, B., Turner, M. W. & Soothill, J. F. (1977). *Lancet* **1**, 321.

Matthews, D. M. (1975). *Physiol. Rev.* **55**, 537.

Matthews, J. D. (1975). *Lancet* **2**, 681.

Mawer, G. E. & Nixon, E. (1969). *Clin. Sci.* **36**, 463.

Mawes, E. B., Backhouse, J., Holman, C. A., Lumb, G. A. & Stanbury, S. W. (1972). *Clin. Sci.* **43**, 413.

Maxfield, E. & Konishi, F. (1966). *J. Am. Dietetic Ass.* **49**, 406.

Mayer, J. (1953). *New Engl. J. Med.* **249**, 13.

Mayer, J. (1966). *Science, N.Y.* **152**, 291.

Mayer, J. (1971). In *Famine*. Swedish Nutrition Foundation. Uppsala: Almqvuist and Wiksell.

Mayer, J. (1972). *Postgrad. Med.* **51**, 66.

Mayer, J. (ed.) (1973). *US Nutrition Policies in the Seventies*. Freeman: San Francisco.

Mayer, J. & Bullen, B. (1960). *Physiol. Rev.* **40**, 369.

Mayer, J. & Bullen, B. (1964). In *Proceedings of the Sixth International Congress of Nutrition*, ed. Mills, C. F. & Passmore, R., p. 27. Edinburgh: Livingstone.

Mayer, J., Marshall, N. B., Vitale, J. J., Christensen, J. H., Mashayekhi, M. B. & Stare, F. J. (1954). *Am. J. Physiol.* **177**, 544.

Mayer, J. & Sidel, W. (1966). *Christian Century*, **83**, 829.

Medical Boards of Finland, Norway and Sweden (1968). *Vår föda* **1**, 3.

Medical Research Council (1956). *Lancet* **1**, 901.

Medical Research Council (1965). *Lancet* **2**, 501.

Medical Research Council (1968). *Lancet* **2**, 693.

Medical Research Council (1970). Report by its Working Party on the relationship between dietary sugar intake and arterial disease. *Lancet* **2**, 1265.

Medvedev, Z. A. (1974). *Gerontologist*, **14**, 381.

Mehta, S., Kalsi, H. K., Jayaraman, S. & Mathur, V. S. (1975). *Am. J. clin. Nutr.* **28**, 977.

Mellanby, E. (1918). *J. Physiol. Lond.* **52**, xi, liii.

Mellanby, E. (1925). *Spec. Rep. Ser. med. Res. Coun. Lond.* No. 93.

Mellanby, E. (1934). *Nutrition and Disease*. Edinburgh: Oliver & Boyd.

Mellanby, E. (1950). A Story of Nutritional Research. Baltimore: Williams & Wilkins.

Mellanby, M. & Mellanby, H. (1954). *Br. med. J.* **2**, 944.

Mellander, O., Vahlquist, B. & Melebin, T. (1959). *Acta Paediat.* **48**, Suppl. 116.

Mellbin, T. & Vuille, J. C. (1973). *Br. J. prev. soc. Med.* **27**, 225.

Mendel, L. B. (1915). *J. Am. med. Ass.* **64**, 1539.

Mendelson, J. H. & Mello, N. K. (1973). *Science*, **180**, 1372.

Merskey, C. & Nossell, H. L. (1957). *Lancet* **1**, 806.

Merson, M. H., Baine, W. B., Gangarosa, E. J. & Swanson, R. C. (1974). *J. Am. med. Ass.* **288**, 1268.

Mertz, W. (1969). *Physiol. Rev.* **49**, 163.

Metropolitan Life Insurance Company (1960). *Statist. Bull.* 41 (Feb.) 6 (Mar.) 1.

Metz, J., Brandt, V. & Stevens, K. (1962). *Br. med. J.* **1**, 24.

Meulengracht, E. (1939). *Br. med. J.* **2**, 321.

Meyer, K. F. (1953). *New Engl. J. Med.* **249**, 843.

Meyer, S. & Calloway, D. H. (1977). *Cereal Chem.* **54,** 110.

M'Gonigle, G. M. C. & Kirby, J. (1936). *Poverty and Public Health.* London: Gollancz.

Miettinen, M., Karvonen, M. J., Turpeinen, O., Elosno, R. & Paavilainen, E. (1972a). *Lancet* **2,** 835.

Miettinen, M., Turpeinen, O., Karvonen, M. J., Elosno, R. & Paavilainen, E. (1972b). *Lancet* **2,** 1418.

Miettinen, M., Turpeinen, O., Karvonen, M. J., Elosno, R. & Paavilainen, E. (1973). *Lancet* **2,** 1267.

Millar, J. H. D., Zilka, K. J., Langman, H. L., Payling-Wright, H., Smith, A. D., Belin, J. & Thompson, R. H. S. (1973). *Br. med. J.* **1,** 768.

Miller, A. T. (1968). *Energy Metabolism.* Philadelphia: Davis.

Millis, J. (1952). *Med. J. Malaya,* **6,** 157.

Mills, A. R. (1974). In *Companion to Medical Studies,* ed. Passmore, R. & Robson, J. S., Vol. 3, Chap. 71. Oxford: Blackwell.

Mills, D. C. B (1970). *Symp. zool. Soc. Lond.* **27,** 99.

Milne, J. S., Lonergan, M. E., Williamson, J., Moore, F. M., McMaster, R. & Percy, N. (1971). *Br. med. J.* **2,** 383.

Milne, M. D., Crawford, M. A., Girdo, C. B. & Loughbridge, L. W. (1960). *Q. Jl Med.* **29,** 407.

Milner, R. D. G. (1970). *Mem. Soc. Endocr.* **18,** 191.

Ministry of Agriculture, Fisheries and Food (1970). *Manual of Nutrition.* London: HMSO.

Ministry of Agriculture, Government of Norway (1975). Norwegian Food and Nutritional Policy. White Paper no. 32 (1975–76). Oslo. (English edition available free of charge from the Ministry of Agriculture Government of Norway, Oslo-Dep., Oslo 1, Norway.)

Ministry of Health (1964). *Report of the Working Party on Irradiation of Food.* London: HMSO.

Ministry of Health (1968). *Rep. publ. Hlth med. Subj. Lond.* no. **117.**

Ministry of Health, Scottish Office (1962). *Rep. publ. Hlth med. Subj. Lond.* no. **105.**

Minot, G. R. & Murphy, W. P. (1926). *J. Am. med. Ass.* **87,** 470.

Mirski, A. (1942). *Biochem. J.* **36,** 232.

Mitchell, H. K., Snell, E. E. & Williams, R. J. (1941). *J. Am. chem. Soc.* **63,** 2284.

Mitchell, R. G. (1967). In *World Review of Nutrition and Dietetics,* ed. Bourne, G. H., vol. 8, p. 207. London: Pitman.

Mitra, K. (1941). *Indian J. med. Res.* **29,** 143.

Mitra, K. (1942). *Indian J. med. Res.* **30,** 91.

Modlin, M. (1967). *Ann. R. Coll. Surg. Engl.* **40,** 155.

Mohabbat, O., Srivasta, R. N., Younos, M. S., Sediq, G. C., Merzad, A. A. & Aram, G. N. (1976). *Lancet* **2,** 269.

Molenaar, I., Hulstaert, C. E., Vos, J. & Hommes, F. A. (1973). *Proc. Nutr. Soc.* **32,** 249.

Montgomery, R. D., Cruickshank, E. K., Robertson, W. B. & McMenemey, W. H. (1964). *Brain* **87,** 425.

Moore, C. V. (1961). *Harvey Lectures,* Series **55,** 67.

Moore, C. V. (1973). In *Modern Nutrition and Health and Disease,* 5th edn, ed. Goodhart, R. & Shils, M., p. 297. Philadelphia: Lea & Febiger.

Moore, F. D. (1959). *The Metabolic Care of the Surgical Patient.* Philadelphia: Saunders.

Moore Lappé, F. & Collins, J. (1977). *Food First.* Boston: Houghton Mifflin.

Moore, T. (1957). *Vitamin A.* New York: Elsevier.

Mordasini, R., Klose, G. & Greten, H. (1978). *Metabolism* **27,** 71.

Morgan, M. Y. & Sherlock, S. (1977). *Br. med. J.* **1,** 939.

Morgan, T., Adam, W., Gillies, A., Wilson, M., Morgan, G. & Carney, S. (1978). *Lancet* **1,** 227.

Morin, Y. L., Foley, A. R., Martineau, G. & Roussel, J. (1967). *Can. med. Ass. J:* **97,** 883.

Morley, D. (1973). *Paediatric Priorities in the Developing World.* London: Butterworth.

Morley, D. & Cutting, W. (1974). *Lancet* **1,** 711.

Morris, G. K. & Feeley, J. C. (1976). *Bull. Wld Hlth Org.* **54,** 79.

Morris, J. N. (1951). *Lancet* **1,** 1, 6.

Morris, J. N. (1975). *Uses of Epidemiology,* 3rd edn. Edinburgh: Churchill Livingstone.

Morris, J. N. & Crawford, M. D. (1958). *Br. med. J.* **2,** 1485.

Morris, J. N., Heady, J. A., Raffle, P. A. B., Roberts, C. G. & Parke, J. W. (1953). *Lancet* **2,** 1053, 1111.

Morris, J. N., Kagan, A., Pattison, D. C., Gardner, M. J. & Raffle, P. A. B. (1966). *Lancet* **2,** 5543.

Morris, J. N., Marr, J. W. & Clayton, D. G. (1977). *Br. med. J.* **2,** 1307.

Morris, J. N., Marr, J. W., Heady, J. A., Mills, G. L. & Pilkington, T. R. W. (1963). *Br. med. J.* **1,** 571.

Morrison, L. M. (1960). *J. Am. med. Ass.* **173,** 884.

Morton, I. D. (1977). In *Physical, Chemical and Biological Changes in Food Caused by Thermal Processing,* ed. Høyem, T. & Kvåle, O., p. 135. London: Applied Science.

Mourant, A. E., Tills, D. & Domaniewska-Sobczak, K. (1976). *Hum. Genet.* **33,** 307.

Moynahan, E. J. (1974). *Lancet* **2,** 399.

Muehrcke, R. C. (1956). *Br. med. J* **1,** 1327.

Muenter, M. D., Perry, H. O. & Ludwig, J. (1971). *Am. J. Med.* **50,** 129.

Muller, D. P., Lloyd, J. K. & Bird, A. C. (1977). *Archs Dis. Childh.* **52,** 209.

Müller, E. A. & Franz, H. (1952). *Arbeitsphysiologie* **14,** 499.

Munro, H. N. (1976). In *Fat Content and Composition of Animal Products,* p. 24. Washington, D.C.: National Academy of Sciences.

Munro, H. N. & Allison, J. B. (1964). *Mammalian Protein Metabolism*. New York: Academic Press.

Munro, H. N., Fenstrom, J. D. & Wurtman, R. J. (1975). *Lancet* **1**, 722.

Murphy, E. L. (1975). In *Nutritional Improvement of Food Legumes by Breeding. PAG Symposium*. ed. Milner, M. New York: Wiley.

Murphy, E. W., Willis, B. W. & Watt, B. K. (1975). *J. Am. diet. Assn* **66**, 345.

Murphy, K. J. (1971). *Med. J. Aust.* **1**, 1119.

Murray, M. J., Murray, A., Murray, N. J. & Murray, M. B. (1978). *Am. J. clin. Nutr.* **31**, 57.

Murray, M. M., Ryle, J. A., Simpson, B. W. & Wilson, D. C. (1948). *MRC Memo.* no. 18.

Murthy, H. B. N., Reddy, S. K., Swaminathan, M. & Subrahmanyan, V. (1955). *Br. J. Nutr.* **9**, 203.

Mustafa, K. Y., Mahmoud, N. A., Gumaa, K. A. & Gader, A. M. A. *Br. J. Nutr.* **40**, 583.

Mylotte, M., Egan-Mitchel, B., McCarthy, C. F. & McNicholl, B. (1973). *Br. med. J.* **1**, 703.

Nagarajan, V. (1971). In *A Decade of Progress, 1961-70*, p. 23. New Delhi: Indian Council of Medical Research.

Naismith, D. J. (1973). *Nutr. Rep. Int.* **7**, 383.

Naismith, D. J. (1977). In *Scientific Foundations of Obstetrics and Gynaecology*, ed. Philipp, E. E., Barnes, J. & Newton, M. London: Heinemann.

Naismith, D. J. & Ritchie, C. D. (1975). *Proc. Nutr. Soc.* **34**, 116$_A$.

Nakagawa, I. Ohguri, S., Sasaki, A., Kajimoto, M., Sasaki, M. & Takahashi, T. (1975). *J. Nutr.* **105**, 1241.

Narang, R. K., Mehta, S. & Mathur, V. S. (1977). *Am. J. clin. Nutr.* **30**, 1979.

National Research Council (1943). Recommended Dietary Allowances. *NRC Reprint and Circular Series* no. 115. Washington, D.C.

Neale, G., Antcliff, A. C., Wellbourn, R. B., Mollin, D. L. & Booth, C. C. (1967). *Q. Jl Med.* **36**, 469.

Neel, J. V. (1962). *Am. J. hum. Genet.* **14**, 353.

Nelson, J. W. (1952). *Trans. R. Soc. trop. Med. Hyg.* **46**, 538.

Nelson, W. E. (1971). *Textbook of Pediatrics*, 9th edn. Philadelphia: Saunders.

Nestel, P. J., Havenstein, N., Whyte, H. M., Scott, T. J. & Cook, L. J. (1973). *New Engl. J. Med.* **288**, 379.

Nesterov, A. I. (1964). *Arthritis Rheum.* **7**, 29.

Newey, H. & Smyth, D. H. (1967). *Proc. Nutr. Soc.* **26**, 5.

Nicholls, A. & Scott, J. T. (1972). *Lancet* **2**, 1223.

Nicholls, L. & Nimalasuriya, A. (1939). *J. Nutr.* **18**, 385.

Nicol, B. M. (1949). *Br. J. Nutr.* **3**, 25.

Nicol, B. M. (1952). *Br. J. Nutr.* **6**, 34.

Nicol, B. M. (1956). *Br. J. Nutr.* **10**, 275.

Nicol, B. M. (1953). *Proc. Nutr. Soc.* **12**, 66.

Nielsen, F. H., Giraud, S. H. & Myron, D. R. (1975). *Fedn Proc. Fedn Am. Socs exp. Biol.* **34**, 923.

Nikkilä, E. A. (1974). *Proc. R. Soc. Med.* **67**, 662.

Nikkilä, E. A. & Aro, A. (1973). *Lancet* **1**, 954.

Nisenson, A. (1964). *Pediatrics* **44**, 1014.

Nobbs, B. J. (1974). *Lancet* **1**, 405.

Nordin, B. E. C. (1966). *Clin. Orthop.* **45**, 17.

Nordin, B. E. C. (1971). *Br. med. J.* **1**, 571.

Nordin, B. E. C. (1976). *Calcium, Phosphorus and Magnesium Metabolism*. Edinburgh: Churchill Livingstone.

Nordøy, A. (1976). *Thrombosis and Haemostasis* **35**, 32.

Norris, A. H., Lundy, T. & Shock, N. W. (1963). *Ann. N.Y. Acad. Sci.* **110**, 623.

Norum, K. R., Børsting, S. & Grundt, I. (1970). *Acta med. scand.* **188**, 323.

Nutrition Society (1954). Symposium on The Provisioning of Expeditions in the Field. *Proc. Nutr. Soc.* **13**, 41.

Nutrition Today (1972). **7**, March/April, p. 2.

Nutritional Research Laboratories, Hyderabad (1968). *Annual Report, 1966-1967*. Delhi: Indian Council of Medical Research.

Oakley, W. G., Pyke, D. A. & Taylor, K. W. (1974). *Clinical Diabetes and Its Biochemical Basis*, 2nd edn. Oxford: Blackwell.

O'Brien, D. (1974). In *Companion to Medical Studies*, ed. Passmore, R. & Robson, J. S., vol. 3, chap. 46. Oxford: Blackwell.

O'Brien, J. R., Etherington, M. D., Jamieson, S., Vergroesen, A. J., ten Hoor, F. (1976). *Lancet* **2**, 995.

Office of Health Economics (1968). Paper no. 26. *Old Age*. 162 Regent Street, London.

Ogryzlo, M. A. (1965). *Arthritis Rheum.* **8**, 799.

Okungbowa, P., Ma, M. C. F. & Truswell, A. S. (1976). *Proc. Nutr. Soc.* **36**, 26$_A$.

Olson, J. A. & Lakshmanan (1970). In *The Fat Soluble Vitamins*, ed. De Luca, H. F. & Suttie, J. W., p. 213. University of Wisconsin Press.

Oomen, H. A. P. C. (1958). *Fedn Proc. Fedn Am. Socs exp. Biol.* **17**, suppl. 2, iv.

Oomen, H. A. P. C. (1969). *Am. J. clin. Nutr.* **22**, 1098.

Oomen, H. A. P. C. & Grubber, G. J. H. (1977). *Tropical Leaf Vegetables in Human Nutrition*. Amsterdam: Koniuklijk Instituut voor de Tropen.

Oomen, H. A. P. C., McLaren, D. S. & Escapini, H. (1964). *Trop. geogr. Med.* **16**, 271.

Opie, L. H. & Walfish, P. G. (1963). *New Engl. J. Med.* **268**, 757.

Orr, E. (1977). *Fd Nutr. (FAO)* **3**, 2.

Orr, J. B. (1936). *Food, Health and Income*. London: Macmillan.

Orr, J. B. & Gilks, J. L. (1931). *Spec. Rep. Ser. med. Res. Coun. Lond.* No. **155**.

Orr, M. L. & Watt, B. K. (1957). *Amino Acid Content to Foods*. Home Economics Research Report, no. 4. Washington.

Osborne, T. B. & Mendel, L. B. (1913). *J. biol. Chem.* **15**, 311.

Osuntokun, B. O. (1968). *Brain* **91**, 215.

Osuntokun, B. O., Durowoju, J. E., McFarlane, H. & Wilson, J. (1968). *Br. med. J.* **2**, 647.

Osuntokun, B. O., Monekosso, G. L. & Wilson, J. (1969). *Br. med. J.* **1**, 547.

Ouellette, E. M., Rosett, H. L., Rosman, N. P. & Weiner, L. (1977). *New Engl. J. Med.* **297**, 528.

Owen, O. E. Morgan, A. P., Kemp, H. G., Sullivan, J. M., Herrera, M. G. & Cahill, C. F. (1967). *J. clin. Invest.* **46**, 1589.

Owen, O. E. & Reichard, G. A. (1975). *Israeli J. med. Sci.* **11**, 560.

PAG (1974). *PAG Bull.* **4**, 17.

Painter, N. S., Almeida, A. Z. & Colebourne, K. W. (1972). *Br. med. J.* **2**, 137.

Painter, N. S. & Burkitt, D. P. (1971). *Br. med. J.* **2**, 450.

Palmer, J. K. (1971). In *The Biochemistry of Fruits and their Products*, ed. Hulme, A. C., vol. 2., p. 65. New York: Academic Press.

Panel on Composition and Nutritive Value of Flour (1956). *Report of the Panel on Composition and Nutritive Value of Flour*. Cmd. 9757. London: HMSO.

Parfitt, A. M., Higgins, B. A., Nassim, J. R., Collins, J. A. & Hilb, A. (1964). *Clin. Sci.* **27**, 463.

Pařísková, J. (1977). *Body Fat Physical Fitness*. The Hague: Martinus Nijhoff.

Pařísková, J. & Rogozkin, V. A. (1978). *Nutrition, Fitness and Health*. Baltimore: Univ. Press.

Parsons, D. S. (1967). *Proc. Nutr. Soc.* **26**, 47.

Parsons, F. M., Edwards, G. F., Anderson, C. K., Ahmad, S., Clark, P. B., Hetherington, C. & Young, G. A. (1974). *Lancet* **1**, 243.

Passmore, R. (1951). *Lancet* **2**, 303.

Passmore, R. (1953). *Lancet* **1**, 638.

Passmore, R. (1961). *Nutr. Dieta* **3**, 1.

Passmore, R. & Draper, M. H. (1970). In *Biochemical Disorders in Human Disease*, 3rd edn, ed. Thompson, R. H. S. & Wootton, I. D. P. London: Churchill.

Passmore, R. & Durnin, J. V. G. A. (1955). *Physiol. Rev.* **35**, 801.

Passmore, R., Hollingsworth, D. H. & Robertson, J. (1979). *Br. med. J.* **1**, 527.

Passmore, R., Meiklejohn, A. P., Dewar, A. D. & Thow, R. K. (1955a). *Br. J. Nutr.* **9**, 27.

Passmore, R., Meiklejohn, A. P., Dewar, A. D. & Thow, R. K. (1955b). *Br. J. Nutr.* **9**, 20.

Passmore, R., Nicol, B. M., Rao, M. N., Beaton, G. H. & De Maeyer, E. M. (1974). *Handbook on Human Nutritional Requirements*. FAO Nutritional Studies no. 28. Rome: FAO.

Passmore, R. & Ritchie, F. J. (1957). *Br. J. Nutr.* **11**, 79.

Passmore, R. & Robson, J. S. (eds) (1974). *A Companion to Medical Studies*, vol. 3, 12, 37, Edinburgh: Blackwell.

Passmore, R. & Swindells, Y. E. (1963). *Br. J. Nutr.* **17**, 331.

Passmore, R., Thomson, J. G. & Warnock, G. M. (1952). *Br. J. Nutr.* **6**, 253.

Patwardhan, V. N. (1952). *Nutrition in India*. Bombay: Hind Kitabs.

Paul, A. A. & Southgate, D. A. T. (1978). *The Composition of Foods*. London: HMSO.

Paul, O., Lepper, M. H., Phelan, W. H., Dupertuis, G. W., MacMillan, A., McKean, H. & Park, H. (1963). *Circulation* **28**, 20.

Pauling, L. (1974). *Am. J. Psychiat.* **131**, 1251.

Pauling, L. (1976). *Vitamin C, the Common Cold and the 'Flu*. San Francisco: Freeman.

Paulsrud, J. R., Pensler, L., Whitten, C. F., Stewart, S. & Holman, R. T. (1972). *Am. J. clin. Nutr.* **25**, 897.

Pawan, G. L. S. (1973). *Proc. Nutr. Soc.* **32**, 15A.

Payne, P. R. & Waterlow, J. C. (1971). *Lancet* **2**, 210.

Peacock, M., Knowles, F. & Nordin, B. E. C. (1968). *Br. med. J.* **2**, 729.

Pearce, M. L. & Dayton, S. (1971). *Lancet* **1**, 464.

Peers, F. G. & Linsell, C. A. (1973). *Br. J. Cancer*, **27**, 473.

Pell, S. & D'Alonzo, C. A. (1970). *J. Am. med. Ass.* **214**, 1833.

Pelletier, O. & Brassard, R. (1977). *Am. J. clin. Nutr.* **30**, 21.

Pendreigh, D. M., Heasman, M. A., Howith, M. F., Kennedy, A. C., MacDougall, A. I., MacLeod, M., Robson, J. S. & Stewart, D. K. (1972). *Lancet* **1**, 304.

Penick, S. B. & Stunkard, A. J. (1970). *Med. Clins N. Am.* **54**, 745.

Péquignot, G. (1962). *Münchner med. Wschr.* **103**, 1464.

Peraita, M. (1942). *Arch. Psychiat. Nervenkr.* **114**, 611.

Perez, C., Scrimshaw, N. S. & Muñoz, J. A. (1960). In *Endemic Goitre*. WHO Monograph Series no. 44. Geneva: WHO.

Perheentupa, J. & Paivio, K. (1967). **2**, 528.

Périssé, J., Sizaret, F. & François, P. (1969). *FAO Nutr., Newsl.*, **7**, 1.

Perkins, E. G. (1960). *Fd Technol.* **14**, 508.

Perley, M. & Kipnis, D. M. (1966). *New Engl. J. Med.* **274**, 1237.

Perryman, J. (1973). In *US Nutrition Policies in the Seventies*, ed. Mayer, J., p., 216. San Francisco: Freeman.

Peters, H. A. (1976). *Fedn Proc. Fedn Am. Socs exp. Biol* **36**, 2400.

Peters, J. P. & van Slyke, D. D. (1932). *Quantitative Clinical Chemistry*. vol. 2, p. 665. Baltimore: Williams & Wilkins.

Peters, R. A. (1963). *Biochemical Lesions and Lethal Synthesis*. Oxford: Pergamon Press.

Phansalkar, S. V. & Patwardhan, V. N. (1955). *Indian J. med. Res.* **43**, 265.

Pharoah, P. O. D., Buttfield, I. H. & Hetzel, B. S. (1971). *Lancet* **1**, 308.

Phillips, W. E. J., Murray, T. K. & Campbell, J. S. (1970). *Can. med. Ass. J.* **102**, 1085.

Phoon, W. H. & Pincherle, G. (1972). *Br. J. ind. Med.* **29**, 334.

Pickering, G. W. (1968). *High Blood Pressure*. London: Churchill.

Pickering, G. W., Roberts, J. A. F. & Sowry, G. S. C. (1954). *Clin. Sci.* **13**, 267.

Picou, E., Halliday, D. & Garrow, J. S. (1966). *Clin. Sci.* **30**. 345.

Pierce, N. F. & Hirschorn, N. (1977). *WHO Chron.* **31**, 87.

Pimstone, B. L., Wittman, W., Hansen, J. D. L. & Murray, P. (1966). *Lancet* **2**, 799.

Pingle, U. & Ramasastri, B. V. (1978). *Br. J. Nutr.* **39**, 119.

Pinter, K. G., McCracken, B. H., Lamar, C. & Goldsmith, G. A. (1964). *Am. J. clin. Nutr.* **15**, 293.

Pirie, N. W. (1962). *Jl R. statist. Soc.* A **125**, 399.

Pirie, N. W. (1975). *Nature, Lond.* **253**, 239.

Plagnol. H. & Dutrenit, J. (1956). *Méd. trop.* **16**, 690.

Platt, B. S. (1964). *Rep. publ. Hlth med. Subj. Lond.* no. 111. Ministry of Health.

Platt, B. S., Eddy, T. P. & Pellett, P. L. (1963). *Food in Hospitals*. Oxford Univ. Press.

Platt, B. S. & Lu, G. D. (1936). *Q. Jl. Med.* **5**, 355.

Politzer, W. M. & Schneider, T. (1962). *S. Afr. med. J.* **36**, 608.

Pongpanich, B., Srikrikkich, N., Dhanamitta, S. & Valyasevi, A. (1974). *Am. J. clin. Nutr.* **27**, 1399.

Popkin, J. S., Clow, C. L. Scriver, C. R. & Grove, J. (1974). *Lancet* **1**, 721.

Pories, W. J., Hanzel, J. H., Rob, C. G. & Strain, W. H. (1967). *Ann. Surg.* **165**, 432.

Porter, A. (1889). *The Diseases of the Madras Famine, 1877-78*. Madras: Government Press.

Poskitt, E. M. E. & Cole, T. J. (1977). *Br. med. J.* **1**, 7.

Poskitt, E. M. F. & Parkin, J. M. (1972). *Archs Dis. Childh.* **47**, 626.

Postmus, S. (1958). *Trop. geogr. Med.* **10**, 363.

Prasad, A. S. D., Miale, A., Farid, Z., Stanstead, H. H. & Shubert A. R. (1963). *J. Lab. clin. Med.* **61**, 537.

Preece, M. A. & 8 others (1975). *Q. Jl Med.* **44**, 575.

Press, M., Kikuchi, H., Shimoyama, T. & Thompson, G. R. (1974). *Br. med. J.* **2**, 247.

Price Evans, D. A. (1973). *Lancet* **2**, 1096.

Pringle, J. M. D. (1947). *Listener* **38**, 245.

Prinsloo, J. G., du Plessis, J. P., Kruger, H., de Lange, D. J. & de Villiers, L. S. (1968). *Am. J. clin. Nutr.* **21**, 98.

Prinsloo, J. G. & Kruger, H. (1970). *S. Afr. med. J.* **44**, 49.

Priola, R. C. & Lieber, C. S. (1976). *Am. J. clin. Nutr.* **29**, 90.

Prior, I. A. M. (1972). *Nutrition Today* **6**, 2.

Provis, H. S. & Ellis, R. W. B. (1955). *Archs Dis. Childh.* **30**, 328.

Pugh, G. & Ward, M. (1953). In *The Ascent of Everest*, p. 275, Hunt, Sir John. London: Hodder & Stoughton.

Pugh, L. G. C. (1958). *J. Physiol. Lond.* **141**, 233.

Purvis, R. J. & 6 others (1973). *Lancet* **2**, 811.

Pyke, M. (1970). In *Food Cultism and Nutritional Quackery*. Swedish Nutrition Foundation Symposium no. 8.

Pyke, M. (1971). *Food and Society*, p. 102. London: Murray.

Quaade, F. (1974). *Lancet* **1**, 267.

Quackenbush, F. W., Finch, J. G., Rabourn, W. J., McQuistan, M., Petzold, E. N. & Kargl, T. E. (1961). *Agric. food Chem.* **9**, 132.

Rab, S. & Baseer, A. (1976). *Lancet* **2**, 1211.

Rabinowich, I. M. (1935). *Can. med. Ass. J.* **33**, 136.

Rabinowitz, D. & Zierler, K. L. (1961). *Lancet* **2**, 690.

Rabinowitz, D. & Zierler, K. L. (1962). *J. clin. Invest.* **41**, 2173.

Raica, N. J., Scott, J., Lowry, L. & Sauberlich, H. E. (1972). *Am. J. clin. Nutr.* **25**, 291.

Rajalakshmi, R., Ali, S. Z. & Ramakrishnan, C. V. (1967). *J. Neurochem.* **14**, 29.

Rajalakshmi, R., Deodhar, A. D. & Ramakrishnan, C. V. (1965a). *Acta paediat., Stockh.* **54**, 375.

Rajalakshmi, R., Govindarajan, K. R. & Ramakrishnan, C. V. (1965b). *J. Neurochem.* **12**, 261.

Ramalingaswami, V. (1972). quoted *Lancet* **2**, 1132.

Ramalingaswami, V., Do, M. G. Guleria, J. S., Malhotra, K. K., Soud, S. K., Prakash, O. M. & Sinah, R. V. N. (1971). In *Famine. Symposia of the Swedish Nutrition Foundation* no. 9.

Ramalingaswami, V. & Nayak, N. C. (1970). *Progress in Liver Disease*, **3**, 222.

Ramsbottom, J. (1953). *Proc. Nutr. Soc.* **12**, 39.

Rand, W. M., Scrimshaw, N. S. & Young, V. R. (1977). *Am. J. clin. Nutr.* **30**, 1129.

Randle, P. J., Garland, P. B., Newsholme, E. A. & Hales, C. N. (1965). *Ann. N.Y. Acad. Sci.* **131**, 324.

Randle, P. J., Garland, P. B., Hales, C. N. & Newsholme, E. A. (1963). *Lancet* **1**, 785.

Rao, K. S. J., Srikantia, S. G. & Gopalan, C. (1969). *Archs Dis. Childh.* **43**, 365.

Raoult, A., Thomas, J., Thiery, G., Perrin, G. & Perrellon, G. (1957). *Bull. méd. Afr. occid. fr.* (N.S.). **2**, 5.

Räsänen, L., Wilska, M., Kautero, R. L., Näntö, V., Ahlström, A. & Hallman, N. (1978). *Am. J. clin. Nutr.* **31**, 1050.

Ravi Subbiah, M. T. (1971). *Mayo Clin. Proc.* **46**, 549.

Redgrave, T. G. (1970). *J. clin. Invest.* **49**, 465.

Reh, E. (1962). Manual on Household Food Consumption Surveys. *Nutritional Studies*, no. 18. Rome: FAO.

Reinhold, J. G. Nasr, K., Lahimgarzadeh, A. & Heydayati, H. (1973). *Lancet* **1**, 283.

Reizenstein, P. G., Matthews, C. M. E. & Ek, G. (1964). In *Proceedings of the Sixth International Congress of Nutrition*, ed. Mills, C. F. & Passmore, R., p. 416. Edinburgh: Livingstone.

Renaud, S., Kinlough, R. L. & Mustard, J. F. (1970). *Lab. Invest,* **22**, 339.

Renold, A. E. & Cahill, G. F. (1965). *Adipose Tissue*. Washington: American Physiological Society.

Renwick, J. H. (1972). *Br. J. prev. soc. Med.* **26**, 67.

Reynolds, E. H. (1973). *Lancet* **1**, 1376.

Rhodes, J. (1972). *Gastroenterology* **63**, 171.

Richards, J. R. & Kinney, J. M. (ed.) (1977). *Nutritional Aspects of Care in the Critically Ill.* Edinburgh: Churchill Livingstone.

Richards, P., Metcalfe-Gibson, A., Ward, E. E., Wrong, O. & Houghton, B. J. (1967). *Lancet* **2**, 845.

Rickes, E. L., Brink, N. G., Koniuszy, F. R., Wood, T. R. & Folkers, K. (1948). *Science, N.Y.* **107**, 396.

Ricketts, H. T. (1970). *Diabetes* **19**, suppl. 2, iii.

Rietz, P., Gloor, U. & Wiss, O. (1970). *Int. Z. Vitaminforsch.* **40**, 351.

Rietz, P., Wiss, O. & Weber, F. (1974). *Vitams Horm.* **32**, 237.

Rifkind, B. M. & Gale, M. (1967). *Lancet* **2**, 640.

Ringer, K. (1977). *Am. J. pub. Hlth* **67**, 550.

Rinzler, S. H. (1968). *Bull. N.Y. Acad. Med.* **44**, 936.

Rissanen, V. & Pyörälä, K. (1974). *Atherosclerosis* **19**, 221.

Ritchie, Jean A. S. (1971). *Learning Better Nutrition.* FAO Nutritional Studies no. 20, Rome: FAO.

Ritzel, G. (1961). *Helv. med. Acta* **28**, 63.

Rivers, J. & Yudkin, J. (1972). *Lancet* **2**, 1026.

Rivlin, R. S. (ed.) (1975). *Riboflavin.* New York and London: Plenum Press.

Robboy, M. S., Sato, A. S. & Schwabe, A. D. (1974). *Am. J. clin. Nutr.* **27**, 362.

Roberts, W. C., Levy, R. I. & Fredrickson, D. S. (1970). *Archs Path.* **90**, 46.

Robertson, W. G., Gallagher, J. C., Marshall, D. H., Peacock, M. & Nordin, B. E. C. (1974). *Br. med. J.* **4**, 436.

Robertson, W. G., Peacock, M. & Nordin, B. E. C. (1969). *Lancet* **2**, 21.

Robinson, D. S. (1955a). In *Adipose Tissue,* ed. Renold, A. E. & Cahill, G. F., p. 295. Washington: American Physiological Society.

Robinson, D. S. (1955b). *Q. Jl exp. Physiol.* **40**, 112.

Robinson, M. (1958). *Lancet* **1**, 178.

Robinson, M. F. (1976). *J. hum. Nutr.* **30**, 79.

Robinson, M. F. & Watson, P. E. (1965). *Br. J. Nutr.* **19**, 225.

Robinson, Marion F., McKenzie, Joan M., Thompson, Christine P. & Van Rij, Anita L. (1973). *Br. J. Nutr.,* **30**, 195.

Robson, J. R. K., Larkin, F. A., Sandretto, A. M. & Tadayyon, B. (1972). *Malnutrition. Its Causation and Control* (with special reference to protein calorie malnutrition), vol. 2, p. 349. New York & London: Gordon & Breach.

Rodahl, K. & Moore, T. (1943). *Biochem. J.* **37**, 166.

Rodger, F. C. (1952). *Archs Ophthal. N.Y.* **47**, 570.

Rodger, F. C., Saiduzzafar, H., Grover, A. D. & Fazal, A. (1963). *Br. J. Nutr.* **17**, 475.

Rodriquez, M. S. & Irwin, M. (1972). *J. Nutr.* **102**, 909.

Roe, D. A. (1971). *N.Y. St. J. Med.* **2**, 770.

Roe, D. A. (1973). *A Plague of Corn: The Social History of Pellagra.* Ithaca & London: Cornell University Press.

Roholm, K. (1973). *Fluorine Intoxication.* London: H.K. Lewis.

Rose, C. S. & 8 others (1976). *Am. J. clin. Nutr.* **29**, 847.

Rose, G. A., Thomson, W. B. & Williams, R. T. (1965). *Br. med. J.* **1**, 1531.

Rose, G. & 7 others (1974). *Lancet* **1**, 181.

Rose, K. (1959). *Proc. Nutr. Soc.* **18**, 162.

Rose, W. C., Wixom, R. L., Lockhart, H. B. & Lambert, G. F. (1955). *J. biol. Chem.* **217**, 987.

Rosengarten, F., Jr (1969). *The Book of Spices.* Philadelphia: Livingstone.

Rosenheim, O. & Drummond, J. C. (1920). *Lancet* **1**, 862.

Ross, M. H. (1976). In *Nutrition and Ageing,* ed. Winick, M. New York: Wiley.

Rosso, P., Hormazabal, J. & Winick, M. (1970). *Am. J. clin. Nutr.* **23**, 1275.

Rothman, K. J., Glass, R. L., Espinal, F., Velez, H. & Maija, R. (1972). *J. dent. Res.* **51**, 1686.

Rotter, J. I., Rimoin, D. L., Gursky, M. S., Terasaki, P. & Sturdevant, R. A. L. (1977). *Gastroenterology* **73**, 438.

Rowland, M. G. M., Cole, T. J. & Whitehead, R. G. (1977). *Br. J. Nutr.* **37**, 441.

Roy, R. (1976). *Wastage in the UK Food System.* London: Earth Resources Ltd.

Royal College of Physicians (1976). *Fluoride, Teeth and Health.* London: Pitman.

Royal Society (1972). *Metric Units, Conversion Factors and Nomenclature in Nutritional and Food Sciences.* London.

Rubin, E. & Lieber, C. S. (1968). *New Engl. J. Med.* **278,** 869.

Rubin, E. & Lieber, C. S. (1974). *New Engl. J. Med.* **290,** 128.

Ruck, N. (1973). *Proc. Nutr. Soc.* **33,** 17A.

Ruddell, W. S. J., Bone, E. S., Hill, M. J. & Walters, C. L. (1978). *Lancet* **1,** 521.

Ruderman, N. B. (1975). *A. Rev. Med.* **126,** 245.

Ruffin, J. M. & Smith, D. T. (1934). *Am. J. med. Sci.* **187,** 512.

Rugg-Gunn, A. J., Edgar, W. M., Geddes, D. A. M. & Jenkins, G. N. (1975). *Br. dent. J.* **139,** 351.

Runcie, J. & Thomson, T. J. (1970). *Br. med. J.* **3,** 432.

Russell, G. F. M. (1967). *J. psychosom. Res.* **11,** 141.

Russell, G. F. M. (1970). In *Modern Trends in Psychological Medicine,* No. 2, ed. Price, J. H., p. 131. London: Butterworth.

Saarni, M., Palva, I. & Ahrenberg, P. (1977). *Lancet* **1,** 806.

Sabry, Z. I., Campbell, J. A., Campbell, M. E. & Forbes, A. L. (1974). *Nutrition Today,* **9,** Jan/Feb, 5.

Salaman, R. N. (1948). *History and Social Influence of the Potato.* Cambridge Univ. Press.

Salcedo, J., Bamba, M. D., Carasco, E. O., Jose, F. R. & Valenzuela, R. C. (1948). *J. Philipp. med. Ass.* **25,** 519.

Salen, G., Ahrens, E. H., Jr & Grundy, S. M. (1970). *J. Lipid Res.* **10,** 304.

Salens, L. B., Knittle, J. L. & Hirsh, J. (1968). *J. clin. Invest.* **47,** 153.

Saltin, B. & Hermansen, L. (1967). In *Nutrition and Physical Activity,* ed. Blix, G. Uppsala: Almqvist & Wiksell.

Sampliner, R. E., Bennett, P. H., Comess, L. J., Rose, F. A. & Burch, T. A. (1970). *New Engl. J. Med.* **283,** 1358.

Sanger, F. (1964). The chemistry of insulin. In *Nobel Lectures. Chemistry. 1942-1962,* pp. 544-556. Amsterdam: Elsevier.

Sargeant, K., Allcroft, R. & Carnagham, R. B. A. (1961). *Vet. Rec.* **73,** 865.

Sarkar, S. N. (1948). *Nature, Lond.* **162,** 265.

Sauberlich, H. E., Skala, J. H. & Dowdy, R. P. (1974). *Laboratory Tests for the Assessment of Nutritional Status.* Cleveland, Ohio: CRC Press.

Saunders, S. J., Barbezat, G. O., Wittmann, W. &

Hansen, J. D. L. (1967a). *Am. J. clin. Nutr.* **20,** 760.

Saunders, S. J., Truswell, A. S., Barbezat, G. O., Wittman, W. & Hansen, J. D. L. (1967b). *Lancet* **2,** 795.

Schachter, S. (1968). *Science, N.Y.* **161,** 751.

Scheinen, A., Mäkinen, K. K. & Ylitalo, K. (1974). *Acta odontol. scand.* **32,** 383.

Schlierf, G., Stossberg, V. & Reinheimer, W. (1971). *Nutr. Metabol.* **13,** 80.

Schmitt, W. R. (1965). *Ann. N.Y. Acad. Sci.* **118,** 645.

Schneider, H. A. (1946). *Vitams Horm.* **4,** 35.

Schoub, B. D., Prozesky, O. W., Lecatsas, G. & Oosthuizen, R. (1978). *J. med. Microbiol.* **11,** 25.

Schrager, J. & Oates, M. D. G. (1978). *Br. med. Bull.* **34,** 79.

Schreibman, P. H., Wilson, D. E. & Arky, R. A. (1969). *New Engl. J. Med.* **281,** 981.

Schrire, V. (1966). *Clinical Cardiology,* 2nd edn. London: Staples Press.

Schroeder, H. A. (1965). *J. chron. Dis.* **18,** 217.

Schroeder, H. A. (1971). *Am. J. clin. Nutr.* **24,** 562.

Schulze, A. & Truswell, A. S. (1977). *Proc. Nutr. Soc.* **36,** 25A.

Schwartz, K. & Milne, D. B. (1972). *Bioinorganic Chemistry* **1,** 331.

Schwarz, K. & Foltz, C. M. (1957). *J. Am. chem. Soc.* **79,** 3292.

Scott, D. (1958). *Acta med. scand.* **162,** 69.

Scrimshaw, N. S. (1975). In *Protein-Calorie Malnutrition,* ed. Olson, R. E. New York: Academic Press.

Scrimshaw, N. S. (1976). *New Engl. J. Med.* **294,** 136, 198.

Scrimshaw, N. S., Taylor, C. E. & Gordon, J. E. (1968). *Interactions of Nutrition and Infection.* WHO Monograph series, no. 57.

Scriver, C. R. (1967). *Am. J. Dis. Child.* **113,** 109.

Scriver, C. R. (1973). *Metabolism* **22,** 1253.

Scriver, C. R., Mackenzie, S., Clow, C. L. & Delvin, E. (1971). *Lancet* **1,** 310.

Scriver, C. R. & Rosenberg, L. E. (1973). *Amino Acid Metabolism and Its Disorders.* Philadelphia & London: Saunders.

Sebrell, W. H. & Butler, R. E. (1938). *Pub. Hlth Rep. Wash.* **53,** 2282.

Seftel, H. C., Malkin, C., Schamaman, A., Abrahams, C., Lynch, S. R., Charlton, R. W. & Bothwell, T. H. (1966). *Br. med. J.* **1,** 642.

Seldin, D. W. & Wilson, J. D. (1966). In *The Metabolic Basis of Inherited Disease,* 2nd edn, ed. Stanbury, J. B., Wyngaarden, J. B. & Fredrickson, D. S., p. 1230. New York: Blakiston.

Select Committee on Nutrition and Human Needs, US Senate (1977). *Dietary Goals for the United States,*

2nd edn. Washington, D.C.: US Government Printing Office.

Sellmeyer, E., Bhettay, E., Truswell, A. S., Meyers, O. L. & Hansen, J. D. L. (1972). *Archs Dis. Childh.* **47**, 429.

Seltzer, H. S., Allen, E. W., Herron, A. L., Jr & Brennan, M. L. (1967). *J. clin. Invest.* **46**, 323.

Selzer, C. C. & Mayer, J. (1965). *Postgrad. Med.* **38**, A101.

Shah, D. R. & Singh, S. V. (1967). *J. Ass. Physns India,* **15**, 1.

Shakir, A. & Morley, D. (1974). *Lancet* **1**, 758.

Sharman, I. M., Down, M. G. & Norgan, N. G. (1976). *J. sports Med.* **16**, 215.

Sharman, I. M., Down, M. G. & Sen, R. N. (1971). *Br. J. Nutr.* **26**, 265.

Shaw, J. H. & Sweeney, E. A. (1973). In *Modern Nutrition in Health and Disease,* 5th edn, ed. Goodhart, R. S. & Shils, M. E. Philadelphia: Lea & Febiger.

Shearman, D. J. C. (1978). *Br. med. J.* **1**, 283.

Shearman, D. J. C., Delamore, I. W. & Gardner, D. L. (1966). *Lancet* **1**, 845.

Sheldon, J. H. (1927). *Q. Jl Med.* **21**, 123.

Sherman, H. C. (1920a). *J. biol. Chem.* **41**, 97.

Sherman, H. C. (1920b). *J. biol. Chem.* **44**, 21.

Sherman, H. C. (1941). *Chemistry of Food and Nutrition,* 6th edn, p. 253. New York: Macmillan.

Shils, M. (1973). In *Modern Nutrition in Health and Disease,* ed. Goodhart, R. & Shils, M. Philadelphia: Lea & Febiger.

Shils, M. E. (1976). In *Nutrition Reviews' Present Knowledge in Nutrition,* 4th edn, p. 247. New York: Nutrition Foundation.

Shimazono, N. (1973). *Bibl. Nutr. & Dieta* no. 18, p. 267.

Shorland, F. B., Czochanska, Z. & Prior, I. A. M. (1969). *Am. J. clin. Nutr.* **22**, 594.

Shreeve, W. W. (1965). *Ann. N.Y. Acad. Sci.* **131**, 464.

Shukla, A., Forsyth, H. A., Anderson, C. M. & Marwah, S. M. (1972). *Br. med. J.* **4**, 507.

Silverstone, J. T., Gordon, R. P. & Stunkard, A. J. (1969). *Practitioner* **202**, 682.

Simmonds, R. (1931). *Handbook of Diets.* London: Heinemann.

Simpson, I. A. & Chow, A. Y. (1956). *J. trop. Pediat.* **2**, 3, 69.

Sims, E. A. H. (1976). *Clinics Endocr. Metab.* **5**, 377.

Sims, E. A. H. Goldman, R. F., Gluck, C. M., Horton, E. S., Kelleher, P. C. & Rowe, D. W. (1968). *Trans. Am. Ass. Physns* **81**, 153.

Sinclair, H. M. (1953). *The Work of Sir Robert McCarrison.* London: Faber.

Sinclair, H. M. (1956). *Lancet* **1**, 381.

Sinclair, H. M. & Hollingsworth, D. F. (1969). *Hutchison's Food and the Principles of Nutrition,* 12th edn. London: Arnold.

Singh, A. & Jolly, S. S. (1961). *Q. Jl Med.* **30**, 357.

Sinshina, S., Suskind, R., Edelman, R., Charupatana, C. & Olson, R. E. (1973). *Lancet* **1**, 1016.

Sipple, H. L. & McNutt, K. W. (ed). (1974). *Sugars in Nutrition.* New York: Academic Press.

Sircus, W. (ed.) (1973). *Clinics in Gastroenterology,* **2**, 217.

Sixth Marabou Symposium (1979). Food and Cancer. *Näringsforskning,* **22**, suppl. 15.

Skerfring, S. (1969). In *Nutrition in Preschool and School Age.* Symposia of the Swedish Nutrition Foundation, ed. Blix, G., VII, p. 113. Uppsala: Almqvist & Wiksell.

Slack, J. (1969). *Lancet* **2**, 1380.

Sleeman, W. H. (1844). *Rambles and Recollections of an Indian Official* (new edition 1893), ed. Smith, V. A. London: Westminster Press.

Slover, H. T. (1971). *Lipids* **6**, 291.

Smith, C. L., Kelleher, J., Losowsky, M. S. & Morrish, N. (1971). *Br. J. Nutr.* **26**, 89.

Smith, D. A. & Woodruff, M. F. A. (1951). *Spec. Rep. Ser. med. Res. Coun. Lond.,* no. **274.**

Smith, E. B. & Slater, R. (1970) *Atherosclerosis* **11,** 417.

Smith, E. B., Slater, R. S. & Chu, P. K. (1968). *J. Atheroscler. Res.* **8**, 399.

Smith, E. L. & Parker, L. F. J. (1948). *Biochem. J.* **43**, viii.

Smith, F. R. & 7 others (1973). *Am. J. clin. Nutr.* **26**, 973.

Smith, I. & Wolff, O. H. (1974). *Lancet* **1**, 1229.

Smith, L. A. (1972). *New Engl. J. Med.* **286**, 1371; **287**, 412.

Smythe, P. M. & 8 others (1971). *Lancet* **2**, 931.

Snell, E. E. & Wright, L. D. (1941). *J. biol. Chem.* **139**, 675.

Society of Actuaries (1959). *Build and Blood Pressure Study.* Chicago.

Soler, N. G., Pentecost, B. L., Bennett, M. A., FitzGerald, M. G., Lamb, P. & Malins, J. M. (1974). *Lancet* **1**, 475.

Solomons, N. W., Rosenburgh, I. H. & Stanstead, H. H. (1976). *Am. J. clin. Nutr.* **29**, 371.

Somogyi, J. C. (1974). In *Guide Lines for the Preparation of Tables of food Composition,* ed. Southgate, D.A.T., p. 1. Basle: Karger.

Soskin, S. & Levine, R. (1952). *Carbohydrate Metabolism,* 2nd edn. Chicago Univ. Press.

South African Medical Journal (1972). **46**, 1109.

Southgate, D. A. T. (1969). *J. Sci. Fd Agric.* **20**, 331.

Southgate, D. A. T. (1973). In *Nutritional Problems in a Changing World,* ed. Hollingsworth, D. & Russell, M., p. 199. London: Applied Science.

Southgate, D. A. T. (ed.) (1974). *Guide Lines for the Preparation of Tables of Food Composition.* Basle: Karger.

Southgate, D. A. T. (1977). *Nutr. Revs.* **35**, 31.

Southgate, D. A. T., Bailey, B., Collinson, E. & Walker, A. F. (1978). *J. hum. Nutr.* **30**, 303.

Southgate, D. A. T. & Durnin, J. V. G. A. (1970). *Br. J. Nutr.* **24**, 517.

Speke, J. H. (1863). *Journal of the Discovery of the Source of the Nile*, p. 231. Edinburgh: Blackwood.

Spencer, H., Kramer, L. & Norris, C. (1975). *Fedn Proc. Fedn Am. Socs exp. Biol.* **34**, 888.

Spencer, I. O. B. (1968). *Lancet* **1**, 1288.

Spicer, A. (ed.) (1975). *Bread, Social, Nutritional and Agricultural Aspects.* London: Applied Science.

Spillane, J. D. & Scott, G. I. (1945). *Lancet* **2**, 261.

Spring, J. & Buss, D. H. (1977). *Nature, Lond.* **270**, 567.

Srikantia, S. G., Reddy, M. V. & Krishnaswamy, K. (1968). *Electroencephal. clin. Neurophysiol.* **25**, 386.

Stahmann, M. A., Huebner, C. F. & Link, K. P. (1941). *J. biol. Chem.* **138**, 513.

Stamp, T. C. B., Round, J. M., Rowe, D. J. F. & Haddad, J. G. (1972). *Br. med. J.* **4**, 9.

Stanbury, J. B. (1966). In *Metabolic Basis of Inherited Disease*, 2nd edn. ed. Stanbury, J. B., Wyngaarden, J. B. & Fredrickson, D. S., p. 215. New York: McGraw-Hill.

Stanbury, J. B. (ed.) (1969). *Endemic Goitre.* Pan American Health Organisation Scientific Publication No. 193. Washington, D.C.

Stanbury, J. B. (1970). *WHO Chron.* **24**, 537.

Stanbury, J. B., Erasmus, A. M., Hetzel, B. S., Pretell, E. A. & Querido, A. (1974). *WHO Chron.* **28**, 220.

Stanbury, J. B., Wyngaarden, J. B. & Fredrickson, D. S. (1972). *The Metabolic Basis of Inherited Diseases*, 3rd edn. New York: McGraw-Hill.

Stanstead, H. H., Carter, J. P. & Darby, W. J. (1969). *Nutrition Today* **4**, 20.

Starzl, T. E., Chase, H. P., Putnam, C. W. & Porter, K. A. (1973). *Lancet* **2**, 940.

Stauffacher, W., Orci, L., Marliss, E. & Cameron, D. P. (1972). *Acta Diabetologica Latina* **9**, suppl. 1, 579.

Steel, J. E. (1970). *Med. J. Aust.* **2**, 119.

Stefanik, P. A., Heald, F. P. & Mayer, J. (1959). *Am. J. clin. Nutr.* **7**, 55.

Stein, Z., Susser, M., Saenger, G. & Marolla, F. (1972). *Science, N.Y.* **178**, 708.

Stephen, J. M. L. (1968). *Br. J. Nutr.* **22**, 153.

Stephen, J. M. L. & Stephenson, P. (1971). *Archs Dis. Childh.* **46**, 185.

Stephen, J. M. L. & Waterlow, J. C. (1968). *Lancet* **1**, 118.

Stetten, D. & Boxer, G. E. (1944). *J. biol. Chem.* **155**, 231.

Stewart, J. C., Vidor, G. I., Buttfield, I. H. & Hetzel, B. S. (1971). *Aust. N.Z. J. Med.* **3**, 203.

Stewart, J. S., Roberts, P. D. & Holfbrand, A. V. (1970). *Lancet* **2**, 542.

Stoch, M. B. A. & Smythe, P. M. (1963). *Archs Dis. Childh.* **38**, 546.

Stock, A. L. & Wheeler, E. F. (1972). *Br. J. Nutr.* **27**, 439.

Stoffee, W. P., Goldsmith, R. S., Pencharz, P. B., Scrimshaw, N. S. & Young, V. R. (1976). *Metabolism* **25**, 281.

Stone, D. B. (1961). *Am. J. med. Sci.* **241**, 64.

Stone, D. B. & Connor, W. E. (1963). *Diabetes* **12**, 127.

Stordy, B. J., Marks, V., Kalucy, R. S. & Crisp, A. H. (1977). *Am. J. clin. Nutr.* **30**, 138.

Story, J. A. & Kritcheusky, D. (1976). *J. Nutr.* **106**, 1292.

Stott, H. H. (1972). *S. Afr. med. J.* **46**, 1572.

Strachan, R. W. & Henderson, J. G. (1965). *Q. Jl Med.* **34**, 303.

Strang, J. M. & Evans, F. A. (1929). *J. clin. Invest.* **6**, 277.

Strauss, M. B. (1935). *Am. J. med. Sci.* **189**, 378.

Streiff, R. R. (1970). *J. Am. med. Ass.* **204**, 105.

Strong, J. A., Passmore, R. & Ritchie, F. J. (1958). *Br. J. Nutr.* **12**, 105.

Strong, J. A., Shirling, D. & Passmore, R. (1967). *Br. J. Nutr.* **21**, 909.

Strong, R. P. (1942). *Stitt's Diagnosis, Prevention and Treatment of Tropical Disease*, 6th edn. London: H. K. Lewis.

Stuart, H. C. & Stevenson, S. S. (1959). In *Textbook of Pediatrics*, 7th edn, ed. Nelson, W., p. 12. Philadelphia: Saunders.

Stuart, K. L. (1968). *Q. Jl Med.* **37**, 463.

Stuart, R. B. (1967). *Behav. Res. Ther.* **5**, 357.

Stuart, R. B. & Davis, B. (1972). *Slim Chance in a Fat World.* Champagne, Ill.: Research Press.

Stunkard, A. J. (1976). *The Pain of Obesity.* Palo Alto, Calif.: Bull Publ. Co.

Stunkard, A. J., Levine, H. & Fox, S. (1970). *Archs intern. Med.* **125**, 1067.

Stunkard, A. J. & McLaren Hume, M. (1959). *Archs intern. Med.* **103**, 79.

Suckling, P. V. & Campbell, J. A. H. (1957). *J. trop. Pediat.* **2**, 173.

Sullivan, J. F., Wolpert, P. W., Williams, R. & Egan, J. D. (1969). *Ann. N.Y. Acad. Sci.* **162**, 947.

Sullivan, L. W., Lubby, A. L. & Streiff, R. R. (1966). *Am. J. clin. Nutr.* **18**, 311.

Susser, M. & Stein, Z. (1962). *Lancet* **1**, 115.

Sutor, D. J. & Wooley, S. E. (1971). *Gut* **12**, 55.

Svanberg., U., Gebre-Medhin, M., Ljungqvist, B. & Olsson, M. (1977). *Am. J. clin. Nutr.* **30** 499.

Swaminathan, M. (1938). *Nature, Lond.* **141**, 830.

Swan, D. C., Davidson, P. & Albrink, M. J. (1966). *Lancet* **1**, 60.

Swann, M. M. (1969). Chairman of the Joint Committee. *Report on the Use of Antibiotics in Animal Husbandry and Veterinary Medicine.* London: HMSO.

Swanson, P., Roberts, H., Willis, E., Pesek, I. & Mairs, P. (1955). In *Weight Control*, ed. Eppright, E. S., Swanson, P. & Iverson, C. A., p. 80. Iowa: Iowa State College Press.

Swedish Nutrition Foundation (1971). *Famine.* Uppsala: Almqvist and Wiksell.

Sweeney, E. A. Shaffir, A. J. & de Leon, R. (1971). *Am. J. clin. Nutr.* **24**, 29.

Swindells, Y. E. (1972). *Br. J. Nutr.* **27**, 65.

Sydenstricker, V. P., Sebrell, W. H., Cleckley, H. M. & Kruse, H. D. (1940). *J. Am. med. Ass.* **114**, 2437.

Sydenstricker, V. P., Singal, S. A., Briggs, A. P., de Vaughn, N. M. & Isbell, H. (1942). *J. Am. med. Ass.* **118**, 1199.

Symposium on Jejunostomy for Obesity (1977). *Am. J. clin. Nutr.* **30**, 1.

Tada, K., Yokoyama, Y., Nakagawa, H. & Arakawa, T. (1968). *Tohoku J. exp. Med.* **95**, 107.

Taggart, N. (1962). *Br. J. Nutr.* **16**, 223.

Taggart, P. & Carruthers, M. (1971). *Lancet* **1**, 363.

Taitz, L. S. & Byers, H. D. (1972). *Archs Dis. Childh.* **47**, 257.

Takaki, K. (1885). *Sei-i Kwai med. J.* **4**, suppl. 29.

Takaki, K. (1906). *Lancet* **1**, 1369, 1451, 1520.

Talbot, L. M. (1964). In *Proceedings of the Sixth International Congress of Nutrition*, ed. Mills, C. F. & Passmore, R., p. 243. Edinburgh: Livingstone.

Tamura, T. & Stokstad, E. L. R. (1973). *Br. J. Haemat.* **25**, 513.

Tanner, J. M. (1962). *Growth and Adolescence.* Oxford: Blackwell.

Tanner, J. M., Whitehouse, R. H. & Tahaishi, M. (1966). *Archs Dis. Childh.* **41**, 454.

Tanphaichitr, V. (1976). In *Nutrition Reviews' Present Knowledge in Nutrition*, p. 141. New York: Nutrition Foundation.

Tanphaichitr, V., Vimokesant, S. L., Dhanamitta, S. & Valyasevi, A. (1970). *Am. J. clin. Nutr.* **23**, 1017.

Tappel, A. (1973). *Nutrition Today*, July/August, p. 4.

Tarján, R. (1973). *Bibl. Nutr. & Dieta* No. 18. p. 280.

Taylor, C. E., Kielmann, A. A., De Sweemer, (1978). *Indian J. med. Res.* In press.

Terris, M. (1963). *Goldberger on Pellagra.* Baton Rouge, Louisiana: State University Press.

Thaler, H. (1977). *Nutr. Metab.* **21**, 186.

Thanangkul, O. & Whitaker, J. A. (1966). *Am. J. clin. Nutr.* **18**, 275.

Thomas, B. J., Truswell, A. S. & Brown, A. M. (1974a). *Nutrition, Lond.* **28**, 297.

Thomas, B. J., Truswell, A. S. & Brown, A. M. (1974b). *Nutrition, Lond.* **28**, 357.

Thompson, J. C. (1946). *Proc. Nutr. Soc.* **4**, 171.

Thompson, J. N., Beare-Rogers, J. L., Erdödy, P. & Smith, D. C. (1973). *Am. J. clin. Nutr.* **26**, 1349.

Thompson, R. H. S. & Cumings, J. N. (1970). In *Biochemical Disorders in Human Disease*, 3rd edn, ed. Thompson, R. H. S. & Wootton, I. D. P., p. 451. London: Churchill.

Thomson, A. D., Baker, H. & Leevy, C. M. (1971). *Gastroenterology* **60**, 756.

Thomson, A. M. (1958). *Br. J. Nutr.* **12**, 446.

Thomson, A. M. (1959). *Br. J. Nutr.* **13**, 509.

Thomson, A. M. & Billewicz, W. Z. (1957). *Br. med. J.* **1**, 243.

Thomson, A. M., Billewicz, W. Z. & Passmore, R. (1961). *Lancet* **1**, 1027.

Thomson, A. M., Chun, D. & Baird, D. (1963). *J. Obstet. Gynaec. Br. Commonw.* **70**, 871.

Thomson, A. M., Hytten, F. E. & Billewicz, W. Z. (1970). *Br. J. Nutr.* **24**, 565.

Thomson, J. (1954). *Hlth Bull. Edinb.* **12**, 25.

Thomson, J. (1955). *Hlth Bull. Edinb.* **13**, 16.

Thomson, T. J., Runcie, J. & Miller, V. (1966). *Lancet* **2**, 992.

Thorn, J., Robertson, J. & Buss, D. H. (1978). *Br. J. Nutr.* **39**, 391.

Thurnham, D. I., Migasena, P., Vndhivai, N. & Supawan, V. (1972). *Br. J. Nutr.* **28**, 91.

Tiller, J. R., Schilling, R. S. F. & Morris, J. N. (1968). *Br. med. J.* **4**, 407.

Tillotson, J. A. & Baker, E. M. (1972). *Am. J. clin. Nutr.* **25**, 425.

Time (1972). 18 December, p. 47.

Toepfer, E. W., Mertz, W., Roginski, E. E. & Polansky, M. M. (1973). *J. agric. Fd. Chem.* **21**, 69.

Tolan, A., Robertson, J., Orton, C. R., Head, M. J., Christie, A. A. & Millburn, B. A. (1974). *Br. J. Nutr.* **31**, 185.

Tomkin, G. H. (1973). *Br. med. J.* **3**, 673.

Topley, E. (1968). *Trans. R. Soc. trop. Med. Hyg.* **62**, 579.

Tougaard, L., Sorensen, E., Brochner-Mortensen, J., Christensen, M. S., Radbro, P. & Sorenson, A. W. (1976). *Lancet* **1**, 1044.

Toverud, G. (1949). *Proc. R. Soc. Med.* **42**, 249.

Townley, R. R. W., Bhathal, P. S., Cornell, H. J. & Mitchell, J. D. (1973). *Lancet* **1**, 1363.

Trant, H. (1954). *Lancet* **2**, 703.

Trevelyan, G. M. (1942). *British Social History*, p. 341. London: Longmans Green.

Trout, K. W., Bertrand, C. A. & Williams, M. H. (1956). *J. Am. med. Ass.* **162**, 970.

Trowell, H. C. (1960). *Non-infective Disease in Africa.* London: Arnold.

Trowell, H. C. (1972a). *Atherosclerosis* **16**, 138.

Trowell, H. C. (1972b). *Am. J. clin. Nutr.* **25**, 926.

Trowell, H. C. (1973). *Proc. nutr. Soc.* **32**, 150.

Trowell, H. C. (1974). *Lancet* **2**, 998.

Trowell, H. C. (1975). *Diabetes* **24**, 762.

Trowell, H. C., Davies, J. N. P. & Dean, R. F. A. (1954). *Kwashiorkor.* London: Arnold.

Truswell, A. S. (1974). *Proc. Nutr. Soc.* **33**, 203.

Truswell, A. S. (1976). *Proc. Nutr. Soc.* **35**, 1.

Truswell, A. S. (1977). *Seventh Int. Congress of Dietetics,* Sydney. Abstracts, p.129

Truswell, A. S. (1978a). *Am. J. clin. Nutr.* **31**, 977.

Truswell, A. S. (1978b). *Näringsforskning* **22**, suppl. 15, 65.

Truswell, A. S. (1978c). In *Diet of Man: Needs and Wants,* ed. Yudkin, J., p. 5. London: Applied Science.

Truswell, A. S. & Brock, J. F. (1962). *Am. J. clin. Nutr.* **10**, 142.

Truswell, A. S. & Hansen, J. D. L. (1969). *S. Afr. med. J.* **43**, 280.

Truswell, A. S. & Hansen, J. D. L. (1976). In *Kalahari Hunter-Gatherers,* ed. Lee, R. B. & De Vore, p.167. Cambridge, Mass.: Harvard Univ. Press.

Truswell, A. S., Hansen, J. D. L. & Konno, T. (1972b). *S. Afr. med. J.* **46**, 2083.

Truswell, A. S., Hansen, J. D. L. & Wannenburg, P. (1968). *Am. J. clin. Nutr.* **21**, 1314.

Truswell, A. S., Hansen, J. D. L., Watson, C. E. & Wannenburg, P. (1969). *Am. J. clin. Nutr.* **22**, 568.

Truswell, A. S., Hansen, J. D. L., Wittman, W., Wannenburg, P. Roberts, B. & Watson, C. E. (1966). *S. Afr. med. J.* **40**, 887.

Truswell, A. S. & Kay, R. M. (1976). *Lancet* **1**, 367.

Truswell, A. S., Kennelly, B. M., Hansen, J. D. L. & Lee, R. B. (1972a). *Am. Heart J.* **84**, 5.

Truswell, A. S. & Mann, J. I. (1972). *Atherosclerosis* **16**, 15.

Truswell, A. S., Thomas, B. J. & Brown, A. M. (1975). *Br. med. J.* **4**, 7.

Truswell, A. S., Wittman, W. & Hansen, J. D. L. (1964). In *The Role of the Gastrointestinal Tract in Protein Metabolism,* ed. Munro, H. N., p. 211. Oxford: Blackwell.

Tweedle, D. & Johnson, I. D. (1971). *Br. J. Surg.* **58**, 771.

Udal, J. A. (1965). *J. Am. med. Ass.* **194**, 127.

Underwood, E. J. (1977). *Trace Elements in Human and Animal Nutrition,* 4th edn. New York: Academic Press.

United Nations (1954). *Population Growth and the Standard of Living in Under-developed Countries.* New York: UN Population Studies, No. 20.

University Group Diabetes Program (1970). *Diabetes,* **19**, Suppl. 2.

US Department of Health, Education and Welfare (1972). *Ten-State Nutrition Survey, 1968-70,* DHEW Publication no. (HSM) 72-8134. Center for Disease Control, Atlanta, Georgia.

Vagenakis, A. G., Burger, A., Portnay, G. I., Rudolph, M., O'Brien, J. T., Azizi, F., Arky, R. A., Nicod, P., Ingbar, S. H. & Braverman, L. E. (1975). *J. clin Endocrinol. Metab.* **41**, 191.

Vahlquist, B. (ed.) (1972). *Nutrition. A Priority in African Development.* Stockholm: Almqvist & Wiksell.

Valyasevi, A., Dhanamitta, S. & Van Reen, R. (1969). *Am. J. clin. Nutr.* **22**, 218.

Valyasevi, A., Dhanamitta, S. & Van Reen, R. (1973). *Am. J. clin. Nutr.* **26**, 1207.

van der Meer, M. A. (1972). *Voeding* **33**, 277.

Van der Weele, D. A. & Sanderson, J. D. (1976). In *Hunger: Basic Mechanisms and Clinical Implications,* ed. Novin, D., Wyrwicka, W. & Bray, G. A. New York: Raven Press.

Van Eekelen, M. & Kooy, R. (1933). *Acta brev. neerl. Physiol.* **3**, 169.

van Eytten, C. H. (1969). In *Toxic Constituents of Plants Foodstuffs,* ed. Liener, I. E., p. 103. New York & London: Academic Press.

Van Handel, E. & Zilversmit, D. B. (1957). *J. Lab. clin. Med.* **50**, 152.

Van Slyke, D. D. & Meyer, G. M. (1912). *J. biol. Chem.* **12**, 399.

Van Soest, P. J. & Robertson, J. B. (1977). *Nutr. Rev.* **35**, 16.

van Stuyvenberg, J. H. (ed.) (1969). *Margarine. An Economic, Social and Scientific History.* Liverpool: Liverpool Univ. Press.

Vas, K. (1977). *Fd Nutr.* **3**, 2.

Vaughan Jones, R. (1961). *Br. med. J.* **1**, 1276.

Vedder, E. B. (1913). *Beriberi.* London: Bale & Danielson.

Vergroesen, A. J. & de Boer, J. (1971). *Voeding* **32**, 278.

Vergroesen, A. J., de Deckere, E. A. M., ten Hoor, F., Hornstra, T. & Houtsmuller, U. M. T. (1975). In *The Essential Fatty Acids,* Nutrition Society of Canada, Miles Symposium.

Verney, E. B. (1957). *Lancet* **2**, 1237, 1295.

Victor, M., Adams, R. D. & Collins, G. H. (1971). *The Wernicke-Korsakoff Syndrome.* Philadelphia: Davis.

Vigersky, R. A. (ed.) (1977). *Anorexia Nervosa.* New York: Raven Press.

Vikki, P., Kreula, M. & Pironen, E. (1962). *Ann. Acad. Sci. fenn.* A II, **110**, 1.

Viswanathan, M. (1973). *J. Ass. Physns India* **21**, 887.

Voit, C. (1881). *Physiologie des Stoffwechsels,* p. 519.

Voors, A. W. (1969). *Lancet* **2**, 1337.

Wadhura, P. S., Young, E. A., Schmidt, K., Elson, C. E. & Pringle, D. J. (1973). *Am. J. clin, Nutr.* **26**, 823.

Wagner, M. & Hewitt, M. I. (1975). *J. Am. Dietetic Ass.* **67**, 344.

Wahren, J., Felig, P. & Hagenfeldt, J. (1976). *J. clin. Invest.* **57**, 987.

Wald, G. (1941). *J. opt. Soc. Am.* **31**, 235.

Walker, A. R. P. (1951). *Lancet* **2**, 244.

Walker, A. R. P. & Arvidsson, U. B. (1954). *Metabolism* **3**, 385.

Walker, A. R. P., Arvidsson, U. B. & Draper, W. L. (1954). *Trans. R. Soc. trop. Med. Hyg.* **48**, 395.

Walker, A. R. P., Fox, F. W. & Irving, J. T. (1948). *Biochem. J.* **42**, 452.

Walker, A. R. P., Walker, B. F. & Richardson, B. D. (1971). *Postgrad. med. J.* **47**, 320.

Walsh, B. M. & Walsh, D. (1973). *Br. J. prevent. soc. Med.* **27**, 28.

Walter, R. (1748). *Lord Anson's Voyage Round the World, 1740–44.* Abridged and annotated by Pack, S. W. C. London: Penguin Books, 1947.

Walters, J. H. (1953). *Q. Jl Med.* **22**, 195.

Walters, J. H. & Waterlow, J. C. (1954). *Spec. Rep. Ser. med. Res. Coun. Lond.*, no. **285**.

Wannamacher, R. W. Jr, Pekarek, R. S., Bartelloni, P. J., Vollmer, R. T. & Beisel, W. R. (1972). *Metabolism* **21**, 67.

Warburg, O. & Christian, W. (1932). *Biochem. Z.* **254**, 438.

Ward, B. (1969). *Economist* **233**, 56.

Waterlow, J. C. (1968). *Lancet* **2**, 1091.

Waterlow, J. C. (1973a) *Lancet* **1**, 425.

Waterlow, J. C. (1973b). *Lancet* **2**, 87.

Waterlow, J. C. (1975). *Nature, Lond.* **253**, 157.

Waterlow, J. C. & Alleyne, G. A. O. (1971). *Adv. Protein Chem.* **25**, 117.

Waterlow, J. C., Golden, M. H. N. & Patrick, J. (1978). In *Nutrition in the Clinical Management of Disease,* ed. Dickerson, J. W. T. & Lee, H. A. London: Arnold.

Watson, W. C., Buchanan, K. D. & Dickson, C. (1963). *Br. med. J.* **2**, 709.

Watt, B. K. & Merrill, A. L. (1963). *US Dept. Agric. Handbook,* no. 8.

Wayne, E. J., Koutras, D. A. & Alexander, W. D. (1964). *Clinical Aspects of Iodine Metabolism.* Oxford: Blackwell.

Weaver, A. L. (1964). *Proc. Staff Meet. Mayo Clin.* **39**, 485.

Weijers, H. A. (1950). *Thesis.* University of Utrecht.

Weinzier, R. L., Seeman, A., Herrera, M. G., Assal, J.-P., Soeldner, J. S. & Gleason, R. E. (1974). *Ann. intern. Med.* **80**, 332.

Weir, J. B. de V. (1949). *J. Physiol.* **109**, 1.

Weiss, D., Whitten, B. & Leddy, D. (1972). *Science, N.Y.* **178**, 69.

Weiss-Fogh, T. (1967). In *Nutrition and Physical Activity.* Swedish Nutrition Symposium, vol. 5, ed. Blix, G., p. 84.

Wene, J. C., Connor, W. E. & Den Besten, L. (1975). *J. clin. Invest.* **56**, 127.

Wenlock, R. W. & Buss, D. H. (1977). *J. hum. Nutr.* **31**, 405.

Wenlock, R. W., Buss, D. H. & Dixon, E. J. (1979). *Br. J. Nutr.* **39**, 253.

Wertheimer, E. & Shapiro, B. (1948). *Physiol. Rev.* **28**, 451.

West Derbyshire Medical Society (1966). *Lancet* **2**, 959.

West, K. M. (1973). *Ann. intern. Med.* **79**, 425.

West, K. M. (1974). *Diabetes* **23**, 848.

West, K. M. (1975). *Diabetes* **24**, 641.

West, K. M. & Kalbfleisch, J. M. (1971). *Diabetes* **20**, 99.

West, T. E. T., Joffe, M., Sinclair, L. & O'Riordan, J. L. H. (1971). *Lancet* **1**, 675.

Wharton, B. A., Balmer, S. E., Somers, K. & Templeton, A. C. (1969). *Q. Jl Med.* **38**, 107.

Wharton, B. A. & Berger, H. M. (1976). *Br. med. J.* **2**, 1326.

Whedon, G. D. (1964). In *Proceedings of the Sixth International Congress of Nutrition,* ed. Mills, C. F. & Passmore, R., p. 425. Edinburgh: Livingstone.

Wheeler, E. F., El-Neil, H., Wilson, J. O. C. & Weiner, J. S. (1973). *Br. J. Nutr.* **30**, 127.

Which? (1976). Breakfast Cereals. April, p. 91.

Whichelow, M. J. (1975). *Archs Dis. Childh.* **50**, 669.

White, P. L. (1973). *J. Am. med. Ass.* **224**, 1521.

White, P. L., Mahan, L. K. & Moore, M. F. (1972). *Conference on Guidelines for Nutritional Education in Medical Schools and Postdoctoral Training Programs* (June 1972). Available from American Medical Association, Chicago.

Whitehead, R. G. (1978). *Jl R. Soc. Encouragement of Arts* **76**, 552.

Whitehead, T. P., Browning, D. M. & Gregory, A. (1973). *J. clin. Path.* **26**, 435.

Whitehouse, R. M., Tanner, J. M. & Healy, M. J. R. (1974). *Ann. hum. Biol.* **1**, 103.

Whyte, H. M. (1958). *Aust. Ann. Med.* **7**, 36.

Wicks, A. C. B., Castle, W. M. & Gelfand, M. (1973). *Diabetes* **22**, 733.

Widdowson, E. M. (1955). *Proc. Nutr. Soc.* **14**, 142.

Widdowson, E. M. (1965). *Lancet* **2**, 1099.

Widdowson, E. M. & McCance, R. A. (1943). *Lancet* **1**, 230.

Widdowson, E. M. & McCance, R. A. (1954). *Spec. Rep. Ser. med. Res. Coun. Lond.* no. 287.

Widdowson, E. M. & McCance, R. A. (1960). *Proc. R. Soc.* **152**, 188.

Widdowson, E. M., McCance, R. A., Harrison, G. E. & Sutton, A. (1963). *Lancet* **2**, 1250,

Widdowson, E. M., McCance, R. A. & Spray, C. M. (1951). *Clin. Sci.* **10**, 113.

Widdowson, E. M. & Shaw, W. T. (1973). *Lancet* **2**, 905.

Widdowson, E. M. & Thrussell, L. A. (1951). *Spec. Rep. Ser. med. Res. Coun. Lond.* no. 275.

Wilkinson, A. W. (1961). *Lancet* **2**, 783.

Wilkinson, A. W. (1973). *Body Fluids in Surgery*, 4th edn. Edinburgh: Churchill Livingstone.

Wilkinson, A. W. & Cuthertson, D. P. (ed.) (1976). *Surgical Metabolism*. London: Pitman.

Wilkinson, P. W., Noble, T. G., Gray, G. & Spence, O. (1973). *Br. med. J.* **2**, 15.

Williams, C. D. (1933). *Archs Dis. Childh.* **8**, 423.

Williams, C. D. (1954). *Report on Vomiting Sickness in Jamaica*. Kingston, Jamaica: Government Printer.

Williams, R. D., Mason, H. L., Smith, B. F. & Wilder, R. M. (1942). *Archs intern. Med.* **69**, 721.

Williams, R. H. (1943). *New Engl. J. Med.* **228**, 247.

Williams, R. J. (1939). *Science, N.Y.* **89**, 486.

Williams, R. J. (1956). *Biochemical Individuality*, p. 135. New York: Wiley.

Williams, R. R. & Cline, J. K. (1936). *J. Am. chem. Soc.* **58**, 1504.

Williams, R. R. & Spies, T. (1938). *Vitamin B$_1$ in Medicine*. New York.

Williams, T. F., Winters, R. W. & Burnett, C. H. (1966). In *The Metabolic Basis of Inherited Disease*, 2nd edn, ed. Stanbury, J. B., Wyngaarden, J. B. & Fredrickson, D. S., p. 1179. New York: Blakiston.

Williamson, A. D. & Leong, P. C. (1949). *Med. J. Malaya* **4**, 83.

Wills, L. (1931). *Br. med. J.* **1**, 1059.

Wills, L. (1933). *Lancet* **1**, 1283.

Wills, M. R., Day, R. C., Phillips, J. B. & Bateman, E. C. (1972). *Lancet* **1**, 771.

Wilson, C. W., Loh, H. S. & Foster, F. G. (1976). *Eur. J. clin. Pharmacol.* **6**, 26.

Wilson, D. (1972). In *Nutrition, National Development and Planning*, ed. Berg, A. Scrimshaw, N. S. & Call, D. L., p. 138. Cambridge, Mass.: MIT Press.

Wilson, D. C. (1929). *Indian J. med. Res.* **17**, 338, 881, 903.

Wilson, D. E. & Leeds, R. S. (1972). *J. clin. Invest.* **51**, 1051.

Wilson, W. H. (1921). *J. Hyg. Camb.* **20**, 1.

Winick, M. (1976). *Malnutrition and Brain Development*. Oxford Univ. Press.

Wintrobe, M. M. (1956). *Clinical Haematology*, 4th edn, p. 773. London: Kimpton.

Wogan, G. N. (1975). *Cancer Res.* **35**, 3499.

Wokes, F. & Picard, C. W. (1955). *Am. J. clin. Nutr.* **3**, 383.

Wolbach, S. B. (1953). *Proc. Nutr. Soc.* **12**, 247.

Wolbach, S. B. & Howe, P. R. (1925). *J. exp. Med.* **42**, 753.

Wolf, H. (1971). *Am. J. clin. Nutr.* **24**, 792.

Wolff, O. H. & Lloyd, J. K. (1973). *Proc. Nutr. Soc.* **32**, 195.

Wood, F. W. (1975). *Br. Nutr. Found. Bull.* no. 15, p. 176.

Wood, P. D. S., Stern, M. P., Silvers, A., Reaven, G. M. & von der Groeben, J. (1972). *Circulation* **45**, 114.

Woodham-Smith, C. (1962). *The Great Hunger: Ireland 1845-9*. London: Hamish Hamilton.

Woodruff, A. W. (1961). In *Recent Advances in Human Nutrition*, ed. Brock, J.-F., p. 415. London: Churchill.

Woods, H. F. & Alberti, K. G. M. M. (1972). *Lancet* **2**, 1354.

Working Party on the Monitoring of Foodstuffs for Mercury and Other Heavy Metals (1971). *First Report*, London: HMSO.

World Health Organisation (1953). *Bull. Wld Hlth Org.* **9**, 293.

World Health Organisation (1960). *Endemic Goitre*. WHO Monograph Series no. 44.

World Health Organisation (1965). *Tech. Rep. Ser. Wld Hlth Org.* no. 310.

World Health Organisation (1966a). *Tech. Rep. Ser. Wld Hlth Org.* no. 316.

World Health Organisation (1966b). *The Prevention and Control of Cardiovascular Diseases* (Bucharest Conference). Copenhagen. Euro. **179**, 4.

World Health Organisation (1967). *Tech. Rep. Ser. Wld Hlth Org.* no. 348.

World Health Organisation (1968). *Wld Hlth Org. statist. Rep.* **20**, 145.

World Health Organisation (1970). *Fluorides and Human Health*. WHO Monograph Series no. 59.

World Health Organisation (1972). *Tech. Rep. Ser. Wld Hlth Org.* no. 503.

World Health Organisation (1973). *Tech. Rep. Ser. Wld Hlth Org.* no. 532.

World Health Organisation (1975). *Tech. Rep. Ser. Wld Hlth Org.* no. 580.

World Health Organisation (1976a). *Tech. Rep. Ser. Wld Hlth Org.* no. 590.

World Health Organisation (1976b). *Tech. Rep. Ser. Wld Hlth Org.* no. 593.

World Health Organisation (1977). *Fd Nutr.* **3**, 2.

World Health Organisation (1978). *A Growth Chart for International Use in Maternal and Child Health Care*. Geneva: WHO.

Wretlind, A. (1975). *Bibl. Nutritio et Dieta* **21**, 177.

Wretlind, A., Hejda, S., Isaksson, B., Kübler, W., Truswell, A. S. & Vivanco, F. (1977). *Nutr. Metab.* **21**, 244.

Wynder, E. L. & Hill, P. (1972). *Prev. Med.* **1**, 161.

Wyngaarden, J. B. (1974). *Am. J. Med.* **56**, 651.

Yana, K., Rhoads, G. G. & Kagan, A. (1977). *New Engl. J. Med.* **297**, 405.

Youmans, J. B. (1936). *Int. Clin.* **4**, 120.

Youmans, J. B. (1957). *J. med. Ass. St. Ala.* **26**, 161.

Young, A. (1771). *The Farmer's Tour through the East of England,* vol. 4, p. 120. London.

Young, C. M., Blondin, J., Tensuan, R. & Fryer, J. H. (1963). *Ann. N.Y. Acad. Sci.* **110**, 589.

Young, G. A., Chem, C. & Hill, G. L. (1978). *Am. J. clin. Nutr.* **31**, 429.

Young, G. M., Hutter, L. F., Scanlan, S. S., Rand, C. E., Lutwak, L. & Simko, V. (1972). *J. Am. diet. Ass.* **61**, 391.

Young, R. (1977). *Proc. R. Soc. Edinb.* B **75**, 199.

Young, V. R. & Scrimshaw, N. S. (1968). *Br. J. Nutr.* **22**, 9.

Young, V. R., Stoffee, W. P., Pencharz, P. B., Winterer, J. C. & Scrimshaw, N. S. (1975). *Nature, Lond.* **253**, 192.

Yudkin, J. (1967). *Am. J. clin. Nutr.* **20**, 108.

Yudkin, J. & Roddy, J. (1964). *Lancet* **2**, 6.

Zalusky, R. & Herbert, V. (1961). *New Engl. J. Med.* **265**, 1033.

Zarembski, P. M. & Hodgkison, A. (1962). *Br. J. Nutr.* **16**, 627.

Zimmet, P., Taft, P., Guinea, A., Guthrie, W. & Thoma, K. (1977). *Diabetologia* **13**, 11.

Zlotlow, M. J. & Settipane, G. A. (1977). *Am. J. clin Nutr.* **30**, 1023.

Zöllner, N., Griebsch, A. & Gröbner, W. (1972). *Ernährungs-Umschau,* **3**, 79.

Zöllner, N., Wolfram, G. & Keller, C. (ed.) (1977). Second European Nutrition Conference: Round Table on Comparison of Dietary Recommendations in Different European Countries. *Nutr. Metab.* **21**, 210.

Zuelzer, W. W. & Ogden, F. N. (1946). *Am. J. Dis. Child.* **71**, 211.

Zuntz, N. (1897). *Pflügers Arch. ges. Physiol.* **68**, 191.

Zuskin, E., Lewis, A. J. & Bouhuys, A. (1973). *J. Allergy clin. Immunol.* **51**, 218.

Index